BRIEF CONTENTS

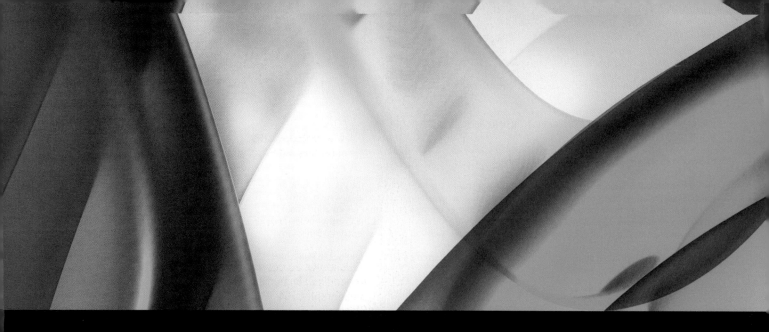

PHARMACOLOGY

EDITION 11

A PATIENT-CENTERED NURSING PROCESS APPROACH

LINDA E. MCCUISTION, PhD, MSN, RN
Mandeville, Louisiana

KATHLEEN VULJOIN-DIMAGGIO, MSN, RN
Professor Emerita, University of Holy Cross New Orleans, New Orleans, Louisiana

MARY B. WINTON, PhD, RN, ACANP-BC
Associate Professor, Tarleton State University, Stephensville, Texas

JENNIFER J. YEAGER, PhD, RN
Associate Professor, Tarleton State University, Stephensville, Texas

ELSEVIER

Elsevier
3251 Riverport Lane
St. Louis, Missouri 63043

PHARMACOLOGY: A PATIENT-CENTERED NURSING PROCESS APPROACH,
ELEVENTH EDITION   ISBN: 978-0-323-79315-5

Notice

Practitioners and researchers must always rely on their own experience and knowledge in evaluating
and using any information, methods, compounds or experiments described herein. Because of rapid
advances in the medical sciences, in particular, independent verification of diagnoses and drug dosages
should be made. To the fullest extent of the law, no responsibility is assumed by Elsevier, authors, editors
or contributors for any injury and/or damage to persons or property as a matter of products liability,
negligence or otherwise, or from any use or operation of any methods, products, instructions, or ideas
contained in the material herein.

Previous editions copyrighted 2021, 2018, 2015, 2012, 2009, 2003, 2000, 1997, 1993.

Director, Content Development: Laurie Gower
Senior Content Strategist: Yvonne Alexopoulos
Senior Content Development Manager: Luke Held
Publishing Services Manager: Catherine Jackson
Senior Project Manager: Kate Mannix
Design Direction: Brian Salisbury

Printed in the United States

Last digit is the print number: 9 8 7 6 5 4 3 2 1

Working together
to grow libraries in
developing countries

ELSEVIER • Book Aid International

www.elsevier.com • www.bookaid.org

LINDA E. MCCUISTION

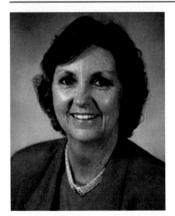

Dr. Linda E. McCuistion received a Diploma of Nursing from the Lutheran Hospital School of Nursing in Fort Wayne, Indiana; Bachelor of Science in Nursing from William Carey College in Hattiesburg, Mississippi; Masters in Nursing from Louisiana State University Medical Center, New Orleans; and PhD in Curriculum and Instruction from the University of New Orleans. She was licensed as an Advanced Practice Nurse in Louisiana and has many years of nursing experience that include acute care and home health nursing. For 20 years, Linda was a Nursing Professor at University of Holy Cross in New Orleans, Louisiana. She received an Endowed Professorship Award in 2000 and 2003. Linda also worked as a nursing professor at South University, Richmond, Virginia.

Linda has served as a past president, vice president, and faculty advisor of the Sigma Theta Tau International Honor Society in Nursing, Xi Psi chapter-at-large. She is a past associate editor of the *NODNA Times,* a New Orleans District Nurses Association newsletter. She has been a member of Phi Delta Kappa and the American Society of Hypertension.

Linda was coordinator for the Graduate Plus internship program, a preceptorship program for new nursing graduates in the state of Louisiana. She has served as a legal nurse consultant; a member of a medical review panel; advisory board member, consultant, and reviewer of a software preparation company focused on the state licensure examination; advisory board member for a school for surgical technicians; and consultant to a local hospital to improve the quality of nursing care and assist acute care facilities in preparation for accreditation.

Linda was chosen as a "Great One-Hundred Nurse" by the New Orleans District Nurses Association in 1993. She is also listed in the 2005/2006 edition of the Empire Who's Who Executive and Professional Registry.

Linda has given numerous lectures and presentations regionally and nationally on a variety of nursing topics. She has published articles in nursing journals and has authored many chapters in several nursing textbooks, including *Pharmacotherapeutics: Clinical Decision Making in Nursing* (1999), *Saunders Manual of Medical-Surgical Nursing: A Guide for Clinical Decision Making* (2002), and *Saunders Nursing Survival Guide: Pathophysiology* (2007). She is author and coauthor of many chapters and coeditor of *Saunders Nursing Survival Guide: Pharmacology* (2007).

Linda enjoys cruises, the beach, and other travel. When at home, she enjoys family, friends, golf, crafts, reading, writing, and her King Charles Cavalier Spaniel, Prince.

KATHLEEN VULJOIN DIMAGGIO

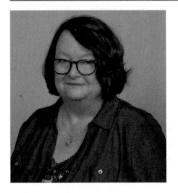

Kathleen Vuljoin DiMaggio received her Bachelor of Science in Nursing from Our Lady of Holy Cross College of New Orleans and her Master of Science in Nursing from Loyola University of New Orleans, with a focus on Healthcare Systems Management. She completed a preceptorship in palliative care at Ochsner Foundation Hospital through Loyola University. She received Level I designation from the National Hospice and Palliative Care Organization in hospice management and development. She is certified with the Louisiana Department of Health and Hospitals Developmental Disabilities as a Registered Nurse Instructor in medication administration. Kathleen has more than 23 years of clinical nursing experience and more than 12 years of baccalaureate nursing education. Her professional practice experience includes medical-surgical nursing and home health and hospice nursing. She has experience in nursing management and has worked as director of nursing for a facility specializing in developmental disabilities. In addition, Kathleen has worked as director of nursing in home health and hospice care. She has worked in quality improvement, disease management, and case management.

Kathleen has served as a volunteer for Junior Achievement of New Orleans, has volunteered for a local hospice agency, and has served in the homeless ministry through her church.

Kathleen is a member of the American Nurses Association, Louisiana State Nurses Association, Academy of Medical-Surgical Nurses, Sigma Theta Tau International Honor Society of Nursing, and Alpha Sigma Nu Jesuit Honor Society.

Kathleen is a recipient of the 2011 and 2015 Endowed Professorship from Eminent Eye, Ear, Nose and Throat Hospital. She has received the Order of St. Louis Award through the Archdiocese of New Orleans and has also received the Florence Nightingale Society Award for Nursing. Kathleen received outstanding faculty of the year award in 2017 from the University of Holy Cross New Orleans. She received the distinction of Professor Emerita from University of Holy Cross New Orleans in May 2018.

Kathleen enjoys spending time with family and friends. She enjoys crocheting, quilting, cooking, and reading.

MARY B. WINTON

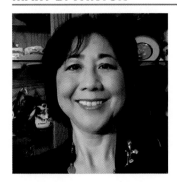

Dr. Mary B. Winton received her Associate Degree in Nursing from Tarleton State University in Stephenville, Texas, a member of the Texas A&M University System; her Bachelor and Master of Science in Nursing from the University of Texas at Arlington; and her PhD in Nursing from the University of Texas at Tyler. Additionally, she is board certified through the American Nurses Credentialing Center as an Acute Care Adult Nurse Practitioner. Mary has many years of hospital nursing experience in areas including critical care, emergency, and medical-surgical nursing as both a nurse and as a nursing supervisor. Additionally, she was employed with a hospitalist group as an Acute Care Nurse Practitioner for many years. She is currently an Associate Professor in the College of Health Sciences and Human Services, School of Nursing, at Tarleton State University. Mary has experience in teaching graduate-level pharmacology, pathophysiology, health assessment, and nursing informatics, and she has vast experience teaching at all levels of the undergraduate nursing program, including nursing pathophysiology, pharmacology, and health assessment.

Mary has served as faculty advisor for the Student Nurses Association at Tarleton. She has been a member of several organizations, including Sigma Theta Tau International Honor Society in Nursing, Tau Chi chapter; American Nurses Association/Texas Nurses Association; Critical Care Nursing Education; and Rural Nurse Organization. She is actively involved in various university, college, school, and departmental committees.

During her career as a nurse educator, Mary was the recipient of the Texas A&M Student Evaluation Teaching Excellence Award and the O.A. Grant Excellence in Teaching Award. She was also a recipient of the AACN 2020-2021 *Scholarship of Teaching and Learning Excellence Award*. She has also taught English as a Second Language at her church of membership.

Mary's research interests include health disparity among minorities, especially among Korean immigrants; student learning outcomes; and the use of technology in classrooms. She has presented at several conferences and has published on the health care of Korean immigrants.

During her spare time, Mary enjoys spending time with her husband, daughters, and grandchildren. She also enjoys traveling, reading, crocheting, and snow skiing.

JENNIFER J. YEAGER

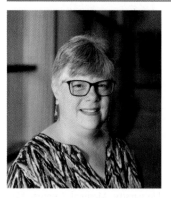

Dr. Jennifer J. Yeager graduated from the University of Portland, Oregon, in 1987 with her Bachelor of Science in Nursing degree; she attended the university on an Air Force ROTC nursing scholarship. After graduation, she began her nursing career as an Air Force officer, assigned to Wilford Hall USAF Medical Center in San Antonio, Texas. The Air Force provided Jennifer with excellent experience as a transplant/nephrology nurse; after 6 years on active duty, she entered the civilian world as a transplant coordinator at Methodist Medical Center in Dallas, Texas. While there, Jennifer began her Master of Science in Nursing degree at the University of Texas at Arlington; she completed her degree as an Adult/Gerontological Nurse Practitioner with Educator Role in 1998. After completing ANCC certification in both specialty areas, she went to work in the Baylor Health Care System as a nurse practitioner in Long-Term Care and Elder House Calls.

Jennifer moved to Stephenville, Texas in 2007 and began teaching at Tarleton State University. She completed her PhD in Nursing at the University of Texas at Tyler in Fall 2013. She teaches a variety of courses, both graduate level and undergraduate.

Jennifer's research interests revolve around simulation; in 2021, in collaboration with co-workers in other disciplines, she published two journal articles related to pandemic simulation.

To relax, Jennifer enjoys spending time with her family, including multiple dogs. She is a strong advocate for dog rescue organizations and participates in Texas Transports with her husband, transporting shelter dogs to no-kill rescues within the state. Her passion for dogs extends to Animal Assisted Therapy. Xander, her American Staffordshire Terrier, is not only a rescue but also a certified therapy dog who joins her at Tarleton to work with nursing students to reduce anxiety before exams and simulations.

IN RECOGNITION

Joyce LeFever Kee taught a pharmacology course to student nurses for 10 years from 1980 to 1990 at the University of Delaware. At the time, there were very few pharmacology texts available, and what was published was not appropriate for some BSN and ADN nursing programs. Daniel Ruth from W.B. Saunders approached Kee in 1990 to write a pharmacology book for nurses. With experience in teaching the subject, Kee developed the contents and format for a pharmacology text.

The chapter Drug Action: Pharmaceutic, Pharmacokinetics, and Pharmacodynamics Phases became the first chapter in the first edition. These drug phases appear both in the Prototype Drug Charts and within the contents in most of the current chapters. There are many drug tables Kee developed that have been updated by coauthors through the years. The important part that Kee established in the chapters were the five steps of the Nursing Process.

Dr. Evelyn R. Hayes joined Kee starting with the first edition. Hayes developed certain chapters and took the responsibility to work with contributors for the book such as the six chapters on Reproductive and Gender-Related Agents among others.

Linda McCuistion joined Kee and Hayes in 2005. McCuistion has updated many of Kee's chapters with new drugs and content.

CONTRIBUTORS

Christina DiMaggio Boudreaux, RN, BSN, IBCLC
Director of Nursing
Elba Medical Distributors
Metairie, Louisiana

Linda Laskowski-Jones, MS, APRN, ACNS-BC, CEN, NEA-BC, FAWM, FAAN
Vice President, Emergency and Trauma Services
Christiana Care Health System
Newark, Delaware

Jared Robertson III, RN, MN
Certified Registered Nurse Anesthesiologist
U.S. Army
Pass Christian, Mississippi

Sharon K. Broscious, RN, PhD
Program Director, Undergraduate Nursing
South University
Savannah, Georgia

Delinda Martin, RNC, DNP
Associate Professor of Nursing
University of Holy Cross
New Orleans, Louisiana

The eleventh edition of *Pharmacology: A Patient-Centered Nursing Process Approach* is written for nursing students who can benefit from presentation of the principles of pharmacology in a straightforward, student-friendly manner. It focuses on need-to-know content and helps students learn to administer drugs safely and eliminate medication errors through extensive practice of dosage calculations and evidence-based application of the nursing process.

ORGANIZATION

Pharmacology: A Patient-Centered Nursing Process Approach is organized into 18 sections and 58 chapters. **Section I** is an introduction to pharmacology and includes thoroughly updated chapters on drug action, the drug approval process, cultural and pharmacogenetic considerations, drug interactions, over-the-counter drugs, ethical considerations, pediatric and geriatric considerations, drugs for substance use disorder, complementary and alternative therapies, life span issues, patient collaboration in community settings, the nursing process, patient-centered care, and the role of the nurse in drug research. This section will introduce the Next Generation NCLEX (NGN) Clinical Judgment Measurement Model (CJMM). Its focus is to develop clinical reasoning and clinical judgment skills in students' decision making. This edition contains several unfolding and single episode case studies presented using the CJMM six cognitive skills and contrasts these skills with the Nursing Process.

Section II focuses on patient safety and quality in pharmacotherapy, medication administration, and it features a comprehensive review of drug dosage calculations for adults and children that is a unique strength of this book. This unit, tabbed for quick reference, includes Systems of Measurement With Conversion Factors, Calculation Methods: Enteral and Parenteral Drug Dosages, Calculation Methods: Drugs That Require Reconstitution, Calculation Methods: Insulin Dosages, and Calculation Methods: Intravenous Flow Rates. Five methods of dosage calculation are presented with color coding for easy identification: basic formula, ratio and proportion/fractional equation, dimensional analysis, body weight, and body surface area. Integral to the sections on dosage calculations are clinical practice problems that feature actual drug labels in full color, which provide extensive practice in real-world dosage calculations. With this wide array of practice problems in a variety of health care settings, this unit eliminates the need to purchase a separate dosage calculations book.

Section III addresses nutrition, fluids, and electrolytes with separate chapters that cover vitamin and mineral replacement, fluid and electrolyte replacement, and nutritional support.

Sections IV through XVIII make up the core of *Pharmacology: A Patient-Centered Nursing Process Approach* and cover the drug classifications that students must understand to practice effectively. Each drug family chapter includes a chapter outline, learning objectives, at least one prototype drug chart, a drug table, and an extensive nursing process section.

- The **prototype drug charts** are a unique tool that students can use to view the many facets of a prototype drug through the lens of the nursing process. Each prototype drug is one of the common drugs in its drug class. The charts include drug class, contraindications, dosage, drug-lab-food interactions, pharmacokinetics, pharmacodynamics, therapeutic effects/uses, side effects, and adverse reactions. With these charts, students can see how the steps of the nursing process correlate with these key aspects of drug information and therapy.

- The **drug tables** provide a quick reference to routes, dosages, uses, and key considerations for the most commonly prescribed medications for a given class. They list the drug's generic names, dosages, uses and considerations, and specific information on half-life and protein binding.

- The **Clinical Judgment [Nursing Process]** provide a convenient summary of related concepts for concept-based curricula, patient assessments, patient problems, plan of care, and outcomes. These sections also include cultural content, nursing interventions, suggestions for patient teaching, and relevant herbal information.

ADDITIONAL FEATURES

Throughout this edition, we have retained, enhanced, and added a variety of features that teach students the fundamental principles of pharmacology and the role of the nurse in drug therapy:

- **Review questions** at the end of each chapter help prepare students for the NCLEX® examination with its increasing emphasis on pharmacology; answers are listed upside down below the questions for quick feedback.

- **Patient safety boxes** include information on medication safety, complementary and alternative therapies, and more.

- **Critical thinking case studies**, **critical thinking unfolding case studies**, and **critical thinking single episode case studies** have been added to several chapters in this edition. These case studies follow the new Next-Generation NCLEX® Exam Clinical Judgment Model and will challenge students in forming clinical judgment skills.

- **Complementary and alternative therapies** appear throughout the text to provide students with a quick reference to information on popular herbs and their side effects, drug interactions, and more.

- **Anatomy and physiology** is contained in all drug therapy chapters, including illustrated overviews of normal anatomy and physiology. These introductions give students the foundation for understanding how drugs work in various body systems.

- **High-alert drugs** (!) and **safety concerns** (⚡) are identified within the text with distinctive icons that make it easy to find crucial information.

TEACHING AND LEARNING RESOURCES

The eleventh edition of *Pharmacology: A Patient-Centered Nursing Process Approach* is the core of a complete teaching and learning package for nursing pharmacology. Additional components of this package include resources designed specifically for students, resources designed specifically for faculty members, and resources designed for both students and faculty.

FOR STUDENTS

A comprehensive *Study Guide,* available for purchase separately, provides thousands of study questions and answers, including clinically based situational practice problems, drug calculation problems and questions (many with actual drug labels), and case studies to help students master textbook content. Answers are provided at the end of the *Study Guide.*

A completely updated Evolve website (http://evolve.elsevier.com/McCuistion/pharmacology) provides additional resources for students, including the following:

- **Review questions for the NCLEX® Examination** organized by chapter
- **Downloadable key points** for content review on the go

- **Pharmacology animations** and **videos**
- **Unfolding case studies** with review questions

FOR FACULTY MEMBERS

The updated faculty Evolve website (http://evolve.elsevier.com/McCuistion/pharmacology) includes all of the student resources mentioned previously plus the following instructor-only resources:

- NEW! Additional Next-Generation NCLEX® pharmacology case studies.
- *TEACH for Nurses* **Lesson Plans** focus on the most important content from each chapter and provide innovative strategies for student engagement and learning. The lesson plans include strategies for integrating nursing curriculum standards (QSEN, concept-based learning, and BSN essentials), links to all relevant student and instructor resources, and an original instructor-only case study in each chapter.
- **ExamView Test Bank** features more than 1000 NCLEX® Examination–format questions that include alternate-item questions as well as rationales and page references for each question.

- **PowerPoint Collection** features customizable slides with images, integrated audience response system questions, and NCLEX-style questions.
- **Image Collection** provides approximately 125 full-color images from the book.

This textbook may be supplemented with the drug content found on government agency websites, which supply the latest information regarding changes to drug brand names.

It is our hope that *Pharmacology: A Patient-Centered Nursing Process Approach* and its comprehensive ancillary package will serve as a dynamic resource for teaching students the basic principles of pharmacology as well as their vital role in drug therapy.

Linda E. McCuistion
Kathleen Vuljoin DiMaggio
Mary B. Winton
Jennifer J. Yeager

ACKNOWLEDGMENTS

We wish to extend our sincere appreciation to the many professionals who assisted in the preparation of the eleventh edition of *Pharmacology: A Patient-Centered Nursing Process Approach* by reviewing chapters and offering suggestions.

We wish to especially thank Joyce LeFever Kee, who originated this pharmacology textbook, and her coauthor Evelyn R. Hayes, who worked tirelessly on many editions of this book.

We wish to thank the current contributors: Christina DiMaggio Boudreaux, Linda Laskowski-Jones, and Jared Robertson.

We wish to thank those who created and updated the previous established chapters: Margaret Barton-Burke, Joseph Boullata, Jacqueline Rosenjack Burchum, Katherine L. Byar, Michelle M. Byrne, Karen Carmody, Robin Webb Corbett, Sandy Elliott, Linda Goodwin, Janice Heinssen, Marilyn Herbert-Ashton, Judith W. Herrman, Kathleen J. Jones, Bettyrae Jordan, Robert J. Kizior, Paula R. Klemm, Anne E. Lara, Linda Laskowski-Jones, Ronald J. LeFever, Patricia S. Lincoln, Patricia O'Brien, Laura K. Williford Owens, Byron Peters, Lisa Ann Plowfield, Larry D. Purnell, Nancy C. Sharts-Hopko, Jane Purnell Taylor, Donald L. Taylor, Lynette M. Wachholz, Marcia Welsh, Gail Wilkes, and M. Linda Workman.

Of course, we are deeply indebted to the many patients and students we have had throughout our many years of professional nursing practice. From them we have learned many fine points about the role of therapeutic pharmacology in nursing practice.

Our deepest appreciation goes to pharmaceutical companies for use of their drug labels. Pharmaceutical companies that extended their courtesy to this book include the following:

- Abbott Laboratories
- AstraZeneca Pharmaceuticals
- Aventis
- Bayer Corporation
- Bristol-Myers Squibb (including Apothecon Laboratories and Mead Johnson Pharmaceuticals)
- DuPont/Merck Pharmaceuticals
- Eli Lilly and Company
- Elkins-Sinn, Inc.
- Glaxo-Wellcome
- Marion Merrell Dow, Inc.
- McNeill Laboratory, Inc.
- Merck and Co., Inc.
- Parke-Davis Co.
- Pfizer Inc.
- Rhone-Poulenc Rorer
- SmithKline Beecham Pharmaceutical
- Wyeth-Ayerst Laboratories

Thanks to Becton, Dickinson and Company for the syringe displays. Thanks to CareFusion Corporation for the photos of the infusion pumps.

Our sincere thanks to Elsevier, especially Yvonne Alexopoulos, Senior Content Strategist; Luke Held, Senior Content Development Manager; and Kate Mannix, Senior Project Manager, for their suggestions and wonderful assistance.

Linda E. McCuistion
Kathleen Vuljoin DiMaggio
Mary B. Winton
Jennifer J. Yeager

CONTENTS

UNIT IX Immunologic Drugs

Clinical Judgment Management Model (CJMM) and the Nursing Process

http://evolve.elsevier.com/McCuistion/pharmacology

OBJECTIVES

- Explain the primary change in the Next Generation NCLEX (NGN).
- Explain Concept and how it relates to patient care and the nursing process.
- Explain the steps of the nursing process and how each step relates to the CJMM.
- Define the six cognitive skills in the Clinical Judgment Measurement Model (CJMM).

- Develop a set of patient-centered outcomes.
- Discuss at least eight principles for health teaching related to drug therapy.
- Define the nurse's role as related to planning medication administration.

OUTLINE

In everyday practice, nurses have many important tasks, with drug administration at the top of their list. It is estimated that about 40% of the nurse's time is spent administering medication. Knowledge of medications is essential to patient safety. Nurses are often the first line of defense against drug errors in patient care. Federal, state, and local authorities issue regulations and guidelines for practice, and each state has a nurse practice act that defines the scope and function under which the nurse practices. Health care institutions also have policies that help nurses follow federal and state guidelines and regulations.

The National Council of State Boards of Nursing's (NCSBN) research has led to the development of the Next Generation NCLEX (NGN). The NGN is designed to measure new graduates' competence in clinical judgment. This chapter introduces the NCSBN's Clinical Judgment Measurement Model (CJMM) as it relates to the nursing process.

EXPLANATION OF TERMS

Nursing Process

The nursing process is used by nurses for the appropriate delivery of patient care. It is a systematic, rational method that addresses health needs and aids in developing a plan of care that includes drug administration. The nursing process supports the nurse in delivering prioritized patient care.

The National Council of State Boards of Nursing (NCSBN) defines the nursing process as "a scientific, clinical reasoning approach to client care." Much study by the NCSBN reveals that nurses use clinical judgment skills more than the nursing process. The steps in the nursing process include (1) assessment, (2) analysis, (3) planning, (4) intervention, and (5) evaluation (NCSBN 2018). Analysis includes both defining and ranking the patient's problems according to priority.

Patient Problems

Patient problems and needs are the basis for the patient plan of care. The problems presented in this chapter closely identify with the use of NANDA-1 language. However, nursing problems replace the use of nursing diagnoses. When using patient problem terminology, the language better defines nursing clinical practice. Patient problems are in the Analyze Cues (Interpret patient problems) and Prioritize Hypothesis (Rank patient problems by priority) in the Clinical Judgment Measurement Model. In the Nursing Process, patient problems are in the Analysis phase (see Box 1.1).

The Nursing Alliance For Quality Care (NAQC)

The Nursing Alliance for Quality Care (NAQC) is an organization that supports quality patient-centered health care. The NAQC in partnership with the American Nurses Association (ANA) has published guidelines that support the core principles of patient-centered quality care. These guidelines aim to foster the patient relationship as the cornerstone of patient safety and quality. The NAQC's mission is to advance the highest quality, safety, and value of consumer-centered health care for all individual patients, their families, and their communities. NAQC believes it is the nurse's role to cultivate successful patient and family engagement. Family engagement is an essential component in reducing drug errors. The nurse serves as a patient advocate by supporting the patient's right to practice informed decision making and by maintaining patient-centered engagement in the health care setting. These guidelines include nurses at all levels of education and across all health care settings. NAQC principles are fundamental to patient-centered practice and safety in pharmacotherapy.

CLINICAL JUDGMENT [NURSING PROCESS]

The NCSBN defines clinical judgment as the observed outcome of critical thinking and decision making (NCSBN, 2018). This edition will offer students a variety of case studies related to pharmacology that encourage the use of clinical judgment skills based on the NCSBN's Clinical Judgment Measurement Model (CJMM; Fig. 1.1). The unfolding case studies are somewhat complex in the information presented and encourage the use of clinical reasoning and clinical judgment skills in the student as the questions are answered.

The student will use CJMM's six cognitive skills: (1) Recognize Cues, (2) Analyze Cues, (3) Prioritize Hypothesis, (4) Generate Solutions, (5) Take Action, and (6) Evaluate Outcomes (see Box 1.1, which compares the Clinical Judgment Measurement Model and the Nursing Process).

Concept

The focus of *concept* is on the patient-centered model of care instead of the disease-centered model of care. Concept influences the organization of patient information and the delivery of the patient's care using the nursing process according to the patient's problems. Nursing care

---

BOX 1.1   Steps of the Clinical Judgment Measurement Model and the Nursing Process

Clinical Judgment Measurement Model	Nursing Process
Recognize Cues	Assessment
Analyze Cues	Analysis (Interpret problems)
Prioritize Hypothesis	Analysis (Rank problems)
Generate Solutions	Planning
Take Action	Interventions
Evaluate Outcomes	Evaluations

The NCSBN clinical judgment measurement model

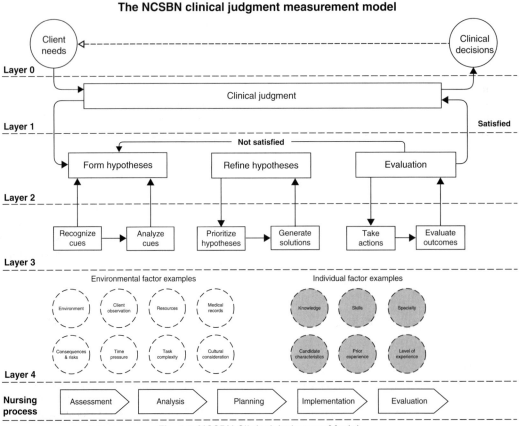

Fig. 1.1 NCSBN Clinical Judgment Model

plans using a nursing diagnosis organize information according to the patient's medical diagnosis.

The Concept centers its focus for nursing care around the reason the care is being provided to the patient. It is a more holistic view of the patient rather than the disease model. The term *Concept* includes health, illness, and health promotion of the patient. This involves preventive, primary, acute, and chronic health care for the ill patient.

Concepts are related to the patient's problems, the medications, or topics of care listed within the nursing process. A definition will immediately follow each concept (e.g., Concept: Safety—protecting the patient from possible injury by practicing safe medication administration.)

By focusing on the Concept, the nurse will provide patient education, restorative health needs, medication administration, and possibly emergency care. The nurse's attention is on promoting the patient's good health needs.

RECOGNIZE CUES [ASSESSMENT]

The nurse gathers cues (information) from the patient about their health and lifestyle practices. Cues are important facts about the patient that aid the nurse in making clinical care decisions. The nurse asks the patient direct questions about their illness. The data collected may be obtained from many different sources, including a systematic physical assessment of the patient's body systems and the medical record, which includes patient history, vital signs, and labs. With the patient's permission, information can be obtained from their family members. Also, other attending health care professionals can be consulted. The data collected are both subjective and objective data. Important cues are identified based on relevant (directly related) or irrelevant (unrelated) information concerning the patient's history, condition, and medical situation. It is vital to determine which data are most relevant to the patient's interventions and outcomes and of immediate concern for the delivery of priority care. This phase is paramount because the nurse will use the information gathered to form the basis of the patient's plan of care, which includes drug administration.

Subjective Data

Subjective data include information provided verbally by the patient, family members, friends, or other sources. The patient must verbalize subjective data, which are imperceptible by the nurse's senses. Subjective data are based on what patients or family members communicate to the nurse. The nurse may ask open-ended questions, allowing the patient to answer directly, such as, "Please tell me about your current medications." The nurse may help the patient explain or describe subjective data but must never speak for the patient. Subjective data comprise what the patient personally has to say about their medications, health problems, and lifestyle. Examples of pertinent information that the nurse can use to help solicit a response from the patient include the following:

- Inquire about the patient's current health history, including family history.
- Question whether or not the patient has problems swallowing (dysphagia).
- Have the patient verbalize signs and symptoms of their illness.
- Discuss the patient's current health concerns:
  - Knowledge of medications and side effects
  - Over-the-counter (OTC) remedies, nutritional supplements, herbal remedies, and contraceptives
  - Knowledge of side effects to report to the physician
  - Attitudes and beliefs about taking medications
  - Allergies

- Financial barriers
- Use of tobacco, alcohol, and caffeine
- Cultural dietary barriers
- The patient's home safety needs
- Caregiver needs and support system

Enhancing the patient's adherence to their drug therapy regimen is an essential component of health teaching. The patient's attitudes and values about taking medication is an important consideration when determining readiness to learn. Attitudes and values should be considered when planning interventions to support the patient's decision to adopt healthy behaviors related to their medications. In addition, the patient's social support system should be emphasized. This special support system is unique to the individual and may be composed of persons who assist in preparing, organizing, and ordering medications. A support system can alert a patient to side effects, encourage actions that promote medication compliance, and notify the health care provider if a problem arises.

Objective Data

Objective data are what the nurse directly observes about the patient's health status. It involves collecting the patient's health information by using personal senses: seeing, hearing, smelling, and touching. Objective data collection provides additional information about the patient's symptoms and also targets the organs most likely to be affected by drug therapy. For example, if a drug is nephrotoxic, the patient's creatinine clearance should be assessed.

The following are examples of objective data assessed by the nurse concerning medication administration:

- Physical health assessment
- Laboratory and diagnostic test results
- Data from the physician's notes (i.e., health history)
- Measurement of vital signs
- The patient's body language

ANALYZE CUES [ANALYSIS] AND PRIORITZE HYPOTHESIS [ANALYSIS]

Analyze Cues and Prioritize Hypothesis are part of the Analysis phase of the Nursing Process. This involves identifying, organizing, and prioritizing the patient's problems from the data collected. Analyze Cues (facts) interprets the patient's problem(s). Prioritize Hypothesis organizes and ranks the problem(s).

Analyze Cues [Analysis]

Consider the cues (facts) in the context of the patient history and determine what kind of care the patient should receive. Ask yourself the following question, "How do these cues relate to the patient's condition or history?" Identify cues that support or contraindicate a problem or condition. Certain cues will be more concerning than others. This process will help identify potential complications and identify the patient's actual problems.

Prioritize Hypothesis [Analysis]

Once the cues (facts) are analyzed, the hypothesis (problem) is determined. The problems are organized, prioritized, and ranked according to acuity. There may be the need to collect additional patient assessment data.

When the cues show an abnormality, it serves as the defining characteristic of the patient's problem(s). Consider all possibilities about what is occurring in the patient's situation, including patient urgency and risk. Think about how the relevant cues relate to the patient's condition or history. Determine which cues are most likely serious and why. Rank the problems according to priority (urgency, likelihood, risk, difficulty, and time). More than one applicable patient problem may be generated.

Patient Problem(s)

Some common patient problems related to drug therapy include:

- Abdominal pain
- Confusion
- Decreased adherence
- Need for health teaching
- Cognitive decline
- Nonadherence

Use of the patient problem(s) is beneficial to the patient because its focus is on the individual patient's care as related to a diagnosis derived from the patient's diagnostic illness. Its focus is patient-centered and not disease-oriented.

GENERATE SOLUTIONS [PLANNING]

This phase identifies expected outcomes and uses the patient's problem(s) to define a set of interventions to achieve the most desirable outcomes. The interventions are specific, evidence-based actions related to the expected outcomes. Consider which actual or potential actions should be avoided or contraindicated, as certain actions may be harmful to the patient in some situations.

Outcomes are patient centered, describe a specific activity, and include a time frame for achievement and reevaluation. Generate Solutions [Planning] includes the development of nursing interventions that assist the patient in meeting medication outcomes. To develop patient-centered expected outcomes, collaboration with the patient and/or family is necessary. Effective expected outcomes have the following qualities:

- The expected outcome is realistic, measurable, and includes reasonable deadlines.
- The expected outcome is acceptable to both the patient and nurse.
- The expected outcome is dependent on the patient's decision making ability.
- The expected outcome is shared with the health care team.
- The expected outcome identifies components for evaluation.

Examples of well-written comprehensive expected outcomes include the following:

- The patient will independently administer the prescribed dose of 4 units of regular insulin by the end of the fourth session of instruction.
- The patient will prepare a 3-day medication recording sheet that correctly reflects the prescribed medication schedule by the end of the second session of instruction.

TAKE ACTION [NURSING INTERVENTIONS]

This phase provides nursing education, drug administration, patient care, and other interventions necessary to accomplish the expected outcomes. The nurse decides which actions will address the highest priority of care. Actions may include, but are not limited to, additional assessment, patient health teaching, documentation, requesting prescriptions from the provider, implementation of nursing skills, consultation with health care team members, and drug administration.

Patient Teaching

It is important for the nurse to keep in mind factors that help promote patient learning: the patient's *readiness* to learn and investment in their learning. If the patient buys into wanting to practice good health

---

> ### BOX 1.2 Patient Teaching Card
>
> **Name of drug:** Acetaminophen 325–650 mg
> **Reason for taking the drug:** Minor aches, pains, and fever
> **Dosage:** One or two tablets as needed every 4 to 6 hours; maximum dose is 3250 mg daily unless under health care provider supervision, then 4 g daily may be used.
> **Time to take the drug:** 8:00 a.m./2:00 p.m./8:00 p.m.
> **Possible side effects:** Nausea, upper stomach pain, itching, loss of appetite, dark urine, and jaundice
> **Possible adverse effects:** Overdosage can affect the liver and cause hepatotoxicity.
> **Notify health care provider:** If side effects occur
> **Health care provider's telephone #:** _____
> **Warning:**
> - *Never* take this medication with alcohol.
> - If pregnant or nursing, notify the health care provider before taking the medication.
> - Do not take this medication with other over-the-counter (OTC) drugs or supplements without notifying the health care provider.

---

principles, learning can be successful. The nurse and patient together must become fully engaged in the learning process.

Timing is another important factor. What is the best time for the patient to learn? Is the patient a morning or night person? People seem to learn best if the time between the learning and implementation is short. The environment should be conducive to learning with a temperature that is comfortable and an environment that is quiet. It is important for the nurse to recognize that certain barriers to learning exist. Pain is an obstacle, and the patient's teaching should be postponed until pain is relieved. Be mindful of language barriers. If the patient does not speak the same language as the nurse, an interpreter may be needed.

Patient teaching is essential to the patient's recovery. It allows the patient to become informed about his or her health problems and to participate in creating interventions that can lead to good health outcomes. It is within the scope and practice of the nurse to embrace patient education and to use health-teaching strategies.

Nurses have a primary role in teaching both patients and families about drug administration. It is important that teachings are tailored to the patient's educational level and that the patient trusts the nurse for learning to begin. With the patient's consent, it is always important to include a family member or friend in the teaching to provide support to the patient with reminders and encouragement; they can also detect possible side effects that may occur in the patient.

General

The following are important principles to remember when teaching patients about their medications:

- Maintain the Health Insurance Portability and Accountability Act (HIPAA) when discussing the patient's medical records and personal health information with their family and friends.
- Prior to the teaching, assess the patient for health literacy skills such as the ability to read, write, listen, speak, communicate, and interact with others.
- Always allow the patient time to perform a repeat demonstration if taught a skill or a moment to teach-back the information learned. This confirms learning has taken place.
- Instruct the patient to take the drug as prescribed. Consistency in adhering to the prescribed drug regimen is important.
- Provide simple written instructions with the doctor and pharmacy names and telephone numbers.

- Advise the patient to notify their health care provider if any of the following occur:
  - The dose, frequency, or time of the drug is adjusted.
  - A female patient becomes pregnant.
  - An OTC medication or supplement is added.

Side Effects

Give the patient instructions that will help minimize any side effects (e.g., avoid direct sunlight with drugs that can cause photosensitivity or sunburn). Advise patients of any expected changes in the color of urine or stool, and counsel the patient who has dizziness caused by orthostatic hypotension to rise slowly from a sitting to a standing position.

Self-Administration

Perform an ongoing health literacy assessment of the patient's motor skills and abilities. Remember that modifications may be necessary to the teaching plan based on the assessment.

Instruct the patient according to the prescribed route: eye or nose instillation, subcutaneous injection, suppository, oral/mucosal (e.g., swish-and-swallow suspensions), and inhaled via a metered-dose inhaler with or without a spacer. Include a return demonstration in the instructions when appropriate.

The use of drug cards is a helpful teaching tool (see Box 1.2). Drug cards can be obtained from the health care provider, pharmacy, or drug manufacturer, or simply designed by the patient or caretaker. They are helpful components for teaching. Drug cards may include: the name of the drug; the reason for taking the drug; the drug dosage; times to take the drug; possible side effects; adverse effects; when to notify the care provider; and specific facts about what should or should not be done when taking the medication (e.g., take with food, do not crush tablets).

Diet

Advise the patient about foods to include in their diet and foods to avoid. Many foods interact with certain drugs. Depending on the nature of the interaction, certain foods have the ability to decrease drug absorption, increase the risk of drug toxicity, or create other problems that are important safety concerns.

Important Nursing Considerations

The nurse must keep in mind the patient's cultural needs to individualize the teaching plan. Begin by identifying your own cultural beliefs, practices, and values to keep them separate from those of the patient. If a language barrier exists, arrange for an interpreter who speaks the patient's language. Research shows that family members are not recommended as an effective interpreter because they may hinder communication. Ask the patient if there is something special you should know concerning his or her cultural needs.

Additional suggestions include the following:

- Space instruction over several sessions, and be flexible in the timing of medication teaching as desired by the patient.
- Allow time for patients to respond to questions. Ask open-ended questions, and have patients demonstrate their understanding of treatments rather than verbalizing them.
- Review community resources related to the patient's plan of care including medications.
- Collaborate with the patient and family and other health care staff and agencies to meet the patient's health care needs.
- Identify patients at risk for noncompliance with their drug regimen. Alert the health care provider and pharmacist so they can develop a plan to minimize the number of drugs and the number of times drugs are administered.
- Evaluate the patient's understanding of the medication regimen on a regular basis.

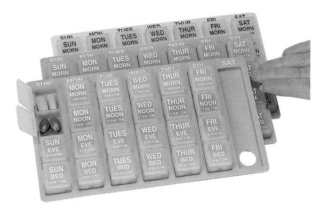

Fig. 1.2 Medication box and pill organizer. (Courtesy Apothecary Products, Inc., Burnsville, MN.)

BOX 1.3 Important Points for Patients and Families to Remember

- Medications should be taken as prescribed by your health care provider. If problems arise with the dose or timing or if side effects occur, contact your medical provider.
- If drugs are placed in a drug box, keep the original labeled containers.
- Keep all drugs out of the reach of children.
- Before using any over-the-counter (OTC) drugs, including vitamins and nutritional supplements, check with your health care provider. This includes the use of aspirin, ibuprofen, and laxatives. Consider consulting the pharmacist before buying or using a product.
- Bring all drugs with you when you visit the health care provider.
- Know the purpose of each medication and which side effect necessitates a call to the health care provider.
- Do not drink alcoholic beverages around the time you take your medications. Alcohol is absolutely contraindicated with certain medications, and it may alter the action and absorption of the medications.
- Be aware that smoking tobacco also can alter the absorption of some medications (e.g., theophylline-type drugs, antidepressants, pain medications). Consult your health care provider or pharmacist for specific information.

- Empower the patient to take responsibility for their drug management.
- General points to remember and tips for successful patient education are presented in Box 1.3.

Many people take multiple drugs simultaneously several times each day, which presents a challenge to patients, their families, and nurses. This complex activity of taking several drugs can be segmented into several simple tasks that include the following:

- Drug boxes (Fig. 1.2) obtained from a local pharmacy may be used to prepare and organize medications. These boxes have labeled compartments for each day of the week and several rows of compartments for drugs taken multiple times a day. The boxes sort the drugs according to the time of day each pill is to be taken. They can simplify the task of taking medications. However, it is important to remember the pill boxes must be filled correctly. A trusted relative or friend can always assist the patient when filling the boxes.
- Multidose pill packets are available from many local pharmacies. The pharmacy will package the patient's prescription medications into easy-to-open packages. Many pharmacies can provide a 30-day supply of the patient's prescription medications, individually packaged and labeled according to dose, date, and time at no extra cost.
- A recording sheet may be helpful. When the drug is administered, the patient or family member marks the sheet, which is designed to meet the patient's individual needs. For example, the time can

BOX 1.4   Medication Recording Sheet

Medication	Dosage Daily	DAYS OF WEEK S	M	T	W	Th	F	S
Captopril	12.5 mg							
Digoxin	0.25 mg							
Furosemide	40 mg							

be noted by the patient, or it can be entered beforehand, with the patient marking the designated time the dose is taken (Box 1.4).

- Alternatives to recording sheets are also available, and alarm reminder devices may be used.

Throughout the teaching plan, the nurse promotes patient independence (e.g., self-administering, safely storing, and ordering of the drug regimen). Always keep in mind patients' expected outcomes when teaching. Box 1.5 presents a checklist for health teaching in drug therapy.

EVALUATE OUTCOMES [EVALUATION]

The nurse evaluates whether the patient's interventions and outcomes have been met and compares the patient's response with the expected outcomes. What signs point to improvement, decline, or appear unchanged in the patient? Determine whether the nursing interventions were effective, ineffective, or made no difference. If the interventions and expected outcomes are unmet, the nurse

BOX 1.5   Checklist for Health Teaching in Drug Therapy

- Assess the patient's health literacy skills to ensure that the patient has the capacity to obtain, process, and understand basic health information.
- Reinforce the importance of drug adherence.
- Always complete a health history and physical assessment on the patient.
- Assess all of the drugs on the patient's profile for possible drug interactions.
- Explain the reason the patient is taking the drug, the time it should be administered, and whether it should be taken with or without food.
- Review the side effects and adverse reactions, and make sure the patient has the doctor's telephone number and knows when to notify the health care provider or pharmacist.
- Distinguish whether the patient needs baseline or monthly laboratory work to monitor drug levels.
- Keep in mind that patient validation of learning may include a return demonstration of psychomotor skills (insulin administration).
- Show the patient how to record drug administration on a sheet of paper by indicating day and time drug is taken.
- Discuss the patient's financial resources and, if needed, consult a social worker for resources.
- Discuss the patient's support system such as family or friends as caregivers.
- Provide the patient with a list of community resources.

will revise the interventions and expected outcomes to ensure success. If the interventions and expected outcomes are met, the nurse will document the successful attainment in the patient's plan of care.

▊ CRITICAL THINKING CASE STUDY

A 66-year-old man just arrived on the medical surgical unit after an emergency appendectomy. He is complaining of incisional pain, nausea, and headache. His blood pressure is 150/80, heart rate is 70 beats per minute, and his temperature is 100.8°F.

1. Identify the patient's highest priority assessment needs.

2. Formulate a nursing problem based on the patient's assessment data.
3. Name two nursing interventions that will achieve a positive outcome.
4. Evaluate the effectiveness of the interventions.
5. Have the expected outcomes been met?

▊ REVIEW QUESTIONS

1. During a medication review session, a patient states, "I do not know why I am taking all of these pills." Based on this piece of subjective data, which problem will the nurse identify?
   a. Pain
   b. Knowledge
   c. Fatigue
   d. Anxiety
2. The nurse is developing a list of the patient's expected outcomes. Which is the best expected outcome for this patient?
   a. The patient will self-administer albuterol by taking a deep breath before inhaling.
   b. The patient will self-administer albuterol by the end of the second teaching session.
   c. The patient will independently self-administer the prescribed dose of albuterol by the end of the second teaching session.
   d. The patient will organize their medications according to the time each medication is due.
3. When developing an effective medication teaching plan, which component will the nurse identify as *most* essential?

   a. Written instructions
   b. The patient's readiness to learn
   c. Use of colorful charts
   d. A review of community resources
4. When developing an individualized medication teaching plan, which topics will the nurse include? (Select all that apply.)
   a. Adherence to the prescribed drug regimen
   b. Always using the prescribed drug route
   c. Knowing adverse side effects to report to doctor
   d. Always doubling the next dose if drug is missed
   e. Telling the doctor when taking over-the-counter (OTC) supplements
5. The Nursing Alliance for Quality Care's main focus is for health care providers to strive for which goal?
   a. Quality in medication administration
   b. Confidentiality as determined by the patient
   c. Development of a patient relationship/family engagement
   d. Patient independence within the family of origin

6. Which teaching strategy is most likely to succeed in health teaching with the patient and family?
   a. Know the reason why each drug was ordered.
   b. Have patients learn the generic name of each pill.
   c. A repeat demonstration should follow the nurse's teaching.
   d. Have the patient identify the number and color of the pills.

7. Prioritize the steps of Clinical Judgment [Nursing Process]
   a. Generate Solutions [Planning]
   b. Analyze Cues [Analysis]
   c. Recognize Cues [Assessment]
   d. Prioritize Hypothesis [Analysis]
   e. Evaluate Outcomes [Evaluation]
   f. Take Action [Intervention]

2

Drug Development and Ethical Considerations

OBJECTIVES

- Identify the three core ethical principles.
- Relate the core ethical principles that govern informed consent and risk-benefit ratio.
- Discuss the 2015 American Nurses Association Code of Ethics and its nine provisions.
- Describe the objectives of each phase of human clinical experimentation.
- Discuss federal legislation acts related to US Food and Drug Administration drug approvals.
- Explain the Canadian schedules for drugs sold in Canada.
- Describe the function of state nurse practice acts.
- Differentiate between chemical, generic, and brand names of drugs.
- Define "over the counter" as it relates to drugs.

OUTLINE

Approval of new drugs by the US Food and Drug Administration (FDA) has been steady since the early 2000s, reaching an all-time high in 2014 with the approval of 44 new drugs. To facilitate this increase, in 2004 the FDA established its Critical Path Initiative, a national strategy "to drive innovation in the scientific processes through which medical products are developed, evaluated, and manufactured." One focus of this initiative is on "improving the prevention, diagnosis, and treatment of rare and neglected disorders." Initiative successes include developing biomarkers and other scientific tools, streamlining clinical trials, and ensuring product safety.

The process of drug discovery and manufacturing takes 10 to 12 years, with a cost of more than $1 billion for each drug. Out of every 5000 to 10,000 compounds that begin preclinical testing, only one makes it through the FDA approval process. The steps of the process are shown in Fig. 2.1. Drug research and development is a complex process that is of particular interest and importance to professional nursing practice.

This chapter is devoted to a description of basic ethical principles that govern drug development and the nurse's role in this process.

CORE ETHICAL PRINCIPLES

Three core ethical principles are relevant to research involving human subjects: respect for persons, beneficence, and justice. Derived from the Belmont Report, the World Medical Association Declaration of Helsinki set out ethical principles for medical research that involves human subjects. These ethical principles are integral to the issues of informed consent and risk-benefit ratio in such research.

Respect for Persons

Patients should be treated as independent persons capable of making decisions in their own best interests. Patients with diminished decision-making capacity are entitled to protection. When making health care decisions, patients should be made aware of alternatives available to them as well as the consequences that stem from those alternatives. The patient's choice should be honored whenever possible. It is imperative that nurses recognize when patients are not capable of making decisions in their own best interest and are therefore entitled to protection. The nurse can assist with the determination of decision-making capacity through frequent assessment of the patient's cognitive status.

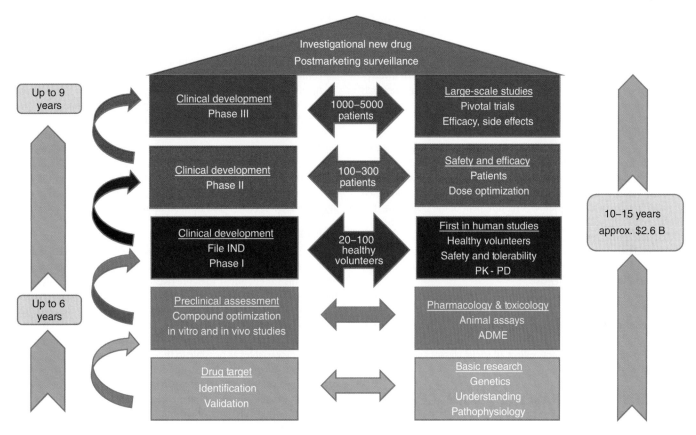

Fig. 2.1 The drug discovery and development process. *ADME,* Absorption, distribution, metabolism, and excretion; *FDA,* Food and Drug Administration; *IND,* investigational new drug; *PD,* pharmacodynamics; *PK,* pharmacokinetics. (From Wecker, L., Taylor, D. A., Theobald, R. J. [2019]. *Brody's human pharmacology* [6th ed.]. Philadelphia: Elsevier.)

Autonomy is an integral component of respect for persons. Autonomy is the right to self-determination. In health care settings, health care personnel must respect the patient's right to make decisions in their own best interest, even if the decision is not what the health care personnel want or think is best for the patient. Generally, patients can refuse any and all treatments (right of autonomy) except when the decision poses a threat to others—such as with tuberculosis, when taking medications is legally mandated. Autonomy is as relevant to the conduct of research as it is in health care decision making; patients have the right to refuse to participate in a research study and may withdraw from studies at any time without penalty.

Informed Consent

Informed consent has its roots in the 1947 Nuremberg Code. The two most relevant aspects of the Code are the right to be informed and that participation is voluntary, without coercion. If coercion is suspected, the nurse is obligated to report this suspicion promptly. Informed consent has dimensions beyond protection of the individual patient's choice:

- It is a mutual sharing of information, a process of communication.
- It expresses respect for the person.
- It gains the patient's active involvement in their care.
- It respects the patient's right to self-determination.

It is the role of the health care provider, *not* the nurse, to explain the study to the patient and what is expected of the patient and to respond to questions from the patient. When giving written consent, the patient must be alert and able to comprehend; consent forms should be written

> **BOX 2.1 Sample Inclusion and Exclusion Criteria**
>
> **Inclusion**
> - Persons between the ages of 18 and 65
> - Persons weighing between 50 and 100 kg
> - Persons on a stable dose (i.e., no dose change in the previous 3 months) of cardiac medications (e.g., anticoagulants, angiotensin-converting enzyme inhibitors [ACEIs], angiotensin II–receptor blockers [ARBs], beta blockers, and diuretics)
> - Persons adhering to a no-added-salt diet
>
> **Exclusion**
> - Women who are pregnant or nursing
> - Women of childbearing age who do not use oral contraceptives
> - Persons with symptomatic cardiac disease, hepatic dysfunction, chronic kidney disease, neurologic disorders, or musculoskeletal disorders
> - Persons with clinically significant abnormal laboratory values (chemistry and hematology)

at or below the eighth-grade reading level, and words should be kept to fewer than three syllables.

Nurses are patient advocates. In collaboration with the health care provider and the pharmacist, the nurse must be knowledgeable about all aspects of a drug study—including all inclusion and exclusion criteria for participants (Box 2.1), study protocol, and study-related documentation—to promote participant safety and quality study results.

Fig. 2.2 shows a sample of an informed consent form for a clinical drug trial, and Box 2.2 shows an informed consent checklist.

Beneficence

Beneficence is the duty to protect research subjects from harm. It involves ensuring the risks and possible benefits from participating in a research study are clearly defined and ensuring the benefits are greater than the risk.

Risk-Benefit Ratio

The risk-benefit ratio is one of the most complex problems faced by the researcher. All possible consequences of a clinical study must be analyzed and balanced against the inherent risks and the anticipated benefits. Physical, psychological, and social risks must be identified and weighed against the benefits. A requirement of the Department of Health and Human Services (DHHS) is that institutional review boards (IRBs) determine that risks to subjects be reasonable in relation to the anticipated benefits, if any, for subjects. No matter how noble the intentions, the calculation of risks and benefits by the researcher cannot be totally accurate or comprehensive.

Justice

Justice requires that the selection of research subjects be fair. Research must be conducted so that the distribution of benefits and burdens is equitable (i.e., research subjects reflect all social classes and racial and ethnic groups).

OBJECTIVES AND PHASES OF PHARMACEUTICAL RESEARCH

The FDA requires clinical research to follow the Good Clinical Practice (GCP) Consolidated Guideline, an international ethical and scientific quality standard for designing, conducting, monitoring, auditing, recording, analyzing, and reporting clinical research. It is the foundation of clinical trials that involve human subjects. Additional guidance and information sheets are available from the FDA on multiple topics related to clinical research.

Preclinical Trials

Before the implementation of clinical research, the FDA requires preclinical trials to determine a drug's toxic and pharmacologic effects through in vitro and in vivo animal testing in the laboratory. Through these trials, drug developers are able to determine genotoxicity, the ability of a compound to damage genetic information in a cell, in addition to drug absorption, distribution, metabolism, and excretion.

Human Clinical Experimentation

Historically, drug research was done only with Caucasian males, causing uncertainty as to the validity of research results for people of other ethnicities and for women and children. In 1993 Congress passed the National Institutes of Health (NIH) Revitalization Act, which helped establish guidelines to include women and minorities in clinical research. Additionally, the Best Pharmaceuticals for Children Act (BPCA) of 2002 and the Pediatric Research Equity Act (PREA) of 2003 encourage pharmaceutical companies to study their drugs in children.

Clinical experimentation in drug research and development encompasses four phases, each with its own objectives (see Fig. 2.1). A multidisciplinary team approach that includes nurses, physicians, pharmacologists, statisticians, and research associates is required to ensure safety and quality in all phases of clinical research. A brief description of each phase follows.

Phase I: Researchers test a new drug or treatment in a small group of people for the first time to evaluate its safety, determine a safe dosage range, and identify side effects.

Phase II: The drug or treatment is given to a larger group of people to see whether it is effective and to further evaluate its safety.

Phase III: The drug or treatment is given to large groups of people to confirm its effectiveness, monitor side effects, compare it with commonly used treatments, and collect information that will allow the drug or treatment to be used safely.

Phase IV: Studies are done after the drug or treatment has been marketed to gather information on the drug's effects in various populations and to assess any side effects associated with long-term use.

Pharmaceutical companies are eager to bring new drugs to market. To reduce delays in the FDA approval process, in 1992 Congress passed the Prescription Drug User Fee Act, which provided the FDA with funds to expedite the review process. As a result, the average drug approval time has decreased from 30 months to 12.

Clinical Research Study Design

An appropriate experimental design is important to answer questions about drug safety and efficacy. Studies are designed to determine the effect of the independent variable (treatment, such as with a drug) on the dependent variable (outcome, such as clinical effect). Intervening (extraneous) variables are factors that may interfere with study results, and these may include age, sex, weight, disease state, diet, and the subject's social environment. It is important to control for as many of the intervening variables as possible to increase study validity.

The *experimental group* in drug trials is the group that receives the drug being tested. The *control group* in drug trials may receive no drug; a different drug; a placebo (pharmacologically inert substance); or the same drug with a different dose, route, or frequency of administration.

AMERICAN NURSES ASSOCIATION CODE OF ETHICS

The American Nurses Association (ANA) Code of Ethics "was developed as a guide for carrying out nursing responsibilities in a manner consistent with quality in nursing care and the ethical obligations of the profession." It was first adopted in 1950 and most recently was revised with interpretive statements in 2015. The ANA Code of Ethics is founded on the principles first identified by Florence Nightingale, who believed that a nurse's ethical duty was first and foremost to care for the patient. The 2015 update addresses advances in nursing leadership, social policy and global health, and the challenges nurses face related to social media, electronic health records, and the nurse's expanded role in clinical research.

The Nurse's Role in Clinical Research

Nurses are at the forefront of clinical research. Regardless of the setting (inpatient or outpatient), nurses are likely to encounter patients eligible to participate, considering participation, or actively participating in clinical research. As such, nurses are responsible for both the safety of the patient and the integrity of the research protocol.

DRUG STANDARDS AND LEGISLATION

Drug Standards

The set of drug standards used in the United States is the United States Pharmacopeia (USP). The *United States Pharmacopeia and the National Formulary* (USP-NF), the authoritative source for drug standards (dosage, forms, drug substances, excipients, biologics, compounded preparations, and dietary supplements), is published annually. Experts in nursing, pharmaceutics, pharmacology, chemistry, and microbiology all contribute. Drugs included in the USP-NF have met high standards for therapeutic use, patient safety, quality, purity, strength, packaging safety, and dosage form. Drugs that meet these standards have the initials "USP" following their official name, denoting global recognition of high quality.

Sample Informed Consent Form for Randomized Clinical Trial of a Drug

Title of study: Comparison of a new drug [A] with an existing drug [B] used in treatment of disease X

Principal investigator: Dr. ABC

Institute: Department of Pediatrics, Aga Khan University

Introduction:

I am Dr. [SAK] from Department of Pediatrics, the Aga Khan University and doing a research on treatment of disease [X, for example malaria]. There is a new drug [A] which is being recommended for its treatment. I want to see if the new drug [A] is as good as or better than the commonly used drug [B] for the treatment of disease [malaria]. Since you are a patient of (or suffering from) disease [malaria], I would like to invite you to join this research study.

Background information

Disease X (Malaria) is a common disease in Pakistan, Asia and Africa, caused by a germ (parasite) spread by mosquito. It causes high grade fever. Some patients may have complications and even die. The commonly used drugs are losing their effectiveness and germs are getting resistant to it. A new drug known as [A] is supposed to be effective in treatment of disease (malaria) but there is not enough evidence that it is as good as other drugs used for treatment of disease (malaria).

Purpose of this research study

The purpose of study is to find out if the new drug is as good as or better than other drugs used for treatment of malaria in our population and; also to see if germs are not resistant to it.

Procedures

In this study, all patients aged 15 to 50 years of age, presenting at the clinic with fever for less than one week duration and having no other diagnosis will be registered and screened for malaria. For diagnosis of disease (malaria), one ml of blood will be taken from the patients and checked for presence of germs (malarial parasite). Those patients having positive test for the disease (malaria), will be included in the study. They will be divided randomly in to two groups by a computer draw. One group will get the new drug (A) and the other group will get the commonly used drug (B). Neither the doctor nor the patient will know which drug he/she is getting for treatment of his/her disease. A record will be kept for the duration of fever and other symptoms including any other side effect. Other necessary treatment will also be provided if needed.

Possible risks or benefits

No significant side effects have been reported for this new drug (A). However, some patients may feel nausea or may have vomiting. Drawing of blood may cause some discomfort or blue discoloration at the site of bleeding. Lowering of white blood cells and platelet is a common feature of the disease.

There is no direct financial or other benefit for the participant of the study. However, all the investigations will be done free of cost to the patients and; the drugs (A) or (B) will be provided free. Treatment of any side effect will also be provided free of cost. Sponsor of the study will bear the cost of drugs, investigations and treatment of side effects related to the study drugs.

Right of refusal to participate and withdrawal

You are free to choose to participate in the study. You may refuse to participate without any loss of benefit which you are otherwise entitled to. You child will receive the same standard care and treatment which is considered best for him irrespective of your decision to participate in the study. You may also withdraw any time from the study without any adverse effect on management of your child or any loss of benefit which you are otherwise entitled to. You may also refuse to answer some or all the questions if you don't feel comfortable with those questions.

Confidentiality

The information provided by you will remain confidential. Nobody except principal investigator will have an access to it. Your name and identity will also not be disclosed at any time. However the data may be seen by Ethical review committee and may be published in journal and elsewhere without giving your name or disclosing your identity.

Available Sources of Information

If you have any further questions you may contact Principal Investigator (Dr. SAK), department of pediatrics at Aga Khan University on following phone number 486xxxx

Fig. 2.2 Sample informed consent for a clinical trial of a drug. (From Sample Informed Consent for a Randomized Clinical Trial of a Drug. [n.d.] Aga Khan University. http://www.aku.edu/research/urc/ethicalreviewcommittee/sampleconsentforms/Pages/sampleconsentforms.aspx.)

1. **AUTHORIZATION**

I have read and understand this consent form, and I volunteer to participate in this research study. I understand that I will receive a copy of this form. I voluntarily choose to participate, but I understand that my consent does not take away any legal rights in the case of negligence or other legal fault of anyone who is involved in this study. I further understand that nothing in this consent form is intended to replace any applicable Federal, state, or local laws.

Participant's Name (Printed or Typed):
Date:

Participant's Signature or thumb impression:
Date:

Principal Investigator's Signature:
Date:

Signature of Person Obtaining Consent:
Date:

Fig. 2.2, cont'd

◎ CLINICAL JUDGMENT [NURSING PROCESS]

Clinical Research

Concept: Safety
- Protection of the patient from potential or actual harm; it is a basic human need.

Recognize Cues [Assessment]
- Identify patients who are eligible to participate in or who are participating in clinical research.
- Assess response to the study agent and identify adverse events (an unfavorable or unintended sign, symptom, or disease that was not present at the time of study enrollment and is associated with the treatment or procedure).

Analyze Cues and Prioritize Hypothesis [Patient Problems]
- Need for health teaching
- Potential for decreased adherence

Generate Solutions [Planning]
- Have a process in place to identify persons who are eligible to participate in clinical research or to identify participants actively participating in clinical research studies.
- Have a process in place to facilitate education and informed consent of eligible study participants.
- Plan educational programming for staff who provide direct care to study participants.

- Plan participant care to ensure integrity and compliance with study protocol.

Take Action [Nursing Interventions]
- Support the process of informed consent in a culturally competent manner.
  - Provide an interpreter when necessary.
  - Provide enough time for the person to read the consent and ask questions.
  - Serve as a witness to informed consent.
- After reviewing the study protocol, administer study agent(s).
- Accurately document all participant care, assessment findings, and study agent administration.
- Accurately and safely collect biospecimens.
- Act as advocate, educator, and collaborator in the research process.
  - Ensure safe care.
  - Ensure integrity of study data.
  - Communicate clearly.

Evaluate Outcomes [Evaluation]
- Determine whether the potential participant understands what it means to participate in the study by asking open-ended questions.
- Monitor response to the study agent or other interventions.
- Determine whether participants understand how to take their study agents, what to do if they miss a dose, how to store the study agent, and when to call their health care provider.

The *International Pharmacopeia,* first published in 1951 by the World Health Organization (WHO), provides a basis for standards in strength and composition of drugs for use throughout the world. The book is published in English, Spanish, and French.

Federal Legislation

Federal legislation attempts to protect the public from drugs that are impure, toxic, ineffective, or not tested before public sale. The primary purpose of the legislation is to ensure safety. America's first law to regulate drugs was the Food and Drug Act of 1906, which prohibited the sale of misbranded and adulterated drugs but did not address drug effectiveness and safety.

1912: The Sherley Amendment

The Sherley Amendment prohibited false therapeutic claims on drug labels. It came about as a result of Mrs. Winslow's Soothing Syrup,

BOX 2.2 Informed Consent Checklist: Basic Elements

- A statement that the study involves research
- An explanation of the purposes of the research
- The expected duration of the subject's participation
- A description of the procedures to be followed
- Identification of any experimental procedures
- A description of any reasonably foreseeable risks or discomforts to the subject
- A description of any benefits to the subject or to others that may reasonably be expected from the research
- A disclosure of appropriate alternative procedures or courses of treatment, if any, that might be advantageous to the subject
- A statement describing the extent, if any, to which confidentiality of records identifying the subject will be maintained
- For research that involves more than minimal risk, an explanation as to whether any compensation will be paid and whether any medical treatments are available if injury occurs, and if so, what the treatments consist of or where further information may be obtained
- An explanation of whom to contact for answers to pertinent questions about the research and research subjects' rights and whom to contact in the event of a research-related injury to the subject
- A statement that participation is voluntary, refusal to participate will involve no penalty or loss of benefits to which the subject is otherwise entitled, and the subject may discontinue participation at any time without penalty or loss of benefits to which the subject is otherwise entitled

From Office for Human Research Protections (OHRP). (2014). U.S. Department of Health & Human Services. Retrieved from http://www.hhs.gov/ohrp/policy/consentckls.html.

a product advertised to treat teething and colic, which contained morphine and led to the death of many infants. Under the Sherley Amendment, the government had to prove intent to defraud before a drug could be removed from the market.

1914: The Harrison Narcotics Tax Act

The Harrison Narcotics Tax Act required prescriptions for drugs that exceeded set narcotic limits. It also mandated increased record keeping by physicians and pharmacists.

1938: The Federal Food, Drug, and Cosmetic Act

The Federal Food, Drug, and Cosmetic Act of 1938 empowered the FDA to ensure a drug was safe before marketing. It is the FDA's responsibility to ensure that all drugs are tested for harmful effects; it also required that drugs be labeled with accurate information and have detailed literature in the drug packaging that explains adverse effects. The FDA can prevent the marketing of any drug it judges to be incompletely tested or dangerous. Only drugs considered safe by the FDA are approved for marketing.

1951: Durham-Humphrey Amendment

The Durham-Humphrey Amendment distinguished between drugs that could be sold with or without prescription by a licensed health care provider.

1962: Kefauver-Harris Amendment to the 1938 Act

The Kefauver-Harris Amendment resulted from the widely publicized thalidomide tragedy of the 1950s in which European patients who took the sedative-hypnotic thalidomide during the first trimester of pregnancy gave birth to infants with extreme limb deformities. The Kefauver-Harris amendment tightened controls

on drug safety, especially experimental drugs, and required that adverse reactions and contraindications be labeled and included in the literature. The amendment also included provisions for the evaluation of testing methods used by manufacturers, the process for withdrawal of approved drugs when safety and effectiveness were in doubt, and the establishment of effectiveness of new drugs before marketing.

1965: Drug Abuse Control Amendments

Enacted in 1965, the Drug Abuse Control Amendments attempted to control the abuse of depressants, stimulants, and hallucinogens.

1970: The Comprehensive Drug Abuse Prevention and Control Act

In 1970 Congress passed the Comprehensive Drug Abuse Prevention and Control Act. This act, designed to remedy the escalating problem of drug abuse, included several provisions: (1) promotion of drug education and research into the prevention and treatment of drug dependence; (2) strengthening of enforcement authority; (3) establishment of treatment and rehabilitation facilities; and (4) designation of schedules, or categories, for controlled substances according to abuse liability.

Based on their abuse potential and acceptable medical use practices, controlled substances are categorized into five schedules, which are listed in Table 2.1. Schedule I drugs are not approved for medical use and have high abuse potential; schedule II through V drugs have acceptable medical use and decreasing potential for abuse leading to psychological and/or physiologic dependence.

Nurses are key to creating a culture of safety and accountability related to controlled substances. As such, nurses must:
- Verify orders before drug administration.
- Account for all controlled drugs.
- Maintain a controlled substance log that ensures all required information is documented accurately.
- Document all discarded or wasted medication; wastage must be witnessed by another nurse.
- Ensure timely documentation in the patient record after drug administration, including patient response to drug administration.
- Keep all controlled drugs in a locked storage area; keep narcotics under double lock. Be certain that only authorized persons have access to the keys, including keys for patient-controlled analgesia and epidural pumps. Medication may also be administered via an automated dispensing cabinet, with bioidentical identifiers used for access.
- The ANA recognizes the significant threat to patient safety and liability to health care organizations caused by nurse drug diversion and recommends that all states have a peer-to-peer assistance program for addicted nurses. Reporting is mandatory if suspected or known diversion occurs.

1983: The Orphan Drug Act

The Orphan Drug Act was designed to promote the development and manufacture of drugs used in the treatment of rare diseases (orphan drugs). The act's three primary incentives are (1) federal funding of grants and contracts to perform clinical trials of orphan products; (2) a 50% tax credit for costs of clinical testing; and (3) exclusive rights to market the drug for 7 years from the marketing approval date.

1994: Dietary Supplement Health and Education Act

The Dietary Supplement Health and Education Act established labeling requirements for dietary supplements and authorized the FDA to promote safe manufacturing practices. It classified dietary supplements as food.

TABLE 2.1   Schedule Categories of Controlled Substances

Schedule	Examples	Description
I	Some examples of drugs listed in Schedule I are heroin, lysergic acid diethylamide (LSD), *cannabis*, peyote, methaqualone, and methylenedioxymethamphetamine (MDMA).	Substances in this schedule have no currently accepted medical use in the United States, a lack of accepted safety for use under medical supervision, and a high potential for abuse.
II	Examples of Schedule II drugs include combination products with less than 15 milligrams of hydrocodone per dosage unit, cocaine, methamphetamine, methadone, hydromorphone, meperidine, oxycodone, fentanyl, dextroamphetamine, dextroamphetamine/amphetamine, and methylphenidate.	Substances in this schedule have a high potential for abuse that may lead to severe psychological or physical dependence.
III	Examples of Schedule III drugs include products containing less than 90 mg of codeine per dosage unit (acetaminophen with codeine), ketamine, anabolic steroids, and testosterone.	Substances in this schedule have a potential for abuse less than substances in Schedules I or II, and abuse may lead to moderate or low physical dependence or high psychological dependence.
IV	Examples of Schedule IV substances include alprazolam, carisoprodol, diazepam, lorazepam, zolpidem, and tramadol.	Substances in this schedule have a low potential for abuse relative to substances in Schedule III.
V	Examples of Schedule V drugs include cough preparations containing not more than 200 mg of codeine or per 100 mL (codeine/guaifenesin), diphenoxylate/atropine, difenoxin/atropine, and pregabalin.	Substances in this schedule have a low potential for abuse relative to substances listed in Schedule IV and consist primarily of preparations containing limited quantities of certain narcotics.

From United States Drug Enforcement Administration. (2018). Drug scheduling. Retrieved January 2, 2019 from https://www.dea.gov/drug-scheduling.

1996: Health Insurance Portability and Accountability Act

The Health Insurance Portability and Accountability Act (HIPAA) of 1996 protects health insurance coverage for workers who change or lose their jobs and sets the standard for the privacy of individually identifiable health information. The act provides patients more control over their health information, including boundaries on the use and release of health records.

1997: The Food and Drug Administration Modernization Act

The five provisions in the Food and Drug Administration Modernization Act are (1) review and use of new drugs is accelerated; (2) drugs can be tested in children before marketing; (3) clinical trial data are necessary for experimental drug use for serious or life-threatening health conditions; (4) drug companies are required to give information on off-label (non–FDA-approved) use of drugs and their costs; and (5) drug companies that plan to discontinue drugs must inform health professionals and patients at least 6 months before stopping drug production.

2002: Best Pharmaceuticals for Children Act

The BPCA gives manufacturers a 6-month extension of patents to evaluate drugs on the market for their safety and efficacy in children.

2003: Pediatric Research Equity Act

The Pediatric Research Equity Act authorizes the FDA to require that drug manufacturers test certain drugs and biologic products for their safety and effectiveness in children, noting that "children are not small adults." Additionally, studies that involve children must be conducted with the same drug and in the same disease process as adults.

2007: Food and Drug Administration Amendments Act

The Food and Drug Administration Amendments Act allows the FDA to do more comprehensive reviews of potential new drugs, mandates postmarketing safety studies, and affects the distribution of drugs found to be not as safe as premarket studies indicated.

2010: Patient Protection and Affordable Care Act

The Patient Protection and Affordable Care Act was signed into law in 2010 and became effective January 1, 2014. Essential provisions of the reform include (1) quality, affordable health care for all Americans; (2) improved quality and efficiency of health care; (3) prevention of chronic disease and improved public health; (4) improved access to innovative medical therapies; and (5) community living services and supports.

2012: Food and Drug Administration Safety and Innovation Act

The Food and Drug Administration Safety and Innovation Act was signed into law on July 9, 2012. It strengthens the FDA's ability to safeguard and advance public health by:

- Collecting fees from industry to fund reviews of drugs with the "breakthrough therapy" designation, medical devices, generic drugs, and biosimilar biologic products
- Expediting development of innovative, safe, and effective products
- Increasing stakeholder engagement in FDA processes
- Enhancing the safety of the global drug supply chain

NURSE PRACTICE ACTS

All states and territories have rules and regulations in place to provide guidance and govern nursing practice, which includes drug administration by nurses. Generally, nurses cannot prescribe or administer drugs without a health care provider's order. Practicing nurses should be knowledgeable about the nurse practice act in the state where they are licensed. (Information can be found through the National Council of State Boards of Nursing at www.ncsbn.org.) Nurses are responsible for knowing their state's law and administrative code. Nurses who administer a drug without a licensed health care provider's order are in violation of the Nurse Practice Act and can have their licenses revoked.

In a civil court, the nurse can be prosecuted for giving the wrong drug or dosage, omitting a drug dose, or giving the drug by the wrong route.

CANADIAN DRUG REGULATION

In Canada, before approval and becoming available to patients, drugs must be reviewed for safety, efficacy, and quality by the Health Products and Food Branch (HPFB) of Health Canada. Health Canada

TABLE 2.2 Canadian Controlled Drugs and Substances Schedule

Schedule	Examples	Description
I	Codeine, hydrocodone, oxycodone, coca, cocaine, levomethorphan, ketamine, sufentanil, methamphetamine, amphetamine, gamma hydroxybutyrate (GHB)	Opium poppy, coca leaves, phenylpiperidines, phenazepines, amidones, methadols, phenalkoxams, thiambutenes, moramides, morphinans, benzazocines, ampromides, benzimidazoles, phencyclidine, fentanyls, tilidine, methamphetamine, amphetamine, flunitrazepam, and GHB and its derivatives, alkaloids, and salts
II	Nabilone	Synthetic cannabinoid receptor type 1 agonists
III	Thirty-three compounds including methylphenidate, lysergic acid diethylamide (LSD), psilocybin, and mescaline	
IV	Twenty-six parent compounds including chlorphentermine, butorphanol, nalbuphine, meprobamate, and zolpidem	Barbiturates, thiobarbiturates, benzodiazepines, and their salts and derivatives; anabolic steroids and their derivatives
V		Propylhexedrine and any of its salts
VI	Class A includes 23 compounds such as ephedrine, ergotamine, and pseudoephedrine Class B includes six compounds such as acetone and sulfuric acid	Part 1 – Class A precursors Part 2 – Class B precursors Part 3 – Preparations and mixtures

For more detailed information, please see the Justice Laws Website at https://laws-lois.justice.gc.ca/eng/acts/c-38.8/page-14.html#h-95541.

is a federal department tasked with the mission of improving the quality of life of all Canadians. (Further information can be found at www.hc-sc.gc.ca.)

In 1996 the Canadian government passed the Controlled Drugs and Substances Act. This act broke controlled drugs and substances into eight schedules and two classes of precursors (Table 2.2). In 2012 the Safe Streets and Communities Act was passed in Canada, which reclassified amphetamines—including methylenedioxyamphetamine (MDA) and methylenedioxymethamphetamine (MDMA)—and also flunitrazepam and gamma hydroxybutyrate (GHB) from Schedule III to Schedule I drugs. This change imposed stiffer penalties for dealers and those in possession of the drugs.

INITIATIVES TO COMBAT DRUG COUNTERFEITING

Distribution of counterfeit drugs is a worldwide problem; it is estimated that more than 10% of all drugs available are counterfeit. Counterfeit drugs may contain the incorrect ingredients, insufficient amounts of active ingredients, or no active ingredients. Additionally, they may contain impurities and contaminants or may be distributed in fake packaging.

The most common drugs counterfeited are those used to treat erectile dysfunction, high cholesterol, hypertension, infections, cancer, and HIV/AIDS. The high cost of drugs, combined with the need for prescription drugs to treat chronic diseases—as well as the desire by consumers to misuse drugs (e.g., steroid-containing drugs for body building)—generates a constant demand easily filled by criminals via rogue Internet drug sites. The FDA and consumer groups are working on strategies to combat this problem, including tougher oversight of distributors, a rapid alert system, and better-informed consumers.

The role of the nurse is critical in consumer education. The nurse must advise patients to report any differences in taste or appearance of a drug or in its packaging. Patients should be alert to slight variations in packaging or labeling (e.g., color, package seal), note any unexpected side effects, and buy drugs from reputable sources. Reputable online pharmacies carry the designation of Verified Internet Pharmacy Practice Site (VIPPS; a list of VIPPS-verified pharmacies can be found at www.nabp.net) and display an approval seal. If any suspicion of counterfeit arises, the patient, family, or nurse should contact the FDA at www.fda.gov/Safety/MedWatch/HowToReport.

DRUG NAMES

Drugs have several names. The chemical name describes the drug's chemical structure. The generic name is the official, *nonproprietary* name for the drug; this name is not owned by any drug company and is universally accepted. Nearly 80% of all prescription drugs in the United States are ordered by generic name. The brand (trade) name, also known as the *proprietary* name, is chosen by the drug company and is usually a registered trademark. Drug companies market a compound using its brand name. For example, Lunesta is the (proprietary) brand name of a drug whose generic name is eszopiclone.

Throughout this text, only generic names for each drug will be used because many brand names may exist for a single generic name—for example, the generic drug ibuprofen carries the brand names Advil, Medipren, Motrin, and Nuprin. Generic names are given in lowercase letters, whereas brand names always begin with a capital letter. An example of a generic and brand-name drug listing is *furosemide (Lasix)*.

Generic drugs must be approved by the FDA before they can be marketed. If the generic drug is found to be *bioequivalent* to the brand-name drug, the generic drug is considered *therapeutically equivalent* and is given an "A" rating. If there is less than a 20% variance in drug absorption, distribution, metabolism, and excretion, a generic drug is considered *equivalent* to the brand-name drug.

A list of FDA-approved drug products can be found at www.accessdata.fda.gov/scripts/cder/drugsatfda. The FDA also publishes a list of approved generic drugs that are bioequivalent to brand-name drugs. Generic drugs have the same active ingredients as brand-name drugs but are usually less expensive because manufacturers do not have to do extensive testing; these drugs were clinically tested for safety and efficacy by the pharmaceutical company that first formulated the drug. However, all drugs have varying inert fillers, binders, and excipients used to shape tablets and control how fast or slow the drug is released in the body, and these factors may result in variations in drug bioavailability.

Health care providers and patients must exercise care when choosing generic drugs because of possible variations in their action or in the patient's response to them. To maintain stable drug levels, patients should be cautioned *not* to change generic drug manufacturers; this is particularly true when patients are prescribed phenytoin or warfarin. Nurses should check with the health care provider or the pharmacist when generic drugs are prescribed. Health care providers must note on prescriptions whether the pharmacist may substitute the generic drug when the brand name is prescribed.

OVER-THE-COUNTER DRUGS

Although all drugs carry risk, over-the-counter (OTC) drugs have been found to be safe and appropriate for use without the direct supervision of a health care provider. They are available for purchase without a prescription in many retail locations. Other OTC drugs (e.g., pseudoephedrine, emergency contraception) are available with some restrictions and must be kept behind the pharmacy counter; before dispensing, patient age and identify are verified and education is provided.

More than $23 billion is spent annually on OTC drugs, which include vitamin supplements, cold remedies, analgesics, antacids, laxatives, antihistamines, sleep aids, nasal sprays, weight-control drugs, drugs for dermatitis and fungal infections, fluoride toothpaste, corn and callus removal products, and herbal products. Information related to OTC drugs available on the market can be found at http://www.drugs.com/otc.

In 2002 the FDA standardized OTC labeling to provide consumers with better information and to describe the benefits and risks associated with taking OTC drugs. It is an important nursing responsibility to ensure that patients are able to read and understand OTC labels. All OTC drugs must have labels that provide the following information in this specific order (Fig. 2.3).

- The product's active ingredients, including the amount in each dosage unit
- The purpose of the product
- The uses (indications) for the product
- Specific warnings, including when the product should not be used under any circumstances, substances or activities to avoid, side effects that could occur, and when it is appropriate to consult with a doctor or pharmacist
- Dosage instructions that include when, how, and how often to take the product
- The product's inactive ingredients and important information to help consumers avoid ingredients that may cause an allergic reaction

Nurses must be aware of OTC drugs and the implications of their use. OTC drugs provide both advantages and potential serious complications for the consumer. The nurse needs to emphasize that many of these drugs are potent and can cause moderate to severe side effects, especially when taken with other drugs. Additionally, many OTC drugs contain the same active ingredients, potentially leading to overdose. Self-diagnosis and self-prescribing OTC drugs may mask the seriousness of clinical conditions. See Box 2.3 for nursing considerations related to OTC drugs.

Many individuals routinely reach for aspirin, acetaminophen, and ibuprofen to relieve discomfort or pain without being aware of potential drug interactions and/or side effects. For example, ibuprofen can increase fluid retention, which can worsen heart failure; use of ibuprofen on a daily basis may decrease the effectiveness of antihypertensive drugs. Ibuprofen has also been linked with cardiovascular events, such as myocardial infarction and stroke; this risk increases with long-term use.

Acetaminophen has been associated with kidney disease, anemia and thrombocytopenia, myocardial infarction, stroke, and hypertension. Additionally, metabolism of the drug results in the development of toxic metabolites, which can cause liver damage. Patients may also develop allergic reactions (anaphylaxis) or potentially fatal skin reactions (Stevens-Johnson Syndrome [SJS] or toxic epidermal necrolysis [TEN]) when taking acetaminophen. Because of the potential for harm caused with high doses or long-term use, since 2011 the FDA has limited the dose of acetaminophen to 325 mg when packaged in combination with other drugs.

Some OTC drugs, such as cough medicine, are a combination product of two to four drugs. It is conceivable that there could be a drug-drug interaction with a cough medicine and one of the drugs prescribed by the patient's health care provider.

Patients with asthma should be aware that aspirin can trigger an acute asthma episode. Patients may be allergic to aspirin, or aspirin may act as a deregulator of leukotrienes. Aspirin is also not recommended for children with influenza symptoms or chickenpox because it has been associated with Reye syndrome. Patients with kidney disease should avoid aspirin, acetaminophen, and ibuprofen because these can further decrease kidney function, especially with long-term use. Also, patients taking moderate to high doses of aspirin, ibuprofen, or naproxen concurrently with an oral anticoagulant may be at increased risk for bleeding.

The previous examples are not all inclusive. Caution is advised before using any OTC preparation, including antacids, decongestants, and laxatives. Patients should check with their health care providers and read drug labels before taking OTC medications so they are aware of possible contraindications and adverse reactions.

The acronym *SAFER* is a mnemonic for the instructions that the FDA recommends before taking any medicine: **s**peak up, **a**sk questions, **f**ind the facts, **e**valuate your choices, and **r**ead labels.

DRUG RESOURCES

Many drug references are available, including nursing texts that identify related nursing implications and areas for health teaching. Some recommended resources follow.

American Hospital Formulary Service (AHFS) Drug Information is published by the American Society of Health-System Pharmacists in Bethesda, Maryland. It provides accurate and complete drug information for both the health care provider and the consumer on nearly all prescription drugs marketed in the United States. This text contains drugs listed according to therapeutic drug classification. The information given for each drug includes chemistry and stability, pharmacologic actions, pharmacokinetics, uses, cautions, contraindications, acute toxicity, drug interactions, dosage and administration, and preparations.

This reference is updated yearly with monthly supplements that provide information on new drugs such as dosage forms and strengths, uses, and cautions. The text is unbiased. Drug information from the AHFS is available online or in print format.

United States Pharmacopeia—Drug Information (USP-DI) is available in most hospitals and pharmacies either online or in print format. It provides drug information for the health care provider, including pharmacology, precautions to consider, side effects and adverse effects, patient consultation, general dosing information, and dosage forms. The USP-DI also contains patient information presented in a way that is easily understood. The topics include administration of drugs, drug effects, indications, adverse reactions, dosage guidelines, and what to do for missed doses.

The *Medical Letter* on drugs and therapeutics is a nonprofit publication for physicians, nurse practitioners, and other health professionals. Each biweekly issue provides reviews of new FDA-approved drugs and comparisons of drugs available for common diseases.

Prescriber's Letter is a newsletter published monthly by the Therapeutic Research Center in Stockton, California. It provides

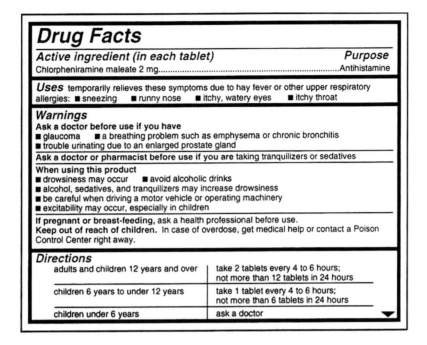

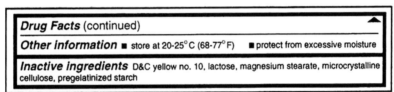

Fig. 2.3 Sample over-the-counter drug label. (From US Food and Drug Administration. [2014]. The current over-the-counter medicine label: Take a look. http://www.fda.gov/drugs/emergencypreparedness/bioterroris-manddrugpreparedness/ucm133411.htm.)

BOX 2.3   Nursing Considerations Related to Over-the-Counter Drugs

Nurses should advise patients of the following when over-the-counter (OTC) drugs are considered:

- Always read the instructions on the label.
- Do not take OTC medicines in higher dosages or for a longer time than the label states.
- If you do not get well, stop treating yourself and talk with a health care professional.
- Side effects from OTCs are relatively uncommon, but it is your job to know what side effects might result from the medicines you are taking.
- Because every person is different, your response to the medicine may be different than another person's response.
- OTC medicines often interact with other medicines and with food or alcohol, or they might have an effect on other health problems you may have.
- If you do not understand the label, check with the pharmacist.
- Do not take medicine if the package does not have a label on it.
- Throw away medicines that have expired (are older than the date on the package).
- Do not use medicine that belongs to a friend.
- Buy products that treat only the symptoms you have.
- If cost is an issue, generic OTC products may be cheaper than brandname items.

- Avoid buying these products online, outside of well-known Internet insurance company sites, because many OTC preparations sold through the Internet are counterfeit products. These may not be what you ordered and may be dangerous.

Parents should know the following special information about using OTCs for children:

- Parents should never guess about the amount of medicine to give a child. Half an adult dose may be too much or not enough to be effective. This is very true of medicines such as acetaminophen (Tylenol) or ibuprofen (Advil), in which repeated overdoses may lead to poisoning of the child, liver destruction, or coma.
- If the label says to take 2 teaspoons and the dosing cup is marked with ounces only, get another measuring device. Don't try to guess about how much should be given.
- Always follow the age limits listed. If the label says the product should not be given to a child younger than 2 years, do not give it.
- Always use the child-resistant cap, and relock the cap after use.
- Throw away old, discolored, or expired medicine or medicine that has lost its label instructions.
- Do not give medicine containing alcohol to children.

From Edmunds, M. W. (2016). *Introduction to clinical pharmacology* (8th ed). St. Louis, MO: Mosby.

concise updates and advice concerning new FDA-approved drugs, various uses of older drugs, and FDA warnings.

MedlinePlus is a service of the US National Library of Medicine. Available at www.nlm.nih.gov/medlineplus/druginformation.html, it offers extensive information on prescribed drugs, as well as herbs and supplements, indexed by generic and brand names.

A good source for OTC drug information is *The Handbook of Nonprescription Drugs,* published by the American Pharmacists Association in Washington, DC. This resource is available online and in text. The Internet can be another great resource, but only if credible websites are used.

CRITICAL THINKING CASE STUDY

A 53-year-old male is seen by his health care provider for chronic pain in his knees. He states the pain is a dull, constant ache in both knees that happens in the evenings after he's been working as a cashier all day.

1. It is important for the nurse to gather what information about the patient's medications?
2. The patient has taken ibuprofen for an extended period of time to control his pain. What risk does this over-the-counter (OTC) drug pose for him?
3. What patient education should the nurse provide concerning OTC drugs?
4. The patient is advised by his health care provider to stop taking ibuprofen and begin taking acetaminophen. Before leaving the office, he asks the nurse how he will be able to remember the possible side effects of this drug. The nurse tells him he can read the label on his bottle. What is the standardized order of information on OTC drug labels?

REVIEW QUESTIONS

1. The nurse in the clinical research setting is knowledgeable about ethical principles and protection of human subjects. What principle is demonstrated by ensuring the patient's right to self-determination?
   a. Beneficence
   b. Respect for persons
   c. Justice
   d. Informed consent
2. The research nurse is meeting with a patient and determines, based on the assessment, that the patient meets inclusion criteria for clinical research. The patient agrees to participate in the clinical trial. The nurse advises the patient that which member of the health care team has the responsibility to explain the study and respond to questions?
   a. Registered nurse
   b. Pharmacist
   c. Research associate
   d. Health care provider
3. The clinical research nurse knows that only a small proportion of drugs survive the research and development process. An appreciation of the process and associated costs grows when the nurse is aware that approximately one in how many potential drugs is approved by the US Food and Drug Administration?
   a. 100
   b. 1000
   c. 10,000
   d. 100,000
4. The nurse is interviewing a patient in a Phase I clinical trial. Which patient statement indicates an understanding of this trial phase?
   a. I am doing this to be sure this drug is safe.
   b. I am doing this to be sure this drug is effective.
   c. I hope this drug is better than the current treatment.
   d. I can be part of demonstrating a cure.
5. The foundation of clinical trials, Good Clinical Practice, is a helpful resource for nurses. The nurse is correct in choosing Good Clinical Practice as a reference for standards in which areas? (Select all that apply.)
   a. Design
   b. Monitoring and auditing
   c. Analyses
   d. Reporting
   e. Outcomes evaluation

6. The nurse researcher reviews the proposed informed consent form for a future clinical trial. The nurse expects to find which in the document? (Select all that apply.)
   a. Description of benefits and risks
   b. Identification of related drugs, treatments, and techniques
   c. Description of outcomes
   d. Statement of compensation for participants, if any
   e. Description of serious risks
7. The nurse knows that the patient should be informed about the risks and benefits related to clinical research. What ethical principle does this describe?
   a. Respect for persons
   b. Justice
   c. Beneficence
   d. Informed consent
8. The nurse is reviewing a patient's list of medications and notes that several have the highest abuse potential. According to US standards, the highest potential for abuse of drugs with accepted medical uses is found in drugs included in which schedule?
   a. II
   b. III
   c. IV
   d. V
9. The nurse is reviewing the drug approval process in the United States and learns that the Food and Drug Administration Modernization Act of 1997 contains which provisions? (Select all that apply.)
   a. Review of new drugs is accelerated.
   b. Drug companies must provide information on off-label use of drugs.
   c. Privacy of individually identifiable health information must be protected.
   d. Drug companies must offer advanced notice of plans to discontinue drugs.
   e. Drug labels must describe side effects and adverse effects.
10. The patient has questions about counterfeit drugs. Which factors alert the patient or nurse that a drug is counterfeit or adulterated? (Select all that apply.)
    a. Variations in packaging
    b. Unexpected side effects
    c. Different taste
    d. Different chemical components
    e. Different odor

11. The nurse knows the importance of administering the right medication to the patient and that drugs have many names. It is therefore most important that drugs be ordered by which name?
    a. Generic
    b. Brand
    c. Trade
    d. Chemical

12. What provisions from the Controlled Substances Act of 1970 were designed to remedy drug abuse?
    a. The act established treatment and rehabilitation facilities.
    b. The act tightened controls on experimental drugs.
    c. The act required clinical trial data on drugs.
    d. The act required drug companies to give information on off-label use of drugs.

3

Pharmacokinetics and Pharmacodynamics

http://evolve.elsevier.com/McCuistion/pharmacology

OBJECTIVES

- Differentiate the three phases of drug action.
- Describe the four processes of pharmacokinetics.
- Identify the four receptor families.
- Describe the influence of protein binding on drug bioavailability.
- Check drugs for half-life, percentage of protein binding, therapeutic index, and side effects in a drug reference book.
- Differentiate the four types of drug interactions.

- Explain the three mechanisms involved with drug-drug interactions.
- Describe the effects of drug-nutrient interactions.
- Explain the meaning of drug-induced photosensitivity.
- Describe the nursing implications of pharmacokinetics and pharmacodynamics.

OUTLINE

Once a drug is administered, it goes through two phases, the pharmacokinetic phase and the pharmacodynamic phase. The *pharmacokinetic phase,* or what the body does to the drug, describes the movement of the drug through the body. It is composed of four processes: (1) absorption, (2) distribution, (3) metabolism (biotransformation), and (4) excretion (elimination). The *pharmacodynamic phase,* or what the drug does to the body, involves receptor binding, postreceptor effects, and chemical reactions. A biologic or physiologic response results from the pharmacodynamic phase.

PHARMACOKINETICS

Pharmacokinetics is the process of drug movement throughout the body necessary to achieve drug action. The four processes are (1) absorption, (2) distribution, (3) metabolism (or biotransformation), and (4) excretion (or elimination). ·

Drug Absorption

Drug absorption is the movement of the drug into the bloodstream after administration. Approximately 80% of drugs are taken by mouth

(enteral). For the body to use drugs taken by mouth, a drug in solid form (e.g., tablet or capsule) must disintegrate into small particles and combine with a liquid to form a solution, a process known as *dissolution* (drugs in liquid form are already in solution), to be absorbed from the gastrointestinal (GI) tract into the bloodstream. Unlike drugs taken by mouth, eyedrops, eardrops, nasal sprays, respiratory inhalants, transdermal drugs, sublingual drugs, and parenteral drugs do not pass through the GI tract.

Tablets are not 100% drug. Fillers and inert substances—such as simple syrup, vegetable gums, aromatic powder, honey, and various elixirs—called *excipients* are used in drug preparation to allow the drug to take on a particular size and shape and to enhance drug dissolution. Some excipients, such as the ions potassium (K^+) in penicillin potassium and sodium (Na^+) in penicillin sodium, increase the absorbability of the drug. Penicillin is poorly absorbed by the GI tract because of gastric acid. However, by adding potassium or sodium salts, penicillin can be absorbed.

Disintegration is the breakdown of an oral drug into smaller particles. The rate of dissolution is the time it takes the drug to disintegrate and dissolve to become available for the body to absorb it. Drugs in

Passive Transport

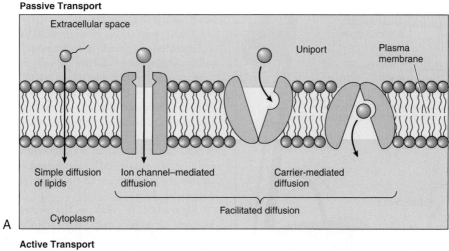

Active Transport

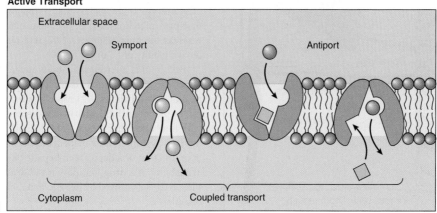

Fig. 3.1 Passive and active transport. *ATP,* Adenosine triphosphate. (From Gartner, L.P. [2017]. *Textbook of histology* [4th ed.]. St. Louis, MO: Elsevier.)

liquid form are more rapidly available for GI absorption than are solids. Generally, drugs are both disintegrated and absorbed faster in acidic fluids with a pH of 1 or 2 rather than in alkaline fluids (those with a pH greater than 7). Both the very young and older adults have less gastric acidity; therefore drug absorption is generally slower for those drugs absorbed primarily in the stomach.

Enteric-coated (EC) drugs resist disintegration in the gastric acid of the stomach, so disintegration does not occur until the drug reaches the alkaline environment of the small intestine. EC tablets can remain in the stomach for a long time; therefore their effect may be delayed in onset. EC tablets or capsules and sustained-release (beaded) capsules should not be crushed because crushing alters the place and time of absorption of the drug. Food in the GI tract may interfere with the dissolution of certain drugs. Some drugs irritate the gastric mucosa, so fluids or food may be necessary to dilute the drug concentration and provide protection.

Most oral drugs enter the bloodstream after absorption across the mucosal lining of the small intestine. The epithelial lining of the small intestine is covered with villi, fingerlike protrusions that increase the surface area available for absorption. Absorption is reduced if the villi are decreased in number because of disease, drug effect, or the removal of some or all of the small intestine.

Absorption across the mucosal lining of the small intestine occurs through passive transport, active transport, or pinocytosis. **Passive transport** occurs through two processes, diffusion and facilitated diffusion. In **diffusion,** drugs move across the cell membrane from an area of higher concentration to one of lower concentration. **Facilitated diffusion** relies on a carrier protein to move the drug from an area of higher concentration to an area of lower concentration. Passive transport does

not require energy to move drugs across the membrane. **Active transport** requires a carrier, such as an enzyme or protein, to move the drug against a concentration gradient. Energy is required for active absorption (Fig. 3.1). **Pinocytosis** is a process by which cells carry a drug across their membranes by engulfing the drug particles in a vesicle.

The mucous membrane that lines the GI tract is composed of lipids (fat) and protein such that lipid-soluble drugs are able to pass rapidly through the mucous membrane. Water-soluble drugs need a carrier, either an enzyme or a protein, to pass through the mucous membrane. Large particles are able to pass through the mucous membrane if they are nonionized (have no positive or negative charge). Drugs that are lipid soluble and nonionized are absorbed faster than water-soluble and ionized drugs.

Blood flow, pain, stress, hunger, fasting, food, and pH affect drug absorption. Poor circulation to the stomach as a result of shock, vasoconstrictor drugs, or disease hampers absorption. Pain, stress, and foods that are solid, hot, or high in fat can slow gastric emptying time, so drugs remain in the stomach longer. Exercise can decrease gastric blood flow by shunting blood flow to peripheral muscles, thereby decreasing blood circulation to the GI tract.

Drugs given intramuscularly are absorbed faster in muscles that have increased blood flow (e.g., deltoid) than in those that do not (e.g., gluteus maximus). Subcutaneous tissue has decreased blood flow compared with muscle, so absorption is slower when drugs are given subcutaneously. However, drugs that are given subcutaneously have a more rapid and predictable rate of absorption than those given by mouth.

Drugs given rectally are absorbed slower than drugs administered by the oral route. Absorption is slower because the surface area in the rectum is smaller than the stomach, and it has no villi. Additionally, the

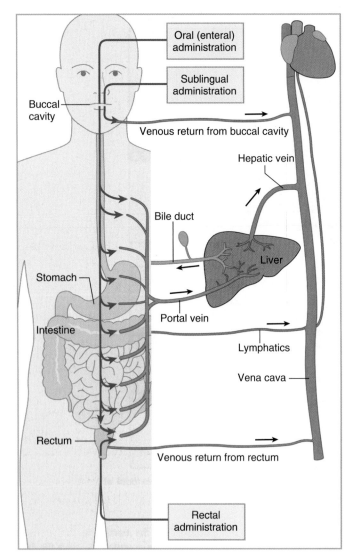

Fig. 3.2 First-pass metabolism. (From Kester, M. [2012]. *Elsevier's integrated review pharmacology* [2nd ed.]. St. Louis, MO: Elsevier.)

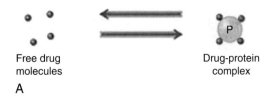

Free drug molecules

Drug-protein complex

A

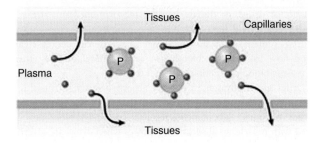

B

Fig. 3.3 Protein binding. *P*, Protein. (From Lilley, L. L., Rainform Collins, S., & Snyder, J. S. [2016]. *Pharmacology and the nursing process* [8th ed.]. St. Louis: Elsevier.)

composition of the suppository base (e.g., fatty bases or water-soluble bases) affects drug absorption.

After absorption of oral drugs from the GI tract, they pass from the intestinal lumen to the liver via the portal vein. In the liver, some drugs are metabolized to an inactive form and are excreted, thus reducing the amount of active drug available to exert a pharmacologic effect. This is referred to as the first-pass effect or first-pass metabolism (Fig. 3.2). Most oral drugs are affected to some degree by first-pass metabolism. Lidocaine and some nitroglycerins, for example, are not given orally because they have extensive first-pass metabolism and most of the drug is inactivated. Drugs that are delivered by other routes (intravenous [IV], intramuscular [IM], subcutaneous [SQ], nasal, sublingual, buccal) do not enter the portal circulation and are not subjected to first-pass metabolism.

Bioavailability refers to the percentage of administered drug available for activity. For orally administered drugs, bioavailability is affected by absorption and first-pass metabolism. The bioavailability of oral drugs is always less than 100% and varies based on the rate of first-pass metabolism (i.e., the bioavailability of rosuvastatin is 20%, whereas the bioavailability of digoxin ranges from 70% to 85%). The bioavailability of IV drugs is 100%.

Factors that alter bioavailability include the (1) drug form, such as tablet, capsule, sustained-release beads, liquid, transdermal patch, suppository, or inhalation; (2) route of administration (e.g., enteral, topical, or parenteral); (3) gastric mucosa and motility; (4) administration with food and other drugs; and (5) changes in liver metabolism caused by liver dysfunction or inadequate hepatic blood flow. A decrease in liver function or a decrease in hepatic blood flow can increase the bioavailability of a drug, but only if the drug is metabolized by the liver. Less drug is destroyed by hepatic metabolism in the presence of a liver disorder.

Drug Distribution

Distribution is the movement of the drug from the circulation to body tissues. Drug distribution is influenced by vascular permeability and permeability of cell membranes, regional blood flow and pH, cardiac output, tissue perfusion, the ability of the drug to bind tissue and plasma proteins (Fig. 3.3), and the drug's lipid solubility. Drugs are easily distributed in highly perfused organs such as the liver, heart, and kidney. Tissues with decreased perfusion, such as muscle, fat, and peripheral organs, result in decreased drug distribution.

Protein Binding

As drugs are distributed in the plasma, many bind with plasma proteins (albumin, lipoproteins, and alpha-1-acid-glycoprotein [AGP]). Acidic drugs such as aspirin and methotrexate and neutral drugs such as nortriptyline bind with albumin or lipoproteins; however, basic drugs (morphine, amantadine) bind to AGP. Drugs that are more than 90% bound to protein are known as *highly protein-bound drugs* (e.g., warfarin, glyburide, sertraline, furosemide, and diazepam); drugs that are less than 10% bound to protein are *weakly protein-bound drugs* (e.g., gentamicin, metformin, metoprolol, and lisinopril). The portion of the drug bound to protein is inactive because it is not available to interact with tissue receptors and therefore is unable to exert a pharmacologic effect. The portion that remains unbound is free, active drug. Free drugs are able to exit blood vessels and reach their site of action, causing a pharmacologic response.

When two highly protein-bound drugs are administered together, they compete for protein-binding sites, leading to an increase in free drug being released into the circulation. For example, if warfarin (99% protein bound) and furosemide (95% protein bound) were administered together, warfarin—the more highly bound drug—could displace furosemide from its binding site. In this situation, it is possible for drug accumulation to occur and for toxicity to result. Another factor that

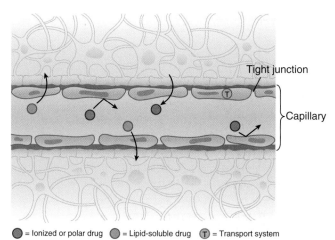

= Ionized or polar drug   = Lipid-soluble drug   (T) = Transport system

Fig. 3.4 Drug movement across the blood-brain barrier.

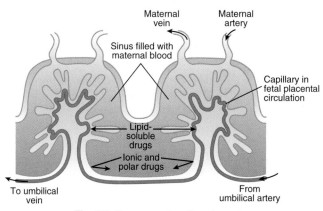

Fig. 3.5 Drug crossing the placenta.

may alter protein binding is low plasma protein levels, which potentially decrease the number of available binding sites and can lead to an increase in the amount of free drug available, resulting in drug accumulation and toxicity. Patients with liver or kidney disease and those who are malnourished may have significantly lower serum albumin levels. Additionally, older adults are more likely to have hypoalbuminemia, particularly if they have multiple chronic illnesses. With these factors in mind, it is important for nurses to understand the concept of protein binding and check their patients' protein and albumin levels when administering drugs.

Blood vessels in the brain have a special endothelial lining where the cells are pressed tightly together (*tight junctions*); this lining is referred to as the blood-brain barrier (BBB). The BBB protects the brain from foreign substances, which includes about 98% of the drugs on the market. Some drugs that are highly lipid soluble and of low molecular weight (e.g., benzodiazepines) are able to cross the BBB through diffusion, and others cross via transport proteins. Water-soluble drugs (e.g., atenolol and penicillin) and drugs that are not bound to transport proteins (free drugs) are not able to cross the BBB, which makes it difficult for these drugs to reach the brain (Fig. 3.4).

During pregnancy, drugs can cross the placenta much as they do across other membranes, and this affects both the fetus and the mother (Fig. 3.5). Drugs taken during the first trimester can lead to spontaneous abortion. During the second trimester, drugs can lead to spontaneous abortion, teratogenesis, or other subtler defects. During the third trimester, drugs may alter fetal growth and development. The risk-benefit ratio should be considered before any drugs are given during pregnancy. During breastfeeding, drugs can pass into breast milk, which can affect the nursing infant. Nurses must teach women who breastfeed to consult

their health care provider before taking any drug—whether over the counter (OTC) or prescribed—or any herb or supplement.

Drug Metabolism

Metabolism, or biotransformation, is the process by which the body chemically changes drugs into a form that can be excreted. The liver is the primary site of metabolism. Liver enzymes—collectively referred to as the *cytochrome P450 system,* or the *P450 system,* of drug-metabolizing enzymes—convert drugs to metabolites. A large percentage of drugs are lipid soluble; thus the liver metabolizes the lipid-soluble drug substance to a water-soluble substance for renal excretion. Liver diseases such as cirrhosis and hepatitis alter drug metabolism by inhibiting the drug-metabolizing enzymes in the liver. When the drug metabolism rate is decreased, excess drug accumulation can occur and can lead to toxicity.

Prodrugs

A prodrug is a compound that is metabolized into an active pharmacologic substance. Prodrugs are often designed to improve drug bioavailability; instead of administering a drug directly, a corresponding prodrug might be used instead to improve pharmacokinetics (absorption, distribution, metabolism, or excretion), decrease toxicity, or target a specific site of action. An example of a prodrug is codeine. Codeine itself has very little intrinsic activity at endogenous opioid receptors. However, drug-metabolizing enzymes in the liver convert codeine into morphine. Morphine, in turn, exhibits greater affinity for opioid receptors.

The drug half-life ($t\frac{1}{2}$) is the time it takes for the amount of drug in the body to be reduced by half. The amount of drug administered, the amount of drug remaining in the body from previous doses, metabolism, and elimination affect the half-life of a drug. For example, with liver or kidney dysfunction, the half-life of the drug is prolonged, and less drug is metabolized and eliminated.

A drug goes through several half-lives before complete elimination occurs, and drug half-life is used to determine dosing interval. This is best understood with an example: ibuprofen has a half-life of about 2 hours. If a person takes 200 mg, in 2 hours, 50% of the drug will be gone, leaving 100 mg. Two hours later, another 50% of the drug will be gone, this time leaving 50 mg; in another 2 hours, 50% more will be gone, so only 25 mg will remain. This process continues such that 10 hours after 200 mg of ibuprofen has been taken, if no additional doses are administered, 6.25 mg of the drug remains.

Half-lives	% of Drug Eliminated From Body
1	50
2	75
3	87.5
4	93.75
5	96.875
6	98.474
7	99.25

Image reproduced with permission from Medscape, *Space out drug discontinuations prior to "drug holiday,"* 2000, available at https://www.medscape.com/viewarticle/413306.

By knowing the half-life, the time it takes for a drug to reach a steady state (plateau drug level) can be determined. A steady state occurs when the amount of drug being administered is the same as the amount of drug being eliminated; a steady state of drug concentration is necessary to achieve optimal therapeutic benefit. This takes about four half-lives, if the size of all doses is the same. For example, digoxin—which has a half-life of 36 hours with normal renal function—takes approximately 6 days to reach a steady-state concentration.

Loading Dose

However, in the case of drugs with long half-lives, it may not be acceptable to wait for a steady state to be achieved. Take, for example, the case of a person with seizures receiving phenytoin. The half-life of phenytoin is approximately 22 hours; if all doses of the drug were the same, a steady state would not be achieved for about 3½ days. By giving a large initial dose, known as a loading dose, that is significantly higher than maintenance dosing, therapeutic effects can be obtained while a steady state is reached. It bears repeating that the loading dose is larger than the dose needed to maintain the drug at steady state; it would produce toxic side effects if given in repeated doses. After the loading dose, maintenance dosing is begun; this is the dose needed to maintain drug concentration at steady state when given repeatedly at a consistent dose and constant dosing interval.

Drug Excretion

The main route of drug excretion, elimination of drugs from the body, is through the kidneys. Drugs are also excreted through bile, the lungs, saliva, sweat, and breast milk. The kidneys filter free drugs (in healthy kidneys, drugs bound to protein are not filtered), water-soluble drugs, and drugs that are unchanged. The lungs eliminate volatile drug substances, and products metabolize to carbon dioxide (CO_2) and water (H_2O).

The urine pH influences drug excretion. Normal urine pH varies from 4.6 to 8.0. Acidic urine promotes elimination of weak base drugs, and alkaline urine promotes elimination of weak acid drugs. Salicylic acid (aspirin), a weak acid, is excreted rapidly in alkaline urine. Treatment of salicylate toxicity includes IV administration of sodium bicarbonate to increase urine pH to 8.0 or higher (alkaline); maintaining alkaline urine promotes the excretion of salicylate at 18 times the normal rate.

Prerenal, intrarenal, and postrenal conditions affect drug excretion. Prerenal conditions, such as dehydration or hemorrhage, reduce blood flow to the kidney and result in decreased glomerular filtration. Intrarenal conditions, such as glomerulonephritis and chronic kidney disease (CKD), affect glomerular filtration and tubular secretion and reabsorption. Postrenal conditions that obstruct urine flow—such as prostatic hypertrophy, stones, and neurogenic bladder—adversely affect glomerular filtration. With any of these situations, drug accumulation may occur, resulting in adverse drug reactions.

Common tests used to determine renal function include creatinine and blood urea nitrogen (BUN). Creatinine is a metabolic by-product of muscle excreted by the kidneys; urea nitrogen is the metabolic breakdown product of protein metabolism. Based on National Kidney Foundation recommendations, the estimated glomerular filtration rate (eGFR) is now calculated as part of routine comprehensive metabolic panels (CMPs) and basic metabolic panels (BMPs). The eGFR is calculated using the person's creatinine level, age, body size, and sex. Decreased eGFR is expected in older adult and female patients because of their decreased muscle mass. It is important for nurses to know their patient's kidney function to ensure correct drug dosage.

PHARMACODYNAMICS

Pharmacodynamics is the study of the effects of drugs on the body. Drugs act within the body to mimic the actions of the body's own chemical messengers. Drug response can cause a primary or secondary physiologic effect or both. A drug's primary effect is the desirable response, and the secondary effect may be desirable or undesirable. An example of a drug with a primary and secondary effect is diphenhydramine, an antihistamine. The primary effect of diphenhydramine is to treat the symptoms of allergy; the secondary effect is a central nervous system (CNS) depression that causes drowsiness. The secondary effect is undesirable when the patient drives a car, but at bedtime it could be desirable because it causes mild sedation.

▶ **Dose-Response Curve**

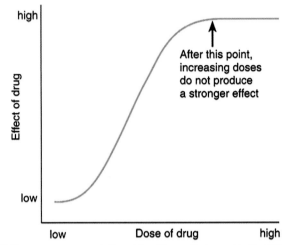

Fig. 3.6 Dose-response relationship. (From Carlson, N. R. [2010]. *Foundations of behavioral neuroscience* [8th ed.]. Upper Saddle River, NJ: Pearson.)

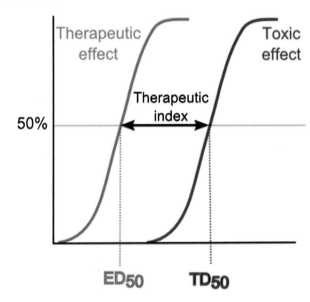

Fig. 3.7 The therapeutic index. The therapeutic index is the ratio between the toxic dose of a drug and the therapeutic dose of a drug. (From Guzman, F. [n.d.]. *Pharmacology corner*. Retrieved from http://pharmacologycorner.com/therapeutic-index/.)

Dose-Response Relationship

The dose-response relationship is the body's physiologic response to changes in drug concentration at the site of action. Two concepts further describe this relationship. Potency refers to the amount of drug needed to elicit a specific physiologic response to a drug. A drug with high potency, such as fentanyl, produces significant therapeutic responses at low concentrations; a drug with low potency, such as codeine, produces minimal therapeutic responses at low concentrations. The point at which increasing a drug's dosage no longer increases the desired therapeutic response is referred to as maximal efficacy (Fig. 3.6).

Closely related to dose-response and efficacy is the therapeutic index (TI), which describes the relationship between the *therapeutic dose* of a drug (ED_{50}) and the *toxic dose* of a drug (TD_{50}). ED_{50} is the dose of a drug that produces a therapeutic response in 50% of the population; TD_{50} is the dose of a drug that produces a toxic response in 50% of the population. The therapeutic index is the difference between these two points (Fig. 3.7). If

Onset-Peak-Duration

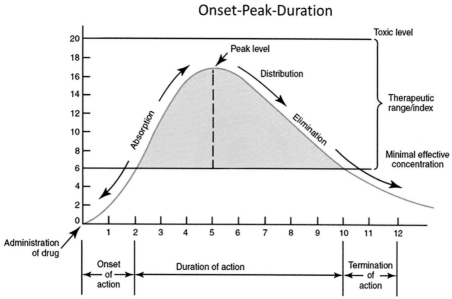

Fig. 3.8 Onset, peak, and duration of action. (From McKenry, L. M., Tessier, E., & Hogan, M. A. [2006]. *Mosby's pharmacology in nursing* [22nd ed.]. St. Louis, MO: Elsevier.)

the ED_{50} and TD_{50} are close, the drug is said to have a narrow therapeutic index. Drugs with a narrow therapeutic index—such as warfarin, digoxin, and phenytoin—require close monitoring to ensure patient safety. To be safe, plasma drug levels of drugs with a narrow therapeutic index must fall within the therapeutic range (also known as the therapeutic window). The therapeutic range is a range of doses that produce a therapeutic response without causing significant adverse effect in patients.

Onset, Peak, and Duration of Action

Other important aspects of pharmacodynamics to understand include a drug's onset, peak, and duration of action. Onset is the time it takes for a drug to reach the minimum effective concentration (MEC) after administration. The MEC is the minimum amount of drug required for drug effect. A drug's peak occurs when it reaches its highest concentration in the blood. Duration of action is the length of time the drug exerts a therapeutic effect. Fig. 3.8 illustrates the areas in which onset, peak, and duration of action occur.

It is necessary to understand this information in relation to drug administration. Some drugs produce effects in minutes, but others may take hours or days. If the drug plasma concentration decreases below the MEC, adequate drug dosing is not achieved; too high of a drug concentration can result in toxicity.

Therapeutic Drug Monitoring

Once a steady state has been achieved, drug concentration can be determined by measuring peak and trough drug levels. Peak and trough levels are requested for drugs that have a narrow therapeutic index and are considered toxic.

The peak drug level is the highest plasma concentration of drug at a specific time, and it indicates the rate of drug absorption. If the peak is too low, effective concentration has not been reached. If the drug is given orally, the peak time is usually 2 to 3 hours after drug administration. If the drug is given intravenously, the peak time is usually 30 to 60 minutes after the infusion is complete. If the drug is given intramuscularly, the peak time is usually 2 to 4 hours after injection. If a peak drug level is ordered, a blood sample should be drawn at the appropriate peak time based on the route of administration.

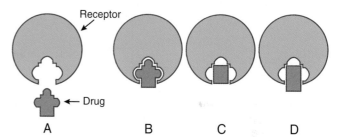

Fig. 3.9 (A) Drugs act by forming chemical bonds with specific receptor sites, similar to a key and lock. (B) The better the fit, the better the response. Drugs with complete attachment and response are called *agonists*. (C) Drugs that attach but do not elicit a response are called antagonists. (D) Drugs that attach and elicit a small response but also block other responses are called partial agonists. (From Clayton, B. D., & Willihnganz, M. J. [2017]. *Basic pharmacology for nurses* [17th ed.]. St. Louis, MO: Elsevier.)

Most drugs only require trough concentration levels to be drawn (the exception is aminoglycoside antibiotics, which require both peak and trough levels). The trough drug level is the lowest plasma concentration of a drug, and it measures the rate at which the drug is eliminated. Trough levels are drawn just before the next dose of drug regardless of route of administration.

Receptor Theory

Drugs act by binding to receptors. Binding of the drug may activate a receptor, producing a response, or it may inactivate a receptor, blocking a response. The activity of many drugs is determined by the ability of the drug to bind to a specific receptor. The better the drug fits at the receptor site, the more active the drug is. Drug-receptor interactions are similar to the fit of the right key in a lock. Fig. 3.9 illustrates drug-receptor binding.

Most receptors, which are protein in nature, are found on cell surface membranes or within the cell itself. Drug-binding sites are primarily on proteins, glycoproteins, proteolipids, and enzymes. The four receptor families (Fig. 3.10) include (1) cell membrane–embedded enzymes, (2) ligand-gated ion channels, (3) G protein–coupled receptor systems, and (4) transcription factors. The ligand-binding domain is the site on the receptor at which drugs bind.

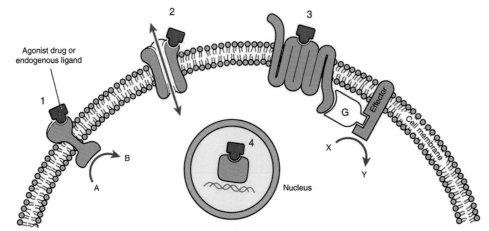

Fig. 3.10 **The four receptor families.** The four receptor families are (1) cell membrane–embedded enzymes, (2) ligand-gated ion channels, (3) G protein–coupled receptor systems, and (4) transcription factors. (From Burchum, J., & Rosenthal, L. [2016]. *Lehne's pharmacology for nursing care* [9th ed.]. St. Louis, MO: Elsevier.)

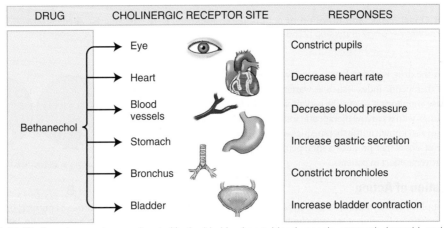

Fig. 3.11 Cholinergic receptors are located in the bladder, heart, blood vessels, stomach, bronchi, and eyes.

- *Cell membrane–embedded enzymes.* The ligand-binding domain for drug binding is on the cell surface. The drug activates the enzyme inside the cell, and a response is initiated.
- *Ligand-gated ion channels.* The channel crosses the cell membrane. When the channel opens, ions flow into and out of the cells. This primarily affects sodium and calcium ions.
- *G protein–coupled receptor systems.* The three components to this receptor response are (1) the receptor, (2) the G protein that binds with guanosine triphosphate (GTP), and (3) the effector, which is either an enzyme or an ion channel. The system works as follows:

$$\text{Drug} \xrightarrow{\text{Activates}} \text{Receptors} \xrightarrow{\text{Activates}} \text{G protein} \xrightarrow{\text{Activates}} \text{Effect}$$

- *Transcription factors.* Found in the cell nucleus on DNA, not on the surface. Activation of receptors through transcription factors regulates protein synthesis and is prolonged. With the first three receptor groups, activation of the receptors is rapid.

Agonists, Partial Agonists, and Antagonists

Drugs that activate receptors and produce a desired response are called agonists. Partial agonists are drugs that elicit only moderate activity when binding to receptors; partial agonists also prevent receptor activation by other drugs. Drugs that prevent receptor activation and block a response are called antagonists. Blocking receptor activation either increases or decreases cellular action, depending on the endogenous action of the chemical messenger that is blocked (see Fig. 3.9).

Nonspecific and Nonselective Drug Effects

Many agonists and antagonists lack specific and selective effects. Receptors produce a variety of physiologic responses, depending on where the receptor is located. Cholinergic receptors are located in the bladder, heart, blood vessels, stomach, bronchi, and eyes. A drug that stimulates or blocks the cholinergic receptors affects all anatomic sites. Drugs that affect multiple receptor sites are considered nonspecific. For example, bethanechol may be prescribed for postoperative urinary retention to increase bladder contraction. This drug stimulates cholinergic receptors located in the bladder, and urination occurs by strengthening bladder contraction. However, because bethanechol is nonspecific, other cholinergic sites are also affected; the heart rate decreases, blood pressure decreases, gastric acid secretion increases, the bronchioles constrict, and the pupils of the eye constrict (Fig. 3.11). These other effects may be either desirable or harmful.

Some drugs affect multiple receptors, and these are considered nonselective drugs. For example, epinephrine, which is used for treatment of anaphylaxis or severe asthma exacerbations, acts on the alpha$_1$, beta$_1$, and beta$_2$ receptors (Fig. 3.12), affecting multiple body systems.

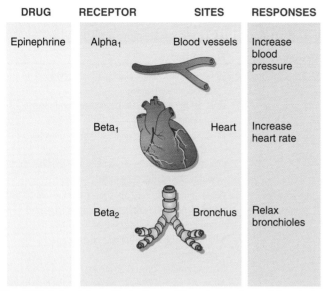

DRUG	RECEPTOR	SITES	RESPONSES
Epinephrine	Alpha$_1$	Blood vessels	Increase blood pressure
	Beta$_1$	Heart	Increase heart rate
	Beta$_2$	Bronchus	Relax bronchioles

Fig. 3.12 Epinephrine affects three different receptors: alpha$_1$, beta$_1$, and beta$_2$.

Mechanisms of Drug Action

Mechanisms of drug action include (1) stimulation, (2) depression, (3) irritation, (4) replacement, (5) cytotoxic action, (6) antimicrobial action, and (7) modification of immune status. A drug that stimulates enhances intrinsic activity (e.g., adrenergic drugs that increase heart rate, sweating, and respiratory rate during fight-or-flight response). Depressant drugs decrease neural activity and bodily functions (e.g., barbiturates and opiates). Drugs that irritate have a noxious effect, such as astringents. Replacement drugs such as insulins, thyroid drugs, and hormones replace essential body compounds. Cytotoxic drugs selectively kill invading parasites or cancers. Antimicrobial drugs prevent, inhibit, or kill infectious organisms. Drugs that modify immune status modify, enhance, or depress the immune system (e.g., interferons and methotrexate).

Side Effects, Adverse Drug Reactions, and Drug Toxicity

Side effects are secondary effects of drug therapy. All drugs have side effects. Even with correct drug dosage, side effects occur that can be predictable and range from inconvenient to severe or life-threatening. In some instances, the side effects may be desirable (e.g., using diphenhydramine at bedtime, when its side effect of drowsiness is beneficial). Chronic illness, age, weight, sex, and ethnicity all play a part in drug side effects.

It is important to know that the occurrence of side effects is one of the primary reasons patients stop taking their prescribed medications. An important role of the nurse includes teaching patients about a drug's side effects and encouraging them to report side effects. Many can be managed with dosage adjustments, changing to a different drug in the same class, or implementing other interventions.

Adverse drug reactions (ADRs) are unintentional, unexpected reactions to drug therapy that occur at normal drug dosages. The reactions may be mild to severe and include anaphylaxis (cardiovascular collapse). Adverse drug reactions are always undesirable and must be reported and documented because they represent variances from planned therapy.

Drug toxicity occurs when drug levels exceed the therapeutic range; toxicity may occur secondary to overdose (intentional or unintentional) or drug accumulation. Factors that influence drug toxicity include disease, genetics, and age.

Tolerance and Tachyphylaxis

Tolerance refers to a decreased responsiveness to a drug over the course of therapy; an individual with drug tolerance requires a higher dosage of drug to achieve the same therapeutic response. In contrast, tachyphylaxis refers to an acute, rapid decrease in response to a drug; it may occur after the first dose or after several doses. Tachyphylaxis has been demonstrated with drugs such as centrally acting analgesics, nitroglycerin, and ranitidine, to name a few. To provide safe and effective care, nurses must be aware of these potential reasons a patient may fail to respond therapeutically to drug administration.

Placebo Effect

Placebo effect is a drug response not attributed to the chemical properties of the drug. The response can be positive or negative and may be influenced by the beliefs, attitudes, and expectations of the patient. Although the placebo effect is psychological in origin, the response can be physiologic, resulting in changes in heart rate, blood pressure, and pain sensation.

DRUG INTERACTIONS

Seventy percent of Americans are taking one or more prescription drugs. Drug therapy is complex because of the great number of drugs available. Drug-drug, drug-nutrient (e.g., food, supplements, alcohol), drug-disease, and drug-laboratory interactions (when a drug interferes with laboratory testing) are an increasing problem. Because of the possibility of numerous interactions, the nurse must be knowledgeable about drug interactions and must closely monitor patient response to drug therapy. Thorough and timely communication among members of the health team is essential. Patients at high risk for interactions include those who have chronic health conditions, take multiple medications, see more than one health care provider, and use multiple pharmacies. Older adults are at especially high risk for drug interactions because 20% of older adults take five or more medications. Multiple drug interaction checker websites are available on the Internet for both health care personnel and consumer use, such as Drugs.com at www.drugs.com/drug_interactions.html or *Web*MD at www.webmd.com/interaction-checker.

A drug interaction is defined as an altered or modified action or effect of a drug as a result of interaction with one or multiple drugs. It should not be confused with drug incompatibility or an adverse drug reaction, an undesirable drug effect that ranges from mild untoward effects to severe toxic effects that include hypersensitivity reaction and anaphylaxis. Drug incompatibility is a chemical or physical reaction that occurs among two or more drugs in vitro. In other words, the reaction occurs between two or more drugs within a syringe, IV bag, or other artificial environment outside of the body.

Drug interactions can be divided into two categories, pharmacokinetic and pharmacodynamic interactions.

Pharmacokinetic Interactions

Pharmacokinetic interactions are changes that occur in the absorption, distribution, metabolism, and excretion of one or more drugs.

Absorption

When a person takes two drugs at the same time, the rate of absorption of one or both drugs can change. A drug can block, decrease, or increase the absorption of another drug. It can do this in one of three ways: (1) by increasing or decreasing gastric emptying time, (2) by changing the gastric pH, or (3) by forming drug complexes.

Drugs that increase the speed of gastric emptying, such as laxatives, may cause an increase in gastric and intestinal motility and a decrease in drug absorption. Most drugs are absorbed primarily in the small intestine; exceptions include barbiturates, salicylates, and theophylline, which undergo gastric absorption. Opioids and anticholinergic drugs such as atropine decrease gastric emptying time and GI motility, causing an increase in absorption rate. For drugs that undergo gastric absorption, the amount or extent of absorption increases the longer the drug remains in the stomach.

When the gastric pH is decreased, a weakly acidic drug such as aspirin is less ionized and is more rapidly absorbed. Drugs that increase the gastric pH decrease absorption of weak-acid drugs. Antacids such as magnesium hydroxide and aluminum hydroxide raise the gastric pH and block or slow absorption. Some drugs may react chemically. For example, tetracycline and the heavy metal ions calcium, magnesium, aluminum, and iron found in antacids or iron supplements may lead to the formation of a drug complex and thus prevent the absorption of tetracycline. This phenomenon may also be observed when products that contain calcium, magnesium, or iron are ingested with fluoroquinolone antibiotics such as ciprofloxacin. Consequently, dairy products, multivitamins, and antacids should be avoided 1 hour before and 2 hours after tetracycline or ciprofloxacin administration. The nonabsorbable cholesterol-lowering drug cholestyramine binds with multiple drugs and fat-soluble vitamins (e.g., vitamin K) in the GI tract, resulting in reduced absorption. Vitamin supplementation may be necessary when cholestyramine is prescribed.

At times, the formation of drug complexes is desired; for example, in the case of acute iron poisoning. In this situation, the chelating agent deferoxamine is administered; it binds to the excess iron in the blood so it can be excreted from the body via the kidneys.

GI bacteria account for 70% of the body's microbes. They play a major role in the absorption of drugs and nutrients and in the metabolism of bilirubin, bile acids, cholesterol, and steroid hormones as well as the synthesis of vitamins B and K. GI bacteria help maintain homeostasis and factor into the overall health and immune status of an individual. Alteration of bacteria normally found in the GI tract (caused by patient genotype, antibiotic treatment, diet, and environment) can affect drug pharmacokinetics. Orally administered drugs can be metabolized by intestinal microbial enzymes, resulting in toxic compounds or reduced drug absorption, which lead to decreased therapeutic response. For example, administration of antibiotics can alter the synthesis of vitamin K, interfering with therapeutic blood levels of the anticoagulant warfarin.

Metabolism

Many drug interactions of metabolism occur with the induction or inhibition of the hepatic microsomal system. A drug can increase the metabolism of another drug by stimulating liver enzymes. These enzymes produce a cascade effect in drug function. Drugs that promote induction of enzymes are called *enzyme inducers*. Some drugs—such as phenobarbital, carbamazepine, and rifampin—are enzyme inducers. Phenobarbital increases the metabolism of most antipsychotics and methylxanthine; phenobarbital, carbamazepine, and rifampin increase the metabolism of warfarin. Increased metabolism promotes drug elimination and decreases plasma concentration of the drug; the result is a decrease in therapeutic drug action. Care must be taken when enzyme inducers are discontinued because less drug is eliminated by hepatic metabolism, and toxicity can result.

Some drugs are enzyme inhibitors. The antiulcer drug cimetidine is an enzyme inhibitor that decreases metabolism of certain drugs (e.g., theophylline, warfarin, phenytoin) and causes an increase in the plasma concentration of these drugs. To avoid toxicity, dosage of these drugs must be reduced. If cimetidine or any enzyme drug inhibitor is discontinued, the dosage of other drugs affected by its administration should be adjusted, and blood levels should be closely monitored.

TABLE 3.1 Drugs: Enzyme Inducers and Enzyme Inhibitors	
Drug Category	**Drug Effect**
Drug enzyme inducer	Onset and termination of drug effect is slow, approximately 1 week. Drug dosage may need to be increased with use of drug inducer. Drug dosage should be adjusted after termination of drug inducer. Monitor serum drug levels, especially if the drug has a narrow therapeutic drug range.
Drug enzyme inhibitor	Onset of drug effect usually occurs rapidly. Half-life ($t\frac{1}{2}$) of the second drug may be increased, causing a prolonged drug effect. Interaction may occur related to the dosage prescribed. Disease entities affect drug dosing. Monitor serum drug levels, especially if the drug has a narrow therapeutic range.

The use of tobacco and alcohol may have variable effects on drug metabolism. Polycyclic aromatic hydrocarbons found in cigarette smoke induce production of the specific family of enzymes responsible for theophylline metabolism. Chronic cigarette smoking leads to an increase in hepatic enzyme activity and can increase theophylline clearance. Patients with asthma who smoke and take theophylline to manage their disease may require an increase in theophylline dosage. With chronic alcohol use, hepatic enzyme activities are increased; with acute alcohol use, metabolism is inhibited.

Natural or herbal products can also affect drug metabolism. St. John's wort, an OTC herbal product used to manage symptoms of depression, induces the metabolism of certain drugs (e.g., warfarin, digoxin, and theophylline). This action potentially decreases the effectiveness of these medications, possibly necessitating a dose increase to sustain efficacy. Flavonoids, a group of naturally occurring compounds found in the juice and pulp of citrus fruits, are potent inhibitors of the metabolism of certain drugs (e.g., carbamazepine, calcium channel blockers, and drugs for erectile dysfunction). Patients who are stabilized on therapeutic doses of these drugs may subject themselves to adverse effects from greater-than-expected drug levels if they eat or drink grapefruit products concurrently with the drug. Table 3.1 describes the effects of drug enzyme inducers and inhibitors.

Excretion

Most drugs are filtered through the glomeruli and are excreted in the urine. With some drugs, excretion occurs in the bile, which passes into the intestinal tract. Drugs can increase or decrease renal excretion and can have an effect on the excretion of other drugs. Drugs that decrease cardiac output decrease blood flow to the kidneys; decreased blood flow results in decreased glomerular filtration rate, which can decrease or delay drug excretion.

Diuretics promote water and sodium excretion from the renal tubules. Furosemide acts on the loop of Henle, and hydrochlorothiazide acts on the distal tubules. Both diuretics decrease reabsorption of water, sodium, and potassium. The renal loss of potassium can result in *hypokalemia,* which can alter the action of some drugs; for example, it can enhance the action of digoxin and can lead to toxicity.

Two or more drugs that undergo the same route of excretion may compete with one another for elimination from the body. Probenecid, a drug for gout, decreases penicillin excretion by inhibiting the secretion of penicillin in the renal tubules of the kidneys. In some cases, this effect may be desirable to increase or maintain the plasma concentration of penicillin—which has a short half-life—for a prolonged period of time.

Changing urine pH affects drug excretion. The antacid sodium bicarbonate causes the urine to be alkaline. Alkaline urine promotes the excretion of drugs that are weak acids (e.g., aspirin, barbiturates). Drugs that acidify the urine, such as ascorbic acid, promote the excretion of drugs that are weak bases (e.g., amphetamine).

With decreased renal or hepatic function, there is usually an increase in free drug concentration. It is essential to closely monitor these patients for drug toxicity when they take multiple drugs. Checking serum drug levels, a practice known as therapeutic drug monitoring (TDM), is especially important for drugs that have a narrow therapeutic range and are highly protein bound. Digoxin and phenytoin are two drugs that require TDM.

Pharmacodynamic Interactions

Pharmacodynamic interactions are those that result in additive, synergistic, or antagonistic drug effects.

Additive Drug Effects

When two drugs are administered in combination and the response is increased beyond what either could produce alone, the drug interaction is called an additive effect; it is the sum of the effects of the two drugs. Additive effects can be desirable or undesirable. For example, a desirable additive drug effect occurs when a diuretic and a beta blocker are administered for the treatment of hypertension. In combination, these two drugs use different mechanisms to have a more pronounced blood pressure–lowering effect. As another example, aspirin and codeine are two analgesics that work by different mechanisms but can be given together for increased pain relief.

An example of an undesirable additive effect is that from two vasodilators, hydralazine prescribed for hypertension and nitroglycerin prescribed for angina. The result could be a severe hypotensive response. Another example is the interaction of aspirin and alcohol. Aspirin is directly irritating to the stomach; it causes platelet dysfunction, and it inhibits prostaglandin-mediated mucus production of the gastric mucosa that protects the underlying tissues of the stomach. Alcohol disrupts the gastric mucosal barrier and suppresses platelet production. Both aspirin and alcohol can prolong bleeding time and, when taken together, may result in gastric bleeding.

Synergistic Drug Effects and Potentiation

When two or more drugs are given together, one drug can have a synergistic effect on another. In other words, the clinical effect of the two drugs given together is substantially greater than that of either drug alone. An example of this is the use of two cytotoxic drugs to reduce individual drug dosing, thereby decreasing side effects. An example of an undesirable effect occurs when alcohol and a sedative-hypnotic drug such as diazepam are combined. The resultant effect of this example is increased CNS depression.

Some antibiotics have an enzyme inhibitor added to the drug to potentiate the therapeutic effect. Examples are ampicillin with sulbactam and amoxicillin with clavulanate, in which sulbactam and clavulanate potassium are bacterial enzyme inhibitors. Ampicillin and amoxicillin can be given without these inhibitors; however, the desired therapeutic effect may not occur because of the bacterial beta-lactamase, which inactivates the drugs and causes bacterial resistance. The combination of the antibiotic with either sulbactam or clavulanate inhibits bacterial enzyme activity and enhances the effect, or broadens the spectrum of activity, of the antibacterial agent.

Antagonistic Drug Effects

When drugs with antagonistic effects are administered together, one drug reduces or blocks the effect of the other. In some situations, antagonistic effects are desirable. In morphine sulfate overdose, naloxone is given as an antagonist to block the narcotic effects of morphine sulfate. This is a beneficial drug interaction of an antagonist. Likewise, in the case of heparin overdose, protamine sulfate is administered to block the effects of heparin.

The most common symptoms of drug-drug interactions include nausea, heartburn, headache, and lightheadedness. Patients should contact their pharmacist or health care provider if they experience any unusual reaction. The most feared interactions are those that result in a dramatic drop in blood pressure or cause a rapid or irregular heart rate. Also of concern are drug interactions that produce toxins capable of damaging vital organs such as the heart or liver. Fortunately, most interactions are not severe or life-threatening. Patients should be aware that prescription drugs, OTC drugs, and herbal products can interact with each other. It is a myth that interactions occur only with prescription medications. Severe adverse reactions are highlighted with a boxed warning in the product literature.

DRUG-NUTRIENT INTERACTIONS

Food may increase, decrease, or delay the body's pharmacokinetic response to drugs. A classic drug-food interaction occurs when a monoamine oxidase inhibitor (MAOI) antidepressant (e.g., phenelzine) is taken with tyramine-rich foods such as cheese, wine, organ meats, beer, yogurt, sour cream, or bananas. Tyramine is a potent vasoconstrictor, and when taken in conjunction with an MAOI, the result could be a hypertensive crisis. These foods must be avoided when taking MAOIs.

Grapefruit alters the metabolism of many drugs through inhibition of the CYP450-3A4 drug-metabolizing enzyme. This is important because the CYP3A4 substrate is involved in metabolism of roughly 50% of the drugs on the market; grapefruit is known to affect more than 44 drugs, inhibiting metabolism and potentially causing serious adverse drug reactions.

Nutritional deficiencies such as protein-energy malnutrition (PEM) may alter pharmacokinetic processes and drug responses, resulting in toxicity. There are two forms of PEM, kwashiorkor and marasmus. Persons with either form of PEM may have altered pharmacokinetics, such as decreased drug absorption and decreased protein binding, altered volume of distribution and biotransformation, and decreased drug elimination. Because of the risk for toxicity, persons with PEM require careful monitoring and possible changes in drug dosing.

DRUG-LABORATORY INTERACTIONS

Drugs often interfere with clinical laboratory testing by cross-reaction with antibodies, interference with enzyme reactions, or alteration of chemical reactions. Drug-laboratory interactions may lead to misinterpretation or invalidation of test results, resulting in additional health care costs associated with unnecessary repeat laboratory testing or additional testing. Drug-laboratory interactions may also lead to missed or erroneous clinical diagnosis. Health care personnel and consumers can find information related to drug-laboratory interactions on several websites on the Internet, such as RxList at http://www.rxlist.com/script/main/hp.asp.

DRUG-INDUCED PHOTOSENSITIVITY

A drug-induced photosensitivity reaction is a skin reaction caused by exposure to sunlight. It is caused most often by the interaction of a

⊚ CLINICAL JUDGMENT [NURSING PROCESS]

Pharmacokinetics and Pharmacodynamics

Concept: Caring Intervention
- Nursing intervention designed to meet the physical and emotional needs of the patient.

Concept: Clinical Decision Making
- Process used by nurses to identify patient problems and intervene to achieve desired outcomes.

Concept: Safety
- Protecting the patient from potential or actual harm; is a basic human need.

Recognize Cues [Assessment]
- Assess family patterns, economic issues, and cultural patterns that influence compliance with the medical regimen.
- Assess language spoken, literacy level, cognitive level, and use of glasses or other aids.
- Check peak levels and trough levels of drugs as appropriate.
- Detect possible interactions and cumulative or other adverse effects among prescribed medications, self-administered over-the-counter (OTC) products, culturally based home treatments, herbal remedies, and foods.
- Determine whether the patient participates in traditional health practices or complementary and alternative medical practices.
- Determine renal function by checking for adequate urine output; the guideline is 30 mL/h for adults.
- Determine the potential for drug interaction problems related to an increased or decreased absorption rate of drugs.
- Determine whether the patient smokes cigarettes.
- Identify all of the patient's current drugs, including prescription and OTC drugs, supplements, herbs, and teas.
- Inquire about the patient's preferences regarding touch, modesty, and personal space.
- Perform a physical examination to identify problems that may affect pharmacokinetics and pharmacodynamics.
- Review all literature provided by drug companies and pharmacies; be sure to check the protein-binding percentage of the drug and any need for therapeutic monitoring.
- Take a thorough patient history to identify factors that may affect drug pharmacokinetics and pharmacodynamics.

Analyze Cues and Prioritize Hypothesis [Patient Problems]
- Anxiety
- Need for health teaching
- Potential for decreased adherence
- Coping

Generate Solutions [Planning]
- The patient will demonstrate behaviors that decrease the risk for injury.
- The patient will describe the rationale for the therapeutic regimen.
- The patient will discuss blocks to implementing a therapeutic regimen or related fears.
- Effective communication techniques will be used.
- The patient will follow a mutually agreed on health maintenance plan.
- The patient will be aware of drug interactions, will avoid drugs that may cause a severe reaction, and will know what to report immediately to the health care provider.
- The patient will effectively manage the therapeutic regimen.
- The patient will not take any OTC drugs without consultation with the health care provider.
- The patient's health care needs will be met within a culturally competent framework.
- The patient will express confidence in his or her personal ability to manage the health situation and remain in control of life.

Take Action [Nursing Interventions]
- Advise patients not to eat high-fat foods before ingesting an EC tablet; high-fat foods decrease the drug absorption rate.
- Allow patients adequate time with significant members of the social group.
- Incorporate traditional health practices with mainstream prescriptive therapies when appropriate.
- Anticipate unique responses to drugs based on social, cultural, and biologic influences.
- Consult a pharmacist about the use of a drug interaction computer program.
- Consult with persons who are knowledgeable about both the patient's culture and mainstream culture.
- Contact the health care provider to assess the need for a drug dose adjustment if one has not been ordered after a drug enzyme inducer has been discontinued.
- If negative side effects of prescribed drugs are a problem, explain that many side effects can be controlled or eliminated.
- Include significant members of the social group in the planning and implementation of patient care.
- Monitor the therapeutic range of drugs that are more toxic or that have a narrow therapeutic range.
- Notify the health care provider of drugs ordered that have antagonistic or opposite effects, such as beta stimulants and beta blockers.
- Recognize drugs of the same category that might have an additive effect. The additive drug effect might be undesirable and could cause a severe physiologic response.
- Recognize the need for patients to exercise control in their environment.
- Reconcile all drugs at discharge and provide a list to the patient; ensure that accurate drug information is available to all health care personnel involved in patient care.
- Simplify therapy.
- Use appropriate persons as translators.
- Use therapeutic communication.
- Facilitate adherence to mainstream prescriptive therapies within the patient's social and cultural contexts.
- Provide health information written in the patient's primary language. Medline, an online service of the National Institutes of Health, offers a variety of patient education materials in a number of languages online at www.nlm.nih.gov/medlineplus/languages/languages.html.
- Advise patients not to take OTC drugs with prescribed drugs without first notifying the health care provider.
- Encourage the patient to use one pharmacy.
- Include significant members of the social group, when appropriate, in the drug regimen.
- Remind patients to be cautious about taking herbal products, especially if taking OTC or prescription medications; advise that they check with their health care provider first.
- Use illustrations to explain the drug regimen.

Evaluate Outcomes [Evaluation]
- Assess for signs and symptoms of drug side effects and toxicity.
- Evaluate physical, social, and psychological outcomes of prescriptive therapies.
- Evaluate the effectiveness of the drugs.
- Monitor for patient adherence to prescriptive therapies.

drug and exposure to ultraviolet A (UVA) light, which can cause cellular damage; however, ultraviolet B (UVB) light may also contribute to drug-induced photosensitivity reactions.

The two types of photosensitivity reactions are photoallergic and phototoxic. A *photoallergic reaction* occurs when a drug (e.g., sulfonamide) undergoes activation in the skin by ultraviolet light to a compound that is more allergenic than the parent compound. Because it takes time to develop antibodies, photoallergic reactions are a type of delayed hypersensitivity reaction. With a *phototoxic reaction,* a photosensitive drug undergoes photochemical reactions within the skin to cause damage. This type of reaction is not immune mediated. The onset of a phototoxic reaction with erythema can be rapid, occurring within 2 to 6 hours of sunlight exposure.

Both types of reactions are the result of light exposure, but they differ according to the wavelength of light and the photosensitive drug. A phototoxic reaction may be the result of the drug dose, whereas a photoallergic reaction is not and only requires previous exposure, or sensitization, to the offending agent.

Most photosensitive reactions can be avoided by using sunscreen with a sun protection factor (SPF) greater than 15; avoiding excessive sunlight, especially at the height of the daylight hours; and wearing protective clothing. Decreasing the drug dose may decrease the risk of photosensitivity if treatment is required. It may be necessary, however, to discontinue use of the offending drug.

CRITICAL THINKING CASE STUDY

The nurse is caring for a patient who was admitted to the hospital with severe migraines. He has been taking warfarin, a highly protein-bound anticoagulant, for atrial fibrillation. After a thorough evaluation, the neurologist has ordered valproic acid, an antiseizure medication. Valproic acid is also highly protein bound.

1. What patient problem would be appropriate for this patient?

2. What information needs to be included in the interdisciplinary health/teaching plan for this patient?

3. During a teaching session, the patient shares that he plans to start taking over-the-counter products to boost his energy. What is the nurse's best response to the patient's comment? Explain your answer.

REVIEW QUESTIONS

1. Which components of pharmacokinetics does the nurse need to understand before administering a drug? (Select all that apply.)
   a. Drugs with a smaller volume of drug distribution have a longer half-life.
   b. Oral drugs are dissolved through the process of pinocytosis.
   c. Patients with kidney disease may have fewer protein-binding sites and are at risk for drug toxicity.
   d. Rapid absorption decreases the bioavailability of the drug.
   e. When the drug metabolism rate is decreased, excess drug accumulation can occur, which can cause toxicity.

2. The nurse will question the health care provider if a drug with a half-life (t½) of more than 24 hours is ordered to be given more than how often?
   a. Once daily
   b. Every other day
   c. Twice weekly
   d. Once weekly

3. The nurse is explaining drug action to a nursing student. Which statement made by the nurse is correct?
   a. Water-soluble and ionized drugs are quickly absorbed.
   b. A drug not bound to protein is an active drug.
   c. Most receptors are found under the cell membrane.
   d. Toxic effects can result if the trough level is low.

4. A Native American patient is newly diagnosed with type 2 diabetes mellitus and is prescribed the antidiabetic drug metformin 500 mg by mouth with morning and evening meals. Which statement best indicates to the nurse that the patient will adhere to the therapeutic regimen?
   a. I will no longer put sugar on my cereal because that will help me be healthier.
   b. If I take this medicine, I will feel better soon and won't have to take it anymore.
   c. To reduce the possibility of damage to my body, I must take the medicine as scheduled.
   d. I have diabetes because of my ancestry, so there's not much I can do about it.

5. The nurse is aware that the rate of absorption can be changed by which actions? (Select all that apply.)
   a. Modifying gastric emptying time
   b. Changing gastric pH
   c. Decreasing inflammation
   d. Forming drug complexes
   e. Eating too slowly

6. The nurse is meeting with a community group about drug safety. The nurse must emphasize that patients at high risk for drug interactions include which groups? (Select all that apply.)
   a. Older patients
   b. Patients with chronic health conditions
   c. Patients taking three or more drugs
   d. Patients dealing with only one pharmacy
   e. Patients covered by private insurance

7. The nurse recognizes that when a patient takes a hepatic enzyme inducer, the dose of warfarin is usually modified in which way?
   a. It is increased.
   b. It is decreased.
   c. It remains the same.
   d. It is unpredictable.
8. The nurse is describing to a patient the synergistic effects of two of his medications. Which statement by the nurse is correct about synergistic drug effects?
   a. Two drugs have antagonistic effects on each other.
   b. The action of a drug is nullified by another drug.
   c. One drug acts as an antidote to the side effects of another drug.
   d. A greater effect is achieved when two drugs are combined.
9. A patient asks the nurse about drug interactions with over-the-counter preparations. Which is the nurse's best response?
   a. Discuss this with the health care provider.
   b. There are not many interactions, so don't worry about it.
   c. Read the labels carefully, and check with your health care provider.
   d. Avoid over-the-counter preparations.
10. Codeine is an example of a(n) _____ as the cytochrome P450 system metabolizes the drug to facilitate receptor affinity.
    a. agonist
    b. prodrug
    c. antagonist
    d. enzyme

4

Pharmacogenetics

http://evolve.elsevier.com/McCuistion/pharmacology

OBJECTIVES

- Define terminology related to pharmacogenetics.
- Discuss the role of pharmacogenetics in drug therapy.
- Discuss the role of nurse as advocate related to pharmacogenetics.
- Anticipate potential unique responses to drugs based on biologic variations.
- Discuss the legal and ethical issues related to pharmacogenetics.
- Identify barriers to the implementation of pharmacogenetics.

OUTLINE

Each person responds to drugs differently; drugs are not "one size fits all" (Fig. 4.1). Most current drug prescribing occurs through trial and error (Fig. 4.2), typically based on age, weight, sex, and liver and kidney function. For drugs with established therapeutic monitoring parameters, dosing is also adjusted based on plasma drug levels.

Nearly 50% of persons stop taking their prescribed drugs due to side effects or failure of the drug to work as desired. Frequently, a person may try as many as four different drugs before finding one that works for them.

The Centers for Disease Control and Prevention (CDC) estimates nearly one million visits to the emergency department (ED) occur annually due to adverse drug reactions. A quarter of these visits result in hospitalization. Treatment of adverse drug reactions cost Americans more than $3.5 billion a year in health care expenditures. Anticoagulants, antibiotics, diabetes drugs, and opioid analgesics top the list of drugs leading to ED visits.

Pharmacogenetics is the study of how a patient's genome affects his or her response to medications (Table 4.1). Using pharmacogenetics helps individualize drug treatment regimens to optimize therapy and decrease adverse drug reactions, thus promoting adherence and reducing overall health care costs. Nurses need to understand the issues related to pharmacogenetics, such as the role of genetic counseling and the legal and ethical questions surrounding genetic testing (Table 4.2). Nurses also need to have a basic understanding of pharmacogenetic technology to advocate and educate patients and their families so they can make the best decisions and pave the way for the best outcomes.

BRIEF HISTORY

For thousands of years, people have been breeding animals and growing plants to achieve specific characteristics. Genetic differences in humans have been recognized for centuries. In 1865 Gregor Mendel was the first to explain the difference between dominant and recessive genes in inheritance, using pea flowers as an example (Fig. 4.3). More recently, in 1953 James Watson and Francis Crick discovered that deoxyribonucleic acid (DNA), the main constituent of chromosomes and the carrier of genetic information, was composed of a double-stranded helix of nucleotides (Fig. 4.4). Advances in genetics came rapidly after this discovery. In 2003 the Human Genome Project completed mapping of the roughly 25,000 genes in human DNA (Box 4.1).

In 2015 the Precision Medicine Initiative launched. This initiative sought to expand the treatment and prevention of disease by taking into account a person's genes, environment, and lifestyle. The ultimate goal of the initiative is to expand the use of precision medicine, truly treating the right patient, with the right drug, at the right dose.

CLINICAL USES

Mapping of the human genome has instilled hope for improving diagnosis and treatment of disease, predicting disease potential based on genetic predisposition, and personalizing medicine based on genetic profiles (Box 4.2). However, as with drugs not being "one size fits all," use of pharmacogenetics is not appropriate for all patients. Those who can benefit most are patients taking multiple prescription drugs or those who are on a complex treatment regimen, those who are not responding well to current therapy or who have had previous adverse drug reactions, and patients taking any drug with pharmacogenetic information included in a boxed warning (e.g., abacavir, clopidogrel) or in the prescribing information (e.g., aripiprazole, citalopram, warfarin). Pharmacogenetic testing is not available for all drugs. One single test cannot determine how a patient will respond to all drugs; if pharmacogenetic testing is appropriate, more than one test may be needed.

INDIVIDUAL VARIATION IN METABOLISM OF SELECT DRUGS

Mercaptopurine. The US Food and Drug Administration (FDA) recommends genetic testing before the administration of mercaptopurine to patients with acute lymphoblastic leukemia. Genetic variation in thiopurine S-methyltransferase (TPMT) and nudix

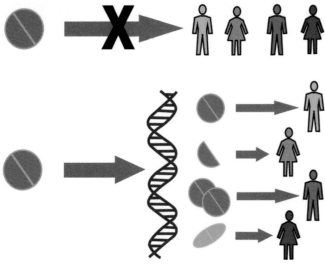

Fig. 4.1 One size does not fit all. The study of variability in drug response due to heredity. (From Pharmacogenomics Laboratory, Indiana University School of Medicine. [2016]. Pharmacogenetics brochure. *Ignite*. https://gmkb.org/?utm_source=ignite-genomics.org&utm_medium=referral.)

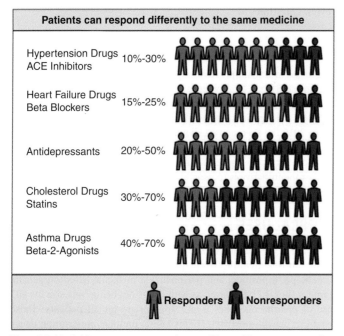

Patients can respond differently to the same medicine

Hypertension Drugs ACE Inhibitors	10%-30%
Heart Failure Drugs Beta Blockers	15%-25%
Antidepressants	20%-50%
Cholesterol Drugs Statins	30%-70%
Asthma Drugs Beta-2-Agonists	40%-70%

Responders   Nonresponders

Fig. 4.2 Variable response to drugs. (From Pharmacogenomics Laboratory, Indiana University School of Medicine. [2016]. Pharmacogenetics brochure. *Ignite*. https://gmkb.org/?utm_source=ignite-genomics.org&utm_medium=referral.)

hydrolase 15 (NUDT15) can interfere with the metabolism of the drug, leading to an increased severity in side effects and increased risk of myelosuppression and infection.

Irinotecan. Genetic testing is recommended for patients with colon cancer receiving irinotecan as part of their treatment protocol. Persons with variation in the UGT1A1 gene may be unable to eliminate the drug, leading to severe diarrhea and severe neutropenia, resulting in life-threatening infections.

Abacavir. Between 6% and 10% of patients prescribed this drug for the treatment of human immunodeficiency virus (HIV) develop potentially fatal multiorgan hypersensitivity. Genetic testing has identified the allele HLA-B*5701 in relation to hypersensitivity. The FDA now recommends genetic testing before initiating drug therapy or restarting the drug.

TABLE 4.1	Terminology
Pharmacogenetics[a]	The study of variability in drug response due to heredity.
Pharmacogenomics[a]	The study of the combination of pharmacology and genomics to develop effective and safe medications to compensate for genetic differences in patients that cause varied responses to a single therapeutic regimen.
Allele	One of two or more versions of a gene; an individual inherits two alleles for each gene, one from each parent; if the two alleles are the same (e.g., CYP2C19*1/*1), the individual is homozygous for that gene; if the alleles are different (e.g., CYP2C19*1/*2), the individual is heterozygous.
Extensive metabolizers	Have an ordinary response to drugs.
Gene	A region of DNA containing genetic information. Is the basic physical and functional unit of heredity.
Genome	The totality of genetic information found in an organism's DNA and/or ribonucleic acid (RNA).
Genomics	The study of the combination of the environment, personal factors as well as all genetic variation.
Genotype	An individual's collection of genes.
Intermediate metabolizers	Decreased efficiency in drug metabolism and therefore an increased concentration of the parent drug with decreased formation of metabolites and a possible decrease in responsiveness.
Personalized medicine	The tailoring of medical treatment to the individual characteristics of each patient, which include genetic predisposition to disease, environmental and personal factors, and pharmacogenetics tailored to improve patient outcomes.
Phenotype	Clinical presentation or observable characteristics of an individual with a particular genotype.
Polymorphisms	Natural variations in a gene, DNA sequence, or chromosome that have no adverse effects on the individual and occur with high frequency in the general population.
Poor metabolizers	Significant decrease in drug metabolism, and as a result tend to have higher levels of the parent drug but with little to no therapeutic benefit and an increased risk for adverse drug responses.
Ultrarapid metabolizers	Increased efficiency in drug metabolism resulting in a possible decrease in effectiveness at established doses. Increased risk for adverse drug responses because of increased metabolite or active drug production.

[a]Often used interchangeably.

From: Chang, K. L., Weitzel, K., & Schmidt, S. (2015). Pharmacogenetics: Using genetic information to guide drug therapy. *American Family Physician, 92*(7), 588-594. www.aafp.org/afp; McClary, L. M. (2020). *Essentials of medical genetics for nursing and health professionals: An interprofessional approach.* Burlington, MA: Jones & Bartlett Learning; Montgomery, S., Brouwer, W. A., Everett, P. C., Hassen, E., Lowe, T., McGral, S. B., ... Eggert, J. (2017). Genetics in the clinical setting: What nurses need to know to provide the best patient care. *American Nurse Today, 12*(10), 10-16.

TABLE 4.2 Available Pharmacogenetic Testing

Drug	Associated Diseases/Conditions	Gene(s) Tested
Warfarin	Excessive clotting disorder	*VKORC1* and *CYP2C9*
Thiopurines (e.g., azathioprine, mercaptopurine, and thioguanine)	Autoimmune/childhood leukemia	*TPMT*
Clopidogrel	Cardiovascular	*CYP2C19*
Irinotecan	Cancer	*UGT1A1*
Abacavir	HIV	*HLA-B*5701*
Carbamazepine, phenytoin	Epilepsy	*HLA-B*1502*
Some antidepressants, some antiepileptics (e.g., phenytoin, phenobarbital, carbamazepine, valproic acid)	Psychiatric, epilepsy	*CYP2D6, CYP2C9, CYP2C19, CYP1A2, SLC6A4, HTR2A/C*
Tamoxifen	Cancer	*CYP2D6*
Some antipsychotics (e.g., haloperidol, mephobarbital, thioridazine)	Psychiatric	*DRD3, CYP2D6, CYP2C19, CYP1A2*
Methylphenidate	Attention deficit disorder	*DRD4*
Opioids	Pain management	*OPRM1*
5-Fluorouracil	Cancer	*DPYD* variants and *TYMS* gene mutations testing
Selective serotonin reuptake inhibitors (SSRIs)	Depression	*5-HTT*
Some statins (e.g., simvastatin)	High cholesterol	*SLCO1B1*

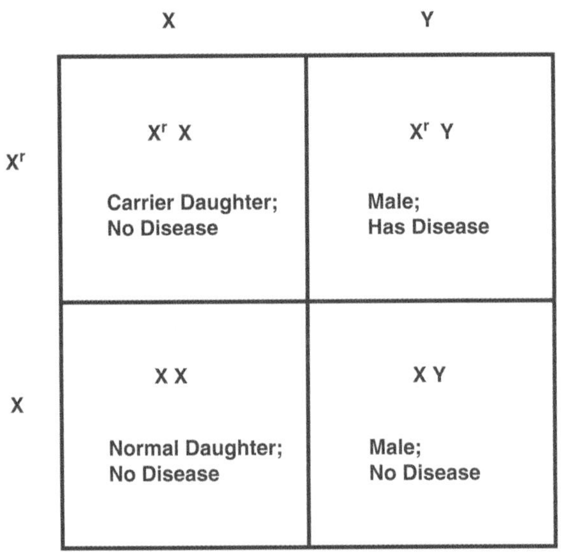

	X	Y
X^r	X^r X **Carrier Daughter; No Disease**	X^r Y **Male; Has Disease**
X	X X **Normal Daughter; No Disease**	X Y **Male; No Disease**

Fig. 4.3 Punnett Square.

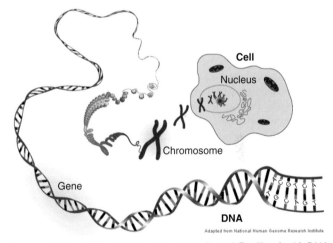

Fig. 4.4 DNA. (From Chromosome Analysis and Fertility. [n.d.] *DNAdirect.* https://services.dnadirect.com/grc/patient-site/chromosome-analysis-infertility/chromosome-analysis-and-fertility.html.)

Warfarin. This drug is a vitamin K antagonist used for prophylaxis and treatment of venous thromboembolism and for persons with atrial fibrillation or heart valve replacement, among other uses. It has a narrow therapeutic range. From 10% to 16% of persons prescribed warfarin experience life-threatening bleeding. Alterations in CYP2C9 and vitamin K epoxide reductase (VKOR) enzymes result in decreased clearance and increased blood levels, thereby increasing the risk for bleeding. Warfarin labeling contains dosing information based on CYP2C9 and VKORC1 genotypes.

Clopidogrel. Persons with genetic variation in the CYP2C19 enzyme, which is necessary to convert the prodrug clopidogrel, an inhibitor of platelet aggregation, to the active metabolite, may be at risk for clot formation due to failure to convert the prodrug to active drug. Point-of-care buccal swab genetic testing has been available since 2013 to help guide treatment. The test determines whether a person has the normal (also referred to as *wild type*) enzyme or a mutation in CYP2C19 enzyme.

Opioids. Codeine and tramadol are prodrugs that do not exhibit analgesic properties until converted to active drug by the CYP2D6 enzyme in the liver. Nearly 10% of the population lack this drug-metabolizing enzyme and therefore do not achieve pain relief with codeine or tramadol. Additionally, this enzyme has several polymorphisms that alter drug metabolism. Persons with two variant alleles are considered poor metabolizers and will not achieve pain relief with codeine or tramadol. People of Asian, Caucasian, and Middle Eastern descent are most likely to have this variant. Persons with two *wild-type* alleles are designated ultrarapid metabolizers and are at risk for toxicity, sedation, and respiratory depression due to higher rates of conversion of codeine or tramadol to active drug.

Mental Health Drugs. Many drugs used to treat depression (e.g., tricyclic antidepressants and selective serotonin reuptake inhibitors) and other psychiatric disorders (i.e., aripiprazole for use in bipolar disorder and schizophrenia, and atomoxetine for use in ADHD) are metabolized by the CYP 2D6 enzyme. This enzyme has 90 known variants that slow drug metabolism, potentially leading to toxic drug concentrations. Additionally, a couple of known variants increase enzymatic activity, leading to subtherapeutic drug levels. Another variant results in an inactive form of the enzyme, resulting in severe adverse reactions to the drugs.

BOX 4.1   Genes

- Each gene has a specific genetic code.
  - This code is a sequence of nucleotides (A, T, G, or C).
- For each nucleotide position in the gene, one of the four nucleotides is the predominant nucleotide in the general population.
  - This predominant nucleotide is usually referred to as *wild type*.
- If an individual has a nucleotide that is different from wild type in one copy of his or her genes, that person is said to have a heterozygous variant.
- If an individual has the same variant nucleotide in both copies of his or her genes, that person is said to have a homozygous variant.

From American Association for Clinical Chemistry: Lab Tests Online. (2019). *Pharmacogenetic tests.* https://labtestsonline.org/tests/pharmacogenetic-tests.

BOX 4.2   Clinical Application of Pharmacogenetics

- Improve quality outcomes
- Customize patient plans of care
- Decrease adverse effects of drug therapy
- Predict patient response to drug therapy
- Save time and money by reducing "trial and error" in drug prescribing
- Decrease treatment failures

Carbamazepine. Persons with the human leukocyte antigen (HLA) B*1502 variant should avoid using carbamazepine due to increased risk of developing Stevens-Johnson syndrome or toxic epidermal necrolysis. Persons of Asian descent are most likely to carry this genetic variant.

LEGAL AND ETHICAL ISSUES

Legal and ethical considerations encompass the principles of privacy, autonomy, and justice:

- Privacy
  - Who has access to patient genetic information?
  - Who owns the genetic information?
  - Concerns about patient "labeling" based on genetic code.
- Autonomy
  - A patient may consent to or refuse genetic testing.
  - Patients may change their minds about obtaining genetic testing.
- Justice
  - Equal and fair treatment of all.
  - Not everyone has access to the same level of care, nor can everyone afford care.

The health care community must not allow genetic profiling to occur. Within an ethnic group, not everyone shares the same genetic variations. Therefore we must guard against denial of treatment based on race and ethnicity in the absence of available pharmacogenetic testing. It is vital to remember that medical conditions are not the result of genetics alone but the fusion of life choices and environment as well.

People have voiced concerns regarding the use of genetic information. Many decline to have genetic testing performed due to fears their employers or insurance companies will unfairly use the results. In response to these concerns, in 2008 the Genetic Information Nondiscrimination Act (GINA) was enacted, which prohibits insurance companies from requiring genetic testing to obtain health insurance and from using genetic information to determine coverage and premiums. The protections provided by GINA allow people to have genetic tests as recommended by their providers without fear that the results will adversely affect insurance or employment decisions. However, these protections do not extend to life insurance, disability insurance, and long-term care insurance, nor do they apply to military members, Indian Health Services, the Veterans Health Administration, or the Federal Employees Health Benefits Program.

Implementation of pharmacogenetics, in conjunction with other patient factors and clinical information, can improve patient safety, quality of care, morbidity, and mortality, and decrease cost. The hope for the future of pharmacogenetics is ensuring delivery of the right drug, at the right dose, to the right patient, via the right route, administered at the right time.

◎ CLINICAL JUDGMENT [NURSING PROCESS]

Pharmacogenetics

Concept: Safety
- Protection of the patient from potential or actual harm; it is a basic human need.

Recognize Cues [Assessment]
- Assess family history back three generations; does anyone in the family have a history of adverse reactions to drugs or treatment failures?
- Asses patient knowledge concerning genetics and genetic testing; explore concerns they may have.
- Determine patient ethnicity.
- Assess patient for therapeutic response to drug regimen.
- Determine side effects and adverse responses to drug therapy.

Analyze Cues and Prioritize Hypothesis [Patient Problems]
- Anxiety
- Coping
- Need for health teaching

Generate Solutions [Planning]
- Integrate patient preferences and family implications into developing evidence-based plans of care.
- Incorporate the patient's preferred language, values, traditions, religion, and health beliefs into plans of care.

Take Action [Nursing Interventions]
- Refer identified patients to genetic counseling as needed.
- Ensure patients know to report genetic findings to all of their health care providers to reduce duplicate testing and promote optimal prescribing.
- Encourage behavior change to reduce the environmental effect on a person's genetic makeup; refer to appropriate services as needed to facilitate positive treatment outcomes.
- Guide patients in the implications and uses of genetic results.
- Ensure the provision of holistic nursing care; practice with compassion and respect for the inherent dignity, worth, and unique attributes of every person, regardless of genetic makeup.

Evaluate Outcomes [Evaluation]
- Evaluate the effectiveness of pharmacogenetic interventions and treatment on patient outcomes.

Additional Resources
Clinical Pharmacogenetics Implementation Consortium: https://cpicpgx.org/
Clinical Genome Resource: https://www.clinicalgenome.org/
Genetic Alliance: http://www.geneticalliance.org/
National Human Genome Research Institute: https://www.genome.gov/
Pharmacogenomics Knowledgebase: https://www.pharmgkb.org/

CRITICAL THINKING CASE STUDY

The patient is prescribed tramadol 100 mg every 6 hours as needed for moderate to severe pain after vertebral fracture. After routinely receiving the drug over 24 hours without relief, the prescriber increases the dose to 150 mg every 4 hours. The patient continues to complain of pain, rated at 8 out of 10, on routine dosing.

1. Which liver enzyme converts tramadol to its active metabolite?
2. Which polymorphism is suspected in this patient?
3. How do patients with this polymorphism metabolize their drugs? This leads to which potential side effects?

REVIEW QUESTIONS

1. Which class of drug is clopidogrel?
   a. low-molecular-weight heparin
   b. vitamin K antagonist
   c. direct thrombin inhibitor
   d. inhibitor of platelet aggregation
2. Patients with HIV should receive genetic testing for the allele HLA-B*5701 before being treated with:
   a. abacavir
   b. tenofovir
   c. lamivudine
   d. rilpivirine
3. Which are the clinical applications of pharmacogenetics? (Select all that apply.)
   a. Improve quality outcomes
   b. Customize patient plans of care
   c. Decrease adverse effects of drug therapy
   d. Reduce cost
   e. Decrease treatment failures
4. Which action should be taken with a patient prescribed mercaptopurine who has a deficiency of TPMT or NUDT15?
   a. The dose of mercaptopurine should be increased.
   b. The dose of mercaptopurine should be decreased.
   c. No change should be made to their dose of mercaptopurine.
   d. The dose of mercaptopurine should be decreased with TPMT deficiency and increased with NUDT15 deficiency.
5. Which factors are taken into account in personalized medicine? (Select all that apply.)
   a. Pharmacogenetic profile
   b. Lifestyle choices
   c. Environmental factors
   d. Provider decision making
   e. Life expectancy

5

Complementary and Alternative Therapies

http://evolve.elsevier.com/McCuistion/pharmacology

OBJECTIVES

- Discuss at least five important points associated with the use of complementary and alternative medicine.
- Compare at least six common herbs and their associated toxicity.
- Differentiate at least eight of the most common herbal therapies and the potential use for each.

- Describe the recommendations for labels on herbal products.
- Discuss the nursing implications, including patient teaching, related to herbal products.

OUTLINE

Complementary and alternative medicine (CAM) is used by 40% of adults to either augment or replace traditional medical therapies. CAM practices include, but are not limited to, botanicals, nutritional products, and herbal supplements. It is critical for nurses to know about alternative medicine and to note its use in their assessment. CAM products can have both positive and negative effects, and they can interact with prescription and over-the-counter (OTC) medications. Nurses are in an excellent position to educate patients about these interactions.

Botanicals are additive substances that come from plants; an herb is any plant that is used for culinary or medicinal purposes. Plants have been the source of old and new drugs for some time: foxglove is the source of digitalis, from snakeroot we get reserpine, willow bark is the source of aspirin, and Taxol comes from the Pacific yew tree, just to name a few. The therapeutic value of plants is the basis of phytomedicine. Research into the effects of CAM continues to grow.

Many Americans use botanical dietary supplements for therapeutic or preventive reasons, and herbal therapy has surged in popularity; marketing and media have fueled the demand, with advertisements and promotions on television, in magazines, and on the Internet. In the United States alone, sales have topped the $6 billion mark and are expected to continue to grow.

Few pharmacy schools in the United States offer courses in botanical remedies, but herbal therapy is being addressed in the professional literature with increasing frequency and seriousness. Health care providers and consumers are asking questions about herbal therapy's effectiveness, potential toxicity, and reactions with conventional medications. Consumers are right to question advertisements that imply that herbs will cure anything. Herbs can be useful, but they can also be ineffectual or even dangerous.

 COMPLEMENTARY AND ALTERNATIVE THERAPIES

Patient Responsibility

To optimize the therapeutic regimen, the patient has the responsibility to (1) consult with the health care provider before taking any herbal preparation, (2) report all herbal preparations taken to all health care providers, (3) inform health care providers of any allergy or sensitivity to any herbal products, (4) use caution if pregnant or lactating, and (5) not take a greater dose than recommended.

In 1992 the US Congress instructed the National Institutes of Health (NIH) to develop an Office of Alternative Medicine to support studies of alternative therapies. This office is now called the *National Center for Complementary and Integrative Health* (NCCIH) and lists current clinical trials with herbal products on their website (www.nccam.nih.gov/research/clinicaltrials). The Natural Standard research collaboration

TABLE 5.1   Definitions of Herbal Preparations

Preparation	Definition
Decoction	A tea made from boiling plant material—usually the bark, rhizomes, roots, or other woody parts—in water. May be used therapeutically. Natural dyes are often made this way.
Infusion	A tea made by pouring water over plant material (usually dried flowers, fruit, leaves, and other parts, although fresh plant material may also be used); the mixture is then allowed to steep. The water is usually boiling, but cold infusions are also an option. May be used therapeutically; hot tea is an excellent way to administer herbs.
Tincture	An extract of a plant made by soaking herbs in a dark place with a desired amount of either glycerin, alcohol, or vinegar for 2–6 weeks. The liquid is strained from the plant material and then may be used therapeutically.
Liniment	Extract of a plant added to either alcohol or vinegar and applied topically for therapeutic benefits.
Poultice	A therapeutic topical application of a soft, moist mass of plant material (such as bruised fresh herbs), usually wrapped in a fine woven cloth.
Essential oils	Aromatic volatile oils extracted from the leaves, stems, flowers, and other parts of plants. Therapeutic use generally includes dilution of the highly concentrated oil.
Herb-infused oils	A process of extraction in which the volatile oils of a plant substance are obtained by soaking the plant in a carrier oil for approximately 2 weeks and then straining the oil. The resulting oil is used therapeutically and may contain the plant's aromatic characteristics.
Percolation	A process to extract the soluble constituents of a plant with the assistance of gravity. The material is moistened and evenly packed into a tall, slightly conical vessel; the liquid (*menstruum*) is then poured onto the material and allowed to steep for a certain length of time. A small opening is then made in the bottom, which allows the extract to slowly flow out of the vessel. The remaining plant material (the *marc*) may be discarded. Many tinctures and liquid extracts are prepared this way.

also reviews global literature on herbal studies. These studies are important because CAM cannot be patented, so their manufacturers generally cannot justify the expenses associated with safety and efficacy testing in an already booming conventional medicine economy.

This chapter describes selected aspects of herbal therapy, including (1) the Dietary Supplement Health and Education Act of 1994, (2) varieties of herbal preparations, (3) the most commonly used herbs, (4) herbs used to treat selected common ailments, (5) potential hazards of herbs, (6) tips for consumers and health care providers, and (7) herbal resources.

DIETARY SUPPLEMENT HEALTH AND EDUCATION ACT OF 1994

In 1994 the US Congress enacted the Dietary Supplement Health and Education Act (DSHEA), which defined dietary supplements as the following:
- Is intended to supplement the diet
- Contains one or more dietary ingredients (including vitamins, minerals, herbs or other botanicals, amino acids, and certain other substances) or their constituents
- Is intended to be taken by mouth, in forms such as tablet, capsule, powder, softgel, gelcap, or liquid
- Is labeled as being a dietary supplement

Although dietary supplements are regulated through the US Food and Drug Administration (FDA), oversight is limited compared with prescription drugs (see http://www.fda.gov/Food/DietarySupplements/default.htm). Manufacturers are required to ensure that their products are safe and that the label information is truthful and not misleading; however, they are not required to demonstrate product safety before the product is sold. Packaging of all dietary supplements must bear the wording "This statement has not been evaluated by the US Food and Drug Administration (FDA). This product is not intended to diagnose, treat, cure, or prevent any disease."

Additionally, all labels are required to have the following five components:
1. Name of the supplement
2. Amount of the supplement (net quantity)
3. Nutrition labeling
4. Ingredient list
5. Name and place of the manufacturer, packer, or distributor

Manufacturers of dietary supplements are allowed to make three types of claims: (1) health claims, (2) structure and function claims, and (3) nutrient content claims. To make these claims, manufacturers must have supporting data. The Federal Trade Commission (FTC) is responsible for regulating the truth in advertising related to dietary supplements. Herbal supplements can be marketed with suggested dosages. The physiologic effects of the product can be noted, but no claims can be made about preventing or curing specific conditions. For example, a product label cannot claim that the agent "prevents heart disease," but it can say that the agent "helps increase blood flow to the heart." Health maintenance claims (e.g., "maintains a healthy immune system") and claims for relief of minor symptoms related to life stages (e.g., "alleviates hot flashes") are acceptable because they do not relate to disease. Herbal products using a "may be beneficial" disclaimer, rather than claims of definite benefit, are appropriate legally. Dietary supplement manufacturers are still required to substantiate any claims they make. Consumers are reminded that premarket testing for safety and efficacy is not required, and manufacturing is not standardized.

CURRENT GOOD MANUFACTURING PRACTICES

The FDA proposed standards for marketing and labeling dietary supplements in 2003. Known as the Current Good Manufacturing Practices (CGMPs), these standards are multifaceted and require that package labels give the quality and strength of all contents and that products be free of contaminants and impurities (Table 5.1). Manufacturing quality control procedures are part of the CGMPs.

Additionally, a *seal of approval* is awarded to products that meet criteria similar to that of the CGMPs by four organizations: the US Pharmacopeial Convention (USP), ConsumerLab.com, National Products Association, and NSF International. The fee-based tests provide information on an herbal product's identity, potency, dissolution, purity, and labeling accuracy. However, the seal of approval is no indication of the product's safety or efficacy.

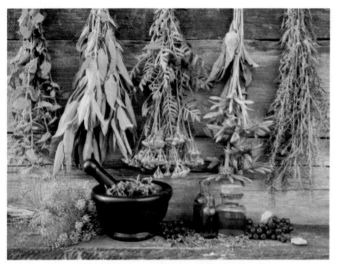

Fig. 5.1 Medicinal herbs. (Copyright © marilyna/iStock/Thinkstock.com.)

COMMONLY USED HERBAL REMEDIES

Most herbal therapies are used to maintain or improve health (Fig. 5.1). This section discusses the most commonly used herbs. The NCCIH (https://nccih.nih.gov/) is an excellent resource for information on herbal therapies not discussed here.

Astragalus *(A. membranaceus and A. mongholicus)*

Astragalus membranaceus and *Astragalus mongholicus* have been used as an adjunct to boost the immune system, such as for hepatitis and cancer, and to limit the effects of cold and flu symptoms. There is no strong evidence to support the use of astragalus to support the immune system; however, preliminary evidence supports such benefits. Astragalus is considered safe, but little is known about its side effect profile because it is commonly used as adjunctive therapy. The herb may interact with drugs used to alter immune function, such as cyclosporine. Persons using CAM need to be aware that not all species of astragalus are safe for human consumption; some species contain the neurotoxin swainsonine, and others contain toxic levels of selenium.

Chamomile *(Matricaria recutita and Chamomilla recutita)*

Chamomile is used primarily to treat sleeplessness, anxiety, and stomach or intestinal ailments. Little research has been conducted on chamomile; however, early studies indicate some benefit in the use of chamomile for some skin conditions and oral ulcers secondary to chemotherapy or radiation treatment. Side effects include allergic reaction from mild skin reactions to anaphylaxis. Allergic reactions are more likely to occur in persons who are allergic to ragweed or other members of the daisy family.

Cinnamon *(Cinnamomum zeylanicum and C. cassia)*

Cinnamon has a long history of use as a treatment for bronchitis, gastrointestinal (GI) problems, anorexia, and diabetes. However, little evidence is available to support any of these claims. Although some people have allergic reactions to cinnamon, in general it is usually safe if taken in amounts of no more than 6 g per day. Both species of cinnamon contain coumarin; however, cassia cinnamon contains much larger amounts and may decrease blood clotting.

Echinacea *(Echinacea purpurea)*

Echinacea is commonly used for colds, flu, and infections. It has also been used for skin problems, such as acne. It is thought to stimulate the immune system to fight infection. Research regarding the benefits of echinacea as treatment for cold and flu symptoms is inconclusive. Few side effects are reported by persons taking the herb; the most common are GI effects and allergic reactions, particularly in those who are allergic to ragweed.

Garlic *(Allium sativum)*

Garlic is reported to lower cholesterol, decrease blood pressure, and reduce heart disease. It has also been used to prevent cancer of the stomach and colon. Inconclusive evidence supports the use of this herb as a treatment for elevated cholesterol, hypertension, and heart disease; no evidence supports its use in the prevention of cancer. Garlic has few side effects but may cause heartburn and upset stomach; it has also been associated with body odor. Because it also reduces blood clotting, patients should be advised to notify their health care provider about taking garlic if they are having surgery or dental work. Patients should be cautioned not to take garlic if they have a bleeding disorder or if they are taking the drug saquinavir (a protease inhibitor used in the treatment of human immunodeficiency virus [HIV]). Garlic reduces the effectiveness of saquinavir.

Ginger *(Zingiber officinale)*

Ginger has been used to treat postoperative, pregnancy-related, and chemotherapy-related nausea as well as motion sickness and diarrhea. In addition, it may provide relief from pain, swelling, and stiffness of both osteoarthritis and rheumatoid arthritis. Available research suggests it is effective for the short-term treatment of nausea associated with pregnancy. Evidence is inconclusive concerning its use for motion sickness, as treatment of chemotherapy-induced or postoperative nausea, and in the treatment of arthritis. Side effects of ginger include gas, bloating, heartburn, and nausea.

Ginkgo *(Ginkgo biloba)*

Ginkgo has been used for thousands of years to treat ailments such as asthma, bronchitis, fatigue, and tinnitus. In more recent times, it has been used to improve memory, prevent Alzheimer disease and other dementias, decrease intermittent claudication, and as a treatment for sexual dysfunction and multiple sclerosis. In a study following older adult subjects for an average of 6 years, ginkgo was shown to be ineffective in the prevention of Alzheimer and other dementias. Other studies have shown it to be ineffective in improving memory in older adults. There is conflicting evidence of the benefit of ginkgo for treatment of intermittent claudication and tinnitus. Side effects include headache, nausea, GI upset, dizziness, and allergic reactions that include severe reactions leading to death. In patients taking blood thinners, ginkgo has been shown to increase bleeding risk. Animal studies have shown that rats and mice given ginkgo develop tumors; however, more research is needed to determine whether this is true for humans.

Ginseng *(Panax ginseng)*

Ginseng has been said to boost the immune system, increase a person's sense of well-being, and increase stamina. It has also been used to treat erectile dysfunction, hepatitis C, and menopausal symptoms and to lower glucose and blood pressure. The active component in the herb is thought to be a chemical called *ginsenoside*. Some evidence supports the use of ginseng in the treatment of hypertension and as an immune system booster. Short-term use of the herb appears to be safe; however, long-term use is associated with side effects such as headaches, GI problems, and allergic reactions. There have also been reports of breast tenderness, menstrual irregularities, and high blood pressure, although it is not known whether it is the herb causing these effects or other components. Patients with diabetes should use caution when taking ginseng, especially if used in conjunction with other herbs or drugs, because hypoglycemia may result.

Green Tea *(Camellia sinensis)*

Tea has been used for medicinal purposes for thousands of years. It has been said to improve mental alertness, relieve headaches, protect against heart disease and cancer, and promote weight loss. The topical drug sinecatechins contains extracts of green tea leaves and carries FDA approval as treatment of genital warts. Green tea contains caffeine, which may improve alertness. Studies looking at the protective effects of green tea on heart disease are inconclusive, as are the studies looking at the protective effects of green tea on cancer. Green tea is presumed to be safe in quantities up to eight cups per day; however, drinking more than six cups per day while pregnant or breastfeeding may increase the risk of birth defects. Nursing mothers should be aware the caffeine in green tea passes into breast milk. Liver dysfunction has been reported by persons taking green tea in pill form. Persons with liver disease should not use the product. High doses of green tea reduce the effectiveness of nadolol.

Hawthorn *(Crataegus laevigata* and *C. monogyna)*

Hawthorn has predominantly been used in the treatment of heart disease (e.g., heart failure and angina). It has also been used to treat digestive issues and kidney disease. Although some evidence supports its use in mild heart failure, study results are conflicting. Side effects of hawthorn include nausea, headache, and dizziness. Hawthorn may interact with multiple drugs, including those used for erectile dysfunction (hypotension), nitrates (dizziness and lightheadedness), and antihypertensives (hypotension).

Licorice Root *(Glycyrrhiza glabra* and *G. uralensis)*

Licorice has been used to treat stomach ulcers, bronchitis, sore throat, and viral hepatitis. However, there is not enough research to show the benefit of licorice in the treatment of any condition. In large amounts, licorice can elevate blood pressure, cause salt and water retention, and lower potassium levels. When taken with diuretics, corticosteroids, or other medications that lower potassium, life-threatening hypokalemia may result. People with heart disease or hypertension and those who are pregnant (some data associate licorice with preterm labor) should not take licorice in large amounts.

Kava Kava *(Piper methysticum)*

Kava kava (also referred to as "kava") has been used to aid relaxation and treat anxiety. Research indicates there may be a small benefit in treating anxiety, but flawed research designs have yielded equivocal results. Additionally, the risk of severe liver damage related to ingesting kava outweighs any benefit. Combining kava with alcohol increases the risk for liver damage. Side effects of long-term kava use include dry, scaly, yellowing skin; it is also associated with heart problems and eye irritation.

Milk Thistle *(Silybum marianum)*

Milk thistle has been used widely to treat cirrhosis, chronic hepatitis, and gallbladder disorders. It has also seen use in the treatment of elevated cholesterol and insulin resistance in type 2 diabetes. Although laboratory study has indicated that milk thistle may promote the growth of liver cells and may fight oxidation and inhibit inflammation, two rigorous human studies found no benefit compared with standard therapy and no change in viral activity or inflammation. Milk thistle may cause stomach upset, and in persons allergic to ragweed, milk thistle may trigger an allergic reaction. When combined with drugs for diabetes, milk thistle may lead to hypoglycemia. Nurses should caution patients with diabetes using milk thistle to closely monitor their blood sugars and to watch for symptoms of hypoglycemia.

Peppermint *(Mentha piperita)*

Peppermint has been used to treat a wide variety of ailments, from nausea, indigestion, and irritable bowel syndrome (IBS) to cold symptoms, headaches, and muscle and nerve pain. Some evidence supports the use of peppermint in the treatment of IBS and possibly the use of peppermint oil to relieve indigestion; however, no current evidence supports the use of peppermint to treat other ailments. Side effects include possible allergic reaction and heartburn.

Saw Palmetto *(Serenoa repens)*

Saw palmetto has been used to treat urinary symptoms related to benign prostatic hypertrophy, chronic pelvic pain, decreased libido, migraine, and hair loss. Based on high-quality research and comprehensive reviews of the literature, the evidence does not support the use of saw palmetto for the treatment of any adverse health issue. Side effects include digestive issues and headache. No drug interactions are reported.

St. John's Wort *(Hypericum perforatum)*

St. John's wort has been used extensively throughout history to treat mental disorders and nerve pain. It has also been used as a treatment for malaria, sleep disorders, and wounds. The results of research concerning St. John's wort are mixed; there may be some benefit in patients with mild depression, but it has been reported to be no more effective than placebo in patients with moderate to severe depression. Patients must be cautioned see their health care provider before starting St. John's wort because it interacts with multiple drugs, sometimes in life-threatening ways. Drug interactions include antidepressants (which can lead to serotonin syndrome), birth control pills, cyclosporine, digoxin, indinavir, irinotecan, drugs for seizure control, and anticoagulants. Side effects include sensitivity to sunlight, anxiety, dry mouth, dizziness, GI problems, fatigue, headache, and sexual dysfunction.

Turmeric *(Curcuma longa)*

Turmeric has been used for heartburn, stomach ulcers, gallstones, inflammation, and cancer. However, little research has been conducted on the use of turmeric to treat health conditions. Preliminary research in the laboratory suggests that it may have antiinflammatory, anticancer, and antioxidant properties, but human studies have not been conducted to confirm such properties outside of the laboratory. Turmeric is generally safe, although high doses may cause nausea or diarrhea. Persons with gallbladder disease should avoid the herb because it may worsen their condition.

Valerian *(Valeriana officinalis)*

Valerian has seen wide use in the treatment of insomnia; it has also been used to treat anxiety, headaches, depression, irregular heartbeat, and tremors. Although early research indicates valerian may be useful in the treatment of insomnia, there is not enough evidence to recommend the herb for this treatment. Multiple research studies are in progress, but no available evidence supports the use of valerian for any other medical condition at this time. Valerian is generally safe when used for short periods of time (4–6 weeks). Side effects include fatigue, headaches, dizziness, and stomach upset.

POTENTIAL HAZARDS OF HERBS

> Do not use elderberry or other dietary supplements for prevention or treatment of COVID-19. They have not been shown to be effective.

Consumers and health care providers must be alert to potential hazards with herbal therapy; although herbs are natural substances, *natural* does not mean safe. Patients may not disclose use of herbal products to health care providers for a variety of reasons, including the sense that the health care provider is biased against or not knowledgeable about herbal products or the belief that these products are not considered medications. However, it is essential that health care providers obtain a complete listing of all of the herbal preparations the patient takes in all forms—teas, infusions, tinctures, tablets, and dried herbs—the reason they are taken, and their perceived effectiveness to ensure that they do not interfere with the use and actions of prescribed medications (a 2018 listing of drug-herb interactions can be found at https://www.standardprocess.com/MediHerb-Document-Library/Catalog-Files/herb-drug-interaction-chart.pdf). This assessment should be updated regularly along with information on the patient's OTC and prescription drug use.

Health care providers must be alert for possible herb-drug interactions. For example, Asian ginseng induces the drug-metabolizing enzyme CYP3A; when taken in combination with other CYP3A substrates with a narrow therapeutic index, drug levels and therapeutic response should be monitored carefully. Goldenseal has a high potential for herb-drug interaction because it is a potent inhibitor of both CYP3A4 and CYP2D6. St. John's wort has significant documented interactions with cyclosporine, indinavir, oral contraceptives, warfarin, digoxin, and benzodiazepines, among other drugs; it is also a potent inducer of CYP-450 enzymes and intestinal p-glycoprotein.

Some herbal products can also directly affect laboratory test results. Two Chinese alternative therapies, Danshen and Chan Su, are known to interfere with tests to determine digoxin levels. It is *extremely important* that patients taking digoxin avoid these two products!

Not all compounds are safe via all routes. For example, comfrey has both internal and external preparations. Internal use is discouraged because hepatic damage may be fatal. For external use, comfrey is used as an ointment for relief of swelling associated with abrasions and sprains.

Many products have significance for patients facing surgery because they may interfere with the absorption, breakdown, and excretion of anesthetics, anticoagulants, and other surgery-related medications. The American Society of Anesthesiologists suggests patients discontinue herbal therapy beginning 2 to 3 weeks before surgery.

 COMPLEMENTARY AND ALTERNATIVE THERAPIES

Anticoagulants

The following commonly used herbal products have been reported to interfere with anticoagulants: bilberry, cat's claw, chamomile (German), Dong Quai, feverfew, garlic, ginseng, ginger, ginkgo, licorice, and St. John's wort.

TIPS FOR CONSUMERS AND HEALTH CARE PROVIDERS

The following are guidelines for prudent use of herbs:
- Do not take herbs without talking to your health care provider first if you are taking any prescription drugs.
- Do not take herbal supplements if you are pregnant, attempting to become pregnant, or are nursing.
- Do not give herbs to infants or young children.
- Follow the label instructions!
- If you experience any side effects that concern you, stop taking the herb and contact your health care provider.
- *Natural* does not mean safe!
- Herbal supplements may contain many compounds, and all of the ingredients may not be known; what is on the label may not be what is in the bottle.

HERBAL RESOURCES

It is the responsibility of consumers to educate themselves about herbs before use and to purchase products only from reputable dealers. Determination of the purity and concentration of a particular product can be done only through assays, a costly process; thus most products have not had appropriate human toxicologic analysis. Many herbal resources are available on the Internet and from print sources, and the reader must evaluate each independently and decide whether the information is credible and appropriate.

◎ CLINICAL JUDGMENT [NURSING PROCESS]
Complementary and Alternative Therapies

Concept: Culture
- Patient beliefs and health care practices exhibited by an identified group that are passed down through generations

Concept: Safety
- Protection of patients from potential or actual harm; is a basic human need

Concept: Health, Wellness, and Illness
- A continuum of states that patients may experience throughout life. In the provision of holistic nursing care, it is important that nurses understand both conventional drug therapy and complementary and alternative practices.

Recognize Cues [Assessment]
- Assess for the influence of cultural beliefs, norms, and values in the patient's therapeutic regimen.
- Using culturally sensitive, nonjudgmental, and unbiased questioning, assess the following:
  - Which herbs are being used and how long ago were they started?
  - Why is the herb being used?
  - Who recommended the herb?
  - How often and how much of the herb is being taken?

- Assess use of other prescribed and over-the-counter (OTC) drugs and supplements, and include the reason for and duration of use.
- Assess for potential or actual side effects of any drug, herb, or supplement being used.
- Assess for potential or actual drug-drug, drug-herb, or drug-supplement interactions.
- Assess the patient's readiness to learn and literacy skill.

Analyze Cues and Prioritize Hypothesis [Patient Problems]
- Need for health teaching

Generate Solutions [Planning]
- The patient and family will verbalize understanding of herbal therapy, prescription and OTC drugs, interaction between herbal therapy and prescription and OTC drugs, and strategies for optimal participation in the therapeutic regimen.

Take Action [Nursing Interventions]
- Engage patients in the care planning process; provide information supportive of self-management and mutual goal setting; support patients and family choices.
- Consult a dietitian and other specialists as necessary.

⊚ CLINICAL JUDGMENT [NURSING PROCESS]—CONT'D

Complementary and Alternative Therapies

- Use an individualized, culturally appropriate approach when discussing the therapeutic regimen.
- Use open-ended questions.
- Due to inconsistencies in manufacturing, advise patients to continue with the same brand of herbal therapy, and advise them to notify their health care provider if considering changing brands or preparations.
- Advise patients to first notify their health care provider before substituting any herbal product for a prescription or OTC medication.
- Encourage patients to read labels and heed the recommended information displayed on the label.
- Teach patients about foods that enhance or diminish the action of specific herbs.

- Advise patients about foods to avoid, if any, while taking herbs.
- Advise patients of potential side effects of herbal therapy.
- Counsel patients about symptoms that require prompt reporting to the health care provider.

Evaluate Outcomes [Evaluation]

- Evaluate perceived effectiveness of herbal remedies for alleviating symptoms.
- Evaluate adherence to the therapeutic regimen.
- Evaluate drug-herb interactions or side effects.
- Evaluate the patient's use of resources.

CRITICAL THINKING CASE STUDY

A 55-year-old male is seen in follow-up after being diagnosed with type 2 diabetes. He was prescribed metformin 500 mg twice daily at his last visit. When talking to the patient, he admits he never filled his prescription but took his neighbor's advice instead and began taking cinnamon. He states he Googled the spice and found that it is effective at lowering blood sugar. Upon further questioning, he states he just grabs a spoon from the drawer and uses his wife's baking cinnamon and mixes a heaping spoonful in his morning tea.

1. What additional information is needed before developing a mutually agreed-upon plan of care?
2. What information should the patient be given concerning the use of cinnamon to treat diabetes?

REVIEW QUESTIONS

1. What provisions of the Dietary Supplement Health and Education Act (DSHEA) of 1994 are most important for the nurse to know related to patient health teaching? (Select all that apply.)
   a. Clarified marketing regulations
   b. Reclassified herbs as dietary supplements
   c. Stated that herbal products can be marketed with suggested dosages
   d. Required that package labels give quality and strength of all contents
   e. Stated that herbs can be used as drugs

2. The nurse discovers that a patient has recently decided to take four herbal preparations. Which action will the nurse take first?
   a. Discuss the cost of herbal products.
   b. Instruct the patient to inform the health care provider of all products taken.
   c. Instruct the patient to stop taking all herbal products immediately.
   d. Suggest that the patient taper off use of herbal products over the next 2 weeks.

3. Labeling of herbal products is important. Which is an appropriate claim for an herbal product?
   a. Prevents diabetes
   b. Helps increase blood flow to the extremities
   c. Cures Alzheimer disease
   d. Is safe for all

4. The nurse is reviewing a patient's current drug list. Which herbal products interfere with the action of anticoagulants? (Select all that apply.)
   a. Astragalus
   b. Garlic
   c. Ginger
   d. Licorice root
   e. Ginkgo

5. A patient being seen at a cardiovascular clinic mentions he takes garlic, which is reported to decrease cholesterol, blood pressure, and heart disease. Which patient statements indicate a need for further teaching? (Select all that apply.)
   a. I can just take garlic for my heart problems.
   b. Garlic may provide some decrease in blood pressure.
   c. Garlic is very effective in preventing depression.
   d. Garlic will not cure impotence.
   e. I will need to stop taking my garlic pills before dental work.

6

Pediatric Considerations

OBJECTIVES

- Apply principles of pharmacokinetics and pharmacodynamics to pediatric drug administration.
- Differentiate components of pharmacology unique to pediatric patients.
- Synthesize knowledge about pediatric drug safety and administration with current or potential nursing practice.

OUTLINE

A nurse who is providing care to children must make certain adaptations in assessment, treatment, and evaluation of nursing care because of the physiologic, psychological, and developmental differences inherent in the pediatric population. This is especially true in the science of pharmacology, in both the administration of drugs to children and evaluation of the therapeutic and adverse effects of a drug. This chapter addresses pediatric nursing adaptations and discusses the effect of a child's growth and development on many aspects of pharmacology: pharmacokinetics, pharmacodynamics, dosing and monitoring, methods of drug administration, and nursing implications.

Pediatric pharmacology is limited to available research in the provision of dosing protocols, safe practices, key assessments, and important nursing implications. Most available information about drugs is derived from studies that use adult samples, small sample sizes, or samples with healthy children. Few studies have been conducted to determine the effectiveness of drugs in the pediatric population. Generalizing the results of studies using adult patients to pediatric populations may result in serious errors and ignores the effect of growth and development on pharmacology.

Research related to pediatric patients is limited because of several factors. Research risks and obtaining informed consent make it difficult to recruit a pediatric sample. Parents and guardians are reluctant to provide permission for children to participate in research studies because of the risk involved and the potentially invasive nature of data gathering. Pharmaceutical companies invest fewer resources in pediatric drug research because of the smaller market share afforded to pediatric drugs. However, many contend that lack of pediatric data reflects lack of due diligence, especially when drugs are administered to pediatric patients without supporting research data on which to base safe practices. As a result, less is known about the effects, uses, and dosages of pediatric drugs, and nurses must investigate pediatric drugs carefully to provide knowledgeable nursing care for children.

⚡ PATIENT SAFETY

Preventing Drug Administration Errors in Pediatric Pharmacology

- Owing to developmental factors and smaller body size, infants and young children may receive drug dosages much different from those of adults. Careful calculations, double-checking math, and checking with another registered nurse can prevent errors in drug administration.
- Ensure that families understand the units of measurement for a drug. Confusion may occur with the discussion of metric, household, and other measurement systems.
- For safety when administering injectable drugs to children, use the smallest syringe that ensures the most exact measurement of the drug.
- Use the correct drug and procedure to ensure safe dosing. Dilutions, different concentrations, and different solutions of a prescribed drug can complicate administration of appropriate pediatric dosages.
- Infants and children may not be able to confirm identity, allergies, or drugs. The nurse must be positive of such information before drug administration.
- Nurses must be vigilant for severe side effects or adverse reactions to drugs because information on pediatric drug response is limited.
- Regulatory agencies caution that drug administration errors are more common in pediatric patients, which warrants increased precautions in drug administration.

Closely aligned with the conflicts that affect pediatric pharmacologic research are those associated with drug labeling and dosing instructions. Because many drugs have not undergone the clinical trials required for federal approval, they have not been approved for pediatric use. Safe use for children may be guided by small studies or the judgment of the clinician and may be based on anecdotal evidence rather than scientific study. These conflicts have generated new legislation designed to protect pediatric patients and provide health care professionals with better information and resources.

Despite the permanent reauthorization of the Pediatric Research Equity Act (PREA) in 2012, which requires drug manufacturers to study pediatric drug use and offers incentives for pediatric pharmacology research, only half of all drugs carry federally approved indications for use in children. This means many drugs prescribed for children are being prescribed off-label, which means the drug is being used for some purpose for which it has not been approved. Current research agendas reinforce the need for pediatric drug research and establishment of safe guidelines for pediatric drug dosing, administration, and evaluation.

PHARMACOKINETICS

Significant differences exist in drug pharmacokinetics for pediatric patients versus adults. These distinctions stem from differences in body composition and organ maturity and appear to be more pronounced in neonates and infants but less significant in school-age and adolescent children. Pharmacokinetics may be defined as the study of the time course of drug absorption, distribution, metabolism, and excretion.

Absorption

The degree and rate of drug absorption are based on factors such as age (Table 6.1), health status, weight, and route of administration. As children grow and develop, the absorption of drugs generally becomes more effective; therefore less developed absorption in neonates and infants must be considered in dosage and administration. In contrast, poor nutritional habits, changes in physical maturity, and hormonal differences during the adolescent years may cause slowing of drug absorption. Hydration status, presence of underlying disease, and gastrointestinal (GI) disorders in the child may be significant factors in the absorption of drugs.

Drug absorption is initially influenced by the route of administration. For oral drugs, conditions in the stomach and intestine such as gastric acidity, gastric emptying, gastric motility, GI surface area, enzyme levels, and intestinal flora all mediate drug absorption. Lack of maturation of the GI tract is most pronounced in infancy, making the neonatal and infancy periods those most affected by changes in absorption physiology. Gastric pH is alkaline at birth; acid production begins in the neonatal period, and gastric acid secretion reaches adult levels around 2 to 3 years of age. A low pH, or acidic environment, favors acidic drug absorption, whereas a high pH, or alkaline environment, favors basic drug formulations; therefore differences in pH may hinder or enhance drug absorption. Gastric emptying and GI motility are unpredictable in neonates and infants; however, it approaches that of adults between 6 and 8 months of age. Gastric emptying is affected by feeding, and breastfed infants have faster gastric emptying than formula-fed infants. Unpredictable GI motility may hinder or enhance absorption of oral drugs, depending on the usual site of chemical absorption.

TABLE 6.1	Pediatric Age Classification
Classification	**Age**
Term neonate	Birth at 38 or more weeks' gestation to 27 days
Infant/toddler	28 days to 23 months
Children	24 months to 11 years
Adolescent	12 years to 16 or 18 years (regional difference)

From US Food and Drug Administration. (2014). Pediatric exclusivity study age group (C-DRG-00909). Retrieved from http://www.fda.gov/Drugs/DevelopmentApprovalProcess/FormsSubmissionRequirements/ElectronicSubmissions/DataStandardsManualmonographs/ucm071754.htm.

Intestinal surface area in neonates does not reach that of adults until 20 weeks; before this, the reduced surface area leads to reduced drug absorption. Immature enzyme function may also affect drug absorption; neonates have inadequate production of bile salts and pancreatic enzymes, which leads to reduced absorption of lipid-soluble drugs. Intestinal microbial colonization begins in the first few hours after birth and is influenced by gestational age and whether the neonate is breast- or formula-fed; GI microbial colonization reaches adult levels in adolescence. All of these factors must be considered when assessing the effectiveness of drugs administered by the oral route.

For drugs administered via the subcutaneous (subcut) or intramuscular (IM) routes, absorption occurs at the tissue level. The level of peripheral perfusion and effectiveness of circulation affects drug absorption. Conditions that alter perfusion—dehydration, cold temperatures, and alterations in cardiac status—may impede absorption of drugs in the tissues. Intravenous (IV) drugs are administered directly into the bloodstream and are immediately absorbed and distributed.

The skin of infants and young children is thinner than that of adults; additionally, the ratio of body surface area to body mass of infants and children is proportionately higher than for adults such that many drugs are more readily absorbed in children, and toxicity may result.

Distribution

Drug distribution is affected by factors such as body fluid composition, body tissue composition, protein-binding capability, and effectiveness of various barriers to drug transport. In neonates and infants, the body is about 75% water, compared with 60% in adults. This increased body fluid proportion allows for a greater volume of fluid in which to distribute drugs, which results in a lower drug concentration. Until about age 2 years, the pediatric patient requires higher doses of water-soluble drugs to achieve therapeutic levels. Younger patients also have higher levels of extracellular fluids, which increase the tendency for children to become dehydrated and changes the distribution of water-soluble drugs. Compared with older children, neonates and infants have fat stores with an increased ratio of water to lipids, which alters the distribution of some lipid-soluble drugs. Close monitoring of drug levels (e.g., antiepileptic drugs) can help ensure drug safety.

To varying degrees, drugs become bound to circulating plasma proteins in the body. Only drugs that are free, or unbound, are available to cross the cell membrane and exert their effect. Neonates and infants have decreased protein concentrations compared with adults, and they have fewer protein receptor sites with an affinity for drug binding in the first 12 months after birth; this results in higher levels of unbound drug and an increased risk of drug toxicity.

In neonates, high bilirubin levels may pose a health risk related to drug administration. Bilirubin molecules may bind with protein receptor sites, which makes the sites unavailable to drugs or displaces drugs from binding sites, allowing large amounts of drug to remain free and available for effect. When drugs are prescribed to neonates, dosages must be decreased and closely monitored to both avoid adverse effects and ensure therapeutic effectiveness.

Anatomic barriers to drug distribution, such as the blood-brain barrier (BBB), must be considered when drugs are administered to pediatric patients. This barrier in neonates is relatively immature and allows drugs to pass easily into central nervous system (CNS) tissue, thereby increasing the likelihood for toxicity. As a child matures, the BBB becomes more impervious to drugs, and drug dosages must be titrated accordingly.

Metabolism

The metabolism of drugs depends greatly on the maturation level of the pediatric patient and varies from child to child. Metabolism is carried out primarily in the liver, with the kidneys and lungs playing a small part in metabolism. Infants have reduced hepatic blood flow and drug-metabolizing enzymes; however, by the time they reach 1 year of age, hepatic blood flow has reached that of an adult. Although drug-metabolizing enzymes reach an adult level at around 11 years of age, it is important to understand that the isoenzymes involved in the cytochrome P450 system—CYP1, CYP2, and CYP3—develop at different rates and demonstrate individual variation. Drug prescribing should be based on therapeutic effect and drug concentration. Such differences in drug metabolism, as with other pharmacokinetic factors, reinforce the importance of the nurse evaluating therapeutic effects and monitoring the adverse effects of drugs.

Excretion

Renal excretion is the predominant means of drug elimination. The glomerular filtration rate (GFR) in term neonates is roughly 30% that of adults. During infancy, the GFR rises, and by 12 months it reaches adult levels. Nurses must carefully monitor renal function, urine flow, and drug effectiveness to evaluate the effect of drug administration on patient status.

PHARMACODYNAMICS

Pharmacodynamics refers to the mechanisms of action and effects of a drug on the body and includes the onset, peak, and duration of effect of a drug. It can also be described as the intensity and time course of therapeutic and adverse effects of drugs. The variables of pharmacokinetics—absorption, distribution, metabolism, and excretion—all affect the parameters of pharmacodynamics. These processes determine the time a drug begins to function, reaches its peak, and sustains its length of action. Variables such as organ function, developmental factors, and administration issues affect drug pharmacodynamics and drug half-life in pediatric patients, and these have an effect on drug dosing.

NURSING IMPLICATIONS

Pediatric Drug Dosing and Monitoring

Because of the changes in pharmacokinetics and pharmacodynamics inherent in pediatric patients, a key nursing role is to monitor the patient for therapeutic effect and adverse reactions. The processes described earlier in the chapter may be measured using plasma or serum drug levels, which indicate the amount of drug in a patient's body. The therapeutic ranges established for many drug levels are based on adult studies; therefore close monitoring of serum drug levels can assist in establishing appropriate dosages, schedules, and routes of administration. Monitoring can also assist in indicating when the dose is subtherapeutic or becomes toxic. Serum blood levels are not available for all drugs, so patient clinical responses to drugs are especially important when monitoring drug effects.

The calculation of pediatric dosages is based in part on US Food and Drug Administration (FDA) recommendations; as a result of the Best Pharmaceuticals for Children Act (BPCA) and PREA, pediatric dosing is now available for more than 450 drugs. For those drugs without pediatric dosing schedules, dosing is based on approved protocols, research studies, and provider experience. Drugs for pediatric patients are ordered based on either the child's weight in kilograms (mg/kg) or body surface area (BSA; or mg/m²). Body surface is based on a percentage of adult surface area (1.73 m²). Dosing must also consider the individual child's status, including age, organ function, health, and route of administration.

Pediatric Drug Administration

Developmental and cognitive differences must always be considered in pediatric drug administration. It is important for the nurse to differentiate the child's developmental age from chronologic age, because this difference has an effect on the child's response to drug administration. The pediatric patient's ability to understand the process, the reason for drug administration, and the need to cooperate with the procedure must always figure prominently in the nurse's plan of care. The child's temperament may influence understanding and level of cooperation. The concept of family-centered care is essential to ensuring safety during and after health care interventions, especially drug administration. Teaching is directed toward both family members or caregivers and patients, commensurate with the cognitive level of the child. When possible, family members or caregivers should be solicited to assist in drug administration. These significant persons in the child's life, individuals who see the child on a day-to-day basis, are usually in the best position to evaluate the effectiveness of a drug and observe for adverse reactions. Some adverse drug reactions in children, such as ringing in the ears and nausea, may be difficult to evaluate; those closest to the child may be in the best position to assess for these reactions. However, family members or caregivers may request not to participate in invasive procedures such as injections. This request should be respected, and family members or caregivers should be encouraged to provide comfort to the child after drugs are administered. Family members or caregivers should always be supported in their caring function so that the child feels safe and secure.

Pediatric patients must be assessed for the ability to understand the reason for the drug, the need for the drug despite unpleasant taste or method of administration, and the need to complete all doses and courses of the drug. When the family is taught about pediatric drug administration, education for the child at a developmentally appropriate level must also be included. Communication with the child and family members or caregivers must always consider level of knowledge, developmental age, cultural factors, and anxiety levels. The nurse should use optimal interpersonal skills to ensure the best outcome in drug administration to pediatric patients.

The primary concerns in drug administration to infants are maintaining safety and providing care while ensuring as much comfort as possible. Family members or caregivers must be able to practice and repeat the psychomotor skills associated with drug administration. The following are tips to enhance safe drug administration and facilitate comfort:

- Toddlers may react violently and negatively to drug administration. Simple explanations, a firm approach, and enlisting the imagination of a toddler through play may enhance success.
- Preschoolers are fairly cooperative and respond well to age-appropriate explanations. Allowing some level of choice and control may facilitate success with preschool children.
- School-age children, although often cooperative, may fear bodily injury and should be permitted even more control, involvement in the process, and information.
- Age-appropriate fears related to pain, changes in body image, and injury are prevalent among older school-age and adolescent patients. The nurse should establish a positive rapport with the patient, develop the plan of care in collaboration with the patient, and ensure privacy in all aspects of drug administration.

Atraumatic care principles should be used when possible. Donna Wong's Principle of Atraumatic Care is the philosophy of providing therapeutic care through the use of interventions that eliminate or minimize the psychological and physical distress experienced by children and families. Atraumatic care is achieved by decreasing the separation of children from their family members or caregivers, identifying family and patient stressors, decreasing pain, and providing care within the framework of a collaborative partnership.

Most pediatric drugs are administered via the oral route (Table 6.2). This route is the least invasive and easiest to use and can be used by

TABLE 6.2 Dosage Form Variability for Pediatric Age Groups

Age	Dosage Form
Neonates: 0–4 weeks	Indication dependent
Infants: 1 month–2 years	Liquids—small volumes (syrups, solutions)
Children: 2–5 years	Liquids; effervescent tablets dispersed in liquids; sprinkles on food
Children: 6–11 years	Solids (chewable tablets, orally disintegrating tablets, oral films)
Adolescents: 12–18 years	Solids (typical adult dosage forms—tablets, capsules)

From Federal Drug Administration (FDA), Pinto, J. C. (n.d.). Pediatric formulation development: A quality perspective. Retrieved from https://cersi.umd.edu/sites/cersi.umd.edu/files/Pediatric%20Fomrulations%20-%20Clinical%20Investigators%20Workshop%20Julia%20 Pintov2.pptx.

family members or caregivers. Topical, rectal, and parenteral routes are also used to deliver drugs to pediatric patients for whom the oral route is contraindicated. Because of tissue differences among children, the IV route is more predictable than other routes.

Most oral drugs administered to children under 6 years of age are given using an oral syringe. Oral syringes ensure more exact dosing and are relatively easy to use. Syringes may be marked to ensure correct dosages. The syringe is inserted into either side of the mouth and is pointed toward the buccal mucosa. Depositing the drug too close to the front of the mouth increases the likelihood that it will be spit out. Pointing the syringe directly toward the back of the mouth may increase the risk for gagging or choking. Infants may suck drugs from a bottle nipple into which the measured drug has been squirted from an oral syringe. Preschool and school-age children are usually able to inject oral drugs into their own mouths, enhancing their sense of control over what can be an anxiety-provoking situation.

Nurses may need to crush pills or dissolve the contents of capsules in fluid for administration to pediatric patients. The nurse should work closely with the pharmacist and in compliance with hospital policies to determine the advisability of crushing or dissolving a drug before administration; some drugs, particularly timed-release and enteric-coated drugs, should *not* be crushed or dissolved. Some drugs may be made more palatable by adding jam, yogurt, or honey (although infants younger than 1 year should not be given honey because of the risk of botulism). Small volumes (10 mL) should be used to dilute drugs so the patient is ensured the full dose. For children who require tube feeding, oral drugs can be administered via nasogastric, orogastric, or gastrostomy tubes, if the drugs can be crushed or dissolved before administration.

When drug injection or venipuncture is necessary, topical anesthetic protocols may be followed to reduce the pain associated with the procedure. Agents such as eutectic mixture of local anesthetics (EMLA), topical liposomal 4% lidocaine cream (LMX4), or a vapocoolant spray may be effective in reducing the pain and fear associated with invasive procedures, such as injection or venipuncture, in children.

Based on the cognitive level of the child, other nonpharmacologic methods of pain and anxiety control such as distraction, diversion, relaxation, and creative imagery can also be used to decrease the perception of pain. Injections should *never* be given to a sleeping child with the intent to surprise the child with a quick procedure. The child may subsequently experience a lack of trust and may be reluctant to sleep in the future.

IV infusion sites must be protected, especially in infants and toddlers, who do not understand the rationale or importance of maintaining the IV site. Commercial products are available to protect the IV site and maintain an intact IV infusion set. Stocking-like covers may hide the IV site from infants before they master the concept of object permanence. The patency of an IV site should be checked before each drug administration to avoid infiltration and extravasation. Any injection site on a preschooler should be covered with a bandage, preferably a decorated one, so that the child does not fear "leakage" from the area. Selection of injection and IV sites is made based on developmental variables, site of preference, and access to administration sites. The ventrogluteal or vastus lateralis are preferred sites for pediatric IM injections. The length of the needle depends on the child's muscle mass, subcutaneous tissue, and the site of injection. Children may prefer subcutaneous injections in the leg or upper arm rather than in the abdomen. IV sites may be difficult to find in children. The amount of fatty tissue, hydration status of the child, and ability to isolate and immobilize veins are all mitigating factors.

When administering drugs to children, follow these basic principles: honesty, respect, age-appropriate teaching and explanations, attention to safety, atraumatic care, use of the least amount of restraint necessary (e.g., swaddling a neonate), providing positive reinforcement for age-appropriate cooperation, refraining from use of negative messages or behaviors, and upholding family-centered principles. These standards may be used throughout the pediatric life span and highlight the need for nursing interventions that are sensitive, individualized, and caring.

CONSIDERATIONS FOR THE ADOLESCENT PATIENT

Adolescent patients need individualized nursing care specific to their developmental stage. Age-oriented developmental considerations include physical changes, cognitive level and abilities, emotional factors, and effect of chronic illness.

Physically, adolescence is a highly diverse period of growth and development. Growth rates during these years may be affected by nutrition, factors within the environment, genetics and heredity, and sex. A group of adolescents of similar ages may manifest very different sizes, height-to-weight proportions, timing of secondary sex characteristics, and other indicators of physical maturity. These differences may warrant individualization of drug dosage based on weight or body surface area, even when the adolescent meets or exceeds the size of standard adults. For example, an adjustment may be required in the dosage of a lipid-soluble drug because of the changes in lean-to-fat body mass, especially in young adolescent males, which coincide with physical maturation. Hormonal changes and growth spurts may necessitate changes in drug dosages; many children with chronic illnesses require dosage adjustments in the early teen years as a result of these transitions. Sleep requirements and metabolic rates may greatly increase during the teen years, along with appetite and food consumption, which may affect the scheduling of and response to drugs. Although adolescents' physical appearance and organ structure and function resemble those of adults, their bodies continue to grow and change; this requires increased vigilance in monitoring therapeutic and toxic drug levels.

The cognitive level and abilities of adolescents may pose additional considerations. Cognitive theorists have posited that adolescents progress from concrete to abstract reasoning. Individuals who are still in the concrete operational stage may have difficulty comprehending how a drug exerts its effects on the body and the importance of meticulous dosing and administration. Adolescents may also have difficulty understanding such concepts as drug interactions, side effects, adverse reactions, and therapeutic levels. For example, the patient taking birth control pills may or may not be able to comprehend the reduced action of birth control pills caused by antibiotics taken during an acute infection and may fail to take extra precautions to prevent pregnancy.

An understanding of the adolescent brain and the ongoing development of social, reasoning, and decision-making skills can be used to guide nursing assessment and interventions with the pediatric patient. As adolescents learn to reason in an abstract manner, teaching may be based on more complex information. Potentially, adolescent perception of invulnerability and difficulty relating future consequences to current actions may dictate that the nurse adapt teaching to address specific adolescent thought processes. An adolescent who is told that an insulin injection schedule must be followed to avoid long-term complications may not understand the rationale for treatment if it is only substantiated by abstract, future-oriented risks. The same patient may find the relationship between using insulin to maintain normoglycemia and the ability to participate in sports more immediate and relevant. Allowing the adolescent to verbalize concerns about the drug and its regimen may offer opportunities for clarifying misconceptions and teaching new concepts.

Emotional development of the adolescent also occurs on an individual basis. The adolescent years are characterized by sensation seeking, risk taking, questioning, formation of identity, and increasing influences exerted by peer groups. To avoid potential drug interactions, the nurse should assess for high-risk behaviors that include use of alcohol, tobacco, and recreational drugs. Other issues, including sexual practices and stressful family and social situations, may affect the patient's response to drugs. Nurses must be respectful of the emotional needs of adolescents while attending to the mental health issues that may surface during these years. A comprehensive history must be solicited from adolescent patients to ensure appropriate drug administration. The nurse must also be conscious of the need to exercise care in offering confidentiality in the event that information needs to be divulged to other health care providers, family members, or caregivers to ensure patient safety.

As adolescents attain greater levels of independence from their parents, self-care behaviors increase. The nurse should assess the patient's abilities to self-administer drugs and monitor therapeutic and adverse reactions. Adolescents spend less time with family members and caregivers and may need increased instruction about their drug regimen and the key observations that are needed. Although adolescents frequently display "breaking away" behaviors in response to parental bonds, they often continue to use family members or caregiver drug habits as models for their own drug behaviors.

For the pediatric patient with a chronic illness, issues may change during adolescence. Engaging peers in the plan of care for drug administration, allowing the adolescent to make safe choices and have flexibility within that plan, setting up mutual drug contracts, and permitting the patient to design his or her own adult-monitored drug regimen may facilitate adherence. The nurse can facilitate required adaptations and support both the patient and family members during these times.

FAMILY-CENTERED COLLABORATIVE CARE

In working with pediatric patients, key developmental differences must be considered when administering and monitoring drugs. The nursing process provides the framework to guide nursing practice in administering drugs, planning and evaluating nursing care, providing patient and family teaching, and incorporating the family in all aspects of treatment.

Family and patient teaching is a key role for the nurse. Issues such as indications for the drug, the side effects, the dose, how to measure the dose, how to administer the dose, the therapeutic effect, adverse effects to monitor for, the duration, and the frequency are all important information needed by the family or caregiver. Specifics such as the need for refrigeration, the need to shake the medicine, the difference between household and prescriptive measurements, and other issues should be addressed to ensure patient safety. Adherence to the drug regimen is of paramount importance with children and families; providing written instructions or a drug calendar may facilitate this through concrete reminders.

Nurses should also be aware of the tendency for parents to treat infants and children with over-the-counter (OTC) analgesics. Parents may provide frequent analgesia to their children and may be largely unaware of the potential for misuse and overuse in the pediatric population. Additional concern has arisen regarding the inappropriate use of OTC cough and cold remedies with children. Deaths and significant illness have been attributed to lack of label recommendations, misuse of adult drugs, poor drug instructions, and overdose, which warrants rigid restrictions on the use of these drugs in the pediatric population.

◎ CLINICAL JUDGMENT [NURSING PROCESS]

Pediatrics

Concept: Safety
- Protection of the patient from potential or actual harm; is a basic human need

Concept: Health, Wellness, and Illness
- Health, wellness, and illness are a dynamic response to a continuum of biopsychosocial states experienced through all stages of life.

Concept: Illness
- Illness is an abnormal process where function is altered in comparison to previous status.

Recognize Cues [Assessment]
- Assess the context and meaning of illness.
- Assess the influence of cultural beliefs and values on the knowledge base.
- Assess developmental age, health status, nutritional status, and hydration status.
- Assess family member and caregiver health literacy level and the child's cognitive level.
- Assess family patterns, economic issues, and cultural patterns that influence adherence to a therapeutic regimen.

- Assess learning style.
- Assess readiness to learn.
- Assess the allergy history of the child and determine family allergy history.
- Identify all of the patient's drugs (prescriptions, over-the-counter [OTC], and herbal).
- Record the age, weight, and height of the child. Drug calculations are based on these three factors.

Analyze Cues and Prioritize Hypothesis [Patient Problems]
- Need for health teaching
- Anxiety

Generate Solutions [Planning]
- Family members and caregivers, as well as the pediatric patient if appropriate, will recognize the need for drug administration.
- Family members and caregivers, as well as the pediatric patient if appropriate, will describe the rationale for drug therapy.
- Family members and caregivers, as well as the pediatric patient if appropriate, will incorporate the drug treatment regimen into their lifestyle.

◎ CLINICAL JUDGMENT [NURSING PROCESS]—CONT'D

Pediatrics

- Family members and caregivers, as well as the pediatric patient if appropriate, will demonstrate safe drug administration practices.
- Family members and caregivers, as well as the pediatric patient if appropriate, will state with confidence their ability to manage the treatment regimen and remain in control of their life.
- The pediatric patient will remain free of drug-related injuries.

Take Action [Nursing Interventions]

- Assist the patient, family members, and caregivers with appropriate follow-up resources and support.
- Avoid the use of restraints.
- Engage the patient, family members, and caregivers as partners in the educational process.
- Follow all rights of safe drug administration.
- Help patients, their family members, and caregivers manage complex drug schedules.
- Reconcile the drug list at discharge and provide the list to the patient, family members, and caregivers as appropriate.
- Support patient, family member, and caregiver priorities, preferences, and choices.
- Use at least two methods of patient identification.

- Use open-ended questions and encourage two-way communication.
- Consider the use of alternative settings for teaching the chronically ill pediatric patient, his or her family members, and caregivers.
- Provide a developmentally appropriate environment when addressing the health education needs of adolescents.
- Provide educational materials in the preferred language of patients, family members, and caregivers.
- Provide information to support self-efficacy, self-regulation, and self-management of the drug regimen.
- Use educational strategies that are interactive and engaging for younger children and toddlers.
- Use family-centered approaches when teaching children and adolescents.
- Use strategies to promote motivation and sustain learning.

Evaluate Outcomes [Evaluation]

- Evaluate the child's physiologic and psychological response to the drug regimen.
- Evaluate the family member's knowledge about the drug, the dosage, the schedule for administration, and the side effects.
- Evaluate the therapeutic and adverse effects of the drug(s).

▌ CRITICAL THINKING CASE STUDY

A 9-month-old infant weighing 20 pounds comes to the emergency department with a 3-day history of vomiting, fever greater than 102.5°F, and significant pain. Physical assessment reveals acute otitis media, for which the health care provider prescribed amoxicillin susp 400 mg twice a day for 10 days and ibuprofen 2.5 mL every 6 hours.

1. Which nursing assessments must take place before administration of amoxicillin?
2. How will the nurse instruct the family member administer the drugs safely?

▌ REVIEW QUESTIONS

1. A 4-year-old patient is discharged on an oral liquid drug suspension of 4 mL per dose. Which device will the nurse recommend to ensure the highest level of accuracy in home administration of the drug?
   a. Measuring spoon
   b. Graduated medicine cup
   c. Household teaspoon
   d. Oral syringe
2. The nurse understands the differences between drug excretion in children and that in adults. With this knowledge, what does the nurse consider when administering drugs to children?
   a. Most children need a higher dose of drug, so the nurse will contact the physician for an increase in the ordered dose.
   b. Children excrete drugs rapidly, so the nurse must assess carefully for therapeutic effects of the drug.
   c. The most important assessment is to evaluate for drug accumulation, because the excretion of drugs is slower in children.
   d. Excretion of most drugs is the same in children as in adults, but assessments are important to avoid side effects.
3. A parent is learning to administer drug to a school-age child. Which strategy will the nurse teach the parent to achieve cooperation in a child of this age?
   a. Enlisting physical restraint
   b. Establishing drug contracts
   c. Providing age-appropriate explanations
   d. Tolerating violent reactions

4. A nurse caring for a child with developmental delay prepares to teach the patient about prescribed drugs. Which actions are essential to ensure patient safety? (Select all that apply.)
   a. Assess the child's developmental age.
   b. Assess for side effects the same as those experienced by adults.
   c. Consider the actions and uses of the drug.
   d. Focus on the child's chronologic age.
   e. Involve the family in teaching sessions.
5. The Principle of Atraumatic Care includes: (Select all that apply.)
   a. Reducing any pain associated with drug administration.
   b. Development of a collaborative partnership with the family during drug administration.
   c. Restraining infants during drug administration.
   d. Keeping the child apart from family members when administering drugs.
   e. Reducing the child's stress during drug administration.
6. Which of the following strategies are helpful when working with adolescent patients to promote adherence? (Select all that apply.)
   a. Allow flexibility in the treatment plan.
   b. Use future-oriented examples and consequences to support the need for drug therapy.
   c. Guarantee the adolescent patient privacy when obtaining history.
   d. Set up a mutually developed drug contract.
   e. Understanding the adolescent's sexual practices is not necessary to promote adherence.

7

Drug Therapy in Older Adults

http://evolve.elsevier.com/McCuistion/pharmacology

OBJECTIVES

- Explain how the physiologic changes associated with aging affect drug therapy.
- Describe two ways the Beers criteria can be used to improve the care of older adults.
- Discuss issues that affect older adults' adherence to therapeutic regimens.
- Describe nursing implications related to drug therapy in the older adult.

OUTLINE

By 2030, all of the baby boomers will be older than 65. By 2034, adults over the age of 65 will outnumber those under 18. There are expected to be more than 94.7 million older adults by the year 2060, with 19 million over 85 years of age. These numbers are staggering, more so considering 92% of older adults have at least one chronic illness, and more than 75% of older adults have two chronic illnesses. Typically, persons with two or more chronic conditions take five or more prescription drugs.

More than half of all older adults use at least one over-the-counter (OTC) drug, and nearly three-quarters of older adults use at least one supplement to augment their prescription drugs; however, older adults are more likely to experience adverse reactions or drug interactions related to OTC drugs and supplements, many times resulting in hospitalization.

Administration of drugs in the older adult population requires special attention to age-related factors that influence drug absorption, distribution, metabolism, and excretion. Drug dosages are often adjusted according to the older adult's weight, laboratory results (e.g., liver enzymes and glomerular filtration), and comorbid health problems. Because of altered organ function in the older adult, the effects of drug therapy must be closely monitored to prevent adverse reactions and possible toxicity.

Drug toxicity may develop in the older adult for drug doses within the therapeutic range for the younger adult. These therapeutic drug ranges are usually safe for young and middle-aged adults but are not always within the safe range for older adults. It has been suggested that drugs for older adults should initially be prescribed at low dosages with a gradual increase in dosage based on therapeutic response; this practice is commonly stated as *start low and go slow*. This approach to drug prescribing reduces the chance of drug toxicity.

Common characteristics in older adults that increase the risk for problems with drug administration include lack of coordinated care, recent discharge from the hospital, self-treatment, multiple diagnoses, sensory and physical changes associated with aging, multiple health care providers, and cognitive impairment.

PHYSIOLOGIC CHANGES

Physiologic changes associated with aging can influence absorption, distribution, metabolism, and excretion of drugs as well as pharmacodynamic responses at receptors and target organs. These physiologic changes include the following:

- A reduction in total body water and lean body mass, resulting in increased body fat, which alters the volume of distribution of drugs
- A reduction in kidney mass and lower kidney blood flow, leading to a reduced glomerular filtration rate (GFR) and reduced clearance of drugs excreted by the kidneys
- A reduction in liver size and blood flow, resulting in reduced hepatic clearance of drugs

A decline in the physiologic processes that maintain equilibrium in the older adult may mean a higher incidence of adverse effects. Examples of this include:

- Postural hypotension in response to drugs that reduce blood pressure
- Volume depletion and electrolyte imbalance in response to diuretics
- Excessive bleeding with anticoagulant and antiplatelet drugs
- Altered glycemic response to antidiabetic drugs

- Gastrointestinal (GI) irritation with nonsteroidal antiinflammatory drugs (NSAIDs)

Physiologic changes with aging affect the determination of risk versus benefit underlying drug choice, dose, and frequency.

PHARMACOKINETICS

Pharmacologic processes have not received adequate study in the older adult; therefore a thorough understanding of pharmacokinetics is necessary for the safe administration of drugs in this population.

Absorption

Adults experience several GI changes with aging that may influence drug absorption. These include a decrease in small bowel surface area, slowed gastric emptying, reduced gastric blood flow, and a 5% to 10% decrease in gastric acid production. These changes are not always clinically relevant; however, calcium carbonate is affected by the decreased gastric acidity. Older adults should be prescribed calcium citrate, which requires a less acidic environment for dissolution. Other common problems that occur in older adults that can significantly influence drug absorption include swallowing difficulties, poor nutrition, and dependence on feeding tubes.

Distribution

Aging can significantly alter drug distribution. With aging, adults experience a decline in muscle mass and a 20% to 40% increase in fat. The increase in body fat means lipid-soluble drugs have a greater volume of distribution, increased drug storage, reduced elimination, and a prolonged period of action. Older adults have a 10% to 15% reduction in total body water, which affects water-soluble drugs, and a 10% reduction in albumin. Reduced albumin levels can result in decreased protein binding of drugs and increased free drug available to exert therapeutic effects, but it also increases the risk for drug toxicity.

Metabolism

Hepatic blood flow in the older adult may be decreased by 40%; aging also results in a 15% to 30% decrease in liver size and a reduction in cytochrome P450 (CYP450) enzyme activity, which is responsible for the breakdown of drugs. Drug clearance by hepatic metabolism can be reduced by these age-related changes. A reduction in hepatic metabolism can decrease first-pass metabolism and can prolong drug half-life, resulting in increased drug levels and potential drug toxicity. Nurses must be aware of these metabolic changes and must monitor response to drug therapy to avoid adverse reactions.

To assess liver function, liver enzymes must be checked. Elevated levels of alanine aminotransferase (ALT) and aspartate aminotransferase (AST) may indicate possible liver dysfunction. However, an older adult can have normal liver function test (LFT) results and still have impaired hepatic enzyme activity.

Excretion

Renal excretion of drugs decreases with age. Excretion is altered by age-related changes in kidney function, such as decreased renal size and volume, which differ for each individual. However, it is generally accepted that the GFR declines by 1 mL/min after 40 years of age (normal GFR is 100–125 mL/min). Despite a decline in kidney function, an individual's creatinine may remain normal as he or she ages due to a decline in muscle mass and activity. Changes in kidney function affect many drugs, leading to a prolonged half-life and elevated drug levels. Changes in kidney function require dosage adjustment, especially if the drug has a narrow therapeutic range.

GFR can be calculated using the Cockcroft-Gault formula, which is the formula recommended by the US Food and Drug Administration (FDA) and therefore used by pharmaceutical manufacturers when determining dosage adjustments:

$$C_{Cr} = [(140 - Age) \times Weight / (72 \times S_{Cr}) \times 0.85 \text{ (If female)}]$$

where:

C_{Cr} (creatinine clearance) = mL/min
Age = years
Weight = kg
S_{Cr} (serum creatinine) = mg/dL

However, it can also be estimated by many calculators found on the Internet (www.globalrph.com/crcl.htm).

Nurses must have a general understanding of drug classifications that require dosage adjustment in patients with chronic kidney disease (CKD). The mnemonic *BANDD CAMP* (Table 7.1) may be helpful in

TABLE 7.1 Drug Classes That Require Dosage Adjustment in Chronic Kidney Disease

	Drug Class	Adjust Dose	Avoid in Stages 4 and 5
B	Beta blockers	Acebutolol, atenolol, bisoprolol, nadolol, sotalol	Sotalol
A	ACEIs/ARBs	All ACEIs	Olmesartan
N	NSAIDs, opioids	Codeine, morphine, oxycodone, tramadol	All NSAIDs, meperidine
D	Diuretics	Potassium-sparing diuretics, thiazide diuretics	Potassium-sparing diuretics, thiazide diuretics
D	Diabetic medications	Gliclazide, acarbose, insulin, gliptins	Glyburide, metformin, exenatide
C	Cholesterol medications	Pravastatin, rosuvastatin, fibrates	—
A	Antimicrobials (dose reductions are often delayed for 24–48 h to allow for aggressive dosing and for the drug to reach steady state)	Antibiotics: Most antibiotics except cloxacillin, clindamycin, metronidazole, erythromycin, azithromycin Antifungals: Fluconazole, itraconazole Antivirals: Acyclovir, famciclovir, valacyclovir	Nitrofurantoin
M	Miscellaneous	Allopurinol, colchicine, digoxin, H$_2$RAs	New anticoagulants
P	Psychotropics	Lithium, gabapentin, pregabalin, topiramate, vigabatrin, bupropion, duloxetine, paroxetine, venlafaxine	—

ACEI, Angiotensin-converting enzyme inhibitor; *ARB*, angiotensin II receptor blocker; *h*, hours; *H$_2$RA*, histamine-2 receptor antagonist; *NSAID*, nonsteroidal antiinflammatory drug.
From Meyer, D., Damm, T., & Jensen, K. (2012). *Drug dosage adjustments in chronic kidney disease: The pharmacist's role*. Saskatchewan Drug Information Services College of Pharmacy and Nutrition, University of Saskatchewan. Retrieved from www.rxfiles.ca/rxfiles/uploads/documents/ltc/HCPs/CKD/SDIS.Renal_newsletter.pdf

remembering the drug classifications; however, nurses should not rely on their memory for drug administration. Package inserts, up-to-date drug reference books, and reputable websites (www.globalrph.com/index_renal.htm) maintain current dosing information.

PHARMACODYNAMICS

Pharmacodynamic responses to drugs are altered with aging as a result of changes in the number of receptor sites, which affects the affinity of certain drugs. These changes are seen most clearly in the cardiovascular system and central nervous system (CNS).

Older adults experience a loss of sensitivity in adrenergic receptors, affecting both agonists and antagonists; this results in a reduced response to beta blockers and beta$_2$ agonists. Older adults also experience a blunting in compensatory reflexes leading to orthostatic hypotension and falls.

With age, there is a reduction in dopaminergic and cholinergic receptors, neurons, and available neural connections in the brain. There is reduced blood flow to the brain, and the blood-brain barrier also becomes more permeable. This puts the older adult at risk for CNS drug side effects, which include dizziness, seizures, confusion, sedation, and extrapyramidal effects.

NURSING IMPLICATIONS: OLDER ADULT DRUG DOSING AND MONITORING

Polypharmacy

Polypharmacy refers to the use of more medications than is medically necessary. There is little agreement on the actual number of drugs that constitutes polypharmacy, but researchers use five drugs because this number has been associated with increased incidence of adverse drug reactions, geriatric syndromes, and increased mortality.

Risk factors associated with polypharmacy include advanced age, female sex, multiple health care providers, use of herbal therapies and OTC drugs, multiple chronic diseases, and the number of hospitalizations and care transitions. Polypharmacy can cause an increase in geriatric syndromes (cognitive impairment, falls, decreased functional status, urinary incontinence, pressure injury, delirium, and weight loss) as well as an increased incidence of adverse drug reactions and poor adherence.

Pharmacotherapy in older adults is complex. To reduce the risk for and incidence of polypharmacy, nurses must be involved in the coordination of care for older adults. Older adults should be encouraged to use only one pharmacy and should give the pharmacist a list of all the drugs taken—prescribed, herbal, and OTC. A properly informed pharmacist will be able to conduct a clinical review of the patient's drugs to ensure the appropriateness of therapy. A pharmacist can also confirm patient understanding of individual therapy and can monitor responses to drug therapy. All of this is done to improve the overall quality of life of patients in their care.

Beers Criteria for Potentially Inappropriate Medication Use in Older Adults

The American Geriatrics Society Beers Criteria for Potentially Inappropriate Medication Use in Older Adults is a document developed by an interdisciplinary expert panel in geriatric care to aid health care providers in the safe prescription and administration of drugs to older adults (available free from https://www.pharmacytoday.org/article/S1042-0991(19)31235-6/pdf). First developed in 1991, it has been revised four times, most recently in 2019. The 2019 Beers Criteria addressed drugs that may exacerbate a disease or syndrome, drugs to

be used with caution in older adults, those with clinically important drug interactions, and drugs that should not be prescribed or have their dose reduced due to kidney dysfunction. As in previous editions, it continues to provide safety information based on best available evidence to use in decision making for drug therapy. Although the document provides information on drugs to avoid in older adults and drugs to use with caution, it is not designed for use in isolation. All drug therapy decisions should be made taking into consideration an individual's preferences, values, and needs. It is very important that the nurse advocate for the patient in these areas to ensure safety and promote adherence.

Adverse Drug Events

No drug is safe. Every year, more than 775,000 emergency department (ED) visits occur due to adverse drug events (ADEs), and more than 125,000 people are hospitalized due to ADEs. Older adults are twice as likely as younger adults to visit the ED with ADEs and are seven times as likely to be hospitalized. Most visits and hospitalizations occur due to reactions to blood thinners, drugs used to treat diabetes and seizures, cardiac drugs, and drugs used for pain control.

According to the World Health Organization, ADEs are "unintended and undesired effects of a [drug] at the normal dose." There are five types of ADEs: (1) adverse drug reactions, (2) medication errors, (3) therapeutic failures, (4) adverse drug withdrawal events, and (5) overdoses. Older adults have multiple risk factors for ADEs, including frailty, multiple comorbidities, polypharmacy, and cognitive issues.

Adherence

Adherence to a drug regimen is a problem for all patient age groups, but it is especially troublesome in older adult patients. Older adults may fail to ask questions during interactions with health care providers, which leads to the drug regimen not being fully understood or precisely followed. Failure to adhere to a drug regimen can cause underdosing or overdosing that could be harmful to the patient's health. Table 7.2 lists barriers to effective drug use by older adults.

Failure to adhere to a drug regimen can lead to ADEs, resulting in hospital admission, readmission to health care institutions, and even death. Complex drug regimens may be difficult for older adults to follow. Education is the cornerstone of adherence, and this includes education of the patient, family, and formal and informal caregivers.

Working with older adult patients is an ongoing nursing responsibility. The nurse should plan strategies with the patient and family or friends to encourage adherence with prescribed regimens. Daily contact may be necessary at first. Simply ordering the drug does not mean that the patient is able to get the drug or take it correctly. Older adults should have their prescriptions filled at one pharmacy if possible so a relationship can be established with a pharmacist and drug interactions can be identified and monitored closely.

The Medicare Modernization Act of 2003 made it possible for older adults to obtain prescription drug coverage through Medicare, with initial enrollment beginning in 2006. Older adults who are eligible for Medicare Part A or Part B are eligible for the optional Medicare Prescription Drug Plan (Part D) or coverage through a Medicare Advantage Plan (Part C). Each of these plans has its own formulary, copay rate, and in-network pharmacies. No plan is perfect for every older adult; the nurse, as advocate, must be able to assist the older adult to find the plan that is right for him or her and to make the most of the policy.

However, not all older adults have insurance that includes prescription drug coverage, nor are they able to afford their drugs even with insurance. Nurses need to assess the patient's ability to obtain prescriptions before sending the patient home. Options for assistance

TABLE 7.2   Barriers to Effective Drug Use by Older Adults

Causes	Nursing Actions
Taking too many drugs at different times	Develop a chart indicating times to take drugs. Provide space to place a mark for each drug taken. Coordinate the drug regimen with activities of daily living (e.g., meals) and events. Use an organizer container (daily or weekly). Have the patient bring all drugs—including over-the-counter drugs and herbal, vitamin, and mineral supplements—to all health appointments.
Failure to understand the purpose or reason for a drug	Explain the purpose, drug action, and importance of the drug. Provide time for questions and reinforcement. Reinforce with written information.
Impaired memory	Encourage family members or friends to monitor the patient's drug regimen.
Decreased mobility and dexterity	Advise family members or friends to have drugs and water or other fluid accessible and to assist older adults as needed.
Visual and hearing disturbances	Suggest eye and ear examinations (glasses or hearing aids).
High cost of prescriptions	Contact the social services department of your institution and compassionate care programs as appropriate.
Childproof drug bottles	Suggest that the patient request non-childproof bottle caps.
Side effects or adverse reactions from the drug	Educate the patient and family about side effects to report to the health care provider.

are available, and the nurse can assist patients in navigating the system to obtain their drugs for free or at a reduced cost (see Partnership for Prescription Assistance at www.pparx.org and Extra Help at www.ssa.gov/medicare/prescriptionhelp).

Health care professionals—nurses, pharmacists, and health care providers—need to work collaboratively to enhance safety and adherence of older adult patients and to avoid errors and unwarranted concerns. Nurses are in a unique position to educate patients and to monitor the effectiveness of therapeutic regimens. A handout of tips for patients on talking with their pharmacist is available at https://www.fda.gov/downloads/Drugs/ResourcesForYou/UCM163351.pdf.

HEALTH TEACHING WITH THE OLDER ADULT

Specific factors that enhance educational readiness and promote adherence in the older adult include the following:

- Ensure that the patient is wearing eyeglasses and has working hearing aids in place if needed. Check sensory aids to be sure they are clean and working.
- Speak in a tone of voice that the patient can hear; sit facing the patient, and limit distractions.
- Treat the patient with respect; never infantilize (also referred to as "elderspeak"); expect that the patient can learn.

- Use large print and dark type against a light background; use a font with serifs, or "feet and tails" (like this font), which makes letters close together easier to read.
- Review all drugs at each patient visit; ask the patient to bring all drugs to each appointment, and advise use of only one pharmacy.
- Advise the patient to complete the *vial of life* (medical information for emergency personnel to use in the provision of care; www.vialoflife.com) and keep it on the refrigerator door where safety personnel will know to look for it.
- Instruct the patient to keep a list of all drugs taken, bring it to all health appointments, and carry it when out of the house.
- Encourage a simple dosing schedule when possible.
- Suspect recently prescribed drug(s) if new confusion or disorientation occurs.
- Encourage the patient to report if a drug is not improving the condition for which it was prescribed.
- Consider use of memory aids such as pill organizers or planners, alarms, blinking lights, or prerecorded messages.

The National Institutes of Health (NIH) websites on aging are excellent resources for both health care providers and older adults and their families. The website for health care providers is www.nia.nih.gov; it has sections on health information, research, grants, training, news, and events. The website for older adults is https://www.nia.nih.gov/health.

◉ CLINICAL JUDGMENT [NURSING PROCESS]

Older Adult

Concept: Communication
- A process by which information is exchanged using multiple methods.

Concept: Safety
- Protecting the patient from potential or actual harm; considered a basic human need.

Recognize Cues [Assessment]
- Assess for allergies.
- Assess for sensory and cognitive barriers.
  - Assess the patient's use of eyeglasses, and check the date of the last eye examination.
  - Is the patient confused or disoriented? If so, is this state transitory?
- Assess laboratory test results and follow up as appropriate.

- Decreased kidney and liver function can increase the half-life of drugs.
- Assess weight and vital signs.
- Determine all drugs the patient takes, including illicit, prescription, and over-the-counter (OTC) drugs and supplements.
  - Assess patient adherence to the drug regimen.
  - Assess patient knowledge of the purpose of each drug, how it works, and its possible side effects.
- Discern whether the patient has difficulty opening drug containers and whether the patient is experiencing side effects or adverse reactions.
- Discern whether the patient lives alone, with or without social support, and whether assistance is needed with drugs, including costs or the transportation to acquire them.
- Obtain a history of chronic conditions.

Continued

◎ CLINICAL JUDGMENT [NURSING PROCESS]—CONT'D

Older Adult

Analyze Cues and Prioritize Hypothesis [Patient Problems]
- Need for health teaching
- Changes in elimination
- Potential for decreased adherence

Generate Solutions [Planning]
- The patient will collaborate with health care providers to develop a therapeutic regimen that is congruent with health goals and lifestyle.
- The patient will describe why the drug is needed, how the drug is administered, common adverse reactions, and drug interactions.
- The patient will identify measures to prevent constipation.
- The patient will list resources that can be used for more information or support.
- The patient will verbalize the ability to manage the therapeutic regimen.

Take Action [Nursing Interventions]
- Ascertain whether financial problems are preventing the patient from purchasing prescribed drugs. Assistance programs are available.
- Communicate with the pharmacist or health care provider when a drug dose is in question. Check drug references for recommended drug dosages for older adults.
- Establish a collaborative partnership with the patient to meet health-related goals.
- Monitor the patient's laboratory results to ensure that blood urea nitrogen (BUN), serum creatinine, estimated glomerular filtration rate (eGFR), and liver enzymes are within normal range and that drug levels are within the therapeutic range. Discuss findings with the health care provider.
- Observe the patient for adverse reactions when multiple drugs are being taken.
- Recognize a change in usual behavior or an increase in confusion. One of the first signs of drug toxicity is a change in mental status. Report changes to the health care provider.

- Remind the patient and family to tell the pharmacist about OTC preparations the patient is taking when picking up prescriptions.
- Advise patients and family to request a non-childproof cap from the pharmacy if the patient has arthritis in the hand joint or has difficulty opening childproof bottle caps. The patient may need to sign for this at the pharmacy, and safety of children or pets in the environment must be ensured.
- Advise patients to keep a record of their drugs and when they are to be taken. Consider offering them a sample log for recording information. This removes barriers, increases drug adherence, and avoids drug errors.
- Advise patients to use one pharmacy to fill prescriptions, and instruct them to inform the pharmacist of all illicit, prescription, and OTC drugs and supplements taken.
- Be available to answer patient questions. Be supportive of the older adult and the family. Discuss problems related to the drugs.
- Counsel patients not to share prescribed drugs with others or to take drugs prescribed for another person.
- Explain to patients and family the importance of adherence to the drug regimen. Emphasize the importance of taking drugs as prescribed.
- To promote adherence, provide additional time for verbal and written explanations.
- Review drugs with patients and family, including the reason the drug was prescribed, route of administration, frequency, common side effects, and when to notify the health care provider.
- Recognize that language difficulties may interfere with older adults' understanding of the prescribed drug regimen; provide educational material in the patient's preferred language.

Evaluate Outcomes [Evaluation]
- Evaluate adherence to the drug regimen, and answer any questions the older adult may have.
- Evaluate therapeutic drug response, and ascertain side effects or adverse reactions.

■ CRITICAL THINKING CASE STUDY

A 78-year-old woman comes to the clinic for a new patient examination. She reports that she smokes *cannabis* several times a week and also takes alprazolam 0.5 mg three times per day, a combination tablet of metoprolol tartrate 50 mg/hydrochlorothiazide 25 mg daily, aspirin 81 mg daily; garlic soft gels 1000 mg twice a day; and ibuprofen 400 mg four times a day.

1. Do any of these drugs appear on the 2019 American Geriatrics Society Beers Criteria for Potentially Inappropriate Medication Use in Older Adults? If so, what do the criteria say about them?
2. What interactions exist among the drugs and supplements this patient is taking?
3. What is the evidence for taking garlic to reduce cholesterol?

■ REVIEW QUESTIONS

1. A patient has nine drugs prescribed to take daily. Which are common reasons for nonadherence to the drug regimen in an older adult? (Select all that apply.)
   a. Taking multiple drugs at one time
   b. Impaired memory
   c. Decreased dexterity
   d. Increased mobility
   e. Increased visual acuity

2. The nurse is reviewing a patient's list of drugs. The nurse understands that the older adult's slower absorption of oral drugs is primarily because of which phenomenon?
   a. Decreased cardiac output
   b. Increased gastric emptying time
   c. Decreased gastric blood flow
   d. Increased gastric acid secretion

3. The older adult patient has questions about oral drug metabolism. Information on what subject is most important to include in this patient's teaching plan?
   a. First-pass effect
   b. Enzyme function
   c. Glomerular filtration rate
   d. Motility

4. An older patient has just started on hydrochlorothiazide and is advised by the health care provider to eat foods rich in potassium. What is the nurse's best recommendation of foods to consume?
   a. Cabbage and corn
   b. Bread and cheese
   c. Avocados and mushrooms
   d. Brown rice and fish

5. The nurse is developing teaching materials for an 82-year-old man with macular degeneration, who is being discharged on two new drugs. Which strategies would be best to use to impart the information? (Select all that apply.)
   a. Limit distractions in the room when teaching.
   b. Wait until discharge to teach so information is fresh in the memory.
   c. Augment teaching with audio material.
   d. Use "Honey" and other terms of familiarity when addressing him to promote trust.
   e. Use large, dark print on a light background for written material.

6. Which changes with aging alter drug distribution? (Select all that apply.)
   a. An increase in muscle mass and a decrease in fat
   b. A decrease in muscle mass and an increase in fat
   c. A decrease in serum albumin levels
   d. An increase in total body water
   e. A decrease in kidney mass

7. Which factors contribute to polypharmacy in older adults? (Select all that apply.)
   a. Multiple health care providers
   b. Multiple chronic diseases
   c. Use of a single pharmacy
   d. Care coordination by a nurse
   e. Few hospitalizations

8. Which is the best measure for the nurse to use to determine a patient's kidney function?
   a. Creatinine clearance
   b. Estimated glomerular filtration rate
   c. Serum creatinine level
   d. Blood urea nitrogen level

Drugs in Substance Use Disorder

http://evolve.elsevier.com/McCuistion/pharmacology

OBJECTIVES

- Define substance use disorder and differentiate among mild, moderate, and severe cases.
- Describe the short- and long-term effects of drug use.
- Identify the physical and psychological assessment findings associated with drugs most commonly used.
- Explain the rationale for the use of drug-assisted treatments during toxicity, withdrawal, and maintenance of abstinence from commonly misused drugs.

- Analyze Cues and Prioritize Hypotheses [Patient Problems] during the treatment of patients with drug toxicity and withdrawal.
- Take Appropriate Action [Nursing Interventions] during the management of surgical experiences and pain in patients with substance use disorder.
- Describe the nurse's role in recognizing and promoting the treatment of nurses with substance use disorder.
- Utilize Clinical Judgment [Nursing Process] in the care of patients with substance use disorders.

OUTLINE

Although most drugs are used safely and within prescribed guidelines, it is possible for all drugs to be misused. It has been reported that more than 40 million Americans 12 years of age and older use tobacco, alcohol, or illicit drugs. Drug use is a serious and complex social and health issue with negative consequences for both the individual and society that include family dysfunction, loss of employment, failure in school, domestic violence, and child abuse. The economic cost of drug use is staggering: $600 billion annually in costs related to lost productivity, health-related issues, and crime.

SUBSTANCE USE DISORDER

Context

Since 1975, the Monitoring the Future project has been tracking drug use in adolescents and young adults. Current data from the survey indicate that 26.4% of children have tried illicit drugs by the eighth grade, 40% by the tenth grade, and 51.8% by the twelfth grade. Tenth graders had tried alcohol (49.8%), *cannabis* (28.8%), amphetamines (6.6%), and prescription and over-the-counter (OTC) drugs such as oxycodone or cough medicine (2.6%–5.9%). Between 15% and 39% used more than one drug, known as polydrug use.

Many factors play into the decision to use drugs and whether an individual develops substance use disorder. Cognitive development at the time drugs are introduced plays a major role; adolescents are in a

period of brain development where they are especially vulnerable to stress and risk-seeking behaviors. Other risk factors are also related to substance use disorder:

- *Family-related risk factors:* Between 16% and 29% of children who suffer neglect or abuse—physical, sexual, and emotional—have tried or use drugs.
- *Social risk factors:* Deviant peer relationships (i.e., the adolescent associates with abusers and uses drugs to feel accepted), peer pressure, popularity, and bullying have all been correlated to drug use. Gang affiliation is associated with higher drug use and delinquent behavior.
- *Individual risk factors:* Individuals with attention-deficit/hyperactivity disorder (ADHD) are three times as likely as the general population to use drugs such as nicotine, alcohol, and drugs other than *cannabis*; depression is associated with alcohol use, particularly among young men.

It should be noted that positive family relationships are a protective factor that has been related to a decrease in drug use among adolescents.

Definition

According to the *Diagnostic and Statistical Manual of Mental Disorders* (5th edition [DSM-5]), substance use disorder occurs "when the recurrent use of alcohol and/or drugs causes clinically and functionally

TABLE 8.1 Substance Use Disorder Categories

Criteria	Subcomponents

• Mild substance use disorder (2–3 criteria required)
 • Moderate substance use disorder (4–5 criteria required)
 • Severe substance use disorder (6–7 criteria required)
	• The substance is often taken in larger amounts or over a longer period than was intended.
	 • There is a persistent desire or unsuccessful effort to cut down on or control use of the substance.
	 • A great deal of time is spent in activities necessary to obtain the substance, use the substance, or recover from its effects.
	 • Craving, or a strong desire or urge to use the substance, is present.
	 • Recurrent use of the substance results in a failure to fulfill major role obligations at work, school, or home.
	 • Continued use of the substance occurs despite having persistent or recurrent social or interpersonal problems caused or exacerbated by the effects of its use.
	 • Important social, occupational, or recreational activities are given up or reduced because of use of the substance.
	 • Recurrent use of the substance occurs in situations in which it is physically hazardous.
	 • Use of the substance is continued despite knowledge of having a persistent or recurrent physical or psychological problem that is likely to have been caused or exacerbated by the substance.
	 • Tolerance[a] occurs, as defined by either of the following:
	   • A need for markedly increased amounts of the substance to achieve intoxication or desired effect
	   • A markedly diminished effect with continued use of the same amount of the substance
	 • Withdrawal[a] occurs, as manifested by either of the following:
	   • The characteristic withdrawal syndrome for that substance is evident as specified in the DSM-5.
	   • The substance or a closely related substance is taken to relieve or avoid withdrawal symptoms.

[a]Does not apply when used appropriately under medical supervision. *DSM-5, Diagnostic and Statistical Manual of Mental Disorders,* 5th edition. From Horvath, A. T., Misra, K., Epner, A. K., & Cooper, G. M. (n.d.). *The diagnostic criteria for substance use disorders (addiction).* Retrieved from https://www.mentalhelp.net/addiction/diagnostic-criteria/; and National Institute on Drug Abuse. (2014). *The science of drug abuse and addiction: The basics.* Retrieved from www.drugabuse.gov/publications/media-guide/science-drug-abuse-addiction-basics.

significant impairment, such as health problems, disability, and failure to meet major responsibilities at work, school, or home." Substance use disorder is categorized along a continuum from mild to severe, based on the number of diagnostic criteria met (Table 8.1). The terms *abuse* and *dependence* are no longer used due to the violence and stigma associated with the term *abuse* and the ambiguity associated with the term *dependence*; gambling is the only condition in the category of behavioral addiction (continued involvement in an activity despite the substantial harm it causes; Table 8.2). Excessive caffeine use is not considered a substance use disorder, even though there appears to be a withdrawal syndrome with cessation of use.

Neurobiology

Drugs that are misused typically increase the availability of dopamine and other neurotransmitters in the limbic system of the brain. This area contains the brain's reward circuit, a structure that regulates our ability to feel pleasure and other emotions, both positive and negative. The drugs interfere with the way neurons in the brain normally send, receive, and process information by mimicking the brain's own neurotransmitters; however, drugs do not copy neurotransmitters exactly, which results in faulty transmission or excessive stimulation. Most of the drugs facilitate an increase of dopamine in the system, leading to mood elevation or euphoria—factors that provide strong motivation to repeat the experience. Some drugs increase the availability of other neurotransmitters, such as serotonin and gamma-aminobutyric acid (GABA), but dopamine's effect on the reward system appears to be pivotal to substance use disorder.

Repeated use of drugs remodels the neural circuitry of the brain cells and reduces the responsiveness of receptors. This decreased responsiveness leads to **tolerance**, the need for a larger dose of a drug to obtain the original euphoria. Drug use results in levels of dopamine that do not naturally occur; tolerance also reduces the sense of pleasure from experiences that previously resulted in positive feelings,

such as food, sex, or relationships. Without the drug, the individual may experience depression, anxiety, and/or irritability (Table 8.3; see also Table 8.2).

Current research is focused on epigenetics, the study of environmental influences on genetics. How a person responds to their social and cultural environment affects drug use. Altering environmental factors that increase the risk for drug use can discourage drug-seeking behavior. Studies have shown that drug use alters DNA proteins, those that affect both gene expression and function, and this influences drug-seeking behavior. Understanding these processes may lead to new treatments for substance use disorders.

Types of Substance Use Disorders

Alcohol Use Disorder

People drink for many reasons, including socializing, celebrating, and relaxing; people also drink to cope, because of low self-esteem and a need for approval, or because of peer pressure. Alcohol affects everyone differently, depending on the amount consumed, the frequency of consumption, age, health status, and family history. People of all ages drink. Recent data indicate 29% of high school students drink, with 14% stating they binge drink. Alcohol use is the underlying cause in 95,000 deaths per year.

Alcohol use inhibits the effects of GABA, thereby reducing neurotransmission in the brain. Short-term effects of alcohol use include nausea, vomiting, headaches, slurred speech, impaired judgment, memory loss, hangovers, and blackouts. Box 8.1 discusses alcohol toxicity.

Long-term problems associated with heavy drinking include stomach ailments, heart problems, cancer, brain damage, serious memory loss, immune system compromise, and liver cirrhosis. Persons with alcohol use disorder (AUD) increase their chances of dying from automobile accidents, homicide, and suicide. Spouses and children of persons with AUD may face family violence, and children may suffer

TABLE 8.2 Terminology Related to Substance Use Disorder

Term	Definition
Abstinence	Refraining from drug use
Craving	Strong desire for a drug or for the intoxicating effects of that drug
Intoxication	A condition that results in disturbances in the level of consciousness, cognition, perception, judgment, affect or behavior, or other psychophysiological functions and responses
Stabilization	Acute treatment for substance use disorder involving supervision, observation, support, intensive education, and counseling that involves multidisciplinary treatment interventions
Tolerance	Requiring a significantly increased amount of a drug to achieve the desired effect
Withdrawal syndrome	A group of symptoms of varying severity that occur upon cessation or reduction of use of a drug that has been taken repeatedly, usually for a prolonged period and/or in high doses; may be accompanied by signs of physiologic disturbance
Remission	None of the 11 criteria for substance use disorder for at least 3 months (early remission, 3–12 months; sustained remission, after 12 months)
Controlled environment	Environment where access to any drug is restricted (e.g., treatment center or halfway house)
Impaired control	Diminished ability of an individual to control his or her use of a drug in terms of onset, level, or termination
Social impairment	Recurrent drug use despite problems at work or school, interpersonal problems, or the cessation of social and recreational activities
Risky use	Recurrent drug use despite the difficulty it is causing (e.g., driving while intoxicated, liver damage)
Recovery	A process of change through which an individual improves health and wellness, lives a self-directed life, and strives to reach full potentials
Relapse	A return to drug use after a period of abstinence, often accompanied by reinstatement of substance use disorder

From Substance Abuse and Mental Health Services Administration. (2015). *Substance use disorders.* Retrieved May 17, 2016, from www.samhsa.gov/disorders/substance-use; and World Health Organization. (n.d.). *Lexicon of alcohol and drug terms published by the World Health Organization.* Retrieved May 18, 2016, from http://www.who.int/substance_abuse/terminology/who_lexicon/en/.

physical and sexual abuse and neglect and may develop psychological problems. Women who drink during pregnancy run a serious risk of their fetus developing fetal alcohol spectrum disorder. To intervene promptly and avoid long-term problems associated with AUD, nurses should question all patients about their drinking habits with every encounter, using plain language, without bias (Fig. 8.1).

Treatment. AUD can be treated through a variety of options. However, very few people with the disorder seek care. Alcohol treatment centers offer inpatient-type care, where the person undergoes stabilization in a controlled environment that includes group therapy. Persons with AUD are provided the tools they need to become abstinent and go into remission. Outpatient treatment is also available. People with AUD who participate in outpatient therapy are given the tools to become abstinent and go into remission (Table 8.4).

Drug-Assisted Treatment. Several drugs have been approved by the US Food and Drug Administration (FDA) to treat AUD. Disulfiram, acamprosate, and naltrexone are the most commonly used (Table 8.5). Disulfiram inhibits aldehyde dehydrogenase, the enzyme involved in metabolizing alcohol. It is best used in people who are newly abstinent. Disulfiram is administered in tablet form; dosage ranges from 125 to 500 mg daily. It is contraindicated in persons who are intoxicated and should not be taken within 12 hours of alcohol consumption (including use of mouthwash, cough medicine, or eating desserts that contain alcohol or eating foods cooked in alcohol). Side effects occur within 10 minutes of alcohol consumption and can last for more than an hour. These side effects include nausea, headache, vomiting, chest pains, and difficulty breathing. Disulfiram keeps patients from drinking because of the unpleasant side effects that occur if alcohol is consumed while taking the drug. Patients who have recently been treated with metronidazole or paraldehyde should not take disulfiram because these same side effects will occur as if they had been drinking. Because of the risk for drug toxicity, disulfiram should *never* be used in combination with eliglustat or ritonavir.

Other side effects of disulfiram include rash, drowsiness, impotence, acne, and a metallic aftertaste. Serious reactions include psychosis, hepatotoxicity, peripheral neuropathy, and optic neuritis. Patients taking disulfiram should have baseline liver function studies obtained; liver function studies should be repeated after 2 weeks of therapy. For disulfiram to be effective, persons with AUD also need to participate in behavior modification, psychotherapy, and counseling. Whether disulfiram will harm the fetus is unknown; however, it is excreted into breast milk. Therefore a decision should be made to either discontinue breastfeeding or discontinue the drug, taking into account the importance of the drug to the mother.

Acamprosate is a GABA analogue thought to work in the brain to restore the balance between neuronal excitation and inhibition via GABA and glutamate. It should only be used in persons who are abstinent; however, acamprosate may be continued through a relapse. Usual dosing is 666 mg orally three times per day. Dosing is adjusted in kidney disease, and a serum creatinine level should be obtained at baseline. Persons with a creatinine clearance of 30 mL/min to 50 mL/min should only take 333 mg three times per day. Acamprosate is contraindicated in people with a creatinine clearance less than 30 mL/min. Common side effects include pain, loss of appetite, nausea, diarrhea, dizziness, anxiety, pruritus, depression, insomnia, xerostomia, and paresthesia. Patients should be assessed for suicidal ideation before beginning treatment. This drug is used in conjunction with behavior modification and counseling. Naltrexone increases acamprosate levels. No dosage adjustment is needed, but patients should be monitored closely. It is not known if acamprosate will harm the fetus or if it is excreted into breast milk. Therefore a decision should be made to either discontinue breastfeeding or discontinue the drug, taking into account the importance of the drug to the mother.

Naltrexone is a competitive opioid antagonist with a high affinity for mu receptors. Oral forms absorbed through the gastrointestinal (GI) tract undergo up to 40% first-pass metabolism. Onset occurs in 15 to 30 minutes with peak occurring in 1 hour. Naltrexone is used in

TABLE 8.3 Most Commonly Used Illicit Drugs

Drug	Street Name	Desired Effects by the User	Short-Term Effects	Long-Term Health Effects	Treatment
Dimethyltriptamine (DMT) is a synthetic drug that produces intense, short-lived, hallucinogenic experiences. It is smoked, consumed orally, or injected.	Businessman's Special, DMT, Dimitri	Brief yet intense visual and auditory hallucinations that have been described by users as an alternate reality, otherworldly, or a near-death experience.	Intense visual hallucinations, depersonalization, auditory distortions, and an altered perception of time and body image, usually peaking in about 30 minutes when drunk as tea. Physical effects include hypertension, increased heart rate, agitation, seizures, dilated pupils.	Unknown	There are no FDA-approved medications to treat addiction to DMT. More research is needed to find out if DMT is addictive and, if so, whether behavioral therapies are effective.
Mescaline (peyote) is a hallucinogen found in disk-shaped "buttons" in the crown of several cacti, including peyote. Swallowed (chewed or soaked in water and drunk).	Big Chief, Buttons, Cactus, Mescalito	Rich visual hallucinations; "trips" for the users may be pleasurable and enlightening or anxiety-producing and unpleasant (known as a "bad trip"). There is no way to know how a user's experience may ultimately play out.	Enhanced perception and feeling; hallucinations; euphoria; anxiety; increased body temperature, heart rate, blood pressure; sweating; problems with movement.	Unknown	There are no FDA-approved medications to treat addiction to mescaline. More research is needed to find out if behavioral therapies can be used to treat addiction to hallucinogens.
Psilocybin. Swallowed (eaten, brewed as tea, or added to other foods).	Little Smoke, Magic Mushrooms, Purple Passion, Sacred Mush, Sewage Fruit, Shrooms, Zoomers	Psilocybin effects are similar to those of other hallucinogens, such as mescaline from peyote or LSD. The psychological reaction to psilocybin use includes visual and auditory hallucinations and an inability to discern fantasy from reality. Panic reactions and psychosis also may occur, particularly if large doses of psilocybin are ingested.	Hallucinations, altered perception of time, inability to tell fantasy from reality, panic, muscle relaxation or weakness, problems with movement, enlarged pupils, nausea, vomiting, drowsiness.	Risk of flashbacks and memory problems	There are no FDA-approved medications to treat addiction to psilocybin. More research is needed to find out if psilocybin is addictive and whether behavioral therapies can be used to treat addiction to this or other hallucinogens.
Salvia. Smoked, chewed, or brewed as tea.	Chia seeds, Diviner's Sage, Magic Mint, Sally-D, Ska Pastora	Altered perceptions, distorted reality, visual and auditory hallucinations, loss of control over body movements; however, users may experience anxiety and fear from a "bad trip."	Short-lived but intense hallucinations; altered visual perception, mood, body sensations; mood swings, feelings of detachment from one's body; sweating.	Unknown	There are no FDA-approved medications to treat addiction to salvia. More research is needed to find out if salvia is addictive, but behavioral therapies can be used to treat addiction to dissociative drugs.

Continued

TABLE 8.3   Most Commonly Used Illicit Drugs—cont'd

Drug	Street Name	Desired Effects by the User	Short-Term Effects	Long-Term Health Effects	Treatment
Inhalants are compounds that can be breathed in without smoking or using heat to vaporize them. Includes solvents, aerosols, and gases found in household products such as spray paints, markers, glues, and cleaning fluids; also nitrites (e.g., amyl nitrite), which are prescription medications for chest pain.	Poppers, Snappers, Whippets, Laughing Gas, Air Blast, Aimies, Bullets, Moon Gas, Snotballs, Toilet Water, White Out	Generally, people experience mild highs that last for a short time—normally on the order of minutes—so they tend to be taken repeatedly to extend the high.	Confusion; nausea; slurred speech; lack of coordination; euphoria; dizziness; drowsiness; disinhibition, lightheadedness, hallucinations, delusions; headaches	Liver and kidney damage; bone marrow damage; limb spasms due to nerve damage; brain damage from lack of oxygen that can cause problems with thinking, movement, vision, and hearing; sudden death due to heart failure (from sniffing butane, propane, and other chemicals in aerosols); death from asphyxiation or suffocation, convulsions or seizures, coma, or choking	There are no FDA-approved drugs to treat inhalant addiction. More research is needed to find out if behavioral therapies can be used to treat inhalant addiction.
Ketamine is a dissociative drug used as an anesthetic in veterinary practice. Dissociative drugs are hallucinogens that cause the user to feel detached from reality. It is typically injected or snorted, but it can be smoked or taken in pill form.	Cat Valium, K, Special K, Vitamin K, Lady K	Ketamine produces an abrupt high that lasts for about an hour. Large doses of ketamine can result in what some describe as the "K-hole," which can include intense and unpleasant visual and auditory hallucinations coupled with marked derealization and a frightening detachment from reality.	Problems with attention, learning, and memory; dreamlike states, hallucinations; sedation; confusion and problems speaking; loss of memory; problems moving to the point of being immobile; raised blood pressure; unconsciousness; slowed breathing that can lead to death	Ulcers and pain in the bladder; kidney problems; stomach pain; depression; poor memory	There are no FDA-approved drugs to treat ketamine addiction. More research is needed to find out if behavioral therapies can be used.
Cocaine is a powerfully addictive stimulant drug made from the leaves of the coca plant. It is usually snorted, smoked, or injected.	Blow, Bump, C, Nose, Candy, Charlie, Coke, Crack, Flake, Rock, Snow, Toot, Dust, Sneeze, White Rock, Sniff	Users claim to feel euphoric or high when using crack; some paradoxical drawbacks exist to using crack for any length of time—the initial euphoria can quickly turn to feelings of depression and paranoia. People who experience drug-induced paranoia might imagine someone is following them or trying to get into their house or that others are trying to attack them.	Narrowed blood vessels; enlarged pupils; increased body temperature, heart rate, and blood pressure; headache; abdominal pain and nausea; euphoria; increased energy and alertness; insomnia, restlessness; anxiety; erratic and violent behavior, panic attacks, paranoia, psychosis; heart rhythm problems, heart attack, inflammation of the heart muscle, deterioration of the ability of the heart to contract, and aortic ruptures; stroke, seizure, coma	Loss of sense of smell, nosebleeds, nasal damage and trouble swallowing from snorting; infection and death of bowel tissue from decreased blood flow; poor nutrition and weight loss from decreased appetite. Movement disorders, including Parkinson's disease, may also occur after many years of cocaine use. Smoking cocaine damages the lungs and can worsen asthma.	There are no FDA-approved drugs to treat cocaine addiction. CBT, a community reinforcement approach, plus vouchers, contingency management, motivational incentives, the matrix model (an intensive, structured, 16-week outpatient treatment program), and 12-step therapy may facilitate recovery.

Methamphetamine is a central nervous system stimulant drug with high potential for addiction, easily made in small clandestine laboratories, with relatively inexpensive over-the-counter ingredients such as pseudoephedrine, a common ingredient in cold medicines. It is typically swallowed, snorted, smoked, or injected.	Crank, Chalk, Crystal, Scooby Snax, Pookie, Quartz, Dunk, Gak, Rocket Fuel, Trash, Ice, Meth, Speed ("crystal meth" is methamphetamine in the form of a rock-like crystal.)		Decreased appetite; increased breathing, heart rate, blood pressure, temperature; irregular heartbeat	Anxiety, confusion, insomnia, mood problems, violent behavior, paranoia, hallucinations, delusions, weight loss, severe dental problems ("meth mouth"), intense itching leading to skin sores from scratching	There are no FDA-approved drugs to treat methamphetamine addiction. CBT, contingency management, or motivational incentives along with matrix model 12-step therapy may facilitate recovery.
MDMA is an abbreviation for 3,4-methylenedioxymethamphetamine. It is a synthetic chemical with complex effects that mimic both methamphetamine stimulants and mescaline hallucinogens. It is typically swallowed or snorted.	Adam, Candy, E-bomb, Thizz, Love Drug, Skittles, Sweets, Vitamin E or X, Molly, E, X, XTC, Rolls, Beans	A perceived increase in energy levels and a euphoric state of being; distorted perception of time; higher pleasure from and desire for physical touch; increased levels of sexuality and sexual arousal; elevated alertness, increased energy and focus.	Lowered inhibition, enhanced sensory perception; confusion, depression, sleep problems, anxiety; increased heart rate and blood pressure; muscle tension, teeth clenching; nausea; blurred vision; faintness; chills or sweating Taking more than one dose at a time or taking a series of pills over time to maintain the desired effects (*piggybacking*) can lead to overdose, which presents with high blood pressure, seizures, loss of consciousness, and a sharp rise in body temperature that leads to liver, kidney, or heart failure and death	Long-lasting confusion, depression, problems with attention, memory, and sleep; increased anxiety, impulsiveness, aggression; loss of appetite; decreased libido	There are no FDA-approved drugs to treat MDMA addiction. More research is needed to find out if behavioral therapies can be used; however, psychosocial and behavioral interventions and participation in a 12-step group or other support fellowship may be effective.
Synthetic cathinones (bath salts) are typically made from a synthetic version of an amphetamine-like stimulant in the cathinone class, α-PVP. Bath salts can be swallowed, snorted, or injected.	Bloom, Cloud Nine, Cosmic Blast, Flakka, Ivory Wave, Lunar Wave, Scarface, Vanilla Sky, White Lightning, Salting, Wicked X, Bubbles, Bath Blow, Blue Silk	Use results in a flood of dopamine in the brain leading to an intense feeling of euphoria.	Increased heart rate and blood pressure, euphoria, increased sociability and sex drive, paranoia, agitation, hallucinations, psychotic or violent behavior, nosebleeds, sweating, nausea and vomiting, insomnia, irritability, dizziness, depression, suicidal thoughts, panic attacks, reduced motor control, cloudy thinking	Breakdown of skeletal muscle tissue, kidney failure, death	There are no FDA-approved drugs to treat addiction to synthetic cathinones. Behavioral therapy includes CBT, contingency management, and motivational incentives such as motivational enhancement therapy (MET) and behavioral treatments geared to teens.

Continued

TABLE 8.3 Most Commonly Used Illicit Drugs—cont'd

Drug	Street Name	Desired Effects by the User	Short-Term Effects	Long-Term Health Effects	Treatment
Kratom comes from the leaves of a tropical deciduous tree, *Mitragyna speciosa*, that contains mitragynine, a psychoactive opioid. The leaves may be chewed, eaten (mixed in food or brewed as tea), or smoked.	Herbal Speedball, Biak-biak, Ketum, Kahuam, Thang, Thom	Kratom is consumed for mood-lifting effects and pain relief and as an aphrodisiac.	Sensitivity to sunburn, nausea, itching, sweating, dry mouth, constipation, increased urination, loss of appetite *Low doses*: Increased energy, sociability, alertness *High doses*: Sedation, euphoria, decreased pain	Anorexia, weight loss, insomnia, skin darkening, dry mouth, frequent urination, constipation; with long-term use at high doses, hallucination and paranoia	No clinical trials have been conducted on medications for kratom addiction. More research is needed to find out if behavioral therapies can be used.
Heroin is an opioid drug processed from morphine, a naturally occurring opiate extracted from the seedpod of certain varieties of poppy plants. It can be injected, smoked, or snorted.	Brown Sugar, Chiva, Dope, H, Horse, Junk, Skag, Skunk, Smack, White Horse	Heroin binds to opioid receptors in the body, prompting a release of dopamine and creating intensely pleasurable feelings.	Euphoria, warm flushing of skin, dry mouth, heavy feeling in the hands and feet, clouded thinking, alternating wakeful and drowsy states, itching, nausea and vomiting, slowed breathing and heart rate	Collapsed veins, abscesses, infection of the lining and valves in the heart, constipation and stomach cramps, liver or kidney disease, pneumonia, and hypoxic brain injury	Medications approved to treat heroin addiction and aid withdrawal include methadone, buprenorphine, and naltrexone. Behavioral therapy includes contingency management, motivational incentives, and 12-step facilitation therapy.
Phencyclidine (PCP) is a dissociative drug that causes the user to feel detached from reality. It can be injected, snorted, swallowed, or smoked.	Angel Dust, Hog, Embalming Fluid, Rocket Fuel, Sherms	Produces visual and auditory distortions and perceptual changes that result in an individual feeling detached from themselves or the world around them; users may feel that their body is not their own.	Delusions, hallucinations, paranoia, problems thinking, a sense of distance from one's environment, anxiety *Low doses*: A slight increase in breathing rate, increased blood pressure and heart rate, shallow breathing, face redness and sweating, numbness of the hands or feet, problems with movement *High doses*: Lowered blood pressure, pulse rate, breathing rate; nausea and vomiting; blurred vision; flicking up and down of the eyes; drooling; loss of balance, dizziness; violence or suicidal thoughts; seizures, coma, death	Impaired memory, thinking, and decision-making abilities; speech problems; severe depression, suicidal thoughts; higher anxiety, paranoia, and isolation; extreme weight loss; "flashback" phenomena and continuous hallucinations and delusional thinking even when not using the substance	There are no FDA-approved drugs to treat addiction to PCP. More research is needed to find out if behavioral therapies can be used to treat addiction to dissociative drugs.
Synthetic cannabinoids; may be smoked or swallowed.	K2, Spice, Black Mamba, Bliss, Bombay Blue, Fake Weed, Genie, Moon Rocks, Skunk, Smacked, Yucatan, Zohai	Euphoric feelings, altered perception, feelings of relaxation	Increased heart rate, vomiting, agitation, confusion, hallucinations, anxiety, paranoia, increased blood pressure	Kidney failure and heart attacks; severe and lasting heart conditions, seizure activity in frequent users.	There are no FDA-approved drugs to treat synthetic cannabinoid addiction. More research is needed to find out if behavioral therapies can be used.

Substance	Street Names	Why Used	Health Effects	Addiction Potential	Treatment Options
Rohypnol (flunitrazepam); an intermediate-acting benzodiazepine typically swallowed (as a pill or dissolved in a drink) or snorted	Circles, Date Rape Drug, Forget-Me Pill, La Rocha, Mexican Valium, Mind Eraser, Pingus, R2, Rib, Roaches, Roachies, Roapies, Rochas Dos, Roofies, Rope, Rophies, Rowie, Ruffies	Because of the strong amnesia produced by the drug, it has been used for its ability to sedate and incapacitate unsuspecting rape victims when placed in their drinks. It has also been used illegally to lessen the depression caused by the use of stimulants, such as cocaine and methamphetamine, and by heroin and cocaine users to produce profound intoxication and boost the high of heroin.	Drowsiness, sedation, sleep; amnesia, blackout; decreased anxiety, muscle relaxation, impaired reaction time and motor coordination; impaired mental functioning and judgment; confusion; aggression; excitability; slurred speech; headache; slowed breathing and heart rate; in combination with alcohol, severe sedation, unconsciousness, and slowed heart rate and breathing can lead to death.	Unknown	There are no FDA-approved drugs to treat addiction to flunitrazepam. More research is needed to find out if behavioral therapies can be used to treat addiction.
GHB (gamma-hydroxybutyrate) is a depressant approved for use in the treatment of narcolepsy. It is swallowed.	G, Gamma-oh, GEEB, Georgia Home Boy, Goop, Grievous Bodily Harm, Liquid Ecstasy, Liquid X, Soap, Scoop	Euphoria, increased sex drive, and tranquility; has been used for sexual assault as victims become incapacitated due to the sedative effects and they are unable to resist. GHB may also induce amnesia in its victims.	Euphoria, drowsiness, decreased anxiety, confusion, memory loss, hallucinations, excited and aggressive behavior, nausea, vomiting, unconsciousness, slowed heart rate and breathing, lower body temperature *High doses*: Even without other illicit substances or alcohol, high doses may result in profound sedation, seizures, coma, severe respiratory depression, and death.	Unknown	Withdrawal may be treated with benzodiazepines. More research is needed to find out if behavioral therapies can be used to treat GHB addiction.
LSD (lysergic acid diethylamide) is a hallucinogen that is swallowed or absorbed through mouth tissues	Acid, Blotter, Tabs, Boomers, Cid, Golden Dragon, Looney Tunes, Lucy Mae, Microdot, Yellow Sunshine	Users experience impaired depth and time perception and a distorted perception of the size and shape of objects, movements, color, sound, touch, and body image; sensations may seem to "cross over," giving the feeling of hearing colors or seeing sounds (synesthesia, also called "tripping").	Rapid emotional swings; distortion of a person's ability to recognize reality, think rationally, or communicate with others; raised blood pressure, heart rate, body temperature; insomnia; loss of appetite, dry mouth, sweating, numbness, weakness, tremors, dizziness, enlarged pupils	Frightening flashbacks (called *hallucinogen persisting perception disorder* [HPPD]); ongoing visual disturbances, disorganized thinking, paranoia, and mood swings	There are no FDA-approved drugs to treat addiction to LSD. More research is needed to find out if behavioral therapies can be used to treat addiction.

α-PVP, Alpha-pyrrolidinopentiophenone; *CBT*, cognitive behavioral therapy; *FDA*, US Food and Drug Administration.
Information obtained from DrugAbuse.com. (n.d.). http://drugabuse.com/library/drugs-a-z/; www.drugs.com. (2016). *Drugs A–Z*. Retrieved May 15, 2016, from www.drugs.com; and National Institute on Drug Abuse. (2016). *Commonly abused drugs*. Retrieved December 19, 2020, from www.drugabuse.gov/drugs-abuse/.

BOX 8.1 Alcohol Toxicity

Alcohol toxicity is a life-threatening condition that can occur by drinking large amounts of alcohol over a short period of time. A standard drink contains 10 g of alcohol. This is equal to 10 ounces of beer with 5% alcohol, 3.25 ounces of wine with 12% alcohol, or 1 ounce of hard liquor with 40% alcohol (or 80 "proof"). Roughly 20% of alcohol is absorbed from the stomach, and the remainder is absorbed in the small intestine. Food intake slows absorption. Alcohol is metabolized in the liver and is excreted by the lungs and kidneys, and the average person can only metabolize 10 g of alcohol per hour.

Complications of alcohol toxicity include aspiration of vomitus, asphyxiation, severe dehydration, seizures, hypothermia, brain damage, and death. Treatment involves airway management and supplemental oxygenation, correction of hypoglycemia if present, supportive care, and intravenous (IV) hydration. If the person chronically uses alcohol, thiamine 100 mg may be administered intramuscularly to prevent neurologic damage. Patients with impaired hepatic function may require hemodialysis to remove alcohol from the blood; however, this invasive treatment is only used in persons whose condition is rapidly deteriorating.

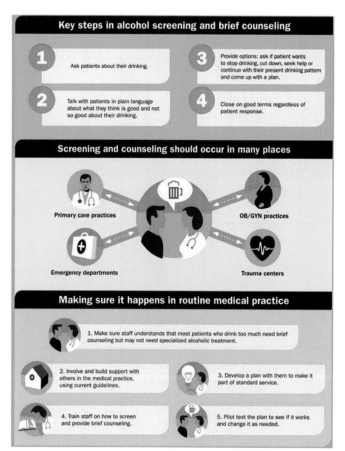

Fig. 8.1 Alcohol screening and brief counseling. (From National Center for Chronic Disease Prevention and Health Promotion, Division of Population Health. [2014]. *Alcohol screening and counseling.* Retrieved August 26, 2019 from https://www.cdc.gov/vitalsigns/alcohol-screening-counseling/index.html.)

persons who are abstinent. If there is concern about comorbid opioid use disorder (OUD), a naloxone challenge test may be done before initiating treatment, in which a test dose of 25 mg is administered orally, and the patient is observed for an hour. If no withdrawal is observed, dosing may begin the next day at 50 mg per day for 12 weeks or less. Dosing using 380 mg intramuscularly (IM) once every 4 weeks can

be used for maintenance therapy. Common side effects include insomnia, nausea, vomiting, anxiety, headache, abdominal pain, myalgia, arthralgia, rash, dizziness, fatigue, constipation, and increased creatine phosphokinase (CPK). Serious reactions include suicidality, depression, hepatotoxicity, and hypersensitivity reaction. Patients should be assessed for suicidal ideation before beginning treatment. This drug should *not* be taken in conjunction with any drugs that bind to opioid receptors because withdrawal may be precipitated in persons with OUD. It is not known if naltrexone will harm the fetus, and it is excreted into breast milk. Therefore a decision should be made to either discontinue breastfeeding or discontinue the drug, taking into account the importance of the drug to the mother.

Cannabis Use Disorder

Cannabis is the most commonly used recreational drug in the United States. More than 4.2 million people 12 years of age and older meet the criteria for *cannabis* use disorder. *Cannabis* use disorder is more common among people in their late teens and early 20s. Users report feeling an alteration in their senses and an altered sense of time as well as changes in mood. *Cannabis* goes by many street names, including Marijuana, Blunt, Bud, Dope, Ganja, Grass, Green, Herb, Joint, Mary Jane, Pot, Reefer, Sinsemilla, Skunk, Smoke, Trees, and Weed; names for various forms of hashish include Boom, Gangster, Hash, and Hemp. *Cannabis* contains more than 60 related psychoactive chemicals known as *cannabinoids*; however, the most abundant of these is delta-9-tetrahydrocannabinol (THC).

When smoked, THC rapidly crosses the blood-brain barrier and binds to cannabinoid receptors in many areas of the brain, overwhelming the endocannabinoid system and making it difficult for the user to respond appropriately to incoming stimuli. The drug impairs short-term memory, learning, and ability to focus, and it can cause problems with balance and coordination. In addition, *cannabis* increases heart rate and may cause hallucinations, anxiety, panic attacks, and psychosis in some people. When smoked, *cannabis* may harm the lungs, and concurrent use of alcohol increases blood pressure in addition to heart rate and further slows mental processes and reaction times. Box 8.2 discusses issues associated with vaping *cannabis*.

Long-term use of *cannabis* is associated with chronic cough, frequent respiratory infections, and exposure to cancer-causing compounds because the smoke has many of the same irritating and lung-damaging properties as tobacco. Ingestion of the drug increases the heart rate for hours, increasing risk for heart attack and stroke. When repeated use begins in adolescence, there is an association with decreased motivation and decreased performance on memory-related tasks. The drug has also been linked to mental health problems and increased symptoms in persons with schizophrenia. Babies born to women who use *cannabis* have behavioral issues and problems with attention, memory, and problem solving.

Many have supported the nationwide legalization of *cannabis* to treat medical conditions; however, rigorous scientific evidence to show that the benefits of *cannabis* outweigh its health risks is limited and does not support approval. Despite the current evidence, 33 states and the District of Columbia have legalized medical use of *cannabis* to treat pain (e.g., cancer pain, headaches, glaucoma, and nerve pain), muscle spasms related to multiple sclerosis, chemotherapy-induced nausea and vomiting, anorexia and weight loss associated with human immunodeficiency virus (HIV), seizure disorders, and Crohn disease. The District of Columbia and 15 states—Alaska, California, Colorado, Illinois, Maine, Massachusetts, Michigan, Nevada, Oregon, Vermont, New Jersey, Arizona, South Dakota, Montana, and Washington—have legalized the recreational use of *cannabis*, leading to sales of $12.2 billion in 2019, which is projected to increase to $31.1 billion by 2024.

TABLE 8.4 Nonpharmacological Therapy for Substance Use Disorders: Individual and Group Counseling

Therapy	Description
Cognitive behavioral therapy (CBT)	CBT teaches people to recognize and stop negative patterns of thinking and behavior and helps enhance self-control. For instance, therapy might help a person become aware of the stressors, situations, and feelings that lead to substance use so that the person can avoid them or act differently when they occur.
Contingency management	This approach is based on frequent monitoring of behavior and removal of rewards for drug use and was designed to provide incentives to reinforce positive behavior and help the person remain abstinent from drug use.
Motivational enhancement therapy (MET)	MET helps people with substance use disorders develop internally motivated changes and commit to specific plans to engage in treatment and seek recovery. It is often used early in the process to engage people in treatment.
Twelve-step facilitation therapy	Seeks to guide and support engagement in 12-step programs such as Alcoholics Anonymous or Narcotics Anonymous.

From Substance Abuse and Mental Health Services Administration. (2015). *Treatments for substance use disorders.* Retrieved June 3, 2016, from www.samhsa.gov/treatment/substance-use-disorders.

TABLE 8.5 Pharmacokinetics of Drug-Assisted Treatments

Drug Name	Absorption	Distribution	Metabolism	Excretion
Acamprosate	Peak plasma time: 3–8 h Bioavailability: 11%, decreased by food but not clinically important	Protein binding: Negligible	Not metabolized	In urine as unchanged drug Half-life: 20–33 h
Buprenorphine	Extensive first-pass effect if taken orally; 31% bioavailability (SL) Time to peak plasma varies from 40 min-3.5 h.	Highly lipophilic Highly protein bound (96%)	Extensive hepatic	In bile and feces, 70%; urine, 30% Half-life: SL, 37 h
Disulfiram	Absorbed from the GI tract (80%–90%), onset is 3–12 h after administration Effects may persist up to 14 d after the last dose	Highly lipophilic	Hepatic	In urine primarily but also in feces (5%–20% unchanged) and lungs
Methadone	Oral administration: Bioavailability ranges from 36%–100%, and peak plasma concentrations are achieved between 1 and 7.5 h.	Lipophilic; 85%–90% protein bound	Hepatic, into inactive metabolite	Renal and fecal Half-life is highly variable.
Naloxone	Onset: Administered IV, 2 min; subcut and IM, 5 min; Intranasal route: 1 mg in each nostril × 1 Duration of action is 30–60 min.	Plasma protein binding occurs but is relatively weak	Hepatic	In urine Half-life is 1–1.5 h.
Naltrexone	96% absorbed from the GI tract; extensive first-pass metabolism; 5%–40% reaches the systemic circulation Onset is 15–30 min; duration is 24 h and is dose dependent	Protein bound: 21%–28%	Hepatic, into active metabolite	In urine
Varenicline	Well absorbed from the GI tract and unaffected by food Time to peak plasma: 3–4 h	Less than 20% protein binding	Minimal hepatic (<10%)	In urine, 92% unchanged Half-life: 24 h

d, Day; *GI*, gastrointestinal; *h*, hours; *IM*, intramuscular; *IV*, intravenous; *min*, minutes; *SL*, sublingual; *subcut*, subcutaneous.
From Drugs.com for Healthcare Professionals. (n.d.). Retrieved from www.drugs.com/professionals.html; and Medscape.com. (n.d.). *Drugs, OTCs & Herbals.* Retrieved from http://reference.medscape.com/drugs.

The economic impact of *cannabis* is expected to reach $77 billion by 2022.

Cognitive behavioral therapy (CBT), contingency management, and motivational enhancement therapy (MET) may be effective in the treatment of *cannabis* use disorder; however, no medications are currently approved or indicated for this use.

Opioid Use Disorder

Opioids (e.g., oxycodone, hydrocodone, morphine, methadone, and fentanyl) are controlled substances legally prescribed to treat moderate to severe pain. These drugs interact with opioid receptors in the brain and nervous system to reduce pain. In addition to reducing pain, this receptor interaction floods the brain's reward system with dopamine, producing a sense of euphoria and tranquility.

Short-term effects of opioid use include drowsiness, mental confusion, nausea, constipation, and dose-dependent respiratory depression. When taken with alcohol, users may experience dangerous slowing of heart rate and breathing leading to coma or death. When taken with serotonergic drugs (e.g., selective serotonin reuptake inhibitors [SSRIs], serotonin-norepinephrine reuptake inhibitors [SNRIs], and antimigraine agents), serotonin syndrome may occur. Symptoms of

BOX 8.2 Vaping *Cannabis*

Use of *cannabis* in e-cigarettes is a public health concern. Recent reports indicate 8.9% of middle- and high-schoolers have vaped *cannabis*. Johns Hopkins School of Medicine researchers note that "compared with smoking *cannabis*, vaping it increased the rate of short-term anxiety, paranoia, memory loss and distraction when doses were the same" in infrequent users. Persons who vape the drug may also experience nausea, vomiting and hallucination for hours after use (McMains, 2018).

Additional concerns surround the farming and manufacturing processes of *cannabis* oil. Not only is there little oversight of *Cannabis* farmers and the chemicals used to eliminate mites, mold, and mildew on the plants and to make the buds denser, there is no oversight on the process and chemicals used to extract the substance, referred to as butane hash oil (BHO), that is often made in "the basement or backyard." Although California and Oregon are trying to regulate the industry, "black market" cartridges show up in dispensaries. Lewis (2017) stated, "You don't know what's in the oil you're vaping, and you don't know how it's going to affect your health."

E-cigarettes with *cannabis* oil in the cartridge heat the liquid until it vaporizes. They generate very little odor and the cartridges look like a flash drive, making it nearly impossible to tell if the user is vaping tobacco or *cannabis*. Nurses who work with children and adolescents must be diligent in asking about the use of *cannabis* oil in e-cigarettes and providing counseling concerning the dangers of using them.

Excerpts from McMains, V. (2018). *Vaping marijuana might be too much for first-timers.* Retrieved January 3, 2019 from https://www.futurity.org/vaping-cannabis-anxiety-1925032-2/; and, Lewis, A. C. (2017). *Are weed vape pens safe?* Retrieved January 3, 2019 from https://www.rollingstone.com/culture/culture-features/are-weed-vape-pens-safe-202125/.

BOX 8.3 Naloxone Use by Laypersons

When administered by laypersons trained to recognize opioid overdose, the use of intranasal naloxone can reverse the symptoms of overdose, thereby reducing mortality.

Naloxone distribution programs provide kits to opioid users and their friends and family. This practice is endorsed by the American Medical Association, the American Public Health Association, the United Nations Office on Drugs and Crime, and the World Health Organization.

The overdose kits contain naloxone, gloves, a breathing shield, and instructions. Fig. 8.2 shows proper use of intranasal naloxone. When overdose is identified, the layperson should call 911 and give naloxone. Once the drug is administered, it acts in two to three minutes. Rescue breathing should be performed while waiting for the drug to take effect.

There are minimal risks associated with the use of naloxone by laypersons. If the recipient is not using opiates, it may make them uncomfortable, but it will not harm them (unless pregnant, nursing, or allergic to naloxone). It only works to reverse the effects of opioids, not other drugs such as benzodiazepines, bath salts, cocaine, methamphetamine, or alcohol.

NIDA. 2017, March 30. Naloxone for Opioid Overdose: Life-Saving Science. Retrieved from https://www.drugabuse.gov/publications/naloxone-opioid-overdose-life-saving-science on 2020, December 19

Bar-Ilan University. (2020, August 3). Properly equipped laypersons can potentially reverse opioid overdose mortality. EurekAlert! https://www.eurekalert.org/pub_releases/2020-08/bu-plc073020.php

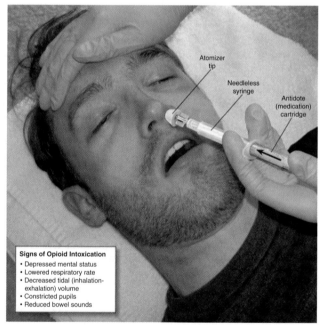

Fig. 8.2 Properly equipped laypersons can potentially reverse opioid overdose mortality.

serotonin syndrome include agitation, hallucinations, coma, tachycardia, hypertension, hyperthermia, and rigidity.

In addition to the oral route, when misused, opioids are smoked, snorted, or administered parenterally. Prescription opioids are also known by numerous street names, including Vikes, Cody, China White, Fizzies, M, Demmies, Blue Heavens, Juice, Smack, Hillbilly Heroin, and Roxy.

Nonmedical use of prescription opioid drugs has reached epidemic proportions; more than 1.9 million people in the United States meet criteria for OUD. Close to 19,000 people with OUD die each year, secondary to overdose of prescription opioids. More than 50% of people who misuse prescription opioids obtain them from a friend or relative for free, and 22.1% obtain them from a doctor. With repeated use, tolerance to the euphoric effects of the drug increase, and users may not be able to obtain the drug from friends, relatives, or any doctor; this causes them to turn to the street for drugs. Some users switch from prescription drugs to cheaper and riskier substitutes, like heroin.

The FDA has toughened the safety warnings on opioids, including adding a boxed warning about the potentially lethal risks associated with misuse. The safety warning includes a caution regarding the use of opioids during pregnancy and the risk of neonatal opioid withdrawal syndrome (NOWS), which can be life-threatening.

Contingency management therapy or 12-step facilitation therapy may be useful in treating prescription opioid addiction. Treatment approaches are tailored to each patient and are often combined with medication therapy.

Drug-Assisted Treatment. Naloxone (see Table 8.5) is the drug of choice in the treatment of respiratory depression associated with opioid overdose. Naloxone is a short-acting opioid antagonist that competitively attaches to opioid receptors in the central nervous system (CNS), thereby blocking activation by opioid drugs. In emergency situations, it is administered intravenously (IV); however, it may also be administered IM or subcutaneously (subcut). In persons with suspected OUD, dosing begins at 0.1 to 0.2 mg every 2 to 3 minutes until the patient responds Properly equipped laypersons can also potentially reverse opioid mortality (Box 8.3 and Fig. 8.2). Careful monitoring is required to prevent opioid withdrawal. Symptoms of withdrawal include nausea and vomiting, abdominal cramps, hyperthermia, hypertension, and restlessness.

Naltrexone is approved by the FDA to treat OUD. (See the previous discussion under Alcohol Use Disorder.) Dosing begins at 50 mg daily after the patient has been opioid free for 7 to 10 days. It is also available in an injectable, extended-release form, with dosing at 380 mg each month. Once treated with naltrexone, patients may have reduced tolerance to opioids; if they relapse after a period of abstinence and resume opioid use at previous doses, they may experience life-threatening consequences, including respiratory arrest and circulatory collapse.

Since the 1950s, methadone has been prescribed to treat persons with OUD. When taken as prescribed and combined with counseling and behavioral therapies, administration of this long-acting opioid drug is safe and effective. Methadone has a boxed warning concerning the risk of cardiac and respiratory-related deaths due to QT prolongation and cardiac arrhythmias. Methadone used for stabilization and maintenance of persons with OUD may only be administered by programs certified by the Substance Abuse and Mental Health Services Administration (SAMHSA) and approved by state authority. Opioid treatment programs must follow federal guidelines and standards for medically monitored withdrawal and treatment.

Methadone works by changing the way a person's brain responds to pain; it is an opioid receptor agonist at the mu receptor and an antagonist at the N-methyl-D-aspartate (NMDA) receptor. Taken daily, it blocks the sense of euphoria and tranquility caused by opioid use and prevents opioid withdrawal and craving. Concurrent administration of rifampin, phenytoin, St. John's wort, phenobarbital, and carbamazepine can reduce serum methadone levels and precipitate withdrawal. Administration with zidovudine may lead to toxicity.

Initial dosing ranges from 20 mg to 30 mg, followed by 5 mg to 10 mg, adjusting the methadone dose to suppress withdrawal and block the euphoric effects of opioids. Maximum dosage is 40 mg on the first day of stabilization. Maintenance therapy is based on patient assessment and ranges from 80 to 120 mg a day. Tapering methadone should only be done under medical supervision, with dose reductions of less than 10% every 14 days.

Common methadone side effects include lightheadedness, constipation, dizziness, sedation, nausea, and vomiting. Patients should be educated to prevent theft and misuse of methadone by friends, family, and others. Whether methadone will harm the fetus is unknown, but it is excreted into breast milk; therefore a decision should be made to either discontinue breastfeeding or discontinue the drug, taking into account the importance of the drug to the mother.

Buprenorphine is a long-acting, mixed narcotic agonist-antagonist. It binds to various opioid receptors in the brain, producing partial antagonism at mu receptors and antagonism at kappa receptors, resulting in decreased withdrawal symptoms and cravings. Although it does produce some euphoria, there is a ceiling effect; increasing the dose beyond a moderate level (8–16 mg) does not increase euphoria, so it has a low potential for misuse. To further deter people from misusing buprenorphine, naloxone is added. Because of the almost complete first-pass metabolism of naloxone, it has minimal pharmacologic activity when the drug is used appropriately as a sublingual tablet. However, if the tablet is crushed and injected, the effects of naloxone lead to opioid withdrawal.

This drug may be administered in qualified outpatient settings (e.g., office, health department, or correctional facility) after providers have received training. When taken as prescribed and used in combination with counseling and behavioral therapies, it is safe and effective. Initial dosing begins when the person with OUD has been opioid free for at least 12 hours and is beginning to experience withdrawal. Dosing starts at 2 to 4 mg sublingual (SL) for the first day and then is raised to 8 to 16 mg SL for 1 to 2 days. Once the patient is stable and is not experiencing cravings or significant side effects, dosing is tailored to the individual. Although the maximum daily dose of buprenorphine is 44 mg, doses higher than 24 mg/day do not provide any clinical advantage.

Side effects of buprenorphine include nausea, vomiting, and constipation; muscle aches and cramps; and cravings, sedation, headache, depression, anxiety, and withdrawal symptoms. Whether buprenorphine will harm the fetus is unknown, but it is excreted into breast milk. Therefore a decision should be made to either discontinue breastfeeding or discontinue the drug, taking into account the importance of the drug to the mother.

Tobacco Use Disorder

In 2019, 50.6 million adults used tobacco products. According to the CDC, "Cigarettes were the most commonly used tobacco product among adults, and e-cigarettes were the most commonly used noncigarette tobacco product (4.5%). The highest prevalence of e-cigarette use was among smokers aged 18–24 years (9.3%), with over half (56.0%) of these young adults reporting that they had never smoked cigarettes." Other tobacco products used include cigars, smokeless tobacco, and pipes.

When smoked, nicotine is absorbed from the lungs into the pulmonary venous circulation. It then enters the arterial circulation and moves quickly to the brain. Once across the blood-brain barrier, nicotine stimulates the release of dopamine, norepinephrine, GABA, glutamate, and endorphins, resulting in stimulation and pleasure and a reduction in stress and anxiety. These sensations fuel the brain's reward circuit.

According to the CDC, more than 480,000 deaths each year are caused by cigarette smoking. Short-term effects of tobacco use include increased blood pressure, breathing, and heart rate. Tobacco use does long-term damage to nearly every organ in the human body, often leading to a variety of cancers, respiratory disorders, heart disease, stroke, immune dysfunction, and type 2 diabetes. Women who smoke while pregnant may experience miscarriage, premature delivery, and stillbirth and may have infants of lower birth weight. Children born to women who used tobacco while pregnant may be born with learning and behavior problems. Persons with tobacco use disorder (TUD) have increased health care utilization and higher health care costs compared with nonusers, and they are frequently absent from work.

Since 2002, the number of persons with TUD in sustained remission has outnumbered those actively using nicotine; the CDC reported that 70% of smokers want to quit. Within 1 to 2 years of quitting, persons with TUD significantly reduce their risk for cancer, heart disease, stroke, and respiratory illness. Quitting is difficult. Persons attempting to quit experience irritability, anger, anxiousness, difficulty thinking, cravings, and increased hunger. Support is a very important part of the process and is often combined with pharmacologic measures.

CBT is a goal-directed and problem-focused therapy designed to help the person with TUD identify negative thought patterns and inaccurate beliefs to learn new ways of coping and develop new ways of thinking. It helps the person increase their self-confidence in the ability to quit. CBT helps people identify their triggers and learn to either avoid them or respond differently to them. It also helps with any ambivalence people may feel about quitting.

Self-help materials in the form of Internet-based aids or cell phone apps are available to assist the person with TUD. For example, the American Lung Association offers *Freedom From Smoking Online* (www.ffsonline.org/?referrer=http://www.lung.org/stop-smoking/join-freedom-from-smoking), which offers modules with lessons and activities that reinforce the person's commitment to quit. Phone apps are available as well. Some require a small fee, such as *Butt Out—Quit Smoking Forever,* which monitors progress and helps the person stay focused on the goal to quit by providing motivational pictures and messages. Other apps are free, such as *Get Rich or Die Smoking,* which shows the person how much money they are saving each day by not smoking. It also monitors their health progress and shows what the person could buy with the money they have saved, and it rewards the app user with trophies.

Telephone-based resources link persons with TUD with counselors trained to assist the caller in developing an individualized plan to quit smoking. Telephone-based counseling is easy to use because it does not require the person to drive or find child care to attend a meeting in person; additionally, it is available nights and weekends.

Combining a nonpharmacologic support measure with drug-assisted treatment is the most effective means to quit smoking.

Drug-Assisted Treatment. Nicotine replacement drugs—sold as a gum, patch, spray, inhaler, or lozenge—mimic the nicotine effects of tobacco by binding to nicotine receptors in the CNS (see Table 8.5). They are used to relieve the withdrawal symptoms associated with smoking cessation and provide some of the stimulation and stress-relief effects the user gained from smoking. Those who choose to use nicotine replacement gums, sprays, inhalers, or lozenges dose themselves when they feel the urge to smoke; those who use the patch have a sustained nicotine level throughout the day (see Nursing Process: Patient-Centered Collaborative Care—Tobacco Use Disorder). Side effects include hypertension, tachycardia, dizziness, insomnia, irritability, anorexia, dyspepsia, nausea, vomiting, hiccups, and cough. In 2013 the FDA relaxed warnings about patients who relapse while using nicotine-replacement products; it was determined there are no significant safety concerns. Nicotine should be used during pregnancy only if the benefit outweighs the risk to the fetus. Nicotine has been shown to cause adverse fetal outcomes in animals; however, nicotine replacement is believed to be safer during pregnancy than smoking. Nicotine is excreted into breast milk and may increase infant heart rate; therefore a decision should be made to discontinue breastfeeding or discontinue the drug, taking into account the importance of the drug to the mother.

Bupropion, an antidepressant drug, increases levels of dopamine and norepinephrine in the brain, mimicking the effects of nicotine. It also has some neuronal nicotinic receptor–blocking activity, reducing reinforcement from the brain's reward circuit. When used for smoking cessation, the dosage is 150 mg ER once daily for 3 days; increase to 150 mg ER twice daily (maximum dose 300 mg ER/day) if tolerated. Treatment should continue for 7 to 12 weeks; however, ongoing treatment for a year has shown benefit.

When starting the drug, smokers continue to smoke for the first week but have a stop date set for the second week. If patients have not quit smoking by week 7, providers may add a nicotine replacement drug. Bupropion should not be used by those who have seizures or eating disorders. Additionally, it should not be taken within 14 days of taking a monoamine oxidase inhibitor (MAOI). Bupropion should not be stopped suddenly; instead, the patient should be weaned off the drug to avoid withdrawal symptoms. The drug can cause a false-positive drug screen; when providing urine for a drug screen, laboratory personnel should be told of bupropion use. Whether bupropion will harm the fetus is unknown, but it is excreted into breast milk; therefore a decision should be made to either discontinue breastfeeding or discontinue the drug, taking into account the importance of the drug to the mother.

Varenicline is a partial alpha-4–beta-2 nicotinic receptor agonist that stimulates dopamine activity in the brain but not to the extent of nicotine, thereby reducing cravings and withdrawal. Dosing begins 1 week before an identified quit date at 0.5 mg daily for 3 days, then 0.5 mg is taken twice daily for 4 days, then maintenance therapy begins at 1 mg twice daily for 11 weeks. Dosage is adjusted for patients with a creatinine clearance (CrCl) less than 30 mL/min (maximum dosage, 0.5 mg twice daily). Common side effects include nausea and vomiting, insomnia, headache, abnormal dreams, constipation or diarrhea, fatigue and malaise, upper respiratory tract infection, dyspnea, chest pain, abdominal pain, xerostomia, appetite changes, rash, and emotional disturbances. ⚡ Varenicline carries a black-box warning for serious neuropsychiatric symptoms including behavior changes, hostility, agitation, depression, and suicidality. Nurses must caution patients and their families about this warning and advise them to contact their provider immediately if suicidal thoughts or actions occur. It is unknown whether varenicline will harm the fetus or if it is excreted in breast milk; therefore a decision should be made to either discontinue breastfeeding or discontinue the drug, taking into account the importance of the drug to the mother.

To advocate for their patients, nurses must keep in mind that 80% of those with TUD who attempt to quit relapse in the first month; only 3% remain abstinent at 6 months. Patients with TUD require multiple attempts at quitting before they achieve sustained remission.

Box 8.4 discusses **e-cigarettes** (electronic cigarettes).

Other Substance Use Disorders

Cough and Cold Products. One in 10 adolescents has used cough and cold products to get high. Cough and cold products contain ingredients that are psychoactive when taken in higher-than-recommended amounts (sometimes up to 25 times the recommended dose). Dextromethorphan (DXM), an antitussive that can be purchased without a prescription, and promethazine-codeine cough syrup, available by prescription only, are the products most frequently misused. Using DXM is known on the street as "robotripping" or "skittling"; when taken in higher-than-recommended amounts, users may experience euphoria, dissociative effects, or hallucinations. Side effects of DXM include nausea and vomiting, stomach pain, confusion, dizziness, double or blurred vision, slurred speech, impaired coordination, tachycardia, drowsiness, numbness, and disorientation. Many of the DXM-containing products used to get high also contain other drugs, such as antihistamines, analgesics, or decongestants. High doses of these drugs can lead to hepatic damage or failure, cardiovascular effects, and coma.

Promethazine-codeine cough syrup can result in relaxation and euphoria when taken in higher-than-recommended amounts; when combined with soda, it is referred to as *Syrup, Sizzurp, Purple drank, Barre,* or *Lean.* Hard candy may be added for flavor. (See the previous section on OUD for information concerning codeine, an opioid drug.)

Teens may also misuse antihistamines, wherein they may take up to 40 tablets of dimenhydrinate or diphenhydramine. Apparently, such excessive doses induce feelings similar to a narcotic high, complete with hallucinations. Misusing these over-the-counter drugs is not without danger. The FDA reports teenagers ending up in emergency rooms or dying after participating in the "Benadryl Challenge" encouraged in videos posted on the social media application TikTok.

There are no FDA-approved drugs to treat substance use disorders related to cough and cold products. More research is needed to find out if behavioral therapies can be used to treat such misuse.

Anabolic-Androgenic Steroids. An anabolic-androgenic steroid (AAS) is a synthetic agent used to treat conditions caused by low levels of testosterone in the body, such as delayed puberty, hypogonadism, and cachexia related to chronic disease states. By binding to androgen receptors, these prescription drugs (e.g., danazol, fluoxymesterone, nandrolone, and oxandrolone) exert *anabolic effects,* such as growth of muscle and bone and red blood cell production, and *androgenic effects,* such as production of primary and secondary sexual characteristics.

BOX 8.4 Electronic Cigarettes (e-Cigarettes)

Electronic cigarettes are a tobacco product often marketed as a tool to stop smoking; however, marketing is also aimed at children and adolescents. A reported 2.4 million middle and high school students use e-cigarettes, also known as *Hookah Pens, e-Hookahs,* and *Vape Pipes.* E-cigarettes aerosolize "e-juice," a mixture of flavorings, propylene glycol (a toxic component of antifreeze), glycerin, and nicotine. The vapor from e-cigarettes contains heavy metals and formaldehyde, a breakdown product of propylene glycol. Because of this, the secondhand aerosol from e-cigarettes is also potentially harmful. Some of the flavors used in e-cigarettes contain carcinogens and other harmful chemicals. For example, the butter flavoring may contain diacetyl, the chemical used to give popcorn a buttery flavor and that causes irreversible lung disease when inhaled, a disease referred to a *popcorn lung.*

According to the Centers for Disease Control and Prevention (CDC), e-cigarettes are no safer than traditional tobacco cigarettes, nor are they a more effective method of quitting smoking than counseling and drug-assisted treatments. When users try to quit e-cigarettes, they experience the same withdrawal symptoms as users of traditional tobacco cigarettes, including irritability, depression, restlessness, and anxiousness. E-cigarettes increase the risk for myocardial infarction due to hypertension, tachycardia, and hardening of the arteries secondary to nicotine. Nicotine has been shown to adversely affect adolescent brain development, leading to cognitive and behavioral issues. There are more than 500 brands of e-cigarettes, each of which contains *some* level of nicotine—even those that claim they do not. E-juice refill cartridges often contain more nicotine than is indicated on the label.

In August 2016 the US Food and Drug Administration (FDA) began regulation of all tobacco products, including e-cigarettes, cigars, hookah tobacco, and pipe tobacco. The sale of all tobacco products, including e-cigarettes, will be prohibited to those under 18 years of age; packaging and marketing of all tobacco products, including e-cigarettes, will require the display of health warnings; and the FDA will be able to stop manufacturers from making statements about their products that have not been proven by research.

In 2019 the CDC released information identifying the additive vitamin E acetate in vaping products as the presumed causative agent in persons presenting with e-cigarette product use lung injury (EVALI). However, the CDC cautioned it was too soon to rule out other chemicals as additional causative agents. By November 2019, nearly 2300 cases of EVALI had been reported to the CDC from 49 states, including 47 deaths. Please refer to https://www.cdc.gov/tobacco/basic_information/e-cigarettes/severe-lung-disease.html for further information and updates.

Nurses who work with children and adolescents must be diligent in asking about the use of e-cigarettes and providing counseling concerning the dangers of using them. Related to this, they must ask about media and Internet usage and teach young people critical viewing skills; that is, they must help young people understand that what appears in the media does not always represent reality; often, it is a representation of someone's or something's special interest. Nurses must urge children and adolescents who use e-cigarettes to quit, and they must provide the help needed to achieve sustained remission.

BOX 8.5 Dehydroepiandrosterone

Dehydroepiandrosterone (DHEA), a precursor to testosterone and estrogen, can be found in many dietary supplements. Many people take supplements that contain DHEA in the belief that it will slow aging, increase energy levels, and build bone and muscle strength. However, there is no evidence to support these claims. Small studies have noted that DHEA may be effective in the relief of mild depression and skin changes associated with aging. Side effects include oily skin and acne, hair loss, nausea, hypertension, menstrual changes, deepening of the voice in women, fatigue, headache, irregular heartbeat, insomnia, and hypercholesterolemia. Long-term effects include stunting of growth, aggressive behavior, mood swings, and hepatic toxicity. Nurses who care for patients who take dietary supplements containing DHEA should be sure to counsel them about the risks and benefits associated with DHEA use.

extreme irritability, delusions, impaired judgment, and infection at the injection site. Long-term effects include kidney damage or failure, liver damage, high blood pressure, enlarged heart, or changes in cholesterol leading to increased risk of stroke or heart attack. Additionally, men may experience shrunken testicles, infertility, baldness, development of breasts, and an increased risk for prostate cancer. Women may experience excess facial and body hair, male-pattern baldness, menstrual cycle changes, enlargement of the clitoris, and deepened voice. Adolescents who use anabolic steroids may experience stunted bone growth and height.

Withdrawal from AAS use may lead to mood swings, fatigue, restlessness, loss of appetite, and decreased sex drive. ⚡ Nurses must be alert when caring for persons withdrawing from AAS use because withdrawal may cause depression lasting up to a year, which can result in suicide attempts. Antidepressants and behavioral therapy may be helpful.

Box 8.5 discusses dehydroepiandrosterone (DHEA) and its risks and benefits.

SPECIAL NEEDS OF PATIENTS WITH SUBSTANCE USE DISORDER

Surgical Patients

Patients with substance use disorder are at high risk for drug interactions, postoperative complications, and death when surgery is required. An assessment of drug use and application of the CAGE questionnaire, a screening tool for alcohol misuse, should be part of all patient histories. Respiratory changes in persons with TUD make introduction of endotracheal and suction tubes more difficult and increase the risk for postoperative respiratory problems. During the postoperative period, nurses should be alert for signs and symptoms of drug interactions with pain medications or anesthesia and for signs of withdrawal.

Special precautions must be taken for the patient with AUD who requires surgery. Alcohol use may be overlooked in an accident victim if there are injuries that cause CNS depression. In addition, many persons are undiagnosed as persons with AUD at the time of admission for elective surgery. The patient with AUD may require an increased level of anesthesia, which can increase the risk for cardiovascular instability in susceptible patients. Delirium may be triggered by surgery and abstinence. After surgery, patients with AUD may develop withdrawal syndrome, indicated by tremors, mild anxiety, gastric distress, and headache; left untreated, withdrawal may progress to withdrawal seizures or delirium tremens (DT), manifested by hallucinations, disorientation, tachycardia, hypertension, hyperthermia, agitation, and diaphoresis. Symptoms may develop anywhere from 6 hours to 5

Anabolic-androgenic steroids have been used to enhance athletic and sexual performance and physical appearance in all age groups. Evidence indicates AAS use by athletes ranges from 1% to 6%. Street names of these drugs include Juice, Gym Candy, Pumpers, Stackers, and Roids. The drug may be taken orally or may be administered IM in doses 10 to 100 times higher than what would be recommended for medical conditions.

Short-term effects of AAS use include headache, acne, fluid retention in the hands and feet, oily skin, yellowing of the skin and whites of the eyes, aggression, extreme mood swings, anger, paranoid jealousy, days after the last drink; left untreated, alcohol withdrawal syndrome can be fatal. Use of a tool, such as the Clinical Institute Withdrawal Assessment of Alcohol Scale, Revised (CIWA-Ar), can improve recognition and treatment of alcohol withdrawal. A copy of this tool can be found at https://www.uptodate.com/contents/image?imageKey=P-C%2F64835&topicKey=EM%2F323&source=see_link. The goal of treatment is the alleviation of symptoms and the provision of supportive care with fluids and nutrition.

Pain Management

Although health care personnel may be reluctant to administer narcotic analgesics to persons with substance use disorder, there is no evidence that providing narcotic analgesia to these patients in any way worsens their disease. *When patients experience pain, the goal is to treat the pain.* All patients should be treated with dignity and respect. Withholding adequate analgesia due to misconceptions leads to unnecessary suffering and harm and is a breach of the ethical principles central to nursing care. Addressing substance use disorder is *not* a priority when a patient is in pain.

When patients acknowledge substance use disorder, it is important to determine which drug is used and the amount taken each day. If the patient misuses opioids, it is often best to avoid further exposure to the drug of choice because recommended opioid doses do not provide adequate pain relief due to tolerance. Paradoxically, significantly increasing the dose of opioid in an effort to achieve pain control can induce hyperalgesia, where patients become abnormally sensitive to pain. Effective doses of other analgesics can be determined whether daily doses of the drug of choice are known. Nonopioid and adjuvant analgesics and nonpharmacologic pain relief measures may also be used, particularly when the person with OUD is on drug-assisted treatment with buprenorphine or naltrexone.

THE NURSE WITH SUBSTANCE USE DISORDER

Substance use disorder is no more prevalent among nurses than it is among the rest of the population. However, nurses care for others during the most vulnerable times of their life; nurses have the lives of others in their hands and are therefore held to a higher standard than other professionals. Drug use is a serious concern in health care professions. The most commonly used drugs include *cannabis*, cocaine, opioids, alcohol, and nicotine. It is estimated that 10% to 15% of nurses have substance use disorder.

Contributing Factors

Factors that contribute to drug use among nurses have been identified as job stress, the emotional demands of nursing, long hours and shift rotations, and easy access to drugs. Additionally, nurses internalize their feelings to stay in control during crisis and have little to no time to decompress. Nurses take care of others before themselves.

Characteristics

Signs and symptoms of substance use disorder may be indicated by changes in personality and behavior, including alterations in job performance, unexplained absence from the unit, arriving to work late and leaving early, poor judgment and errors (e.g., medication errors), alteration of verbal and telephone orders, and illogical documentation.

Signs and symptoms of substance use disorder also include physical changes. Behaviors related to influence of the drug or signs of withdrawal may also be present, such as subtle changes in appearance, self-imposed isolation, inappropriate responses to situations (i.e., both verbal and emotional), confusion, lapses in memory, and decreased levels of alertness.

Discrepancies in controlled-drug handling and records may indicate drug diversion, the deliberate redirecting of a drug from a patient or facility to the employee for personal use. Indications of drug diversion include frequent narcotic wastage, multiple corrections to medication records and other documentation, and frequent reports of uncontrolled pain from patients.

Nurses often enable drug use among coworkers by covering up their mistakes or tardiness, excusing their behavior, or simply ignoring obvious signs and symptoms. When it is recognized that a nurse is impaired, help for the nurse requires sharing observations and concerns with the nurse and supervisor to provide the means for rehabilitation. For more information related to substance use disorder among nurses, please go to the National Council of State Boards of Nursing (NCSBN) website at www.ncsbn.org.

Management

In most states, nurses may enter nondisciplinary programs designed for evaluation and treatment. These programs include compliance monitoring during treatment and recovery as well as abstinence monitoring upon the nurse's return to work. These programs allow nurses to maintain their licenses. The goals of these programs are to protect the safety of the public, to maintain the integrity of the profession, and to ensure that the nurse is offered the possibility of treatment and rehabilitation before the license to practice is revoked or the job is terminated. Further information can be found at www.ncsbn.org/substance-use-in-nursing.htm.

Given the prevalence of drug use, all nurses care for patients who use drugs, regardless of whether the use has been identified as substance use disorder. Therefore it is important for nurses to identify patients who misuse drugs and to intervene. Knowledge of the most commonly misused drugs and their treatments is critical to sustained remission and promotion of healthy lifestyles.

⊙ CLINICAL JUDGMENT [NURSING PROCESS]

Tobacco Use Disorder

Concept: Coping
- Coping is a process involving cognitive and behavioral actions designed to manage internal or external situations that are perceived as difficult and/or beyond the individual's current resources.

Concept: Safety
- Protecting the patient from potential or actual harm; is a basic human need

Recognize Cues [Assessment]
- Ask the patient to identify any barriers or impediments to quitting.

- Assess current smoking status and smoking history.
- Assess for feelings of hopelessness, depression, and apathy.
- Assess health history.
- Assess the patient's decision-making capacity.
- Determine the willingness of the patient to attempt to quit.
- Have the patient identify negative consequences of smoking and the potential benefits of quitting.
- Identify the cultural context of the patient's smoking pattern.
- Identify the patient's locus of control.
- Identify what rewards for quitting are most important to the patient.

⊚ CLINICAL JUDGMENT [NURSING PROCESS]—CONT'D

Tobacco Use Disorder

Analyze Cues and Prioritize Hypothesis [Patient Problems]
- Potential for nonadherence
- Coping/decreased ability to cope
- Need for health teaching

Generate Solutions [Planning]
- The patient begins to identify ways to achieve control over nicotine use.
- The patient demonstrates positive health maintenance behaviors as evidenced by keeping scheduled appointments and participating in a tobacco cessation program.
- The patient identifies and uses available resources.

Take Action [Nursing Interventions]
- Advise the patient to keep a list of "slips" and "near-slips" to learn to avoid their causes.
- Assist the patient with problem solving.
- Define your role as the patient's advocate.

- Encourage the patient to avoid environments and activities previously associated with smoking.
- Enhance the patient's sense of autonomy by involving the patient in decision making.
- Help the patient choose the best method to quit smoking based on patient preferences and anticipated benefits.
- Refer the patient to support groups or programs available in the community.
- Schedule frequent follow-up contacts with the patient to offer encouragement and help the patient deal with relapses.
- Set a quit date with the patient, ideally within 1 to 2 weeks.
- Teach the patient about drug-assisted treatment available to assist in smoking cessation.
- Teach the patient to anticipate the withdrawal symptoms and challenges of quitting.

Evaluate Outcomes [Evaluation]
- To avoid relapse, evaluate the effectiveness of the cessation plan, including the use of drug-assisted treatment and support systems.

▮ CRITICAL THINKING CASE STUDY

A 57-year-old man is admitted to the surgical unit in preparation for back surgery after conservative treatment for a recent back injury failed to relieve his pain. His wife tells the nurse she hopes the surgery will be successful. She confides that her husband has just been sitting around the house drinking more beer than usual because he has not been able to work. The patient appears relaxed and unconcerned about his anticipated surgery. He jokes with the nurse, telling her that he would be cured if "a cute young thing like her would only rub his back."

1. What assessments of the patient's alcohol use should the nurse make and communicate to the surgeon and anesthesiologist before he is further prepared for surgery?
2. During the patient's postoperative period, when will the nurse expect signs of withdrawal syndrome to occur?
3. What early signs and symptoms would alert the nurse to the development of withdrawal syndrome?
4. What goal of treatment during the patient's postoperative period is related to alcohol withdrawal syndrome?

▮ REVIEW QUESTIONS

1. When caring for a patient recovering from an episode of opioid toxicity, the nurse determines that the patient has opioid use disorder based on which finding?
   a. Withdrawal symptoms
   b. A history of daily use
   c. Craving that results in drug-seeking behaviors
   d. Intravenous, rather than oral, use of the drug
2. A patient hospitalized with a fractured femur after an automobile accident develops nausea and vomiting, abdominal cramps, and restlessness. The nurse suspects that the patient is experiencing which reaction?
   a. Opioid withdrawal
   b. Alcohol toxicity
   c. Flashbacks from LSD use
   d. Nicotine withdrawal
3. Which treatments will the nurse anticipate administering to a patient who has been admitted with alcohol toxicity? (Select all that apply.)
   a. Naloxone
   b. Thiamine
   c. Intravenous fluids
   d. Naltrexone
   e. Intravenous glucose solution
   f. Flumazenil

4. The nurse observes another nurse taking oral opioids from the medication room at the hospital. Which is the best action for the nurse who observes drug diversion to take?
   a. Report the finding to the nursing supervisor to enable the nurse's participation in a nondisciplinary program.
   b. Ignore the situation to protect the nurse from dismissal and possible loss of licensure.
   c. Confront the nurse and demand that the drugs be returned before someone notices their absence.
   d. Ask the nurse to request pain medications from a physician rather than stealing them from the hospital.
5. A patient is to start disulfiram to help with alcohol use disorder. The nurse providing medication education about the drug will include which topics in the education plan? (Select all that apply.)
   a. Importance of taking the medication every day
   b. That better results are experienced when a support group helps with treatment adherence
   c. Common food and hygiene products that contain alcohol
   d. That disulfiram treatment should be stopped 1 day before alcohol consumption
   e. That disulfiram works by disrupting the metabolism of alcohol
   f. That use of alcohol with disulfiram may cause nausea and vomiting and may even be fatal

9

Safety and Quality

http://evolve.elsevier.com/McCuistion/pharmacology

OBJECTIVES

- Describe the "Six Rights" of medication administration.
- Verbalize possible safety risks when administering patients' medications.
- Discuss the "Culture of Safety" and include the National Academy of Medicine's *To Err Is Human* and the American Nurses Association's "Just Culture" effect on nursing practice.
- Discuss the Quality and Safety Education for Nurses Institute (QSEN) competencies and how they relate to medication safety.
- Discuss safe disposal of medications.

- Discuss high-alert medications and strategies for safe administration.
- Discuss the Nurse's Bill of Rights and how it applies to medication administration.
- Discuss the US Food and Drug Administration's (FDA) pregnancy safety regulations.
- Apply Clinical Judgment [Nursing Process] to safe administration of medication.

OUTLINE

According to the IQVIA Institute for Human Data Science (2018–2020), spending on prescription medicines continues to increase each year. Medication spending in the United States is expected to increase from $344 billion to $420 billion by 2023, with medication errors listed as the third leading cause of death (https://www.iqvia.com/institute/reports/medicine-use-and-spending-in-usa).

The focus of this chapter is quality and safety in medication administration. It involves a discussion of safety initiatives and interventions that include the "Six Rights" of medication administration, the Nurse's Bill of Rights, the Quality and Safety Education for Nurses Competencies, the Culture of Safety, and The Joint Commission (TJC) National Patient Safety Goals. Also included are high-alert drugs, look-alike and sound-alike drugs, and dosage forms to crush or not to crush.

QUALITY AND SAFETY EDUCATION FOR NURSES

The Institute for Quality and Safety Education for Nurses provides competencies to help guide nurses in safe and comprehensive care. The focus of the competencies is on nurses' education, practice, and scholarship to help improve the quality and safety of the health care system in which nurses work. The competencies are as follows: Patient- and family-centered care (respecting the patients' rights); Collaboration and teamwork (interprofessional teams working together); Evidence-based practice (safe delivery of care based on current research); Quality improvement (improving patients' delivery of care); Safety (minimizing risk to patients); and Informatics (using technology to improve care). They represent six focus areas where quality and safety standards should be practiced. The competencies are vital to safe medication administration in nursing care.

"SIX RIGHTS" OF MEDICATION ADMINISTRATION

The "Six Rights" of medication administration are important goals for medication safety. The nurse following these guidelines will verify the following: (1) the right patient, (2) the right drug, (3) the right dose, (4) the right route, (5) the right time, and (6) the right documentation. The original six rights have included subsequent additions throughout the years in an attempt to maintain safety (e.g., right assessment, right education, right evaluation, and right of the patient to refuse). All interventions are designed to ensure safe medication practices. It is important to remember the nurse collaborates with other health care providers (HCPs; e.g., the physician, the pharmacist, and the nurse practitioner) to provide safe medication administration, and it's the nurse who relays the patient's response to the entire health care team.

Right Patient

The right patient determination is essential. The Joint Commission (TJC) requires at least two forms of identification before drug administration (http://www.jointcommission.org):

- Ask the patient to state their full name and birth date, and compare these with the patient's identification (ID) band and the medication administration record (MAR).
- Many facilities have electronic health records (EHRs) that allow the nurse to directly scan the bar code from the patient's ID band. Once the band is scanned, the patient's medication record appears for the nurse to view (Fig. 9.1). Additional nursing implications include the following:
  - Most hospitals have color-coded ID bands that include bands coded for allergy, do not resuscitate (DNR), fall risk, and restricted extremity. Always check facility policies for the use of color-coded bands and their meanings.
  - Verify the patient's identification by using two methods of identification each time a medication is administered.
  - If the patient is an adult with a cognitive disorder or a child, verify the patient's name with a family member. In the event a family member is unavailable and the patient is unable to self-identify, follow the facility's policy. Many facilities have policies that include a photo ID on the band with the patient's name and birth date affixed to the band.
  - Distinguish between two patients with the same first or last name by placing "name-alert" stickers as warnings on the medical records.

Right Drug

The nurse must accurately determine the right drug before administration. When working with an EHR, after scanning the wristband, the patient's drug profile appears on the computer screen. The nurse's next step is to scan the medication label, and it will automatically validate the time, date, and nurse administering the patient's medication. If it is not the correct medication, the nurse will receive an alert and will be unable to proceed in the MAR until the correct medication is scanned.

Both federal and state legislation governs who may write a prescription order. Medication orders are prescribed by a licensed HCP under authority from the state to prescribe drugs. The disciplines that have prescriptive authority are the medical doctor (MD), dentist (doctor of dental surgery [DDS]), podiatrist (doctor of podiatric medicine [DPM]), certified nurse practitioner (CNP), advanced practice registered nurse (APRN), physician assistant (PA), veterinarian (DVM), chiropractor

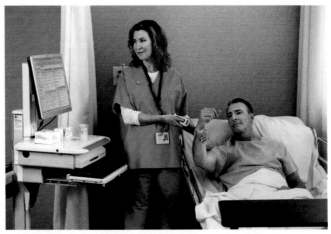

Fig. 9.1 Bar code scanner used to access the patient's medical record. (From Ignatavicius, D. D., Workman, L. M., Rebar, C. R., et al. [2018]. Medical-surgical nursing [9th ed.]. St. Louis: Elsevier.)

(DC), and optometrist (DO). In addition, medical clinical psychiatrists and pharmacists have prescriptive authority with strict guidelines set by the state. Prescriptions may be handwritten by the HCP, delivered as a telephone order (T/O) or verbal order (V/O), or directly entered into the patient's EHR. Handwritten prescriptions are written on a provider's legal prescription pad and are filled by a pharmacist.

Sometimes providers order medications by directly speaking to the nurse. All telephone orders or verbal orders for medications are either handwritten by the nurse taking the order or entered directly into a computer and "read back" to ensure accuracy. The nurse will write the name of the prescribing provider and add a notation that the order was verified. The order will be completed when the doctor affixes their signature onto the order. After dictating a verbal order, the provider must sign it within 24 hours. If the order is a controlled medication, most facilities require two licensed nurses to listen to the order and sign it. Nursing students are not allowed to accept or take provider orders, but they may administer the medication after a registered nurse (RN) has verified it.

Many hospitals are implementing computerized physician order entry (CPOE) systems to handle HCP medication orders. This method of ordering medications can help decrease drug errors by decreasing transcription errors. HCPs using a CPOE will directly input the prescription into the patient's EHR; the order is electronically signed by the HCP and is sent directly to the pharmacy, and it is recorded as part of the patient's MAR. A strong safety feature is the ability to identify drug interactions with the patient's current drugs and any newly prescribed medications.

The use of computerized ordering systems has added speed and a measure of safety to the ordering process. Orders can be written from virtually any location and sent electronically, but the computer will not process the order until all necessary information is provided. Because the order is computerized, illegible orders or signatures are prevented. Before the nurse can administer the medication, both pharmacy and the nurse must validate the accuracy of the patient's prescription order in the EHR.

The components of a drug order are as follows (Fig. 9.2):
- Patient name and birth date
- Date the order is written
- Provider signature or name if an electronic order, T/O, or V/O
- Signature of licensed staff who took the T/O or V/O, if applicable
- HCPs who wish to prescribe controlled drugs must register with the US Federal Drug Enforcement Agency (DEA); when prescribing controlled substances, the HCP's DEA number must be on the prescription

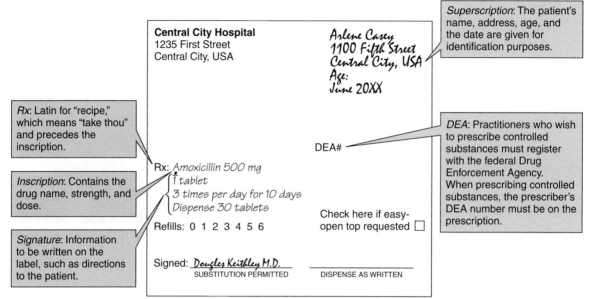

Fig. 9.2 Example of a drug order. (From Medical School Headquarters. [n.d.] Prescription writing 101. Retrieved from http://medicalschoolhq.net/prescription-writing-101.)

- Drug name and strength
- Drug frequency or dose (e.g., once daily)
- Route of administration
- Duration of administration (e.g., ×7 days, ×3 doses, when applicable)
- Number of patient refills
- Number of pills to be dispensed
- Any special instructions for withholding or adjusting dosage based on nursing assessment, drug effectiveness, or laboratory results

It is the nurse's responsibility to administer the drug, as ordered, by the provider, and if the drug order is incomplete, the drug should not be administered. Verification of a questionable order must be done in a timely manner. The HCP is usually contacted, and the conversation is documented. Nurses must become familiar with the components of a drug order and question any incomplete or unclear orders. Nurses are legally liable if they give a prescribed drug and the dosage is incorrect, or if the drug is contraindicated for the patient's health status. Once the drug has been administered, the nurse becomes liable for the predicted effects of that drug.

Medication administration is never considered just a process of "passing" drugs. Nurses must use critical thinking skills and assess whether the medication is correct for the patient's diagnosis. The nurse must ask critical questions: Is the dose appropriate? What is the patient's expected response? Also, the nurse must teach the patient about the drug's side effects and when it is necessary for the patient to notify the HCP.

To avoid drug errors, the drug label should be read three times: (1) when the nurse picks up the drug and removes it from the automatic dispensing cabinet (ADC), (2) as the nurse prepares the drug for administration, and (3) when the nurse administers the drug.

Nursing interventions related to drug orders can ensure correct administration of medications:

- The nurse should verify the identity of the patient by comparing the name on the wristband with the name on the MAR for accuracy.
- Always use two patient identifiers, such as having patients repeat their name and date of birth.
- The nurse must become familiar with the patient's health history and always perform a head-to-toe assessment on the patient, including a complete set of vital signs.

- Always review the patient's laboratory work before the administration of drugs.
- Read the drug order carefully. If the order is unclear, verify it with the HCP before administering the drug.
- Know the patient's allergies.
- Know the reason the patient is to receive the medication.
- Check the drug label by identifying the drug name, the amount of the drug (tablet or volume), and its suitability for administration by the intended route.
- Check dosage calculations.
- Know the date the medication was ordered and ending date. Some agencies have automatic stop orders that are generally facility specific. Examples of such orders include controlled drugs that need to be renewed every 48 hours, antibiotics usually renewed every 7 to 14 days, and cancellation of all medications when the patient goes to surgery.
- All orders—including first-dose, one-time, and as-needed (PRN) medication orders—should be checked against the original orders.

Right Dose

The **right dose** refers to verification by the nurse that the dose administered is the amount ordered, and that it is safe for the patient for whom it is prescribed. The right dose is based on the patient's physical status. Many medications require the patient's weight to determine the right dose. Usually pediatrics, medical-surgical, and critical care situations require weight to complete the drug calculation and determine the correct dose (heparin and digoxin drips are examples of medications calculated according to weight). The nurse determines whether the drug is safe to administer according to the drug's pharmacodynamics (action) and the patient's vital signs.

Before administration, it is important the nurse carefully review the patient's current laboratory results. A chemistry panel includes renal and liver function and sodium and potassium levels. Renal and hepatic functions are important considerations because many drugs are cleared through the kidneys and metabolized by the liver. Also, the nurse should review the hematology laboratory reports, which include a complete blood count (CBC), red blood cells (RBCs), hemoglobin, hematocrit, and platelets. It is most important that the nurse check the

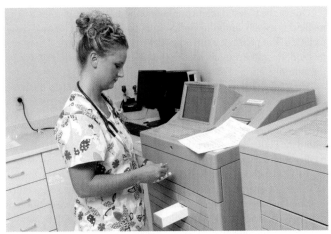

Fig. 9.3 Automated dispensing cabinet used to hold patients' medications for dispensing. (From Potter, P. A., & Perry, A. G. [2009]. *Fundamentals of nursing* [7th ed.]. St. Louis: Elsevier.)

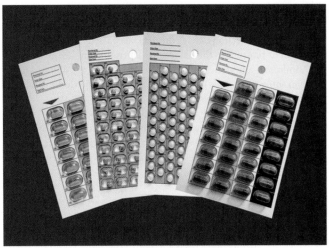

Fig. 9.4 Unit dose sheets. (Courtesy Omnicell, Inc.)

drug's correct dose range in a reliable drug resource book or by consulting with a pharmacist. In most cases, the right dose for a specific patient is within the recommended range for the drug.

Nurses use dimensional analysis or ratio and proportion when calculating a drug dose (Chapter 11). Always recheck the drug calculation, especially if the dose is within a fraction or an extremely large dose. Consult another nurse or the pharmacist when in doubt.

Today, most drugs are dispensed through automated dispensing cabinets (ADCs) (Fig. 9.3), which are computerized drug storage cabinets that store and dispense medications near the point of care while controlling and tracking drug distribution. The patient's drugs are stocked in the cabinet by the pharmacist and are accessed under the patient's name. The nurse can select and pull the patient's drugs from the cabinet. This technology improves patient care by promoting accurate and quick access to medications, locked storage for all medications, and electronic tracking for controlled substances. Automation of drug administration saves time and decreases costs associated with drug administration.

Another method of dispensing drugs is the unit dose method, in which drugs are individually wrapped and labeled for single-dose use for each patient. The unit dose method has reduced dosage errors because no calculations are required. Some facilities still use a multidose vial from the ADC. If this occurs, the nurse must complete a calculation to retrieve the correct amount ordered by the physician from the vial. If there is any medication left in the vial, it is disposed of according to the facility's policy for disposal of drugs.

Long-term care, day care, and assisted living facilities use punch cards to organize medications. This special packaging is obtained from the facility's pharmacy. The pharmacy sends a 30-day supply of medication for each prescription in a punch card, and the nurse administers the medication from the card (Fig. 9.4).

An important nursing intervention related to the right dose includes calculating the drug dose correctly. If in doubt about the amount to be administered, consult with a nurse peer to validate the correct amount. In some settings, two RNs are required to check the dosage for certain medications, such as insulin and heparin.

Right Time

The right time refers to the time the prescribed dose is ordered for administration. Daily drug dosages are given at specified intervals, such as twice a day (bid), three times a day (tid), four times a day (qid), or every 6 hours; this is so the plasma level of the drug is maintained at

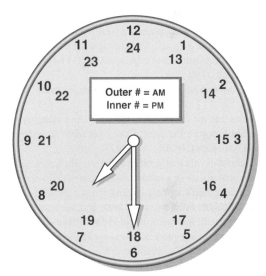

Fig. 9.5 Military time.

a therapeutic level. Every drug cannot be given exactly when ordered; therefore health care agencies have policies that specify a range of times within which drugs can be administered (check your agency's policy). When a drug has a long half-life, it is usually given once a day. Drugs with a short half-life are given several times a day at specified intervals. Some drugs are given before meals, whereas others must be given with meals.

Use of military time, which is based on a 24-hour clock (Fig. 9.5), reduces administration errors and decreases documentation. Many nursing facilities use military time rather than standard time. Nursing interventions related to the right time include the following:

- Administer drugs at the specified times (refer to agency policy).
- Administer drugs that are affected by food, such as tetracycline, 1 hour before or 2 hours after meals.
- Give food with drugs that can irritate the stomach (gastric mucosa)—for example, potassium and aspirin. Some medications are absorbed better after eating.
- Adjust the medication schedule to fit the patient's lifestyle, activities, tolerances, or preferences as much as possible.
- Check whether the patient is scheduled for any diagnostic procedures that contraindicate the administration of medications, such

as endoscopy or fasting blood tests. Determine whether the medication should be given before or after the test based on the policy.

- Check the expiration date. If the date has passed, discard the medication or return it to the pharmacy, depending on the policy.
- Administer antibiotics at even intervals (e.g., every 8 hours rather than three times daily) throughout the 24-hour period to maintain therapeutic blood levels.
- Patients who require dialysis usually have blood pressure medications stopped before dialysis because dialysis can decrease blood pressure. However, some doctors order the medications to be given before dialysis. If any questions arise, check with the HCP before proceeding.

Right Route

The right route is necessary for adequate or appropriate absorption. The right route is ordered by the HCP and indicates the mechanism by which the medication enters the body. The more common routes of absorption include the following: oral (drug in the form of a liquid, elixir, or suspension); pill (tablet or capsule); sublingual (under the tongue for venous absorption); buccal (between the cheek and gum); feeding tube (enteral); topical (applied to the skin); inhalation (aerosol sprays); otic (ear); ophthalmic (eye); nasal (spray instillation); suppository (rectal or vaginal); and through the parenteral routes: (1) intradermal, (2) subcutaneous (subcut or SQ), (3) intramuscular (IM), or (4) intravenous (IV).

Nursing interventions related to the right route include the following:

- Assess the patient's ability to swallow before administering oral medications; ensure the patient does not have an order requiring nothing by mouth (NPO).
- Do not crush or mix medications in other substances without consulting a pharmacist or a reliable drug reference. Do not mix medications in an infant's formula feeding.
- If the medication must be mixed with another substance, explain this to the patient. For example, elderly patients may use applesauce or yogurt to mix their medications to make them easier to swallow. Medications should be administered one at a time in the substance.
- Best Practice Guidelines and TJC state that drugs must be identifiable up until the point of delivery. When administering many drugs at one time, it is *not* recommended to mix drugs together. The correct practice is to administer one pill at a time. When a patient has an enteral tube, it is important to follow these guidelines; this allows the nurse to flush the tube before and after each pill or liquid is administered to prevent the tube from clogging. In the event the patient's drug inadvertently falls to the ground, the nurse will be able to identify, discard, and replace the pill.
- Instruct the patient that medications must be swallowed with water. Juice can interfere with the absorption of certain medications; however, it is recommended that iron be taken with orange juice or vitamin C supplements to aid in its absorption.
- Use aseptic technique when administering drugs. Sterile technique is required with the parenteral routes.
- Administer drugs at the appropriate sites for the route.
- Stay with the patient until oral drugs have been swallowed.

Right Documentation

The right documentation requires the nurse to immediately record the appropriate information about the drug administered. Many systems are available for documenting drug administration. Both paper and computerized MAR systems include: information about the drug to be administered, including (1) the name of the drug, (2) the dose, (3) the route, (4) the time and date, and (5) the nurse's initials or signature.

One of the oldest documentation methods is the paper MAR. This method is usually found in clinics, nursing homes, and assisted living facilities. The pharmacy furnishes a written MAR record. Using this method, the nurse initials next to the patient's name and drug, verifying administration of the drug.

Most large facilities have computerized charting, in which the nurse enters a personal identification and password to enter the system. By scanning the patient's identification band, which includes the patient's bar code information, the nurse accesses the patient's personal MAR within the EHR system. Once the nurse scans the bar code on the patient's medication package, the administration is validated in the computerized MAR. The computerized system interfaces with other departments, including the pharmacy, laboratory, and sometimes the physician's office.

Documentation of the patient's response to the medication is required with a variety of medications such as (1) opioid and nonopioid analgesics (How effective was pain relief?); (2) sedatives (How effective was relaxation?); and (3) antiemetics (Was nausea/vomiting decreased or eliminated?). The nurse continues to assess and evaluate the patient's response to the medication. (For example: Is there any gastrointestinal upset or skin sensitivity?) All information obtained is documented into the patient's medical record. Keep in mind that patient responses are not necessarily verbal; they may be physiologic (e.g., blood pressure decreasing in response to an antihypertensive).

Delay in scanning/charting may result in forgetting to chart the medication, and another nurse can inadvertently readminister the drug, assuming it was not given because it was not charted. Therefore it is important to remember that drugs *must* be charted when the drug is administered. Graphic formats or computerized systems (Fig. 9.6) assist in the accurate and timely recording of drugs administered.

The American Nurses Association (ANA) published a Bill of Rights for nurses containing seven premises concerning workplace expectations and environments that nurses from across the United States recognize as necessary for safe nursing practice. The Bill of Rights supports nurses in workplace situations and includes issues such as unsafe staffing, mandatory overtime, and health and safety issues in the workplace. These issues are essential to meet the responsibilities of patient care, including safe drug administration and the responsibility nurses have to themselves (http://www.nursingworld.org).

Facilities have an obligation to both nurses and patients to educate and provide guidelines and policies concerning patient safety in all aspects of patient care. Many disciplines are involved in medication administration, and the different departments must work together to provide a method of drug delivery and administration in a safe environment for the patient and the nurse. This can be done by having modern equipment, staff education opportunities, policies and procedures, and communication among the different departments involved in drug administration.

JUST AND SAFE CULTURE

The National Coordinating Council for Medication Error Reporting (NCCMERP 2020) defines medication error as "any preventable event that may cause or lead to inappropriate medication use or harm to a patient while the medication is in the control of the health care professional" (http://www.nccmerp.org).

Much progress has been made concerning the area of patient safety to embrace change in the medical culture so reporting of errors does not result in personal blame but a failure of the system. The landmark decision of the National Academy of Medicine (previously known as the Institute of Medicine) report, *To Err Is Human: Building a Safer Health Care System,* has certainly effected a positive change in the development of a "Culture of Safety." The report serves as a basis for creating an awareness of patient safety systems in health care and has led to the

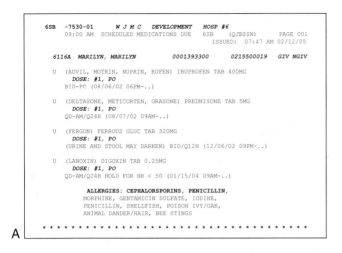

```
6SB  -7530-01    W J M C  DEVELOPMENT   HOSP #6
     09:00 AM SCHEDULED MEDICATIONS DUE  6SB  (QJB$$N)    PAGE 001
                                  ISSUED:  07:47 AM 02/12/05

     6116A  MARILYN, MARILYN      0001393300    0215500019  GIV NGIV

  U  (ADVIL, MOTRIN, NUPRIN, RUFEN) IBUPROFEN TAB 400MG
         DOSE: #1, PO
      BID-PC (08/06/02 06PM-..)

  U  (DELTASONE, METICORTEN, ORASONE) PREDNISONE TAB 5MG
         DOSE: #1, PO
      QD-AM/Q24H (08/07/02 09AM-..)

  U  (FERGON) FERROUS GLUC TAB 320MG
         DOSE: #1, PO
      (URINE AND STOOL MAY DARKEN) BID/Q12H (12/06/02 09PM-..)

  U  (LANOXIN) DIGOXIN TAB 0.25MG
         DOSE: #1, PO
      QD-AM/Q24H HOLD FOR HR < 50 (01/15/04 09AM-..)

         ALLERGIES: CEPHALORSPORINS, PENICILLIN,
         MORPHINE, GENTAMICIN SULFATE, IODINE,
         PENICILLIN, SHELLFISH, POISON IVY/OAK,
         ANIMAL DANDER/HAIR, BEE STINGS

A  * * * * * * * * * * * * * * * * * * * * * * * * * * * * *
```

UNIVERSITY HOSPITAL

Nurse's Signature/Title		Initials
Evelyn Hayes RN		EH
Joyce Kee RN		JK
Rodney Brown LPN		RB
Jody Smith LPN		JS

Allergies: *Codeine*

Continuing Medical Record

		Date	8/14	8/15	8/16	8/17
8/14	Digoxin 0.125 mg po qd	0900	EH	EH	JK	
EH				AR=74	AR=70	AR=70
8/14	Capoten 12.5 mg po bid	0900	EH	EH	JK	
EH		2100	RB	RB	RB	
8/15	8/22	Amoxicillin 250 mg po q6h	0600			JS
EH	LD 0500	x7d	1200		EH	JK
1100			1800		RB	RB
			2400		JS	JS

One-Time/PRN/STAT Medications

Date	Medication/Dosage/Route/Frequency	Time/Initials	Reason	Result
8/14	Nitroglycerin 1/150 gr sublingual PRN	1600 EH	Chest pain	Relief of pain
	Chest pain			

B

Fig. 9.6 Medication record. (A) Computerized format. (B) Written format. Labeling for Human Prescription Drug & Biological Products.

TABLE 9.1   "Do Not Use" Abbreviations

The Joint Commission's "Do Not Use List" of abbreviations is shown below. These abbreviations must be written out to avoid misinterpretation. Please visit http://www.thejointcommission.org and http://www.ismp.org for detailed safety information concerning "Do Not Use" abbreviations.

Do Not Use Abbreviation	Use Instead
q.d., Q.D., QD, qd	Write "daily."
q.o.d., Q.O.D., QOD, qod	Write "every other day."
U, u	Write "unit."
IU	Write "International Unit."
MS	Write "morphine sulfate."
$MgSO_4$, MSO_4	Write "magnesium sulfate."
Lack of leading zero (.X mg)	Use a zero before a decimal point when the dose is less than a whole unit (e.g., write 0.X mg).
Trailing zero (X.0 mg)	Do not use a decimal point or zero after a whole number (write X mg).

Copyright © 2019 The Joint Commission.

processes are caught and resolved. The most common occurrence of sentinel events is medication errors, and of those, the most frequently implicated drug was potassium chloride (KCl). Most often, KCl was mistaken for sodium chloride, heparin, or furosemide.

The Joint Commission National Patient Safety Goals

Additionally, TJC has taken steps to support safety and quality care in the workplace. TJC has developed National Patient Safety Goals, which focus on problems in health care safety and how to solve them. These goals are updated and published annually. Once a goal becomes a standard, the goal number is retired and is not used again, and the standard must be adopted by all TJC-accredited agencies. Two important goals that have already become standards for all TJC-accredited organizations are the "do not use" abbreviations (Table 9.1) and the list of acceptable abbreviations (Table 9.2).

US Food and Drug Administration

Another safety feature is the US Food and Drug Administration's (FDA) black-box warning system. When a prescription drug is known to be effective for some patients, but may cause serious side effects in others, the FDA will require the drug's printed materials to carry a warning about the adverse effects surrounded by a black box. A black-box warning is the strongest form of warning issued by the FDA about a drug (http://fda.gov).

Drug Reconciliation

Drug reconciliation is an important component of the culture of safety. It is defined as the process of identifying the most accurate list of all medications that the patient is taking at transitions in care. This includes admission and discharge from a hospital to another health care setting such as long-term care facility. Correct drug reconciliation is important because it prevents discrepancies that can cause a drug error. One in five patients experience an adverse event when transitioning from hospital to home.

Drug reconciliation was created to provide drug continuity during care transitions, thereby promoting patient safety. For this reason, the nurse should advise patients to do the following:

- Always carry a list of personal drug information in case of an emergency.
- Update this list of drugs whenever a change occurs.
- Bring a list of medications to each HCP appointment.

development of safety tools instrumental in decreasing the number of drug errors. Over the past 18 years, drug administration and the margin of error have shown some improvements with the development of bar coding, CPOE systems, EHRs, and ADCs. However, there is still much work ahead. The ANA's position statement titled "Just Culture" encourages individuals to report drug errors, so the system can be repaired and the problems fixed. "Just Culture" does not hold individual practitioners responsible for a failing system, although it does not tolerate disregard for a patient or gross misconduct (http://www.nursing world.org).

In a true culture of safety, everyone in the organization is committed and driven to keep patients safe from harm. Risk management is a process that identifies weaknesses in the system. It then allows changes to be made to minimize the effects of adverse patient outcomes. Most organizations have a risk management department staffed with nurse managers and risk managers who conduct root cause analysis (RCA), a method of problem solving used to identify potential workplace errors. Such analysis presents opportunities for learning and focuses on strategies that can be put in place to correct problems.

Drug administration is a vulnerable area where the possibility for error is high. If a patient is injured or dies as the result of a drug error, a sentinel event occurs. This is an unanticipated event in a health care setting that results in death or serious harm to a patient unrelated to the natural course of the patient's illness. TJC tracks sentinel events in a database to ensure they are adequately analyzed and that unsafe

TABLE 9.2 Acceptable Abbreviations

These abbreviations are frequently used in drug therapy and a must for nurses to learn. In addition, check your facility's list of medical abbreviations. It is a standard of The Joint Commission that each facility have a list of acceptable medication abbreviations.

Abbreviation	Meaning
Drug Measurements and Drug Forms	
cap	capsule
elix	elixir
ER	extended release
g	gram
gtt	drops
kg	kilogram
L	liter
m^2	square meter
mcg	microgram
mEq	milliequivalent
mg	milligram
mL	milliliter
NKA	no known allergies
NKDA	no known drug allergies
oz	ounce
SR	sustained release
Half-tablet	one-half tablet
supp	suppository
susp	suspension
Tbsp, tbs, or T	tablespoon
Tsp	teaspoon
Routes of Medication Administration	
ID	intradermal
Inj	injection
IM	intramuscular

IV	intravenous
IVPB	intravenous piggyback
KVO	keep vein open
PO	by mouth
SUBCUT	subcutaneous
S/S	sliding scale
TKO	to keep open
vag	vaginal

Times of Administration	
Prior Usage	Current Usage
AD, OS, OU	right ear, left ear, each ear
OD, OS, OU	right eye, left eye, or each eye
ad lib	as desired
bid (twice a day)	BID or bid
D/C	discharge or discontinue
hr (hour)	hr or hrs
hs	bedtime
NPO (nothing by mouth)	NPO
Per os	PO, by mouth, or orally
PCA (patient-controlled analgesia)	PCA
per (through, by [route])	per
prn (as needed)	PRN
qd	daily, every or each day
qh or q1h	every hr or every 1 hr
qid (four times daily)	QID or qid
q2h, q4h, etc.	every 2 hrs, every 4 hrs, etc.
UD	as directed
stat	immediately, at once
tid (three times a day)	TID or tid

Please visit http://www.jointcommission.org and www.ismp.org for detailed safety information concerning "Acceptable Abbreviations."

Disposal of Medications

The FDA and the DEA issue guidelines for appropriate disposal of prescription drugs based on the Secure and Responsible Disposal Act issued by Congress in 2010. This encourages both public and private entities to develop secure, convenient, and responsible methods for collecting and destroying medications and controlled substances. It also recommends a decrease in the amount of controlled substances released into the environment, especially into water and sewage systems.

General guidelines include drug take-back events, mail-back programs, and collection receptacles provided by authorized DEA collection companies for facilities to dispose of unwanted controlled substances. Facilities may contract with an independent or local collection program authorized by the state and the DEA to dispose of medical waste and hazardous materials. The drugs are disposed of in a receptacle that must comply with strict security and record-keeping requirements as established by the FDA and DEA. The company then incinerates the waste.

Consumers who do not have available DEA-authorized collectors or medicine take-back programs can follow these simple steps:

1. Remove medications from the original packaging and mix them (do not crush tablets or capsules) with an unpalatable substance such as dirt, kitty litter, or used coffee grounds. This method is intended to make medications less attractive to people and animals.
2. Place the mixture in a container such as a sealed plastic bag.
3. Throw the container in the household trash.
4. Scratch out all personal information on the prescription label before disposing of the empty container.

Unless specifically instructed, do not flush drugs down the toilet, where they will pollute the environment and pose a danger to humans and animals. (Exceptions to this rule are listed in Box 9.1.) Nurses and patients can consult a pharmacist with questions related to medication disposal. Pharmacists are always available to answer questions on how to properly dispose of unused medications (http://dea.org/disposalact).

Sharps Safety

US hospital-based health care professionals experience more than 385,000 needlestick injuries each year (http://www.cdc.gov/sharpssafety. html). The ANA's campaign for "Safe Needles Save Lives" prompted the Occupational Safety and Health Administration (OSHA) to enforce a

BOX 9.1   Medications Recommended for Disposal by Flushing[a]

Medicine	Active Ingredient
Abstral, tablets (sublingual)	fentanyl
Actiq, oral transmucosal lozenge	fentanyl citrate
Belbuca, soluble film (buccal)	buprenorphine hydrochloride
Buprenorphine; Naloxone, tablets (sublingual)	buprenorphine hydrochloride; naloxone hydrochloride
Butrans, transdermal patch system	buprenorphine
Daytrana, transdermal patch system	methylphenidate
Demerol, tablets	meperidine hydrochloride
Demerol, oral solution	meperidine hydrochloride
Diastat/Diastat AcuDial, rectal gel	diazepam
Dilaudid, tablets	hydromorphone hydrochloride
Dilaudid, oral liquid	hydromorphone hydrochloride
Dolophine hydrochloride, tablets	methadone hydrochloride
Duragesic, patch (extended release)	fentanyl
Embeda, capsules (extended release)	morphine sulfate; naltrexone hydrochloride
Exalgo, tablets (extended release)	hydromorphone hydrochloride
Fentora, tablets (buccal)	fentanyl citrate
Hysingla ER, tablets (extended release)	hydrocodone bitartrate
Kadian, capsules (extended release)	morphine sulfate
Methadone hydrochloride, oral solution	methadone hydrochloride
Methadose, tablets	methadone hydrochloride
Morphabond ER, tablets (extended release)	morphine sulfate
Morphine sulfate, tablets (immediate release)	morphine sulfate
Morphine sulfate, oral solution	morphine sulfate
MS Contin, tablets (extended release)	morphine sulfate
Nucynta ER, tablets (extended release)	tapentadol
Onsolis, soluble film (buccal)	fentanyl citrate
Opana, tablets (immediate release)	oxymorphone hydrochloride
Opana ER, tablets (extended release)	oxymorphone hydrochloride
Oxecta, tablets (immediate release)	oxycodone hydrochloride
Oxycodone, capsules	oxycodone hydrochloride
Oxycodone, oral solution	oxycodone hydrochloride
Oxycontin, tablets (extended release)	oxycodone hydrochloride
Percocet, tablets	acetaminophen; oxycodone hydrochloride
Percodan, tablets	aspirin; oxycodone hydrochloride
Suboxone, film (sublingual)	buprenorphine hydrochloride; naloxone hydrochloride
Targiniq ER, tablets (extended release)	oxycodone hydrohloride; naloxone hydrochloride
Xartemis XR, tablets	oxycodone hydrochloride; acetaminophen
Xtampza ER, capsules (extended release)	oxycodone
Xyrem, oral solution	sodium oxybate
Zohydro ER, capsules (extended release)	hydrocodone bitartrate
Zubsolv, tablets (sublingual)	buprenorphine hydrochloride; naloxone hydrochloride

US Food and Drug Administration. Medications recommended for disposal by flushing: Listed by medicine and active ingredient. Retrieved from https://www.fda.gov/media/85219/download.

[a]The FDA believes the known risk of harm, including death, from accidental exposure to the drugs listed above far outweighs any potential risk to humans or the environment from flushing of these medications (www.fda.gov/2018).

Needlestick Safety and Prevention Act (NSPA). The act requires that employers implement safer medical devices for their employees, provide a safe and secure workplace environment with educational opportunities, and develop written policies to help prevent sharps injuries.

SAFETY RISKS WITH MEDICATION ADMINISTRATION

Every year the United States experiences 1.5 million preventable drug errors. Data support that a hospitalized patient is subject to one medication administration error per day. Most medication errors occur in the transcription stage (56%), followed by the nurse administration stage (41%), and finally the doctor prescribing stage (39%) (https://www.iqvia.com).

Examples of risks to safety include the following:

- *Tablet splitting.* In effort to counteract steeply rising drug costs, some patients are cutting their pills in half. However, this is not recommended by the FDA. The only time tablet splitting is advisable is when it is specified by the pharmacist on the label. Splitting tablets is risky because the patient may not receive an equal distribution of the medication with each dose. Some tablets are not recommended for splitting and are difficult to split. The FDA recommends that a

TABLE 9.3 Abbreviations for Sustained- or Extended-Release Medications

Abbreviation	Meaning
CD	Controlled delivery
CR	Controlled release
DR	Delayed release
ER	Extended release
IR	Immediate release
LA	Long-acting
LAR	Long-acting release
MR	Modified release
PR	Prolonged release
SA	Sustained action (ambiguous, can also mean short acting)
SR	Sustained release
TR	Timed release
XR	Extended release
XT	Extended release
XL	Extended release

patient receive advice directly from the pharmacist to determine whether tablet splitting is appropriate for a particular drug.

- *Buying drugs over the Internet.* Consumers may find it convenient to order drugs over the Internet, but precautions must be taken because drugs sold online may be too old, too strong, or too weak to be effective. Online sources may sell expired medications without the consumer knowing. The FDA suggests drugs obtained from these sites may not be made using safe standards, are unsafe to use with other medications, and may be expired. Patients should look for websites that (1) require a prescription from an HCP; (2) have a licensed pharmacist to answer questions and a contact person to consult if problems arise; (3) are in the United States; and (4) are licensed by the state board of pharmacy. Some sites may sell counterfeit drugs.

Counterfeit Drugs

Counterfeit drugs look like the desired drug but may have no active ingredient, the wrong active ingredient, or the wrong amount of active ingredient. Improper packaging and contamination are also problems. Counterfeit drugs may look remarkably like the real thing. To report suspected counterfeit products, call the FDA Office of Counterfeit Issues at 1-800-551-3989. To reduce the risk of exposure to counterfeit drugs, patients should purchase drugs only from licensed pharmacies.

Dosage Forms: To Crush or Not to Crush

Although some drugs can be crushed, there are many that shouldn't be crushed. Always consult with the pharmacist or, when possible, the HCP before crushing a patient's drug. Also, consult a reliable drug guide to confirm the medication is crushable. Do not crush any extended- or sustained-release drugs because this will change the pharmacokinetic phase of the drug. There is no industry standard for sustained- or extended-release abbreviations, which can cause confusion and drug errors. Table 9.3 includes abbreviations for sustained- and extended-release drugs. For a current complete listing of drugs that should not be crushed, see http://www.ismp.org/do-not-crush.

⚠ High-Alert Medications

High-alert drugs can cause significant harm to the patient. If a high-alert medication is given in error, it can have a major effect on the

patient's organs; this includes cardiac, respiratory, vascular, and neurologic systems. A high-alert drug can also affect the sympathetic and parasympathetic nervous systems. Specific high-alert medications as listed by the Institute for Safe Medication Practices (ISMP) include epinephrine (SQ); epoprostenol (IV); insulin (SQ and IV); magnesium sulfate injection; methotrexate (oral nononcologic use); opium tincture; oxytocin (IV); nitroprusside sodium for injection; potassium chloride concentrate for injection; potassium phosphate injection; promethazine (IV); and vasopressin (IV). Please note that all forms of insulin, subcutaneous and IV, are considered high-alert medications. For additional classes and categories of high-alert medications, visit the Institute for Safe Medication Practice's website at http://www.ismp.org/. Lists are provided to reduce the risk of errors, but specific strategies can optimize safety when dealing with high-alert drugs:

1. Simplify the storage, preparation, and administration of high-alert drugs.
2. All high-alert medications must be confirmed and documented by two nurses before administering.
3. Write policies concerning safe administration.
4. Improve information and education.
5. Limit access to high-alert medications.
6. Use labels and automated alerts.
7. Use redundancies (automated or independent double-checks).
8. Closely monitor the patient's response to the medication (possibly the most important step).

⚡ Look-Alike and Sound-Alike Drug Names

Nurses should be aware that certain drug names sound alike and are spelled similarly. Examples of drugs involved in medication errors and recognized as confusing drug names include *CeleXA* with *CeleBREX*; *diazePAM* with *dilTIAZem*; *ePHEDrine* with *EPINEPHrine*; *glipiZIDE* with *glyBURIDE*; *HumaLOG* with *HumuLIN*; *SOLU-Medrol* with *Solu-CORTEF*; *SOLU-Medrol* with *DEPO-Medrol*; *ZyrTEC* with *ZyPREXA*. The FDA, ISMP, and TJC advocate the use of "tall-man" letters as a safety strategy to reduce confusion between similar-sounding drugs. For example, *risperiDONE* and *rOPINIRole* to call attention to differences in spelling. Tall-man letters should be used for computer listing and storage labeling for look-alike and sound-alike drug names. This is now the standard; the complete list may be found at https://www.ismp.org/confused-drugnames.pdf. Nursing students must become familiar with this list.

Other Factors in the Prevention of Medication Errors

Creating a distraction-free environment is critical to safe administration of medications. Data show that interruptions are responsible for 45% of medication errors (http://www.ismp.org). To avoid drug errors, many facilities are creating medication safety zones by implementing policies that provide for a medication room or safety area. When a nurse enters this safety zone, they are not to be disturbed. The zone offers a quiet atmosphere in which nurses can dispense medications from an ADC system and prepare the medication for administration. The patient's medical record is available to the nurse in the safety zone, which has proper lighting and a design conducive to safe preparation of medications. Overall, the nurse's role is best achieved by the application of the nursing process.

Resources for Preventing Errors in Medication Administration

Several resources address medication errors and their prevention:

- The ISMP provides accurate medication safety information. Also, the ISMP provides knowledge and understanding of the system-based causes of medication errors based largely on interdisciplinary reviews of thousands of reports to its national Medication Error Reporting Program (MERP) as well as hundreds of visits to health care organizations nationwide.

CLINICAL JUDGMENT [NURSING PROCESS]

Medication Safety

Concept: Safety
- Protecting the patient from possible injury by practicing safe medication administration

Recognize Cues [Assessment]
- Assess the patient's vital signs and perform a head-to-toe physical assessment.
- Assess the patient's current laboratory results such as hematology laboratories, chemistry panel, and other pertinent laboratory tests pertaining to the patient's diagnosis and designated medication profile.
- Assess the patient's history, including current diagnostics and ability of the patient to swallow oral medications.
- Assess medication orders for completeness. Know the purpose and the expected effect of the medications and possible interactions, including any over-the-counter (OTC) and herbal preparations. Question the health care provider (HCP) if the prescription is unclear or seems inappropriate for the client's condition.
- ⚡ Use critical thinking skills by applying the assessment data and laboratory values to determine whether it is safe to administer the patient's medications.
- Report any abnormal findings to the provider.
- ⚡ Refuse to give a medication if you believe it to be unsafe, and notify the patient's HCP and the nurse manager.

Analyze Cues and Prioritize Hypothesis [Patient Problems]
- Need for health teaching
- Pain (surgical)
- Decreased adherence

Generate Solutions [Planning]
- ⚡ Calculate doses accurately, and if necessary, verify dosages with a colleague or pharmacist.
- Measure doses accurately and double-check high-alert medications.

- Avoid distractions during drug preparation.

Take Action [Nursing Interventions]
- ⚡ Use relevant resources and calculate doses correctly.
- Avoid skin contamination or inhalation of substances to minimize exposure.
- Always use hand hygiene before administering drugs.
- ⚡ Never administer medications that another nurse has prepared.
- ⚡ Use two forms of identification when identifying the patient.
- ⚡ Administer medications according to the six rights: right patient, right drug, right dose, right time, right route, and right documentation.
- Stay with the patient until the medication is taken.
- Discard needles and syringes in appropriate containers; be alert to sharps safety.
- Use aseptic/sterile technique appropriate for the route of administration.
- Thoroughly document drug administration in a timely manner.
- Document a patient's refusal to take a medication, and notify the HCP.

Patient Teaching
- Counsel patients and families on anticipated effects of the medications.
- Counsel patients on side effects and adverse reactions.
- Advise patients what foods to eat or avoid.
- Advise patients whether to take medications before, with, or after meals to promote optimal absorption.

Evaluate Outcomes [Evaluation]
- Evaluate the patient's response to the medication.
- Assess the patient for side effects. Document and report appropriately.
- Evaluate the patient's understanding of the expected results from the medication and what to report to the HCP.
- Omit or delay doses, as indicated by the patient's condition, and if not administered, report this to the provider.

TABLE 9.4 US Food and Drug Administration Pregnancy Categories

8.1 Pregnancy (Includes Labor and Delivery)	8.2 Lactation (Includes Nursing Mothers)	8.3 Females and Males of Reproductive Potential
Information Included in Subsection		
Pregnancy Exposure Registry	Risk Summary	Pregnancy Testing
Risk Summary	Clinical Considerations	Contraception Recommendations
Clinical Considerations	Data	Infertility Information
Data		

Data from https://www.fda.gov/drugs/labeling/outline-section-81-83drug labeling.

- The FDA database of medication errors and "near misses" assists all health care personnel to identify, implement, and evaluate strategies to prevent medication errors. It is strongly suggested that health care workers report errors and near misses to the FDA. Reports are confidential.
- When the nurse is unsure about a dosage, potential side effects, expected therapeutic effects, contraindications, or adverse reactions, an external resource—a drug reference book, pharmacist, or an acceptable technology resource—should be consulted to determine the correct answer (e.g., Micromedex, Epocrates).

PREGNANCY CATEGORIES AND SUBSECTIONS

The FDA Pregnancy Categories and Subsection Labeling System provides a broad explanation based on current available information of the benefits and risks medications can have to the mother, the fetus, and the breastfeeding child. The subsections are listed as Pregnancy (includes Labor and Delivery); Lactation (includes Nursing Mothers); and Females and Males of Reproductive Potential (Table 9.4). The Pregnancy subsection provides information relevant to the use of the drug in pregnant women, such as dosing, potential risks to the fetus, information about whether a registry collects and maintains data on how pregnant women are affected when they use a medication, and relevant information to help HCPs make prescribing and counseling decisions. The Lactation subsection provides information about using the drug while breastfeeding, such as the amount of the drug in breast milk and potential effects on the breastfed child. The Females and Males of Reproductive Potential subsection includes information about pregnancy testing, contraception, and infertility as it relates to the drug. For more information, see https://www.fda.gov/drugs/labeling/pregnancy-and-lactation-labeling-drugs-final-rule and lactation categories.htm.

GUIDELINES FOR MEDICATION ADMINISTRATION

General guidelines for correct administration of medications are listed in Box 9.2. Nurses should follow these guidelines to enhance safety when administering medications. Application of Clinical Judgment [Nursing Process] to medication administration is presented in Chapter 1.

BOX 9.2 Guidelines for Correct Administration of Medications

Preparation
1. Perform hand hygiene.
2. Access patient's drug administration record (MAR) or electronic health record (EHR).
3. Check patient's drugs with the health care provider's order for accuracy.
4. Obtain the patient's drugs from automatic dispensing cabinet (ADC), remote stock, or pharmacy while checking the drug label with the patient's drug order for accuracy.
5. Check drug allergies.
6. Prepare drugs for only one patient at a time.
7. Calculate the drug dose and perform a double-check of the calculation.
8. Check the expiration date on the drug label, and use the drug only if the date is current.
9. While preparing the drug, check the label against the MAR for accuracy.
10. If a unit dose is prescribed, open the packet at the patient's bedside.
11. If a liquid is prescribed, measure in a calibrated syringe and put it into a drug cup (see Chapter 10; Fig. 10.2).
12. Never leave medications unattended.

Administration
13. Only administer drugs that have been personally prepared.
14. Identify patients by using at least two patient identifiers (e.g., name and birth date). Compare the patient's name and birth date from the MAR, computer printout, or EHR with the information on the patient's identification (ID) bracelet. If possible, ask the patient to state their name and birth date.
15. Assist patient into an appropriate position, depending on the route of administration.
16. Before administering compare label on medication with the MAR to complete the three checks.
17. Explain each drug and its action to the patient.
18. For patients who cannot hold the drug, place the cup to their lips. Introduce one drug at a time, and do not rush the patient.
19. Stay with the patient until all drugs have been taken.
20. Dispose of used supplies and perform hand hygiene.
21. Evaluate the patient's response to the drugs.
22. Educate patients and family members about drug actions and side effects.

Documentation
23. Report any drug errors immediately to the patient's health care provider and to the nurse manager; complete an incident report per your facility's policy.
24. Record effectiveness and results of drugs administered, especially medications administered as needed (prn).
25. Record drugs that were refused and report refusal to the patient's health care provider along with the reason given for the refusal.
26. Record the amount of fluid taken with medications on an input and output chart.

CRITICAL THINKING CASE STUDY

A 70-year-old female patient was admitted to the medical-surgical unit with a diagnosis of heart failure. This morning her blood pressure was elevated. She denies chest pain, but complains of shortness of breath. Her morning weight indicated a 4-lb increase from the previous day. The nurse notified the health care provider (HCP), who ordered a diuretic of furosemide 40 mg PO immediately.

1. How will the nurse identify the patient before administering the drug?
2. What safety measures will the nurse implement to ensure accuracy?

3. The nurse scans the patient's armband and then attempts to scan the drug into the electronic health record (EHR). However, the EHR will not accept the drug scan. When the nurse compares the label with the order, the nurse realizes two 20 mg tablets should have been pulled from the automatic dispensing cabinet (ADC) to complete the order of 40 mg. The nurse only pulled one 20 mg tablet. What is the nurse's next step?
4. Explain the necessary steps when retrieving medications from the ADC and the steps prior to patient administration to avoid drug errors.

REVIEW QUESTIONS

1. The patient asks the nurse how to dispose of old medications. What should the nurse tell the patient? (Select all that apply.)
   a. Mix old drugs with cat litter before disposing.
   b. Flush the medications down the toilet.
   c. Remove personal information from the bottle.
   d. Add water and crush drugs before disposing.
   e. Throw bottle of medications into the trashcan.
2. The nurse educator on the unit receives a list of high-alert drugs. Which strategy is recommended to decrease the risk of errors? (Select all that apply.)
   a. Store drugs on a shelf for quick retrieval.
   b. Limit access to high-alert drugs.
   c. Use special labels for high-alert drugs.
   d. Provide increased training to staff.
   e. Prior to administration, have two nurses confirm and document correct drug and dose.
3. The Joint Commission recommends which of the following abbreviations for the "Do Not Use" list?
   a. qd
   b. NPO
   c. qid
   d. bid
4. A patient refuses to take the prescribed medication. Which is the nurse's best response to this patient?
   a. Leave the medication at the patient's bedside.
   b. Persuade the patient to take the medication.
   c. Tell the patient there is no choice in the matter.
   d. Explain the benefits and side effects of the drug.

5. What information is essential for the nurse to document when giving drugs? (Select all that apply.)
   a. Document all drugs given by the end of a shift.
   b. Document the correct site of an injectable drug.
   c. Document the patient's response to the drug.
   d. Document the blood pressure before giving a drug.
   e. Document the date, time, and dose drug is given.
6. The nurse prepares to administer medications. Which drug orders are complete? (Select all that apply.)
   a. Aspirin 81 mg PO daily
   b. Multivitamin sustained
   c. Vitamin D PO
   d. Ciprofloxacin 500 mg PO tid
   e. Promethazine 25 mg STAT
7. The Quality and Safety Education for Nurses' focus on safety is *best* exemplified by which competency?
   a. Patient advocacy
   b. Technology
   c. Infection control
   d. Collaborative patient and family care

10

Drug Administration

http://evolve.elsevier.com/McCuistion/pharmacology

OBJECTIVES

- Identify the different routes of drug administration.
- Discuss the various sites for parenteral therapy.
- Explain the equipment and technique used in parenteral therapy.
- Explain the Z-track intramuscular injection technique.

- Analyze the nursing interventions related to administration of medications by various routes.
- Apply Clinical Judgment [Nursing Process] to drug administration.

OUTLINE

Administration of medications is a complex but routine nursing activity practiced by nurses daily. Nurses have a significant responsibility in preparing, administering, teaching, and evaluating patients' responses to the medications they administer. Whether in an acute care, clinic, long-term care, or home setting, nurses work closely with patients and their family members. Patients must receive adequate training from the nurse to self-administer medications upon discharge. Nurses share their knowledge about the many aspects of drug administration, including: drug interactions, safety practices, side effects, and dosage calculations. This chapter will explain drug administration routes and procedures.

FORMS AND ROUTES OF DRUG ADMINISTRATION

A variety of forms and routes are used for the administration of drugs. These include sublingual, buccal, oral (tablets, capsules, liquids, suspensions, and elixirs), transdermal, topical, instillation (drops and sprays), inhalation, nasogastric and gastrostomy tubes, suppositories, and parenteral forms (Fig. 10.1).

Tablets and Capsules

- Tablets and capsules are the most common drug forms; they are convenient and less expensive and do not require additional supplies for administration.
- Oral drugs are not given to patients who are vomiting, who lack a gag reflex, or who are comatose.
- Do not mix a drug with large amounts of food or beverage. Patients may not be able to consume and will not get the full dose of medication. Do not mix drugs in infant formula.

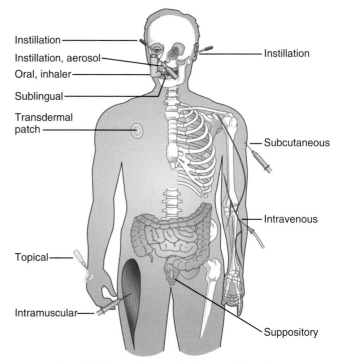

Fig. 10.1 Routes for medication administration.

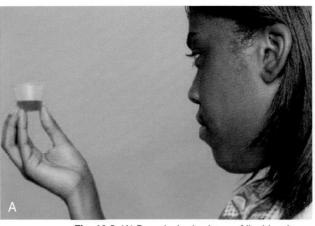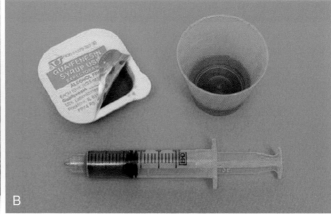

Fig. 10.2 (A) Pour desired volume of liquid so base of meniscus is level with mL increment on plastic dosing cup. (B) Measure liquid medication in a mL syringe and squirt liquid into dosing cup. (From Potter, P. A., & Perry, A. G. [2009]. *Fundamentals of nursing* [7th ed.]. St. Louis: Elsevier.)

- Enteric-coated and timed-release capsules must be swallowed whole to maintain a therapeutic drug level, so the drug is released gradually. If crushed, the initial excessive drug release poses a risk of toxicity such that it could lead to a potentially fatal overdose. Crushing can increase the rate of absorption, and it can cause oropharyngeal irritation. Advise the patient or family member to notify the health care provider (HCP) or pharmacist if the patient is having difficulty swallowing the medication. Instruct the patient to never cut or crush medications unless advised by the HCP or pharmacist that cutting or crushing is safe. In acute care settings, the nurse should follow the agency's policy for changing or altering drugs. Most policies indicate to notify the HCP or pharmacist if the patient is unable to swallow the drug. Many drugs can be given in liquid or intravenous (IV) form, or in a non-extended-release form.
- Extended release medications should never be cut in half or crushed. If patient has difficulty swallowing, inquire whether a liquid form is available.
- Administer irritating drugs with food to decrease gastrointestinal (GI) discomfort.
- Administer drugs on an empty stomach if food interferes with medication absorption.
- Drugs given via sublingual (under the tongue) or buccal (between the cheek and gum) routes remain in place until fully absorbed; therefore no food or fluid should be taken while the medication is in place.
- If patients have difficulty opening child-resistant caps, have them request non-child-resistant caps from the pharmacist.

Liquids

- Forms of liquid medication include elixirs, emulsions, and suspensions. *Elixirs* are sweetened, hydro-alcoholic liquids used in the preparation of oral liquid medications. *Emulsions* are a mixture of two liquids that are not mutually soluble. *Suspensions* are liquids in which particles are mixed but not dissolved.
- Read the labels to determine whether diluting or shaking is required.
- Make sure your facility has plastic dosing cups that measure in milliliters (mL) and not in archaic drams. One dram is equivalent to 3.7 mL. To avoid mix-ups, it is always best to measure the prescribed dose of liquid medication in a syringe calibrated for milliliters and to then squirt the medication into the oral measuring cup. According to the US Pharmacopeia (USP) Convention, a proposed change is required for all facilities to supply dosing cups with legible markings in metric units (Fig. 10.2).

Transdermals

- Transdermal medication is stored in a patch placed on the skin and is absorbed through the skin to produce a systemic effect. A patch may be left in place for as little as 12 hours or as long as 7 days depending on the drug. Transdermal drugs provide more consistent blood levels than oral and injectable forms, and they avoid GI absorption problems associated with oral products. To prevent skin breakdown, transdermal patches should be rotated to different sites and should not be reapplied over the exact same area every time. Additionally, the area should be thoroughly cleansed before administration of a new transdermal patch.
- Perform hand hygiene and apply gloves when administering medicated patches to prevent transfer of medication; advise the patient to do the same for self-administration. Never cut the patch in half.
- Advise patients to secure the patch with tape, being careful not to apply the tape too tightly, which could alter the drug delivery.

Topical

- Topical medications are most frequently applied to the skin by painting or spreading the medication over an area and applying a moist dressing or leaving the area exposed to air. Such medications can be applied to the skin in several ways, such as with a glove, tongue blade, or cotton-tipped applicator. Nurses should never apply a topical medication without first protecting their own skin with gloves.
- Use the appropriate technique to remove the medication from the container, and apply it to clean, dry skin when possible. Do not contaminate the drug in a container; instead, use gloves or an applicator.
- Gloves and applicators that come in contact with a patient should not be reinserted into the container. Estimate the amount needed and remove it from the container, or use a fresh sterile applicator each time the container is entered.

Instillations

Instillations are liquid medications usually administered as drops, ointments, or sprays in the following forms:
- Eyedrops (Box 10.1 and Fig. 10.3)
- Eye ointments (Box 10.2 and Fig. 10.4)
- Eardrops (Box 10.3 and Fig. 10.5)
- Nose drops and sprays (Box 10.4 and Figs. 10.6 and 10.7)

Inhalations

- Metered-dose inhalers (MDIs) are handheld devices used to deliver a number of commonly prescribed asthma and bronchitis

BOX 10.1   Administration of Eyedrops

1. Perform hand hygiene and wear gloves.
2. Instruct patient to lie down or sit back in a chair, and have them look at the ceiling.
3. Remove any discharge by gently wiping from the inner to outer canthus. Use a separate cloth for each eye.
4. Gently draw the skin down below the affected eye to expose the conjunctival sac (see Fig. 10.3).
5. Notify patient immediately before drops are administered so they are prepared to avoid blinking when drops hit the conjunctiva.
6. Administer the prescribed number of drops into the center of the sac. If the drug is placed directly on the cornea, it can cause discomfort or damage. Avoid touching eyelids or eyelashes with the dropper.
   a. Gently press on the lacrimal duct with a sterile cotton ball or tissue for 1 to 2 minutes after instillation to prevent systemic absorption through the lacrimal canal.
   b. Instruct patient to keep their eyes closed for 1 to 2 minutes after application to promote absorption.

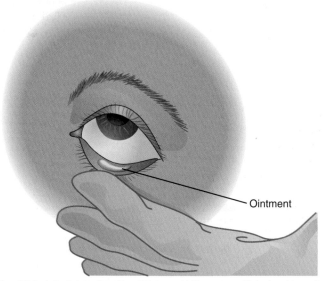

Fig. 10.4 Administering Eye Ointment. Squeeze a ¼-inch-wide strip of ointment into the conjunctival sac.

BOX 10.3   Administration of Eardrops

1. Perform hand hygiene and wear gloves.
2. Ensure the medication is at room temperature.
3. Instruct patient to sit up with the head tilted slightly toward the unaffected side. This position straightens the external ear canal for better visualization. Maintain this position for 2 to 3 minutes to facilitate drops reaching the affected area (see Fig. 10.5).
4. Pull down and back on the auricle for a child younger than 3 years of age. For a child older than 3 years or an adult, pull upward and outward on the auricle.
5. Instill the prescribed number of drops. Take measures to avoid allowing drops to fall directly on the tympanic membrane. Drops should be aimed at the side of the ear canal and should be allowed to run down into the ear.
6. Do not contaminate the dropper.

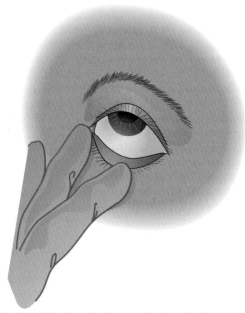

Fig. 10.3 Administering Eyedrops. Gently pull down on the skin below the eye to expose the conjunctival sac. Apply drops to the middle third of the sac, and apply gentle pressure over the lacrimal duct after administration.

BOX 10.2   Administration of Eye Ointment

1. Perform hand hygiene and wear gloves.
2. Instruct patient to lie down or sit, and have them look at the ceiling.
3. Remove any discharge by gently wiping outward from the inner canthus. Use a separate cloth for each eye.
4. Gently draw the skin down below the affected eye to expose the conjunctival sac.
5. Prepare patient by explaining that ointment will be placed in the eye, so they can help by not blinking.
6. Squeeze a strip of ointment (about ¼ inch unless stated otherwise) onto the conjunctival sac (see Fig. 10.4). Medication placed directly on the cornea can cause discomfort or damage. Avoid touching eyelids or eyelashes with the applicator tip.
7. Instruct patients to close their eyes for 2 to 3 minutes.
8. Instruct patients to expect blurred vision for a short time. If possible, apply at bedtime.

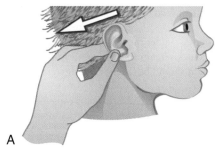

A

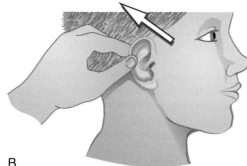

B

Fig. 10.5 Administering Eardrops. (A) Straighten the external ear canal by pulling the auricle down and back in children under 3 years of age. (B) In patients older than 3 years of age, including adults, pull the auricle upward and outward.

BOX 10.4 Administration of Nose Drops and Sprays

1. Perform hand hygiene and wear gloves.
2. Advise patient to blow their nose.
3. Advise patient to tilt the head back for drops to reach the frontal sinus and to tilt the head to the affected side to reach the ethmoid sinus (see Figs. 10.6 and 10.7).
4. Administer the prescribed number of drops or sprays without touching the tip of the medication applicator to the nasal passages.
5. Some sprays have instructions to close one nostril, tilt the head to the closed side, and hold the breath or breathe through the nose for 1 minute.
6. If a patient is using a nasal spray to reach the sinuses, proper head position is with the patient looking down at the feet with the spray tip aimed toward the eye.
7. Advise the patient to keep the head tilted back for 5 minutes after instillation of drops.

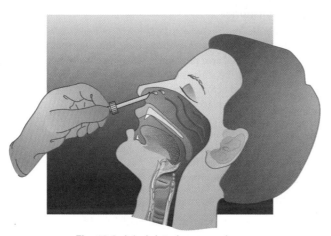

Fig. 10.6 Administering nose drops.

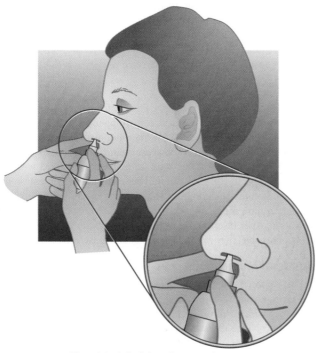

Fig. 10.7 Administering nasal spray.

BOX 10.5 Correct Use of a Metered-Dose Inhaler

1. Explain what a metered dose is, and warn the patient about overuse and side effects of the drug.
2. Explain the steps for administering the drug using a squeeze-and-breathe metered-dose inhaler (MDI), and demonstrate the steps when possible. Consult a pharmacist for details if necessary.
3. Insert the medication canister into the plastic holder.
4. If a spacer is used, insert the MDI into the end of the spacer.
5. Shake the inhaler vigorously five or six times before using. Remove the cap from the mouthpiece.
6. Have the patient breathe out through the mouth and exhale.
7. An MDI may be positioned in one of two ways:
   a. With the mouth closed around the MDI with the opening toward the back of the throat
   b. With the device positioned 1 to 2 inches from the mouth
   c. If a spacer is used, the patient closes the mouth around the mouthpiece of the spacer. Avoid covering the small exhalation slots with the lips.
8. With the inhaler properly positioned, have the patient hold the inhaler with the thumb at the mouthpiece and the index finger and middle finger at the top (see Fig. 10.8).
9. Instruct the patient to take a slow, deep breath through the mouth and during inspiration, to push the top of the medication canister once.
10. Have patient hold the breath for 10 seconds and then exhale slowly through pursed lips.
11. If a second dose is required, wait 1 to 2 minutes, and repeat the procedure by first shaking the canister in the plastic holder with the cap on.
12. When it is first used or if it has not been used recently, test the inhaler by spraying it into the air before administering the metered dose.
13. If a glucocorticoid inhalant is to be used with a bronchodilator, wait 5 minutes before using an inhaler that contains a steroid.
14. Teach patients to self-monitor their pulse rate.
15. Caution against overuse because side effects and tolerance may result.
16. Teach patient to monitor the amount of medication remaining in the canister. Advise patient to ask a health care provider or pharmacist to estimate when a new inhaler will be needed based on the dosing schedule.
17. Teach patient to rinse their mouth after using an MDI. This is especially important when using a steroid drug. Rinsing the mouth helps prevent irritation and secondary infection to oral mucosa.
18. Advise patient to avoid smoking.
19. Teach patient to do daily cleaning of equipment; this should include (1) washing the hands; (2) taking apart all the washable parts of the equipment and washing them with warm water; (3) rinsing; (4) placing the parts on a clean towel and covering them with another clean towel to air dry; and (5) storing the parts in a clean plastic bag once completely dry. Alternate two sets of washable equipment to make this process easier.

drugs to the lower respiratory tract (Box 10.5) via inhalation. When the airway becomes constricted, the drug is needed quickly. When properly used, MDIs get up to 12% to 14% of the drug deep into the lungs with each puff. MDIs act faster than drugs taken by mouth, and fewer side effects occur because the drug goes right to the lungs and not to other parts of the body. Some MDIs have a counter to indicate the number of inhalations used. For those that do not, ask the pharmacist the number of inhalations the inhaler will provide and then count the number of inhalations used. Every effort should be made to have the patient know how much medication is in the canister and to anticipate and obtain refills in a timely manner.

- Take special measures when handling the capsules used in some MDIs to prevent the transfer of medication (e.g., powder from a punctured capsule can get on the nurse's hands and transfer to the eyes or absorb into the skin).

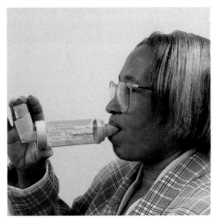

Fig. 10.8 Metered-dose inhaler with spacer. (From Potter, P. A., Perry, A. G., Stockert, P. A., & Hall, A. M. [2017]. *Fundamentals of nursing* [9th ed.]. St. Louis: Elsevier.)

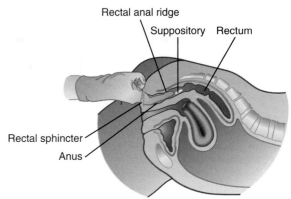

Fig. 10.9 Inserting a rectal suppository.

- **Spacers** are devices used to enhance the delivery of medications from the MDI (Fig. 10.8). A *nebulizer* is a device that changes a liquid medication into a fine mist or aerosol and has the ability to reach the lower, smaller airways. Handheld nebulizers deliver a very fine particle in a spray of medication.
- When administering drugs via an MDI or nebulizer, the preferred patient position is the semi-Fowler or high Fowler position.
- Instruct the patient on the correct use and cleaning of MDIs or nebulizers.

Nasogastric and Gastrostomy Tubes

- Before administering drugs, always check for proper tube placement of any feeding tube that enters the mouth, nose, or abdomen, and always assess the gastric residual. Return any aspirated gastric fluid to the stomach. (Check the agency's policy for tube placement and residual; see Chapter 14.)
- Place patient in a high Fowler position or elevate the head of bed at least 30 degrees to avoid aspiration.
- Make sure the drug is crushable. If it is a capsule, assess whether it can be opened and administered through the tube. The crushed drug should be placed into a plastic dosing cup. A small amount of water is added to liquefy the dry medication.
- Remove the plunger from the syringe and attach it to the feeding tube, pour liquefied medication into syringe, release the clamp, and allow the medication to flow in properly by gravity.
- Ensure proper identification of each drug up until the time of administration. Do this by administering one drug at a time. Flush with 10 to 15 mL of water between each administration to maintain patency of the tubing.
- When finished with drug administration, flush tubing with 30 mL of water or whichever amount is recommended by the agency's policy. Always record the amount of water used with the administration of drugs on the patient's input sheet.
- Clamp the tube and remove the syringe.
- If the patient has a nasogastric tube to suction, clamp the tube for 30 minutes to allow medication to be absorbed before placing the patient back on suction.

Suppositories

A suppository is a solid medical preparation that is cone- or spindle-shaped for insertion into the rectum, globular or egg-shaped for use in the vagina, or pencil-shaped for insertion into the urethra. Suppositories are made from glycerinated gelatin or high-molecular-weight polyethylene glycols and are common vehicles for a variety of drugs. A suppository is a useful route in babies, in uncooperative patients, and in cases of vomiting or certain digestive disorders.

Rectal Suppositories

- Medications administered as suppositories or enemas can be given rectally for local and systemic absorption. The numerous small capillaries in the rectal area promote medication absorption.
- The foil around the suppository is removed, and the suppository may be lubricated before insertion.
- During insertion, place the suppository past the internal anal sphincter; otherwise, the suppository will be expelled before it can dissolve and absorb into the mucosa.
- Some suppositories tend to soften at room temperature and therefore may be refrigerated before use.
- Explain administration procedures to the patient and provide for privacy.
- Use gloves for insertion.
- Instruct the patient to lie in the modified left lateral recumbent position and to breathe slowly through the mouth to relax the anal sphincter.
- Apply a small amount of water-soluble lubricant to the tip of the unwrapped suppository and gently insert the suppository beyond the internal sphincter (Fig. 10.9).
- Ask the patient to remain flat or on one side for at least 30 minutes to prevent expulsion of the suppository.
- Observe for effects of the suppository that correlate with the medication's onset, peak, and duration.

Vaginal Medications

Vaginal drugs are available as suppositories, foams, jellies, or creams. They are individually packaged in foil wrappers and are sometimes stored in the refrigerator to prevent the solid, oval-shaped suppositories from melting. Foams, jellies, creams, and suppositories are generally inserted into the vagina with an applicator supplied with the medication (Fig. 10.10); gloves should be worn, and the patient should be in the lithotomy position. Advise patients to remain lying for a time sufficient to allow medication absorption; times vary depending on the medication. After insertion, provide the patient with a sanitary pad. If the patient is able, they may want to personally insert the vaginal drug.

Parenteral Medications

Safety is a special concern with **parenteral** drugs, which are administered via injection. Manufacturers have responded with safety features to help decrease or eliminate needlestick injuries and possible transfer of blood-borne diseases such as hepatitis and human immunodeficiency virus (HIV); Fig. 10.11 shows examples of safety needles.

Methods of parenteral administration include intradermal, subcutaneous, intramuscular, Z-track technique, and intravenous administration. A description of each follows with special considerations noted for the pediatric patient.

Intradermal (ID)

Action.

- Local effect
- Administered for skin testing (e.g., tuberculin screening, allergy testing, and testing for other drug sensitivities; some immunotherapy for cancer).

Sites.

- Locations are chosen so an inflammatory reaction can be observed. Preferred areas are lightly pigmented, free of lesions, and hairless, such as the ventral midforearm, clavicular area of the chest, or scapular area of the back (Fig. 10.12).

Equipment.

- Needle: 25- to 27-gauge, ¼ to ½ inch long, tuberculin syringe
- Syringe: 1 mL calibrated in increments of (0.01) hundredth mL represented on syringe as 0.1 mL to 1 mL. Syringe holds up to 1 mL of solution; however, tuberculin skin tests require injection of a small amount of solution (usually 0.01 to 0.1 mL) to ensure formation of bleb.

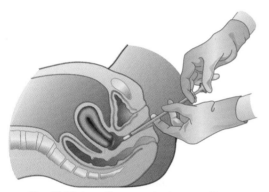

Fig. 10.10 Inserting a vaginal suppository.

Technique.

- Perform hand hygiene and wear gloves.
- Cleanse the area with a circular motion using aseptic technique.
- Hold the skin taut.
- Insert the needle, bevel up, at a 10- to 15-degree angle; the tip of the needle should be visible under the skin (Fig. 10.13).
- Inject the medication slowly to form a bleb (or wheal). A small amount is injected so the volume will not interfere with bleb formation or cause a systemic reaction. If the bleb does not appear, the needle has been injected subcutaneously. Document according to facility policy and inform the HCP. The nurse may need to obtain orders to repeat the procedure.
- Remove the needle slowly, and do not recap it.
- Do *not* massage the area, and instruct the patient not to do so.
- Mark the area with a pen, and ask the patient not to wash it off until the response can be "read" by an HCP.
- It is not recommended to put an adhesive bandage over the testing site because it can alter the results of the test.
- Assess for allergic reaction in 24 to 72 hours; measure the diameter of any local reaction. For tuberculin testing, measure only the indurated area; do not include the area of erythema in the measurement.

Subcutaneous (subcut)

Action.

- Systemic effect
- Sustained effect; absorbed mainly through capillaries; usually slower in onset than with the intramuscular (IM) route.

Sites.

- Locations for subcutaneous injections are chosen for adequate fat-pad size. Areas such as the upper outer aspect of the arms; the abdomen, at least 2 inches from the umbilicus; and the anterior thighs are important subcutaneous sites (Fig. 10.14). Sites should be rotated with subcutaneous injections, such as with insulin and heparin.
- Usually, 0.5 to 1 mL of solution is given subcutaneously. A larger amount (2 mL) of medication may have to be divided and administered at two sites. Larger amounts add to the patient's discomfort and predispose to poor absorption. Refer to agency policy for the maximum amount of medication to be administered via this route.

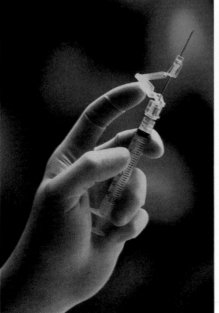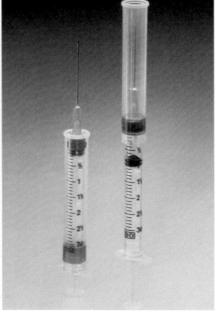

Fig. 10.11 Safety needles.

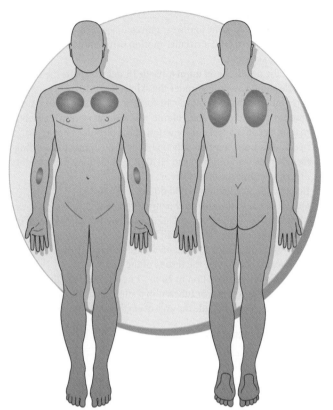

Fig. 10.12 Common sites for intradermal injection.

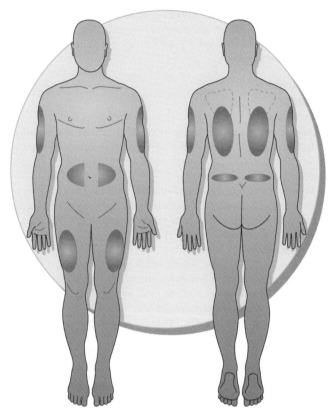

Fig. 10.14 Common sites for subcutaneous injections.

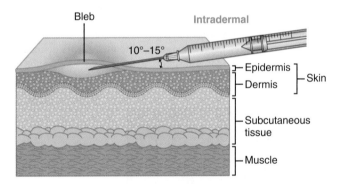

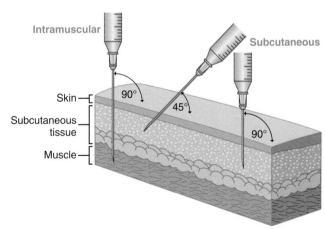

Fig. 10.13 Needle angles for intradermal, subcutaneous, and intramuscular injections.

Equipment.
- Needle: 25- to 27-gauge; ⅜ to ⅝ inch long
- The length of the needle and the angle of the needle insertion are based on the amount of subcutaneous tissue present. The shorter, ⅜-inch needle should be inserted at 90-degree angle, and the longer, ⅝-inch needle is inserted at a 45-degree angle (see Fig. 10.13).
- Syringe: 1 to 3 mL (injection of solution is usually 0.5 to 1 mL)
- Insulin syringe measured in units for use with only insulin

Technique.
- Perform hand hygiene and wear gloves.
- Cleanse the area with a circular motion using aseptic technique.
- Grasp or gently pinch the area of the patient's loose fatty tissue with the fingers of your nondominant hand.
- Insert the needle quickly.
- Release the pinch and use the hand to stabilize the syringe.
- Do not aspirate.
- Inject the medication slowly.
- Remove the needle quickly; do not recap.
- Apply gentle pressure to the injection site to prevent bleeding or oozing into the tissue with subsequent bruising and tissue damage, especially if the patient is on anticoagulant therapy.
- Apply a bandage if needed.

Intramuscular (IM)
Action.
- Systemic effect
- Usually a more rapid effect of drug than with a subcutaneous route
- Used for solutions that are more viscous and irritating for adults, children, and infants
- IM injections are associated with many risks, so the nurse should use accurate, careful technique when administering an IM injection and should check the agency's policy.

TABLE 10.1 Intramuscular Injection Sites: Patient Position, Advantages, and Disadvantages

Site	Patient Position	Anatomic Landmark
Ventrogluteal	Supine, lateral	Locate the ventrogluteal muscle by placing the heel of the hand over the greater trochanter of the patient's hip with the wrists perpendicular to the femur. Use the right hand for the patient's left hip and the left hand for the right hip. Point the thumb toward the patient's groin and the index finger toward the anterior superior iliac spine, and extend the middle finger back along the iliac crest toward the buttock. The index finger, the middle finger, and the iliac crest form a V-shaped triangle; the injection site is the center of the triangle (see Fig. 10.15). The ventrogluteal is the preferred site for most injections given to adults and all children, including infants of any age.
Deltoid	Lateral, prone, sitting, supine	Palpate the lower edge of the patient's acromion process, which forms the base of a triangle in line with the midpoint of the lateral aspect of the upper arm. The injection site is in the center of the triangle, about 1–2 inches below the acromion process. Or locate the site by placing four fingers across the deltoid muscle with the top finger along the acromion process. The injection site is then three finger widths below the acromion process (see Fig. 10.16).
Vastus lateralis	Sitting, supine Flex knee to help relax muscle if supine	Located on the anterior lateral aspect of the thigh, it extends in an adult from a handbreadth above the knee to a handbreadth below the greater trochanter of the femur. Use the middle third of the muscle for injection. With young children or cachectic patients, it helps to grasp the body of the muscle during injection to ensure delivery of the drug into the muscle. Vastus lateralis is frequently used in infants (less than 12 months) receiving immunizations and is often used in older children and toddlers receiving immunizations (see Fig. 10.17).

Sites. Locations are chosen for adequate muscle size and minimal major nerves and blood vessels in the area. Other considerations include the volume of drug administered, needle size, angle of injection, patient position, site location, and advantages and disadvantages of the site. Underweight patients should be evaluated for sites with adequate muscle.

Equipment.

- Needle: 18- to 25-gauge; ⅝ to 1½ inches long. Patient's weight, age, and the amount of adipose tissue influence needle length.

Technique.

- Perform hand hygiene and apply gloves.
- Same as for subcutaneous injection with two exceptions: Flatten the skin area using the thumb and index finger and inject between them, and insert the needle at a 90-degree angle into the muscle (see Fig. 10.13).
- Syringe: 1 to 3 mL, although this varies based on the intended site, the age of the patient, and the developed muscle site. (Check the agency's policy.)

Preferred Intramuscular Injection Sites. Table 10.1 shows the three sites along with the patient positioning and advantages and disadvantages of each injection site.

- *Ventrogluteal* (Fig. 10.15). Located near the gluteus medius, a deep muscle, away from major nerves, this site is well suited for Z-track injections. It is administered with an 18- to 25-gauge, 1½-inch needle. The gauge and length of the needle depend on the medication to be administered and the size of the patient. Slightly angle the needle toward the iliac crest. The ventrogluteal is the preferred site for most injections given to adults and all children, including infants of any age.
- *Deltoid* (Fig. 10.16). This muscle is easy to find, but it is not well developed in many adults. The volume of drug administered is 0.5 to 1 mL, with a 23- to 25-gauge, ⅝- to 1½-inch needle. Place the needle at a 90-degree angle to the skin or slightly toward the acromion. Choose the site carefully; there is risk for injury because of the nerves and arteries that lie within the upper arm along the humerus. Use this site for small medication volumes or when other sites are inaccessible. This site is not used in infants or children due to underdeveloped muscles.

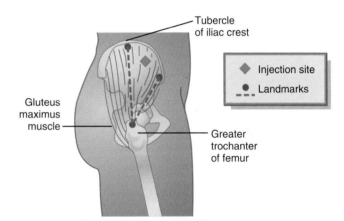

Fig. 10.15 Ventrogluteal injection site.

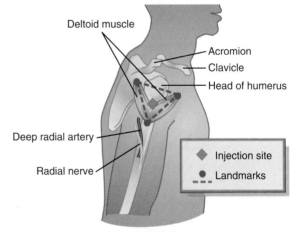

Fig. 10.16 Deltoid injection site.

- *Vastus lateralis* (Fig. 10.17). The vastus lateralis is a good site for multiple injections. It is frequently used in infants (less than 12 months) and is often used in older children and toddlers receiving immunizations. If a long needle is used, insert it with caution to avoid sciatic nerve or femoral structures. The volume of drug administered is 0.5 mL in infants (maximum [max] 1 mL), 1 mL in pediatric patients, and 1 to 1.5 mL in adults (max 2 mL).

Z-track Injection Technique. The Z-track injection technique shown in Fig. 10.18 is recommended when administering IM injections to help minimize local skin irritation by sealing the medication in the muscle tissue. The ventrogluteal site is preferred. Using aseptic technique, draw up the medication. Replace the first needle with a second needle of appropriate gauge and length to ensure the needle will penetrate the muscle. Holding the skin taut, inject the needle at a 90-degree angle deep into the muscle, and if there is no blood return on aspiration, slowly inject the medication. Allow the needle to remain inserted for 10 seconds for the medication to disperse evenly.

Intravenous (IV)

Action.

- Systemic effect
- More rapid than IM or subcutaneous routes

Sites. Accessible peripheral veins are preferred (e.g., cephalic or cubital vein of arm, dorsal vein of hand; Fig. 10.19). When possible, ask the patient about his or her preference, and avoid needless body restriction. In newborns, the veins of the feet, lower legs, and head may also be used after other sites have been exhausted.

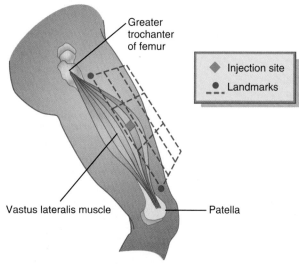

Fig. 10.17 Vastus lateralis injection site in children.

Equipment.

- Needle
  - Adults: 20- to 21-gauge, 1 to 1½ inches
  - Infants: 24-gauge, 1 inch
  - Children: 22-gauge, 1 inch
- Larger bore for viscous drugs and whole blood and a large volume for rapid infusion
- Electronic IV delivery device, an infusion controller, or pump
- May use a mixture of lidocaine/prilocaine anesthetic before starting IV site

Technique.

- Perform hand hygiene and apply gloves.
- Apply a tourniquet.
- Apply anesthetic 30 minutes before the procedure on unbroken skin.
- Cleanse the area using aseptic technique with an appropriate solution.
- Insert catheter, and feed it up into the vein until blood returns. Remove the tourniquet.
- Stabilize the needle or IV catheter, and apply dressing to site.
- Flush the catheter with sodium chloride or sterile water to check for site patency.
- Monitor flow rate, distal pulses, skin color and temperature, and insertion site.
- Consult agency policy regarding IV fluids, intermittent IV (IVPB), and direct IV (IV push) drugs. The pharmacy adds medications to the IV bag to avoid error; except in specialty areas such as critical care, nurses should *never* add medications to the IV bag.

NURSING IMPLICATIONS FOR ADMINISTRATION OF PARENTERAL MEDICATIONS

Sites

- The ventrogluteal site is preferred for IM injections in adults and children, including infants of any age. The gluteal muscle is a deep muscle, situated away from major nerves and blood vessels.
- For infants less than 12 months and toddlers not walking alone, the vastus lateralis is the preferred site for immunizations.

Equipment

- The syringe size should approximate the volume of medication to be administered.

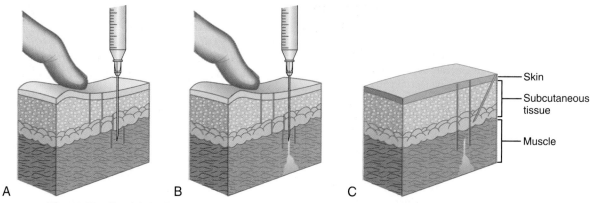

Fig. 10.18 Z-Track Injection. (A) Use a deep muscle, such as in the ventrogluteal injection, and pull skin approximately 1 to 1½ inches laterally to one side and hold it taut with the nondominant hand. (B) Inject the needle at a 90-degree angle deep into the muscle, and if no blood returns on aspiration, slowly inject the medication. (C) Wait 10 seconds before withdrawing the needle and releasing the skin. This technique prevents medication from entering subcutaneous tissue.

- Use the tuberculin syringe for amounts less than 1 mL.
- Use the filter needle to draw up drugs taken from a glass vial or ampule. Change the needle before administration to prevent tissue irritation.

Technique

- Perform hand hygiene and apply gloves.
- Correctly identify the patient.
- Explain the procedure to the patient.
- Position the patient.
- Follow the rights of medication administration (see Chapter 9).
- Inspect the site, choose the correct anatomic markers, and assess skin for breakdown.

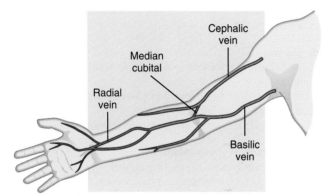

Fig. 10.19 Common sites for intravenous administration.

- Inject the drug slowly to minimize tissue damage.
- Stabilize the skin during needle removal to reduce pain.
- Do not administer injections if sites are inflamed, edematous, or lesioned (e.g., moles, scars).
- Rotate the injection site to enhance absorption of the drug.
- Document the injection site.
- Observe the patient to evaluate drug effectiveness.
- Report any adverse reactions immediately.
- Multiple products are available to reduce the pain of parenteral drug administration (e.g., lidocaine, prilocaine, and benzocaine/tetracaine).

DEVELOPMENTAL NEEDS OF A PEDIATRIC PATIENT

Anticipate patients' developmental needs. Examples of needs associated with administration of medications include the following (see Chapter 6):

- Stranger anxiety (infant): Act to instill a sense of safety and security in the infant.
- Hospitalization, illness, or injury is viewed as punishment (3–6 years of age): Allow control when appropriate; obtain the child's view of the situation; encourage activities, positive relationships, and expression of feelings in an acceptable manner. Include family or support person, if appropriate.
- Fear of the procedure (3–6 years of age): Explain procedures carefully; use less intrusive routes, such as the oral route, whenever possible; allow children to give "play" injections to a doll or stuffed animal.

◎ CLINICAL JUDGMENT [NURSING PROCESS]

Overview of Medication Administration

Concept: Caring Interventions

- The nurse performs caring interventions during medication administration. These interventions ensure safe practice outcomes. The interventions are the result of scientific research and best practice guidelines composed by the professional body of nursing for quality care and safe practice.

Recognize Cues [Assessment]

- Obtain appropriate vital signs and relevant laboratory test results for future comparisons and to evaluate therapeutic response.
- Determine the patient's level of consciousness, risk for aspiration, and ability to take medications.
- Obtain a drug history that includes drug allergies.
- Identify patients at high risk for reactions.
- Assess the patient's capability to follow the therapeutic regimen.
- Assess possible contraindications to certain medication regimens.

Analyze Cues and Prioritize Hypothesis [Patient Problems]

- Potential for injury
- Need for health teaching
- Acute pain
- Decreased mobility

Generate Solutions [Planning]

- Identify patient goals.
- Promote therapeutic response and prevent or minimize adverse reactions.
- Identify strategies to promote adherence to the drug regimen.
- Identify interventions that foster patient independence and safety.

Take Action [Nursing Interventions]

- Prepare equipment and environment and perform hand hygiene.
- Evaluate for allergies and other assessment data.
- View the drug label three times; check the expiration date and apply the rights of medication administration.
- Verify the calculated dose with another registered nurse (RN), licensed personnel, or pharmacy as necessary.
- Measure liquids in a milliliter syringe, and squirt the medication into a plastic measuring cup calibrated in milliliters.
- Avoid contact with topical and inhalation preparations by wearing gloves.
- Verify patient by using two patient identifiers.
- Administer drugs personally prepared.
- Assist the patient into the appropriate position.
- Discard needles and syringes in a sharps container. Do not recap needles.
- Store all drugs properly, especially regarding temperature, light, and moisture.
- The drug must be identifiable up until the time of patient administration.
- Follow agency policy related to discarding drugs and controlled substances.
- Report drug errors immediately.
- Document all appropriate information in a timely manner.
- Record effectiveness of administered drugs, side effects, adverse effects, and if a drug is refused, document patient's reason for refusing the drug. Depending on the drug refused, notify health care provider (HCP).
- Assess patient for pain control.
- If a language barrier exists, request a professional translator.
- Communicate respect for culture and practices of patient and family.

Continued

◎ CLINICAL JUDGMENT [NURSING PROCESS]—CONT'D

Overview of Medication Administration

Patient Teaching
General
- Emphasize safety.
- Monitor the patient's physical abilities regularly as needed.
- Store medications in original, labeled containers with child-resistant caps when needed.
- Provide patient and family with written instructions about the drug regimen; provide audio instructions if the patient or family is visually impaired or unable to read.
- Advise patient and family about expected therapeutic effects, anticipated onset of action, and expected duration of treatment.
- Educate patient and family on possible side effects or signs of an adverse reaction.
- Instruct patient and family about possible laboratory tests that may be required.
- Advise patient of nonpharmacologic measures to promote therapeutic response.
- Encourage patient and family to have an adequate supply of medications available.
- Caution against the use of over-the-counter (OTC) preparations, including herbal remedies, without first contacting the HCP.
- Reinforce the importance of follow-up appointments with the HCP.
- Encourage patient to wear a medical alert band with drugs or allergies indicated.
- As needed, encourage lifestyle changes associated with drug administration (e.g., smoking cessation, exercise, limiting salt or fat intake).

- Encourage use of community resources to assist with patient and family needs.

Diet
- Advise patient and family about possible drug-food interactions and contraindicated foods, if any.
- Advise patient and family about possible drug-alcohol interactions.

Self-Administration
- Advise patient and family regarding drug dose and dosing schedule.
- Teach patient and family about psychomotor skills related to the drug.
- Provide patient and family with contact information for questions and concerns.

Side Effects
- Counsel patient and family about general side effects and adverse reactions of the medications.
- Instruct patient and family to monitor drug effects as appropriate (e.g., check blood pressure if the drug is to treat hypertension).
- Advise patient and family when and how to notify the HCP.

Evaluate Outcomes [Evaluation]
- Evaluate the effectiveness of the drugs administered.
- Identify the expected time frame of the desired response from the drug.
- Determine patient's satisfaction with the therapeutic regimen.

▌ CRITICAL THINKING CASE STUDY

A 66-year-old female new patient with diabetes is planning to be discharged from the hospital on a regular sliding scale of insulin. The nurse is planning the first teaching on how to inject subcutaneous insulin. Please answer the important questions the nurse will include in this patient's teaching.
1. Name three subcutaneous injection sites.

2. How is the skin held when administering a subcutaneous (SUBCUT) injection prior to inserting the needle?
3. What measurement is an insulin syringe calibrated?
4. What happens after the medication is injected into the site?
5. How will the nurse evaluate the effectiveness of the teaching?

▌ REVIEW QUESTIONS

1. The nurse is administering oral medications to a patient. Which are important considerations? (Select all that apply.)
   a. Always administer gastrointestinal (GI)-irritating drugs with food.
   b. Avoid mixing medications into infant formula.
   c. Enteric-coated capsules may be chewed.
   d. Stop oral medications for nausea and vomiting.
   e. Cut all transdermal patches to the correct dose.
2. The clinic nurse is preparing to administer an intradermal injection. Which needle and gauge are most appropriate for this procedure?
   a. ¾- to ⅝-inch needle, 25- to 27-gauge
   b. ⅝- to 1½-inch needle, 18- to 25-gauge
   c. 1- to 1½-inch needle, 20- to 21-gauge
   d. ¼- to ½-inch needle, tuberculin syringe
3. The nurse is administering an intramuscular injection to a 5-year-old child. Choose the correct site the nurse will use.
   a. Ventral forearm
   b. Dorsogluteal

   c. Deltoid muscle
   d. Ventrogluteal
4. The nurse administers a variety of drugs to a patient. Which statement by the patient indicates a need for further teaching?
   a. "I do not eat or drink when I have sublingual nitroglycerin in place."
   b. "I mix the drugs in my dessert and hope I am not too full to finish."
   c. "I keep the drugs in the original containers with label attached to the bottle."
   d. "I store drugs in the medicine cabinet away from children and pets."
5. The nurse is teaching a patient to use an inhaler. What common teaching point is essential for the nurse to include?
   a. Cleaning the metered-dose inhaler is not recommended.
   b. The semi-Fowler or high Fowler position is recommended.
   c. Spacers decrease delivery of medication and are not used.
   d. Nebulizers change the drug to a large-particle powder mist.

6. A 3-year-old patient has an intramuscular medication ordered. What is the most appropriate approach to gain the child's cooperation?
   a. Engage a second nurse to hold the child's body down.
   b. Have the child give a pretend injection to a toy animal.
   c. Restrain the child's lower extremities and give injection.
   d. Request that all family members wait outside of the room.

7. As the nurse prepares to administer oral medications, which nursing intervention is of "most importance" to ensure the patient's safety?
   a. Perform an assessment on the patient for risk of aspiration.
   b. Crush and mix the medications into the patient's meal.
   c. Administer drugs on a full stomach to avoid gastrointestinal (GI) upset.
   d. Administer unpleasant tasting drugs with a glass of water.

8. A patient is to start on a lidocaine transdermal patch. What is essential for the nurse to include in the patient's teaching? (Select all that apply.)
   a. Wear gloves when applying the patch.
   b. Cut the patch in half to decrease the dose.
   c. Wear gloves when removing the patch.
   d. Rotate placement of patch to different sites.
   e. Remove the patch if it becomes loose.

Drug Calculations

OBJECTIVE

- Correctly calculate drug dosages for administration.

OUTLINE

Nurses perform basic mathematical operations on a regular basis when preparing drugs for administration. To accurately calculate drug dosages, a systematic process is used. The same process should be used for every drug calculation so a step is not missed. Missed steps could lead to errors that can cause serious harm or even death to a patient.

This chapter explains five calculation methods. The three methods generally used are (1) the basic formula, (2) a ratio and proportion/fractional equation, and (3) dimensional analysis. The nurse should select one of these methods for the calculation of drug dosages. The other two methods are used to individualize drug dosing by body weight (BW) and body surface area (BSA). Numerous drug labels are used in drug calculation problems to familiarize the reader with the information on a typical drug label. Answers for the practice problems can be found at the end of this chapter.

To calculate correct dosages, knowing how to convert from one unit to another is essential because this is the basis for most drug calculations. Two common systems of measurement, metric and English (household), are shown. However, to calculate dosages, the metric system, also known as the *International System of Units (SI),* is the internationally accepted system of measure. Even though the English system

is more widely used in the United States, it is not the considered form when determining dosages for drug administration. Chapter 9 lists and discusses currently approved abbreviations used in drug dosages.

Keeping in mind that the goal is to prepare and administer drugs in a safe and correct manner, the following recommendations are offered:

- Think. Focus on each step of the problem. This applies to both simple and difficult problems.
- Read accurately. Be attentive to the location of the decimal point and to the operation to be performed, such as conversion from one system of measurement to another.
- Picture the problem.
- Identify an expected range for the answer. The dose should be *reasonable.*
- Seek to understand the problem. Do not merely master the mechanics of the mathematical operations. Seek a second opinion to ensure that the calculation is correct.
- To decrease drug errors, always perform *three checks* before administering a drug: (1) when retrieving the drug from a dispensing system, (2) when preparing the drug, and (3) just before administering the drug to the patient.

SYSTEMS OF MEASUREMENT AND CONVERSION FACTORS

Metric System

The metric system is a decimal system based on the power of 10. The basic units of measure used in dosage calculations include the gram (g, gm, G, Gm) for weight, liter (L) for volume, and meter (m, M) for linear measurement or length. Prefixes such as *nano, micro, milli, centi,* and *kilo* indicate the size of the units in powers of 10 of the base unit and stand for a specific degree of magnitude: for instance, *kilo* stands for thousands, *milli* for one-thousandth, and *centi* for one-hundredth. To convert a quantity, one of the values must be known, such as a gram (g, G), liter (l, L), meter (m), milligram (mg), milliliter (mL), millimeter (mm), or microgram (mcg). Grams, liters, and meters are larger units, whereas milligrams, milliliters, millimeters, and micrograms are smaller units. Because the conversion between degrees of magnitude always involves multiplying by a power of 10, converting from one magnitude to another is relatively easy. Common conversions used to calculate drug dosages using the metric and English systems are listed in Table 11.1.

Grams and milligrams are related by three factors of 10 according to this relationship. In the first illustration that follows, the larger unit (gram) is converted to the smaller unit (milligram). In the second illustration, the smaller unit is converted to the larger unit.

$$1 \text{ g} = 1 \text{ mg} \times 10^3 = 1000 \text{ mg}$$

and

$$1000 \text{ mg} = 1 \text{ g} \times 10^{-3} = 1 \text{ g}$$

The easiest way to convert larger units to smaller units is to move the decimal point the appropriate number of spaces to the *right*. In the next illustration, grams have been converted to milligrams by moving the decimal point three spaces to the right:

$$1 \text{ g} = 1.000 = 1000 \text{ mg}$$

To convert smaller units to larger units, move the decimal point the appropriate number of spaces to the *left*. In the next illustration,

milligrams have been converted to grams by moving the decimal point three spaces to the left (thousandths):

$$1000 \text{ mg} = 1.000 = 1 \text{ g}$$

Remember: When changing larger units to smaller units, move the decimal point to the *right;* when changing smaller units to larger units, move the decimal point to the *left.* There should always be a zero (0) placed before the decimal point, called a *leading zero,* to alert the reader that the number is less than 1. For example, *0.5* clearly indicates a value of ½. If the number was written as *.5,* the reader could mistake the number for *5.* Do not leave extraneous zeroes after a decimal point (trailing zeroes). The reader may perceive a number many times larger than the desired dose. For example, *1.0* could be misread as *10.*

(100,000) Hundred-thousands 6	(10,000) Ten-thousands 5	(1000) Thousands 4	(100) Hundreds 3	(10) Tens 2	(1) Ones (Units) 1	Decimal point ↓ .	(0.1) Tenths 1	(0.01) Hundredths 2	(0.001) Thousandths 3	(0.0001) Ten-thousandths 4	(0.00001) Hundred-thousandths 5

Whole Numbers to the Left   **Decimal Numbers to the Right**

PRACTICE PROBLEMS

Metric System Conversions

Larger to Smaller Units	Smaller to Larger Units
1. Change 2 g to mg	4. Change 1500 mg to g
2. Change 0.5 g to mg	5. Change 3000 mcg to mg
3. Change 2.5 L to mL	6. Change 500 mL to L

TABLE 11.1   Equivalent Units of Measurement

Units	Metric				English
Weight	1 kilogram (kg, Kg)	=	1000 g	=	2.2 lb
	1 gram (g, gm, G, Gm)	=	1000 mg		
	1 milligram (mg)	=	1000 mcg		
	1 microgram (mcg)	=	1000 ng (nanograms)		
Fluid Volume	1 liter (L)	=	1000 mL (milliliters)	=	
	240 mL			=	1 c (cup)
	30 mL			=	1 oz (ounce)
	15 mL			=	1 T (tablespoon)
	5 mL			=	1 t (teaspoon)
	60 gtt (drop)			=	1 t
Length	1 kilometer (km)	=	1000 m		
	1 meter (m, M)	=	100 cm		
	1 centimeter (cm)	=	10 mm		
	2.54 cm	=	1 inch		
	25.4 millimeters (mm)	=	1 inch		

English System

In the United States, English measurements are still widely used for powders and liquids. However, the English measurement is not as accurate as the metric system. Converting English measurements to the metric system will be necessary when calculating dosages. Table 11.1 provides the equivalents of the English measurement to metric system.

When converting larger units to smaller units within the English system, multiply the requested number by the basic equivalent value. When converting smaller units to larger units in the English system, divide the requested number of units by the basic equivalent value.

Examples

Larger to smaller units:
1. Convert 2 T to t.
   The equivalent value of 1 T is 3 t (1 T = 3 t)
   To solve the problem, multiply 2 T with 3 t to get 6 t (2 T × 3 t = 6 t)
2. Convert 2 T to milliliters (mL).
   The equivalent value of 1 T is 15 mL (1 T = 15 mL)
   To solve the problem, multiply 2 T with 15 mL to get 30 mL (2 T × 15 mL = 30 mL).

Smaller to larger units:
1. Convert 6 t to T.
   The equivalent value of 3 t is 1 T (3 t = 1 T).
   To solve the problem, divide 6 t by 3 t to get 2 T (6 t ÷ 3 t = 2 T).
2. Convert 30 mL to T.
   The equivalent value of 15 mL is 1 T (15 mL = 1 T).
   To solve the problem, divide 30 mL by 15 mL to get 2 T (30 mL ÷ 15 mL = 2 T).

Because English measurements are not as accurate as the metric measurements, instruct patients and caregivers to obtain an approved drug-measuring device to dispense liquid medicine, such as the following:

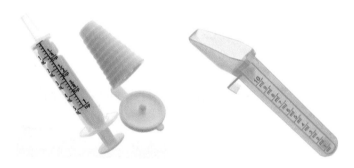

PRACTICE PROBLEMS

English System Conversions

Remember: To change larger units to smaller units, *multiply* the requested number of units by the basic equivalent value. To change smaller units to larger units, *divide* the requested number of units by the basic equivalent value.

Larger to Smaller Units	Smaller to Larger Units
1. Change 3 oz to T	4. Change 3 T to oz
2. Change 5 T to t	5. Change 12 t to T
3. Change 2 T to mL	6. Change 45 mL to t

Other Measuring Systems

Drugs are most commonly measured in grams, milligrams, or micrograms. However, some are measured in units. This includes insulin and heparin. Typically, units are not converted to any other measure.

Insulin is prescribed and measured in US Pharmacopeia (USP) units. Most insulins are produced in concentrations of 100 units per mL. Insulin should be administered with an insulin syringe, which is calibrated to correspond with the concentration of 100 units of insulin per mL in the vial. If the prescribed insulin dosage is 30 units, using an insulin syringe calibrated to 100 units per mL, withdraw insulin from the vial to the 30-unit mark (Fig. 11.1). **!** *(Note that 30 units is not interchangeable with 30 mL or 0.3 mL.)*

U-100 insulin syringes are available in various sizes, such as low-dose insulin syringes that hold a total of 0.3 mL or 0.5 mL. The size of the insulin syringe does not alter the calibration of 100 units per mL. The US Food and Drug Administration (FDA) has now approved a U-500 insulin syringe specifically dedicated to be used with regular U-500 insulin. The U-100 and U-500 insulin syringes are *not* interchangeable. Some insulin is available in insulin pen injectors and insulin pumps. These are further illustrated in Chapter 50.

Administering insulin with a tuberculin syringe is to be *avoided.* Although both syringes have 1-mL capacities, the tuberculin syringe is calibrated in milliliters rather than units. It is critical that the correct type and dose of insulin is administered to avoid severe aberrations of the patient's blood glucose. Chapter 50 provides information on the different types of insulin.

INTERPRETING DRUG LABELS

Pharmaceutical companies usually label their drugs with the brand name, also called the trade name, and the generic name. Labels for generic drugs may have only the generic name of the drug listed. The formulation or the drug amount per tablet, capsule, or unit of liquid (for oral and parenteral doses) is printed on the drug label. Other information found on drug labels includes lot number, expiration date, proper storage of the drug, and whether it is a controlled substance. Examples of drug labels are given as follows.

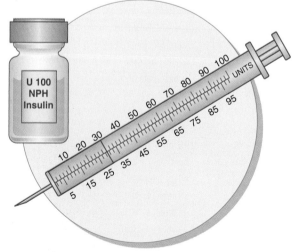

Fig. 11.1 Vial U-100 insulin and U-100 syringe. (From Kee, J. L., & Marshall, S. M. [2013]. *Clinical calculations* [7th ed.]. St. Louis: Elsevier.)

Examples

1. *Tylenol* is the brand (trade) name, *acetaminophen* is the generic name, and the formulation is 500 mg per caplet.

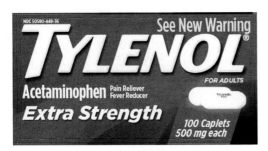

2. This label lists the generic name only (folic acid). The formulation is 5 mg per mL. There are 10 mL in the vial.

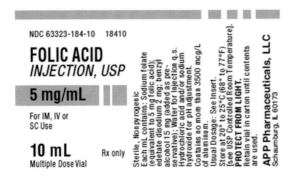

3. This label lists the drug (heparin) and its purpose (heparin lock flush). Note: It is not intended for anticoagulant therapy.

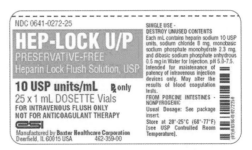

4. The following provides additional information provided on drug labels. *Kadian*[1] is the brand (trade) name and *morphine sulfate*[2] is the generic name. The formulation[3] (unit or form) is 60 mg per capsule, and the container holds 100[4] capsules. It is a Schedule II[5] drug, which is a **controlled substance** because of its potential for abuse. The label indicates how the drug is to be stored,[6] and the lot number[7] also appears.

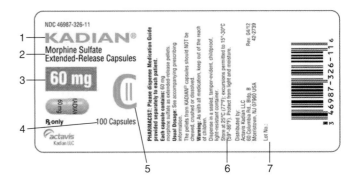

PRECAUTIONS WHEN READING DRUG LABELS

Be aware of drug names that sound or look alike; for example, note the similarity between the trade names *Percodan* and *Percocet*. Percocet, which contains oxycodone and acetaminophen, is the preparation most commonly prescribed.

Percodan contains oxycodone and aspirin, and a patient may be allergic to aspirin or should not take aspirin because of a stomach ulcer. Acetaminophen can cause liver toxicity; in persons with normal liver function, the maximum dosage of acetaminophen is 3000 mg per 24 hours.

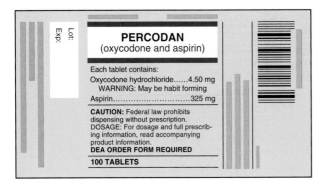

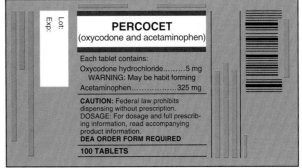

Note the similarity between *quinine sulfate* and *quinidine gluconate.* These drugs differ greatly. Quinine is prescribed for malaria, whereas quinidine is prescribed for cardiac arrhythmias.

To decrease medication errors, the nurse administering the drug should perform a minimum of three label checks with the patient's medication administration record (MAR).

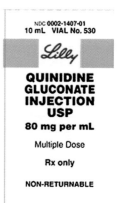

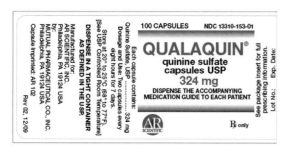

PRACTICE PROBLEMS

Interpreting Drug Labels

1.

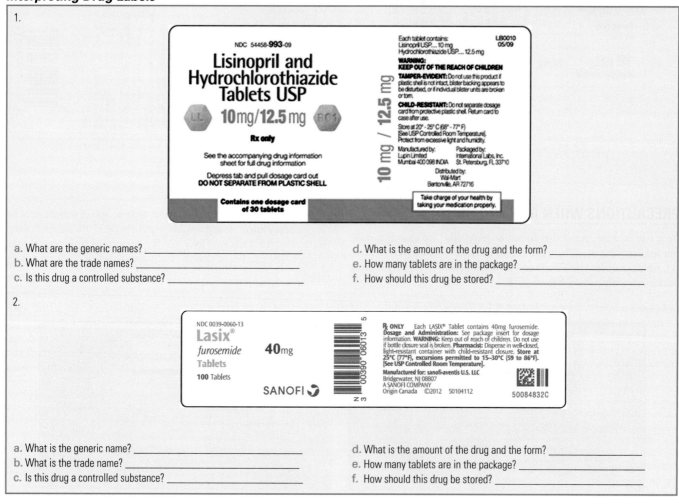

a. What are the generic names? _____

b. What are the trade names? _____

c. Is this drug a controlled substance? _____

d. What is the amount of the drug and the form? _____

e. How many tablets are in the package? _____

f. How should this drug be stored? _____

2.

a. What is the generic name? _____

b. What is the trade name? _____

c. Is this drug a controlled substance? _____

d. What is the amount of the drug and the form? _____

e. How many tablets are in the package? _____

f. How should this drug be stored? _____

PRACTICE PROBLEMS—CONT'D

Interpreting Drug Labels

3.

NDC 59011-451-01
One Pint (473 mL)

Dilaudid® **C II**
hydromorphone HCl
ORAL LIQUID
(1 mg/1 mL)

Each 5 mL (1 teaspoonful)
contains 5 mg hydromor-
phone HCl.
Usual Dose: See package
insert.
Storage: Store at 25°C (77°F);
excursions permitted to
15°-30°C (59°-86°F) [See USP
Controlled Room Temperature].
Shake well before using.
Dispense in a tight,
light-resistant container
as defined in the USP.

a. What is the generic name? _____

b. What is the trade name? _____

c. Is this drug a controlled substance? _____

d. What is the concentration of the drug? _____

e. What is the total volume? _____

f. How should this drug be stored? _____

4.

NDC 63739-931-14   Ⴅonly

HEPARIN
SODIUM INJECTION, USP

10,000 USP Units**/10** mL
(1,000 USP Units/mL)

For IV or SC use

10 mL   Multiple Dose Vial

NOT FOR LOCK FLUSH

Derived from Porcine Intestinal Mucosa
Sterile, Nonpyrogenic
Store at 20° to 25°C (68° to 77°F) [See USP
Controlled Room Temperature].
KEEP THIS AND ALL DRUGS OUT OF THE
REACH OF CHILDREN
Mfd. in INDIA for McKesson Packaging
Services.
M.L. No: 13/MD/AP/2010/F/CC
I05/2013
P1410420

a. What is the generic name? _____

b. What is the concentration of the drug? _____

c. Is the purpose of the drug for heparin locks? _____

d. What route can the drug be given? _____

e. Is the vial for single use or multiple use? _____

DRUG RECONSTITUTION

Drugs that come in powder or liquid form may need reconstitution. The liquid used to reconstitute the drug is called a **diluent**. Diluents can be nonsterile water for enteral administration, sterile water intended for injection, 0.9% saline solution, or a special liquid supplied by the manufacturer. The nurse must follow manufacturer's directions for reconstitution.

1. The following is a label for reconstituting oral cefadroxil.

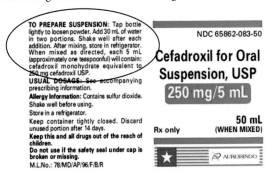

TO PREPARE SUSPENSION: Tap bottle lightly to loosen powder. Add 30 mL of water in two portions. Shake well after each addition. After mixing, store in refrigerator. When mixed as directed, each 5 mL (approximately one teaspoonful) will contain: cefadroxil monohydrate equivalent to 250 mg cefadroxil USP.
USUAL DOSAGE: See accompanying prescribing information.
Allergy Information: Contains sulfur dioxide. Shake well before using.
Store in a refrigerator.
Keep container tightly closed. Discard unused portion after 14 days.
Keep this and all drugs out of the reach of children.
Do not use if the safety seal under cap is broken or missing.
M.L.No.: 78/MD/AP/96/F/B/R

NDC 65862-083-50

Cefadroxil for Oral Suspension, USP
250 mg/5 mL

Rx only   **50 mL** (WHEN MIXED)

★   Αℛ AUROBINDO

Read the left side of the label that says *To Prepare Suspension*. Note that 30 mL of water in two portions is needed to liquefy the powder. This is an oral drug, so drinking water can be used. The nurse is instructed to shake the powder loose to prevent clumping. Add 15 mL of water and shake well. Add another 15 mL of water and shake well. The powder has now been reconstituted into a **suspension**, and each 5 mL of liquid contains 250 mg of cefadroxil. The entire bottle has 50 mL when mixed, a number that is irrelevant when calculating a dose. Now the equation can be set up for calculation of a dosage.

2. The following is a label of a parenteral drug that requires reconstitution.

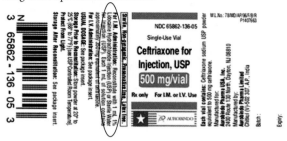

Read the left side of the label. For intramuscular (IM) injection, it states to reconstitute with 1 mL of 1% lidocaine hydrochloride (this diluent is sometimes used when a medication is very painful when given IM) *or* 1 mL sterile water for injection. After this preparation is reconstituted and shaken, each milliliter contains 350 mg. The figure *500 mg* in the center of the label is the dose contained in the *whole vial*. If the medication is to be given intravenously, the instructions are written in the package insert. The nurse will need to read the drug insert to determine proper reconstitution for the intravenous (IV) route.

CALCULATION METHODS

Drug calculations are usually made for one dose. For example, if the prescription states that a patient is to be given 500 mg of a drug three times a day, the nurse would calculate the amount of drug equivalent to 500 mg. Occasionally, nurses calculate the full daily dose, which in this case would be 1500 mg (500 mg times three doses).

The three general methods for dosage calculations are the (1) basic formula (BF), (2) ratio and proportion/fractional equation (RP/FE), and (3) dimensional analysis (DA). These methods are used to calculate most enteral and parenteral drug dosages. The nurse should select one of the methods to calculate drug dosages and use that method consistently. All but the DA require using the same units of measure. It is most helpful to convert to the system used on the drug label. If the drug is prescribed in grams (g, G) and the drug label gives the dose in milligrams (mg), convert grams to milligrams (the measurement on the drug label) and proceed with the drug calculation. If conversion factors are needed during calculation, BF and RP/FE becomes a multistep process, which increases the risk of miscalculation.

PRACTICE PROBLEMS

Drug Reconstitution

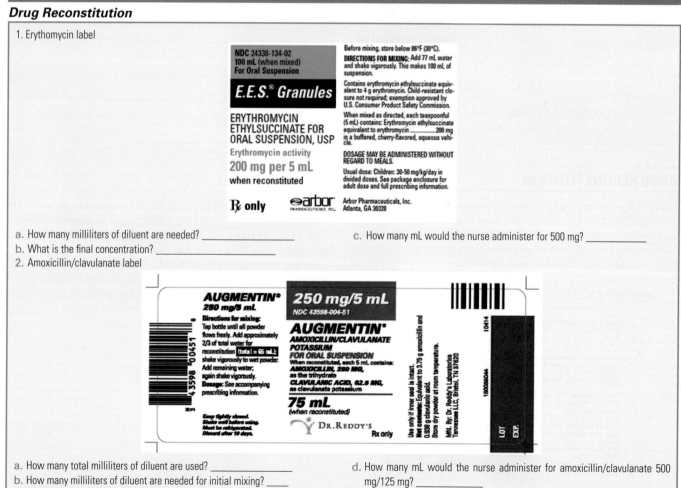

1. Erythomycin label

a. How many milliliters of diluent are needed? _____

b. What is the final concentration? _____

c. How many mL would the nurse administer for 500 mg? _____

2. Amoxicillin/clavulanate label

a. How many total milliliters of diluent are used? _____

b. How many milliliters of diluent are needed for initial mixing? _____

c. What is the final concentration for each drug? _____

d. How many mL would the nurse administer for amoxicillin/clavulanate 500 mg/125 mg? _____

For drugs that require individualized dosing, calculation by BW or by BSA may be necessary. These last two methods are mostly used for the calculation of pediatric dosages and for drugs used in the treatment of cancer (antineoplastic drugs). BW and BSA methods of calculation are also useful for individuals whose BW is low, who are obese, or who are older adults.

✳ Method 1: Basic Formula

The **basic formula (BF)** is easy to recall:

$$\frac{D}{H} \times V = A$$

Where:
D is the *desired* dose (as prescribed)
H is the drug on *hand* (available)
V is the *vehicle* or *volume* of a drug form (tablet, capsule, liquid [mL])
A is the *amount* calculated to be given to the patient.

Examples Using the Basic Formula

1. **Prescribed:** Cefaclor 0.5 g PO bid
   Available:

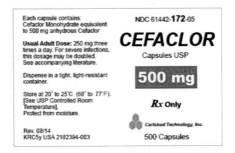

   How many capsules would the patient receive per dose? (This is a two-step process.)

   a. The unit of measure that is prescribed (grams) and the unit of measure on the label (milligrams) are from the same system of measurement—the metric system. Conversion to the same unit as on the label is necessary to solve the problem. Because the label is in milligrams, convert grams to milligrams. To convert grams (large value) to milligrams (smaller value), move the decimal point three spaces to the right as discussed earlier:

$$\frac{D}{H} \times V; \text{ where } D = 500 \text{ mg}, \quad H = 500 \text{ mg},$$
$$\text{and } V = 1 \text{ capsule; then}$$

$$\frac{D}{H} \times V = \frac{500 \text{ mg}}{500 \text{ mg}} \times 1 \text{ capsule} = 1 \text{ capsule}$$

   Answer: 500 mg, or 1 capsule
   The patient would receive 1 capsule per dose.

2. **Prescribed:** Phenobarbital 30 mg PO STAT
   Available:

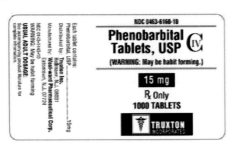

How many tablets would the patient receive per dose?
The dosage is prescribed in milligrams and the unit of measure on the label is also expressed in milligrams. There is no need for conversion.

$$\frac{D}{H} \times V; \text{ then}$$

$$\frac{30 \text{ mg}}{15 \text{ mg}} \times 1 \text{ tablet} = 2 \text{ tablets}$$

Answer: 30 mg = 2 tablets
The patient would receive 2 tablets per dose.

✳ Method 2: Ratio and Proportion/Fractional Equation

Ratio and Proportion: Linear Method

The ratio and proportion (RP) method can be expressed linearly or as a fraction (a fractional equation). The linear setup is as follows:

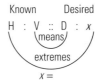

Where:
D is the *desired* dose (as prescribed)
H is the drug on *hand* (available)
V is the *vehicle* or *volume* of a drug form (tablet, capsule, liquid [mL])
x is the *unknown* amount to give to the patient
The double colon symbol (::) stands for "as" or "equal to"

Multiply the extremes and the means ($Hx :: VD$). Solve for x $\left(\dfrac{Hx}{H} :: \dfrac{VD}{H}\right)$; H is the divisor $\left(x = \dfrac{VD}{H}\right)$.

Examples Using Ratio and Proportion: Linear Method.

1. **Prescribed:** Amoxicillin 100 mg PO qid
   Available:

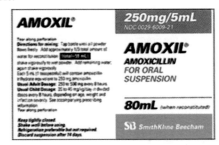

How many milliliters would the patient receive per dose?
Conversion is not needed because both are expressed in the same unit of measure.

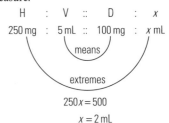

$$250x = 500$$
$$x = 2 \text{ mL}$$

Answer: Amoxicillin 100 mg = 2 mL
The patient would receive 2 mL per dose.

2. **Prescribed:** Aspirin 162 mg PO once daily
   Available:

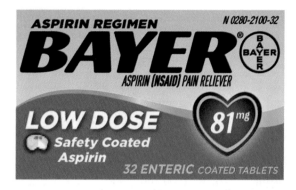

How many tablets would the patient receive per dose?

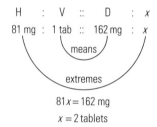

$$81x = 162 \text{ mg}$$
$$x = 2 \text{ tablets}$$

Answer: Aspirin 162 mg = 2 tablets
The patient would receive 2 tablets per dose.

Fractional Equation

The **fractional equation (FE)** setup is written as a fraction and is more commonly used than the linear setup.

$$\frac{H}{V} = \frac{D}{x}; \text{ where } \frac{H \text{ (dosage on hand)}}{V \text{ (vehicle)}} \qquad \frac{D \text{ (desired dosage)}}{x \text{ (unknown)}}$$

Cross-multiply and solve for x, where Hx = VD; then $x = \dfrac{VD}{H}$.

Examples Using the Fractional Equation–Fraction Method.

1. **Prescribed:** Ciprofloxacin 500 mg PO q12h
   Available:

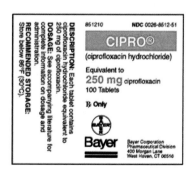

How many tablet(s) should the patient receive per dose?

$$\frac{H}{V} = \frac{D}{x}$$

Where:
H = 250 mg
V = tablet (tab)
D = 500 mg
x = unknown number of tablets

$$\frac{250 \text{ mg}}{1 \text{ tab}} = \frac{500 \text{ mg}}{x \text{ tab}}$$

Cross-multiply and solve for x.

$$250x = 500$$
$$x = 2$$

Answer: 500 mg = 2 tablets
The nurse would administer 2 tablets per dose.

2. **Prescribed:** Citalopram 10 mg PO once daily
   Available:

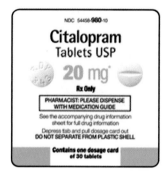

How many tablets would the nurse administer per dose?

$$\left(\frac{H}{V} = \frac{D}{x}\right)$$

$$\frac{20 \text{ mg}}{1 \text{ tab}} = \frac{10 \text{ mg}}{x \text{ tab}}$$

Cross-multiply and solve for x.

$$20x = 10$$
$$x = 0.5 \text{ tablet } \left(^1/_2 \text{ tab}\right)$$

(Note that this tablet is scored to allow it to be split in half.)
Answer: x = 0.5 tablet
The nurse would administer 0.5 tablet per dose.
(For the duration of this chapter, any RP or FE calculation will be shown using the FE method.)

Method 3: Dimensional Analysis

Dimensional analysis (DA) is a calculation method known as *units and conversions*. The D, H, and V are still used in DA. The advantage of DA is that all steps for calculating drug dosages are conducted in one equation without having to remember various formulas. However, conversion factors (CFs) still need to be memorized.

Steps for Dimensional Analysis

1. Identify the unit/form (tablet, capsule, mL) of the drug to be calculated. Place this unit/form to one side of the equal sign (=). *This is your desired unit/form.*
2. Determine the *known* dose and unit/form from the drug label. Place this on the other side of the equal sign.

3. Continue with additional fractions, including conversion factors, using a multiplication operation between each fraction until all but the desired *unit/form* is eliminated.
4. Multiply the numerators and multiply the denominators.
5. Divide the denominator into the numerator.
6. Solve for *x* (the unknown unit/form).

Examples Using Dimensional Analysis.
1. **Prescribed:** Amoxicillin 500 mg PO q8h
   Available: 250 mg per capsule
   How many capsules (cap) would the nurse administer per dose?

$$cap = \frac{1\,cap}{250\,mg}\ (H = on\ hand)$$

a. Notice that the drug form "cap" to the left of the equal sign is the same as the "cap" in the numerator to the right of the equal sign. (We must determine how many capsules need to be administered for the dose to be 500 mg.) The available capsule is 250 mg; this is placed in the denominator.
b. The available strength (250 mg) is the denominator, and the unit/form "mg" must match the next numerator, which is the ordered dose of 500 mg (*desired dose*). The next *denominator* would be *x cap* (*unknown*) or it would be left blank.

$$cap = \frac{1\ cap}{250\ \overline{)mg}} \times \frac{500\ \overline{)mg}}{x\ cap}$$

c. Cancel out the *mg*, multiply the numerators, then multiply the denominators.
d. Solve for *x* by isolating *x*; reduce the resulting fraction. (Reducing fractions could be done earlier.) What remain are *cap* and 2.

$$\frac{500}{250\ x}\ ;\ then\ x = 2\ cap$$

Answer: 2 capsules

When conversions are needed (e.g., between milligrams and grams) a CF is needed to calculate dosages using the BF or RP/FE, requiring a multistep process. When using DA, there should *only* be the one unknown value in the equation (*x*). This will be especially important when calculating dosages that involve milligrams per kilogram (mg/kg) or milligrams per meters squared (mg/m^2).

2. **Prescribed:** Amoxicillin 0.5 g PO q8h
   Available: 250 mg per capsule
   How many capsules would the nurse administer?
   A conversion is needed between grams and milligrams. Following the steps for DA, the equation looks like this:

$$H \times CF \times \frac{D}{unknown} =$$

$$cap = \frac{1\ cap}{250\ mg} \times \frac{1000\ mg}{1\ g} \times \frac{0.5\ g}{x\ cap} = \frac{1000 \times 0.5}{250}$$

$$= \frac{500}{250} = 2\ capsules\ of\ amoxicillin$$

As with other methods of calculation, the three components are *D*, *H*, and *V* as indicated in the previous problem. With DA, the CF is built into the equation and is included when the ordered drug's unit of measurement and the drug available differ. If the same units of measurement are used, the CF is eliminated from the equation, as shown in the first example.

3. **Prescribed:** Acetaminophen 1 g PO q6h PRN for headache
   Available: Acetaminophen 325 mg per tablet

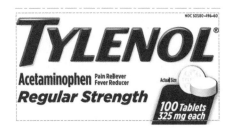

Conversion factor: 1000 mg = 1 g
How many tablet(s) would be given?

$$tap = \frac{1\ tap}{325\ \overline{)mg}} \times \frac{1000\ \overline{)mg}}{1\ \overline{)g}} \times \frac{1\overline{)g}}{x\ tap} = \frac{1000}{325} = 3.07$$

Answer: 1000 mg [1 G] = 3 tablets
The nurse would administer 3 tablets per dose.

✳ Method 4: Body Weight
The **body weight (BW)** method of calculation allows for individualization of the drug dosage and involves the following three steps:
1. Convert pounds to kilograms; 2.2 lb is equivalent to 1 kg.
2. Determine the drug dose for the body weight by multiplying as follows:

$$Drug\ dose \times Body\ weight = Patient's\ dose$$

3. Follow the BF, RP/FE, or DA method to calculate the drug dosage.

Examples of Using Body Weight for Drug Calculation.
1. **Prescribed:** Fluorouracil 12 mg per kg per day IV for a patient who weighs 176 lb
   Available:

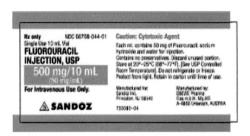

How many milliliters would the nurse administer per day?

Basic Formula
a. The first step is to convert pounds to kilograms by dividing the number of pounds the patient weighs by 2.2 (1 kg = 2.2 lb).

$$176\ lb\,/\,2.2 \% 80\ kg$$

b. The second step is to multiply the ordered dose by the patient's weight in kilograms.

$$mg \times kg = Patient\ dose$$

$$12\ mg \times 80\ kg = 960\ mg\ per\ day$$

c. The third step is to determine the volume in milliliters to administer 960 mg.

$$\frac{D}{H} \times V = \frac{960 \text{ mg}}{50 \text{ mg}} \times 1 \text{ mL}$$
$$= 19.2 \text{ mL}$$

Dimensional Analysis
(Notice that the CFs are included in this one equation.)

$$mL = \frac{1 \text{ mL}}{50 \text{ mg}} \times \frac{12 \text{ mg}}{1 \text{ kg}} \times \frac{1 \text{ kg}}{2.2 \text{ lb}} \times \frac{176 \text{ lb}}{x \text{ mL}}$$
$$= \frac{2112 \text{ mL}}{110}$$
$$= 19.2 \text{ mL}$$

(Since liquid medications can be given in partial amounts, round to the nearest tenth.)

2. **Prescribed:** Cefaclor oral suspension 20 mg per kg per day in three divided doses for a pediatric patient who weighs 66 lb
   Available: Cefaclor oral suspension 125 mg per 5 mL

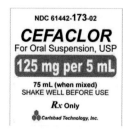

NDC 61442-**173**-02
CEFACLOR
For Oral Suspension, USP
125 mg per 5 mL
75 mL (when mixed)
SHAKE WELL BEFORE USE
Rx Only
Carlsbad Technology, Inc.

How many milliliters would the nurse administer per dose? _____

Basic Formula
a. Convert pounds to kilograms.

$$66 \text{ lb} / 2.2 \text{ lb} \% 30 \text{ kg}$$

b. Multiply the desired dosage with the patient's weight in kg

$$20 \text{ mg} \times 30 \text{ kg} = 600 \text{ mg per day}$$

c. Divide by the number of doses needed for the day.

$$600 \text{ mg} / 3 \text{ doses} = 200 \text{ mg per dose}$$

d. Using the BF, determine the mL per dose.

$$\frac{D}{H} \times V = \frac{200 \text{ mg}}{125 \text{ mg}} \times 5 \text{ mL}$$
$$= 8 \text{ mL}$$

Dimensional Analysis

$$mL = \frac{5 \text{ mL}}{125 \text{ mg}} \times \frac{20 \text{ mg}}{1 \text{ kg}} \times \frac{1 \text{ kg}}{2.2 \text{ lb}} \times \frac{66 \text{ lb}}{3 \text{ doses}}$$
$$= \frac{6600 \text{ mL}}{825 \text{ mg}}$$
$$= 8 \text{ mL per dose}$$

 Method 5: Body Surface Area—West Nomogram

The measurement of body surface area (BSA) is the most precise method for calculating drug dosages. BSA can be measured using the West nomogram or the square root method.

The BSA by the West nomogram (Fig. 11.2A) is measured in square meters (m^2) and is determined by the patient's height and weight. Determine where the height and weight intersect on the nomogram scale; the height and weight can be in inches and pounds or centimeters and kilograms depending on the column used, but the systems of measurement must match. Centimeters and kilograms are both within the metric system and are most commonly used for the calculation of BSA. To calculate a drug dosage, multiply the dose ordered with the patient's BSA.

Examples of Using Body Surface Area: Drug Calculation.
1. Drug dosage will be determined using the West nomogram and the square root calculations for a patient who is 70 inches tall and weighs 160 lb.
   a. Determining Body Surface Area Using the West Nomogram (Using Inches and Pounds): Draw a straight line from *70* in the *inches* column to *160* in the *pounds* column (Fig. 11.2B). Note that the line intersects between 1.9 and 2 square meters.
   b. Determining Body Surface Area Using the West Nomogram (Using Centimeters and Kilograms): The patient is 178 cm tall (1 in = 2.54 cm) and weighs 73 kg (2.2 lb = 1 kg). The height and the weight were rounded to whole numbers. Draw a straight line from 178 in the *centimeters* column to 73 in the *kilograms* column (Fig. 11.2C). Note that the line also intersects between 1.9 and 2. For the purposes of calculation, 1.95 can be used.
   c. Determining Body Surface Area Using the Square Root Method: The most precise way to determine BSA is to use the square root method for the calculation. When calculating the BSA in household measurement (inches and pounds), the following formula applies:

$$BSA = \sqrt{\frac{\text{Height (inches)} \times \text{Weight (pounds)}}{3131 \text{ (constant)}}}$$
$$= \sqrt{\frac{70 \text{ in} \times 160 \text{ lb}}{3131}}$$
$$= \sqrt{\frac{11200}{3131}}$$
$$= \sqrt{3.6}$$
$$= \sqrt{3.6} = 1.9 \text{ m}^2$$

When calculating the BSA using the metric system (centimeters and kilograms), the following formula applies:

$$BSA = \sqrt{\frac{\text{Height (centimeters)} \times \text{Weight (kilometers)}}{3600 \text{ (constant)}}}$$
$$= \sqrt{\frac{178 \text{ cm} \times 73 \text{ kg}}{3600}} = \sqrt{\frac{12994}{3600}} = \sqrt{3.6}$$
$$\sqrt{3.6} = 1.9 \text{ m}^2$$

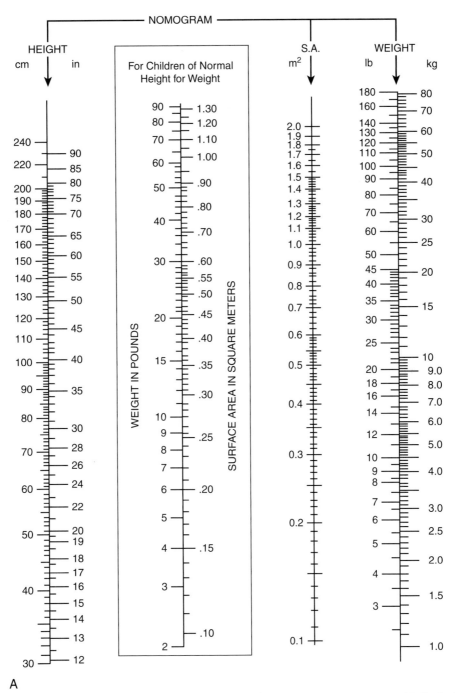

A

Fig. 11.2A West nomogram. The outside columns are used to calculate the meters squared (m²) of adults. The middle column is used to calculate the meters squared of children. (Modified from data by Boyd, E., & West, C. D. [2011]. In R. M. Kliegman, B. F. Stanton, J. W. St. Geme III, et al. [Eds.], *Nelson textbook of pediatrics* [19th ed]. Philadelphia: Saunders.)

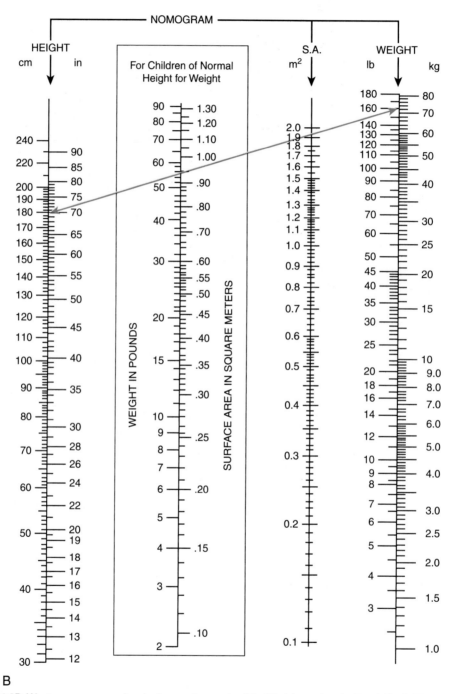

Fig. 11.2B **West nomogram using inches and pounds.** (Modified from data by Boyd, E., & West, C. D. [2011]. In R. M. Kliegman, B. F. Stanton, J. W. St. Geme III, et al. [Eds.], *Nelson textbook of pediatrics* [19th ed]. Philadelphia: Saunders.)

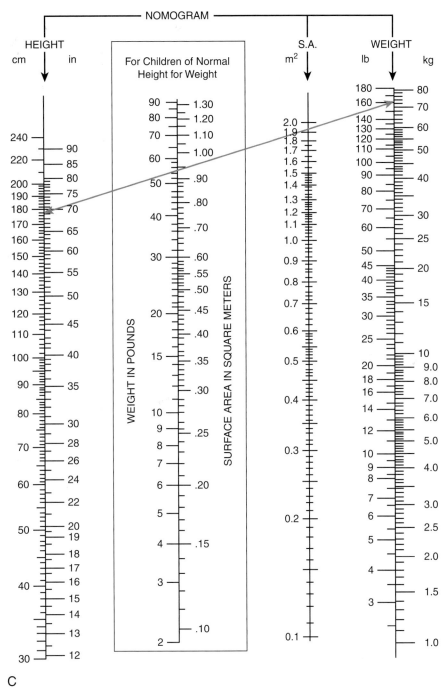

Fig. 11.2C **West nomogram using centimeters and kilograms.** (Modified from data by Boyd, E., & West, C. D. [2011]. In R. M. Kliegman, B. F. Stanton, J. W. St. Geme III, et al. [Eds.], *Nelson textbook of pediatrics* [19th ed.]. Philadelphia: Saunders.)

(Numbers have been rounded to the nearest tenth, which is common for adults.)

Note that both results using the square root method agree and are more precise than using the West nomogram. The variance of 0.05 from the lowest calculated BSA to the highest calculated BSA is negligible.

2. The following drug dosage for this patient is calculated using a BSA of 1.9 m².
   Prescribed: CISplatin 20 mg per m² IV today
   Available:

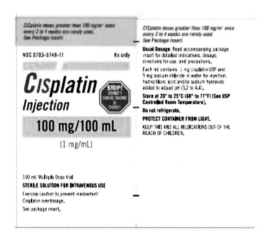

(Note that the label also states 100 mg per 100 mL. Using the lowest numbers listed on a drug label helps prevent errors by eliminating extraneous zeroes.)

a. How many milligrams are prescribed?
   To calculate the child's dose, multiply 20 mg with 1.9 m² to get 38 mg.

b. How many milliliters would the nurse administer?

Basic Formula

$$\frac{D}{H} \times V$$

$$= \frac{38 \text{ mg}}{1 \text{ mg}} \times 1 \text{ mL}$$

$$= 38 \text{ mL}$$

Ratio and Proportion/Fractional Equation

$$\frac{H}{V} = \frac{D}{x}$$

$$\frac{1 \text{ mg}}{1 \text{ mL}} = \frac{38 \text{ mg}}{x}$$

$$x = 38 \text{ mL}$$

Dimensional Analysis

$$mL = \frac{1 \text{ mL}}{1 \text{ mg}} \times \frac{1000 \text{ mg}}{1 \text{ g}} \times \frac{38 \text{ mg}}{x}$$

$$x = 38 \text{ mL}$$

Answer: The nurse would administer 38 mL of CISplatin intravenously.

3. Calculating a pediatric dose based on BSA using the West nomogram and the square root method is illustrated in the following:
   Prescribed: Vincristine 2 mg per m² today
   Available: Vincristine 1 mg per mL

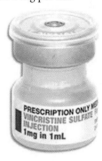

How many milliliters would the nurse administer?

This pediatric patient's height and weight fall within the normal percentile. The child weighs 44 lb (20 kg).

a. Using the center column on the West nomogram, the child's BSA is *0.8 m²*.

b. Use the square root method to calculate BSA using inches and pounds if the child is 36 inches tall.

$$BSA = \sqrt{\frac{36 \text{ in} \times 44 \text{ lb}}{3131}} = \sqrt{\frac{1584}{3131}} = \sqrt{0.51}$$

$$0.71 \text{ m}^2$$

(Rounding numbers to the hundredth place is common when calculating pediatric dosages.)

c. Use the square root method to calculate BSA using centimeters and kilograms.

$$BSA = \sqrt{\frac{91.4 \text{ cm} \times 20 \text{ kg}}{3600}} = \sqrt{\frac{1828}{3600}} = \sqrt{0.51}$$

$$= 0.71 \text{ m}^2$$

d. The more precise number, 0.71 m², will be used to calculate the drug dosage.

Basic Formula

a. Determine desired dose based on the previous BSA.
b. The desired dose is calculated by multiplying 2 mg with 0.71 m² to get 1.42 mg.
c. Solve for the desired unit of measure.

$$\frac{D}{H} \times V$$

$$\frac{1.42 \text{ mg}}{1 \text{ mg}} \times 1 \text{ mL}$$

$$= 1.4 \text{ mL}$$

The dose was rounded to the tenth place to accommodate the calibrations on a syringe.

Dimensional Analysis

a. Determine BSA (we will use the calculated BSA from earlier, 0.71 m²).
b. Solve for the desired unit of measure.

$$mL = \frac{1 \text{ mL}}{1 \text{ mg}} \times \frac{1000 \text{ mg}}{1 \text{ g}} \times \frac{38 \text{ mg}}{x}$$

$$= 1.4 \text{ mL}$$

The dose was rounded to the tenth place to accommodate the calibrations on a syringe.

PRACTICE PROBLEMS

Calculating Dosages Based on Body Weight

1. **Prescribed:** Valproic acid oral solution PO 15 mg per kg per day in two divided doses for a pediatric patient who weighs 66 lb
   Available:

   NDC 0093-9633-16

   VALPROIC ACID
   Oral Solution USP
   250 mg/5 mL

   Each 5 mL contains the equivalent of
   250 mg valproic acid as the sodium salt.

   ℞ only

   USUAL DOSAGE: See package insert for
   prescribing information.

   Store at 20° to 25°C (68° to 77°F) [See
   USP Controlled Room Temperature].

   Dispense in a tight container as defined
   in the USP.

   KEEP THIS AND ALL MEDICATIONS OUT
   OF THE REACH OF CHILDREN.

   L22102   Rev. C 10/2006
   TEVA PHARMACEUTICALS USA
   Sellersville, PA 18960

   16 fl oz

   TEVA

   a. How many kilograms does the child weigh? _____
   b. How many milligrams per *day* would the child receive? _____
   c. How many milligrams per *dose* would the child receive? _____
   d. How many *milliliters* per dose would the child receive? _____

2. **Prescribed:** Gentamicin 2.5 mg per kg q8h IM for a pediatric patient who weighs 33 lb
   Available:

   NDC 63323-173-02   17302

   GENTAMICIN
   INJECTION, USP
   (PEDIATRIC)

   equivalent to 10 mg/mL Gentamicin

   20 mg/2 mL

   For IM or IV Use.
   Must be diluted for IV use.
   2 mL Single Dose Vial
   Preservative Free   Rx only

   a. How many kilograms does the child weigh? _____
   b. How many milligrams per dose would the child receive? _____
   c. How many milliliters per dose would the child receive? _____

PRACTICE PROBLEMS

Calculating Dosages Based on Body Surface Area—Square Root Method

1. **Prescribed:** Carboplatin 300 mg per m² per IV infusion today for a patient 66 inches tall who weighs 176 lb
   Available:

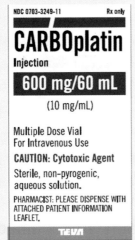

   NDC 0703-3249-11   Rx only

   CARBOplatin

   Injection

   600 mg/60 mL

   (10 mg/mL)

   Multiple Dose Vial
   For Intravenous Use

   CAUTION: Cytotoxic Agent

   Sterile, non-pyrogenic,
   aqueous solution.

   PHARMACIST: PLEASE DISPENSE WITH
   ATTACHED PATIENT INFORMATION
   LEAFLET.

   TEVA

   a. Use the square root method to determine the patient's square meters (BSA) based on inches and pounds.
   b. What is the dosage in milligrams? _____
   c. How many milliliters would the patient receive? _____
2. **Prescribed:** Fluorouracil 350 mg per m² per day IV for a patient 164 cm tall who weighs 66.8 kg.
   a. Use the square root method to determine the patient's square meters (BSA) based on centimeters and kilograms.
   b. How many milligrams would the patient receive? _____

Rounding Rules

Notice when to round. Tablets and caplets can be rounded to the nearest half if they are scored (see the image for citalopram). Some tablets are scored in fourths. In this case the dosage can be rounded to the nearest fourth or quarter tablet. However, tablets and caplets that are extended release, sustained release, controlled release, or enteric coated should not be split because splitting or crushing these preparations destroys the properties that render the drug long-lasting. For this reason, these preparations in addition to capsules are rounded to the nearest whole number. Liquid drugs can be rounded to the nearest tenth; the exception to this rule is when calculating dosages of drops, which are rounded to the nearest whole number.

When rounding, determine how many places beyond the decimal point are appropriate. The general rounding rules are:
1. If a number to the right of the digit that needs to be rounded is less than 5, round down. For example, when rounding 1.343 to the hundredth place, the number becomes 1.34. Rounding 1.343 to the tenth place, it becomes 1.3. Rounding 1.343 to a whole number, it becomes 1.
2. If a number to the right of the digit that needs to be rounded is 5 or greater, round up. For example, when rounding 1.745 to the hundredth place, the number becomes 1.75. Rounding 1.745 to the tenth place, it becomes 1.7. Rounding 1.745 to a whole number, it becomes 2.

CONSIDERATIONS FOR ENTERAL ADMINISTRATION

Most drugs are administered orally. Oral drugs are available in tablet, caplet, capsule, powder, and liquid forms. Oral medications are absorbed by the gastrointestinal (GI) tract, mainly from the small intestine.

Oral medications have several advantages: (1) the patient can often take oral medications without assistance, (2) the cost of oral medications is usually less than that of parenteral preparations, and (3) oral medications are easy to store. The disadvantages include (1) variation in absorption because of food in the GI tract and pH variation of GI secretions, (2) irritation of the gastric mucosa by certain drugs (e.g., potassium chloride), and (3) destruction or partial inactivation of the drugs by liver enzymes. Oral drugs (tablets, capsules, liquids) that may irritate the gastric mucosa should be taken with 6 to 8 ounces of fluids or should be taken with food. Nursing considerations when administering enteral drugs are further illustrated in Chapter 10.

Tablets, Capsules, and Liquids

Tablets come in different forms and drug strengths. Many tablets are scored and thus can be readily broken when half of the drug amount is needed. Capsules are gelatin shells that contain powder or timed-release pellets (beads). Capsules that are sustained release (pellet) or controlled release *should not* be crushed and diluted because the medication will be absorbed at a much faster rate than indicated by the manufacturer. Many medications sold in tablet form are also available in liquid form. When the patient has difficulty taking tablets, the oral liquid form of the medication is given. The liquid form can be in a suspension, syrup, elixir, or tincture. Some liquid medications that irritate the stomach, such as potassium chloride, are diluted. The tincture form is always diluted.

Tablets that are enteric coated (with a hard shell) must *not* be crushed because the medication could irritate the gastric mucosa. Enteric-coated drugs pass through the stomach into the small intestine where the drug's enteric coating dissolves, and then absorption occurs. Fig. 11.3 shows the different forms of tablets and capsules.

Liquid medications are poured into a medicine cup that is calibrated (i.e., ounces, teaspoons, tablespoons, and milliliters). Fig. 11.4 shows the markings on a medicine cup.

Drugs Administered via Nasogastric Tube

Oral medications can be administered through a nasogastric (NG) or other feeding tube for enteral administration. If the patient is receiving a tube feeding, the drug should *not* be mixed with the feeding solution. Mixing the medications in a large volume of tube feeding solution decreases the amount of drug the patient receives for a specific time.

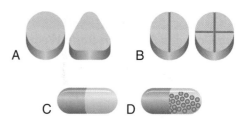

Fig. 11.3 Shapes of tablets and capsules. (A) Nonscored tablets. (B) Scored tablets. (C) Nonextended release capsule. (D) Extended release capsule.

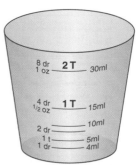

Fig. 11.4 Medicine cup for liquid measurement. (From Kee, J. L., & Marshall, S. M. [2013]. *Clinical calculations* (7th ed.). St. Louis: Elsevier.)

The medication (but *not* timed-release or sustained-release capsules and psyllium hydrophilic mucilloid) should be diluted in 15 to 30 mL of water or other desired fluid unless otherwise instructed. The medication is administered through the tube via a syringe, followed by another 15 to 30 mL of water to ensure that the drug reaches the stomach and is not left in the tube. Nurses should be familiar with the institution's policy prior to administering medications through a feeding tube.

PRACTICE PROBLEMS

Enteral Administration

1. **Prescribed:** Ranitidine 150 mg PO q12h
   Available:

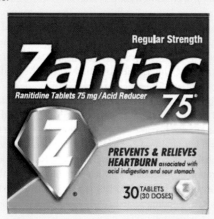

Administer how many tablets per dose? _____

2. **Prescribed:** Doxycycline 100 mg PO q12h
   Available:

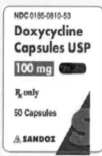

Administer how many capsules per dose? _____

3. **Order:** Warfarin 2 mg PO once daily
   Available:

NDC# 67544-0401-15

Warfarin NA (Coumadin)

2mg   15 Tablets

Store between 20-25 degrees C (68-77 degrees F).
See USP Controlled Room Temperature.
Dispense in a tight light-resistant container as defined by USP.
Keep this and all drugs out of the reach of children.

Mfg. By: Bristol-Myers Squibb Company
Garden City, NY

Repackaged by Aphena Pharma
Cookeville, TN 38506

Warfarin NA (Coumadin) 2mg 15 Tablets

Administer how many tablets per dose? _____

PRACTICE PROBLEMS—CONT'D

4. **Prescribed:** Hydrochlorothiazide 12.5 mg PO every morning
   Available:

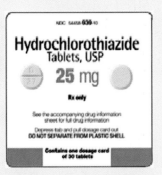

Hydrochlorothiazide
Tablets, USP

25 mg

Rx only

See the accompanying drug information
sheet for full drug information

Depress tab and pull dosage card out
DO NOT SEPARATE FROM PLASTIC SHELL

Contains one dosage card
of 30 tablets

Administer how many tablets per dose? _____

5. **Prescribed:** Lactulose solution 20 g by mouth tid
   Available:

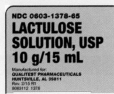

NDC 0603-1378-65
**LACTULOSE
SOLUTION, USP
10 g/15 mL**
Manufactured for:
QUALITEST PHARMACEUTICALS
HUNTSVILLE, AL 35811
Rev. 2/15 R1
6063112 1378

Administer how many milliliters per dose? _____

6. **Prescribed:** Phenytoin oral solution 0.25 g PO bid
   Available:

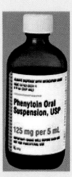

Phenytoin Oral
Suspension, USP

125 mg per 5 mL

Administer how many milliliters per dose? _____

7. **Prescribed:** Valproic acid oral solution PO 15 mg per kg per day in two
   divided doses for a pediatric patient who weighs 66 lb
   Available:

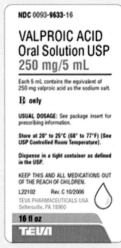

NDC 0093-9633-16

**VALPROIC ACID
Oral Solution USP
250 mg/5 mL**

Each 5 mL contains the equivalent of
250 mg valproic acid as the sodium salt.

℞ only

USUAL DOSAGE: See package insert for
prescribing information.

Store at 20° to 25°C (68° to 77°F) [See
USP Controlled Room Temperature].

Dispense in a tight container as defined
in the USP.

KEEP THIS AND ALL MEDICATIONS OUT
OF THE REACH OF CHILDREN.

L22102   Rev. C 10/2006
TEVA PHARMACEUTICALS USA
Sellersville, PA 18960

16 fl oz

TEVA

a. How many kilograms does the child weigh? _____
b. How many milligrams per *day* would the child receive? _____
c. How many milligrams per *dose* would the child receive? _____
d. How many *milliliters* per dose would the child receive? _____

CONSIDERATIONS FOR PARENTERAL ADMINISTRATION

When medications cannot be taken by mouth because of (1) an inability to swallow, (2) a decreased level of consciousness, (3) an inactivation of the drug by gastric juices, or (4) a desire to increase the effectiveness of the drug, the parenteral route may be the route of choice. Parenteral medications are administered under the skin (intradermally [ID]), into the fatty tissue (subcutaneously [subcut]), within the muscle (intramuscularly [IM]), or in the vein (intravenously [IV]). Nursing considerations when administering parenteral drugs are further discussed in Chapter 10.

Injectable Preparations

The appropriate drug container (vial or ampule) and the correct selection of needle and syringe are essential in the preparation of the prescribed drug dose. The route of administration is part of the medication order.

Syringes

The syringe is composed of a barrel (outer shell), plunger (inner part), and the tip where the needle joins the syringe (Fig. 11.5). Syringes are available in various types and sizes, including tuberculin and insulin syringes. Syringes prefilled with drugs may be glass, plastic, or metal. The tip of the syringe, inside of the barrel, and the plunger should remain sterile.

Vials and Ampules

A vial is usually a small glass vacuum container with a self-sealing rubber top. Some are multiple-dose vials, and when properly stored, they can be used over time. An ampule is a glass container with a tapered neck for snapping open and using only once. Caution is advised when snapping an ampule to prevent skin laceration. Also, glass fragments can occur; therefore a filter needle must be used to withdraw medication. Fig. 11.6 shows a vial and an ampule. Drugs that deteriorate readily in liquid form are packaged in powder form in vials for storage. Once the dry form of the drug is reconstituted (usually with sterile or bacteriostatic water or 0.9% saline), the drug is used immediately or must be refrigerated. Check the accompanying drug circular for specific storage lengths and other instructions. Once the drug in a multidose vial is reconstituted, the vial should be labeled with the date and time of reconstitution and the initials of the person who reconstituted the drug. The shelf life of a reconstituted

drug is determined by the manufacturer and can be found on the drug label or drug circular.

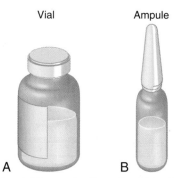

Fig. 11.6 **(A) Vial and (B) ampule.** (From Kee, J. L., & Marshall, S. M. [2013]. *Clinical calculations* [7th ed.]. St. Louis: Elsevier.)

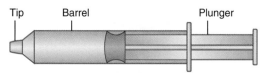

Fig. 11.5 Parts of a syringe. (From Kee, J. L., & Marshall, S. M. [2015]. *Clinical calculations* [8th ed.]. St. Louis: Elsevier.)

PRACTICE PROBLEMS

Subcutaneous and Intramuscular Administration

1. **Prescribed:** NPH insulin 45 units subcutaneous (subcut)
   Available: NPH insulin 100 units per mL and insulin syringe 100 units per mL
   Indicate on the insulin syringe the amount of insulin that should be withdrawn.

2. **Prescribed:** Regular insulin 23 units subcut
   Available: Regular insulin 100 units per mL and insulin syringes 100 units per mL as 1-mL and 0.5-mL syringes
   Specify which insulin syringe is best to use, and indicate on the appropriate syringe the amount of insulin to be withdrawn.

PRACTICE PROBLEMS—CONT'D
Subcutaneous and Intramuscular Administration

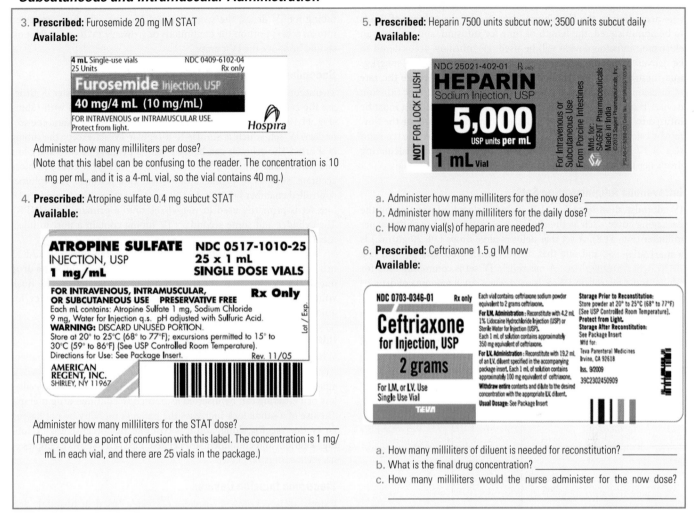

3. **Prescribed:** Furosemide 20 mg IM STAT
   Available:

   4 mL Single-use vials · NDC 0409-6102-04
   25 Units · Rx only
   Furosemide Injection, USP
   40 mg/4 mL (10 mg/mL)
   FOR INTRAVENOUS or INTRAMUSCULAR USE.
   Protect from light. · *Hospira*

   Administer how many milliliters per dose? _____
   (Note that this label can be confusing to the reader. The concentration is 10 mg per mL, and it is a 4-mL vial, so the vial contains 40 mg.)

4. **Prescribed:** Atropine sulfate 0.4 mg subcut STAT
   Available:

   ATROPINE SULFATE NDC 0517-1010-25
   INJECTION, USP · **25 × 1 mL**
   1 mg/mL · **SINGLE DOSE VIALS**
   FOR INTRAVENOUS, INTRAMUSCULAR,
   OR SUBCUTANEOUS USE · **PRESERVATIVE FREE** · **Rx Only**
   Each mL contains: Atropine Sulfate 1 mg, Sodium Chloride 9 mg, Water for Injection q.s. pH adjusted with Sulfuric Acid.
   WARNING: DISCARD UNUSED PORTION.
   Store at 20° to 25°C (68° to 77°F); excursions permitted to 15° to 30°C (59° to 86°F) (See USP Controlled Room Temperature).
   Directions for Use: See Package Insert. · Rev. 11/05
   AMERICAN REGENT, INC. SHIRLEY, NY 11967

   Administer how many milliliters for the STAT dose? _____
   (There could be a point of confusion with this label. The concentration is 1 mg/mL in each vial, and there are 25 vials in the package.)

5. **Prescribed:** Heparin 7500 units subcut now; 3500 units subcut daily
   Available:

   NDC 25021-402-01 · Rx only
   HEPARIN Sodium Injection, USP
   5,000 USP units **per mL**
   1 mL Vial
   NOT FOR LOCK FLUSH
   For Intravenous or Subcutaneous Use · From Porcine Intestines
   Mfd. for: SAGENT Pharmaceuticals · Made in India

   a. Administer how many milliliters for the now dose? _____
   b. Administer how many milliliters for the daily dose? _____
   c. How many vial(s) of heparin are needed? _____

6. **Prescribed:** Ceftriaxone 1.5 g IM now
   Available:

   NDC 0703-0346-01 · Rx only
   Ceftriaxone for Injection, USP
   2 grams
   For I.M. or I.V. Use · Single Use Vial
   Each vial contains: ceftriaxone sodium powder equivalent to 2 grams ceftriaxone.
   For I.M. Administration: Reconstitute with 4.2 mL 1% Lidocaine Hydrochloride Injection (USP) or Sterile Water for Injection (USP). Each 1 mL of solution contains approximately 350 mg equivalent of ceftriaxone.
   For I.V. Administration: Reconstitute with 19.2 mL of an I.V. diluent specified in the accompanying package insert. Each 1 mL of solution contains approximately 100 mg equivalent of ceftriaxone.
   Withdraw entire contents and dilute to the desired concentration with the appropriate I.V. diluent.
   Usual Dosage: See Package Insert
   Storage Prior to Reconstitution: Store powder at 20° to 25°C (68° to 77°F) [See USP Controlled Room Temperature].
   Protect from Light.
   Storage After Reconstitution: See Package Insert
   Mfd for: Teva Parenteral Medicines Irvine, CA 92618 · Iss. 9/2009
   39C2302450909 · **TEVA**

   a. How many milliliters of diluent is needed for reconstitution? _____
   b. What is the final drug concentration? _____
   c. How many milliliters would the nurse administer for the now dose? _____

Intravenous Routes

Intravenous (IV) therapy is used to administer fluids that contain water, dextrose, vitamins, electrolytes, and other drugs. Today an increasing number of drugs are administered by the IV route for direct absorption and fast action. Methods of IV administration include intermittent bolus **(IV push [IVP])**, usually with a syringe; intermittent infusions **(IV piggyback [IVPB])**; and continuous infusions. Drugs given IVP are usually small in volume and are administered over a few seconds to a few minutes. Medications administered by this route have a rapid onset of action, and calculation errors can have serious and even fatal consequences. The nurse must read drug inserts carefully to obtain administration information and must give attention to the amount of drug that can be given per minute. If the drug is pushed into the bloodstream at a rate faster than that specified in the drug literature, adverse reactions can occur.

IVPBs contain a larger volume of diluent and are administered over a longer period (e.g., 30 minutes, 1 hour, 3 hours). Continuous infusions, such as 0.9% saline solution or insulin drip, flow continuously until the container of solution is changed or the order for the infusion is stopped.

Many IV drugs irritate the veins; therefore they are diluted before administration. The amount of diluent used depends on the drug; drugs given by IVP can be diluted in small amounts of diluent, whereas other drugs are diluted in a large volume of fluid given over a specific period, such as 4 to 8 hours. Continuous IV infusion replaces fluid loss, maintains fluid balance, and serves as a vehicle for IV drugs.

The current trend in IV medication administration is the use of premixed IV drugs in 50- to 500-mL containers. These premixed IV medications are prepared by the manufacturer or by the hospital pharmacy. The problems of contamination and drug errors are decreased with the use of premixed IV medications. Each IV solution container has separate tubing to prevent admixture. With the use of premixed IV solution containers, the cost is higher, but the risk of medication error is lower. Because not all medication can be premixed in the solution, nurses will continue to prepare some drugs for IV administration.

Nurses have an important role in the preparation and administration of IV solutions such as 0.9% sodium chloride (normal saline, [NS]), 0.45% sodium chloride (½NS), 5% dextrose in water (D_5W), and lactated Ringer's solution (LR) and also IV drugs. Chapter 12 further discusses different types of IV solutions. The nursing functions and responsibilities during IV preparation include the following:

- Gathering equipment
- Knowing IV sets, including drop factors
- Calculating appropriate IV flow rates
- Mixing and diluting drugs in compatible IV fluids
- Knowing the pharmacotherapeutics, pharmacokinetics, and pharmacodynamics of drugs and their side and adverse effects

Nursing responsibilities continue with an assessment of the patient for expected outcomes and adverse effects of the therapy in addition to assessment of the IV site. The nurse calculates the IV flow rate according to the IV tubing's drop factor, the volume of fluids to be administered, the length of time for infusion, and whether an electronic infusion device will be used. IV infusions are ordered to be delivered in some unit of measure over time (e.g., mL/h, mcg/kg/min, unit/h, drops per minute [gtt/min]). Nurses calculate the rate of infusion in milliliters per hour when using an electronic infusion device. If no infusion device is available, the IV medication must be infused by gravity. The nurse will need to manually regulate the flow rate by calculating the infusion rate in drops per minute. The type and size of IV administration tubing must be known when calculating drops per minute.

Intravenous Administration Sets

IV administration sets (Fig. 11.7) include printed information on the packaging cover, such as the drop factor or the number of drops per milliliter (Fig. 11.8). A set that delivers large drops (10–20 gtt/mL) is a macrodrip set, and one that delivers small drops (60 gtt/mL) is a microdrip (minidrip) set. A macrodrip IV set is commonly used for adults, and a microdrip IV set is used when small amounts of drug or more precise administration is warranted.

At times, primary IV fluids are given at a slow rate, ordered to keep vein open (KVO), also called to keep open (TKO). The reasons for KVO include a suspected or potential emergency situation for rapid administration of fluids and drugs and the need for an open line to give IV drugs at specified hours. For KVO, a microdrip set (60 gtt/mL) and

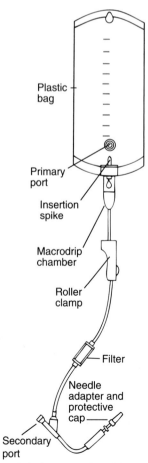

Fig. 11.7 Intravenous infusion sets. (From Morris, D. G. [2014]. *Calculate with confidence* [6th ed.]. St. Louis: Elsevier.)

Labels for Fig. 11.7:
- Plastic bag
- Primary port
- Insertion spike
- Macrodrip chamber
- Roller clamp
- Filter
- Needle adapter and protective cap
- Secondary port

a 250-mL IV solution bag may be used. KVO is usually regulated to deliver 10 to 30 mL/h.

Drugs prescribed as IVPB (Fig. 11.9) are administered via separate tubing for IV drugs, the secondary IV line set, which is connected into an access port on the continuous or primary IV line set; the port should be above the IV pump.

Secondary Intravenous Administration Sets

Two secondary IV administration sets available to administer IV drugs are the calibrated cylinder (volume-controlled chamber) with tubing (Fig. 11.10)—such as the Buretrol, Volutrol, and Soluset—and the secondary IV set, which is similar to a regular IV set except the tubing is shorter. The cylinder can be used with a primary or secondary line and when measurement of small-volume IV therapy needs to be more accurate, such as in pediatric or critical care settings. The volume-controlled chamber holds up to 150 mL of solution. The secondary IV line set is primarily used to piggyback onto a primary line (IVPB). The cylinder and some secondary IV tubing contain a port to inject medications.

When using a calibrated cylinder, such as the Buretrol, add 15 mL of IV solution, such as 0.9% sodium chloride, to flush the drug out of the IV line after the drug infusion is completed. The flush volume is added to the patient's intake. Check hospital policy for guidance.

Intermittent Infusion Adapters and Devices

When continuous IV infusion is to be discontinued but the patient still requires IV access, the IV tubing is removed and a saline lock is attached. Saline locks have ports (stoppers) where needles and needleless or IV tubing can be inserted as needed to continue drug therapy. The use of a saline lock increases the patient's mobility by not having an IV line tagging along, and it is cost effective because less IV tubing, solution, and equipment are needed. Fig. 11.11 shows examples of needleless infusion devices.

Electronic Infusion Devices

Pumps are electronic intravenous devices used in hospitals and some community settings. Such IV pumps are set to deliver a prescribed rate of volume. IV pumps deliver IV solution against resistance. If the flow is obstructed, an alarm sounds; however, the alarm does not sound until the pump has exerted its maximum pressure to overcome resistance. Pumps do not recognize infiltration; therefore the nurse must frequently assess the IV site. When an electronic IV device is used, the flow rate is set in milliliters per hour (mL/h).

IV pumps are recommended for use with all IV therapy; however, some noncritical IV solutions and drugs can be administered using gravity by manually calculating drops per minute. Ongoing nursing assessment is essential with any IV therapy to ensure proper duration of administration.

Several electronic infusion devices are available that include electronic volumetric pumps (IV pumps), syringe pumps, and patient-controlled analgesia (PCA) devices. Fig. 11.12 shows a variety of electronic IV regulators for the administration of IV solutions and drugs.

The objective of PCA is to provide a uniform serum concentration of the medication, thus avoiding drug peaks and valleys. This method is designed to meet the needs of patients who require at least 24 to 48 hours of frequent IM or IV narcotic injections.

Several reasons for the use of PCA include (1) effective pain control without the patient feeling oversedated, (2) considerable reduction in the amount of narcotic used (approximately one-half that of

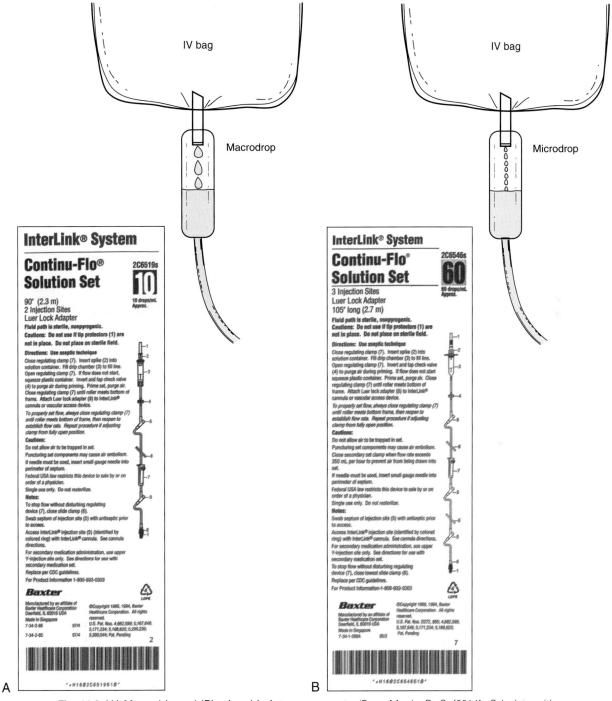

Fig. 11.8 (A) Macrodrip and (B) microdrip intravenous sets. (From Morris, D. G. [2014]. *Calculate with confidence* [6th ed.]. St. Louis: Elsevier.)

IM delivery), and (3) patients' feelings of having greater control over their pain.

Choices are available in the delivery of PCA. The pump can be programmed to administer the prescribed medication (1) at patient demand, (2) continuously, or (3) continuously and supplemented by patient demand (see Chapter 25).

The health care provider's order must include the following:
- Drug prescribed
- Loading dose to obtain a baseline serum concentration of analgesic
- PCA dose, administered each time the patient activates the button

- Lockout interval, the time during which the drug cannot be administered
- Dose limit, the maximum amount the patient can receive during a specified time

Patient Teaching
- Inform the patient that the pain should be tolerable but not necessarily absent.
- Advise the patient of the pump's safety features, including the alarms.

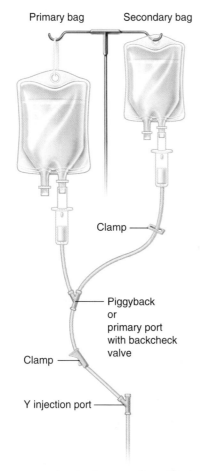

Primary bag   Secondary bag

Clamp

Piggyback
or
primary port
with backcheck
valve

Clamp

Y injection port

Fig. 11.9 Intravenous piggyback setup. (From Morris, D. G. [2014]. *Calculate with confidence* [6th ed.]. St. Louis: Elsevier.)

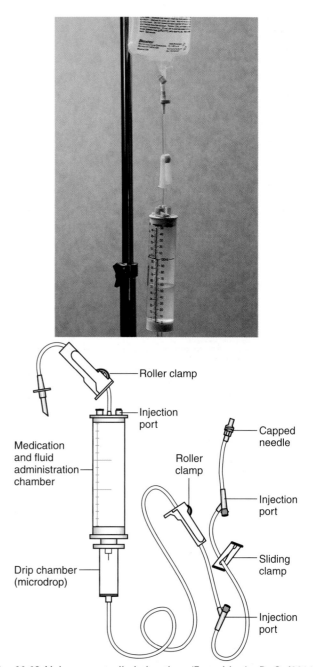

Roller clamp

Injection
port

Medication
and fluid
administration
chamber

Roller
clamp

Capped
needle

Injection
port

Sliding
clamp

Drip chamber
(microdrop)

Injection
port

Fig. 11.10 Volume-controlled chamber. (From Morris, D. G. [2014]. *Calculate with confidence* [6th ed.]. St. Louis: Elsevier.)

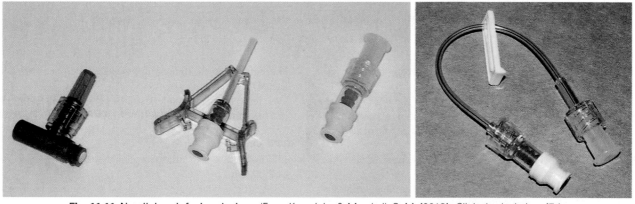

Fig. 11.11 Needleless infusion devices. (From Kee, J. L., & Marshall, S. M. [2013]. *Clinical calculations* [7th ed.]. St. Louis: Elsevier.)

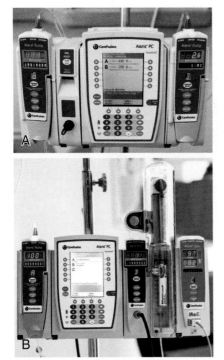

Fig. 11.12 Electronic infusion devices. (A) Alaris system with two channels. (B) Alaris system with PCA module. (Modified from Kee, J. L., & Marshall, S. M. [2013]. *Clinical calculations* [7th ed.]. St. Louis: Elsevier.)

- Instruct the patient in the use of the control button (medication is administered when the button is *released*).
- Instruct the patient to report any side effects or adverse reactions to the drug.
- Have naloxone, the reversal agent for opioids, easily accessible.
- Instruct patients, family members, and caregivers that the PCA button is to be depressed only by the patient.

Safety Considerations for Intravenous Infusions

All IV infusions and sites should be checked frequently. Common problems associated with IV infusions are kinked tubing, infiltration, and so-called free-flow IV rates. If IV tubing kinks, the flow is interrupted and the prescribed amount of fluid will not be given. The access site can also become obstructed, which prevents the flow. When infiltration occurs, IV fluid extravasates into the tissues and not into the vascular space. Trauma occurs to the tissues around the IV site. A free-flow IV rate refers to a rapid infusion of IV fluids that is faster than prescribed, which can cause fluid overload due to rapid infusion. Because of the possibility of a free-flow IV rate, electronic infusion pumps with multiple safety features are commonly used today.

Electronic infusion pumps are not without flaws, and mechanical problems can occur. Also, incorrectly programming an infusion pump can result in an incorrect infusion rate. Frequent monitoring of IV infusions can prevent complications of IV therapy such as fluid overload, thrombus formation, and infiltration.

Safety Considerations When Administering Heparin Sodium

Like insulin, heparin sodium is prescribed in unit dosages. Heparin is a high-alert drug that is available in multiple concentrations from 10 units/mL to 50,000 units/mL. It is important for the nurse to identify the label dosage strength and verify the patient's MAR; significant risk of causing serious injury or death can occur with errors. Heparin labels must be read carefully to ensure the correct drug is being administered. The following four heparin labels are examples of available strengths.

Note that *only one* is indicated for heparin flush (100 units/mL). All other labels indicate "NOT for Lock Flush."

Heparin can be given as a direct IV injection and as a continuous infusion. IV infusion is calculated in units per hour.

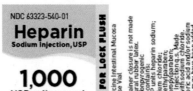

NDC 63323-549-01   504901
HEPARIN LOCK FLUSH SOLUTION, USP
100 USP Units/mL
(Derived from Porcine Intestinal Mucosa)
Preservative Free   Rx only
1 mL Single Dose Vial

NDC 63323-540-01
Heparin Sodium Injection, USP
1,000 USP units per mL
For intravenous or subcutaneous use   1 mL
NOT FOR LOCK FLUSH
From Porcine Intestinal Mucosa
Multi-Dose Vial
Rx only
Fresenius Kabi USA, LLC
Lake Zurich, IL 60047
42586K
25 Vials

NDC 63739-931-14   Rx only
HEPARIN SODIUM INJECTION, USP
10,000 USP Units/10 mL
(1,000 USP Units/mL)
For IV or SC use
10 mL   Multiple Dose Vial
NOT FOR LOCK FLUSH

250 mL SINGLE-DOSE CONTAINER   NDC 0409-7794-52
HEPARIN   RX ONLY
**12,500 USP Units/250 mL
(50 USP Units/mL)**

HEPARIN SODIUM IN 5% DEXTROSE INJECTION
WARNING: CONTAINS SULFITES
EACH 100 mL CONTAINS HEPARIN SODIUM 5,000 USP UNITS (PORCINE INTESTINAL MUCOSA); DEXTROSE, HYDROUS 5 g; CITRIC ACID, ANHYDROUS 51 mg; SODIUM CITRATE, DIHYDRATE 334 mg; SODIUM METABISULFITE 20 mg; ELECTROLYTES: SODIUM 38 mEq/L; CITRATE 42 mEq/L. STERILE. USUAL DOSAGE: SEE INSERT. ADDITIVES SHOULD NOT BE MADE TO THIS SOLUTION. LATEX-FREE. SINGLE DOSE CONTAINER. DISCARD UNUSED PORTION. FOR INTRAVENOUS USE ONLY.
50
100
150
200

OTHER
IM-3490
HOSPIRA, INC., LAKE FOREST, IL 60045 USA   Hospira

CALCULATING INTRAVENOUS FLOW RATE: DROPS PER MINUTE

When an electronic device is not used and the nurse manually regulates the IV rate, the nurse must calculate the number of drops per minute (gtt/min). The flow rate in drops per minute is determined by the size of the IV tubing (gtt/mL) as discussed earlier in this chapter. To convert hours to minutes, multiply the hours with 60 minutes. The drops will always be rounded to a whole number because a partial drop is not deliverable.

Example
Calculating Drops per Minute (gtt/min)

1. **Prescribed:** 500 milliliters of 0.45% sodium chloride (½NS) to be infused over 8 hours. IV tubing reads 10 drops per milliliter. What is the flow rate in drops per minute?
(The question is asking for flow rate with a given drop factor. When drop factor is involved in computing flow rate, solve for drops per minute.)

Basic Formula

$$gtt/min = \frac{amount\ of\ solution\ in\ mL \times gtt\ factor}{Time\ in\ h \times 60\ min}$$

$$gtt/min = \frac{500\ mL \times 10\ gtt/mL}{8\ h \times 60\ min}$$

= 10.4 gtt/min = 10 gtt/min (A partial drop cannot be administered.)

Ratio and Proportion/Fractional Equation

a. Determine milliliters per hour.
b. Determine drops per minute.

$$\frac{500\ mL}{8h} = \frac{x}{1h},\ then\ cross-multiply\ and\ divide$$

62.5 mL/h; then

$$\frac{62.5\ ^{mL}/_h}{60\ min} = \frac{x}{10\ gtt/mL},\ then\ cross-multiply\ and\ divide$$

$62.5 \times 10 = 60\ x$; then solve for x

$x = 10.4$ gtt/min = 10 gtt/min per the rounding rule

Dimensional Analysis

$$\frac{gtt}{min} = \frac{10\ gtt}{mL} \times \frac{500\ mL}{8\ h} \times \frac{1\ h}{60\ min}$$

$$= \frac{10\ gtt}{8} \times \frac{500}{60\ min}$$

$$= \frac{5000\ gtt}{480\ min}$$

$x = 10.41$ gtt/min = 10 gtt/min

2. **Prescribed:** A client is to receive D$_5$ ½NS at 75 mL/h. The drop factor is 20 gtt/mL. What is the flow rate?
(The question is asking for flow rate with a given drop factor. When drop factor is involved in computing flow rate, solve for drops per minute.)

Dimensional Analysis

$$\frac{gtt}{min} = \frac{20\ gtt}{mL} \times \frac{75\ mL}{1\ h} \times \frac{1\ h}{60\ min}$$

$$= 25\ gtt/min$$

3. **Prescribed:** 1 L of 0.9% sodium chloride (NS) to be infused over 12 hours. What is the flow rate with the pictured IV tubing?

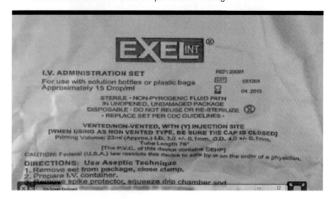

Answer: $gtt/min = \frac{15\ gtt}{1\ mL} \times \frac{1000\ mL}{12\ h} \times \frac{1\ h}{60\ min} = 20.8$

21 gtt/min (per the rounding rule)

CALCULATING INTRAVENOUS FLOW RATE: MILLILITERS PER HOUR

Regardless of the method used to determine the rate, the nurse should have the following information before calculating the flow rate: (1) the volume to be infused, (2) the drop factor of the infusion set, and (3) the time frame or how long to infuse the fluid. As with previous drug calculations, the nurse should select one method, be familiar with it, and consistently use it to calculate IV flow rate. When delivering IV drugs via electronic devices, the flow rate is calculated for milliliters per hour (mL/h).

Example

1. **Prescribed:** 500 mL of 0.45% sodium chloride (½NS) to be infused over 8 hours.
What is the flow rate?

Basic Formula

$$\frac{Amount\ of\ solution}{Hours\ to\ administer} = milliliters\ per\ hour\ (mL/h)$$

$$x\ mL/h = \frac{500\ mL}{8\ h}$$

$$= 62.5\ mL/h$$

If the infusion pump can be programmed to deliver partial milliliters, set the pump to deliver 62.5 mL/h (round to the nearest tenth); if the infusion pump cannot be set to deliver partial milliliters, the nurse would set the pump to infuse at 63 mL/h (round to the nearest whole number, according to the rounding rule).

Ratio and Proportion/Fractional Equation

$$\frac{Total\ volume}{Time\ (h)} = \frac{x\ mL}{1\ h}$$

$$\frac{500\ mL}{8\ h} = \frac{x\ mL}{1\ h}$$

$$8x = 500$$

$$x = 62.5\ mL/h$$

Dimensional Analysis

$$mL/h = \frac{\text{Amount of solution}}{\text{Time in hours}}$$

(DA for this particular problem is set up similar to the BF.)

2. **Prescribed:** 1000 milliliters of 0.9% sodium chloride (NS) to infuse at 75 milliliters per hour.
What is the total infusion time in hours and minutes?

Dimensional Analysis

$$\text{Time (h and min)} = \frac{1\,h}{75\ \cancel{mL}} \times \frac{1000\ \cancel{mL}}{x\ \text{time}}$$

$$\frac{1000}{75} = 13.33\,h\,;\ \text{and}$$

$$0.33\,h \times 60\,\text{min} = 19.8\,\text{min} = 20\,\text{min}$$

Answer: Total infusion time is 13 h and 20 min.

3. Using the total time in Example 2, what time will the infusion complete if the initial infusion was started at 2:00 p.m.?

Convert 2:00 p.m. to military time (1400 h), then add 13 h and 20 min.

$$1400 + 1320 = 2720 = 3{:}20\ \text{p.m. the next day}$$

4. Infuse lactated Ringer's solution (LR) 1000 milliliters over 12 hours.
What is the flow rate?

Answer: $mL/h = \dfrac{1000\,mL}{12\,h} = 83.3\,mL/h$

5. D_5 ½NS has been infusing at 125 mL/h.
After 5½ hours, the IV infiltrated, and the infusion had to be stopped. How many milliliters are left in the IV bag?

Dimensional Analysis

Answer: If $mL = \dfrac{125\,mL}{1\,h} \times \dfrac{5.5\,\cancel{h}}{x\,mL} = 687.5\,mL$ used,

then 1000 mL − 687.5 mL = 312.5 mL left in the bag

CRITICAL THINKING UNFOLDING CASE STUDY

Phase 1:
Question 1:
SLO: Applying the nursing process in preparing medications.
NGN Item Type: Enhanced SATA.
Cognitive Skills: Recognize cues.

The nurse received morning report at 0700 on C.J., a 34-year-old female who weighs 243 pounds and has left leg pain and swelling, in room 18. At 0830, the nurse reviews C.J.'s medication administration record (MAR):

- enoxaparin 1 milligram per kilogram twice daily subcutaneously
- warfarin 7.5 milligram orally every night at bedtime.

While reviewing the patient's information in preparing to administer 0900 medications, the nurse considers the following:

- Name on the MAR is C.J.
- C.J. is in room 18
- Dose of enoxaparin is 110 milligrams at 0900
- Warfarin 7.5 mg at 2100
- Enoxaparin is given subcutaneously
- Warfarin is given orally
- Medication cup is needed for warfarin
- The right medication
- C.J.'s ethnicity is Caucasian

Highlight the information above that the nurse recognizes as part of the six rights of medication administration.

Answers:
- Name on the MAR is C.J.
- C.J. is in room 18
- Dose of enoxaparin is 110 milligrams at 0900
- Warfarin 7.5 mg at 2100
- Enoxaparin is given subcutaneously
- Warfarin is given orally
- Medication cup is needed for warfarin
- The right medication
- C.J.'s ethnicity is Caucasian

Rationale:
Nurses have the duty to ensure patients are safe while administering medications. The six rights of medication administration include (1) the right patient, (2) the right medication, (3) the right dose, (4) the right time, (5) the right route, and (6) the right documentation. C.J. is the right patient. The nurse is preparing to administer 0900 medications; therefore, right medication, dose, route, and time is enoxaparin 110 milligrams subcutaneously at 0900. C.J. weighs 243 pounds, which is equal to 110 kg; therefore, the dose is 110 milligrams. Although knowing the room number is needed, it is not part of the six rights of medication administration. Patients can be reassigned to a different room. Warfarin would not be correct because it is ordered for 2100. The nurse would gather all the necessary supplies needed to administer subcutaneous medications, such as alcohol swabs and the appropriate syringe and needle. The medication cup is not needed for this patient. Ethnicity can affect the drug's pharmacokinetic and pharmacodynamic profile, but it is not considered as one of the six rights to medication administration.

Question 2:
SLO: Applying nursing process in preparing medications.
NGN Item Type: Cloze.
Cognitive Skills: Analyze cues.

C.J., a 34-year-old female, presented to the emergency room with left leg pain and swelling. C.J. is diagnosed with a deep vein thrombosis and was started on enoxaparin 1 mg/kg subcutaneously bid and warfarin 7.5 mg PO daily at 2100.

Choose the most likely options for the missing information in the following statements by selecting from the lists of options provided.

Before administering the medications, the nurse will assess patient's _____1_____ for warfarin and determine the patient's _____2_____ for the proper dose of enoxaparin.

Options for 1	Options for 2
Partial thromboplastin time (PTT)	Blood pressure
Weight	Heart rate
International normalized ratio (INR)	INR
Hemoglobin level	Weight
Blood pressure	PTT

Continued

CRITICAL THINKING UNFOLDING CASE STUDY—CONT'D

Answers:

Options for 1	Options for 2
Partial thromboplastin time (PTT)	Blood pressure
Weight	Heart rate
International normalized ratio (INR)	INR
Hemoglobin level	Weight
Blood pressure	PTT

Rationale:

Warfarin is an anticoagulant prescribed for persons with blood clots, such as deep vein thrombosis. Warfarin affects the coagulation profile, more specifically the prothrombin time (PT) and the international normalized ratio (INR). Warfarin's therapeutic level in patients without mechanical heart valve is an INR value of 2 to 3 seconds. If the INR value is higher than 3 seconds, the warfarin should be held, and it should be documented in the patient's chart that warfarin was held and why. Prior to administering warfarin, the nurse must assess the INR. PTT is a coagulation profile for intravenous heparin. Weight is needed to determine the correct amount of enoxaparin, not warfarin. Hemoglobin level should be monitored on a regular basis to assess for anemia due to blood loss; however, it does not need to be assessed before administering warfarin. Blood pressure should be measured on a regular basis because hypotension can be a sign of decreased fluid volume due to blood loss, but it does not need to be checked just before administering warfarin.

Enoxaparin is also an anticoagulant prescribed for persons with blood clots. Enoxaparin is a low-molecular-weight heparin and is administered subcutaneously. Since the dose of enoxaparin is based on weight, the patient's weight in kilograms is needed. Blood pressure and heart rate are important to obtain but are not required to determine proper dosing. INR is required prior to warfarin, not enoxaparin. PTT is needed when patients are on intravenous heparin, not enoxaparin.

Reference:

Hull, R.D., Garcia, D.A., & Vasquez, S.R. (June 04, 2019). Patient education: Warfarin (beyond the basics). *UpToDate*, retrieved from https://www.uptodate.com/contents/warfarin-beyond-the-basics#topicContent

Question 3:

SLO: Calculating correct dosages.
NGN Item Type: Extended drag and drop.
Cognitive Skills: Generate solutions.

C.J. was diagnosed with a deep vein thrombosis and was prescribed enoxaparin 1 mg/kg subcutaneously bid and warfarin 7.5 mg PO daily at 2100. C.J. weighs 243 lb. The nurse retrieves the packages from the medication dispensing system. **Indicate in the third column which medication label in the first column is appropriate for each calculation in the second column.** Note: You will use the labels in the first column more than once.

Medication Label	Dosage Calculation	Appropriate Medication Label
	mg = 1 mg/kg × 1 kg/2.2 lbs × 243 lb/x = 110 mg	
	tab = 1 tab/2.5 mg × 7.5 mg/x = 3 tabs	

CRITICAL THINKING UNFOLDING CASE STUDY—CONT'D

NDC 65162-**762**-10

Warfarin Sodium Tablets, USP

2 mg   PHARMACIST: Dispense the enclosed Medication Guide to each patient.

HIGHLY POTENT ANTICOAGULANT
WARNING: Serious bleeding results from over dosage. Do not use or dispense before reading directions and warnings in accompanying product information.

Rx only
100 Tablets

amneal

Amerinet Choice
Remove syringe by peeling lid completely off. Then gently lift syringe straight up by grasping middle of syringe. Do not remove syringe by pulling on plunger. See www.amphastar.com

ENOXAPARIN SODIUM INJECTION
40 mg/0.4 mL

---

mL = 1 mL/100 mg × 100 mg/x = 1.1 mL

mL = 1 mL/100 mg × 1mg/kg × 1kg/2.2 lb × 243 lb/x = 1.1 mL

Answers:

Medication Label

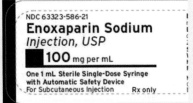

CAMBER
NDC 31722-329-01
Warfarin Sodium Tablets, USP
Crystalline* 2.5 mg
PHARMACIST: Dispense the Medication Guide provided separately to each patient.
HIGHLY POTENT ANTI COAGULANT
WARNING: Serious bleeding results from overdosage. Do not use or dispense before reading directions and warnings in accompanying product information.
Rx Only   100 Tablets

NDC 63323-586-21
Enoxaparin Sodium
Injection, USP
100 mg per mL
One 1 mL Sterile Single-Dose Syringe with Automatic Safety Device
For Subcutaneous Injection   Rx only

Dosage Calculation

mg = 1 mg/kg × 1 kg/2.2 lbs × 243 lb/x = 110 mg

tab = 1 tab/2.5 mg × 7.5 mg/x = 3 tabs

Appropriate Medication Label

No label is needed

CAMBER
NDC 31722-329-01
Warfarin Sodium Tablets, USP
Crystalline* 2.5 mg
PHARMACIST: Dispense the Medication Guide provided separately to each patient.
HIGHLY POTENT ANTI COAGULANT
WARNING: Serious bleeding results from overdosage. Do not use or dispense before reading directions and warnings in accompanying product information.
Rx Only   100 Tablets

Continued

CRITICAL THINKING UNFOLDING CASE STUDY—CONT'D

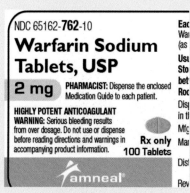

$$mL = 1 \text{ mL}/100 \text{ mg} \times 100 \text{ mg}/x = 1.1 \text{ mL}$$

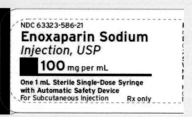

$$mL = 1 \text{ mL}/100 \text{ mg} \times 1\text{mg/kg} \times 1\text{kg}/2.2 \text{ lb} \\ \times 243 \text{ lb}/x = 1.1 \text{ mL}$$

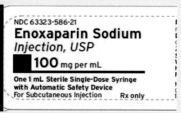

Rationale:

The nurse would correctly read the medication label to determine the amount of the available drug and administer the prescribed amount. To correctly calculate the volume of enoxaparin, the dosage based on the patient's weight must be determined. The calculation mg = 1 mg/kg × 1 kg/2.2 lbs × 243 lb/x = 110 mg does not require a drug label. The calculation tab = 1 tab/2.5 mg × 7.5 mg/x = 3 tabs requires the warfarin label with 2.5 mg/1 tablet, not warfarin 2 mg/tablet label. The calculation mL = 1 mL/100 mg × 110 mg/x = 1.1 mL requires the enoxaparin label with 100 mg/1 mL, not the 40 mg/0.4 mL. However, a nurse could still use the label with 40 mg/0.4 mL; the calculation would then be mL = 0.4 mL/40 mg × 110 mg = 1.1 mL. The last calculation uses dimensional analysis with conversion factors: mL = 1 mL/100 mg × 1 mg/kg × 1kg/2.2 lb × 243 lb/x = 1.1 mL.

Phase 2
Question 4:

SLO: Assessing the actions of the anticoagulants.
NGN Item Type: Extended drag and drop.
Cognitive Skills: Prioritize hypotheses.

C.J., a 34-year-old female, was admitted to the medical-surgical floor for a diagnosis of deep vein thrombosis to the left leg. She has been receiving enoxaparin 81 mg subcutaneously bid and warfarin 7.5 mg PO daily at 2100 without complications. Her international normalized ratio (INR) has been between 2 and 3 for the last 3 days. C.J. weighs 243 lb. On day 5 of hospitalization, C.J. reported shortness of breath and chest pain. A computed tomography (CT) scan revealed a large pulmonary embolus. Enoxaparin and warfarin were discontinued, and the patient was started on heparin intravenously according to the following heparin protocol:

aPTT (sec)	Bolus Dose (units/kg)	Stop Infusion (hr)	Rate Change (units/kg/hr)
Initial dose	80	–	Initial rate: 18
Less than 35	80	–	Increase by 4
35–54	40	–	Increase by 2
55–90	–	–	No change
91–100	–	–	Decrease by 2
101–139	–	1	Decrease by 3
Greater than 139	–	2	Decrease by 4

Indicate at which aPTT value a rate change is needed by placing an "X" in the appropriate space and indicate by how much by identifying the amount of rate change.

	Rate Change Warranted	Amount of Rate Change
aPTT = 40		
aPTT = 150		
aPTT = 34		
aPTT = 58		

Increase by 2 units/kg/hr
No change
Increase by 4 units/kg/hr
Decrease by 4 units/kg/hr

Answer:

	Rate Change Warranted	Amount of Rate Change
aPTT = 40	X	Increase by 2 units/kg/hr
aPTT = 150	X	Decrease by 4 units/kg/hr
aPTT = 34	X	Increase by 4 units/kg/hr
aPTT = 58		No change

Rationale:

The therapeutic range for heparin is between 55 and 90 seconds. When aPTT is below the therapeutic range, patients are at an increased risk for further thrombus formation. When aPTT is higher than the therapeutic range, the patient is at risk for bleeding. According to the heparin protocol, an aPTT of 40 is between 35 and 54, which warrants a rate change by 2 units/kg/hr; an aPTT of 150 is greater than 139, so the infusion should be stopped for 2 hours and then decreased by 4 units/kg/hr upon resuming; an aPTT of 34 seconds is less than 35, so a bolus of 80 units/kg would be administered, followed by an increase in the infusion by 4 units/kg/hr; and an aPTT of 58 is appropriate according to the protocol, so the nurse would continue the infusion at the current rate.

Reference:
Warnock, L.B., & Huang, D. (July 15, 2020). Heparin. *StatPearls* retrieved from https://www.ncbi.nlm.nih.gov/books/NBK538247/

CRITICAL THINKING UNFOLDING CASE STUDY—CONT'D

Question 5:

SLO: Adjusting heparin dose.

NGN Item Type: Cloze.

Cognitive Skills: Generate solutions.

C.J., a 34-year-old female, was admitted to the medical-surgical floor for a diagnosis of deep vein thrombosis to the left leg complicated by a pulmonary embolus. C.J. weighs 243 lb. The patient has been on heparin intravenously according to the following heparin protocol at 18 units/kg/hr:

aPTT (sec)	Bolus Dose (units/kg)	Stop Infusion (hr)	Rate Change (units/kg/hr)
Initial dose	80	–	Initial rate: 18
Less than 35	80	–	Increase by 4
35–54	40	–	Increase by 2
55–90	–	–	No change
91–100	–	–	Decrease by 2
101–139	–	1	Decrease by 3
Greater than 139	–	2	Decrease by 4

After 12 hours of receiving intravenous heparin on the following heparin solution, aPTT was 30 seconds.

250 mL SINGLE-DOSE CONTAINER   NDC 0409-7793-52

HEPARIN

25,000 USP Units/250 mL (100 USP Units/mL)

HEPARIN SODIUM IN 5% DEXTROSE INJECTION

WARNING: CONTAINS SULFITES   50

EACH 100 mL CONTAINS

Choose the most likely option for the missing information in the following statement by selecting from the list of options provided.

Based on the data provided, the nurse would ___Option A_____ heparin with ___Option B_____ and infuse heparin at __Option C_____.

Option A	Option B	Option C
Continue	0 units	18 units/kg/hr
Rebolus	8836 units	24.3 mL/hr
Increase	2 units/kg/hr	22.1 mL/hr
Decrease	4 units/kg/hr	15.5 mL/hr
Stop	1 hr	16.6 mL/hr

Answer:

Based on the data provided, the nurse would ___rebolus_____ heparin with 8836 units_____ and infuse heparin at __24.3 mL/hr_____.

Rationale:

A nurse caring for a patient who is receiving intravenous heparin would monitor their aPTT. C.J. has an aPTT of 30 seconds after 12 hours of receiving heparin, which is subtherapeutic. Based on the heparin protocol, the nurse would *rebolus* heparin at 80 units/kg, which is 8836 units followed by increasing heparin infusion by *4 units/kg/hr* for a total of 22 units/kg/hr. The heparin infusion would resume at *24.3 mL/hr*.

Phase 3:

Question 6:

SLO: Teaching about side effects of heparin.

NGN Item Type: Matrix.

Cognitive Skills: Take action.

C.J. has been receiving intravenous heparin for a pulmonary embolus and is being prepared to transition to an oral anticoagulant. **In the proper column, mark an X indicating whether the teaching is appropriate (correct) or inappropriate (incorrect).**

Health Teaching	Appropriate	Inappropriate
"You will be discharged with intravenous heparin and oral medicine."		
"You will need to continue to monitor for blood in your urine or stool."		
"Notify a health care member for any dizziness."		
"You will need more frequent blood work with the oral medicine."		
"Blood oozing from previous puncture sites is normal."		
"Do not take any over-the-counter medications without talking with your health care provider first."		

Answers:

Health Teaching	Appropriate	Incorrect
"You will be discharged with intravenous heparin and oral medicine."		X
"You will need to continue to monitor for blood in your urine or stool."	X	
"Notify a health care member for any dizziness."	X	
"You will need more frequent blood work with the oral medicine."		X
"Blood oozing from previous puncture sites is normal."		X
"Do not take any over-the-counter medications without talking with your health care provider first."	X	

Rationale:

Intravenous and oral anticoagulants can injure a patient. Ensuring patients understand the benefits and risks and the need for regular monitoring while on anticoagulants is important. Health teaching that is appropriate for C.J. includes the *need to continue to monitor for blood in your urine or stool*. Common side effects of anticoagulants include bleeding in urine or stool or when brushing teeth or uncontrolled bleeding from wounds. Also, nurses would teach patients to *notify a health care member for any dizziness*. Dizziness can be an indication of internal bleeding. Patients who are on anticoagulants should *not take any over-the-counter medications without talking with their health care provider first*. A number of medications, such as aspirin, ibuprofen, and cimetidine, among others, as well as herbal products, can interact with anticoagulants. One of the incorrect responses includes *You will be discharged with intravenous heparin and oral medicine*. Usually, the parenteral anticoagulant (e.g., heparin) is discontinued after 2 to 10 days of starting oral anticoagulant. The number of days for bridging parenteral with oral anticoagulants is dependent on the type of oral

Continued

CRITICAL THINKING UNFOLDING CASE STUDY—CONT'D

anticoagulant and the patient's renal function. Another incorrect response is *You will need more frequent blood work with the oral medicine.* The patient is at risk for bleeding, so a CBC will be periodically monitored rather than every 6 hours. If the patient is prescribed warfarin, then an international normalized ratio (INR) will need periodic monitoring to adjust warfarin dose. *Blood oozing from previous puncture sites is normal* is incorrect. Patients should notify their health care provider if they develop oozing of blood from previous puncture sites or bleeding from gums when brushing teeth.

Reference:

Hull, R.D., Garcia, D.A., & Vasquez, S.R. (June 04, 2019). Patient education: Warfarin (beyond the basics). *UpToDate*, retrieved from https://www.uptodate.com/contents/warfarin-beyond-the-basics#topicContent

Question 7:

SLO: Evaluate patient's assessment findings to determine effectiveness of anticoagulation for pulmonary embolus.

NGN Item Type: Matrix.

Cognitive Skills: Evaluate outcomes.

C.J. has been on parenteral heparin and dabigatran for 4 days for venous thromboembolism (VTE). **For each assessment finding, use an X to indicate whether nursing and collaborative interventions were effective (helped meet expected outcomes), ineffective (did not help meet expected outcomes), or unrelated (not related to expected outcomes).**

Assessment Finding	Effective	Ineffective	Unrelated
Spontaneous oxygen saturation at 95%			
The infusion pump is frequently alarming			
Reports increased swelling to left leg			
aPTT has been 62 seconds for the last 24 hours			
INR is 2.7 seconds			
Reports no evidence of blood in urine or stool			
Denies chest pain			
Multiple petechiae to trunk and arms			

Answers:

Assessment Finding	Effective	Ineffective	Unrelated
Spontaneous oxygen saturation at 95%	X		
The infusion pump is frequently alarming			X
Reports increased swelling to left leg		X	
aPTT has been 62 seconds for the last 24 hours	X		
INR is 2.7 seconds			X
Reports no evidence of blood in urine or stool	X		
Denies chest pain	X		
Multiple petechiae to trunk and arms		X	

Rationale:

Effective outcome includes spontaneous oxygen saturation (SpO_2) of 90% or greater, aPTT between 50 to 90 seconds, patient denying blood in urine or stool, and denying chest pain. If the SpO_2 was less than 90%, the nurse would be concerned about worsening pulmonary embolus. An activated partial thromboplastin time (aPTT) of 62 seconds is within the therapeutic range according to the heparin protocol. Patient would be at an increased risk of blood clots or pulmonary embolus with lower aPTT level. If the aPTT was supratherapeutic, the patient would be at an increased risk of bleeding, and patient may develop blood in urine or stool. Ineffective outcomes include increased swelling to the left leg. This could indicate the thrombus to the leg is worsening. Reports of chest pain could indicate worsening pulmonary embolus, an ineffective outcome. Another ineffective outcome includes the presence of multiple petechiae to the trunk and arms. Petechiae could be an indication of bleeding if the patient is receiving too much anticoagulation. The infusion pump frequently alarming and an INR of 2.7 seconds are unrelated to the expected outcomes of anticoagulant therapy with heparin and dabigatran. INR would be appropriate if the patient was on warfarin.

References:

Hull, R.D., Garcia, D.A., & Vasquez, S.R. (June 04, 2019). Patient education: Warfarin (beyond the basics). *UpToDate*, retrieved from https://www.uptodate.com/contents/warfarin-beyond-the-basics#topicContent

Kang, H. G., Lee, S. J., Chung, J. Y., & Cheong, J. S. (2017). Thrombocytopenia induced by dabigatran: Two case reports. *BMC Neurology, 17*(1), 124. https://doi.org/10.1186/s12883-017-0900-8

Leung, L.L.K. (Nov 11, 2020). Direct oral anticoagulants (DOACs) and parenteral direct-acting anticoagulants: Dosing and adverse effects. *UpToDate,* retrieved from https://www.uptodate.com/contents/direct-oral-anticoagulants-doacs-and-parenteral-direct-acting-anticoagulants-dosing-and-adverse-effects?search=dabigatran&source=search_result&selectedTitle=1~110&usage_type=default&display_rank=1#H27804459

PRACTICE PROBLEMS

Intravenous Administration

1. **Prescribed:** 1000 mL of D_5 ½NS to infuse over 12 hours.
   Available: Microdrip set with a drop factor of 60 gtt/mL
   a. Calculate the IV flow rate in drops per minute. _____
2. **Prescribed:** 3 L of IV solution to infuse over 24 hours: with 1 L of D_5W and 2 L of D_5 ½NS.
   a. One liter is equal to how many milliliters? _____
   b. Each liter should infuse for how many hours? _____
   c. The institution uses a set with a drop factor of 15 gtt/mL. How many drops per minute should the patient receive per liter of fluid? _____
3. **Prescribed:** 250 mL of D_5W over 3 hours.
   a. Determine the flow rate. _____

PRACTICE PROBLEMS—CONT'D

Intravenous Administration

4. **Prescribed:** 1000 mL of D_5 ½NS, 1 vial of multiple vitamin (MVI), and 10 mEq of potassium chloride (KCl) to be infused over 10 hours.
   Available: 1000 mL of D_5 ½NS; MVI 1 vial = 10 mL; KCl 20 mEq/20 mL vial; macrodrip set, 15 gtt/mL; microdrip set, 60 gtt/mL
   a. What is the total volume of the solution? _____
   b. How many drops per minute should the patient receive using the macrodrip set?_____ The microdrip set? _____
   c. The IV pump is set at how many milliliters per hour? _____

5. **Prescribed:** Protamine sulfate 40 mg IV STAT; IV infusion not to exceed 5 mg per min.
   Available:

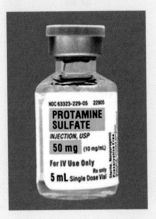

   a. How many milliliters should the patient receive? _____
   b. Over how many minutes should protamine be administered? _____

6. **Prescribed:** Morphine sulfate 5 mg IV q3h PRN.
   Available:

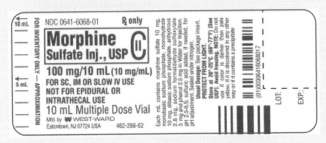

   Instructions are to dilute the dose with 5 mL of NS and to administer 2.5 to 15 mg over 5 minutes.
   a. How many milliliters of morphine should the patient receive? _____
   b. For how many minutes should morphine be administered? _____

7. **Prescribed:** Furosemide 80 mg IV now.
   Available:

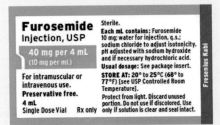

   Drug insert states rate of administration is 20 mg/min.
   a. How many milliliters will the nurse administer? _____
   b. How long should furosemide be given? _____

Continued

PRACTICE PROBLEMS—CONT'D

Intravenous Administration

8. **Prescribed:** Regular insulin 20 units IV for blood glucose over 600.
   Available:

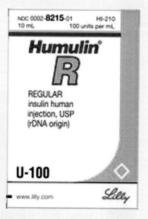

Indicate by shading the appropriate syringe to show the amount of insulin to give.

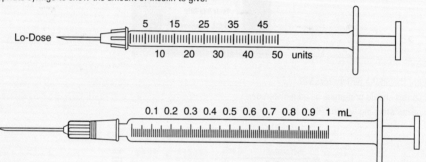

9. **Prescribed:** Digoxin 0.375 mg IV over 5 min.
   Available: Digoxin 0.25 mg/mL
   How many milliliters will the nurse administer? _____
   (When giving drugs by IV, always verify the compatibility of the IV solution and the drug; otherwise, precipitation can result. Incompatibility can be avoided if the IV tubing is flushed with a compatible solution of either normal saline or sterile water before and after administration.)

10. **Prescribed:** 1000 mL D_5W with heparin sodium 20,000 units to infuse at 30 mL/h.
    Calculate the units per hour.

11. **Prescribed:** Heparin sodium 750 units/h.
    Available: Heparin sodium 25,000 units in 500 mL D_5W
    Calculate the milliliters per hour.

12. **Prescribed:** Heparin sodium 80 units/kg IV bolus is ordered followed by heparin sodium infusion at 15 units/kg/h for a patient who weighs 175 lb.
    Available:

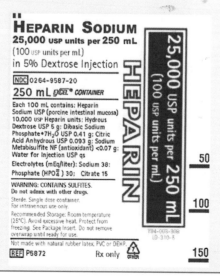

PRACTICE PROBLEMS—CONT'D

Intravenous Administration

    a. Calculate the amount of bolus in units and milliliters to administer.

    b. Calculate flow rate in units per hour.

    c. Calculate flow rate in milliliters per hour.

13. **Prescribed:** Heparin sodium 800 units/h.

    Available: Heparin sodium 40 units/mL

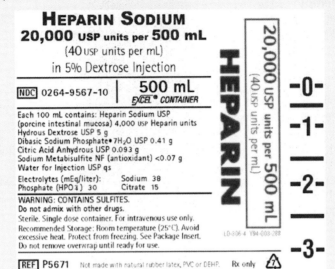

Calculate the flow rate. _____

14. **Prescribed:** 250 mL 0.9% sodium chloride (NS) with heparin sodium 25000 units to infuse at 35 mL/h.

    Calculate units per hour. _____

15. **Prescribed:** Heparin flush Mediport every 3 days.

    Which heparin product is appropriate? _____

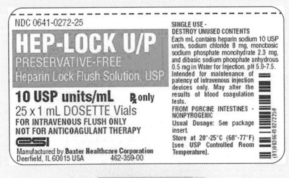

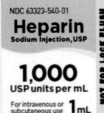

16. **Prescribed:** Bolus with heparin at 80 units/kg, then initiate heparin infusion at 20 units/kg/hour for a patient who weighs 150 lb.

    Available: Heparin sodium 25000 units in 500 mL 5% dextrose in water (D₅W).

    a. Calculate bolus dose in units. _____

    b. Calculate bolus dose in milliliters. _____

    c. What is the flow rate of the heparin infusion? _____

17. **Prescribed:** Infuse heparin sodium 25000 units in 1000 mL of NS at 30 mL/h.

    Calculate units per hour. _____

Continued

Calculating Critical Care Drugs

Most drugs administered in critical care are *titrated* (adjusted) according to the patient's response to the drug therapy. The patient is monitored closely for therapeutic effects and any adverse events. When calculating critical care drugs, any method previously discussed is effective; however, DA is the best method because units and CFs are calculated in one equation.

Example

Calculating Critical Care Therapy

1. **Prescribed:** Infuse dopamine at 5 mcg/kg/min to maintain systolic blood pressure above 110 mm Hg. The patient weighs 130 lb.
   Available: Dopamine hydrochloride (HCl) 200 mg in 250 mL of 5% dextrose in water (D_5W)
   Calculate milliliters per hour.
   Answer:

$$mL/h = \frac{250 \text{ mL}}{200 \text{ mg}} \times \frac{1 \text{ mg}}{1000 \text{ mcg}} \times \frac{5 \text{ mcg}}{1 \text{ kg}} \times \frac{1 \text{ kg}}{2.2 \text{ lb}} \times \frac{130 \text{ lb}}{1 \text{ min}} \times \frac{60 \text{ min}}{1 \text{ h}} = 22.2 \text{ mL/h}$$

   (All the CFs for milligrams per microgram, pounds per kilogram, and units are eliminated except for milliliters and hours.)

2. **Prescribed:** Dobutamine HCl 2 mcg/kg/min, titrated to maintain hemodynamic goals in a patient who weighs 180 lb.
   Available: Dobutamine HCl 250 mg in 500 mL of D_5W
   Calculate micrograms per kilograms per minute.
   Calculate milliliters per hour.
   Answer:

$$mcg/kg/min = \frac{2 \text{ mcg}}{1 \text{ kg}} \times \frac{1 \text{ kg}}{2.2 \text{ lb}} \times \frac{180 \text{ lb}}{x \text{ min}} = 163.6 \text{ mcg/kg/min}$$

$$mL/h = \frac{500 \text{ mL}}{250 \text{ mg}} \times \frac{1 \text{ mg}}{1000 \text{ mcg}} \times \frac{2 \text{ mcg}}{1 \text{ kg}} \times \frac{1 \text{ kg}}{2.2 \text{ lb}} \times \frac{180 \text{ lb}}{1 \text{ min}} \times \frac{60 \text{ min}}{1 \text{ h}} = 19.6 \text{ mL/h}$$

   ! (Be aware of sound-alike drugs, dopamine and dobutamine. *Dopamine* is an adrenergic agonist that affects dopamine receptors. *Dobutamine* is a beta$_1$-adrenergic agonist and does *not* affect dopamine receptors. They both have inotropic properties and are used as vasopressors.)

3. **Prescribed:** Isoproterenol 2 mg in 250 mL of D_5W to infuse at 8 mcg/min.
   Calculate milliliters per hour.
   Answer:

$$mL/h = \frac{250 \text{ mL}}{2 \text{ mg}} \times \frac{1 \text{ mg}}{1000 \text{ mcg}} \times \frac{8 \text{ mcg}}{1 \text{ min}} \times \frac{60 \text{ min}}{1 \text{ h}} = 60 \text{ mL/h}$$

   Additional practice problems for all drug calculations are available in the Study Guide and on the Evolve website.

ANSWERS TO PRACTICE PROBLEMS

Metric System Conversions

Converting From Larger Units to Smaller Units

The gram is three factors of 10 greater than the milligram, so the decimal point is moved three spaces to the right.

1. If 1 g = 1000 mg, then
   2 g = 2.000 = 2000 mg

2. If 1 g = 1000 mg, then
   0.5 g = 0.500 = 500 mg

3. If 1 L = 1000 mL, then
   2.5 L = 2.500 = 2500 mL

Converting From Smaller Units to Larger Units

The milligram is three factors of 10 smaller (less) than the gram, so the decimal point is moved three spaces to the left.

4. If 1000 mg = 1 g, then
   1500 mg = 1500. = 1.5 g

   (Note there are no trailing zeroes [no 00] after the decimal.)

5. If 1000 mcg = 1 mg, then
   3000 mcg = 3.000 = 3 mg

   (Note there are no trailing zeroes [no 000] after the decimal.)

6. If 1000 mL = 1 L, then
   500 mL = 0.500 = 0.5 L

   (Note that a leading zero was placed before the decimal.)

English System Conversions

Converting From Larger Units to Smaller Units

1. If 1 oz = 2 T, then
   3 oz = 3 × 2 T = 6 T
2. If 1 T = 3 t, then
   5 T = 5 × 3 t = 15 t
3. If 1 T = 15 mL, then
   2 T = 2 × 15 mL = 30 mL

Converting From Smaller Units to Larger Units

4. If 2 T = 1 oz, then
   3 T = 3 ÷ 2 T = 1.5 oz
5. If 3 t = 1 T, then
   12 t = 12 ÷ 3 t = 4 T
6. If 15 mL = 1 T and 1 T = 3 t, then
   15 mL = 3 t, so
   (45 mL ÷ 15 mL) × 3 t = 3 × 3 t = 9 t

Interpreting Drug Labels

1. a. Lisinopril and hydrochlorothiazide
   b. There is no trade name
   c. No
   d. Lisinopril 10 mg; hydrochlorothiazide 12.5 mg per tablet
   e. 30 tablets
   f. At room temperature (68°F to 77°F)
2. a. Furosemide
   b. Lasix
   c. No
   d. 40 mg per tablet
   e. 100 tablets
   f. Room temperature (59°F to 86°F)
3. a. Hydromorphone
   b. Dilaudid
   c. Yes, Schedule II
   d. 1 mg per mL (oral)
   e. 473 mL = 473 mg
   f. Room temperature (59°F to 86°F)
4. a. Heparin sodium
   b. 1000 units per mL
   c. No
   d. IV or subcut
   e. Multiple use

Drug Reconstitution

1. a. 77 mL

   b. 200 mg per 5 mL

   c. $mL = \dfrac{5\ mL}{200\ \text{mg}} \times \dfrac{500\ \text{mg}}{x} = 12.5\ mL$

2. a. 65 mL

   b. $65 = 3 = 21.6 \times 2 = 43.3\ mL \left(\dfrac{2}{3} \text{ of } 65\ mL \right)$

   c. Amoxicillin 250 mg and Clavulanic acid 62.5 mg per 5 mL

   d. Amoxicillin: $mL = \dfrac{5\ mL}{250\ \text{mg}} \times \dfrac{500\ \text{mg}}{x\ mL} = 10\ mL$

   Clavulanic acid: $mL = \dfrac{5\ mL}{62.5\ \text{mg}} \times \dfrac{125\ \text{mg}}{x\ mL} = 10\ mL$

   (Note that the amoxicillin and clavulanic acid were both 10 mL; therefore a total of 10 mL will be given for a 500 mg/250 mg dose.)

Calculating Dosages Based on Body Weight

1. a. 66 lb = 2.2 = 30 kg

   b. 15 mg × 30 kg = 450/day

   c. 450 mg = 2 = 225 mg/dose

   d. $mL = \dfrac{5\ mL}{250\ \text{mg}} \times \dfrac{225\ \text{mg}}{x} = 4.5\ mL$

Dimensional Analysis

$$mL = \dfrac{5\ mL}{250\ \text{mg}} \times \dfrac{15\ \text{mg}}{1\ \text{kg}} \times \dfrac{1\ \text{kg}}{2.2\ \text{lb}} \times \dfrac{66\ \text{lb}}{2\ dose} = 4.5\ mL/dose$$

2. a. 33 1b = 2.2 = 15 kg

   b. 2.5 mg × 15 kg = 37.5 mg

   c. $mL = \dfrac{1\ mL}{10\ \text{mg}} \times \dfrac{37.5\ \text{mg}}{x} = 3.8\ mL$

Dimensional Analysis

$$mL = \dfrac{1\ mL}{10\ \text{mg}} \times \dfrac{2.5\ \text{mg}}{1\ \text{kg}} \times \dfrac{1\ \text{kg}}{2.2\ \text{lb}} \times \dfrac{33\ \text{lb}}{x} = 3.8\ mL$$

Calculating Dosages Based on Body Surface Area—Square Root Method

1. a. $BSA = \sqrt{\dfrac{66\ in \times 176\ lb}{3131}} = \sqrt{\dfrac{11616}{3131}} = 1.93\ m^2$

   b. $mg/m^2 = 300\ mg \times 1.93\ m^2 = 579\ mg$

Dimensional Analysis

$$mL = \dfrac{1\ mL}{10\ \text{mg}} \times \dfrac{300\ \text{mg}}{\text{m}^2} \dfrac{\sqrt{\dfrac{66\ in \times 176\ lb}{3131}}\ \text{m}^2}{x} = 57.8\ mL$$

Note that the volume to administer is less since the BSA was not rounded up. Instead, rounding was performed on the final answer.

2. a. $\sqrt{\dfrac{164\ cm \times 66.8\ kg}{3600}}\ m^2 = 1.74\ m^2$

   b. mg = 350 mg × 1.74 m² = 609 mg

Dimensional Analysis

$$\dfrac{mg}{m^2} = \dfrac{350\ \text{mg}}{\text{m}^2} \times \dfrac{\sqrt{\dfrac{66.8\ kg \times 164\ cm}{3600}}\ \text{m}^2}{x} = 611\ mg$$

Note that the mg to administer is more since the BSA was not rounded down. Instead, rounding was performed on the final answer.

Enteral Administration

All answers will be shown using dimensional analysis.

1. $tab = \dfrac{1\ tab}{75\ \text{mg}} \times \dfrac{150\ \text{mg}}{x} = 2\ tabs$

2. $cap = \dfrac{1\ cap}{100\ \text{mg}} \times \dfrac{100\ \text{mg}}{x} = 1\ cap$

3. $tab = \dfrac{1\ tab}{2\ \text{mg}} \times \dfrac{2\ \text{mg}}{x} = 1\ tab$

4. $\text{tab} = \dfrac{1 \text{ tab}}{25 \text{ mg}} \times \dfrac{12.5 \text{ mg}}{x} = 0.5 \text{ tab}$

5. $\text{mL} = \dfrac{15 \text{ mL}}{10 \text{ g}} \times \dfrac{20 \text{ g}}{x} = 30 \text{ mL}$

6. $\text{mL} = \dfrac{5 \text{ mL}}{125 \text{ mg}} \times \dfrac{1000 \text{ mg}}{1 \text{ g}} \times \dfrac{0.25 \text{ g}}{x} = 10 \text{ mL}$

7. a. 66 lb/2.2 = 30 kg

   b. $\dfrac{\text{mg}}{\text{day}} = \dfrac{15 \text{ mg}}{\text{kg}} \times \dfrac{1 \text{ kg}}{2.2 \text{ lb}} \times \dfrac{66 \text{ lb}}{\text{day}} = 450 \text{ mg/day}$

Dimensional Analysis

$\dfrac{\text{mg}}{\text{dose}} = \dfrac{15 \text{ mg}}{\text{kg}} \times \dfrac{1 \text{ kg}}{2.2 \text{ lb}} \times \dfrac{66 \text{ lb}}{2 \text{ doses}} = 225 \text{ mg/day}$

   c. 450 mg ÷ 2 doses = 225 mg / doses

Dimensional Analysis

   d. $\dfrac{\text{mL}}{\text{dose}} = \dfrac{\text{mL}}{250 \text{ mg}} \times \dfrac{15 \text{ mg}}{\text{kg}} \times \dfrac{1 \text{ kg}}{2.2 \text{ lb}} \times \dfrac{66 \text{ lb}}{2 \text{ doses}} = 4.5 \text{ mL/dose}$

Subcutaneous and Intramuscular Administration

1. Answer:

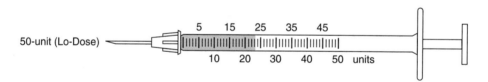

2. Answer: The best syringe is the 50-unit syringe. It is marked in 1-unit increments to withdraw a more precise dose. The 100-unit syringe has 2-unit increments.

3. $\text{mL} = \dfrac{1 \text{ mL}}{10 \text{ mg}} \times \dfrac{20 \text{ mg}}{x} = 2 \text{ mL}$

4. $\text{mL} = \dfrac{1 \text{ mL}}{1 \text{ mg}} \times \dfrac{0.4 \text{ mg}}{x} = 0.4 \text{ mL}$

5.

   a. $\text{mL} = \dfrac{1 \text{ mL}}{5000 \text{ mg}} \times \dfrac{7500 \text{ units}}{x} = 1.5 \text{ mL}$

   (Note that units is spelled out rather than using only U, which could be mistaken for a zero.)

   b. b. $\text{mL} = \dfrac{1 \text{ mL}}{5000 \text{ units}} \times \dfrac{3500 \text{ units}}{x} = 0.7 \text{ mL}$

   (Note "units" is spelled out rather than using "U," which could be mistaken for a zero.)

   c. 1.5 mL + 0.7 mL = 2.2 mL, so 2 vials are needed

6.

a. 4.2 mL

b. 350 mg per mL

c. $mL = \dfrac{1\,mL}{350\,\cancel{mg}} \times \dfrac{1000\,\cancel{mg}}{1\,\cancel{g}} \times \dfrac{1.5\,\cancel{g}}{x} = 4.28\,mL; = 4.3\,mL$ per rounding rule (since the total volume is greater than 3 mL, administer in two seperate injections)

Calculating Intravenous Administration

All answers are provided using dimensional analysis.

1. $gtt/min = \dfrac{60\,gtt}{1\,\cancel{mL}} \times \dfrac{1000\,\cancel{mL}}{12\,\cancel{h}} \times \dfrac{1\,\cancel{h}}{60\,min} = 83\,gtt/min$

2.

a. 1000 mL

b. $\dfrac{24\,hr}{3\,L} = 8\,h/L$

c. $gtt/min = \dfrac{15\,gtt}{1\,\cancel{mL}} \times \dfrac{1000\,\cancel{mL}}{8\,\cancel{h}} \times \dfrac{1\,\cancel{h}}{60\,min} = \dfrac{15000\,gtt}{480\,min} = 31\,gtt/min$

3. $mL/h = \dfrac{250\,mL}{3\,h} = 83.3\,mL/h$

4.

a. 1030 mL; 10 mL of MVI and 20 mL of KCl is added to 1000 mL of IV fluid.

b. Macro drip set: $gtt/min = \dfrac{15\,gtt}{1\,\cancel{mL}} \times \dfrac{1030\,\cancel{mL}}{10\,\cancel{h}} \times \dfrac{1\,\cancel{h}}{60\,min} = \dfrac{15450\,gtt}{600\,min} = 25.75\,gtt/min = 26\,gtt/min$ after rounding to the nearest whole number

Micro drop set: $gtt/min = \dfrac{60\,gtt}{1\,\cancel{mL}} \times \dfrac{1030\,\cancel{mL}}{10\,\cancel{h}} \times \dfrac{1\,\cancel{h}}{60\,min} = \dfrac{61800\,gtt}{60\,min} = 103\,gtt/min$

c. $mL/h = \dfrac{1030\,mL}{10\,h} = 103\,mL/h$

5.

a. 4 mL

b. $\dfrac{1\,min}{5\,\cancel{mg}}\quad\dfrac{40\,\cancel{mg}}{x} = 8\,min$ or 0.5 mL/min

6.

a. $\dfrac{1\,mL}{10\,\cancel{mg}} \times \dfrac{5\,\cancel{mg}}{x} = 0.5\,mL$

b. Because 2.5 to 5 mg can be given over 5 minutes, 5 mg is given over 5 minutes.

7.

a. $\dfrac{1\,mL}{10\,\cancel{mg}} \times \dfrac{80\,\cancel{mg}}{x} = 8\,mL$

b. $\dfrac{1\,min}{20\,\cancel{mg}} \times \dfrac{80\,\cancel{mg}}{x} = 4\,min$ or 2 mL/min

8.

(The top syringe is calibrated in units; the bottom syringe is in milliliters.)

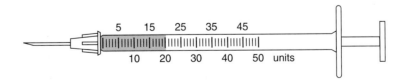

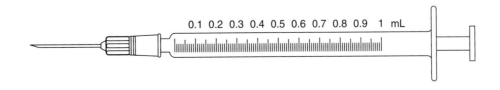

9. $mL = \dfrac{1\,mL}{0.25\,\cancel{mg}} \times \dfrac{0.375\,\cancel{mg}}{x} = 1.5\,mL$

10. $units/h = \dfrac{20000\,units}{1000\,\cancel{mL}} \times \dfrac{30\,\cancel{mL}}{1\,h} = 600\,units/h$

11.
12. $mL/h = \dfrac{500\,mL}{25000\,\cancel{units}} \times \dfrac{750\,\cancel{units}}{1\,h} = 15\,mL/h$

  a. $units = \dfrac{80\,units}{1\,\cancel{kg}} \times \dfrac{1\,\cancel{kg}}{2.2\,\cancel{lb}} \times \dfrac{175\,\cancel{lb}}{x} = 6364\,units\ bolus$

  $mL = \dfrac{1\,mL}{100\,\cancel{units}} \times \dfrac{6364\,\cancel{units}}{x} = 63.6\,mL\ bolus$

  b. $units/h = \dfrac{15\,units}{1\,\cancel{kg}} \times \dfrac{1\,\cancel{kg}}{2.2\,\cancel{lb}} \times \dfrac{175\,\cancel{lb}}{x} = 1193\,units/h$

  c. $mL/h = \dfrac{1\,mL}{100\,\cancel{units}} \times \dfrac{15\,\cancel{units}}{1\,\cancel{kg}} \times \dfrac{1\,\cancel{kg}}{2.2\,\cancel{lb}} \times \dfrac{175\,\cancel{lb}}{x} = 11.9\,mL/h$

13. $mL/h = \dfrac{1\,mL}{40\,\cancel{units}} \times \dfrac{800\,\cancel{units}}{1\,h} = 20\,mL/h$

14. $units/h = \dfrac{25000\,units}{250\,\cancel{mL}} \times \dfrac{35\,\cancel{mL}}{1\,h} = 3500\,units/h$

15.

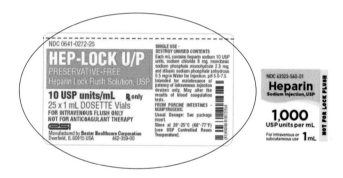

16.

  a. Bolus in units $= \dfrac{80\,units}{1\,\cancel{kg}} \times \dfrac{1\,\cancel{kg}}{2.2\,\cancel{lb}} \times \dfrac{150\,\cancel{lb}}{x} = 5454.5\,units$; round to the nearest whole number $= 5455\,units$

  b. Bolus in milliliters $= \dfrac{500\,mL}{25000\,\cancel{units}} \times \dfrac{80\,\cancel{units}}{1\,\cancel{kg}} \times \dfrac{1\,\cancel{kg}}{2.2\,\cancel{lb}} \times \dfrac{150\,\cancel{lb}}{x} = 109.1\,mL$

  c. Flow rate in mL/h $= \dfrac{500\,mL}{25000\,\cancel{units}} \times \dfrac{20\,\cancel{units}}{1\,\cancel{kg}} \times \dfrac{1\,\cancel{kg}}{2.2\,\cancel{lb}} \times \dfrac{150\,\cancel{lb}}{h} = 27.3\,mL/h$

17. $units/h = \dfrac{25000\,units}{100\,\cancel{mL}} \times \dfrac{30\,\cancel{mL}}{1\,h} = 750\,units/h$

12

Fluid Volume and Electrolytes

http://evolve.elsevier.com/McCuistion/pharmacology

OBJECTIVES

- Describe osmolality and tonicity.
- Describe the classifications of intravenous fluids.
- Discuss the functions of major electrolytes.
- Differentiate between intracellular and extracellular electrolytes.
- Discuss the importance of blood and blood products.
- Apply the Clinical Judgment [Nursing Process] to fluid volume deficit and fluid volume excess.
- Describe major signs and symptoms of deficiency and excess of potassium, sodium, calcium, magnesium, chloride, and phosphorus.
- Explain the methods used to correct potassium, calcium, and magnesium excess and deficiency.

OUTLINE

Fluid and electrolyte balance is necessary to maintain homeostasis. An equal balance of intake and output helps the human body maintain proper equilibrium within all body systems. Intake and output of water are regulated by the kidneys, the pulmonary system, and hormonal and neural functions. Fluid and electrolyte balance is the foundation on which nurses make important decisions concerning patient care.

To function normally, body cells must have fluid and electrolytes in the right compartments and in the right amounts. Total body fluid is contained in two major compartments: the intracellular fluid (ICF) is contained within the body's cells, and the extracellular fluid (ECF) comprises the fluid outside of the cells. The ECF is further divided into three subcompartments: the interstitial compartment bathes and surrounds the tissue cells; the intravascular compartment contains the plasma and blood vessels; and the transcellular compartment, also known as the third space, contains mucus and gastrointestinal (GI), cerebrospinal, pericardial, synovial, and ocular fluids. Table 12.1 shows the sum of fluids within all compartments, which constitutes the total body water (TBW). Fluids move freely between the intracellular and extracellular compartments to maintain balance and homeostasis.

The TBW of a 70-kg (154-lb) man is approximately 60% (40 L) of fluid volume. This percentage varies with age, sex, and percentage of body fat. Neonates are 75% to 80% water, whereas older adults are 45% to 55% water. Women tend to have less body water than men because of hormones and higher amounts of adipose tissue, which contains very little water.

Water that moves through the compartments of the body contains electrolytes. Electrolytes are substances that separate or dissociate into ions (charged particles) in solution, and they are abundant in both ICF and ECF. Ions carry either a positive charge (cation) or a negative charge (anion). Major cations and anions are listed in Table 12.2. Electrolyte balance is essential for normal physiologic functioning and is closely linked with fluid balance. In addition, most electrolytes interact with hydrogen ions to maintain an acid-base balance. Electrolyte balance must be kept within a narrow range to maintain homeostasis. Many illnesses and body system alterations cause electrolyte imbalances.

TABLE 12.1   Adult Body Fluid Volume

Fluid Compartment	Percentage
Intracellular fluid	40%
Extracellular fluid	20%
Interstitial fluid	15%
Intravascular fluid	5%
Transcellular fluid	Approximately 1–2 L total (generally not included in calculations)
Total body fluid	60%

TABLE 12.2   Cations and Anions

Cations	Anions
Potassium (K^+)	Chloride (Cl^-)
Sodium (Na^+)	Bicarbonate (HCO_3^-)
Calcium (Ca^{2+})	Phosphate (PO_4^-)
Magnesium (Mg^{2+})	Sulfate (SO_4^-)

TABLE 12.3   Electrolyte Concentration in Body Fluids

Intracellular Fluid	Extracellular Fluid
Major Cations	*Major Cations*
Potassium	Sodium
Magnesium	Potassium
Sodium	Calcium
	Magnesium
Major Anions	*Major Anions*
Phosphorus	Chloride
	Phosphorus

Electrolytes are important because they carry electrical impulses to other cells in the body.

The major electrolytes in body fluids are sodium, potassium, calcium, magnesium, chloride, phosphorus, sulfate, hydrogen, and bicarbonate ions and many proteins. Electrolyte concentrations differ in ICF and ECF. Table 12.3 lists the major cations and anions found in body fluids.

Administering intravenous (IV) fluids and electrolyte replacements may be thought of as routine nursing care; however, both require as much diligence and critical thinking as administration of any medication. This chapter describes fluid replacement strategies, pharmacologic management of specific electrolyte imbalances, and nursing care of patients with fluid and electrolyte imbalances.

HOMEOSTASIS

Homeostasis maintains a constant internal balance within the body despite the effects of a constantly changing external environment. Two principles stand out when considering homeostasis and fluid and electrolyte balance. The first principle is that anions and cations must be balanced within each compartment and remain electrically neutral. The amount of fluid within each compartment remains constant, and compartments work continuously to maintain fluid balance and replace and exchange ions to maintain neutrality. The second principle is that the fluid compartments remain in osmotic equilibrium except for transient changes.

Movement of fluid and particles between and within compartments is controlled by a number of processes, including osmosis, the movement of water across a semipermeable membrane from areas of low solute concentration to those of high solute concentration; diffusion, movement of molecules from an area of high concentration to one of low concentration; hydrostatic pressure, the force within a fluid compartment; osmolality, which describes the concentration of fluids; and active transport, which requires metabolic activity and expenditure of energy to move a substance across a cell membrane. The number of solutes in a solution is expressed as a unit of measurement called the osmole, which is particularly useful when referencing osmotic solutions.

Osmolality

Osmolality refers to the number of particles dissolved in the serum, primarily sodium, urea (blood urea nitrogen [BUN]), and glucose. It also is a measure of the concentration of solutes per kilogram in urine. Normal serum osmolality ranges from 275 to 295 mOsm/kg. As the number of particles increases, the concentration of the solution also increases. The change in the concentration of particles will affect chemical behavior and movement of water. Sodium is the primary electrolyte in the ECF and keeps water in this compartment.

The following three types of fluid concentration are based on the osmolality of body fluids:
1. Iso-osmolar fluid has the same weight proportion of particles (e.g., sodium, glucose) and water.
2. Hypo-osmolar fluid contains fewer particles than water.
3. Hyper-osmolar fluid contains more particles than water.

Hypo-osmolality of body fluid may be the result of excess water intake or fluid overload (edema) caused by an inability to excrete excess water. *Hyper-osmolality* of body fluid may be caused by severe diarrhea, increased salt and solute (protein) intake, inadequate water intake, diabetes, ketoacidosis, or sweating.

The terms osmolality and tonicity are similar but not identical. Osmolality refers to the concentration of particles in a solution. Tonicity is used primarily as a measurement of the concentration of IV solutions compared with the osmolality of body fluids.

FLUID REPLACEMENT

General Considerations

All routes of fluid intake and loss must be considered when assessing fluid balance. General guidelines can be used as the basis for establishing fluid needs. The recommended water intake for a healthy adult is about 2300 to 2900 mL per day; oral intake accounts for 1200 to 1500 mL, solid foods about 800 to 1100 mL, and oxidative metabolism about 300 mL daily.

Patients lose water daily through various routes: kidneys, skin, lungs, and GI tract. The kidneys, the major organ regulating fluid loss, produce 1200 to 1500 mL of urine daily. *Insensible water loss* is continuous and occurs daily through the skin and lungs without awareness and is not measurable. *Sensible water loss* occurs through the lungs/respiration (500 mL/day), perspiration/skin (500–600 mL/day), and the GI tract/feces (200 mL/day) and is measurable. The minimum urinary output for an adult is 0.5 to 1 mL/kg/h or 35 to 70 mL/h for a 70-kg patient.

Daily water requirements differ according to the patient's age and medical problems. Intravenous fluids (IVFs) are ordered based on an evaluation of the patient's fluid and electrolyte balance, fluid requirements, and fluid needs. Several questions must be addressed: Is the purpose of IV therapy replacement or maintenance? What are the patient's water, electrolyte, and protein requirements? The patient's weight, caloric needs, and body surface area are other important

TABLE 12.4 Crystalloids Intravenous Solutions

Classifications of Crystalloids	Examples of IVF[a]	General Indications and Cautions for Use
Isotonic	LR 0.9% NaCl 5% Dextrose in water (D_5W)	LR provides electrolytes and is used for rehydration in all types of dehydration and FVD. Use cautiously in patients with renal failure (contains K^+). Use cautiously in alkalosis and liver disease; liver converts LR to bicarbonate. **Hydration** Corrects dehydration and sodium depletion Replaces GI losses Dextrose provides some calories ⚡ Use with caution in patients with cardiac or renal disease due to risk for FVE ⚡ Do not administer isotonic solutions to patients with known or suspected increased intracranial pressure
Hypotonic	0.45% NaCl (½ NS) 0.33% NaCl (⅓ NS) 0.225% NaCl (¼ NS)	Replaces cellular fluid by treating intracellular dehydration (diabetic ketoacidosis, hyperosmolar hyperglycemic state) Provides free water to allow excretion of body wastes Dextrose provides some calories ⚡ Do not administer hypotonic solutions to patients with known or suspected increased intracranial pressure (ICP) or patients with liver disease, shock, trauma, or burns (risk of depleting intravascular volume) Monitor for signs of FVD and worsening hypovolemia due to a decrease in vascular volume
Hypertonic	3% NaCl 5% NaCl 5% Dextrose in 0.45% NaCl 5% Dextrose and 0.9% NaCl 5% Dextrose in LR 10% Dextrose in water ($D_{10}W$)	Increases serum osmolality Corrects severe hyponatremia Decreases ICP in patients with cerebral edema Dextrose provides some calories ⚡ Use with caution; may cause intravascular volume overload and pulmonary edema; ⚡ Administer slowly and carefully with infusion control pump and constant monitoring; monitor electrolytes and monitor for signs of FVE. Avoid prolonged use. ⚡ Contraindicated for patients with cardiac or renal disease and for those with dehydration or diabetic ketoacidosis. Higher concentrations of dextrose (>10%) must be given through a central venous access device; may be added to amino acid solutions as total parenteral nutrition.

>, Greater than; <, less than; *FVD*, fluid volume depletion; *FVE*, fluid volume excess; *GI*, gastrointestinal; *IVF*, intravenous fluids; *K*, potassium; *LR*, lactated Ringer's solution; *NaCl*, sodium chloride; *NS*, normal saline.
[a]Examples of IV fluids: Refer to manufacturer's label on individual bags of intravenous fluids (IVFs) for exact osmolarity.

considerations. Illness and surgery increase the amount of fluids lost and affect fluid and electrolyte needs. Ongoing assessment and monitoring of the patient's responses to fluid and electrolyte therapy are vital for patients with fluid and electrolyte imbalances.

Intravenous Solutions

With fluid volume deficit (FVD) from the extracellular body compartment, fluid is lost from the interstitial and vascular spaces. Different types and concentrations of IVFs are available to replace body fluid losses.

Types of Intravenous Solutions

The three general classifications of IV solutions used for fluid replacement are crystalloids (with and without added electrolytes), colloids, and blood and blood products.

Crystalloids. Crystalloid solutions contain fluids and electrolytes and freely cross capillary walls. They do not contain any proteins, which are necessary to maintain the colloidal oncotic pressure that prevents water from leaving the intravascular space. Crystalloids are used as short-term maintenance fluids and to treat dehydration and electrolyte imbalances. Crystalloids cause early plasma expansion but have a shorter duration of action than colloid solutions.

The three major classifications of crystalloid IVFs are isotonic, hypotonic, and hypertonic (Table 12.4):

- Isotonic solutions have the same approximate osmolality as ECF or plasma. Because of the osmotic equilibrium, water does not enter or leave the cell; therefore there is no effect on red blood cells (RBCs). Isotonic solutions are primarily used for hydration and to expand ECF volume, because the fluid remains in the intravascular space.
- Hypotonic solutions exert less osmotic pressure than ECF, which allows water to move into the cell. IV infusions of hypotonic solutions result in an increased solute concentration in the intravascular space, causing fluid to move into the intracellular and interstitial spaces. Excessive infusion of hypotonic solutions may cause hemolysis, decreased blood pressure, and decreased IVF volume.
- Hypertonic solutions exert greater osmotic pressure than ECF, resulting in a higher solute concentration than the serum. When administered, hypertonic IVF fluids pull water from the interstitial space to the ECF via osmosis and cause cell shrinkage. Patients receiving hypertonic solutions must be monitored carefully for signs of circulatory overload (because of the increase in ECF volume).

Parenteral solutions containing dextrose are available in different concentrations and in combination with other solutions, such as normal saline and lactated Ringer's solution. Dextrose solutions provide hydration and some calories and increase glucose levels in the blood. The pharmacist will use dextrose solutions to dilute IV medications for administration. The addition of dextrose to an IV solution affects the tonicity of the solution after it is infused. Five-percent dextrose solutions are hypertonic when added to normal saline or lactated Ringer's solution, but the remaining solution is isotonic because the dextrose is quickly metabolized to carbon dioxide and water.

The Infusion Nursing Society's Practice Guidelines recommend that dextrose solutions higher than 10% should be given via a central vein. An exception is 50% dextrose, which may be given in small amounts via a peripheral vein to correct hypoglycemia. Dextrose can be irritating to veins because of the pH of the solution (3.4–4). If hypertonic solutions are not diluted and are given peripherally, there is a risk of vein irritation, damage, and thrombosis. Long-term use of hypertonic solutions may result in electrolyte depletion, increased intravascular volume, fluid overload, water intoxication, and pulmonary edema. Rapid infusions of dextrose solutions may cause hyperglycemia, which can lead to osmotic diuresis and fluid and electrolyte imbalance.

Sodium solutions are available in various concentrations and tonicities. Isotonic solutions are primarily used for hydration to expand the ECF and during blood product transfusions. Rapid infusion of isotonic saline solutions may lead to hypernatremia, fluid volume excess (FVE), and electrolyte depletion. Long-term use should also be avoided because normal saline provides no calories. Hypotonic solutions are also used for hydration and to treat hyperosmolar diabetes. Hypertonic saline solutions are used to treat severe hyponatremia or hypochloremia; careful monitoring of electrolyte levels is important to avoid excess replacement.

Balanced electrolyte solutions, such as lactated Ringer's solution and Ringer's solution, contain electrolytes (no magnesium) and minimal calories with the addition of dextrose. Their primary use is hydration and electrolyte replacement. However, they do not provide adequate electrolytes for maintenance therapy for patients with limited or no oral intake. Lactated Ringer's solution is similar to plasma in electrolyte content. Lactate is added as a buffering agent and is metabolized to bicarbonate. Complications of infusions of Ringer's and lactated Ringer's include fluid overload, excess electrolytes, and metabolic acidosis with long-term therapy. ⚡ Because lactate is metabolized in the liver, lactated Ringer's is contraindicated for patients with liver disease.

Colloids. Colloid solutions contain protein or other large molecular substances that increase osmolarity without dissolving in the solution. Because of their size, the particles are unable to pass through the semipermeable membranes of the capillary walls and stay within the intravascular compartment; thus colloids are also known as *plasma expanders.* They act by increasing the colloidal oncotic pressure and pulling fluids from the interstitial space into the plasma, increasing blood volume. The composition of colloid solutions includes proteins, carbohydrates, and lipids. Colloids typically have small and large particles, except albumin, whose particles are all one size. Commonly used colloids are shown in Table 12.5.

Blood and Blood Products. Nurses complete a thorough patient assessment before, during, and after administration of blood products. Each facility has a policy and procedure for blood transfusions, and each registered nurse is oriented in the correct procedure. Blood products include packed red blood cells (PRBCs), plasma, platelets, and cryoprecipitate. A unit of PRBCs contains concentrated RBCs with

TABLE 12.5   Common Colloid Solutions

Common Solutions[a]	Indications	Nursing Implications	Adverse Effects and Contraindications
High-molecular-weight dextran 75 Dextran 70 6% in 5% dextrose	Treatment of shock caused by hemorrhage, burns, or trauma Maximum volume expansion effect 1 h after administration with normal renal functioning Increased volume is excreted within 24 h	Administer colloid solutions with an 18-g or larger needle. Dextran solutions are not a substitute for blood products and have no oxygen-carrying capacity but may be used emergently if cross-matching or blood products are unavailable. Monitor pulse, BP, CVP, and urine output every 5–15 min for the first hour, and hourly thereafter Increased volume may cause dilution of Hgb and Hct. Assess fluid volume status; may cause circulatory overload. Monitor for signs and symptoms of FVE.	Bleeding; hypotension; wheezing; urticaria; chest tightness; nausea and vomiting may occur ⚡ Severe anaphylaxis reactions, leading to death Contraindicated for patients with impaired hepatic or renal disease, heart failure, and bleeding disorders ⚡ May interfere with laboratory testing for typing and cross-matching; draw necessary blood samples before administration.
Hydroxyethyl starch 6% (hetastarch) A synthetic polymer closely related to human albumin	Early fluid replacement and treatment of hypovolemic shock and burns Maximum volume expansion occurs shortly after infusion is completed Duration of action is 24–36 h	Hetastarch 6% with 0.9% NaCl is isotonic Hetastarch 6% with 7.2% NaCl is hypertonic Does not interfere with blood typing and cross-matching Assess fluid volume status; may cause circulatory overload	⚡ May cause severe anaphylactic reaction Interferes with platelet function by increasing bleeding time ⚡ Contraindicated for patients with bleeding disorders and renal, cardiac, or liver disease
Albumin 5% Albumin 25% Prepared from human blood and blood products Considered a blood product	Regulates plasma volume and tissue-fluid balance 5% solution is isotonic and is used to treat hypovolemia 25% solution is hypertonic and is generally used for patients with fluid and sodium restrictions	Assess fluid volume status Can cause circulatory overload	⚡ Contraindicated in patients with heart failure or severe anemia ⚡ Hold ACEIs at least 24 h before administering albumin due to the risk of adverse reactions, including hypotension and flushing

ACEI, Angiotensin-converting enzyme inhibitor; *BP,* blood pressure; *CVP,* central venous pressure; *FVE,* fluid volume excess; *g,* gauge; *h,* hour; *Hct,* hematocrit; *Hgb,* hemoglobin; *min,* minute; *NaCl,* sodium chloride.
[a]Common solutions: Refer to manufacturer's label on individual bags of intravenous fluids (IVFs) for exact osmolarity.

most of the plasma and platelets removed; the approximate volume is 350 mL/unit. The approximate volume of a unit of whole blood is 500 mL/unit. Infusing PRBCs over whole blood offers an advantage because packed cells allow an increase in oxygen-carrying capacity with a smaller volume. One unit of whole blood elevates the hemoglobin by approximately 0.5 to 1 g/dL, and one unit of PRBCs elevates the hematocrit by three points.

It is important for nurses to understand the specific blood components before beginning the infusion. Proper product-to-patient identification is paramount in preventing transfusion reactions. Reducing errors during blood administration is a focus of The Joint Commission's 2018 National Patient Safety Goals (http://www.jointcommission.org). Also, the National Healthcare Safety Network's Hemovigilance Module was developed to increase patient safety and decrease costs associated with transfusion-related adverse events (http://www.cdc.gov/nhsn/pdfs/biovigilance/bv-hv-protocol-current.pdf).

The maximum rate of an infusion is 4 hours per unit, beginning with removal of the unit from the refrigerator. If the transfusion is not finished by the 4-hour mark, the transfusion bag must be returned to the blood bank, and a new bag issued to complete the transfusion. *Never* add medications to the unit of blood.

Loop diuretics are often prescribed to patients receiving whole blood or PRBCs to prevent circulatory overload, particularly in patients who are at risk for developing pulmonary edema and FVE. For patients receiving multiple blood transfusions, the serum ionized calcium level should be monitored. Both PRBCs and whole blood products are processed using sodium citrate and citric acid for anticoagulation; multiple blood transfusions can result in a decrease in the plasma calcium levels. Practice guidelines are available from The Joint Commission (see http://www.jointcommission.org/2019/bloodmanagement.pdf). Always confirm with the patient any ethical or legal issues preventing the administration of blood or blood products that might conflict with the patient's personal belief system.

IV fat emulsion, also known as *lipid emulsion,* is a component of parenteral nutrition for patients who are unable to get nutrition through an oral diet (see Chapter 14). Fat emulsion can supply up to 30% of the patient's caloric intake and is usually recommended for patients who are unable to tolerate oral or enteral feedings for 7 days or more. The contents of fat emulsion are primarily soybean or safflower and triglycerides with egg phospholipids added as an emulsifier. Parenteral nutrition provides essential nutrients intravenously, including proteins, carbohydrates, electrolytes, trace minerals, and vitamins. Fat emulsion is often added to parenteral nutrition formulas by the pharmacist. The patient must have a centrally or peripherally inserted vascular access device to receive parenteral nutrition formulas. Nausea, vomiting, and elevated temperature have been reported when fat emulsion is infused too quickly. It is used cautiously in patients at risk for fat embolism, such as with a fractured femur, and in patients with an allergy to eggs or soybeans and those with pancreatitis, bleeding disorders, liver failure, and respiratory disease.

◎ CLINICAL JUDGMENT [NURSING PROCESS]
Fluid Imbalances (Fluid Volume Deficit and Fluid Volume Excess)

Concept: Fluid and Electrolytes
- Patients require the regulation of fluid and electrolytes to maintain homeostasis. Nurses will encounter potential and actual alterations of fluid and electrolyte balance when caring for patients. Nursing assessments and interventions ensure the intake of fluid and electrolytes remains balanced by closely monitoring the patient's intake and output and careful assessment of laboratory values.

Recognize Cues [Assessment]
- Identify patients at risk for fluid volume deficit (FVD) and fluid volume excess (FVE).
- Contributing factors for FVD include prolonged inadequate intake, excessive losses due to bleeding or trauma, and gastrointestinal (GI) losses. Contributing factors for FVE include heart failure, liver disease, kidney failure, excessive sodium intake, and excessive or too rapid infusion of intravenous fluids (IVFs).
- Assess the patient's history to identify factors that may contribute to FVD and FVE.
- Differentiate between causes of FVD, including hypovolemia and dehydration, and causes of FVE, including heart failure and kidney and liver diseases.
- Assess the patient's vital signs and note usual baseline values. Report abnormal findings.
- Assess the patient's laboratory values. A complete blood count, basic metabolic profile, and serum osmolality are good indicators of the patient's hydration status.
- Determine the patient's input and output.
- Obtain urine specific gravity. The normal range is 1.005 to 1.030 g/mL.
- Check the types of IVF ordered per day, including the amount to be infused, the hourly rate, and the solution for tonicity and electrolyte content. Consider if fluid ordered is appropriate for the patient's history and clinical condition. If any questions arise, collaborate with the health care provider (HCP) to determine appropriate fluid replacement for the patient. Excessive administration of IVF containing sodium to patients with altered regulatory mechanisms may precipitate FVE.

- Assess the patient's current weight and baseline weight.

Analyze Cues and Prioritize Hypothesis [Patient Problems]
- Dehydration
- Fluid overload
- Disrupted fluid and electrolyte balance

Generate Solutions [Planning]
- The patient will exhibit balanced fluid volume within 24 hours as evidenced by normal electrolyte panel.
- The patient will have balanced intake and output over a 24-hour period.
- The patient will experience hydration as evidenced by moist mucous membranes, elastic skin turgor, and vital signs within normal limits; adequate urine output; urine specific gravity between 1.005 and 1.010 g/mL; stable weight; and no changes in mental status.
- With FVE, the patient will not exhibit signs of circulatory overload as evidenced by absence of signs and symptoms of edema or anasarca, having clear lung sounds, being free of jugular venous distension, and vital signs within normal limits.
- Patient and family will verbalize an understanding of teaching related to FVD and FVE as evidenced by notifying the doctor of signs and symptoms:
  - FVD signs to notify provider are excessive thirst, confusion, decreased urine output, nausea, vomiting, diarrhea, and weakness.
  - FVE signs to notify provider include weight gain, swelling in body including feet, difficulty breathing, anxiety, and changes in urine output.

Take Action [Nursing Interventions]
General
- Monitor and record vital signs; assess trends and deviation from baseline and document findings. Report significant changes to the HCP.
- Measure and record intake and output every 4 hours. Identify sources of excessive intake or fluid losses.

Continued

⊚ CLINICAL JUDGMENT [NURSING PROCESS]—CONT'D

Fluid Imbalances (Fluid Volume Deficit and Fluid Volume Excess)

- Measure urine specific gravity. Readings greater than 1.025 g/mL indicate concentrated urine, whereas those less than 1.010 g/mL indicate dilute urine.
- Implement strict aseptic technique when inserting intravenous (IV) access devices. Check IV site for patency and signs of complications such as phlebitis and infiltration. Adhere to agency policy regarding site rotation and dressing and tubing changes.
- Avoid contamination when administering IV medications. Follow evidence-based practice guidelines and implement interventions to decrease central line–associated infections.
- Monitor IV infusions at least hourly, and ensure that the prescribed amount infuses hourly. Set the IV pump correctly, and validate the correct drip rate.
- Measure the patient's weight daily and compare it with the baseline measurement. A gain of 1 kg (2.2 lb) is equivalent to 1 L of fluid.
- Use an interpreter if appropriate.
- With the patient's permission, involve the extended family in health teaching and support.

Fluid Volume Deficit

- Administer isotonic IVF as ordered.
- Monitor strict intake and output hourly. Encourage frequent oral intake if the patient can drink liquids. Provide oral care if the patient is unable to perform independently. Moisturize skin to prevent dryness, and reposition the patient every 2 hours, padding bony prominences; monitor frequently for skin breakdown and pressure.
- Monitor for signs and symptoms of FVD because of hypovolemia, including thirst (usually the first sign of dehydration), restlessness, headaches, inability to concentrate, dry mucous membranes, poor skin turgor, tachycardia, changes in mental status, and slightly decreased systolic blood pressure.
- Recognize late symptoms of hypovolemia, which include cyanosis; cold, clammy skin; weak thready pulse; confusion; and oliguria.
- Monitor vital signs for indications of FVD, including increased temperature, weak pulse, tachycardia (early sign), hypotension, and tachypnea.
- Assess for orthostatic hypotension and use safety precautions when transferring the patient from bed to chair, avoiding abrupt changes in position. Other signs and symptoms of FVD include flattened neck veins; weight loss; decreased skin turgor; dry mucous membranes; decreased capillary refill; pale, cool, clammy skin; and muscle weakness.
- Monitor laboratory values associated with FVD daily, including increased hemoglobin and hematocrit; urine specific gravity greater than 1.030 g/mL; and increased sodium, BUN, creatinine, electrolyte levels, and serum osmolality.

Fluid Volume Excess

- Monitor and record vital signs that indicate FVE, including tachycardia, bounding pulse, tachypnea, increased blood pressure, and increased pulse

pressure. Other signs and symptoms of FVE include altered mental status; generalized edema (use +1 to +4 scale to quantify edema); anasarca; constant, irritated cough; dyspnea; orthopnea; crackles; pulmonary congestion; muffled heart sounds; fatigue; increased central venous pressure; jugular vein distension; and increased urine output. Listen to lung sounds for crackles, and monitor respirations. The most consistent sign of FVE is increased body weight.
- Monitor laboratory results associated with FVE daily, including BUN, hemoglobin, hematocrit, sodium, potassium, creatinine, albumin, and urine specific gravity below 1.010. Chest radiography may reveal pulmonary congestion. Monitor intake and output, and note trends that reflect urine output.
- Monitor daily weight for sudden increases.
- Administer diuretics as ordered; implement fluid and sodium restrictions. Recommend a nutritionist consult if warranted. Position the patient with the head of bed elevated 30 to 45 degrees to facilitate respiration. Monitor edematous areas for signs of pressure and altered skin integrity and provide meticulous skin care; reposition the patient at least every 2 hours.

Patient Teaching
General

- Instruct patients that thirst means a mild fluid deficit. Oral fluid intake is the best means of fluid replacement for a patient with FVD.
- Advise patients to report vomiting or diarrhea. When these occur constantly or over several days, severe fluid volume and electrolyte imbalance can result.
- If a patient has FVE, fluid may be restricted. Instruct patients on limited intake of fluids around the clock.
- Assist patients in planning a typical 24-hour fluid intake based on individual fluid needs. Encourage patients to monitor fluid intake and output, and advise them to report to their HCP any abnormal findings such as changes in urination patterns, fatigue, shortness of breath, weight gain (>3 lb in 2 days or 1.4 kg), peripheral edema, or tight shoes and rings.
- Provide (if ordered) and instruct patient in a low sodium diet: Fresh fruits and vegetables, sodium-free herbs and spices, frozen vegetables, broiled meats and chicken. Avoid canned foods, sausage, or deli meats.

Evaluate Outcomes [Evaluation]

- The patient's vital signs should remain within normal limits.
- Fluid intake is balanced with output.
- Urine output is adequate for age, weight, and history.
- The patient and family understand the treatments and are able to verbalize the treatment plan and expected outcomes.
- IVFs are administered as ordered without complications or harm to the patient.

ELECTROLYTES

Potassium

Potassium (K^+) is the primary intracellular cation, and 98% of the body's potassium is found within the cells. Its concentration inside the cell is roughly 150 to 160 mEq/L, which is 25 to 35 times greater than extracellular concentration. Only 2% of potassium is found in the extracellular concentration. Potassium is essential for neuromuscular activity and cellular metabolism. Potassium levels affect cardiac and skeletal muscle activity and play a major role in muscle and nerve cell electrodynamics.

Potassium moves in and out of the cells under the influence of the potassium-sodium pump. It maintains the concentration difference in the

cells by pumping potassium into the cells and pumping sodium out. Acid-base balance also influences potassium levels. *Acidotic* conditions tend to pull potassium out of cells, whereas *alkalotic* conditions tend to put potassium back into cells. The kidneys are the primary route for potassium loss, eliminating about 90% of the daily potassium intake. An inverse relationship exists between sodium and potassium reabsorption in the kidneys. Aldosterone also plays a role in the excretion of potassium.

Daily dietary intake is necessary because potassium is poorly stored in the body. Recommended daily potassium intake is 40 to 80 mEq/day in 1 or 2 divided doses within 24 hours in either potassium-rich foods or a potassium supplement. Foods rich in potassium include tuna, fruits, and vegetables such as mangoes, oranges, avocados, tomatoes, cucumbers, spinach, strawberries, and bananas.

Functions

Potassium is necessary for transmission and conduction of nerve impulses and for contraction of skeletal, cardiac, and smooth muscles. It is also necessary for normal kidney function and for the enzyme action used to change carbohydrates to energy (glycolysis) and amino acids to protein. Potassium promotes glycogen storage in hepatic cells, regulates the osmolality of cellular fluids, and plays a role in acid-base balance.

Hypokalemia

Hypokalemia, or potassium deficit, is generally defined as a serum potassium concentration of less than 3.5 mEq/L. Most cases of hypokalemia are caused by excessive loss rather than deficient intake. Whenever cells are damaged from trauma, injury, surgery, or shock, potassium leaks from the cells into the intravascular fluid and is excreted by the kidneys. With cellular loss of potassium, potassium shifts from the blood plasma into the cells to restore the cellular potassium balance; hypokalemia usually results. GI sources of potassium loss include vomiting, diarrhea, suctioning, recent ileostomy formation, draining fistulae, and diuretic therapy. Between 80% and 90% of potassium in the body is excreted in the urine; another 8% is excreted in the feces. Other causes of potassium loss include burns, total parenteral nutrition therapy, alkalosis, prolonged laxative use, excessive licorice consumption, corticosteroid use, increased aldosterone levels, and decreased magnesium levels.

It is important to recognize the signs and symptoms of hypokalemia. Hypokalemia may not be symptomatic until potassium levels fall below 3.0 mEq/L. Muscle weakness does not usually occur until potassium levels fall below 2.5 mEq/L. Quadricep weakness is one of the earliest signs of hypokalemia. Other early signs include fatigue, muscle weakness, anorexia, nausea, and vomiting. Severe signs and symptoms include paresthesia, leg cramps, decreased bowel motility and paralytic ileus, confusion, rhabdomyolysis and myoglobinuria, atrial and ventricular dysrhythmias, and cardiac arrest. Electrocardiogram (ECG) changes include flattened or inverted T waves and depressed ST segments. If severe enough, hypokalemia can result in cardiac arrest, paralysis, respiratory arrest, and death.

Certain drugs, such as potassium-wasting diuretics and cortisone preparations, promote potassium loss. Patients receiving these drugs should increase their potassium intake by consuming foods rich in potassium or by taking potassium supplements as prescribed by their health care provider (HCP). Keep in mind that potassium-sparing diuretics do not deplete potassium stores, so patients would not be requested to increase potassium intake or to take supplements. Serum potassium levels should be monitored periodically for abnormalities.

Treatment for hypokalemia due to excessive potassium loss depends on the severity of the deficit. Patients with low-normal serum potassium levels may be advised to consume additional foods high in potassium. Management goals for patients with hypokalemia include preventing and treating life-threatening complications, replacing potassium and returning levels to normal, and diagnosing and correcting the cause of the deficiency.

Potassium replacements can be given orally or intravenously (Box 12.1). Table 12.6 lists the potassium preparations used to treat hypokalemia, and see the Prototype Drug Chart: Potassium Chloride, which compares the pharmacokinetics and pharmacodynamics of oral and IV potassium preparations.

Pharmacodynamics. Potassium maintains neuromuscular activity. Onset of action of oral potassium is unknown; with IV potassium, onset is rapid. Duration of action of potassium is also unknown; however, it may vary according to the dose taken. Continuous cardiac monitoring and serum potassium levels should be closely monitored when large doses are administered. To raise the serum potassium level by 1 mEq, the patient should receive 100 to 200 mEq of IV potassium.

Hyperkalemia

Hyperkalemia is defined as a serum potassium level above 5.0 mEq/L. Causes include excessive intake, impaired renal excretion, or a shift from intracellular to extracellular spaces. The most common causes are renal failure and medications that interfere with potassium excretion. Renal disease or kidney failure results in potassium accumulating in the intravascular fluid, which results in hyperkalemia. Persons at risk for developing hyperkalemia include premature infants, older adults, and those with a history of genitourinary disease, adrenal insufficiency, cancer, poorly controlled diabetes, or polypharmacy. Hyperkalemia manifests primarily as cardiac and neuromuscular symptoms. Signs and symptoms include cardiac dysrhythmias that include characteristic changes on the ECG, such as early tachycardia followed by bradycardia; paresthesia of the face, tongue, hands, and feet; and GI hyperactivity, including nausea, diarrhea, and abdominal cramping. Metabolic acidosis may also be present.

Management goals are to eliminate the cause of the excess potassium, shift potassium back into the cells, increase potassium excretion, decrease potassium intake, and prevent further episodes of hyperkalemia. For mild hyperkalemia, foods rich in potassium are usually restricted. Treatment strategies for hyperkalemia are outlined in Box 12.2.

Effect of Drugs on Potassium Balance

Potassium-wasting diuretics are a major cause of hypokalemia. Diuretics are divided into two categories: potassium-wasting and potassium-sparing drugs. Potassium-wasting diuretics cause excretion of potassium and other electrolytes, such as sodium and chloride, in the urine. Potassium-sparing diuretics cause retention of potassium, but sodium and chloride are excreted in the urine.

Laxatives, corticosteroids, antibiotics, and potassium-wasting diuretics are the major drug classifications that can cause hypokalemia. Other drug classifications that may cause hyperkalemia include oral and IV potassium salts, central nervous system (CNS) agents, and potassium-sparing diuretics. Tables 12.7 and 12.8 identify drugs that affect potassium balance.

Sodium

Sodium is the major cation in the ECF. The normal serum sodium level is 135 to 145 mEq/L. A serum sodium level below 135 mEq/L is called hyponatremia, and a serum sodium level above 145 mEq/L is called hypernatremia. Sodium and chloride imbalances typically occur together. The most serious problems associated with serum sodium deficit (hyponatremia) are cerebral edema, altered mental status, confusion, and seizure. In sodium excess imbalances (hypernatremia), a rapid decrease occurs in intracellular water to the brain, which results in cerebral dehydration, seizure, and coma.

The dietary requirement for sodium is 2000 mg to 4000 mg daily. Sodium-rich foods include bacon, luncheon meats, corned beef, decaffeinated coffee, ham, tomato juice, pickles, and soda crackers.

Functions

Sodium is found in most body fluids; it plays a major role in fluid volume balance and is the primary determinant of plasma osmolality. Sodium combines readily with chloride (Cl^-) or bicarbonate (HCO_3^-) to promote acid-base balance. Sodium is important for the maintenance of neuromuscular irritability and for conduction of nerve impulses. In conjunction with neural and hormonal mediators, the kidney maintains normal serum sodium concentrations through renal tubular reabsorption. The serum sodium level reflects the ratio of sodium to water, not necessarily the loss or gain of sodium.

◎ CLINICAL JUDGMENT [NURSING PROCESS]

Potassium

Concept: Fluid and Electrolyte Balance

- Patients require the regulation of fluid and electrolytes to maintain homeostasis. Nurses will encounter potential and actual alterations of fluid and electrolyte balance when caring for patients. Nursing assessments and interventions ensure the intake of fluid and electrolytes remains balanced by closely monitoring the patient's intake and output and careful assessment of laboratory values.

Recognize Cues [Assessment]

- Assess for signs and symptoms of potassium imbalance. Symptoms of hypokalemia include nausea and vomiting; polyuria; cardiac dysrhythmias; abdominal distension; and soft, flabby muscles. Symptoms of hyperkalemia include oliguria, nausea, abdominal cramps, tachycardia and later bradycardia, weakness, and numbness or tingling in the extremities.
- Assess serum potassium level; a normal level is 3.5 to 5.0 mEq/L. Report serum potassium deficits or excesses to the health care provider (HCP).
- Obtain baseline vital signs and electrocardiogram (ECG) readings and report abnormal findings. Vital signs and ECG results can be compared with future readings.
- Check for signs and symptoms of digitalis toxicity when the patient is receiving a digitalis preparation and a potassium-wasting diuretic or a cortisone preparation. A decreased serum potassium level enhances the action of digitalis and increases the likelihood of digitalis toxicity. Signs and symptoms of digitalis toxicity are nausea, vomiting, anorexia, bradycardia (pulse rate <60 or markedly decreased), cardiac dysrhythmias, and visual disturbances.

Analyze Cues and Prioritize Hypothesis [Patient Problems]

- Hypokalemia
- Hyperkalemia
- Dehydration
- Fluid overload

Generate Solutions [Planning]

- The patient's serum potassium level will remain within normal ranges (K+ 3.5 to 5.0 mEq/L).
- The patient will verbalize understanding of the potassium imbalance and state methods to decrease recurrence.
  - Patients with hypokalemia will eat potassium-rich foods.
  - Patients with hyperkalemia will avoid potassium-rich foods.
- At the end of the first teaching, the patient will name four signs and symptoms of hypokalemia and four signs and symptoms of hyperkalemia.
- At the end of the second teaching, the patient will name four signs and symptoms of fluid overload and four signs and symptoms of fluid deficit.

Take Action [Nursing Interventions]

- Administer oral potassium with enough water or orange juice (at least 8 oz) and with meals. Potassium is extremely irritating to the gastric mucosa.
- Administer potassium-containing intravenous (IV) solutions with a calibrated infusion pump. Potassium IV solutions should always be diluted and thoroughly mixed in 100 to 1000 mL of IV solution and must be infused slowly (generally no faster than 10 mEq/h).

- **!** Never administer potassium intramuscularly or as an IV bolus or push. Giving IV potassium directly into the vein causes cardiac dysrhythmias, cardiac arrest, and death. (Potassium chloride is one of the agents used in lethal injection because rapid infusion results in immediate cardiac arrest.)
- Evaluate the amount of urine output. Potassium accumulation occurs if a patient is receiving potassium and urine output is below 25 mL/h or below 600 mL/d. Remember that 80% to 90% of potassium is excreted in the urine. Report results to the health care provider.
- Monitor serum potassium levels frequently in addition to serum creatinine, blood urea nitrogen (BUN), glucose, electrolytes, and arterial blood gases. Report abnormal results to the health care provider.
- Monitor ECG. With hypokalemia, there is a flat or inverted T wave, a depressed ST segment, and a prolonged QT interval. With hyperkalemia, there is a narrow and peaked T wave, a widened QRS complex, a prolonged PR interval, flattened or absent T waves, and a depressed ST segment.
- Monitor the patient's response to activity, and plan frequent rest periods due to muscle weakness associated with potassium imbalances.
- Evaluate the IV site for infiltration if a patient is receiving IV potassium. Potassium can cause extravasation and tissue necrosis if it infiltrates into subcutaneous tissue. Discontinue IV fluids immediately if infiltration occurs.
- Monitor patients receiving medications for hyperkalemia for signs and symptoms of continuing hyperkalemia or iatrogenic hypokalemia.
- Use an interpreter as appropriate.
- Involve the extended family in health teaching and support.

Patient Teaching
General

- Advise patients to have the serum potassium level checked at regular intervals as prescribed by the HCP when taking medications that affect potassium levels.
- Instruct patients to drink a full glass of water when taking oral potassium supplements. Potassium preparations can be taken during or after a meal. Explain to patients that potassium is very irritating to the stomach.
- Encourage patients to comply with the prescribed potassium dose, regular laboratory tests, and medical follow-up related to the health problem and drug regimen.
- Instruct patients on the signs and symptoms of hypokalemia and hyperkalemia to report to their physician.

Diet

- Instruct patients who are taking medications that promote potassium loss to eat potassium-rich foods.
- Instruct patients at risk for potassium imbalances regarding dietary sources of potassium and the potassium content of foods.

Evaluate Outcomes [Evaluation]

- Evaluate the patient's serum potassium level and ECG.
  - The cardiac rhythm is normal baseline without dysrhythmias.
  - The serum potassium level is within normal range.
  - Report to the HCP if the level does not return to normal, in which case the potassium replacements and diet may need modification.

BOX 12.1 Oral and Intravenous Potassium Preparations

Potassium (K⁺) Preparations

Potassium preparations are individualized according to the needs of the patient. Requirement estimation is based on clinical condition, which includes electrocardiogram (ECG), plasma concentrations, and patient's response.

- *Potassium Acetate:* Available for intravenous (IV) administration. NOTE: Potassium chloride is typically used for the acute treatment of hypokalemia; however, potassium acetate may be used if correction of acidemia is needed.
- *Potassium Bicarbonate:* Available in oral/granule dosing. NOTE: Potassium chloride is typically used for replacement; however, bicarbonate is recommended when potassium depletion occurs in the setting of metabolic acidosis (pH less than 7.4).
- *Potassium Phosphate:* Available in oral dose and solution for injection. NOTE: Guidelines generally recommend the use of potassium phosphate for potassium serum concentration less than 4 mg/dL and sodium phosphate for potassium serum concentration more than 4 mg/dL. Potassium phosphate is usually appropriate as most conditions associated with hypophosphatemia are also associated with hypokalemia.
- *Potassium Gluconate:* Available as elixir or tablet. Potassium gluconate is a dietary supplement used to maintain potassium balance (i.e., hypokalemia prevention).
- *Potassium Chloride:* Available as a liquid, powder, tablet, capsule, controlled-release microencapsulated tablet, enteric-coated tablet, and effervescent tablet and parenteral use.
  - Potassium chloride is used for the treatment of hypokalemia and to maintain acid-base balance.

Nursing Implications for Oral Preparations

- Tablets and capsules should be administered with or after meals followed by a large glass of water while the patient is sitting up to decrease gastrointestinal irritation. The patient should remain upright at least 30 minutes after administration. Use of tablets and capsules should be reserved for patients who cannot tolerate liquid preparations.
  - Dissolve effervescent tablets in 3 to 8 oz of cold water. Ensure the tablet is fully dissolved.
  - Powders and liquid solutions should be diluted in 3 to 8 oz of cold water or juice.
  - Dilute liquid forms before administering via an enteral feeding tube.
- Do not chew or crush enteric-coated or extended-release tablets or capsules they must be swallowed.
- Advise patients not to suck on tablets to avoid oral ulceration.

- Advise patients to avoid salt substitutes.
- Patients on K⁺ therapy should have levels drawn to monitor progress.
- Explain to patients the need to take medications as directed, especially when concurrent digoxin or diuretics are taken.

Nursing Implications for Intravenous Potassium Administration[a]

- IV therapy is indicated for patients who are unable to tolerate oral therapy or, in addition to oral therapy, for patients with severe hypokalemia.
- [!] Medication errors involving too rapid infusion or bolus of IV administration of K⁺ chloride or K⁺ acetate have resulted in fatalities.
- [!] *Never* administer potassium via IV push or bolus.

Potassium Acetate (Continuous IV)[a]

- [!] Do not administer undiluted. Each single dose *must* be diluted and thoroughly mixed in 100 to 1000 mL normal saline (preferred), Ringer's, or lactated Ringer's solutions. Usually limited to 10 mEq/100 mL or 40 mEq/1000 mL via a peripheral line. Pain is associated with peripheral infusion; administer central vein when possible.
- [!] Rate: Infuse slowly at a rate up to 10 mEq/h in adults. Check hospital policy for maximum infusion rates. (The maximum rate in a monitored setting is 40 mEq/h in adults).

Potassium Chloride (Continuous IV)[a]

- [!] Do not administer undiluted; fatalities have occurred. Concentrated products have black caps on vials or black stripes above the constriction on ampules and are labeled with a warning about dilution requirements. Each single dose must be diluted and thoroughly mixed in 100 to 1000 mL of IV solution and is usually limited to 10 mEq/L to 20mEq/L via a peripheral line. Administer central vein when possible.
- [!] Rate: Infuse slowly at a rate up to 10 mEq/h in adults. Check the hospital policy for maximum infusion rates (maximum rate in a monitored setting is 40 mEq/h in adults). Always use an infusion pump.
- Monitor the IV site and infusion carefully to avoid extravasation and infiltration.
- [!] Too rapid an infusion may cause fatal hyperkalemia.
- [!] Symptoms of toxicity: Slow, irregular heartbeat; fatigue; muscle weakness; paresthesia; confusion; dyspnea; peaked T waves; depressed ST segments; prolonged QT segments; widened QRS complexes; loss of P waves; and cardiac arrhythmias.

[a]The Institute for Safe Medication Practices (ISMP) has listed potassium as a high-alert medication because of the high risk of causing significant harm to a patient when administered in error.

TABLE 12.6 Potassium Chloride Supplements

Preparation	Drug
Capsules, tablets, oral solution	Normal dose: 40–80 mEq/d Hypokalemia: 40–100 mEq/d Divide larger doses 2–3/d
Powder for oral solution	40–100 mEq/d in 2–5 divided doses; limit single doses to 40 mEq/dose; *max:* 200 mEq/24 h
Intravenous (IV) potassium	IV: Infusion rate 10 mEq/h. Never administer undiluted (Na + Cl is preferred diluent). Doses >10 mEq/h: ECG monitoring and repeat serum lab values necessary. Central line infusion required.

d, Daily; *g,* grams; *h,* hour; *L,* liter; *max,* maximum; *mL,* milliliters; *mEq,* milliequivalent

Hyponatremia

Hyponatremia is caused by a loss of sodium-containing fluids, deficient intake, or water gain. Sodium loss can result from vomiting, diarrhea, nasogastric suctioning, burns, wound drainage, trauma, renal failure, heart failure, third spacing, syndrome of inappropriate antidiuretic hormone (SIADH), excessive hypertonic IVF, surgery, and thiazide diuretics.

Hyponatremia may occur with hypovolemia and hypervolemia symptoms will depend on the onset and degree of deficit. Signs and symptoms of hyponatremia due to water shifting into cells are primarily neuromuscular and GI and include muscle weakness, decreased deep tendon reflexes, headaches, lethargy, confusion, seizures, coma, abdominal cramps, nausea and vomiting, pale skin, and dry mucous membranes.

Oral sodium replacement is the preferred treatment if the patient can tolerate oral intake or if the deficit is mild. Sodium may also be replaced

◎ CLINICAL JUDGMENT [NURSING PROCESS]
Sodium

Concept: Fluid and Electrolyte Balance

- Patients require the regulation of fluid and electrolytes to maintain homeostasis. Nurses will encounter potential and actual alterations of fluid and electrolyte balance when caring for patients. Nursing assessments and interventions ensure the intake of fluid and electrolytes remains balanced by closely monitoring the patient's intake and output, and careful assessment of laboratory values.

Recognize Cues [Assessment]

- Assess the patient for signs and symptoms of sodium imbalance. Symptoms of *hyponatremia* are muscle weakness, headaches, lethargy, confusion, seizures, abdominal cramps, nausea and vomiting, tachycardia and hypotension, pale skin, and dry mucous membranes. Symptoms of *hypernatremia* are flushed, dry skin; agitation; elevated body temperature; rough, dry tongue; nausea and vomiting; anorexia; tachycardia; hypertension; muscle twitching; and hyperreflexia.
- Check the serum sodium level. Report critically low sodium levels (<125 mEq/L) to the health care provider (HCP) because prompt medical care is required.
- Obtain a history of health problems that may lead to sodium loss or excess.

Analyze Cues and Prioritize Hypothesis [Patient Problems]

- Hypernatremia
- Hyponatremia
- Confusion
- Dehydration

- Disrupted fluid and electrolyte balance

Generate Solutions [Planning]

- The patient's serum sodium level will reach normal range (135–145 mEq/L in 3–5 days).

Take Action [Nursing Interventions]

- Monitor the prescribed medical regimen for correction of hyponatremia or hypernatremia.
- Instruct patients on the signs and symptoms of hyponatremia and hypernatremia, and instruct them to notify their HCP if any of these occur.
- Monitor serum sodium levels and report abnormal levels.
- Use an interpreter if the patient has a language barrier.
- Involve the extended family in health teaching and support.

Patient Teaching

- Instruct patients with hypernatremia to avoid foods high in sodium, to avoid using salt when cooking, and to refrain from adding extra salt to their food at the table.
- Emphasize the importance of reading labels on food products.

Evaluate Outcomes [Evaluation]

- Evaluate the patient's serum sodium level. Report if the sodium imbalance continues.
- Monitor fluid intake and output carefully; monitor daily weights.
- Assess patients for signs of circulatory overload and deficit.

---

via enteral feeding tubes. For a serum sodium level between 125 and 135 mEq/L, IV normal saline (0.9% sodium chloride) may increase sodium content in vascular fluid. For a serum sodium level below 120 mEq/L, a hypertonic 3% or 5% saline solution may be necessary.

Hypernatremia

Hypernatremia can be caused by sodium gain, sodium retention, or water loss. Causes include excessive oral sodium intake, deficient water intake, hypertonic tube feedings, hypertonic IVF, hyperaldosteronism, Cushing syndrome, corticosteroid use, and acute kidney failure. Other causes include vomiting, diarrhea, burns, diabetes insipidus, and mineralocorticoid excess.

Signs of fluid imbalance depend on the cause; water loss presents with symptoms of FVD, whereas sodium gain presents with symptoms of FVE. Signs and symptoms of hypernatremia are dry, sticky mucous membranes; flushed, dry skin; agitation; elevated body temperature; rough, edematous, dry tongue; nausea and vomiting; anorexia; tachycardia; hypertension; muscle twitching; hyperreflexia; seizures; and coma.

Management of hypernatremia depends on the cause and severity of the deficit. Frequent monitoring of sodium levels is necessary while the underlying cause is being treated. When the serum sodium level is elevated above 145 mEq/L, sodium restriction is indicated. Treatments include administration of IVF and diuretics.

Calcium

Calcium is the most abundant mineral in the body, accounting for approximately 40% of all body minerals and 2% of body weight. The total serum calcium range is 8.6 to 10.2 mg/dL. A calcium deficit (<8.6 mg/dL) is called **hypocalcemia**, and a calcium excess (>10.2 mg/dL) is called **hypercalcemia**. More than 90% of the body's calcium is found in bones and teeth. Of the remaining calcium found in the blood, about 50% is bound to protein, primarily albumin, a serum protein. Another 50% is free and not bound to protein and is called the *ionized form* of calcium; it can leave the vascular space and be active in cellular functions. Normal ionized calcium levels are reported separately (4.64 to 5.28 mg/dL).

Calcium levels are affected by acid-base balance and plasma albumin levels. When an individual is acidotic (decreased plasma pH), there is a decrease in calcium binding to the albumin, which leads to more ionized calcium. During alkalosis (increased plasma pH), increases in calcium binding lead to decreased ionized calcium. Alterations in serum albumin levels affect the interpretation of total calcium levels. Low albumin levels result in a drop in the total calcium level, although the level of ionized calcium is not affected.

Functions

Calcium is necessary for the transmission of nerve impulses and normal contraction of skeletal and heart muscles, regulation of the heart and blood pressure, hormone secretion, maintenance of muscle tone. This cation also maintains normal cellular permeability and promotes blood clotting by converting prothrombin into thrombin. Calcium is also needed for formation of bone and teeth. Two hormones, parathyroid hormone (PTH) and thyrocalcitonin (TCT), along with vitamin D and the blood pH, play an important role in maintaining the balance

PROTOTYPE DRUG CHART

! *Potassium Chloride*

Drug Class	Dosage
Electrolyte replacement	Treatment of hypokalemia (serum K+ level of <3.5 mEq/L) ADULTS: PO: Capsules/tablets/oral solution: 40–100 mEq/day in 2–5 divided doses/with meal not to exceed 200 mEq/day IV: K+ level 2.5–3.5 mEq/L, use 10 mEq/h not to exceed 200 mEq/in 24 h; K+ level <2.5 with ECG changes evident of symptomatic hypokalemia, use 40 mEq/h (with central line, continuous ECG, and lab monitoring) not to exceed 400 mEq in 24 h ! IV: Do not administer undiluted; use solution for IV infusion; infuse slowly at a rate up to 10 mEq/h

Contraindications	Drug-Lab-Food Interactions
Renal insufficiency or failure, Addison disease, hyperkalemia, severe dehydration, acidosis, potassium-sparing diuretics, in patients with known hypersensitivity *Caution:* Cardiac and renal disease, burns, hypomagnesemia, and cirrhosis	Drug: Any disease or condition in which high potassium levels may occur through potassium retention or other processes. Food: Excessive intake of licorice may cause hypokalemia and sodium retention; salt substitutes contain potassium.

Pharmacokinetics	Pharmacodynamics
Absorption: Well absorbed after oral administration Distribution: Enters extracellular fluid and is then actively transported into cells Metabolism: Excreted 80%–90% in urine by the kidneys and 10% in feces Half-life: UK Protein binding: UK	PO: Onset: UK Peak: 1–2 h Duration: UK IV: Onset: Rapid Peak: End of infusion Duration: UK

Therapeutic Effects/Uses

To correct potassium deficit and treat hypokalemic alkalosis, strengthen cardiac and muscular activities, and prevent hypokalemia in at-risk patients
Mechanism of Action: Transmits and conducts nerve impulses; contracts skeletal, smooth, and cardiac muscles

Side Effects	Adverse Reactions
Nausea, vomiting, diarrhea, abdominal cramps, irritability, rash (rare); phlebitis with IV administration	Hyperkalemia (older adults with renal impairment); oliguria, ECG changes (peaked T waves, widened QRS complex, prolonged PR interval), GI ulceration *Life-threatening:* Cardiac dysrhythmias, respiratory distress, ventricular fibrillation, cardiac arrest

A, Adult; *d,* day; *ECG,* electrocardiography; *GI,* gastrointestinal; *h,* hour; *IV,* intravenous; *max,* maximum; *PO,* by mouth; *UK,* unknown; *meq,* milliequivalent; *L,* liter; *K+,* potassium.

BOX 12.2 Hyperkalemia: Treatments and Rationales

Potassium Restriction
- Restriction of potassium intake will slowly lower the serum level.
- For mild hyperkalemia (slightly elevated K+ levels [5.4–5.6 mEq/L]), potassium restriction is normally effective.

Intravenous Sodium Bicarbonate
- Sodium bicarbonate elevates the pH level, potassium moves back into cells and lowers the serum level.
- This is a temporary treatment.

Calcium Gluconate 10%
- 10% IV solution contains 1 g Ca+ gluconate/10 mL and 90 mg (4.5 mEq) of elemental Ca+
- Decreases irritability of myocardium resulting from hyperkalemia
- A temporary treatment that does not promote K+ loss
- Caution: Administering 10% calcium gluconate to a patient on digitalis can cause digitalis toxicity.

Insulin and Glucose
- Administering insulin and glucose will move the potassium back into cells

- A temporary treatment effective for approximately 6 hours, and not always as effective when repeated.

Sodium Polystyrene Sulfonate
- Sodium polystyrene sulfonate is used to treat high levels of potassium in the blood for severe hyperkalemia; may cause hypocalcemia, hypomagnesemia, and sodium retention.
- Can be administered orally or rectally

Oral Administration
- Sodium polystyrene sulfonate: PO (adults) 15 g 1–4 times daily in water (up to 40 g 4 times daily)
- The oral route is the preferred route and is more effective than the rectal route.

Rectal Administration
- Sodium polystyrene sulfonate: (adults) 30–50 g as a retention enema; repeat as needed every 6 hours. Constipation is a common adverse effect. Assess bowel function daily and monitor for fecal impaction. A mild laxative may be prescribed.

Ca+, Calcium; *g,* grams; *h,* hour; *K+,* potassium; *PO,* by mouth; *mEq,* milliequivalent; *mg,* milligram; *mL,* millimeter.

TABLE 12.7   Drugs That Cause Hypokalemia

Substances	Rationale
Acetylsalicylic acid/acetaminophen	Causes changes in acid-base balance.
Antibiotic I: Amphotericin B; polymyxin B; gentamicin; neomycin; amikacin; tobramycin	These have a toxic effect on renal tubules and thus decrease potassium reabsorption.
Antibiotic II: Penicillin; ampicillin; carbenicillin; ticarcillin; nafcillin; piperacillin	These enhance potassium excretion by the presence of nonabsorbable anions.
Alpha-adrenergic blockers Insulin Glucose	These promote movement of potassium into cells, thus lowering the serum potassium level.
Beta$_2$ agonists: terbutaline, albuterol	These promote potassium loss.
Cardiac glycoside: digoxin	Used with caution in patients with electrolyte imbalances; can result in toxicity.
Corticosteroids	Absorption of calcium is reduced.
Cortisone	Cortisone causes electrolyte disturbances.
Dextrose intravenous (IV) solution	Can worsen hypokalemia by stimulating insulin release, which will cause intracellular shifting of potassium.
Diuretics LOOP: furosemide, torsemide THIAZIDE: hydrochlorothiazide	Diuretics deplete potassium through urination.
Laxatives Enemas (hyperosmolar)	Abuse can cause potassium depletion.
Prednisone	Steroids promote potassium loss and sodium retention.
Sodium polystyrene sulfonate enema	Exchanges a potassium ion for a sodium ion.

TABLE 12.8   Drugs That Cause Hyperkalemia

Substances	Rationale
Angiotensin-converting enzyme inhibitors (ACE inhibitors)	ACEs increase the state of hypo-aldosterone (decrease sodium and increase potassium) and impair renal potassium excretion.
Angiotensin receptor blockers (ARBs)	ARBs decrease adrenal synthesis of aldosterone; potassium is retained, and sodium is excreted.
Antifungals	Elevate serum potassium levels.
Beta-adrenergic blockers	Beta blockers decrease cellular uptake of potassium and decrease Na-K-ATPase function.
CNS agents: Barbiturates; sedatives; opioids; heroin, amphetamines	CNS substances are usually characterized by muscle necrosis and cellular shift of potassium from cells to serum.
Digoxin	The therapeutic dose is not affected; however, with overdose, potassium excess may occur.
Heparin	Heparin inhibits adrenal aldosterone production.
LMWH	LMWHs suppress aldosterone and decrease potassium homeostasis; renal excretion of potassium is reduced.
Immunosuppressive drugs: cyclosporine; tacrolimus, cyclophosphamide	Reduce potassium excretion by induction of hypo-aldosterone and loss of potassium from cells.
Nonsteroidal antiinflammatory drugs	NSAIDs impair potassium homeostasis and block cellular potassium uptake.
Potassium chloride (oral or IV); potassium salt substitutes; potassium penicillin; potassium phosphate (KPO_4) enema; potassium-sparing diuretics	Excess ingestion or infusion can cause potassium excess.
Succinylcholine	Succinylcholine allows for leakage of potassium out of the cells.
Transfusion of packed red blood cells	There is evidence that transfusion of PRBCs can lead to increased potassium levels, especially in cases of large volume transfusions

ATPase, Adenosine triphosphates; *CNS,* central nervous system; *IV,* intravenous; *K,* potassium; *LMWH,* low-molecular-weight heparin; *Na,* sodium; *NSAID,* nonsteroidal antiinflammatory drug.

of serum calcium. Calcium functions are closely related to magnesium and phosphorus. Calcium and phosphorus have an inverse relationship; that is, increased calcium levels result in decreased phosphorus levels.

Vitamin D is needed for calcium absorption from the GI tract. Aspirin and anticonvulsants can alter vitamin D, affecting calcium absorption. Loop or high-ceiling diuretics (see Chapter 38), steroids (cortisone), magnesium preparations, and phosphate preparations promote calcium loss. Conversely, thiazide diuretics increase serum calcium levels.

Hypocalcemia

Inadequate calcium intake causes calcium to leave bone to maintain a normal serum calcium level. Because of calcium loss from bones (bone demineralization), pathologic fractures may occur if calcium deficit persists. Common causes of hypocalcemia include hyperphosphatemia, acute pancreatitis, widespread bony metastases, hypoparathyroidism, alkalosis, diarrhea, alcoholism, malnutrition, use of loop diuretics, vitamin D deficiency, and multiple blood transfusions.

Signs and symptoms of hypocalcemia reflect calcium's role in nerve transmission and heart and muscle function. Neurologic and neuromuscular symptoms include anxiety, irritability, and tetany; twitching; hyperactive deep tendon reflexes; spasms of hands, wrist, feet, and ankles; spasmodic contractions; laryngeal spasm; and seizures. Cardiovascular manifestations include decreased cardiac output, dysrhythmias, and ECG changes.

⚡ Calcium preparations can be administered orally or intravenously. The treatment depends on the cause, degree of deficit, and clinical condition of the patient. IV calcium replacement should be administered only to acutely symptomatic patients. Calcium preparations are combined with various salts such as chloride, carbonate, citrate, and gluconate. The two main forms of oral calcium supplements are calcium carbonate, which contains 40% elemental calcium, and calcium citrate, which contains 21% elemental calcium. There is a threefold difference in the primary cation between calcium gluconate,

PROTOTYPE DRUG CHART

⚡ *Calcium*

Drug Class	Dosage
Electrolyte Calcium carbonate (chewable) Calcium citrate (capsule/tablet) Calcium gluconate (IV) Calcium chloride (IV) ⚡ IV form is a high-alert drug.	Calcium carbonate: 250 mg/400 mg/500 mg/750 mg in 1–3 divided doses Calcium citrate: 200 mg/d to 1 g/d divided doses Calcium gluconate: 1-2 g IV q6h (**Note:** 500 mg calcium gluconate is equal to 45 mg [2.25 mEq] elemental calcium) Calcium chloride IV: 1000 mg over 10 min; repeat every 60 min until s/s resolved; 1 g is equal to 270 mg of elemental calcium

Contraindications	Drug-Lab-Food Interactions
Hypercalcemia, patients receiving digitalis glycosides and patients with renal calculi, severe respiratory insufficiency, and cardiac disease	Drug: Increased risk of digoxin toxicity with calcium channel blockers, tetracyclines, fluoroquinolones, phenytoin, iron salts, thiazides, sodium polystyrene sulfonate Food: Cereals, spinach, rhubarb Lab: May affect serum calcium or ionized calcium, sodium, potassium, magnesium, albumin, and parathyroid hormone.

Pharmacokinetics	Pharmacodynamics
Absorption: From GI tract, requires vitamin D Distribution: Readily enters ECF Metabolism and excretion: Excreted mostly in the feces; 20% eliminated by the kidneys Half-life: UK	PO: Onset: UK Peak: UK Duration: UK IV: Onset: Immediate Peak: Immediate Duration: 0.5–2 h

⚡ Safety alert from the Institute for Safe Medication Practices: Errors with IV calcium gluconate (CaGl) and calcium chloride (CaCl) have occurred secondary to confusion over which salt is ordered. Clarify incomplete orders. Confusion has occurred with milligram doses of CaCl and CaGl, which are not equal. Calcium chloride and calcium gluconate IV forms are routinely available on most hospital crash carts; physicians should specify the form of calcium desired, and doses should be expressed in milliequivalents.

Therapeutic Effects/Uses

To correct calcium deficit or tetany symptoms, prevent osteoporosis.
Mechanism of Action: Transmits nerve impulses, contracts skeletal and cardiac muscles, maintains cellular permeability, and promotes strong bones and teeth

Side Effects	Adverse Reactions
PO: Nausea, vomiting, constipation, pain, drowsiness, headache, muscle weakness	Hypercalcemia, ECG changes, metabolic alkalosis, heart block, rebound hyperacidity *Life-threatening:* Renal failure, cardiac dysrhythmias, cardiac arrest

A, Adult; *d*, day; *ECF*, extracellular fluid; *ECG*, electrocardiogram; *GI*, gastrointestinal; *g*, gram; *h*, hour; IV, intravenous; *mg*, milligram; *mEq*, milliequivalent; *PO*, by mouth; *s/s*, signs and symptoms; *UK*, unknown.

which contains 4.65 mEq Ca⁺⁺/gram, and calcium chloride, which contains 13.6 mEq Ca⁺⁺/gram. When ordering IV calcium, this difference has important implications. Calcium chloride is more irritating when given intravenously. Both calcium chloride 10% (CaCl) and calcium gluconate 10% (CaGl) can be used for acute hypocalcemia and during cardiac resuscitation. Calcium gluconate has the same action on the heart as digitalis; it increases the force of systolic contractions. Prototype Drug Chart: Calcium describes the pharmacokinetics and pharmacodynamics of calcium preparations.

The patient's renal functioning should be assessed before administering IV calcium chloride; this solution contains aluminum, which can be toxic if renal insufficiency exists. IV calcium should be administered cautiously in patients who take digitalis because an increase in serum calcium increases the risk of digitalis toxicity. Calcium chloride 10% solution should be administered slowly via an infusion control pump, and the patient should be monitored frequently. Care should be taken

to prevent extravasation; local extravasation may cause tissue necrosis and sloughing. Refer to the agency's policy if infiltration occurs. Too rapid an infusion may cause cardiac syncope and decreased blood pressure from peripheral vasodilation. Oral calcium preparations are available in tablets, capsules, gelcaps, and powders.

Patients with hypocalcemia should be assessed for hypomagnesemia, hypokalemia, and acid-base imbalances, and any abnormalities should be corrected. Hypomagnesemia should be corrected first; low magnesium levels may prevent the patient from responding to treatment for hypocalcemia.

Pharmacokinetics. Vitamin D promotes calcium absorption from the GI tract; phosphorus inhibits calcium absorption. The pH affects the amount of ionized calcium. When pH is decreased (acidic), there is more free ionized calcium because it has been released from protein-binding sites. With an increased pH (alkalosis), more calcium is bound to protein.

◎ CLINICAL JUDGMENT [NURSING PROCESS]

Calcium

Concept: Fluid and Electrolyte Balance

- Patients require the regulation of fluid and electrolytes to maintain homeostasis. Nurses will encounter potential and actual alterations of fluid and electrolyte balance when caring for patients. Nursing assessments and interventions ensure the intake of fluid and electrolytes remains balanced by closely monitoring the patient's intake and output and careful assessment of laboratory values.

Recognize Cues [Assessment]

- Assess the patient for signs and symptoms of calcium imbalance. Signs and symptoms of *hypocalcemia* are tetany, muscle cramps, bleeding tendencies, and cardiac contractions. Signs and symptoms of *hypercalcemia* are flabby muscles, pain over bony areas, and kidney stones of calcium composition.
- Check serum calcium levels; a normal total calcium level is 8.6 to 10.2 mg/dL. Report abnormal test results.
- Assess albumin levels; a normal albumin level is 3.4 to 5.4 g/dL. Low levels of albumin decrease total calcium levels.
- Obtain baseline vital signs and electrocardiogram (ECG) readings. Report abnormal findings.
- ⚠️ Gather a current patient drug history. If the patient is receiving digoxin, calcium enhances the effect of digoxin. An elevated serum calcium level can cause digitalis toxicity, signs and symptoms of which include nausea, vomiting, anorexia, bradycardia (pulse rate <60 or markedly decreased), cardiac dysrhythmias, and visual disturbances. Thiazide diuretics can increase serum calcium levels. Drugs that decrease the effect of calcium are calcium channel blockers, tetracycline, and sodium chloride.

Analyze Cues and Prioritize Hypothesis [Patient Problems]

- Weight loss
- Decreased sensation in upper extremities
- Reduction in motor function
- Hypercalcemia

Generate Solutions [Planning]

- The patient's serum calcium level remains within normal range.
- Tetany symptoms will cease.
- The patient will eat calcium-rich foods or take calcium supplements as ordered.
- Patients with hypercalcemia will avoid calcium-rich foods.

Take Action [Nursing Interventions]

- Monitor vital signs and report abnormal findings. Compare with baseline vital signs.
- Assess patients on digitalis for digitalis toxicity (e.g. bradycardia).
- Administer IVFs slowly with 10% calcium gluconate or chloride. The pharmacist will add or decrease calcium to the solutions as ordered by the provider

and will dilute in compatible solutions (e.g., normal saline [NS], 5% dextrose in water [D_5W], 10% dextrose in water [$D_{10}W$]).

- ⚡ Assess the IV site for infiltration. Calcium can cause tissue necrosis and sloughing if it infiltrates into subcutaneous tissue. Concentrations of calcium chloride (CaCl) of 20 mg/mL are usually recommended for central lines; concentrations of no more than 1 mg/mL given over 10 minutes have been recommended for peripheral lines.
- Monitor serum total calcium and ionized calcium levels.
- Monitor ECGs. In hypocalcemia, the ST segment is lengthened, and the QT interval is prolonged. In hypercalcemia, the ST segment is decreased, and the QT interval is shortened.
- If a language barrier exists, use an interpreter if appropriate.
- Involve the extended family in health teaching and support.

Patient Teaching
General

- Instruct patients to avoid overuse of antacids and chronic use of laxatives. Overuse of certain antacids may cause alkalosis, decreasing calcium ionization. Chronic use of laxatives decreases calcium absorption from the gastrointestinal (GI) tract. Suggest high-fiber foods for improving bowel elimination.
- Encourage patients taking calcium supplements to check with the pharmacist to ensure that the calcium tablet is absorbable.
- Advise patients to take oral calcium supplements with meals or after meals to increase absorption.
- Instruct patients to report symptoms of hypercalcemia, including muscle weakness and pain over bony areas. Remind patients to report any chest pain or urinary problems because calcium can cause ECG changes and renal stones.
- Instruct patients to report symptoms of hypocalcemia, including neuromuscular signs such as numbness, tingling sensations in fingers and toes, and muscle cramps. Wheezing may develop from bronchospasm, dysphagia, voice changes, fatigue, and seizures.

Diet

- Instruct the patient to consume high-calcium foods such as milk and dairy products.
- Remind the patient that foods rich in protein and vitamin D enhance calcium absorption.

Evaluate Outcomes [Evaluation]

- Evaluate the patient's serum calcium and electrolyte levels. Report if the calcium imbalance continues.
- Monitor patients for neuromuscular and cardiac manifestations of calcium imbalance.

Hypercalcemia

Elevated serum calcium may be a result of hyperparathyroidism, malignancy, hypophosphatemia, excessive calcium intake, prolonged immobilization, multiple fractures, drugs such as thiazide diuretics, and steroids. Signs and symptoms of hypercalcemia are fatigue, muscle weakness, depressed deep tendon reflexes, confusion, impaired memory, anorexia, nausea, vomiting, constipation, and kidney stones of calcium composition. The patient may experience ECG changes and exhibit decreased heart rate and dysrhythmias.

Effect of Drugs on Calcium Balance

Phosphate preparations, corticosteroids, loop diuretics, aspirin, anticonvulsants, magnesium sulfate, and plicamycin (an antineoplastic antibiotic) are

a few of the drugs that can lower serum calcium levels. Excess calcium salt ingestion or infusion and thiazide diuretics can all contribute to an increased serum calcium level. Table 12.9 lists some drugs that affect calcium balance.

Clinical Management of Calcium Imbalance

Clinical management of hypocalcemia consists of oral supplements and IV calcium. Table 12.10 lists oral and IV preparations of calcium salts, their dosages, and drug forms. Calcium carbonate can cause GI upset because it produces carbon dioxide. For better calcium absorption, calcium supplements should contain vitamin D, and oral calcium should be taken 30 minutes before meals.

The goal for managing hypercalcemia is to correct the underlying cause of serum calcium excess. IV saline solution and drugs such as

TABLE 12.9 Drugs Affecting Calcium Balance

Substances	Rationale
Drugs That Cause Hypocalcemia	
Bisphosphonates	Used in the treatment of osteoporosis. Prevents bones from leaking calcium, which means less calcium in the bloodstream.
Cinacalcet	Used to decrease parathyroid hormone levels in chronic kidney disease and decrease risk of kidney stones. Decreases calcium levels.
Cisplatin	Chemo medication used to treat cancer. Known to cause low blood calcium levels.
Corticosteroids and mineralocorticoids	Decreases calcium mobilization and inhibits calcium absorption.
Denosumab	A human monoclonal antibody used in the treatment of osteoporosis. Decreases blood calcium levels.
Diuretics: loop	Decreases calcium mobilization and inhibits calcium absorption decreasing calcium.
Estrogen	Can alter vitamin D metabolism needed for calcium absorption decreasing calcium.
Magnesium sulfate	Inhibits parathyroid hormone secretion and decreases serum calcium level
Phenytoin	Decreases vitamin D levels that decrease calcium absorption and lowers calcium levels.
Phosphate preparations: oral, enema, intravenous; sodium phosphate, potassium phosphate	Can increase serum phosphorus level and decrease serum calcium level.
Drugs That Cause Hypercalcemia	
Aminoglycosides	
Calcium acetate Calcium carbonate Calcium salts Vitamin D (calcitriol)	Excess ingestion of calcium and vitamin D and infusion of calcium can increase serum calcium level.
Intravenous fat emulsion	Can increase serum calcium level.
Diuretics: thiazides (chlorthalidone)	Can induce hypercalcemia by preventing calcium release in the urine. Can lead to kidney stones.
Lithium	Increases parathyroid hormone secretion.

TABLE 12.10 Calcium Oral Preparations

Calcium Name	Drug Form	Drug Dose
Calcium carbonate	Chewable	250 mg/400 mg/500 mg/750 mg
Calcium citrate	Caplet Tablet	200 mg/950 mg
Calcium gluconate	Tablet	500 mg

TABLE 12.11 Drugs That Affect Magnesium Balance

Drugs	Rationale
Drugs That Cause Hypomagnesemia	
Diuretics: loop and thiazide	Promote urinary loss of magnesium
Antibiotics: gentamicin, tobramycin, aminoglycosides, amphotericin B	Can cause magnesium loss via kidneys
Laxatives, cisplatin	Abuse can cause magnesium loss via the gastrointestinal tract
Drugs That Cause Hypermagnesemia	
Magnesium salts (oral and enema); magnesium hydroxide; magnesium sulfate; magnesium citrate	Excessive use can increase serum magnesium level. Use of excessive magnesium sulfate in treatment of toxemia can cause hypermagnesemia

calcitonin and loop diuretics can be used to promote rapid urinary excretion of calcium.

⚡ Magnesium

Magnesium is most plentiful in the ICF, and it plays a role in maintaining normal calcium and potassium balance. Magnesium deficit often occurs with hypokalemia and hypocalcemia. The normal serum magnesium level is 1.5 to 2.5 mEq/L. Magnesium deficit is called hypomagnesemia, and magnesium excess is called hypermagnesemia. The daily magnesium requirement is 8 to 20 mEq/day.

Functions

Magnesium promotes transmission of neuromuscular activity and is an important mediator of neural transmission in the CNS. Alterations in serum magnesium levels profoundly affect neuromuscular excitability and contractility. Like potassium, magnesium promotes contraction of the myocardium. Magnesium activates many enzymes for metabolism of carbohydrates and protein and is responsible for transportation of sodium and potassium across cell membranes.

Serum magnesium deficit increases the release of acetylcholine from the presynaptic membrane of the nerve fiber, which increases neuromuscular excitability. Serum magnesium excess has a sedative effect on the neuromuscular system, which can result in loss of deep tendon reflexes. Cardiac (ventricular) dysrhythmias, hypotension, and heart block can occur because of hypomagnesemia.

Hypomagnesemia is probably the most undiagnosed electrolyte deficiency. This is most likely because it is asymptomatic until the serum magnesium level approaches 1 mEq/L. To correct severe hypomagnesemia, IV magnesium sulfate is usually given. For hypermagnesemia, calcium gluconate may be given to decrease the serum magnesium level.

Causes of Magnesium Imbalance

Prolonged parenteral nutrition without magnesium supplements can decrease magnesium levels. Also, diuretics, certain antibiotics, laxatives, and steroids are drug groups that promote magnesium loss. Like hypokalemia, hypomagnesemia enhances the action of digitalis and can cause digitalis toxicity. Chronic alcoholism, prolonged fasting, starvation, or increased renal losses can promote hypomagnesemia.

Magnesium sulfate corrects hypomagnesemia and symptoms of digitalis toxicity. It is common practice after bypass surgery or myocardial infarction for patients to be given magnesium sulfate orally, even when blood levels are normal, to prevent ventricular arrhythmias in the perioperative period.

Excess intake of magnesium salts is the major cause of serum magnesium excess. Commonly used medications that may cause hypermagnesemia include laxatives and antacids. A patient with chronic kidney disease who ingests products that contain magnesium will have a problem with excess magnesium. Patient teaching regarding prolonged or frequent use of laxatives, particularly in older adults, is an important intervention in preventing electrolyte imbalance. Table 12.11 lists some drugs that affect magnesium balance.

◎ CLINICAL JUDGMENT [NURSING PROCESS]

Magnesium

Concept: Fluid and Electrolyte Balance

- Patients require the regulation of fluid and electrolytes to maintain homeostasis. Nurses will encounter potential and actual alterations of fluid and electrolyte balance when caring for patients. Nursing assessments and interventions ensure the intake of fluid and electrolytes remains balanced by closely monitoring the patient's intake and output and careful assessment of laboratory values.

Recognize Cues [Assessment]

- Assess the patient for signs and symptoms of magnesium imbalance. Signs and symptoms of *hypomagnesemia* are tetany-like symptoms caused by hyperexcitability (tremors, twitching of the face) and ventricular tachycardia that leads to ventricular fibrillation and hypertension. Signs and symptoms of *hypermagnesemia* are lethargy, drowsiness, weakness and paralysis, loss of deep tendon reflexes, hypotension, and heart block.
- Check serum magnesium levels for magnesium imbalance. Symptoms of magnesium deficiency may not be seen until the serum level is below 1 mEq/L.
- ⚡ Observe patients taking digitalis preparations for digitalis toxicity. Like potassium deficit, magnesium deficit enhances the action of digitalis, causing digitalis toxicity.

Analyze Cues and Prioritize Hypothesis [Patient Problems]

- Dysrhythmias
- Hypomagnesemia
- Hypermagnesemia

Generate Solutions [Planning]

- The patient's serum magnesium level is within normal range (1.5 to 2.5 mEq/L).
- The patient will not experience life-threatening symptoms of magnesium imbalance such as central nervous symptoms (confusion, coma) and cardiac dysrhythmias (premature ventricular contractions and ventricular fibrillation).

Take Action [Nursing Interventions]

- Communicate to the health care provider (HCP) if a patient is ordered nothing by mouth (NPO) and is receiving intravenous fluids (IVFs) without magnesium salts for a prolonged period.

- Monitor urinary output. Most of the body's magnesium is excreted by the kidneys. Report if urine output falls below 600 mL/day.
- ⚡ Monitor for digitalis toxicity (e.g., nausea, vomiting, bradycardia) in patients who have hypomagnesemia and are taking digoxin. Magnesium deficit enhances the action of digitalis preparations.
- Monitor vital signs and compare with baseline values. Report abnormal findings to the health care provider.
- Monitor serum electrolyte results. Report low serum potassium or calcium levels because low serum magnesium levels may be attributed to hypokalemia or hypocalcemia. When correcting a potassium deficit, potassium is not replaced in cells until magnesium is replaced. ⚡ A serum magnesium level of 1 mEq/L or less can cause cardiac arrest.
- Prepare for emergency reversal of hypomagnesemia deficit by having available intravenous (IV) calcium gluconate.
- Use an interpreter as needed.
- Involve the extended family in health teaching and support.

Patient Teaching

- Advise patients with hypomagnesemia to eat foods rich in magnesium (green vegetables, fruits, fish, grains, and nuts).
- Instruct patients with hypermagnesemia to avoid routine use of laxatives and antacids that contain magnesium. Suggest that patients check drug labels and speak with a pharmacist.
- Instruct patients on signs and symptoms of hypomagnesemia and hypermagnesemia.

Evaluate Outcomes [Evaluation]

- Evaluate the patient's serum magnesium level. Report if the magnesium imbalance continues.
- Have the patient verbalize the signs and symptoms of hypomagnesemia and hypermagnesemia, and instruct them to report these to their health care provider.

Chloride

Chloride is the principal anion of ECF. The chloride ion is a major contributor to acid-base balance, gastric juice acidity, and the osmolality of ECF. A normal serum chloride level is 96 to 106 mEq/L. Hypochloremia is a decreased serum chloride level, and hyperchloremia is an elevated level. With increased serum osmolality (>300 mOsm per kg of water), there are more sodium and chloride ions proportional to the water. Sodium and chloride frequently work in combination. For example, during sodium retention, chloride is also frequently retained, resulting in increased water retention. Clinical manifestations of hypochloremia include tremors, twitching, and slow, shallow breathing. With severe chloride loss, decreased blood pressure is seen. Clinical manifestations of hyperchloremia include weakness; lethargy; deep, rapid breathing; and eventual unconsciousness.

Phosphorus

Phosphorus is the primary anion in ICF and is the second most abundant element in the body. The majority of the body's phosphorus is found as phosphate; therefore these two terms are used interchangeably.

Both phosphorus and calcium levels are regulated by PTH and need vitamin D for absorption from the GI tract. A reciprocal relationship exists between phosphorus and calcium. High serum phosphate levels cause low calcium levels; low calcium levels stimulate the release of PTH, which decreases reabsorption of phosphorus.

A normal serum phosphorus level is 2.4 to 4.4 mEq/L. Regulation of phosphate balance requires adequate renal functioning because the kidneys are the major route of phosphate excretion.

Phosphorus is essential in bone and teeth formation and for neuromuscular activity. Phosphorus is an important component of nucleic acids (DNA and RNA) and assists in energy transfer in cells, helps maintain cellular osmotic pressure, and supports the acid-base balance of body fluids. Clinical manifestations of hypophosphatemia include muscle weakness, tremors, paresthesia, bone pain, hyporeflexia, seizures, hyperventilation, anorexia, and dysphagia. Symptoms of hyperphosphatemia are like those of hypocalcemia and include hyperreflexia, tetany, flaccid paralysis, muscular weakness, tachycardia, nausea, diarrhea, and abdominal cramps. Phosphorus-rich foods include whole-grain cereals, nuts, milk, and meat. Phosphorus deficiency can result from decreased intestinal absorption, malnutrition, alcoholism, vomiting, diarrhea, use of concentrated glucose solutions, respiratory alkalosis, glycosuria, hypokalemia, hypomagnesemia, or use of thiazide diuretics. Hypophosphatemia may lead to hemolytic anemia, platelet dysfunction, and reduced oxygen transport. Hyperphosphatemia is most often related to chronic kidney disease. Increased intake in the form of laxatives may also increase serum levels.

! Treatment of phosphorus imbalance is aimed at eliminating or reducing the cause. Monitoring phosphorus, calcium, and magnesium levels and assessing the patient for signs of electrolyte and acid-base imbalance are important nursing interventions. Phosphorus replacement is guided by the degree of deficit, onset, and patient presentation. Oral intake is the preferred route of replacement. IV phosphorus is available for treatment of patients who are unable to tolerate oral replacements or those with severe deficits. **⚡**

Potassium phosphate is an Institute for Safe Medication Practices (ISMP) high-alert medication used for IV phosphorus replacement. Potassium phosphate must be diluted before use and must be infused slowly using an infusion control pump. Too rapid an infusion may cause potassium toxicity in patients with severe renal or adrenal insufficiency. The IV insertion site must be monitored for infiltration; potassium phosphate may cause tissue necrosis and sloughing if infiltration occurs. Phosphorus, potassium, and calcium levels and renal function should be monitored during and after infusion. Use of potassium phosphate is contraindicated in patients with hyperkalemia or hypocalcemia.

Hyperphosphatemia in patients with chronic kidney disease is treated with restriction of dietary phosphorus, phosphorus-binding medications such as calcium acetate, or dialysis. Hyperphosphatemia can lead to secondary hyperparathyroidism and osteodystrophy.

CRITICAL THINKING UNFOLDING CASE STUDY

Cognitive Skill: Recognize cues (enhanced hot spot)

Question 1:
A 70-year-old active male is admitted to the emergency department from home. The patient's wife tells the nurse he appears to have gained weight (normal weight is 175) and is feeling short of breath (SOB). His vitals are taken and a complete physical assessment is performed. His medication profile includes 25 mg thiazide daily. His wife indicates he has refused to take his prescribed medication because it makes him tired. The nurse documents the following assessment findings.

- Blood pressure 180/90 and heart rate of 100 bpm
- Pain rated 1 on a scale of 0–10
- Tachypnea (28 breaths per minute [bpm])
- Bilateral crackles base of lungs
- Patient reports tiredness and fatigue
- Bowel sounds present x4
- Bilateral pedal edema +3
- Oriented to person, place, and time
- Weight gain of 10 lbs (185 lbs)
- Oxygen saturation 96% (room air)

Highlight or place a check mark next to the assessment findings that require follow-up by the nurse.

Answers:
Blood pressure 180/90 and heart rate of 100 bpm
- Tachypnea (28 bpm)
- Bilateral crackles base of lungs
- Patient reports tiredness and fatigue
- Bilateral pedal edema +3
- Weight gain of 10 lbs (185 lbs)
- Oxygen saturation 96% (room air)

Rationale:
The previous signs are indicative of a patient with fluid overload. The patient stopped taking his prescribed diuretic. This caused increased bodily fluids to build up in his body. This results in an excessive amount of fluid circulating around the heart and lungs. Increased bodily fluids can cause weight gain, increased blood pressure, and increased heart rate. As fluid enters the lungs, the

patient can develop crackles at the lung base, increased respiratory rate, shortness of breath, and decreased oxygen saturation as they struggle to breathe. The most consistent sign of fluid overload is increased body weight.

Reference:
Lewis, et al, Medical Surgical Nursing, 10th ed, pgs 270-299, Fluid & Electrolyte Imbalances.
McCuistion: Ch 12 pgs 133-149 and Clinical Judgment [Nursing Process] care plan (see) Fluid Volume Excess, McCuistion: pgs. 137-138.

Cognitive Skill: Analyze cues (cloze).

Question 2:
A 70-year-old active male is admitted to the emergency department from home. The patient's wife tells the nurse he appears to have gained weight (normal weight is 175) and is feeling short of breath (SOB). His vitals are taken, and a complete physical assessment is performed. His medication profile includes 25 mg thiazide daily. His wife indicates he has refused to take his prescribed medication because it makes him tired. The nurse documents the following assessment findings.

- Blood pressure 180/90 mm Hg and heart rate of 100 bpm
- Pain rated 1 on a scale of 0–10
- Tachypnea (28 bpm)
- Bilateral crackles base of lungs
- Patient reports tiredness and fatigue
- Bowel sounds present ×4
- Bilateral pedal edema +3
- Oriented to person, place, and time
- Weight gain of 10 lbs (185 lbs)
- Oxygen saturation 96% (room air)

Choose the most likely information missing from the statements below by selecting the information from the list of options provided.

Based on the patient's assessment data, the nurse determines that the patient's vital sign findings are due to _____(1)_____. Bilateral crackles at the base of the lungs and oxygen saturation of 96% indicate the need for _____(2)_____. The provider orders the following blood tests to evaluate the patient's health status: _____(3)_____, _____(3)_____, and _____(3)_____.

Continued

CRITICAL THINKING UNFOLDING CASE STUDY—CONT'D

Option 1	Option 2	Option 3
a. Bradycardia	a. Chest x-ray	a. Complete blood count
b. Respiratory failure	b. Fasting blood glucose	b. Urine specific gravity
c. COVID-19	c. Kidney function test	c. Basic metabolic panel
d. Fluid volume excess	d. CPAP	d. Lipid panel
e. Fluid volume deficit	e. Oxygen at 8L/NC	c. Hepatitis level
f. Weight loss	f. Barium swallow test	d. Calcium level

Answers:
Based on the patient's assessment data, it is determined that the patient's vital sign findings are due to Fluid volume excess (d). Bilateral crackles at the base of the lungs and oxygen saturation of 96% indicate the need for chest x-ray (a). The following blood tests are ordered to evaluate the patient's health status: complete blood count (a), basic metabolic panel (c), and urine specific gravity level (b).

Rationale:
Excess body fluids can dilute (and lower) the hemoglobin and hematocrit levels found in the complete blood count. Excess body fluids can dilute (and lower) the potassium and sodium levels found in the basic metabolic panel. Fluid excess can dilute (and lower) the urine specific gravity levels as well. These tests can help identify the patient's problem of fluid volume excess. When a patient has bilateral crackles at the base of the lungs and an oxygen saturation of 96% (room air), and is experiencing tachypnea with a rate of 28 bpm, standard protocol is for the provider to order a chest x-ray. This will indicate if there is fluid in the patient's lungs from fluid overload.

Reference:
Lewis, et al, Medical Surgical Nursing, 10th ed, pgs 270-299, Fluid & Electrolyte Imbalances. McCuistion: CH 12 pgs 133-149 and Clinical Judgment [Nursing Process] care plan (see) Fluid Volume Excess, McCuistion: pgs. 137-138.

Cognitive Skill: Prioritize hypothesis (extended multiple response).

Question 3:
The health care provider admits a 70-year-old active patient to the telemetry unit for monitoring. The patient has a weight gain of 10 pounds with bilateral crackles at the base of the lungs. The provider orders oxygen 2 L NC and the patient's oxygen saturation has increased to 99%, and he is resting comfortably.
   Circle or place a check mark next to the serum lab result that supports the diagnosis of fluid volume overload.
a. Urine specific gravity 1.000 g/mL
b. Hemoglobin 15.5 gd/L
c. Hematocrit 30.5%
d. Potassium 3.2 mEq/L
e. Sodium 120.0 mEq/L
f. Chloride (blood) 85 mEq/L
g. Calcium (total) 9.0 mg/dL
h. Platelet 200,000/μL
i. Creatinine (blood) 0.8 mg/dL
j. Total red blood count $5.0 \times 10^6/\mu L$

Answers:

a. Urine specific gravity 1.000 g/mL	✓
b. Hemoglobin 15.5 gd/L	
c. Hematocrit 30.5%	✓
d. Potassium 3.2 mEq/L	✓
e. Sodium 120.0 mEq/L	✓
f. Chloride (blood) 85 mEq/L	✓
g. Calcium (total) 9.0 mg/dL	
h. Platelet 200,000/μL	
i. Creatinine (blood) 0.8 mg/dL	
j. Total red blood count $5.0 \times 10^6/\mu L$	

Rationale:
Increased body fluids will dilute (and lower) the hemoglobin and hematocrit (normal range: 42%–52%) (complete blood count) as well as the potassium (normal range 3.5–5.0 mEq/L), sodium (normal range: 135–145 mEq/L), and chloride (normal range 96–106 mEq/L) (basic metabolic panel) in the patient's body. It can also dilute (and lower) the urine specific gravity (normal range: 1.005–1.030 g/mL). This can help identify the patient's fluid volume excess.

Reference:
McCuistion: Ch 12, pgs 133-149 and Clinical Judgment [Nursing Process] care plan (see) Fluid Volume Excess, McCuistion: pgs. 137-138. Lewis, Sharon, et al, (2017) Medical Surgical Nursing (10th ed) Appendix C. (CH 16)

Cognitive Skill: Generate solutions (drag & drop)

Question 4:
The health care provider admits a 70-year-old active patient to the telemetry unit for monitoring. The patient has a weight gain of 10 pounds with bilateral crackles at the base of the lungs. The provider orders oxygen 2 L NC, and the patient's oxygen saturation has increased to 99% and he is resting comfortably. In addition, the provider has changed his medication from 25 mg of thiazide to furosemide 20 mg and has added potassium 20 mEq daily.
   Indicate which patient teaching is appropriate by placing the appropriate response in the column to the far right.

Nurse's Teaching	Patient Question	Which teaching response is appropriate for each patient question?
1. While in the hospital your provider has placed you on fluid restriction of 1000 mL/day. You must record your intake and output daily.	"I will forget. Can you show me how to record?"	
2. The provider has placed you on a low-sodium diet.	"What is a low-sodium diet?"	

CRITICAL THINKING UNFOLDING CASE STUDY—CONT'D

Nurse's Teaching	Patient Question	Which teaching response is appropriate for each patient question?
3. You must weigh yourself every day and notify your provider for a weight gain >3 lbs in 2 days.	"Why every day?"	
4. Your provider has stopped thiazide 25 mg and has started you on furosemide 20 mg/d and potassium 20 mEq/d.	"Why have my medications been changed?"	
5. Do not add extra salt to your food and make low-sodium choices.		
6. Use this list to record your fluid intake (remember 237 mL = 1 cup). This container is used to measure your urine output daily. Record the output on this list.		
7. Furosemide is a loop diuretic. It will decrease the amount of fluid in your body and lower your blood pressure. It also depletes the level of potassium (K+) in your blood so a K+ supplement is necessary. You must take this medication as prescribed by the provider.		
8. If a weight gain occurs, it is important to notify your provider immediately to avoid fluid volume overload.		

Answers:

Nurse's Teaching	Patient Question	Which teaching response is appropriate for each patient question?
1. While in the hospital your provider has placed you on fluid restriction of 1000 mL/day. You must record your intake and output daily.	"I will forget. Can you show me how to record?"	6. Use this list to record your fluid intake (remember 237 mL = 1 cup). This container is used to measure your urine output daily. Record the output on this list.
2. The provider has placed you on a low-sodium diet.	"What is a low-sodium diet?"	5. Do not add extra salt to your food and make low-sodium choices.

Nurse's Teaching	Patient Question	Which teaching response is appropriate for each patient question?
3. You must weigh yourself every day and notify your provider for a weight gain >3 lbs in 2 days.	"Why every day?"	8. If a weight gain occurs, it is important to notify your provider immediately to avoid fluid volume overload.
4. Your provider has stopped thiazide 25 mg and has started you on furosemide 20 mg/d and potassium 20 mEq/d.	"Why have my medications been changed?"	7. Furosemide is a loop diuretic. It will decrease the amount of fluid in your body and lower your blood pressure. It also depletes the level of potassium (K+) in your blood so a K+ supplement is necessary. You must take this medication as prescribed by the provider.

Rationale:
These questions are important for the nurse to validate the patient's understanding of care for fluid volume excess. Intake and output records provide valuable information about fluid and electrolyte problems. They reveal sources of excess fluid intake and/or fluid losses. Sodium is an essential mineral important to fluid and electrolyte balance and blood pressure maintenance. Limiting sodium through a low-sodium diet will prevent the buildup of excessive fluid in the body. Daily weigh-ins serve as the most authentic measure of volume status. If a weight gain occurs of greater than 3 lbs in 2 days, it is necessary to notify the provider immediately to avoid hospitalization. Furosemide is a loop diuretic that decreases the amount of fluid buildup in the body. It can also deplete potassium supply, which is why the doctor ordered a potassium supplement.

Reference:
Lewis, et al, Medical Surgical Nursing, (10th ed) pgs 270-299, Fluid & Electrolyte Imbalances. McCuistion: Ch 12, pgs 133-149 and Clinical Judgment [Nursing Process] care plan (see) Fluid Volume Excess, McCuistion: pgs. 137-138. McCuistion: Ch 38, pgs 501-511.

Cognitive Skill: Take action (extended multiple response).

Question 5:
This 70-year-old male patient is resting comfortably. His oxygen saturation on room air is 99%. His blood pressure is 140/80 mm Hg and heart rate 60 bpm. On auscultation his lungs are bilaterally clear. The nurse is preparing the patient for possible morning discharge. More patient instruction is needed concerning the low-sodium diet. When presented with this list, the patient is asked to check off the best food choices for a low-sodium diet.

Circle or place a check mark next to the best low sodium food choice. Select all that apply.
a. Canned vegetables
b. Fresh fruit
c. Sausage and deli meats
d. Sodium free herbs and spices
e. Frozen vegetables (nothing added)
f. Canned meat or fish
h. Frozen dinners
i. Broiled chicken and meats (plain)

Continued

CRITICAL THINKING UNFOLDING CASE STUDY—CONT'D

j. Breaded meats

Answers:

a. Canned vegetables	
b. Fresh fruit	✓
c. Sausage and deli meats	
d. Sodium free herbs and spices	✓
e. Frozen vegetables (nothing added)	✓
f. Canned meat or fish	
h. Frozen dinners	
i. Broiled chicken and meats (plain)	✓
j. Breaded meats	

Rationale:

The nurse is validating that the patient understands what is contained in a low-sodium diet. Sodium is an essential mineral important to fluid and electrolyte balance and blood pressure maintenance. Limiting sodium intake through a low-sodium diet will prevent the buildup of excessive fluid in the body.

Reference:

Lewis, et al, Medical Surgical Nursing, (10th ed) pgs 270-299, Fluid & Electrolyte Imbalances. McCuistion: Ch 12, pgs 133-149 and Clinical Judgment [Nursing Process] care plan (see) Fluid Volume Excess, McCuistion: pgs. 137-138; also, McCuistion, Ch 41.

Cognitive Skill: Evaluate outcomes (matrix).

Question 6:

After the patient experiences a stable and restful night, the nurse performs a careful morning assessment for possible discharge. The assessment includes information for a health teaching plan for this patient prior to discharge.

For each assessment finding, use an X to indicate whether the nurse's teaching was "Effective" (helped to meet expected outcomes), "Ineffective" (did not help to meet expected outcomes), or "Unrelated" (not related to the expected outcomes).

Assessment Finding	Effective	Ineffective	Unrelated
The patient's lungs are clear (bilaterally), no SOB, oxygen saturation is 100% on room air.			
Patient states, "I will weigh each morning and call the health care provider if I gain more than 3 pounds in 2 days."			
Patient's vital signs are 120/80 mm Hg, pulse 60, weight 175 lb.			
Patient states, "I cannot wait to get home to have bacon and ham with my morning breakfast."			

Assessment Finding	Effective	Ineffective	Unrelated
Patientt states, "My provider says I should exercise by walking. Should I walk in the morning or the evening with my neighborhood friends?"			
Patient states, "I will take my medication as ordered by my provider every morning."			

Answers:

Assessment Finding	Effective	Ineffective	Unrelated
The patient's lungs are clear (bilaterally), no SOB, oxygen saturation is 100% on room air.	X		
Patient states, "I will weigh each morning and call the health care provider if I gain more than 3 pounds in 2 days."	X		
Patient's vital signs are 120/80 mm Hg, pulse 60, weight 175 lbs.	X		
Patient states, "I cannot wait to get home to have bacon and ham with my morning breakfast."		X	
Patient states, "My provider says I should exercise by walking. Should I walk in the morning or the evening with my neighborhood friends?"			X
Patient states, "I will take my medication as ordered by my provider every morning."	X		

Rationale:

The nurse evaluates the patient's expected outcomes to validate their effectiveness prior to discharge. The patient's lungs are clear (bilaterally), no SOB, oxygen saturation is 100% (effective). The patient validates knowledge of importance of daily weigh-ins (effective). The patient's vital signs are within normal range and weight has returned to normal (effective). The patient validates taking his medications as ordered by the provider (effective). The nurse will document the effectiveness of these expected outcomes in the nursing notes. When the patient expresses his desire to eat bacon and ham with breakfast, this is an ineffective outcome. The nurse must provide more teaching on making better low-sodium choices. After additional teaching, the nurse will document the outcome in the nursing notes. It is good that the provider has given permission for the patient to exercise by walking. The time of day the patient chooses to walk is up to the patient and is unrelated.

Reference:

Lewis, et al, Medical Surgical Nursing, pgs 270-299, (10th ed) Fluid & Electrolyte Imbalances. McCuistion: Ch 12 pgs 133-149 and Clinical Judgment [Nursing Process] care plan (see) Fluid Volume Excess, McCuistion: pgs. 137-138.

REVIEW QUESTIONS

1. Three days after a patient's total colectomy and ileostomy, he has a nasogastric tube for continuous suction and a Foley catheter for continuous drainage. The night nurse reports a high output from the ileostomy. The patient's pulse is irregular, and he reports muscle weakness and leg cramping. Based on this situation, the nurse would correctly suspect what type of imbalance?
   a. Hypokalemia
   b. Hyperkalemia
   c. Hypomagnesemia
   d. Hypochloremia

2. A patient is receiving intravenous (IV) potassium supplements. What is the most important nursing implication when administering this drug?
   a. It is administered via a central vascular access device.
   b. It is diluted with IV fluids and delivered by infusion pump.
   c. IV potassium must be chilled before administration.
   d. IV potassium preparations should not contain preservatives.

3. A patient is receiving 10 mEq of potassium chloride in 100 mL of normal saline intravenously (IV) to infuse over 1 hour via infusion pump. The patient has a 22-gauge peripheral IV in his right forearm and reports pain at the insertion site; the nurse notes that the site is reddened, warm, and tender to the touch. Which action would the nurse take?
   a. Aspirate and check for blood return, and then slow the IV rate.
   b. Discontinue the IV, and then have a central line inserted.
   c. Stop the infusion, and discontinue the IV immediately.
   d. Apply warm compresses to the IV site and elevate extremity.

4. The health care provider orders a hypertonic crystalloid IV solution for a 70-year-old patient. Which solution will the nurse hang?
   a. Lactated Ringer's
   b. 0.45% sodium chloride (NaCl)
   c. 0.9% sodium chloride (NaCl)
   d. 5% dextrose in 0.9% sodium chloride (NaCl)

5. A patient is receiving fluid replacement. The nurse's primary Clinical Judgment [Nursing Process] plan of care and Take Action [Nursing Interventions] include which of the following statements? (Select all that apply.)
   a. Measure patient's weight every morning.
   b. Know that thirst means a mild fluid deficit.
   c. Monitor fluid intake and fluid output daily.
   d. Avoid using calcium and chloride supplements.
   e. Review patient's daily electrolyte labs for changes.

6. A patient gained 4.4 lb (2 kg), and it has been determined that the weight gain is caused by fluid retention. The nurse correctly estimates that the weight gain may be equivalent to approximately how much fluid?
   a. 1 L
   b. 2 L
   c. 6 L
   d. 8 L

7. A patient has hypernatremia. Which components are appropriate to include in the Clinical Judgment [Nursing Process] plan of care? (Select all that apply.)
   a. Instruct patient on seizure precautions.
   b. Keep appointments for laboratory tests.
   c. A sign of hypernatremia is hypotension.
   d. Explain the meaning of fluid restriction.
   e. Instruct patient on how to read food labels.

8. The nurse is reviewing the medication list of a patient with hypokalemia. Which products may contribute to the cause of this imbalance? (Select all that apply.)
   a. Cortisone
   b. Licorice
   c. Azithromycin
   d. Estrogen
   e. Digoxin

13

Vitamin and Mineral Replacement

OBJECTIVES

- Discuss four positive reasons for using vitamins.
- Differentiate between water-soluble and fat-soluble vitamins.
- Relate food sources and deficiency conditions associated with each vitamin.

- Explain the body's need for iron supplementation and name four foods that are high in iron.
- Explain the uses for copper, zinc, chromium, and selenium.
- Describe what is important to include in patient teaching related to vitamins A and C.

OUTLINE

Vitamins and minerals are needed in the correct portions for normal body function. Most vitamin and mineral nutrients can be safely obtained through the diet. Overuse of vitamins and minerals occurs easily, especially if the nutrients are coming from pills instead of food. It is important to check all supplements with the patient's health care provider (HCP).

VITAMINS

Vitamins are organic substances necessary for normal metabolic functions and for tissue growth and healing. The body needs only a small number of vitamins daily, which are obtained through the diet. A well-balanced diet has all of the vitamins and minerals needed for body functioning. The intake of vitamins should be increased by people experiencing periods of rapid body growth; those who are pregnant or breastfeeding; patients with debilitating illnesses; those with malabsorptive issues, such as Crohn disease; and those with inadequate diets, which includes alcoholics and some geriatric patients. Children who have poor nutrient intake and are malnourished may need vitamin replacement. People on "fad" or restrictive diets may have vitamin deficiencies, as may those who are unable to afford or do not select a wide variety of foods.

The sale of vitamins in the United States is a multibillion-dollar business. About 77% of US adults use a variety of nutritional supplements (http://www.crnusa.org). Older women and people with higher education are typical users of nutritional supplements. Numerous vitamins and herbal medications are available for specialized needs such as cholesterol, memory, menopause, and prostate support. Before purchasing these agents, the patient should discuss with their HCP the use and health benefits of multiple vitamins and herbal medications. Vitamin supplements are not necessary if the individual is healthy and consumes a well-balanced daily diet on a regular basis.

The Food and Nutrition Board of the National Academy of Medicine has established the Dietary Reference Intakes (DRIs).

The DRI nutrient recommendations include these components:

1. Adequate intake (AI) is the consumption and absorption of sufficient food, vitamins, and essential minerals necessary to maintain health.
2. Estimated average requirement (EAR) is the daily intake of a specific nutrient estimated to meet the requirement in 50% of healthy people in an age- and sex-specific group.
3. Recommended dietary allowance (RDA) is the amount of vitamins, minerals, or other essential nutrients that should be ingested every day by a normal person engaged in average activities. RDAs are increased for patients who are experiencing increased activity, children who are growing, and women who are pregnant and lactating. RDAs assume a state of wellness and are of little use in patients who are ill.
4. Tolerable upper intake level (UL) is the maximum level of continuing daily nutrient intake that is likely to pose no risk to the health of most of those in the age group for which it has been established. Vitamin deficiencies can cause cellular and organ dysfunction that may result in slow recovery from illness. Vitamin supplements are necessary for the vitamin deficiencies described in Table 13.1, but vitamins are frequently taken prophylactically rather than therapeutically.

With the goal of facilitating better nutrition, the US Department of Agriculture (USDA) has developed http://www.choosemyplate.gov. "Choose My Plate" is an interactive tool that helps Americans eat more healthy foods (Fig. 13.1). The website offers a variety of features, including both consumer and professional information.

The Food and Nutrition Board of the National Academy of Medicine publishes the US RDA for daily dose requirements of each vitamin. The US Food and Drug Administration (FDA) requires all vitamin products to be labeled according to the vitamin content and the proportion

TABLE 13.1   Vitamin Deficiencies That Require Use of Vitamin Supplements

Categories	Deficiencies
Inability to metabolize and absorb vitamins	Malabsorption disorders: Diarrhea, infectious and inflammatory diseases (e.g., Crohn disease, celiac disease)
Inability to use vitamins	Liver disease (cirrhosis, hepatitis), renal disease, certain hereditary deficiencies (cystic fibrosis)
Increased vitamin losses	Fever from infectious processes, hyperthyroidism, hemodialysis, cancer, starvation, crash diets
Increased vitamin requirements	Early childhood, pregnancy, debilitating disease (cancer, alcoholism), gastrointestinal surgery, special diets

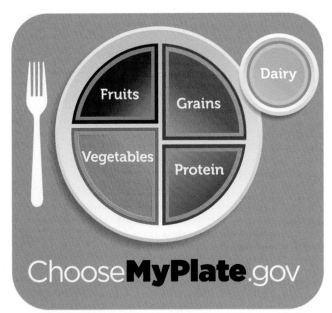

Fig. 13.1 The US Department of Agriculture's Choose My Plate.

of the RDA provided by the vitamin product. Individuals should be encouraged to check the RDA listed on the vitamin label to determine whether the product provides the RDA dose requirements. The RDA may need to be modified for patients who are ill.

Megadoses of vitamins are available and are advertised for specific health conditions, but high doses of some vitamins can be toxic. Patients should be advised to contact their HCP before taking any of these products. Megadoses of fat-soluble vitamins (A, D, E, and K) may cause toxic effects, whereas megadoses of water-soluble vitamins are eliminated via the urine and thus are generally not toxic. Adverse reactions—kidney stones and nerve damage, respectively—have been reported from vitamins C and B_6. However, it is also claimed that B vitamins may positively influence metabolism in older adults.

Table 13.2 lists fat- and water-soluble vitamins, their functions, suggested food sources, and related deficiency conditions.

Fat-Soluble Vitamins

Vitamins fall into two general categories: fat-soluble and water-soluble. The fat-soluble vitamins are A, D, E, and K. They are metabolized slowly; can be stored in fatty tissue, liver, and muscle in significant amounts; and are excreted in the urine at a slow rate. Vitamins A and D are toxic if taken in excessive amounts over time. Current research shows that vitamin D toxicity is quite rare, and its symptoms are nonspecific. Given that many people are found to be vitamin D deficient, it is not uncommon to see high-dose vitamin D therapy (e.g., 50,000 units/week).

Foods rich in vitamins A, D, E, and K are shown in Table 13.2.

Vitamin A

Vitamin A (retinol and beta-carotene) is essential for bone growth and for maintenance of epithelial tissues, skin, eyes, and hair. Vitamin A has antioxidant properties. Excessive doses can become toxic. During pregnancy, the female should maintain the RDA because excessive amounts of vitamin A can cause fetal harm. Prototype Drug Chart: Vitamin A describes the pharmacologic data on vitamin A.

Pharmacokinetics. Vitamin A is absorbed in the gastrointestinal (GI) tract, and 90% is stored in the liver; however, this function can be inhibited with liver disease. Massive doses of vitamin A can cause hypervitaminosis. Signs and symptoms include hair loss, peeling skin, anorexia, abdominal pain, lethargy, nausea, and vomiting.

The RDA for adult males is 900 mcg/d (3000 international units [IU]) by mouth daily. The RDA for adult females is 700 mcg/d (2300 IU) by mouth daily. The UL for adults is 10,000 IU/d by mouth. Vitamin A toxicity affects multiple organs, especially the liver. Mineral oil, cholestyramine, alcohol, and antihyperlipidemic drugs decrease the absorption of vitamin A. Vitamin A is excreted through the kidneys and feces.

Pharmacodynamics. Vitamin A is necessary for many biochemical processes. It aids in the formation of the visual pigment needed for night vision. This vitamin is needed in bone growth and development, and it promotes the integrity of the mucosal and epithelial tissues. An early sign of vitamin A deficiency (hypovitaminosis A) is night blindness. This may progress to dryness and ulceration of the cornea and cause blindness.

Vitamin A taken orally is readily absorbed from the GI tract and peaks in 3 to 5 hours. Its duration of action is unknown. Because vitamin A is stored in the liver, the vitamin may be available to the body for days, weeks, or months.

Vitamin D

Vitamin D has a major role in regulating calcium and phosphorus metabolism, and it is needed for calcium absorption from the intestines. Dietary vitamin D is absorbed in the small intestine and requires bile salts for absorption. There are two compounds of vitamin D: vitamin D_2, *ergocalciferol*, a synthetic fortified vitamin D, and vitamin D_3, *cholecalciferol*, a natural form of vitamin D influenced by ultraviolet sunlight on the skin. Over-the-counter (OTC) vitamin D supplements usually contain vitamin D_3. Once absorbed, vitamin D is converted to calcifediol (also known as *25-hydroxycholecalciferol*) in the liver. Calcifediol is then converted to an active form, calcitriol, in the kidneys. Studies have suggested that vitamin D taken with calcium can reduce the incidence of fractures. Vitamin D deficiency can cause rickets in children and osteomalacia in adults and bone fractures.

Calcitriol, the active form of vitamin D, functions as a hormone, and along with parathyroid hormone (PTH) and calcitonin, it regulates calcium and phosphorus metabolism. Calcitriol and PTH stimulate bone reabsorption of calcium and phosphorus. Excretion of vitamin D is primarily in bile; only a small amount is excreted in the urine. If serum calcium levels are low, more vitamin D is activated; when serum calcium levels are normal, activation of vitamin D is decreased. The normal adult RDA of vitamin D is 15 mcg/d (600 IU/day) by mouth a day.

Tolerable upper intake level is 4000 International units/day (100 mcg/day). Excess vitamin D ingestion (>4000 IU/day) results in hypervitaminosis D and may cause hypercalcemia (an elevated serum calcium level). Anorexia, nausea, and vomiting are early symptoms of vitamin D toxicity.

TABLE 13.2 Vitamins: Functions, Suggested Food Sources, and Deficiency Conditions

Vitamin	Function	Food Sources	Deficiency Conditions
A (Retinol) (fat-soluble)	Required for development and maintenance of healthy eyes, gums, teeth, skin, hair, glands, and immune function.	Darkly colored fruits and vegetables including carrots, cantaloupe, mangoes, spinach, pumpkin, and sweet potatoes. Natural vitamin A is found only in foods of animal origin: Dairy products, meat, fish oil, and fish.	Night blindness is often the first indication of deficiency. Skin lesions and dysfunction of mucous membranes also occur.
B-Complex Vitamin			
B_1 (Thiamine) (water-soluble/B-complex group)	Promotes carbohydrate metabolism (energy) and is required for good function of the nervous system and as a replacement in deficiency.	Enriched, fortified whole-grain products; legumes; cereal grains; pork is the richest source of the natural vitamin.	Beriberi; metabolic disorders; necrotizing encephalomyelopathy; cardiovascular complications; neurologic disorders; ataxia; diplopia; Wernicke encephalopathy and Korsakoff syndrome, significant CNS disorders, and alcoholism.
B_2 (Riboflavin) (water-soluble/In B-complex group)	Promotes body's use of carbohydrates, proteins, and fats; is required for tissue integrity; necessary for normal RBC function.	Milk, enriched flour, green vegetables, yogurt, eggs, nuts, cheese, and meats, especially organ meats (liver and kidney).	Sore throat, dry/cracked skin at the corners of the mouth can signal deficiency, pellagra (dermatitis/mental disturbance), microcytic anemia, and alcoholism.
B_3 (Niacin or nicotinic acid) (water-soluble in B-complex group)	In all body tissues; necessary for energy-producing reactions (lipid metabolism, glycogenolysis, and tissue respiration) and assists nervous system. Large doses decrease lipoprotein and triglyceride synthesis by inhibiting the release of free fatty acids from adipose tissue and decreasing hepatic lipoprotein synthesis.	In many foods: animal and plant protein, liver, peanuts, mushrooms, whole wheat, enriched grains, green vegetables, and unpolished rice.	Pellagra (rough skin), flushing of the face and neck, pruritus, abdominal pain, hepatotoxicity, headache, dizziness, blurred vision, orthostatic hypertension, memory loss, anorexia, insomnia, and alcoholism.
B_6 (Pyridoxine) (water-soluble/in B-complex group)	Required for amino acid, carbohydrate, and lipid metabolism, protein synthesis, and formation of RBCs.	Cereal grains, meat, fish, vegetables, legumes, white potatoes, and organ meats.	Neuritis, convulsions, seborrheic dermatitis, anemia, depression, confusion, and alcoholism.
B_{12} (Cobalamin) (water-soluble)	Functions as nucleic acid to help RBCs; aids in functioning of the nervous system; assists in the making of DNA in our cells.	Liver, kidney, fish, dairy products, eggs, chicken, and meat.	Low levels can cause GI disorders, poor growth, neurologic damage from anemia, and pernicious anemias. Deficiency may be found in strict vegans. Receive laboratory work before treatment: Iron, reticulocyte, Hct, folate and B_{12} concentrations.
Folic acid (vitamin B_9) (Folate) (water-soluble, in B-complex group)	Essential in the synthesis of DNA; assists with intestinal functioning and prevents certain anemias.	Leafy green vegetables, yellow fruits and vegetables, yeast, organ meats, black-eyed peas, lentils.	Decreases occur in WBC count and clotting factors, along with anemias (pernicious, thalassemia, megaloblastic, macrocytic), intestinal disturbances, depression, and alcoholism.
Pantothenic acid (vitamin B_5) (Folate) (water-soluble)	Essential nutrient in multiple biochemical processes: gluconeogenesis, carbohydrate metabolism, fatty acid synthesis, biosynthesis of steroid hormones, and acetylcholine.	Present in peas, beans, lean meat, fish, poultry, eggs, milk, and whole-grain cereals (most foods).	Unlike other vitamins, pantothenic acid has no RDA. It is questionable whether a true deficiency state can be produced in the absence of other deficiencies, perhaps due to the widespread availability of pantothenic acid in foods. Deficiency states have been observed in conjunction with other B complex vitamin deficiencies.
Biotin (vitamin H; coenzyme R; classified as a B vitamin) (water-soluble)	Responsible for metabolism and synthesis of fats, carbohydrates, and amino acids in energy production.	Eggs (egg yolk), milk, liver, kidney, nuts, soybean, and oat bran.	Natural deficiency is unknown in humans. There is a risk of hypersensitivity as with all medications: Chest pain, shortness of breath, hives, and skin rash.
C (Ascorbic acid) (water-soluble)	Free radical antioxidant, essential for tissue repair and growth, required for formation of collagen.	Citrus fruits, cantaloupe, tomatoes, leafy green vegetables, green peppers, potatoes, strawberries, kiwi fruit.	Deficiency leads to poor wound healing, bleeding gums, scurvy, and faulty bone and tooth development. Deficiency is prevalent in critical illness. High doses of vitamin C used in treatment of sepsis, trauma, and burns with beneficial effects and no adverse reactions.

TABLE 13.2 Vitamins: Functions, Suggested Food Sources, and Deficiency Conditions—cont'd

Vitamin	Function	Food Sources	Deficiency Conditions
D (cholecalciferol—vitamin D_3 and ergocalciferol, vitamin D_2) (fat-soluble).	Promotes phosphorus and calcium balance, important for strong teeth and bones.	Vitamin D–fortified milk, cereal, eggs, fatty fish, and liver.	Rickets can occur in children; osteomalacia in adults.
E (Alpha-tocopherol) (fat-soluble)	Promotes formation and functioning of RBCs, muscles, and other tissues. Acts as an antioxidant and plays a role in antiinflammatory processes, inhibition of platelet aggregation, and immune enhancement.	Whole-grain cereals, wheat germ, sunflower seeds, milk, eggs, meat, avocados, asparagus, broccoli, spinach, and vegetable oils.	Breakdown of RBCs can occur with deficiency. Also, peripheral neuropathies, ataxia, retinopathy, and impairment of the immune response.
K (Phytonadione) (fat-soluble)	Essential for blood clotting (the "coagulations vitamin")	Leafy green vegetables (broccoli, brussel sprouts, collard greens, lettuce, spinach), liver, cheese, egg yolk, vegetable oil (soybean and canola).	Increased clotting time leads to increased bleeding and hemorrhage.

CNS, Central nervous system; *GI*, gastrointestinal; *HCT*, hematocrit, *RBC*, red blood cell; *RDA*, required dietary allowance, *WBC*, white blood cell; *HCT*, hematocrit.

📄 PROTOTYPE DRUG CHART

Vitamin A

Drug Class	Dosage
Vitamin A (retinol) Fat-soluble vitamin	*Daily requirements[a]:* A: 700 mcg/day (females); 900 mcg/day (males) NOTE: Pregnancy: 770 mcg/day RDA *Vitamin A in excess of RDA can cause fetal harm. Tolerable upper limit (UL) of vitamin A 3000 mcg/d* *Severe deficiency:* A: IM 30,000 mcg/day × 3 days; then 15,000 mcg/day IM × 14 days, then follow-up with oral supplement

Contraindications	Drug-Lab-Food Interactions
Hypervitaminosis A Vitamin A in pregnancy: avoid amounts > RDA Hypersensitivity to ingredients in preparations (Polysorbate-80)	Drugs: Mineral oil (may decrease absorption of vitamin A); castor oil (toxic effect); oral contraceptives and warfarin (increase vitamin A levels): Cholestyramine and colestipol may decrease absorption Lab: May increase BUN, calcium, cholesterol, and triglycerides; may lower erythrocyte and leukocyte counts Food: None known

Pharmacokinetics	Pharmacodynamics
Absorption: PO: 1 h (GI absorption requires bile acids, fat, lipase, and protein) Distribution: PB: UK Metabolism: mostly through the liver; t½: UK Excretion: Small amounts excreted in urine	PO: Onset: quickly Peak: 3–5 h Duration: UK

Therapeutic Effects/Uses

Treatment of vitamin A deficiency, biliary tract or pancreatic disease, colitis, cirrhosis, celiac disease, skin disorders, prevention of night blindness, and promotion of bone development

Mechanism of Action: Essential for developmental growth, bone and teeth development, vision, integrity of skin and mucous membranes, and reproduction

Side Effects	Adverse Reactions
Headache, fatigue, drowsiness, irritability, anorexia, vomiting, diarrhea, dry skin, visual changes	Anaphylactic shock and anaphylactoid reactions, increased intracranial pressure, hypervitaminosis A, thrombocytopenia, cholestasis, hepatomegaly, metabolic acidosis, hypotension

A, Adult; *BUN*, blood urea nitrogen; *C*, child; *GI*, gastrointestinal; *IM*, intramuscular; *PB*, protein binding; *PO*, by mouth; *t½*, half-life; *UK*, unknown; *RDA*, recommended daily allowance.

[a]For daily requirements, see: www.nal.usa.gov/fnic.

Vitamin E

Vitamin E has antioxidant properties that protect cellular components from being oxidized and protect red blood cells (RBCs) from hemolysis. Vitamin E depends on bile salts, pancreatic secretion, and fat for its absorption. Vitamin E is stored in all tissues, especially the liver, muscle, and fatty tissue. About 75% of vitamin E is excreted in bile.

Although early evidence had suggested the potential for vitamin E to reduce cardiovascular disease (CVD), more recent outcome studies have not shown CVD benefits with vitamin E. Currently, the American Heart Association guidelines do not recommend vitamin E therapy as a preventative measure for CVD. Vitamin E has been of interest for its antioxidant properties, and it has been used off-label for various conditions, including Alzheimer disease.

The RDA of vitamin E in adults, including pregnant and lactating females, is 22.4 IU/day (15 mg/day) and should not exceed the UL of 1000 mg/day (1500 IU/day) in oral intake. The dosage is determined by nutritional intake or degree of deficiency by the HCP. Side effects of large doses of vitamin E may include fatigue, weakness, nausea, GI upset, headache, bleeding, and breast tenderness. Vitamin E may prolong the prothrombin time (PT), and patients taking warfarin should have their PT monitored closely. Iron and vitamin E should not be taken together because iron can interfere with the body's absorption and use of vitamin E.

Vitamin K

Vitamin K occurs in three forms. Vitamin K_1 (phytonadione) is the most active form and is a synthetic type of vitamin K made by plants, and it represents the bulk of dietary vitamin K. Vitamin K_2 (menaquinone) is synthesized by probiotic bacteria in the digestive tract. Vitamin K_3 (menadione) is another synthetic form of vitamin K. After vitamin K is absorbed, it is stored primarily in the liver and in other tissues. Half of vitamin K comes from the intestinal flora, and the remaining portion comes from the diet. The RDA for an adult male is 120 mcg/day, and for an adult female the RDA is 90 mcg/day. The National Academy of Medicine has not been able to determine a tolerable upper level for vitamin K, so always speak to an HCP before increasing the dose of vitamin K.

Vitamin K is needed for synthesis of prothrombin and clotting factors VII, IX, and X. For oral anticoagulant overdose, vitamin K_1 (phytonadione) is the only vitamin K form available for therapeutic use and is most effective in preventing hemorrhage. Vitamin K is used for two purposes: as an antidote for oral anticoagulant overdose and to prevent and treat the hypoprothrombinemia of vitamin K deficiency. Spontaneous hemorrhage may occur with vitamin K deficiency due to lack of bile salts and malabsorption syndromes that interfere with vitamin K uptake (e.g., celiac disease). Vitamin K deficiency is uncommon in adults, but certain people are at increased risk: those taking anticoagulant therapy such as warfarin, people receiving antibiotic therapy, and those who have fat malabsorption syndrome. Some of the side effects of vitamin K deficiency are increased bruising, bleeding from mucous membranes, and dark, tarry stools. When vitamin K levels are too high, people can form excessive blood clots quickly, which can cause stroke, heart attack, and blocked blood flow anywhere in the body.

Newborns are vitamin K deficient; thus a single dose of phytonadione is recommended immediately after delivery. This practice is common in the United States but is controversial in other countries because it can elevate the bilirubin level and can cause hyperbilirubinemia with a risk of kernicterus. Oral and parenteral forms of phytonadione are available; intravenous (IV) administration is dangerous and may cause death.

Water-Soluble Vitamins

Water-soluble vitamins are the B-complex vitamins and vitamin C. This group of vitamins is not usually toxic unless taken in extremely excessive amounts. Water-soluble vitamins are not stored by the body, so consistent, steady supplementation is required. Water-soluble vitamins are readily excreted in the urine. Protein binding of water-soluble vitamins is minimal. Foods that are high in vitamin B are grains, cereals, breads, and meats. There are reports that B vitamins may promote a sense of well-being and increased energy as well as decreased anger, tension, and irritability. Citrus fruits and green vegetables are high in vitamin C. If the fruits and vegetables are cut or cooked, a large amount of vitamin C is lost.

Vitamin B Complex

Vitamin B_1 (thiamine), vitamin B_2 (riboflavin), vitamin B_3 (nicotinic acid, or niacin), and vitamin B_6 (pyridoxine) are four vitamins in the vitamin B complex group that are water-soluble. Vitamin B complex is a common group of vitamins administered in the clinical setting, especially to patients with alcoholism.

Thiamine deficiency can lead to the polyneuritis and cardiac pathology seen in Beriberi or Wernicke encephalopathy that progresses to Korsakoff syndrome, conditions most commonly associated with alcohol abuse. Wernicke-Korsakoff syndrome is a significant central nervous system (CNS) disorder characterized by confusion, nystagmus, diplopia, ataxia, and loss of recent memory. If not treated, it can cause irreversible brain damage. IV administration of thiamine is recommended for treatment of Wernicke-Korsakoff syndrome. Thiamine must be given before giving any glucose to avoid aggravation of symptoms.

Riboflavin may be given to manage dermatologic problems such as scaly dermatitis, cracked corners of the mouth, and inflammation of the skin and tongue. To treat migraine headache, riboflavin is given in larger doses than for dermatologic concerns.

Niacin is given to alleviate pellagra and hyperlipidemia, for which large doses are required. Chapter 44 offers a discussion of niacin use to reduce cholesterol levels. However, large doses may cause GI irritation and vasodilation, resulting in a flushing sensation.

Pyridoxine is administered to correct vitamin B_6 deficiency. It may also help alleviate the symptoms of neuritis caused by isoniazid (INH) therapy for tuberculosis. Vitamin B_6 is essential as a building block of nucleic acids, in red blood cell (RBC) formation, and in synthesis of hemoglobin. Pyridoxine is used to treat vitamin B_6 deficiency caused by lack of adequate diet, inborn errors of metabolism, or drug-induced deficiencies secondary to INH, penicillamine, or cyclosporine (or hydralazine) therapy. It is also used to treat neonates with seizures refractive to traditional therapy. Vitamin B_6 deficiencies may occur in patients with alcoholism along with deficiencies of other B-complex vitamins. Patients with diabetes or alcoholism may benefit from daily supplementation. Pyridoxine is readily absorbed in the jejunum and is stored in the liver, muscle, and brain. It is metabolized in the liver and excreted in the urine.

Vitamin C

Vitamin C (ascorbic acid) is absorbed from the small intestine. Vitamin C aids in the absorption of iron and in the conversion of folic acid. Vitamin C is not stored in the body and is excreted readily in the urine. A high serum vitamin C level that results from excessive dosing of vitamin C is excreted by the kidneys unchanged. Vitamin C is used in the treatment of scurvy, which is rare in developed countries but seen in individuals who consume few fruits and vegetables. Also, scurvy is seen in people who are on restricted diets or who abuse alcohol or drugs.

The RDA of vitamin C (adult dose) is 75 mg/day for women and 90 mg/day for men to prevent deficiency. Some individuals take greater amounts. Massive doses of vitamin C can cause GI upset. Prototype Drug Chart: Vitamin C details pharmacologic data on vitamin C.

PROTOTYPE DRUG CHART

Vitamin C

Drug Class	Dosage
Water-soluble vitamin	*Daily requirements*[a]: A: PO 75 mg/d (female); 90 mg/d (men); (male smokers PO 125 mg/d, female smokers PO 110 mg/d) *Severe deficit:* Scurvy A: PO: 500 mg to 1000 mg/d 2–4 weeks. IV: 200 mg/day × 1 week; if treatment unresolved may continue dose until symptoms resolve

Contraindications	Drug-Lab-Food Interactions
Caution: Acute and chronic oxalate nephropathy has been reported with prolonged administration of high doses of ascorbic acid; tartrazine hypersensitivity (FDC yellow dye #5); use cautiously in recurrent kidney stones. Can increase risk of iron toxicity in patients with hemochromatosis, sickle cell anemia, thalassemia.	Decreases ascorbic acid uptake when taken with salicylates; may decrease effect of oral anticoagulants (warfarin); may decrease elimination of aspirins Lab: May decrease bilirubin and urinary pH; may increase uric acid and uric oxalate Food: None known

Pharmacokinetics	Pharmacodynamics
Absorption: PO: Quickly Distribution: PB: 25% Metabolism: t½: UK Excretion: In the urine; unchanged with high doses	PO: Absorbed orally through active transport Onset: >2 d Peak: UK Duration: UK

Therapeutic Effects/Uses
To prevent and treat vitamin C deficiency (scurvy), to increase wound healing, and for burns; preserves integrity of blood vessels. Mechanism of Action: A water-soluble vitamin, it is essential for collagen formation and tissue repair (bones, skin, blood vessels) and for synthesis of lipids, protein, and carnitine

Side Effects	Adverse Reactions
Oral: Nausea, vomiting, diarrhea, heartburn, headache Parenteral: Flushing, headache, dizziness, soreness at injection site	Kidney stones, crystalluria, hyperuricemia, hemolytic anemia *Life-threatening:* Sickle cell crisis, deep venous thrombosis

A, Adult; *bid,* twice a day; *C,* child; *IM,* intramuscular; *IV,* intravenous; *PB,* protein binding; *PO,* by mouth; *RDA,* recommended dietary allowance; *t½,* half-life; *UK,* unknown.
[a]For daily requirements, see: www.nal.usa.gov/fnic..

Pharmacokinetics. Vitamin C is absorbed readily through the GI tract and is distributed throughout the body fluids. The kidneys completely excrete vitamin C mostly unchanged.

Pharmacodynamics. Vitamin C is needed for carbohydrate metabolism and protein and lipid synthesis. Collagen synthesis also requires vitamin C because it is part of the intercellular matrix that binds cells together and aids in wound healing. Smoking decreases serum vitamin C levels. Vitamin C in doses greater than 500 mg aids iron absorption; however, it may decrease the effect of oral anticoagulants.

The use of large doses of vitamin C is questionable. Large doses of any vitamin can cause toxicity. Most authorities believe that vitamin C does not prevent the common cold, cure advanced cancer, or treat schizophrenia. Moreover, large doses of vitamin C can cause nausea, abdominal cramps, and diarrhea. If taken with aspirin or sulfonamides, it may cause crystal formation in the urine. Vitamin C directly irritates the intestinal mucosa in the GI tract. This is why the Food and Nutrition Board has set 2 g/day as the adult UL for vitamin C. Large doses of vitamin C can decrease the effect of oral anticoagulants. If large doses of any vitamin are to be discontinued, a gradual reduction of the dosage is necessary to avoid vitamin deficiency.

Folic Acid (Folate)

Folic acid is absorbed from the small intestine, and the active form of folic acid—folate—is circulated to all tissues. One-third of folate is stored in the liver, and the rest is stored in the tissues. It is excreted 80% in bile and 20% in urine.

Folic acid is essential for body growth. It is needed for DNA synthesis, and without folic acid, cellular division is disrupted. Adults' (oral dose) RDA is 0.4 mg/day. The tolerable UL for folic acid (oral) is 1 mg/day. Chronic alcoholism, poor nutritional intake, malabsorption syndromes, pregnancy, and drugs that cause inadequate absorption (phenytoin, barbiturates) or folic acid antagonism (methotrexate, triamterene, trimethoprim) are causes of folic acid deficiencies. Symptoms of folic acid deficiencies include anorexia, nausea, stomatitis, diarrhea, fatigue, alopecia, and blood dyscrasias (megaloblastic anemia, leukopenia, thrombocytopenia). These symptoms are usually not noted until 2 to 4 months after folic acid storage is depleted.

Folic acid deficiency during the first trimester of pregnancy can affect the development of the CNS of the fetus. This may cause neural tube defects (NTDs) such as spina bifida, defective closure of the bony structure of the spinal cord, or anencephaly, which is lack of brain mass formation. The US Public Health Services recommends that all women who may become pregnant consume 600 mcg (0.6 mg) of supplemental folic acid each day in addition to the folate they get with food. Synthetic folate is more stable than folic acid obtained from food: bioavailability is greater than 85% with synthetic folate and less than 59% for food-sourced folic acid.

Excessive doses of folic acid may mask signs of vitamin B_{12} deficiency, which is a risk in older adults. Patients taking phenytoin to control seizures should be cautious about taking folic acid. This vitamin can lower the serum phenytoin level, which could increase the risk of seizures; the phenytoin dose would need to be adjusted in such patients. This is a complex interaction that is not fully understood, but it is thought that 1 mg or less per day of folic acid is safe in patients with controlled epilepsy.

Vitamin B_{12}

Vitamin B_{12}, like folic acid, is essential for DNA synthesis. Vitamin B_{12} aids in the conversion of folic acid to its active form. With active folic acid, vitamin B_{12} promotes cellular division. It is also needed for normal hematopoiesis (development of RBCs in bone marrow) and to maintain nervous system integrity, especially of the myelin. RDA is 2.4 mcg/day for adults, 2.6 mcg/day for pregnant women, and 2.8 mcg/day for lactating women.

The gastric parietal cells produce an intrinsic factor that is necessary for the absorption of vitamin B_{12} through the intestinal wall. Without the intrinsic factor, little or no vitamin B_{12} is absorbed. After absorption, vitamin B_{12} binds to the protein transcobalamin II and is transferred to the tissues. Most vitamin B_{12} is stored in the liver and is slowly excreted, and it can take 2 to 3 years for stored vitamin B_{12} to be depleted and for a deficit to be noticed.

Adults who are deficient in vitamin B_{12} may receive it orally 1000 to 2000 mcg/day. Vitamin B_{12} deficiency is uncommon unless there is a disturbance of the intrinsic factor and intestinal absorption. Pernicious anemia (lack of the intrinsic factor) is the major cause of vitamin B_{12} deficiency, but deficiency can also develop in strict vegetarians who do not consume meat, fish, or dairy products. Other possible causes of vitamin B_{12} deficiency include malabsorption syndromes (cancer, celiac disease, and certain drugs), gastrectomy, Crohn disease, and liver and kidney diseases. Vitamin B_{12} deficiency is commonly seen with the use of metformin and proton pump inhibitors (e.g., omeprazole). Symptoms may include numbness and tingling in the lower extremities, weakness, fatigue, anorexia, loss of taste, diarrhea, memory loss, mood changes, dementia, psychosis, megaloblastic anemia with macrocytes (overenlarged erythrocytes [RBCs]) in the blood, and megaloblasts (overenlarged erythroblasts) in the bone marrow.

◎ CLINICAL JUDGMENT [NURSING PROCESS]

Vitamins

Concept: Health, Wellness, and Illness
Health, wellness, and illness reflect the many stages of a person's life. Health looks at the absence of illness. Wellness is a balance of well-being throughout the life span. Illness refers to disease, disorder, morbidity, or sickness that impairs a person's normal body functioning. This may apply to physical problems experienced by the patient.

Recognize Cues [Assessment]
- Check the patient for vitamin deficiency before the start of therapy and regularly thereafter. Explore such areas as inadequate nutrient intake, debilitating disease, and gastrointestinal (GI) disorders.
- Obtain a 24- and 48-hour diet history analysis.
- When possible, obtain laboratory results to assess serum blood levels.

Analyze Cues and Prioritize Hypothesis [Patient Problems]
- Weight loss
- Hypokalemia
- Need for health teaching

Generate Solutions [Planning]
- The patient will verbalize the food groups included in ChooseMyPlate.gov at the end of the teaching session.
- The patient will explain the importance of vitamin C supplements before discharge.
- The patient will verbalize which foods contain fat-soluble vitamins A, D, E, and K before the next teaching.
- The patient will verbalize which foods contain water-soluble vitamins B, C, folic acid, and B_{12} before discharge.

Take Action [Nursing Interventions]
- Administer vitamins with food to promote absorption.
- Store vitamins in light-resistant containers.
- Use the supplied calibrated dropper for accurate dosing when administering vitamins in drop form. Solutions may be administered mixed with food or drink.
- Administer vitamins intramuscularly for patients who are unable to take vitamins by the oral route (e.g., those with GI malabsorption syndrome).

- Monitor serum blood levels of patient's suspected vitamin or mineral deficiency.
- Determine the patient's preferred and meaningful foods and incorporate them into the food and supplement plan.
- Use interpreters as appropriate if patient has a language barrier.

Patient Teaching
General
- Advise patients to take the prescribed amount of vitamins.
- Counsel patients to read vitamin labels carefully and discuss with a health care provider (HCP) before taking any vitamin or supplement.
- Advise patients to consult with an HCP or pharmacist regarding interactions with prescription and over-the-counter medications.
- Discourage patients from taking a large-dose vitamins over a long period of time.
- Instruct patient to only take supplements prescribed by HCP.
- Instruct patient when stopping long-term use of high-dose vitamin therapy, a gradual decrease in vitamin intake is advised to avoid vitamin deficiency and always notify HCP.
- Instruct patients that skipping vitamins for short-term use is not a cause of concern because deficiencies occur over long-term omissions.
- Advise patients to check expiration dates on vitamin containers before purchasing. Potency of vitamins is reduced after the expiration date.
- Counsel patients to avoid taking mineral oil with vitamin A on a regular basis because it interferes with absorption of the vitamin; mineral oil also interferes with vitamin K absorption. If needed, take mineral oil at bedtime and vitamins in the morning.
- Instruct patients there is no scientific evidence that large doses of vitamin C will cure a cold.
- Alert patients not to take large doses of vitamin C with aspirin or sulfonamides because crystals may form in the kidneys and urine.
- Alert patients to avoid excessive intake of alcoholic beverages. Alcohol can cause vitamin B complex deficiencies.

Diet
- Advise patients to eat a well-balanced diet. Vitamin supplements are not necessary if the person is healthy and receives proper nutrition on a regular basis.

CLINICAL JUDGMENT [NURSING PROCESS]—CONT'D

Vitamins

- Educate patients about foods rich in vitamin A, including: milk, butter, eggs, and leafy green and yellow vegetables. Foods rich in various vitamins are listed in Table 13.2.
- Have the patient keep a diet chart for a full week to determine typical nutrition.
- Have the patient verbalize important foods that contain fat- and water-soluble vitamins.

Side Effects

- Advise patients that nausea, vomiting, headache, loss of hair, and cracked lips (symptoms of hypervitaminosis for vitamin A) should be reported to the HCP. Early symptoms of hypervitaminosis vitamin D are anorexia, nausea, and vomiting.

Evaluate Outcomes [Evaluation]

- Evaluate the patient's understanding of the purpose and use of vitamins.
- Evaluate the effectiveness of the patient's diet.
- Determine whether the patient with malnutrition is receiving appropriate vitamin therapy.

To correct vitamin B_{12} deficiency, cyanocobalamin in crystalline form can be given intramuscularly for severe deficits. It cannot be given intravenously because of possible hypersensitivity reactions. Cyanocobalamin can be given orally and is commonly found in multivitamin preparations. It can also be given as a subcutaneous injection.

MINERALS

Various minerals—such as iron, copper, zinc, chromium, and selenium—are needed for body function.

Iron

Iron (ferrous sulfate, gluconate, or fumarate) is vital for hemoglobin regeneration. Sixty percent of the iron in the body is found in hemoglobin, and one of the causes of anemia is iron deficiency. A normal diet contains 5 to 20 mg of iron per day. Foods rich in iron include liver, lean meats, egg yolks, dried beans, green vegetables (e.g., spinach), and fruit. Food and antacids slow the absorption of iron, and vitamin C increases iron absorption.

During pregnancy, iron requirements increase due to the expansion of maternal blood volume and production of RBCs by the fetus. The iron needs of pregnant women are too great to be met through their diet; therefore supplementation is needed. About 27 mg/day is recommended during pregnancy and for 2 to 3 months after delivery.

The required iron dose for males is 8 mg/day. The dose for females is 18 mg/day or 8 mg/day for women over 50 years of age. Maximum Dose Limit: Dosage with iron must be individualized according to the patient's age, dietary intake requirements, and the degree of iron deficiency. Excess accumulation may occur if iron therapy is continued after the correction of the dietary deficiency. Prototype Drug Chart: Iron describes the pharmacologic data on iron.

Pharmacokinetics. Iron is absorbed by the intestines and enters the plasma as hemoglobin, or it may be stored as ferritin. Although food decreases absorption by 25% to 50%, it may be necessary to take iron preparations with food to avoid GI discomfort. Vitamin C at doses greater than 500 mg may slightly increase iron absorption, whereas tetracycline, quinolone antibiotics (ciprofloxacin, levofloxacin, etc.), and antacids can decrease absorption.

Pharmacodynamics. Iron replacement is given primarily to correct or control iron-deficiency anemias, which are diagnosed by a laboratory blood smear. Clinical signs and symptoms for deficiency include fatigue, weakness, shortness of breath, pallor, and, in cases of severe anemia, increased GI bleeding.

The onset of action for iron therapy takes days, and its peak action does not occur for days or weeks; therefore the patient's symptoms are slow to improve. Increased hemoglobin and hematocrit levels occur within 3 to 7 days.

About 30% to 50% of adults on parenteral nutrition have been shown to have iron deficiency.

Iron toxicity is a serious cause of poisoning in children. As few as 10 tablets of ferrous sulfate (3 g) taken at one time can be fatal within 12 to 48 hours; hemorrhage from the ulcerogenic effects of unbound iron leads to shock. Therefore parents should be strongly cautioned against leaving iron tablets that look like candy within a child's reach. (Most iron products are distributed in bubble packs.) There is also danger of children and adults overdosing on multivitamins that contain iron.

COMPLEMENTARY AND ALTERNATIVE THERAPIES

Iron

Chamomile, feverfew, peppermint, and St. John's wort interfere with the absorption of iron and other minerals.

Copper

Copper is needed for the formation of RBCs and connective tissues. Copper is a cofactor of many enzymes, and its function is in the production of the neurotransmitters, norepinephrine, and dopamine. Excess serum copper levels may be associated with Wilson disease, an inborn error of metabolism that allows for large amounts of copper to accumulate in the liver, kidneys, brain, and cornea (brown or green Kayser-Fleischer rings).

A prolonged copper deficiency may result in anemia that cannot be corrected by taking iron supplements. Abnormal blood and skin changes caused by a copper deficiency include a decrease in white blood cell count, glucose intolerance, and a decrease in skin and hair pigmentation. Mental retardation may also occur in the young. Copper deficiency in patients receiving parenteral nutrition ranges from 30% to 56% and includes both adults and children.

The RDA for copper is 900 mcg/day. Most adults consume about 1 mg/day. Foods rich in copper are shellfish (crab, oysters), liver, nuts, seeds (sunflower, sesame), legumes, and cocoa.

Zinc

Zinc is a trace element and important to many enzymatic reactions. It is essential for biologic functions and, in animals, is important in

📄 PROTOTYPE DRUG CHART

Iron

Drug Class	Dosage
Ferrous sulfate, ferrous gluconate, ferrous fumarate Mineral to decrease anemia Note: Various iron products are not exchangeable on a milligram-to-milligram basis because each contains different amounts of elemental iron.	*Daily oral requirements*[a]: A: 18 mg/d (female); 8 mg/d (men); 15 mg/d first trimester, 27 mg/d last two trimesters (pregnancy); lactation 9–10 mg/d. *Deficiency:* 60 mg of elemental iron 1–3 times/d × 4 wk (repeat labs)
Contraindications	**Drug-Lab-Food Interactions**
Hemolytic anemia, hemosiderosis (iron overload disorder), peptic ulcer, ulcerative colitis *Caution:* Bronchial asthma, iron hypersensitivity	Increased effect of iron with vitamin C; decreased effect of tetracycline, antacids, penicillamine Lab: May increase bilirubin; may decrease calcium Food: None known
Pharmacokinetics	**Pharmacodynamics**
Absorption: PO: 10%–30% intestines Distribution: PB: UK Metabolism: t½: 6 h Excretion: In urine, feces, and sweat	PO: Onset: 4 d Peak: 7–14 d Duration: 3–4 mo
Therapeutic Effects/Uses	
To prevent and treat iron-deficiency anemia Mechanism of Action: Enables RBC development and oxygen transport via hemoglobin	
Side Effects	**Adverse Reactions**
Nausea, vomiting, diarrhea, constipation, epigastric pain; elixir may stain teeth.	May aggravate existing GI conditions and may cause pallor or drowsiness *Life-threatening:* Iron poisoning (mostly in children) may result in cardiovascular collapse, metabolic acidosis Toxicity: Nausea, vomiting, diarrhea (green then tarry stools), hematemesis, pallor, cyanosis, shock, coma

A, Adult; *bid*, two times a day; *C*, child; *GI*, gastrointestinal; *PB*, protein binding; *PO*, by mouth; *RBC*, red blood cell; *t½*, half-life; *UK*, unknown.
[a]For daily requirements, see: www.nal.usa.gov/fnic.

growth, appetite, testicular maturation, skin integrity, mental activity, wound healing, and immunocompetence. Zinc deficiency is associated with diets high in unrefined cereal and unleavened bread, total parenteral nutrition (TPN), intestinal disease (i.e., Crohn's disease, pancreatic insufficiency), alcoholism, pregnancy, or acrodermatitis enteropathy, an autosomal recessive disease characterized by zinc malabsorption. Some believe zinc can alleviate symptoms of the common cold and shorten its duration, although studies have disputed this claim. Large amounts of zinc can be toxic. Zinc in lozenge form can cause nausea and can leave an unpleasant taste, and zinc in nasal sprays has caused patients to lose their sense of smell. Patients should always check with an HCP before taking zinc. The adult RDA is 8 to 11 mg/day. Foods rich in zinc include beef, lamb, eggs, and leafy and root vegetables.

Large doses, more than 150 mg, may cause a copper deficiency, a decrease in high-density lipoprotein (HDL) cholesterol ("good" cholesterol), and a weakened immune response. Zinc can inhibit tetracycline absorption. Patients taking zinc and an antibiotic should not take them together; zinc should be taken at least 2 hours after taking an antibiotic. About 10% of adults on long-term parenteral nutrition develop a zinc deficiency. Zinc is the most common deficiency likely to occur in parenteral nutrition because zinc is lost in the patient's stool.

Chromium

Chromium, in its trivalent state (i.e., Cr^{3+}), is an essential trace element required for proper carbohydrate, lipid, and nucleic acid metabolism in the human body. Overt signs and symptoms of chromium deficiency are usually only observed in adult patients eating diets high in refined foods or who are receiving long-term TPN without chromium supplementation. Chromium supplementation should only be expected to improve disorders that are due to chromium deficiency.

Limited studies have reported that chromium helps normalize blood glucose by increasing the effects of insulin on the cells. However, the importance of chromium deficiency in the average patient with type 2 diabetes has not been established. In addition, there are claims that chromium weight loss and muscle building. Multiple studies have concluded that there is no evidence that chromium supplementation increases muscle mass to a level greater than that which is produced with a healthy diet and exercise alone. Multivitamin and mineral preparations contain chloride salt of chromium. Some signs and symptoms of chromium deficiency are low blood sugar, dizziness, a need for frequent meals, sleepiness at odd times, a craving for sweet food, and excessive thirst. In chromium excess or toxicity, patients may experience GI bleeding, coagulopathy, seizures, and pulmonary dysfunction.

There is no RDA for chromium; however, 25 to 35 mcg/day is considered within the normal range for adults. Foods rich in chromium include meats, whole-grain cereals, and brewer's yeast.

Selenium

Selenium is an essential nonmetallic element chemically related to sulfur. It is nutritionally essential for humans and is a constituent of more than two dozen selenoproteins (a protein that includes selenocysteine amino acid residue) that play critical roles in reproduction, thyroid hormone metabolism, DNA synthesis, and protection from oxidative damage and infection. Symptoms of selenium deficiency include hypothyroidism, muscle weakness, myalgia, myositis, increased erythrocyte fragility, pancreatic degeneration, macrocytosis, and pseudoalbinism. Selenium works with vitamin E.

It is thought that selenium has an anticarcinogenic effect, and doses lower than 200 mcg may reduce the risk of lung, prostate, and colorectal cancer. However, research has never proven selenium's anticarcinogenic properties. Excess doses of more than 200 mcg might cause weakness, hair loss, dermatitis, nausea, diarrhea, and abdominal pain. Also, there may be a garlic-like odor from the skin and breath.

The RDA for selenium is 55 mcg/day. Foods rich in selenium include meats, especially liver, seafood, poultry, and grains.

CLINICAL JUDGMENT [NURSING PROCESS]

Antianemia Mineral: Iron

Concept: Health, Wellness, and Illness
Health, wellness, and illness reflect the many stages of a person's life. Health looks at the absence of illness. Wellness is a balance of well-being throughout the life span. Illness refers to disease, disorder, morbidity, or sickness that impairs a person's normal body functioning. This may apply to physical problems experienced by the patient.

Recognize Cues [Assessment]
- Obtain a history of current drugs and herbs the patient is taking.
- Obtain a medical history of health problems such as anemia.
- Assess the patient for signs and symptoms of iron-deficiency anemia, such as fatigue, malaise, pallor, shortness of breath, tachycardia, and cardiac dysrhythmia.
- Assess the patient's red blood cell (RBC) count, hemoglobin, hematocrit, iron level, and reticulocyte count before the start of and throughout therapy.

Analyze Cues and Prioritize Hypothesis [Patient Problems]
- Weight loss
- Confusion
- Fatigue
- Constipation

Generate Solutions [Planning]
- The patient will name at least six foods high in iron content.
- The patient will consume foods rich in iron.
- The patient will explain the importance of iron supplements.
- The patient will explain the significance of the red blood count, hemoglobin, and hematocrit labs related to anemia prior to discharge.

Take Action [Nursing Interventions]
- Encourage patients to eat a nutritious diet to obtain sufficient iron. Iron supplements are not needed unless a person is malnourished or pregnant or has abnormal menses.
- Store vitamins in light-resistant containers.
- Administer iron intramuscularly by the Z-track method to avoid leakage of iron into the subcutaneous tissue and skin, resulting in irritation and stains to the skin.
- Discuss importance of keeping appointments with HCP and receiving the required laboratory work before each visit with HCP.
- Use an interpreter if needed.

Patient Teaching
General
- Advise patients to take the tablet or capsule between meals with at least 8 ounces of juice or water to promote absorption. If gastric irritation occurs, instruct the patient to take supplements with food.
- Advise patients to swallow the tablet or capsule whole.
- Encourage patients to maintain an upright position for 30 minutes after taking oral iron preparations to prevent esophageal corrosion from reflux.
- Do not administer the iron tablet within 1 hour of ingesting antacids, milk, or milk products, such as ice cream or yogurt.
- Counsel patients that certain herbal supplements can decrease absorption of iron and other minerals (see Complementary and Alternative Therapies: Iron).
- Advise patients to increase fluids, activity, and dietary bulk to avoid or relieve constipation. Slow-release iron capsules decrease constipation and gastric irritation.
- Instruct adults not to leave iron tablets within reach of children. If a child swallows many tablets, induce vomiting and immediately call the local poison control center.
- Encourage patients to take only the prescribed amount of drug to avoid iron poisoning. Be alert to the iron in multivitamin preparations.
- Be alert that iron content varies among iron salts; therefore do not substitute one for another.
- Advise patients that drug treatment for anemia is generally less than 6 months.

Diet
- Counsel patients to include iron-rich foods in their diet, such as lean meats, egg yolk, dried beans, green vegetables, and fruit.

Side Effects
- Advise patients taking a liquid iron preparation to use a straw to prevent discoloration of tooth enamel.
- Alert patients that the drug turns stools a harmless black or dark green.
- Instruct patients about signs and symptoms of toxicity, including nausea, vomiting, diarrhea, pallor, hematemesis, shock, and coma, and report these occurrences to the health care provider (HCP).

Evaluation Outcomes [Evaluation]
- Evaluate the effectiveness of iron therapy by determining that the patient is not fatigued or short of breath and that the hemoglobin level is within the desired range.

CRITICAL THINKING CASE STUDY

The patient is a 60-year-old female who has been prescribed ferrous sulfate 325 mg/day for anemia. During the nursing assessment, the patient expressed desire to feel better so she can babysit her 2-year-old grandchild.

1. What precautions should the patient take regarding the container of ferrous sulfate? Explain your answer.

2. The patient asks whether she can take iron in the morning before breakfast. How should the nurse respond?
3. The patient asks the nurse whether any side effects are associated with taking iron. What is an appropriate response?
4. The patient asks whether she should include foods high in iron in her daily diet. How should the nurse respond?

REVIEW QUESTIONS

1. The nurse is reviewing a patient's laboratory test results and current medications and notes that the patient's prothrombin time is prolonged. The nurse checks the patient's medication list. What vitamin or mineral might be contributing to this?
   a. Vitamin A
   b. Selenium
   c. Vitamin D
   d. Vitamin E

2. A patient comes to the office with a chief complaint of hair loss and peeling skin. The nurse notes many vitamins and minerals are on the medication list. The patient reports using vitamins to treat liver disease. The patient's complaint may be caused by an excess of which vitamin or mineral?
   a. Vitamin A
   b. Zinc
   c. Vitamin C
   d. Vitamin D

3. The nurse routinely includes health teaching about vitamins to patients. Vitamin D has a major role in which process?
   a. Prevention of night blindness and improve vision
   b. Regulating calcium and phosphorous metabolism
   c. Important for growth and development in children
   d. Responsible for DNA and prothrombin synthesis

4. The nurse is doing preconception counseling with a patient. The patient asks why she must take folic acid (folate) during pregnancy. What is the nurse's response?
   a. Folic acid prevents neural tube defects in the developing fetus.
   b. Folic acid is known to lower blood glucose in diabetic patients.
   c. Folic acid in the gastrointestinal system prevents celiac disease.
   d. Folic acid will prevent migraine headaches in pregnant women.

5. A prenatal patient tells the nurse that she is not taking vitamins because she heard that vitamins may cause damage to the fetus. What is the nurse's best response?
   a. Vitamins are beneficial to the pregnant mother and baby.
   b. Take extra vitamins now to make up for missed doses.
   c. Megadose of vitamins can be harmful in the first trimester.
   d. Taking vitamin doses above the RDA is not recommended.

6. A patient asks the nurse for information about fat-soluble vitamins. What is the nurse's best response?
   a. Fat-soluble vitamins are metabolized rapidly.
   b. Fat-soluble vitamins cannot be stored in the liver.
   c. Fat-soluble vitamins are excreted slowly in urine.
   d. Fat-soluble vitamins can never be toxic.

7. A patient complains of night blindness. The nurse correctly recommends which foods?
   a. Skim milk and peas
   b. Fortified milk and eggs
   c. Nuts and yeast
   d. Enriched breads and cereals

8. A patient diagnosed with alcoholism has questions about his medications. The nurse correctly explains that alcoholism can be associated with deficiency of which vitamin?
   a. A (beta carotene)
   b. B (B-complex)
   c. D (ergocalciferol)
   d. K (phytonadione)

9. Which vitamin plays a major role in regulating calcium and phosphorus absorption?
   a. A
   b. B
   c. C
   d. D

10. A patient takes iron on a daily basis. Which comment from the patient suggests the need for health teaching related to iron?
    a. I will swallow the tablet whole.
    b. I will take the tablet before I go to bed.
    c. I will drink a cup of water after swallowing the iron tablet.
    d. I will keep the tablets out of children's reach.

11. A patient asks the nurse, "What does copper do for me? I think it must be bad for me." What is the nurse's "best" response?
    a. Copper is needed for red blood cell formation.
    b. Be sure to include nuts and seeds in your diet.
    c. Why do you think copper is bad for you?
    d. Only take your prescribed dose of copper 5 mg/d.

Nutritional Support

http://evolve.elsevier.com/McCuistion/pharmacology

Nutrients are substances that nourish and aid in the development of the body. Nutrients provide energy, promote growth and development, and regulate body processes. Inadequate nutrient intake can cause malnutrition. Patients experiencing chronic or critical illnesses that result in surgery are at risk for malnutrition. Without adequate nutritional support, the body's metabolic processes slow down or stop. This can greatly diminish the body's organ functioning and cause a poor immune response. There are two routes for administering nutritional support: enteral nutrition (EN), which involves the gastrointestinal (GI) tract and can be given orally or by tube feeding; and total parenteral nutrition (TPN), which administers high-caloric nutrients through large veins.

The length of time a person may survive without nutrients is influenced by body weight, composition, genetics, health, and hydration. Patients who are critically ill may only tolerate a lack of nutrient support for a short period before organ failure occurs. Recovery is more rapid for patients who have experienced trauma, burns, or critical illness if nutrition is started within 24 to 48 hours of admission to the hospital. Early administration of EN restores intestinal motility, maintains GI function, reduces the movement of bacteria and other organisms, improves wound healing, decreases the incidence of infection, and ultimately decreases the length of the hospital stay. Early nutritional support improves the patient's general health and produces favorable outcomes.

In addition to nutrients, both hydration and electrolyte balance must be considered. If all three are not addressed, preventable complications like constipation, urinary tract infection, and pressure ulcers can occur. The requirements for fluid balance are usually between 30 and 35 mL/kg/day. A healthy person requires 2000 calories per day; critically ill patients require 50% more than the normal energy requirement (approximately 3000 calories per day). If a patient has a 10% weight loss within the past 3 to 6 months, and has had little or no nutrition for more than 5 days, nutritional supplementation should be considered. Nutrition and hydration are essential components necessary for everyday life.

DIFFERENT TYPES OF NUTRITIONAL SUPPORT

Oral Feeding

Many patients require nutritional supplementation due to malnutrition or anorexia (e.g., a deficiency of certain nutrients, vitamins, or minerals). Many factors may affect a patient's appetite: psychological stress about their illness, family problems, finances, and employment issues are just a few of the many challenges a patient may experience. If the patient can swallow and has a working GI tract, oral nutritional supplementation between meals can help increase caloric intake. Many commercially available products may be used to supplement intake. These are marketed as puddings, bars, and supplemental nutritional drinks.

Enteral Nutrition

Enteral nutrition involves the delivery of nutrition or fluid via a tube into the GI tract, which requires a functional, accessible GI tract. Depending on the different pathologies present, EN may be used for short-term nutritional supplementation, such as with reduced appetite or swallowing difficulties. It can also be used for long-term nutritional supplementation for malabsorption disorders or increased catabolism.

Routes for Enteral Feedings

A multidisciplinary team approach is used when a decision is required regarding which feeding route to use. Many factors are considered: the patient's condition, preferences, the length of the feeding, physiologic conditions, tolerance, and the integrity of the patient's GI tract.

The GI routes used for enteral tube feedings are the nasogastric, nasoduodenal/nasojejunal, gastrostomy, or jejunostomy routes (Fig. 14.1). The nasogastric and gastrostomy routes deliver food directly to the stomach. The nasoduodenal/nasojejunal and the jejunostomy

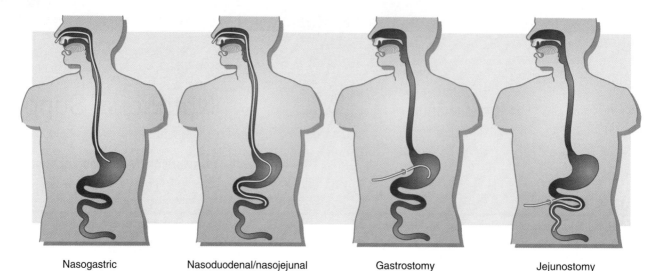

Nasogastric   Nasoduodenal/nasojejunal   Gastrostomy   Jejunostomy

Fig. 14.1 Types of Gastrointestinal Tubes Used for Enteral Feedings. A *nasogastric* tube is passed from the nose into the stomach. A weighted *nasoduodenal/nasojejunal* tube is passed through the nose into the duodenum/jejunum. A *gastrostomy* tube is introduced through a temporary or permanent opening on the abdominal wall (stoma) into the stomach. A *jejunostomy* tube is passed through a stoma directly into the jejunum.

routes deliver food after the stomach or below the pyloric sphincter and are used for patients at risk for aspiration. These GI routes deliver food by a tube inserted through the nose (nasogastric, nasoduodenal/ nasojejunal) or directly into the GI tract (gastrostomy or jejunostomy) through the abdominal wall. The nasogastric, nasoduodenal, and nasojejunal routes are for short-term nutrition of less than 4 weeks' duration. If long-term nutrition is required, the patient may receive a gastrostomy or a jejunostomy tube placed in the stomach or small bowel by a surgical, endoscopic, or fluoroscopic procedure.

The gastrointestinal tubes are small in diameter, are made of urethane or silicone, and are flexible and long. They are radiopaque, which makes their position easy to identify by x-ray. These tubes easily clog, especially when using thick feedings and when the patient's medications are crushed and put down the tube. Always flush the tube before and after medication administration and when determining residual volume, so the tube remains patent and does not clog. If the tube becomes clogged, a new tube may have to be placed, which results in extra discomfort to the patient. It is important to note that these tubes can become dislodged, knotted, or kinked during patient coughing or vomiting. The gastrostomy tube, also known as the *percutaneous endoscopic gastrostomy* (PEG) tube, and the jejunostomy (J) tube are placed surgically, endoscopically, or radiologically. With the PEG tube, the patient must have an intact GI system. For patients with chronic reflux, a J-tube is placed either endoscopically or with laparoscopic surgery. Usually, the doctor orders intravenous (IV) antibiotics to decrease the risk of infection. After placement, always check your facility's policy before initiating the tube feeding, and use correct nursing procedure when putting medication and food through the tubes. Before the initial feeding, the policy in most facilities is to confirm correct placement of the tube with an x-ray.

Enteral Solutions

Many different types of enteral formulas are used for enteral feedings. These solutions differ according to their various nutrients, caloric values, and osmolality. The four groups of enteral solutions are (1) polymeric; (2) modular components; (3) semi-elemental or elemental; and (4) specialty formulas designed to meet specific nutritional needs

in certain illnesses such as diabetes, renal, respiratory, oncology, etc. (Table 14.1). Some of the modular components of enteral solutions include (1) carbohydrates in the form of dextrose, sucrose, lactose, starch, or dextrin (the first three are simple sugars that are absorbed quickly); (2) protein in the form of intact or hydrolyzed proteins or free amino acids; and (3) lipids in the form of corn, soybean, or safflower oil (some have a higher oil content than others). With all EN, sufficient water is needed to maintain hydration.

Methods for Delivery

Enteral feedings are given by continuous infusion pump, intermittent infusion by gravity, intermittent bolus by syringe, and cyclic feedings by infusion pump. Continuous feedings are prescribed for the critically ill and for those who receive feedings into the small intestine. The enteral feedings are given by an infusion pump, which is set to control the flow at a slow rate over 24 hours. Intermittent enteral feedings are administered every 3 to 6 hours over 30 to 60 minutes by gravity drip or infusion pump. At each feeding, 300 to 400 mL of solution is administered. Intermittent infusion is considered an inexpensive method for administering EN. The bolus method was the first method used to deliver enteral feedings, and with this method, 250 to 400 mL of solution is rapidly administered through a syringe into the tube four to six times a day. This method takes about 15 minutes each feeding, but it may not be tolerated well by the patient because a massive volume of solution is given in a short period. The bolus method may cause nausea, vomiting, aspiration, abdominal cramping, and diarrhea. This method is usually reserved for ambulatory individuals. The cyclic method is another type of continuous feeding infused over 8 to 16 hours daily (day or night). Administration during daytime hours is suggested for patients who are restless or for those who have a greater risk for aspiration. The nighttime schedule allows more freedom during the day for patients who are ambulatory.

Complications

Dehydration can occur in patients receiving EN. Diarrhea is a common complication that can lead to dehydration. High-protein formulas can also cause dehydration, and hyperosmolar solutions can draw water

TABLE 14.1 Preparations for Enteral Feeding

Category	Characteristics	Recommended Usage
Polymeric • Isotonic • High protein • High energy • Fiber content	Mimics macronutrients as found in whole food Available with different protein contents, energy densities, and fiber Meets RDA or micronutrients in 1–1.5 L/day	Isotonic, polymeric formula is regarded as a safe option when initiating enteral feeding Supplements prescribed for patients without malabsorptive disorders Fiber can be added to decrease incidence of diarrhea May be used as tube feeding, meal replacement, or oral supplement Blenderized forms are infrequently used because they are more likely to clog the feeding tubes because of their high viscosity
Modular	Carbohydrates Protein Lipid	Contains specific nutrients, usually a single macronutrient (carbohydrates, proteins, or lipids) Tailored to the individual's needs
Semi-elemental or elemental	Macronutrients are hydrolyzed to aid in absorption Available in different energy and protein densities	Patients with impaired GI functioning/malabsorption Patients post GI surgery with reduced nutrient absorption capability and/or prolonged bowel rest Patients with pancreatic dysfunction
Specialty formulas • Diabetes • Renal (low sodium) • Respiratory • Oncology/immune modulating	Modified macronutrient composition to promote glycemic control Available in different energy and protein products Polymeric formula with reduced sodium content Higher energy and protein content to limit excessive fluid administration Modified macronutrient content to reduce CO_2 production Contains omega-3-fatty acids for antiinflammatory properties Contains pharmacologically active substances aimed at modulating the immune response and improving outcome	Used for patients with diabetes mellitus, if adequate blood glucose control cannot be achieved through polymeric formula Uses high fiber and fat content products in patients with gastroparesis For use in patients with persistent hypernatremia Patients with renal impairment can be managed with polymeric products with added protein content Should be used with caution in critically ill, septic patients, due to immune-nutritional components Used in patients with excess CO_2 production Potential benefit of patients undergoing elective surgery; however, cannot be recommended for routine use among critically ill patients

CO_2, Carbon dioxide; *GI*, gastrointestinal; *L*, liter; *RDA*, recommended dietary allowance.
Data from http://www.nutritioncare/aspen.org and http://www.saspen.com/Websites/saspen/files/Content/6280465/1252-8445-1-PB.pdf.

out of the cells to maintain serum osmolality. Fluid intake is monitored, and if appropriate, fluid is added to the patient's daily regimen of feedings. Unless contraindicated, it is recommended that 30 to 35 mL/kg/day be maintained for fluid balance in most patients.

Aspiration pneumonitis is one of the most serious and potentially life-threatening complications of tube feedings. It can occur when the contents of the tube feeding enter the patient's lungs from the GI tract. Consequences range from coughing and wheezing to infection, tissue necrosis, and respiratory failure. An important nursing intervention is to check the agency's policy for specific guidelines before initiating EN. It is imperative that the nurse check for gastric residual by gently aspirating the stomach contents before initiating enteral feeding and thereafter every 4 hours between feedings. Usually, if the residual is greater than 150 mL (check the agency policy), the nurse will hold the feeding, and the residual is checked again in 1 hour. If the residual still exceeds this amount, the provider is notified. Large residuals mean the patient may have an obstruction and is not digesting the feeding. This is important to correct before continuing the feeding.

Another common problem of enteral feeding is diarrhea. Rapid administration of feedings, contamination of the formula, low-fiber formulas, tube movement, and various drugs can all cause diarrhea. Check for drugs that can cause diarrhea; these may be antibiotics or sorbitol in liquid medications. Diarrhea can usually be managed or corrected by decreasing the rate of infusion, diluting the solution with water, changing the solution, discontinuing the drug, increasing the patient's daily water intake, or administering an enteral solution that contains fiber. Constipation is another common problem that frequently occurs. It can be easily corrected by changing the formula, increasing water, or requesting a laxative.

Monitoring is essential when the patient is receiving EN. Recommended parameters to monitor include blood chemistry, blood urea nitrogen (BUN), creatinine, and electrolytes; glucose; triglycerides; serum proteins; intake and output; and weight. Frequency of monitoring is patient dependent and should be implemented during the entire EN process.

Enteral Safety

The nurse has an important role in administering tube feedings safely. Some of the important safety concerns are patient position, aspiration risk, residual volumes, and tube position. Following are important safety pointers for patients receiving enteral nutrition.

• The head of the bed should be elevated to 30 to 45 degrees during the feeding, and if intermittent, keep the head of the bed elevated for 30 to 60 minutes after the feeding. By elevating the head of the bed, the risk of aspiration is decreased.

- Ensure the patient has audible bowel sounds by performing a GI assessment with auscultation. This ensures a working GI tract.
- Always check the gastric residual volume before initiating tube feedings and every 4 to 6 hours if the feedings are continuous.
- Confirm the position of the newly inserted tubing before beginning the initial feeding. This is a required policy for most agencies.
- Initially, after the tube is placed, most agencies require an x-ray to confirm placement. Always follow the agency's policy and procedure for initial confirmation of placement.
- Before each enteral feeding, the nurse should check placement to confirm the tubing has not moved or shifted from the GI tract. Some agencies require pH testing of gastric secretions, whereas others recommend listening for gurgling sounds after inserting air into the tubing. Each of these measures has limitations, so more than one bedside test may be used for confirmation. Check the agency's guidelines.

The American Society for Parenteral and Enteral Nutrition (ASPEN) works to improve the quality of nutrition through its guidelines and standards. ASPEN advocates for high-priority issues about nutrition. They work in conjunction with the National Institutes of Health (NIH) and the Center for Medicare and Medicaid Services (CMS) to improve funding and education in the field of enteral and parenteral nutrition (PN). ASPEN was first to issue guidelines for the use of parenteral and enteral nutrition in adults and pediatric populations, and it continues to update, educate, and monitor use of safe practices. Another agency that advocates for safety in both EN and PN is the National Institute for Health and Care Excellence (NICE), which dedicates itself to the practice of health care in society and provides guidance and quality standards for public health care issues that include but are not limited to EN and PN. NICE set the standard that all patients should be screened for malnutrition and treated by a multidisciplinary team of health care professionals. It also stipulates that patients and caregivers should be given adequate training for self-care if they so desire.

The Joint Commission issued an alert on the seriousness of tube misconnections, which can result in severe injury or death to the patient. One situation involved a feeding administration tube that was inadvertently connected to a tracheostomy tube, which caused serious harm to the patient. It is most important to trace all lines from the site of origin back to the patient to avoid dislodgement and misconnection errors.

◎ CLINICAL JUDGMENT [NURSING PROCESS]

Enteral Nutrition

Concept: Caring Intervention

- Caring interventions are interventions performed by the nurse, so the nurse can perform care for the physical and emotional needs of the clients and families. These interventions help the nurse achieve specific patient outcomes, and they are based on the professional guidelines of nursing practice.

Recognize Cues [Assessment]

- Confirm the feeding tube is securely in place.
- Assess the patient's tolerance of enteral feeding, including possible gastrointestinal (GI) disturbance (nausea, cramping, diarrhea).
- Determine urine output and record it for future comparisons.
- Obtain the patient's weight and use it for future comparisons.
- Listen for bowel sounds. Report diminished or absent bowel sounds immediately to the health care provider. Also palpate the abdomen for distension.
- Assess baseline laboratory values and compare these with future laboratory results.

Analyze Cues and Prioritize Hypothesis [Patient Problems]

- Dysphagia
- Dehydration
- Diarrhea
- Constipation

Generate Solutions [Planning]

- The patient will not aspirate during enteral feedings, especially those given via GI route.
- The patient will receive adequate nutritional support through enteral feedings.
- The patient will be free from complications of diarrhea.

Take Action [Nursing Interventions]

- Perform hand hygiene and apply clean gloves.
- Check the tube placement by aspirating gastric secretions or by injecting air into the tube to listen by stethoscope for air movement in the stomach. (Follow agency guidelines.)
- Determine gastric residual before the enteral feeding. When the residual is more than 100 to 150 mL, hold the feeding for 1 hour and recheck the residual.

If it is still more than 100 to 150 mL, notify the health care provider. (Always check your agency's policy.)

- Check the continuous route for gastric residual every 4 to 6 hours.
- Always raise the head of the bed to a 30- to 45-degree angle during infusion of feedings. If elevating the head of the bed is contraindicated, position the patient on the right side.
- Deliver enteral feedings according to the method ordered: bolus, continuous, intermittent, or cyclic.
- Flush the feeding tube as appropriate: for intermittent feeding, flush with 30 mL before and after; for continuous feeding, flush with 30 mL every 4 hours. When administering drugs through the tube, use a 30-mL flush of water at the beginning and end of administration; flush with 15 mL of water between administration of each drug.
- Monitor for adverse effects of enteral feedings, such as diarrhea. To manage or correct diarrhea, decrease the enteral feeding flow rate, and as diarrhea lessens, slowly increase the feeding rate. The enteral solution may be diluted, with the provider's order, and then gradually increased to full strength. Determine whether side effects of drugs could be causing diarrhea.
- Monitor vital signs and report abnormal findings.
- Give additional water during the day to prevent dehydration. Consult with the health care provider.
- Weigh the patient to determine weight gain or loss. Compare with the patient's baseline weight. Patients should be weighed at the same time each day with the same scale and the same amount of clothing.
- Change the feeding bag daily. Do not add the new solution to the old solution in the feeding bag. The nutritional solution should be at room temperature.
- Use an interpreter if patient has a language barrier.

Patient Teaching

- Instruct patients to report any problems related to enteral feedings, such as diarrhea, sore throat, and abdominal cramping.

Evaluate Outcomes [Evaluation]

- Determine that the patient is receiving the prescribed nutrients daily and is free of complications associated with enteral feedings.

Enteral Medications

Many mistakes can occur during enteral tube feedings. These mistakes are often the result of administering drugs that are incompatible with administration through a tube, failure to prepare the drug properly, and use of faulty techniques. These problems can result in an occluded feeding tube, reduced drug effect, or drug toxicity and can cause patient harm or death.

When administering nonliquid drugs through an enteral tube, the nurse should always ensure that the drug is crushable. (For a current and complete listing of drugs that should not be crushed, see http://www.ismp.org/tools/donotcrush.pdf or consult with a pharmacist.) Also, validate with the pharmacist that the drug will dissolve in water and that it can be absorbed through the enteral route. Drugs that cannot be dissolved are timed-release, enteric-coated, and sublingual forms and bulk-forming laxatives; these medications should *not* be crushed. Prepare each medication separately so that the medication is identifiable up until the time of delivery. Open capsules separately and check with the pharmacist about whether the capsule contents can be crushed. Crush the solid dosage forms after ensuring the medications are crushable, and dissolve each medication separately in about 15 mL of water. The drug must be in liquid form or dissolved in water before administration through enteral tubing. Properly dilute liquid medication with water when administering it through the feeding tube. *Never* mix medications with feeding formulas. Before and after the drug is administered, flush with about 15 mL of water. Proper flushing ensures that the drug has been delivered and the tube is clear. Once the tube has been flushed, the feeding can be restarted after the drug is given.

Many drugs can be given to patients who require tube feeding to aid in absorption and digestion and to promote gastric emptying; these include pancreatic enzymes, probiotics, antiemetics, proton pump inhibitors, and drugs to prevent gastric ulcers.

It is essential to know the importance of temporarily stopping the infusion when certain types of drugs are administered. Some medications require that the feeding is stopped for as long as 30 minutes to allow for adequate absorption.

Parenteral Nutrition

The terms parenteral nutrition, total parenteral nutrition, and hyperalimentation (HA) are used synonymously. PN is the administration of nutrients by a route other than the GI tract (e.g., the bloodstream). If a patient is not eligible for EN because of a nonfunctioning GI tract or intestinal failure, PN is delivered intravenously. The word "total" suggests that the patient is receiving all of the required nutrients, fluid, and electrolyte requirements in the bag. In some circumstances, PN and EN may be given concurrently. The delivery of both EN and PN is used when the GI tract is partially functioning or if the patient is being weaned off of PN. PN has many risks, so the option of EN should be fully explored before starting PN. Suggested indications for patients who require PN are those with bowel obstruction, prolonged paralytic ileus, inflammatory bowel disease, or severe pancreatitis, and those who require bowel rest after complex GI surgery. Also, patients with greater nutritional needs sometimes require PN, such as those who have sustained severe trauma or burns and the severely malnourished.

Solutions for PN include amino acids, carbohydrates, electrolytes, fats, trace elements, vitamins, and water. PN is individualized according to the patient's general health. Each element of the prescription can be manipulated according to changes in the patient's clinical requirements. The entire process requires a multidisciplinary team approach that involves the nurse, nutritionist, and pharmacist with the patient's provider leading the care team. Commercially prepared PN base solutions are available and contain dextrose and protein in the form of amino acids. The pharmacist can add prescribed electrolytes, vitamins, and trace elements to customize the solution to meet the patient's needs. Calories are provided by carbohydrates in the form of dextrose and by fat in the form of fat emulsion. Carbohydrates provide 60% to 70% of calorie (energy) needs. Amino acids (proteins) provide about 3.5% to 20% of a patient's energy needs. PN has a high glucose concentration. Fat emulsion (lipid) therapy provides an increased number of calories, usually 30%, and is a carrier of fat-soluble vitamins. The recommended energy intake is 25 to 35 cal/kg/day in a nonobese patient. Solutions differ for pediatric patients, who have varied fluid needs and require more energy per kilogram.

High glucose concentrations are irritating to peripheral veins, so PN is administered through either a peripherally inserted central catheter (PICC) via the cephalic or basilica vein, or a central venous catheter via the subclavian or internal jugular vein; this depends on the tonicity of the concentration. The rapid blood flow of the central veins allows placement of the catheter in the vena cava, which has the greatest blood flow of any vein in the body and reduces the risk of thrombophlebitis. If the treatment is used for short-term therapy (<4 weeks), a PICC line is inserted. If the treatment will last longer than 4 weeks, a central line catheter is placed. PN must always be administered by an infusion pump to allow for an accurate flow rate. PN enhances wound healing and provides the necessary nutrients to prevent cellular catabolism. Policies and procedures for PN therapy may vary by region and facility and must be researched and followed accordingly.

Complications

Complications associated with PN can result from catheter insertion and PN infusion. See Table 14.2 for a list of PN complications.

Air embolism occurs when air enters into the central line catheter system. To prevent air embolism during dressing, cap, and tubing changes, ask the patient to turn his or her head in the opposite direction of the insertion site and to take a deep breath, hold it, and bear down. This is called the Valsalva maneuver, and it will increase intrathoracic venous pressure while preventing the risk of air embolism. Always keep the clamp on the central line tubing closed except when in use.

Use strict aseptic technique when changing IV tubing and dressings at the insertion site. PN solution has a high concentration of glucose and is an excellent medium for bacterial growth. Monitor the patient's temperature closely, and if fever occurs, suspect sepsis. Always follow the facility's policy for the correct protocol in changing the PN solutions (12 to 24 hours), IV tubing (24 hours), and central line dressing (48 hours). Keep the prepared PN solutions refrigerated, and administer the full amount within the designated time according to the agency's policy.

Hyperglycemia occurs primarily because of the hypertonic dextrose solution, but it also occurs when the infusion rate for PN is too rapid. In some cases the pharmacist can add insulin to the PN solution if ordered by the provider. Assess the patient carefully for glucose intolerance. The infusion is started at a slow rate of 40 to 60 mL/h as prescribed. Monitor the patient's blood glucose level every 4 to 6 hours until stable and then every 24 hours or according to the facility's policy. Many providers will order sliding-scale insulin for their patients receiving PN.

The sudden interruption of PN therapy can cause hypoglycemia; therefore it is wise to keep a bag of 10% dextrose in the patient's room. If the next bag of PN is late in arriving from the pharmacy, the bag of dextrose can be hung to avoid hypoglycemia. Gradually decrease the infusion rate when PN is discontinued, and monitor the patient's blood glucose level.

TABLE 14.2 Complications of Total Parenteral Nutrition

Complication	Explanation/Cause	Symptoms
Catheter Insertion		
Pneumothorax	An abnormal collection of air or gas in the pleural space that causes the lung to collapse **Cause:** Punctured lung or lung injury during procedure or trauma	Sharp chest pain, decreased breath sounds, tachycardia, absence of breath sounds on the affected side
Hemothorax	A collection of blood in the space between the chest wall and the lung (the pleural cavity) **Cause:** Trauma is the most common cause	Anxiety; chest pain; low blood pressure; pale, cool, and clammy skin; rapid heart rate; rapid, shallow breathing; restlessness; shortness of breath
Total Parenteral Nutrition Infusion		
Air embolism	A pathologic condition caused by a gas bubble in the vascular system **Cause:** Disconnected IV tubing; the catheter system opens, and air enters IV tubing during changes	Coughing, shortness of breath, chest pain, cyanosis, hypotension, apprehension
Infection	The result of the body's inability to fight off foreign microorganisms that may cause damage or disease if left untreated **Cause:** Poor aseptic technique or catheter or solution contamination	Fever/temperature greater than 100°F (37.7°C), chills, increased WBC, redness or drainage
Hyperglycemia	High blood glucose **Cause:** Fluid infused too rapidly, insufficient insulin coverage, infection	Nausea, headache, weakness, thirst, elevated blood glucose (>200 mg/dL), restlessness, confusion, Kussmaul respirations
Hypoglycemia	Low blood glucose **Cause:** Fluids discontinued abruptly, too much insulin being administered	Diaphoresis, shakiness, weakness, low blood glucose level (<70 mg/dL), hunger, anxiety
Hypervolemia	Condition characterized by excessive fluid volume **Cause:** Increased IV rate, renal dysfunction, heart failure, hepatic failure	Weight gain greater than desired; jugular venous distension; full, bounding pulse; lung crackles; headache; hypertension

C, Centigrade; *F*, Fahrenheit; *IV*, intravenous; *mg/dL*, milligrams per deciliter; *WBC*, white blood cell.

◎ CLINICAL JUDGMENT [NURSING PROCESS]

Total Parenteral Nutrition

Concept: Caring Intervention
- Caring interventions are interventions performed by the nurse, so the nurse can perform care for the physical and emotional needs of the clients and families. These interventions help the nurse achieve specific patient outcomes, and they are based on the professional guidelines of nursing practice.

Recognize Cues [Assessment]
- Obtain baseline vital signs for future comparisons.
- Confirm baseline weight.
- Determine laboratory results (electrolytes, glucose, protein [prealbumin], and white blood cell levels frequently change during parenteral [PN] therapy). Early laboratory results are useful for future comparisons.
- Check urine output and report abnormal findings.
- Carefully read the label on the bag of PN solution. Compare the ingredients with the health care provider's order.
- Assess the PN insertion site for erythema, edema, swelling, tenderness, and drainage.

Analyze Cues and Prioritize Hypothesis [Patient Problems]
- Decreased gas exchange
- Disrupted fluid and electrolyte balance
- Dehydration
- Wound infection
- Need for health teaching

Generate Solutions [Planning]
- The patient's nutrient needs will be met via PN by patient achieving a weight gain of 3 to 5 lb.
- Refrigerate PN solution that is not in use. Because of its high glucose concentration, the formula is an excellent medium for bacterial growth. Always check your agency's policy concerning storing of PN.
  - Avoid infection by closely monitoring the patient's temperature and ensuring a normal temperature is maintained (98.6°F [37°C]).
  - Do not draw blood from or administer medications through the central line, and do not check central venous pressure via the PN line. Results could be invalid.

Take Action [Nursing Interventions]
- Maintain sterile technique when accessing central line.
- Perform a full set of vital signs and report changes.
- Determine body weight and compare it with the baseline weight.
- Monitor lab results—especially hematology labs, electrolytes, protein, and glucose—and report abnormal findings.
- Compare laboratory results with baseline findings to assess any changes.
- Measure fluid intake and output. Volume deficit or excess may occur due to the hyperosmolar content of the PN solution.
- Monitor temperature changes for possible infection or a febrile state. Use aseptic technique when changing dressings and solution bags.

◎ CLINICAL JUDGMENT [NURSING PROCESS]—CONT'D

Total Parenteral Nutrition

- Check the blood glucose level according to your agency's policy. Initially, glucose levels may be high.
- Monitor the flow rate of PN. Start with 60 to 80 mL/h, and increase slowly to the ordered level to avoid hyperglycemia.
- If PN finishes before the next time it is due to be administered, hang a bag of dextrose 10% to avoid hypoglycemia.
- During tubing and dressing changes, have the patient perform a Valsalva maneuver (taking a deep breath, holding it, and bearing down). Always clamp tubing during bag and tubing changes to prevent air embolus.
- Check for signs and symptoms of overhydration—coughing, dyspnea, engorged neck veins, or chest rhonchi—and report any findings.
- Follow your agency's policy for dressing and tubing changes.
- Respect the patient's beliefs about refusing PN.
- Explain reasons for adequate nutrition, and find ways to meet nutritional needs.
- Use an interpreter as appropriate if a language barrier exists.

Patient Teaching

- Provide emotional support to patients and family before and during PN therapy.
- Be available to discuss the patient's concerns or refer the patient to the appropriate health care provider.
- Instruct patients to notify their health care provider immediately if they experience discomfort or reactions.
- Keep the patient informed of the progress and effectiveness of PN.

Evaluate Outcomes [Evaluation]

- Evaluate the patient's positive and negative response to PN therapy.
- Determine periodically whether the patient's serum electrolytes, protein, and glucose levels are within desired ranges.
- Evaluate nutritional status by weight changes, energy level, feelings of well-being, symptom control, and healing.
- Evaluate patient and family understanding of the purpose and possible complications of PN therapy.

CRITICAL THINKING SINGLE EPISODE CASE STUDY

Cognitive Skill: Prioritize hypothesis (Cloze)

Objective: Prioritize care for a patient with a central line receiving parenteral nutrition (PN).

A 50-year-old female patient who hasn't eaten in five days after complex GI surgery has received a central line and an order for parenteral nutrition. The nurse reviews the patient's morning labs and notes the patient has a potassium level of 3.2 mEq/L. Choose the priority nursing interventions for the information missing from the statements below by selecting from the list of options provided.

Upon receipt of the PN order, the nurse reviews the label of contents to confirm ___(1)___ is included in the bag. Next, a full set of vital signs is performed including ___(1)___ and _____(1)_____. The nurse assesses the central line for patency while maintaining _____(1)_____. The nurse instructs the patient on how to perform the _____(2)_____ and explains this is always done when accessing the central line prior to hanging the PN and when tubing is changed because it prevents the risk of _____(2)_____. Finally, the patient is instructed to notify the nurse if they begin to experience _____(2)_____, _____(2)_____, or _____(2)_____.

Options for 1	Options for 2
Sodium	Coughing
Aseptic technique	Valsalva maneuver
Potassium	Fatigue
Weight	Air embolism
Temperature	Dry skin
Vitamin B complex	Shortness of breath
Clean technique	Nausea
Apical pulse	Chest pain
Magnesium	Increase in mucous secretion

Answers:

Upon receipt of parenteral nutrition, the nurse reviews the label of contents to confirm potassium is included in the bag of PN. Next, a full set of vital signs is performed including temperature and weight. The nurse assesses the central line for patency while maintaining aseptic technique. The nurse instructs the patient on how to perform the Valsalva maneuver and explains this is always done when accessing the central line prior to hanging the PN and when tubing is changed because it prevents the risk of air embolism. Finally, the patient is instructed to notify the nurse if they begin to experience coughing, shortness of breath, or chest pain.

Rationale:

The nurse should carefully read the label on the bag of PN solution and compare the electrolyte ingredients to the patient's most current laboratory results. This patient has a low potassium level of 3.2 mEq/L. The nurse would expect to see potassium included on the PN label. Sodium, vitamin B complex, and magnesium are not indicated for this patient. Always maintain excellent aseptic technique when changing IV tubing and dressings at the insertion site. PN solution has a high concentration of glucose and is a medium for bacterial growth, which can result in infection. Instruct the patient in the Valsalva maneuver, which can prevent air embolism. The patient is asked to turn their head in the opposite direction of the insertion site and take a deep breath, hold it, and bear down. This increases intrathoracic venous pressure while preventing the risk of air embolism. Air embolism is a condition caused by a gas bubble that enters the vascular system. This can easily occur when the catheter system is open to hang a new bag of PN or change the tubing. Symptoms of air embolism include coughing, shortness of breath, and chest pain. Fatigue, dry skin, nausea, and increase in mucous secretions are not symptoms related to air embolism.

Reference:

Chapter 14, pgs 163-169, Table 14.2, Clinical Judgment [Nursing Process] page 168; Lewis, et al 10th ed., Medical Surgical Nursing, Ch39 pgs 869-871.

REVIEW QUESTIONS

1. The nurse is determining a patient's gastric residual before administering an enteral feeding; the last feeding was 240 mL. The patient will be discharged on enteral feedings. It is important to include in the teaching plan that a residual of more than which amount would indicate delayed gastric emptying (based on the last feeding)?
   a. 60 mL
   b. 125 mL
   c. 150 mL
   d. 75 mL

2. What are the four categories for enteral nutrition formulas? (Select all that apply.)
   a. Macro formula
   b. Elemental or semi-elemental formula
   c. Malabsorptive formula
   d. Diabetes specialty formula
   e. Polymeric formula
   f. Modular formula
   g. Nutrient formula

3. The nurse is reviewing the plan of care for a patient receiving enteral therapy. What is the most common complication of enteral therapy?
   a. Aspiration
   b. Constipation
   c. Diarrhea
   d. Muscle weakness

4. Which is appropriate nursing care for a patient receiving total parenteral nutrition (TPN) in an acute care setting? (Select all that apply.)
   a. Monitor patient's blood glucose level.
   b. Measure patient's fluid intake and output closely.
   c. Administer blood through the TPN line.
   d. Monitor the TPN insertion site for erythema.
   e. Monitor the patient's monthly weight.
   f. Sterile technique isn't necessary when accessing the patient's central TPN line.
   g. Determining a baseline weight of the patient prior to TPN is not important.

5. A patient has been on TPN for 1 month, and there is an order to discontinue TPN tomorrow. The nurse contacts the health care provider because sudden interruption of TPN therapy may cause which condition?
   a. Dehydration
   b. Tremors
   c. Urinary retention
   d. Hypoglycemia

6. A patient is receiving TPN at home. The visiting nurse assists the family with the care plan, which includes changing the TPN solution and tubing. What is the recommended initial frequency for changing the tubing?
   a. Every 24 hours
   b. Every 36 hours
   c. Every 48 hours
   d. Every 72 hours

7. The nurse is reviewing the care plan with a patient using enteral nutrition (EN). Which interventions by the nurse are appropriate for this strategy? (Select all that apply.)
   a. Check the continuous route for gastric residual every 2 to 4 hours.
   b. Elevate the bed to a 30- to 45-degree angle before administering EN.
   c. Change the enteral feeding bag and tubing every 3 to 4 days.
   d. Report absent bowel sounds to the health care provider.
   e. Explain that diarrhea is never a result of the EN therapy.
   f. Assessing patient's blood pressure is unnecessary.
   g. Additional water administration is not required.

8. The nurse is to administer enteral medications to a patient who cannot swallow and is receiving continuous enteral feedings. Which is correct concerning administration of the enteral medications?
   a. All ordered medications are added to the enteral feeding solution.
   b. Dilute liquid medications before administering through the feeding tube.
   c. Extra amounts of water are used to dissolve timed-release medications.
   d. Undiluted hyperosmolar medications may be given to patients on fluid restriction.

15

Adrenergic Agonists and Antagonists

http://evolve.elsevier.com/McCuistion/pharmacology

OBJECTIVES

- Explain major responses to stimulation of adrenergic receptors.
- Differentiate between selective and nonselective adrenergic agonists.
- Contrast the uses of alpha and beta antagonists.
- Compare general side effects of adrenergic agonists and adrenergic antagonists.

- Describe nursing interventions, including patient teaching, associated with adrenergic agonists and adrenergic antagonists.
- Apply the Clinical Judgment [Nursing Process] for the patient taking beta-adrenergic antagonists.
- Compare the indications of adrenergic agonists and adrenergic antagonists.

OUTLINE

This chapter discusses two groups of drugs that affect the sympathetic nervous system—adrenergic agonists, or sympathomimetics, and *adrenergic antagonists,* also called *adrenergic blockers* or sympatholytics—along with their dosages and uses.

The *central nervous system* (CNS) is the body's primary nervous system and consists of the brain and spinal cord. The *peripheral nervous system* (PNS), located outside the brain and spinal cord, is made up of two divisions: the autonomic and the somatic. After interpretation by the CNS, the PNS receives stimuli and initiates responses to these stimuli.

The *autonomic nervous system* (ANS), also called the *visceral system,* acts on smooth muscles and glands. Its functions include control and regulation of the heart, respiratory system, gastrointestinal (GI) tract, bladder, eyes, and glands. The ANS is an involuntary nervous system, over which we have little or no control: we breathe, our hearts beat, and peristalsis continues without our realizing it. However, unlike the ANS, the *somatic nervous system* is a voluntary system that innervates skeletal muscles, over which there is control.

The two sets of neurons in the autonomic component of the PNS are the (1) afferent, or *sensory,* neurons and the (2) efferent, or *motor,* neurons. The *afferent neurons* send impulses to the CNS, where they are interpreted. The *efferent neurons* receive the impulses (information) from the brain and transmit these impulses through the spinal cord to the effector organ cells. The efferent pathways in the ANS are divided into two branches: the sympathetic and the parasympathetic nerves. Collectively, these two branches are called the *sympathetic nervous system* and the *parasympathetic nervous system* (Fig. 15.1).

The sympathetic and parasympathetic nervous systems act on the same organs but produce opposite responses to provide homeostasis (balance; Fig. 15.2). Drugs act on the sympathetic and parasympathetic nervous systems by either stimulating or depressing responses.

SYMPATHETIC NERVOUS SYSTEM

The sympathetic nervous system is also called the *adrenergic system.* *Norepinephrine* is the neurotransmitter that innervates smooth muscle. The adrenergic receptor organ cells are of four types: alpha$_1$, alpha$_2$, beta$_1$, and beta$_2$ (Fig. 15.3). Norepinephrine is released from the terminal nerve ending and stimulates the cell receptors to produce a response.

ADRENERGIC AGONISTS

Drugs that stimulate the sympathetic nervous system are called *adrenergic agonists, adrenergics,* or *sympathomimetics* because they mimic

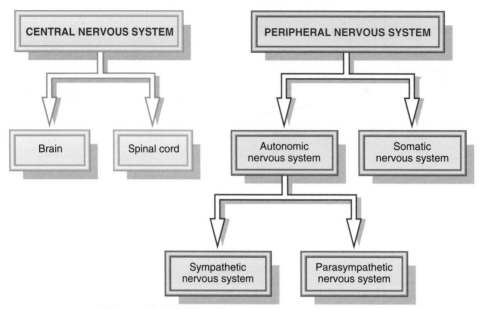

Fig. 15.1 Subdivisions of the peripheral nervous system.

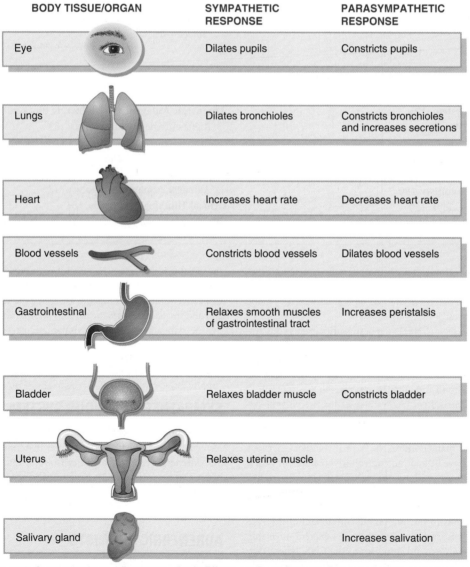

BODY TISSUE/ORGAN	SYMPATHETIC RESPONSE	PARASYMPATHETIC RESPONSE
Eye	Dilates pupils	Constricts pupils
Lungs	Dilates bronchioles	Constricts bronchioles and increases secretions
Heart	Increases heart rate	Decreases heart rate
Blood vessels	Constricts blood vessels	Dilates blood vessels
Gastrointestinal	Relaxes smooth muscles of gastrointestinal tract	Increases peristalsis
Bladder	Relaxes bladder muscle	Constricts bladder
Uterus	Relaxes uterine muscle	
Salivary gland		Increases salivation

Fig. 15.2 Sympathetic and Parasympathetic Effects on Body Tissues. The sympathetic and parasympathetic nervous systems have opposite responses on body tissues and organs.

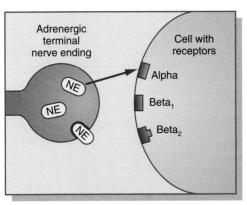

Fig. 15.3 Sympathetic transmitters and receptors. *NE*, norepinephrine.

TABLE 15.1	**Effects of Adrenergic Agonists at Receptors**
Receptor	**Physiologic Responses**
Alpha₁	Increases force of heart contraction; vasoconstriction increases blood pressure; mydriasis (dilation of pupils) occurs; secretion in salivary glands decreases; urinary bladder relaxation and urinary sphincter contraction increases
Alpha₂	Inhibits release of norepinephrine; dilates blood vessels; produces hypotension; decreases gastrointestinal motility and tone
Beta₁	Increases heart rate and force of contraction; increases renin secretion, which increases blood pressure
Beta₂	Dilates bronchioles; promotes gastrointestinal and uterine relaxation; promotes increase in blood glucose through glycogenolysis in the liver; increases blood flow in skeletal muscles

the sympathetic neurotransmitters norepinephrine and epinephrine. They act on one or more adrenergic receptor sites located in the effector cells of muscles such as the heart, bronchiole walls, GI tract, urinary bladder, and ciliary muscles of the eye. There are many adrenergic receptors. The four main receptors are alpha₁, alpha₂, beta₁, and beta₂, which mediate the major responses described in Table 15.1 and illustrated in Fig. 15.4.

The alpha-adrenergic receptors are located in the blood vessels, eyes, bladder, and prostate. When the alpha₁ receptors in vascular tissues (vessels) of muscles are stimulated, the arterioles and venules constrict; this increases peripheral resistance and blood return to the heart, circulation improves, and blood pressure is increased. When too much stimulation occurs, blood flow is decreased to the vital organs.

The alpha₂ receptors are located in the postganglionic sympathetic nerve endings. When stimulated, they inhibit the release of norepinephrine, which leads to a decrease in vasoconstriction. This results in vasodilation and a decrease in blood pressure.

The beta₁ receptors are located primarily in the heart but are also found in the kidneys. Stimulation of the beta₁ receptors increases myocardial contractility and heart rate.

The beta₂ receptors are found mostly in the smooth muscles of the lung and GI tract, the liver, and the uterine muscle. Stimulation of the beta₂ receptor causes (1) relaxation of the smooth muscles of the lungs, which results in bronchodilation; (2) a decrease in GI tone and motility; (3) activation of glycogenolysis in the liver and increased blood glucose; and (4) relaxation of the uterine muscle, which results in a decrease in uterine contraction (Fig. 15.5; see also Table 15.1).

Other adrenergic receptors are dopaminergic and are located in the renal, mesenteric, coronary, and cerebral arteries. When these receptors are stimulated, the vessels dilate and blood flow increases. Only dopamine can activate these receptors.

Inactivation of Neurotransmitters

After the neurotransmitter (e.g., norepinephrine) has performed its function, the action must be stopped to prevent prolonging the effect. Transmitters are inactivated by (1) *reuptake* of the transmitter back into the neuron (nerve cell terminal), (2) enzymatic *transformation* or degradation, and (3) *diffusion* away from the receptor. The mechanism of norepinephrine reuptake plays a more important role in inactivation than does the enzymatic action. After the reuptake of

the transmitter in the neuron, the transmitter may be degraded or reused. The two enzymes that inactivate norepinephrine are monoamine oxidase (MAO), which is *inside* the neuron, and catechol-O-methyltransferase (COMT), which is *outside* the neuron.

Drugs can prolong the action of the neurotransmitter (e.g., norepinephrine) by either inhibiting reuptake, which prolongs the action of the transmitter, or inhibiting the degradation by enzymatic action.

Classification of Sympathomimetics

The sympathomimetic (adrenergic agonist) drugs that stimulate adrenergic receptors are classified into three categories according to their effects on organ cells. Categories include (1) direct-acting sympathomimetics, which directly stimulate the adrenergic receptor (e.g., epinephrine or norepinephrine); (2) indirect-acting sympathomimetics, which stimulate the release of norepinephrine from the terminal nerve endings (e.g., amphetamine); and (3) mixed-acting (both direct- and indirect-acting) sympathomimetics, which stimulate the adrenergic receptor sites and stimulate the release of norepinephrine from the terminal nerve endings (e.g., ephedrine (Fig. 15.6).

Pseudoephedrine is an example of a mixed-acting sympathomimetic. It acts indirectly by stimulating the release of norepinephrine from the nerve terminals, and it acts directly on the alpha₁ and beta₁ receptors. Pseudoephedrine, like epinephrine, increases heart rate. It is not as potent a vasoconstrictor as epinephrine, and the risk of hemorrhagic stroke and hypertensive crisis is less. Pseudoephedrine, an over-the-counter (OTC) drug but controlled, is helpful to relieve nasal and sinus congestion without rebound congestion. This drug is contraindicated in hypertension, closed-angle glaucoma, bronchitis, emphysema, and urinary retention, and should be used with caution in diabetes mellitus.

Catecholamines are the chemical structures of a substance, either endogenous or synthetic, that can produce a sympathomimetic response. Examples of endogenous catecholamines are epinephrine, norepinephrine, and dopamine. The synthetic catecholamines are isoproterenol and dobutamine. Noncatecholamines such as phenylephrine, metaproterenol, and albuterol stimulate the adrenergic receptors. Most noncatecholamines have a longer duration of action than the endogenous or synthetic catecholamines.

Many of the adrenergic agonists stimulate more than one of the adrenergic receptor sites. An example is epinephrine, which acts on alpha₁-, beta₁-, and beta₂-adrenergic receptor sites. The responses from these receptor sites include increase in blood pressure, pupil dilation,

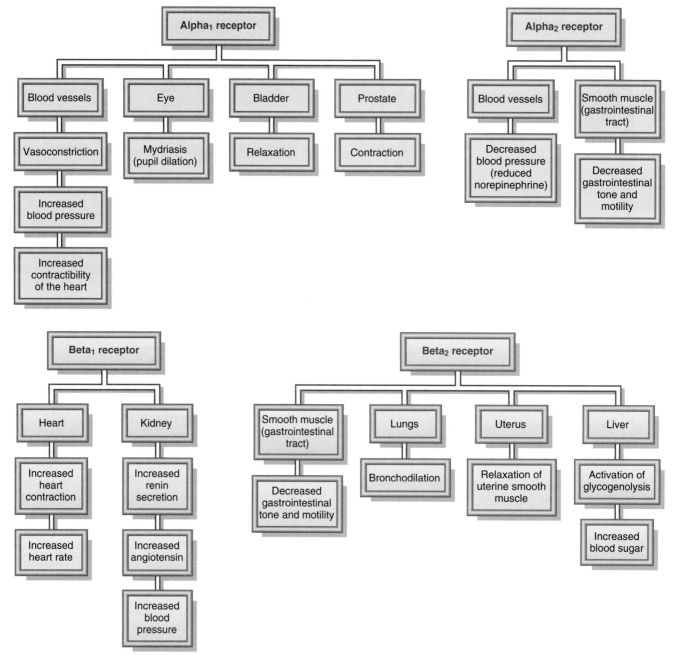

Fig. 15.4 Effects of activation of alpha$_1$, alpha$_2$, beta$_1$, and beta$_2$ receptors.

increase in heart rate (tachycardia), and bronchodilation. In anaphylactic shock, epinephrine is useful because it increases blood pressure, heart rate, and airflow through the lungs. Because epinephrine affects different adrenergic receptors, it is nonselective. Additional side effects result when more responses occur than are desired. Pseudoephedrine is commonly used for illegal production of amphetamine and methamphetamine. National regulatory measures control pseudoephedrine drug sales with individual limits of 3.6 g/day and 9 g within 30 days. Identifications are scanned with each purchase. The database is linked nationally and keeps a 2-year tally. **Prototype Drug Chart: Epinephrine** lists the pharmacologic behavior of epinephrine.

Albuterol sulfate, a beta$_2$-adrenergic agonist, is **selective** for beta$_2$-adrenergic receptors, so the response is relaxation of bronchial smooth muscle and bronchodilation to prevent and treat bronchospasm. A patient with asthma may tolerate albuterol better than isoproterenol, which activates beta$_1$ and beta$_2$ receptors, because albuterol's action is more selective; it activates only the beta$_2$ receptors of smooth muscle in the lungs and uterus, and in the vasculature that supplies the skeletal muscles. By using selective sympathomimetics, fewer undesired adverse effects will occur. However, high dosages of albuterol may affect beta$_1$ receptors, causing an increase in heart rate.

Tremors, headache, and nervousness are the most common side effects of oral or inhalation albuterol. Other side effects include tachycardia, palpitations, dizziness, dysrhythmia, nausea, vomiting, and urinary retention. Beta antagonists (beta blockers) may inhibit the action of albuterol.

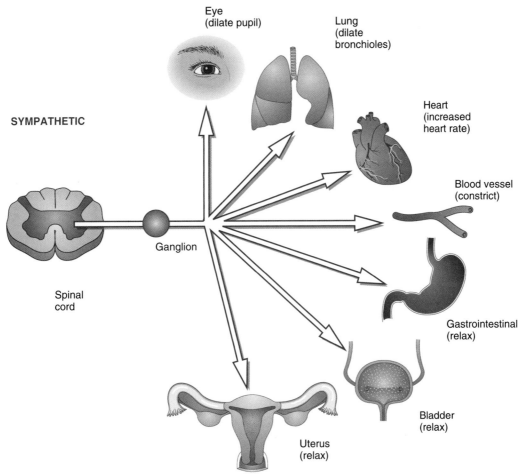

Fig. 15.5 Sympathetic Responses. Stimulation of the sympathetic nervous system or use of sympathomimetic (adrenergic agonist) drugs can cause the pupils and bronchioles to dilate, heart rate to increase, blood vessels to constrict, and muscles of the gastrointestinal tract, bladder, and uterus to relax, thereby decreasing contractions.

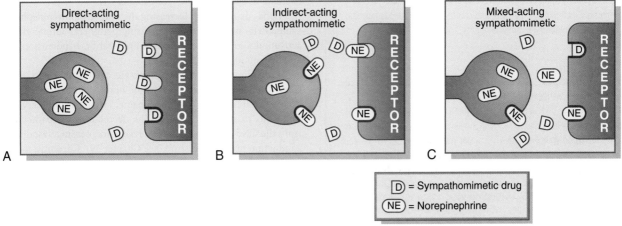

Fig. 15.6 (A) Direct-acting sympathomimetics. (B) Indirect-acting sympathomimetics. (C) Mixed-acting sympathomimetics.

📋 PROTOTYPE DRUG CHART

⚠ *Epinephrine*

Drug Class	Dosage
Sympathomimetic: adrenergic agonist	Anaphylaxis: A: IM/subcut: 0.3 mg EpiPen auto injector, may repeat in 5–20 min; *max:* 2 doses IV: 0.1–0.25 mg of 0.1 mg/mL solution, may repeat q5–15min PRN; may follow with 1–4 mcg/min infusion

Contraindications	Drug-Lab-Food Interactions
Caution: Parkinsonism, closed-angle glaucoma, cerebrovascular disease, labor, hypertension, cardiac disease, hyperthyroidism, diabetes mellitus, renal dysfunction, hypovolemia, renal disease, breastfeeding, pregnancy	Drug: Increased effects with TCAs and MAOIs; methyldopa and beta blockers antagonize epinephrine effects; digoxin may cause dysrhythmias with epinephrine Lab: Increased blood glucose, serum lactic acid

Pharmacokinetics	Pharmacodynamics
Absorption: Subcut/IM/IV: Rapidly; inactivated in GI tract Distribution: PB: UK Metabolism: t½: <5 min IV Excretion: In urine and breast milk	Subcut: Onset: 5–10 min Peak: 20 min Duration: 1–4 h IM: Onset: variable Duration: 1–4 h IV: Onset: Immediate Peak: 2–5 min Duration: 5–10 min Inhaled: Onset: 1 min Peak: 3–5 min Duration: 1–3 hours

Therapeutic Effects/Uses

To treat nasal congestion, allergic reaction, anaphylaxis, asthma exacerbation, bronchospasm, angioedema, status asthmaticus, cardiac arrest, cardiac resuscitation

Mechanism of Action: Acts on alpha and beta receptors; promotion of CNS and cardiac stimulation and bronchodilation; strengthens cardiac contraction, increases cardiac rate and cardiac output; reduces mucosal congestion by inhibiting histamine release; reverses anaphylactic reactions

Side Effects	Adverse Reactions
Nausea, vomiting, restlessness, tremor, agitation, headache, pallor, oliguria, weakness, dizziness, hypo/hyperglycemia, paresthesia	Palpitations, tachycardia, hypertension, dyspnea, MI, renal insufficiency, injection site reaction *Life threatening:* Dysrhythmias, pulmonary edema

<, Less than; *A,* adult; *CNS,* central nervous system; *GI,* gastrointestinal; *h,* hours; *IM,* intramuscular; *IV,* intravenous; *MAOI,* monoamine oxidase inhibitor; *max,* maximum; *min,* minute; *PB,* protein binding; *PRN,* as needed; *q5min,* every 5 minutes; *subcut,* subcutaneous; *t½,* half-life; *TCA,* tricyclic antidepressant; *UK,* unknown.

Epinephrine

Pharmacokinetics. Epinephrine is usually administered intramuscularly, intravenously, or endotracheally. It is not given orally because it is rapidly metabolized in the GI tract and liver, which results in unstable serum levels. Subcutaneous administration is not recommended as absorption is slower and less dependable for anaphylaxis. The half-life of epinephrine is less than 5 minutes intravenously (IV), and the percentage by which the drug is protein bound is unknown. Epinephrine is metabolized by the liver and is excreted in the urine.

Pharmacodynamics. Epinephrine is frequently used in emergencies to treat anaphylaxis, a life-threatening allergic response. Epinephrine is a potent inotropic (myocardial contraction-strengthening) drug that increases cardiac output, promotes vasoconstriction and systolic blood pressure elevation, increases heart rate, and produces bronchodilation. High doses can result in cardiac dysrhythmia, which necessitates electrocardiogram (ECG) monitoring. Epinephrine can also cause renal vasoconstriction, thereby decreasing renal perfusion and urinary output.

The onset of action and peak concentration times are rapid. The use of decongestants with epinephrine has an additive effect. When epinephrine is administered with digoxin, cardiac dysrhythmia may occur. Beta blockers can antagonize the action of epinephrine. Tricyclic antidepressants (TCAs) and monoamine oxidase inhibitors (MAOIs) allow epinephrine's effects to be intensified and prolonged.

Side Effects and Adverse Reactions

Undesired side effects frequently result when the adrenergic drug dosage is increased or when the drug is nonselective. Side effects commonly associated with adrenergic agonists include hypertension, tachycardia, palpitations, restlessness, tremors, dysrhythmia, dizziness, urinary retention, nausea, vomiting, dyspnea, and pulmonary edema.

Names of adrenergic drugs, the receptors they activate, dosage information, and common uses are listed in Table 15.2. Epinephrine is also discussed in Chapter 55 as one of the drugs used during emergencies.

CENTRAL-ACTING ALPHA AGONISTS

Clonidine and Methyldopa

Clonidine is a selective alpha₂-adrenergic agonist used primarily to treat hypertension. Alpha₂ drugs are central acting and produce vasodilation by stimulating alpha₂ receptors in the CNS, leading to a decrease in blood pressure (see Chapter 39).

Alpha₂ drugs act by decreasing the release of norepinephrine from sympathetic nerves and by decreasing peripheral adrenergic receptor activation. Clonidine may produce bradycardia, hypotension, sedation, and dry mouth at very low doses.

Methyldopa is an alpha-adrenergic agonist that acts within the CNS. This drug is taken up into the brain stem neurons and is converted to alpha-methylnorepinephrine, an alpha₂-adrenergic agonist that leads to alpha₂ activation. The decrease of sympathetic outflow from the CNS reduces peripheral resistance, causing vasodilation and a reduction in blood pressure (see Chapter 39). Currently, methyldopa is not used much as an antihypertensive due to the development of other antihypertensives that have fewer side effects.

Side Effects and Adverse Reactions

Additional undesired side effects of central-acting alpha-adrenergic agonists include headache, nasal congestion, drowsiness, nightmares, constipation, and edema. Ejaculation dysfunction and elevated hepatic enzymes may also occur.

⚠ TABLE 15.2 Adrenergic Agonists: Alpha₁, Beta₁, and Beta₂

Drug	Route and Dosage	Uses and Considerations
Epinephrine; alpha₁, beta₁, and beta₂	See Prototype Drug Chart: Epinephrine	
Ephedrine hydrochloride, ephedrine sulfate; alpha₁, beta₁, and beta₂	Hypotension: A: IV: 5–10 mg, may repeat PRN; *max:* 50 mg	For hypotension. May cause restlessness, headache, dizziness, dysrhythmia, bradycardia, tachycardia, hypertension, tolerance, tachyphylaxis, and palpitations. PB: UK; t½: 3–6 h
Norepinephrine bitartrate; alpha₁ and beta₁	Acute hypotension: A: IV: Initially 8–12 mcg/min inf, titrate to maintain adequate BP; *max:* 3.3 mcg/kg/min continuous infusion	For acute hypotension and cardiogenic and septic shock. Monitor blood pressure and rhythm every 2–5 min during infusion. May cause anxiety, headache, bradycardia, hypertension, pulmonary edema, dyspnea, and tissue necrosis. PB: 25%; t½: 2.4 minutes
Dopamine hydrochloride; alpha₁ and beta₁	A: IV/inf: Initially 2–5 mcg/kg/min; gradually increase; *maint:* 5–20 mcg/kg/min; *max:* 50 mcg/kg/min	For hypotension, heart failure, septic shock, and cardiogenic shock. May cause hypotension, hypertension, bradycardia, tachycardia, dysrhythmia, palpitations, headache, angina, dyspnea, nausea, vomiting, and tissue necrosis. PB: UK; t½: 2 min
Midodrine hydrochloride; alpha₁	A: PO: 10 mg tid; *max:* 30 mg/d	For orthostatic hypotension. Do not administer within 4 h of bedtime. May cause hypertension, paresthesias, pruritus, abdominal pain, urinary retention/urgency, dysuria, and piloerection. PB: UK; t½: 25 min
Phenylephrine hydrochloride; alpha₁	Nasal decongestion: A: PO: 10–20 mg q4–6h PRN; *max:* 60 mg/d Intranasal: A: 2–3 sprays each nostril q4h PRN; *max:* 3 sprays each nostril in 4-h period for 3 d	For sinus and nasal congestion, hypotension or shock, pupillary dilation. Have patient blow nose before drug is administered intranasally. May cause headache, blurred vision, nasal irritation, nausea, tachycardia, bradycardia, dysrhythmias, and tissue necrosis. PB: UK; t½: 2.1–3.4 h
Pseudoephedrine hydrochloride; alpha₁, alpha₂, and beta₁	Regular release: A: PO: 60 mg q4–6h; *max:* 240 mg/d 12 h Extended release: A: PO: 120 mg q12h; *max:* 240 mg/d 24 h Extended release: A: PO: 240 mg qd; *max:* 240 mg/d	For nasal congestion. May cause hypertension, tachycardia, palpitations, dizziness, headache, seizure, nausea, urinary retention, restlessness, insomnia, and dysrhythmias. PB: UK; t½: 9–16 h
Albuterol; beta₂	Bronchospasm prophylaxis: Immediate release: A: PO: 2–4 mg q6–8h; *max:* 32 mg/d Extended release: A: PO: 4–8 mg q12h; *max:* 32 mg/d	For prophylaxis and treatment of bronchospasm. May cause headache, nasopharyngitis, tremor, dizziness, nausea, vomiting, muscle cramps, infection, palpitations, tachycardia, and hypertension. PB: 10%; t½: 2.7–6 h
Metaproterenol sulfate; beta₂	A: PO: Initially 10 mg tid/qid; *maint:* 20 mg tid/qid; *max:* 80 mg/d	For acute bronchospasm, asthma, and COPD. May cause headache, tachycardia, palpitations, tremor, nausea, diarrhea, hypokalemia, and dysrhythmias. PB: UK; t½: 6 h
Dobutamine hydrochloride; beta₁	A: IV: Initially 0.5–1 mcg/kg/min; titrate dose gradually so HR does not elevate >10% of baseline; AHA recommends effective dose of 2–20 mcg/kg/min; *max:* 20 mcg/kg/min	For heart failure, cardiogenic shock, and for cardiac surgery. May cause dysrhythmia, tachycardia, angina, palpitations, headache, nausea, hypertension, hypokalemia, and dyspnea. PB: UK; t½: 2 min
Terbutaline sulfate; beta₂	A: PO: 2.5–5 mg tid; *max:* 15 mg/d A: subcut: Initially 0.25 mg, may repeat in 15–30 min PRN; *max:* 0.5 mg in 4 h	For acute bronchospasm. May cause nervousness, tremors, dizziness, drowsiness, headache, hyperhidrosis, nausea, vomiting, hypo/hyperglycemia, palpitations, tachycardia, weakness, and hypokalemia. PB: 25%; t½: 2.9–14 h
Central-Acting Alpha Agonists Clonidine hydrochloride Alpha₂	Immediate release tablets: A: PO: Initially 0.1 mg bid; *maint:* 0.2–0.6 mg/d; *max:* 2.4 mg/d A: Transdermal: 1 patch q7d	For hypertension. May cause dizziness, drowsiness, confusion, fatigue, pruritus, nausea, vomiting, abdominal pain, constipation, dry mouth, orthostatic hypotension, bradycardia, anxiety, and edema. PB: 20%–40%; t½: 12–16 h, transdermal 20 h
Methyldopa Alpha₂	A: PO: Initially 250 mg bid-tid; *maint:* 500–2000 mg/d in 2–4 divided doses; *max:* 3 g/dOlder A: PO: 250–1000 mg/d; *max:* 1 g/d	For hypertension. May cause dizziness, drowsiness, hypotension, depression, bradycardia, peripheral edema, angina, constipation, and erectile/ejaculatory dysfunction. PB: 10%–15%; t½: 2 h

>, Greater than; <, less than; *A*, adult; *AHA*, American Heart Association; *BP*, blood pressure; *COPD*, chronic obstructive pulmonary disease; *d*, day; *GI*, gastrointestinal; *h*, hour; *HR*, heart rate; *IM*, intramuscularly; *inf*, infusion; *IV*, intravenously; *max*, maximum; *MDI*, metered-dose inhaler; *min*, minute; *OTC*, over the counter; *PSVT:* paroxysmal supraventricular tachycardia; *PB*, protein binding; *PO*, by mouth; *PRN*, as needed; *q4h*, every 4 hours; *qid*, four times a day; *subcut*, subcutaneous; *t½*, half-life; *tid*, three times a day; *UK*, unknown; *y*, years.

⊚ CLINICAL JUDGMENT [NURSING PROCESS]

Adrenergic Agonists

Concept: Perfusion
- The passage of blood flow through arteries and capillaries, which deliver oxygen and nutrients to body cells

Recognize Cues [Assessment]
- Record baseline vital signs for future comparisons.
- Assess the patient's drug history.
- Determine patient's health history. Most adrenergic agonists are contraindicated if the patient has a cardiac dysrhythmia, narrow-angle glaucoma, or cardiogenic shock.
- Determine baseline glucose level.

Analyze Cues and Prioritize Hypothesis [Patient Problems]
- Dyspnea
- Decreased gas exchange
- Hypotension
- Decreased tissue perfusion
- Hypoxemia

Generate Solutions [Planning]
- Patient's vital signs will be within acceptable ranges.
- Patient will experience therapeutic effects by improved blood pressure, breathing pattern, and cardiac output.

Take Action [Nursing Interventions]
- Administer intravenous (IV) epinephrine 1 mg (10 mL of a 1:10,000 concentration per American Heart Association [AHA] guidelines) for cardiac resuscitation; may repeat every 3 to 5 minutes. Follow each dose with a 20-mL saline flush to ensure proper delivery. Normally, epinephrine is administered 1 mg IV over 1 minute or more.
- ⚡ Monitor IV site frequently when administering norepinephrine bitartrate or dopamine because extravasation of these drugs causes tissue damage and necrosis within 12 hours. These drugs should be diluted sufficiently in IV fluids.
- Administer antidote, phentolamine mesylate 5 to 10 mg, diluted in 10 to 15 mL of normal saline infiltrated into the area for IV extravasation of norepinephrine and dopamine.
- Record patient's vital signs. Report signs of increasing blood pressure and increasing heart rate. If the patient receives an alpha-adrenergic agonist intravenously for shock, check the blood pressure every 3 to 5 minutes or as indicated to avoid severe hypertension.
- Monitor electrocardiogram (ECG) for dysrhythmia when adrenergic agonists are given intravenously.
- Report side effects of adrenergic drugs such as tachycardia, palpitations, dysrhythmias, tremors, dizziness, and increased blood pressure.
- Check patient's urinary output and assess for bladder distension. Urinary retention can result from a high drug dose or continuous use of adrenergic agonists.
- Offer food to the patient when giving adrenergic agonists to avoid nausea and vomiting.

- Evaluate blood glucose levels in patients with diabetes mellitus for potential elevation.

Patient Teaching
General
- Advise the patient to read labels on all over-the-counter (OTC) drugs for cold symptoms and diet pills. Many of these have properties of sympathetic drugs (adrenergic agonists, sympathomimetics) and should not be taken if a patient is hypertensive or has diabetes mellitus, cardiac dysrhythmia, or coronary artery disease.
- Explain that continuous use of nasal sprays or drops that contain adrenergic agonists may result in rebound nasal congestion (inflamed and congested tissue).

Self-Administration
- Encourage the patient to take medication as prescribed.
- Advise the patient and family on proper administration of the drug and allow a return demonstration. Cold medications by spray or drops in the nostrils should be used with the head in an upright position. Use of nasal spray while lying down can cause systemic absorption. Coloration of nasal spray or drops might indicate deterioration.
- Notify the health care provider if an EpiPen is needed more than twice a week.
- Encourage the patient to have an EpiPen readily available at all times and to store additional medication in a cool, dark place. Refrigeration is not recommended.
- ⚡ Teach the patient and family that the EpiPen must be used immediately upon the initial occurrence of difficulty breathing, wheezing, hoarseness, hives, itching, or swelling of the lips and tongue.
- Teach the patient to administer the EpiPen properly. Inspect the solution for particles or discoloration before administration. Do not use if particles are pink to brown in color. Take care to inject subcutaneously and not intradermally, and be sure to apply sufficient pressure to activate the EpiPen while holding the device in place for 5 to 10 seconds. The EpiPen should be inserted into the outer thigh. After administration, massage the injection site for 10 seconds to promote absorption and reduce vasoconstriction and tissue irritation.

Side Effects
- ⚡ Encourage the patient to report side effects such as rapid heart rate, palpitations, rash, itching, flushing, chest pain, irregular heartbeat, vomiting, or numbness of fingers and toes to a health care provider because the dose may require adjustment.

Evaluate Outcomes [Evaluation]
- Evaluate the patient's response to the adrenergic agonist.
- Evaluate vital signs and report abnormal findings. Epinephrine stimulates alpha₁ (increases blood pressure), beta₁ (increases heart rate), and beta₂ (dilates bronchial tubes) receptors. Albuterol stimulates beta₂ receptors.
- Report possible drug-drug interactions. Beta blockers decrease the effect of epinephrine and albuterol. OTC cold and allergy drugs, caffeine, alcohol, herbs, and dietary supplements may lead to interactions.

ADRENERGIC ANTAGONISTS (ADRENERGIC BLOCKERS)

Drugs that block the effects of adrenergic neurotransmitters are called *adrenergic antagonists, adrenergic blockers,* or *sympatholytics.* They act as antagonists to adrenergic agonists by blocking the alpha- and beta-receptor sites. Most adrenergic antagonists (adrenergic blockers) block either the alpha receptor or the beta receptor. They block the effects of the neurotransmitter either directly by occupying the receptors or indirectly by inhibiting the release of the neurotransmitters norepinephrine and epinephrine. Table 15.3 lists the effects of alpha blockers and beta blockers at receptors.

TABLE 15.3 Effects of Adrenergic Blockers at Receptors

Receptor	Responses
Alpha$_1$	Vasodilation: decreases blood pressure; reflex tachycardia might result; mydriasis (constriction of pupil) occurs; suppresses ejaculation; reduces contraction of smooth muscle in bladder neck and prostate gland
Beta$_1$	Decreases heart rate; reduces force of contractions
Beta$_2$	Constricts bronchioles; contracts uterus; inhibits glycogenolysis, which can decrease blood glucose

Alpha-Adrenergic Antagonists

Drugs that block or inhibit a response at the alpha-adrenergic receptor site are called *alpha-adrenergic antagonists, adrenergic blockers,* or *alpha blockers.* Alpha-blocking agents are divided into two groups: *selective* alpha blockers block alpha$_1$, and *nonselective* alpha blockers block alpha$_1$ and alpha$_2$. Because alpha-adrenergic antagonists can cause orthostatic hypotension and reflex tachycardia, many of these drugs are not as frequently prescribed as beta antagonists.

Alpha antagonists (alpha blockers) promote vasodilation, causing a decrease in blood pressure. If vasodilation is long-standing, orthostatic hypotension can result. Dizziness may also be a symptom of a decrease in blood pressure. As blood pressure decreases, pulse rate usually increases to compensate for the low blood pressure and inadequate blood flow. Alpha antagonists can be used to treat peripheral vascular disease such as Raynaud disease. Vasodilation occurs, permitting more blood flow to the extremities. These drugs are also helpful in decreasing symptoms of benign prostatic hyperplasia (BPH). Alpha antagonists are also discussed in Chapter 39.

Beta-Adrenergic Antagonists

Beta-adrenergic antagonists, more commonly called *beta blockers,* decrease heart rate, and a decrease in blood pressure usually follows. Some beta blockers are nonselective, blocking both beta$_1$ and beta$_2$ receptors. Not only does the heart rate decrease because of beta$_1$ blocking, but bronchoconstriction also occurs. Nonselective beta blockers block both beta$_1$ and beta$_2$ and should be used with extreme caution in any patient who has chronic obstructive pulmonary disease (COPD) or asthma.

Propranolol hydrochloride was the first beta blocker prescribed to treat angina, cardiac dysrhythmia, hypertension, and heart failure. This medication may also be given for migraine prophylaxis. Propranolol has many side effects, partly because of its nonselective response in blocking both beta$_1$ and beta$_2$ receptors.

A selective adrenergic antagonist has a greater affinity for certain receptors. If the desired effect is to decrease pulse rate and blood pressure, a selective beta$_1$ blocker such as atenolol or metoprolol tartrate may be ordered.

Intrinsic sympathomimetic activity (ISA) is a term used to describe the ability of certain beta blockers to bind with a beta receptor to prevent strong agonists from binding to that receptor, producing complete activation. Nonselective beta blockers that have ISA include carvedilol, penbutolol, and pindolol. The selective blocker (blocks beta$_1$ only) that has ISA is acebutolol, and such an agent may be recommended for hypertensive patients who are experiencing bradycardia.

PROTOTYPE DRUG CHART

❗ *Atenolol*

Drug Class	Dosage
Beta$_1$-adrenergic blocker	Hypertension: A: PO: Initially 25–50 mg/d; may increase to 100 mg/d after 7–14 d; *max:* 100 mg/d

Contraindications	Drug-Lab-Food Interactions
Hypersensitivity, bradycardia, heart block greater than first degree, cardiogenic shock, uncompensated cardiac failure *Caution:* Renal dysfunction, diabetes mellitus, bronchospasm, myasthenia gravis, pheochromocytoma, pulmonary edema, acute bronchospasm, pregnancy, lactation	Drug: Increased absorption with atropine and other anticholinergics, decreased effects with NSAIDs, increased risk of hypoglycemia with insulin and sulfonylureas, increased hypotension with prazosin and terazosin, increased lidocaine and verapamil levels with toxicity

Pharmacokinetics	Pharmacodynamics
Absorption: 50% absorbed in GI tract Distribution: PB: 10% Metabolism: t½: 6–7 h Excretion: Urine and feces	PO: Onset: 1 h Peak: 2–4 h Duration: 24 h

Therapeutic Effects/Uses

To treat hypertension, angina, and prophylaxis and treatment of acute myocardial infarction

Mechanism of Action: Selectively blocks beta$_1$-adrenergic receptor sites, decreases sympathetic outflow to the periphery, suppresses renin-angiotensin-aldosterone system

Side Effects	Adverse Reactions
Drowsiness, dizziness, headache, depression, fatigue, nausea, diarrhea, erectile dysfunction	Bradycardia, tachycardia, hypotension, chest pain, heart failure, dyspnea *Life-threatening:* Bronchospasm, renal failure, dysrhythmia, thrombocytopenia

A, Adult; *d,* day; *GI,* gastrointestinal; *h,* hour; *max,* maximum; *NSAID,* nonsteroidal antiinflammatory drug; *PB,* protein binding; *PO,* by mouth; *t½,* half-life.

Atenolol, a selective beta$_1$ blocker, decreases sympathetic outflow to the periphery and suppresses the renin-angiotensin-aldosterone system (RAAS) response. It is contraindicated in bradycardia, heart block, cardiogenic shock, acute heart failure, asthma, and sick sinus syndrome. Beta blockers should be used with caution in patients with COPD. Electrolyte imbalances, such as hypokalemia and hypomagnesemia, should be corrected before initiating beta blocker therapy. Prototype Drug Chart: Atenolol describes the pharmacologic behavior of atenolol.

Beta blockers are useful in treating mild to moderate hypertension, angina, heart failure, and myocardial infarction (MI). Beta blockers should not be abruptly discontinued but rather should be tapered off

❗ TABLE 15.4   Adrenergic Antagonists

Drug	Route and Dosage	Uses and Considerations
Phentolamine mesylate; alpha$_1$	A: Subcut: 5–10 mg in 10 mL NS injected into extravasation area to prevent dermal necrosis	Antidote for dopamine, dobutamine, phenylephrine, epinephrine, norepinephrine, and necrosis from extravasation. May cause pain at injection site. PB: UK; t½: 19 min
Doxazosin mesylate; alpha$_1$	Hypertension: A: PO: Initially 1 mg/d at bedtime; *max:* 16 mg/d	For hypertension and BPH. May cause dizziness, headache, asthenia, fatigue, edema, visual impairment, erectile dysfunction, and orthostatic hypotension. PB: 98%; t½: 22 h
Prazosin hydrochloride; alpha$_1$	A: PO: Initially 1 mg bid/tid; *maint:* 6–15 mg/d in divided doses; *max:* 20 mg/d Older A: PO: Initially 1 mg qd/bid; *max:* 20 mg/d	For hypertension. May cause headache, dizziness, drowsiness, fatigue, weakness, orthostatic hypotension, peripheral edema, nausea, and palpitations. PB: 97%; t½: 2–4 h
Terazosin hydrochloride; alpha$_1$	Hypertension: A: PO capsules: Initially 1 mg at bedtime; *maint:* 1–5 mg/d; *max:* 20 mg/d	For hypertension and BPH. May cause nasal congestion, dizziness, drowsiness, headache, peripheral edema, orthostatic hypotension, nausea, weakness, palpitations, and erectile dysfunction. PB: 90%–94%; t½: 12 h
Carvedilol; alpha$_1$, beta$_1$, and beta$_2$	Heart failure: Regular release: A: PO: 3.125 mg bid for 2 wk; *max:* 50 mg/bid Extended release: A: Initially 10 mg/d; *max:* 80 mg/d	For hypertension and HF. May cause drowsiness, dizziness, orthostatic hypotension, bradycardia, weight gain, dyspnea, fatigue, headache, diarrhea, peripheral edema, hyperglycemia, diarrhea, erectile dysfunction, and weakness. PB: 98%; t½: 7–11 h
Labetalol; alpha$_1$, beta$_1$, and beta$_2$	Chronic hypertension: A: PO: Initially 100 mg bid; dose may be increased q2–3d; *maint:* 200–400 mg bid; *max:* 2400 mg/d	For acute/chronic hypertension. May cause orthostatic hypotension, nasal congestion, dizziness, fatigue, nausea, paresthesia, erectile/ejaculation dysfunction, hyperhidrosis, and depression. PB: 50%; t½: 6–8 h
Propranolol hydrochloride; beta$_1$ and beta$_2$	Hypertension: Immediate release: A: PO: Initially: 40 mg bid; may increase q3–7d; *maint:* 160–480 mg/d in 2–3 divided doses; *max:* 640 mg/d Extended release: A: PO: Initially 80 mg/d, may increase q3–7d; *maint:* 120–160 mg/d; *max:* 640 mg/d	For hypertension, angina, MI, HF, dysrhythmia, and migraine prophylaxis. May cause agitation, fatigue, dizziness, visual impairment, erectile dysfunction, bradycardia, hyperkalemia, and seizures. PB: 90%; t½: 2–6 h
Nadolol; beta$_1$ and beta$_2$	A: PO: Initially 40 mg/d; *maint:* 40–80 mg/d; *max:* 320 mg/d for hypertension and 240 mg/d for angina	For hypertension and angina. May cause dizziness, drowsiness, fatigue, bradycardia, hypotension, palpitations, and erectile dysfunction. PB: 30%; t½: 10–24 h
Pindolol; beta$_1$ and beta$_2$	A: PO: Initially 5 mg bid; *maint:* 10–30 mg in 2–3 divided doses; *max:* 60 mg/d	For hypertension. May cause bradycardia, hypotension, edema, fatigue, myalgia, dizziness, visual impairment, and dyspnea. PB: 40%–60%; t½: 3–4 h
Sotalol; beta$_1$ and beta$_2$	Atrial flutter/fibrillation: A: PO: 80 mg bid; may increase gradually; *max:* 320 mg/d	For ventricular dysrhythmias, atrial flutter, and atrial fibrillation. May cause headache, dizziness, dyspnea, asthenia, bradycardia, palpitations, hypotension, HF, hyperhidrosis, nausea, vomiting, fatigue, and dysrhythmia exacerbation. PB: 0%; t½: 12 h
Timolol maleate; beta$_1$ and beta$_2$	Hypertension: A: PO: Initially 10 mg bid; *maint:* 10–20 mg bid; *max:* 60 mg/d	For hypertension and glaucoma treatment and for migraine prophylaxis. May cause blurred vision, conjunctivitis, ocular irritation, weakness, dizziness, nausea, bradycardia, dyspnea, HF, pulmonary edema, and dysrhythmias. PB: 10%; t½: 3–4 h
Selective Beta-Adrenergic Blockers		
Metoprolol tartrate; beta$_1$	Angina: Regular release: A: PO: Initially 25–50 mg bid; *maint:* 100–400 mg/d in 2 divided doses; *max:* 450 mg/d Extended release: A: PO: Initially 100 mg/d; *maint:* 100–400 mg/d; *max:* 400 mg/d	For hypertension, angina, HF, and acute MI. May cause bradycardia, dizziness, drowsiness, fatigue, nightmares, diarrhea, depression, insomnia, palpitations, erectile dysfunction, hypotension, flushing, syncope, peripheral insufficiency/edema, HF, and dysrhythmias. PB: 10%–12%; t½: 3–7 h
Atenolol; beta$_1$	See Prototype Drug Chart: Atenolol	
Acebutolol hydrochloride; beta$_1$	Hypertension: A: PO: Initially: 400 mg/d; *maint:* 400–800 mg/d; *max:* 1200 mg/d Older adults: Initially 200 mg/d; *max:* 800 mg/d	For hypertension and dysrhythmias. May cause bradycardia, hypotension, dizziness, fatigue, headache, nausea, diarrhea, constipation, visual impairment, edema, and dyspnea. PB: 26%; t½: 3–4 h

⚠ TABLE 15.4	**Adrenergic Antagonists—cont'd**	
Betaxolol; beta₁	Hypertension: A: PO: Initially 10 mg/d; *max:* 20 mg/d Older adult: Initially 5 mg/d; *max:* 20 mg/d	For hypertension and glaucoma. May cause bradycardia, headache, dizziness, insomnia, fatigue, nausea, arthralgia, edema, and chest pain. PB: 50%; t½: 15 h
Bisoprolol fumarate; beta₁	A: PO: Initially: 2.5–5 mg/d; *max:* 20 mg/d	For hypertension. May cause dizziness, bradycardia, headache, fatigue, arthralgia, diarrhea, orthostatic hypotension, weakness, and peripheral edema. PB: 30%; t½: 9–12 h
Esmolol hydrochloride; beta₁	Paroxysmal supraventricular tachycardia: A: IV: LD: Initially 50 mcg/kg/min continuous infusion; *max:* 500 mcg/kg/min per dose or 300 mcg/kg/min continuous infusion	For paroxysmal supraventricular tachydysrhythmia and hypertension. May cause hypotension, dizziness, drowsiness, bradycardia, diaphoresis, nausea, and injection site reaction. PB: 55%; t½: 9 min

<, Less than; *A*, adult; *bid*, two times a day; *BPH*, benign prostatic hyperplasia; *COPD*, chronic obstructive pulmonary disease; *d*, day; *ER*, extended release; *FDA*, US Food and Drug Administration; *h*, hour; *HF*, heart failure; *IOP*, intraocular pressure; *IV*, intravenous; *LD*, loading dose; *maint*, maintenance; *max*, maximum; *MI*, myocardial infarction; *min*, minute; *NS*, normal saline; *PB*, protein binding; *PO*, by mouth; *q2–3d*, every 2 to 3 days; *qid*, four times a day; *sec*, seconds; *subcut*, subcutaneously; *t½*, half-life; *tid*, three times a day; *UK*, unknown.

◎ CLINICAL JUDGMENT [NURSING PROCESS]

Adrenergic Neuron Antagonists

Concept: Perfusion
- The passage of blood flow through arteries and capillaries, which deliver oxygen and nutrients to body cells

Recognize Cues [Assessment]
- Obtain baseline vital signs and electrocardiogram (ECG) for future comparisons. Bradycardia and a decrease in blood pressure are common cardiac effects of adrenergic neuron blockers.
- Determine what drugs the patient currently takes. Report if any are diuretics, nonsteroidal antiinflammatory drugs (NSAIDs), digoxin, monoamine oxidase inhibitors (MAOIs), or central nervous system (CNS) depressants.
- Obtain a health history. Depression, dysrhythmias, and heart failure may result from taking an adrenergic neuron blocker, and these drugs could potentiate preexisting conditions.

Analyze Cues and Prioritize Hypothesis [Patient Problems]
- Hypertension
- Reduced sexual expression

Generate Solutions [Planning]
- Patient will verbalize that they will adhere to the drug regimen.
- Patient's vital signs will be within the desired range.

Take Action [Nursing Interventions]
- Monitor blood pressure. Report marked decreases in blood pressure
- Monitor apical pulse. Withhold and report if less than 60 beats/min.
- Report any complaints of excessive dizziness, lightheadedness, early morning insomnia, mental depression, or chest pain.
- Assist patient with ambulation to avoid falls from orthostatic hypotension, which is more common with high doses.

- Note any complaint of stuffy nose because vasodilation may result, and nasal congestion can occur.

Patient Teaching
General
- Encourage the patient to adhere to the drug regimen.
- Advise the patient that the therapeutic effects of adrenergic neuron antagonists may not occur for 2 to 3 weeks after initiation of therapy.

Self-Administration
- Teach the patient and family how to take pulse and blood pressure.
- Encourage the patient to take adrenergic neuron antagonists at the same time every day and not to discontinue it without permission from the health care provider.

Side Effects
- ⚡ Encourage the patient to avoid orthostatic (postural) hypotension by slowly rising from supine or sitting positions to standing.
- Inform patients and family of possible psychological changes when taking adrenergic neuron antagonists, which occur because of catecholamine depletion. Psychological changes can include depression, sleep disorders, emotional lability, memory impairment, confusion, nightmares, and hallucinations.
- Warn patients that adrenergic neuron antagonists may cause erectile or ejaculation dysfunction, which is usually dose related.
- ⚡ Advise patients not to drive or operate dangerous equipment until the drug response is known.

Evaluate Outcomes [Evaluation]
- Evaluate effectiveness of the adrenergic neuron blocker. Vital signs must be stable within the desired range.

over 1 to 2 weeks to avoid tachycardia, hypertension, severe angina, dysrhythmia, and MI. The use of beta blockers as antihypertensives, antidysrhythmics, and drugs for angina is discussed in Chapters 37 and 39. Table 15.4 lists the alpha and beta blockers and their dosages, uses, and considerations.

Pharmacokinetics. Atenolol distribution into the CNS by crossing the blood-brain barrier is minimal and is 50% to 60% absorbed by the GI tract. The protein-binding capacity is 10%. Atenolol has a half-life of 6 to 7 hours and is eliminated in urine.

Pharmacodynamics. By blocking beta₁ receptors, atenolol decreases the heart rate, peripheral vascular resistance, force of cardiac contractions, and cardiac output and reduces both systolic and diastolic blood pressure. It is available in tablets and for IV administration. The onset of action of the oral preparation is 1 hour; peak time is 2 to 4 hours, and duration of action is 24 hours. This drug is effective for once-daily dosing, especially for patients who do not adhere to drug dose schedules that require dosing several times a day.

Drug Interactions

Many drugs interact with atenolol. Nonsteroidal antiinflammatory drugs (NSAIDs) decrease the hypotensive effect of atenolol. Hypotension can be potentiated if atenolol is taken with another antihypertensive, although this may be the desired result. When atenolol is given concurrently with atropine and other anticholinergics, absorption is increased.

Side Effects and Adverse Reactions

The side effects commonly associated with beta blockers are bradycardia, hypotension, headache, dizziness, cold extremities, and bronchospasm. Other side effects of beta-adrenergic blockers include cardiac dysrhythmia, flushing, hypotension, fatigue, erectile dysfunction, and depression. Usually the side effects are dose related.

Adrenergic Neuron Antagonists

Drugs that block the release of norepinephrine from the sympathetic terminal neurons are called adrenergic neuron antagonists (adrenergic neuron blockers). The clinical use is to decrease blood pressure. For example, reserpine is an antihypertensive agent that closely resembles alpha- and beta-adrenergic blockers; it also reduces the serotonin and catecholamine transmitters, depletion of which may lead to severe mental depression.

CRITICAL THINKING CASE STUDY

An older adult patient has asthma, and an adrenergic agonist is selected for treatment.

1. What are the drug advantages and disadvantages associated with the use of an adrenergic agonist, such as metaproterenol or albuterol, for this patient? Explain your answer.
2. Is age a factor in drug selection? Explain your answer.

An older adult patient has hypertension and asthma. An adrenergic blocker is selected for treatment.

1. What are the drug advantages and disadvantages associated with the use of doxazosin, prazosin, propranolol, metoprolol, and atenolol for this patient? Explain your answer.
2. What needs to be included when teaching this patient about the use of an adrenergic blocker?

REVIEW QUESTIONS

1. The nurse will monitor the patient taking albuterol for which conditions? (Select all that apply.)
   a. Palpitations
   b. Hypertension
   c. Hypoglycemia
   d. Bronchospasm
   e. Uterine contractions
   f. Hypotension
   g. Blurred vision
2. Nadolol is prescribed for a patient. The nurse realizes that this drug is a beta-adrenergic blocker and is contraindicated for patients with which condition?
   a. Hypothyroidism
   b. Angina pectoris
   c. Bronchial asthma
   d. Liver dysfunction
3. The nurse realizes that beta$_1$ receptor stimulation is differentiated from beta$_2$ stimulation in that stimulation of beta$_1$ receptors leads to which condition?
   a. Increased bronchodilation
   b. Decreased uterine contractility
   c. Increased myocardial contractility
   d. Decreased blood flow to skeletal muscles
4. A patient is given epinephrine, an adrenergic agonist (sympathomimetic). The nurse should monitor the patient for which condition?
   a. Decreased pulse
   b. Pupil constriction

   c. Bronchial constriction
   d. Increased blood pressure
5. A patient who is taking epinephrine is also taking several other medications. The nurse should realize that there is a possible drug interaction with which drugs? (Select all that apply.)
   a. Albuterol
   b. Metoprolol
   c. Propranolol
   d. Digoxin
   e. Methyldopa
6. A patient is prescribed metoprolol to treat hypertension. It is important for the nurse to monitor the patient for which condition? (Select all that apply.)
   a. Bradycardia
   b. Hypotension
   c. Diaphoresis
   d. Agitation
   e. Erythema
7. The nurse is administering atenolol to a patient. Which concurrent drugs does the nurse expect to most likely cause an interaction? (Select all that apply.)
   a. Ginseng
   b. Insulin
   c. Atropine
   d. Haloperidol
   e. Methyldopa

16

Cholinergic Agonists and Antagonists

http://evolve.elsevier.com/McCuistion/pharmacology

OBJECTIVES

- Compare the responses of cholinergic agonist and antagonist drugs.
- Differentiate between direct-acting and indirect-acting cholinergic agonists.
- Contrast the major side effects of cholinergic agonists and antagonists.
- Differentiate the uses of cholinergic agonists and antagonists.
- Apply the Clinical Judgment [Nursing Process], including patient teaching, associated with cholinergic agonists and antagonists.
- Apply the Clinical Judgment [Nursing Process] for the patient taking neostigmine, a reversible cholinesterase inhibitor.

OUTLINE

The two groups of drugs discussed in this chapter affect the parasympathetic nervous system. They include cholinergic agonists—muscarinic agonists or parasympathomimetics—and the cholinergic antagonists (blocking agents)—muscarinic antagonists, parasympatholytics, or more commonly called anticholinergics.

PARASYMPATHETIC NERVOUS SYSTEM

The parasympathetic nervous system is called the *cholinergic system* because the neurotransmitter at the end of the neuron that innervates the muscle is acetylcholine.

The cholinergic receptors at organ cells are either nicotinic or muscarinic, meaning that they are stimulated by the alkaloids nicotine and muscarine, respectively (Fig. 16.1).

Acetylcholine stimulates the receptor cells to produce a response, but the enzyme acetylcholinesterase may inactivate acetylcholine before it reaches the receptor cell.

Drugs that mimic the neurotransmitters norepinephrine and acetylcholine produce responses opposite to each other in the same organ. For example, an *adrenergic drug* (sympathomimetic) *increases* the heart rate, whereas a *cholinergic drug* (parasympathomimetic) *decreases* the heart rate (see Fig. 15.2 in Chapter 15). However, a drug that mimics the sympathetic nervous system and a drug that blocks the parasympathetic nervous system can cause similar responses in the organ. For instance, the sympathomimetic and the parasympatholytic (blocks impulses from PNS) drugs both *increase* heart rate; the adrenergic blockers and the cholinergic drugs both *decrease* heart rate.

Many name classifications are given to drugs that mimic or block both the sympathetic and the parasympathetic nervous systems (Table 16.1).

CHOLINERGIC AGONISTS

Drugs that stimulate the parasympathetic nervous system are called *cholinergic agonists,* or *parasympathomimetics,* because they mimic the parasympathetic neurotransmitter acetylcholine. The neurotransmitter located at the ganglions and the parasympathetic terminal nerve endings is acetylcholine (ACh). It innervates cholinergic receptors in organs, tissues, and glands. The two types of cholinergic receptors are muscarinic receptors, which stimulate smooth muscle and slow the heart rate, and nicotinic receptors (neuromuscular), which affect the skeletal muscles. Many cholinergic agonists are nonselective because they can affect both the muscarinic and the nicotinic receptors. However, there are selective cholinergic agonists for the muscarinic receptors that do *not* affect the nicotinic receptors. Fig. 16.2 illustrates the effects of parasympathetic, or cholinergic, stimulation.

There are two types of cholinergic agonists: direct-acting cholinergic agonists act on receptors to activate a tissue response (Fig. 16.3A), and indirect-acting cholinergic agonists inhibit the action of the enzyme cholinesterase (ChE), also called acetylcholinesterase (AChE), by forming a chemical complex that allows acetylcholine to persist and attach to the receptor (Fig. 16.3B). Drugs that inhibit ChE are called *cholinesterase inhibitors, acetylcholinesterase inhibitors,* or *anticholinesterases.* ChE may destroy acetylcholine before it reaches the receptor or after it has attached to the site. By inhibiting or destroying the ChE, more acetylcholine is available to stimulate the receptor and to remain in contact with it longer.

Cholinesterase inhibitors can be separated into reversible and irreversible inhibitors. The *reversible inhibitors* bind the ChE for several minutes to hours, and the *irreversible inhibitors* bind the enzyme permanently. The resulting effects vary with how long the ChE is bound.

The major responses of cholinergic agonists are to stimulate bladder and gastrointestinal (GI) tone; constrict the pupils of the eyes, known as miosis; and increase neuromuscular transmission. Other effects of cholinergic agonists include decreased heart rate and blood pressure and increased salivary, GI, and bronchial secretions. Table 16.2 lists the responses of direct- and indirect-acting cholinergic agonists.

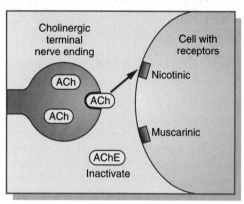

Fig. 16.1 Parasympathetic transmitters and receptors. *ACh,* Acetylcholine; *AChE,* acetylcholinesterase.

Direct-Acting Cholinergic Agonists

Many drugs classified as direct-acting cholinergic agonists are primarily selective to the muscarinic receptors but are nonspecific because the muscarinic receptors are located in the smooth muscle of the GI and genitourinary tracts, glands, and heart. Bethanechol chloride, a direct-acting cholinergic agonist, acts on the muscarinic (cholinergic) receptor and is used primarily to increase urination in the treatment of urinary retention and neurogenic bladder. Metoclopramide hydrochloride (HCl) is a direct-acting cholinergic agonist that is usually prescribed to treat gastroparesis, nausea, and gastroesophageal reflux disease (GERD). In low doses, metoclopramide enhances gastric motility and thus accelerates gastric emptying time. Prototype Drug Chart: Bethanechol Chloride details the pharmacologic behavior of bethanechol, a classic cholinergic agonist.

Pharmacokinetics. Bethanechol chloride is poorly absorbed from the GI tract. The percentage of protein binding and the half-life are unknown. The drug is most likely excreted in the urine.

Pharmacodynamics. The principal use of bethanechol is to promote urination by stimulating the muscarinic cholinergic receptors in the detrusor muscle to contract the bladder and produce urine output. Because of the increased tone of the detrusor

---

📄 PROTOTYPE DRUG CHART

Bethanechol Chloride

Drug Class	Dosage
Cholinergic: Parasympathomimetic	Urinary retention A: PO: Initially 5–10 mg q1h until effective response or 50 mg given; *maint:* 10–50 mg tid/qid; *max:* 200 mg/d A: Subcut: 5 mg tid/qid; *max:* 40 mg/d

Contraindications	Drug-Lab-Food Interactions
Contraindicated: Intestinal or urinary tract obstruction, IBS, bradycardia, hypotension, asthma, peptic ulcer, hyperthyroidism, seizures, parkinsonism *Caution:* COPD, older adults	Drug: Decreases bethanechol effect with antidysrhythmics (e.g., procainamide); ganglionic blocking agents (e.g., mecamylamine) cause significant hypotension after severe abdominal symptoms. False test results (amylase, lipase) may result. Atropine, flavoxate, and opiates counteract bethanechol action. Lab: Increases AST, bilirubin, amylase, lipase

Pharmacokinetics	Pharmacodynamics
Absorption: Poorly absorbed PO Distribution: PB: UK Metabolism: t½: UK Excretion: In urine	PO: Onset: 0.5–1.5 h Peak: 1–2 h Duration: 1–6 h Subcut: Onset: 5–15 min Peak: 15–30 min Duration: 2 h

Therapeutic Effects/Uses

To treat urinary retention and neurogenic bladder
Mechanism of Action: Stimulates the cholinergic (muscarinic) receptors; promotes contraction of the bladder; increases GI secretions and peristalsis, pupillary constriction, and bronchoconstriction

Side Effects	Adverse Reactions
Nausea, vomiting, diarrhea, abdominal cramps, hypersalivation, diaphoresis, headache, dizziness, flushing, urinary urgency and frequency, miosis, lacrimation	Tachycardia, hypotension *Life-threatening:* Bronchospasm, wheezing, seizures

A, Adult; *AST,* aspartate aminotransferase; *COPD,* chronic obstructive pulmonary disease; *d,* day; *GI,* gastrointestinal; *h,* hour; *IBS,* irritable bowel syndrome; *maint,* maintenance; *max,* maximum; *min,* minute; *PB,* protein binding; *PO,* by mouth; *q3–4d,* every 3 to 4 days; *qid,* four times a day; *subcut,* subcutaneous; *t½,* half-life; *tid,* three times a day; *UK,* unknown.

TABLE 16.1 Autonomic Nervous System Stimulants: Sympathetic and Parasympathetic

Sympathetic Stimulants
Sympathomimetics (Adrenergics, Adrenomimetics, or Adrenergic Agonists)
Action:
- Increase blood pressure
- Increase pulse rate
- Relax bronchioles
- Dilate pupils of eyes
- Relax uterine muscles
- Increase blood glucose

Sympathetic Depressants
Sympatholytics (Adrenergic Blockers, Adrenolytics, or Adrenergic Antagonists)
Action:
- Decrease pulse rate
- Decrease blood pressure
- Constrict bronchioles

Direct-Acting Parasympathetic Stimulants
Parasympathomimetics (Cholinergics or Cholinergic Agonists)
Action:
- Decrease blood pressure
- Decrease pulse rate
- Constrict bronchioles
- Constrict pupils of eyes
- Increase urinary contraction
- Increase peristalsis

Indirect-Acting Cholinesterase Inhibitors (Anticholinesterase)
Action:
- Increase muscle tone

Parasympathetic Depressants
Parasympatholytics (Anticholinergics, Cholinergic Antagonists, or Antispasmodics)
Action:
- Increase pulse rate
- Decrease mucous secretions
- Decrease gastrointestinal motility
- Increase urinary retention
- Dilate pupils of eyes

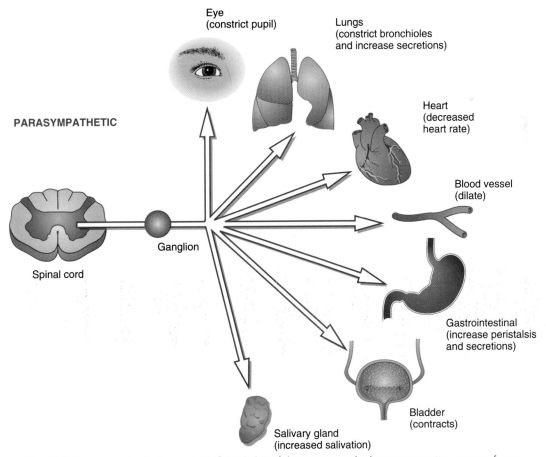

Fig. 16.2 Parasympathetic Responses. Stimulation of the parasympathetic nervous system or use of parasympathomimetic drugs will cause the pupils to constrict, bronchioles to constrict and bronchial secretions to increase, heart rate to decrease, blood vessels to dilate, peristalsis and gastric secretions to increase, the bladder muscle to contract, and salivary glands to increase salivation.

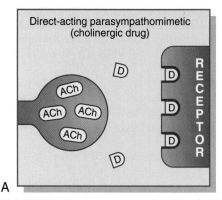
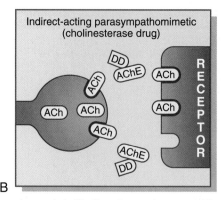

Fig. 16.3 (A) Direct-acting parasympathomimetic (cholinergic agonist). Cholinergic agonists resemble acetylcholine and act directly on the receptor. (B) Indirect-acting parasympathomimetic (cholinesterase inhibitor). Cholinesterase inhibitors inactivate the enzyme acetylcholinesterase (cholinesterase), thus permitting acetylcholine to react to the receptor. *ACh,* Acetylcholine; *AChE,* acetylcholinesterase or cholinesterase; *D,* cholinergic agonist; *DD,* cholinesterase inhibitor (anticholinesterase).

TABLE 16.2	Effects of Cholinergic Agonists
Body Tissue	**Response**
Cardiovascular[a]	Decreased heart rate, lowered blood pressure because of vasodilation, and slowed conduction of atrioventricular node
Gastrointestinal[b]	Increased tone and motility of smooth muscle of stomach and intestine, increased peristalsis, and relaxed sphincter muscles
Genitourinary	Contraction of muscles of the urinary bladder, increased tone of ureters, relaxed bladder sphincter muscles, and stimulated urination
Ocular[b]	Increased pupillary constriction or miosis (pupil becomes smaller) and increased accommodation (flattening or thickening of eye lens for distant or near vision)
Glandular[a]	Increased salivation, perspiration, and tears
Bronchial (lung)[a]	Stimulation of bronchial smooth muscle contraction and increased bronchial secretions
Striated muscle[b]	Increased neuromuscular transmission and maintenance of muscle strength and tone

[a]Tissue responses to large doses of cholinergic agonists.
[b]Major tissue responses to normal doses of cholinergic agonists.

muscle, the onset of action is 30 minutes after taking an oral dose of bethanechol, and the duration is 1–6 hours. Bethanechol also increases peristalsis in the GI tract and gastric emptying time, and the drug should be taken on an empty stomach 1 to 2 hours before meals to minimize nausea and vomiting.

Side Effects and Adverse Reactions

Mild to severe side effects of most muscarinic agonists, such as bethanechol, include hypotension, tachycardia, excessive salivation, increased gastric acid secretion, abdominal cramps, diarrhea, and bronchospasm. This group of agents should be prescribed cautiously for patients with low blood pressure and chronic obstructive pulmonary disease (COPD). Muscarinic agonists are contraindicated for patients with intestinal or urinary tract obstruction, severe bradycardia, or active asthma.

Direct-Acting Cholinergic Agonists: Eye

Pilocarpine is a direct-acting cholinergic agonist that constricts the pupils of the eyes, thus opening the Schlemm canal to promote drainage of aqueous humor (fluid). This drug is used to treat glaucoma by relieving (intraocular) fluid pressure in the eye and to promote miosis in eye surgery and examinations. Pilocarpine also acts on the nicotinic receptor, as does carbachol. Both agents are discussed in more detail in Chapter 44. An oral form of pilocarpine is used to relieve xerostomia (dry mouth).

Indirect-Acting Cholinergic Agonists

The indirect-acting cholinergic agonists do not act on receptors; instead, they inhibit or inactivate the enzyme cholinesterase, permitting acetylcholine to accumulate at the receptor sites (see Fig. 16.3B). This action gives them the name *cholinesterase inhibitors, acetylcholinesterase inhibitors,* or *anticholinesterases,* of which there are two types: reversible and irreversible.

The function of the enzyme cholinesterase is to break down acetylcholine into choline and acetic acid. A small amount of cholinesterase can break down a large amount of acetylcholine in a short period. A cholinesterase inhibitor drug binds with cholinesterase, allowing acetylcholine to activate the muscarinic and nicotinic cholinergic receptors. This action permits skeletal muscle stimulation, which increases the force of muscular contraction. Because of this action, cholinesterase inhibitors are useful to increase muscle tone for patients with myasthenia gravis (a neuromuscular disorder). By increasing acetylcholine, additional effects occur, such as increases in GI motility, bradycardia, miosis, bronchial constriction, and increased micturition.

The primary use of *reversible* cholinesterase inhibitors is to treat myasthenia gravis; another use is to treat Alzheimer disease. The primary clinical indication for *irreversible* cholinesterase inhibitors is glaucoma.

Reversible Cholinesterase Inhibitors

Reversible cholinesterase inhibitors are used to produce pupillary constriction in the treatment of glaucoma and to increase muscle strength in patients with myasthenia gravis. Drug effects persist for several hours. Drugs used to increase muscular strength in myasthenia gravis include neostigmine (short acting), pyridostigmine bromide (moderate acting), ambenonium chloride (long acting), and edrophonium chloride (short acting, for diagnostic purposes). These drugs are discussed in more detail in Chapter 21. A reversible

CLINICAL JUDGMENT [NURSING PROCESS]

Cholinergic Agonist, Direct Acting: Bethanechol

Concept: Elimination

- The excretion of metabolic waste products from the body, such as urination

Recognize Cues [Assessment]

- Assess baseline vital signs for future comparisons.
- Assess urine output (should be >1500 mL/day).
- Obtain patient history of health problems such as peptic ulcer, urinary obstruction, or asthma. Cholinergic agonists can aggravate symptoms of these conditions.

Analyze Cues and Prioritize Hypothesis [Patient Problems]

- Hypotension
- Urinary retention
- Potential for falls
- Fatigue

Generate Solutions [Planning]

- Patient will void with more frequency after taking cholinergic agonists.

Take Action [Nursing Interventions]

- Monitor vital signs. Heart rate and blood pressure decrease when large doses of cholinergics are taken. Orthostatic hypotension is a side effect of cholinergic agonists, such as bethanechol.
- Record fluid intake and output. Decreased urinary output should be reported because it may be related to urinary obstruction.
- Give cholinergic agonists 1 hour before or 2 hours after meals to minimize nausea and vomiting. If a patient complains of gastric pain, the drug may be given with meals.
- Check serum amylase, lipase, aspartate aminotransferase (AST), and bilirubin levels. These laboratory values may increase slightly in a patient taking cholinergic agonists.

- Observe the patient for side effects such as gastric pain or cramping, diarrhea, increased salivary or bronchial secretions, tachycardia, and orthostatic hypotension.
- Auscultate breath sounds for rales, crackling sounds from fluid congestion in the lungs, or rhonchi, rough sounds resulting from mucous secretions in the lungs. Cholinergic agonists can increase bronchial secretions.
- ⚡ Have intravenous (IV) atropine sulfate (0.6 to 1.2 mg) available as an antidote for cholinergic overdose. Early signs of overdosing include flushing, salivation, sweating, nausea, and abdominal cramps.
- Increase bathing frequency and linen change when needed. Diaphoresis (excessive perspiration) may occur.
- ⚡ Monitor for possible cholinergic crisis (overdose), including symptoms of muscular weakness and increased salivation.

Patient Teaching

- Teach patients to take the cholinergic agonist as prescribed. Compliance with the drug regimen is essential.
- Direct patients to report severe side effects, such as profound dizziness or a decrease in heart rate below 60 beats/min.
- ⚡ Teach patients to arise from a lying position slowly to avoid dizziness. This is most likely a result of orthostatic hypotension.
- Encourage patients to maintain effective oral hygiene if excess salivation occurs.
- Advise patients to report any difficulty in breathing as a result of respiratory distress.

Evaluate Outcomes [Evaluation]

- Determine the effectiveness of the cholinergic agonist or anticholinesterase drug.
- Evaluate the stability of patient vital signs, and note the presence of side effects or adverse reactions.

---

anticholinesterase drug is physostigmine, which is used as an antidote for atropine to reverse anticholinergic toxicity. Ophthalmic agents are further discussed in Chapter 44.

Side Effects

Common side effects from reversible cholinesterase inhibitors are hypotension, bradycardia, sweating, hypersalivation, and GI distress, which includes anorexia, nausea, vomiting, abdominal pain, and diarrhea. Reversible cholinesterase inhibitors are contraindicated for patients with asthma, diabetes, cardiovascular disease, and gastrointestinal or genitourinary obstruction. Caution is required for patients who have bradycardia, peptic ulcers, seizures, or dysrhythmia. Cholinesterase inhibitors are contraindicated for patients with intestinal or urinary obstruction.

Irreversible Cholinesterase Inhibitors

Irreversible cholinesterase inhibitors are potent agents because of their long-lasting effects. The enzyme cholinesterase must be regenerated before the drug effect diminishes, a process that may take days or weeks. These drugs are used to produce pupillary constriction.

Table 16.3 lists examples of cholinergic drugs and their standard dosages and common uses.

CHOLINERGIC ANTAGONISTS

Drugs that inhibit the actions of acetylcholine by occupying the acetylcholine receptors are called cholinergic antagonists (blocking agents), muscarinic

antagonists, anticholinergics, cholinergic blocking agents, antispasmodics, or parasympatholytics. The major body tissues and organs affected by the anticholinergic group of drugs are the heart, respiratory tract, GI tract, urinary bladder, eyes, and exocrine glands. By blocking the parasympathetic nerves, the sympathetic (adrenergic) nervous system dominates. Anticholinergics and adrenergic agonists produce many of the same responses.

Anticholinergic and cholinergic agonists have opposite effects. The major responses to anticholinergics are a decrease in GI motility, a decrease in salivation, dilation of pupils—also called mydriasis—and an increase in pulse rate. Other effects of anticholinergics include decreased bladder contraction, which can result in urinary retention, and decreased rigidity and tremors related to neuromuscular excitement. An anticholinergic can act as an antidote to the toxicity caused by cholinesterase inhibitors and organophosphate ingestion. The various effects of anticholinergics are described in Table 16.4.

Muscarinic receptors are a type of cholinergic receptor involved in tissue and organ responses to anticholinergics because anticholinergics inhibit the actions of acetylcholine by occupying these receptor sites. Fig. 16.4 illustrates this action of anticholinergic drugs; these drugs may also block the effect of direct-acting parasympathomimetics, such as bethanechol and pilocarpine, and of indirect-acting parasympathomimetics, such as physostigmine and neostigmine.

Atropine

Atropine sulfate, first derived from the belladonna plant (*Atropa belladonna*) and purified in 1831, is a classic anticholinergic—or muscarinic

TABLE 16.3 Cholinergic Agonists

Drug	Route and Dosage	Uses and Considerations
Direct-Acting Cholinergic Agonists		
Bethanechol chloride	See Prototype Drug Chart: Bethanechol Chloride	
Metoclopramide hydrochloride	Postoperative nausea/vomiting: A: IM/IV: 10 mg near end of procedure, then may repeat q4–6h; *max:* 20 mg single dose	For GERD, gastroparesis, nausea and vomiting. May cause drowsiness, dizziness, fatigue, restlessness, headache, nausea, vomiting, and EPS. PB: 30%; t½: 2.5–6 h
Carbachol	See Chapter 44	See Chapter 44
Pilocarpine hydrochloride	See Chapter 44	See Chapter 44
Cholinesterase Inhibitor		
Donepezil hydrochloride	See Chapter 20	See Chapter 20
Rivastigmine	See Chapter 20	See Chapter 20
Indirect-Acting Cholinergics or Cholinesterase Inhibitors for the Eye		
Echothiophate iodide	See Chapter 44	See Chapter 44
Reversible Cholinergics or Cholinesterase Inhibitors		
Edrophonium chloride	Myasthenia gravis diagnosis: A: IV: 2 mg over 15–30 seconds, then 8 mg if no response in 45 seconds A: IM: Initially 10 mg; if cholinergic reaction, give 2 mg in 30 min to rule out false-negative results	For neuromuscular blockade reversal and to diagnose myasthenia gravis. Monitor pulse, respiratory rate, BP, neurologic static, and ECG frequently during administration. May cause diplopia, hypersalivation, dysphonia, dysphagia, dysarthria, diaphoresis, bradycardia, hypotension, respiratory depression, diarrhea, and seizures. PB: UK; t½: 67–185 min
Neostigmine methylsulfate	Myasthenia gravis: A: PO: Initially 15 mg tid, may gradually increase to *maint:* 15–375 mg/d in divided doses A: Subcut/IM: 0.5 mg q4–6h PRN; *max:* 0.5 mg/dose	For myasthenia gravis, urinary retention, and ileus and for neuromuscular blockade reversal. May cause dizziness, headache, nausea, vomiting, bradycardia, hypotension, tachycardia, muscle cramps, seizures, and dyspnea. PB: 15%–25%; t½: 42–60 min
Physostigmine salicylate	Anticholinergic toxicity: A: IV/IM: 0.5–2 mg/dose, repeat q10–30min PRN; *max:* 1 mg/min IV	For anticholinergic syndrome and glaucoma. May cause diaphoresis, hypersalivation, nausea, vomiting, bradycardia, hypotension, seizures, confusion, muscle paralysis, dyspnea, and bronchospasm. PB: UK; t½: 1–2 h
Pyridostigmine bromide	Neuromuscular blockade reversal: A: IV: 0.1–0.25 mg/kg simultaneously or immediately preceded by atropine 0.6–1.2 mg IV	For myasthenia gravis and neuromuscular blockade reversal and for nerve gas exposure prophylaxis. May cause nausea, vomiting, abdominal cramps, diarrhea, bradycardia, blurred vision, headache, bronchospasm, diaphoresis, hypersalivation, and increased urinary frequency. PB: None; t½: 3 h
Antidote for Irreversible and Reversible Cholinesterase Inhibitors		
Pralidoxime chloride	Cholinesterase inhibitor toxicity: A: IV: 1–2 g in 100 mL of saline solution infused over 15–30 min; follow with 250 mg q5min PRN; *max:* 2 g/dose	For cholinesterase inhibitor toxicity and organophosphate pesticide toxicity. May cause dizziness, blurred vision, headache, drowsiness, tachycardia, hypertension, and hypertonia. PB: None; t½: 74–77 min

A, Adult; *bid,* two times a day; *BP,* blood pressure; *d,* day; *ECG,* electrocardiogram; *EPS,* extrapyramidal syndrome symptoms; *GERD,* gastroesophageal reflux disease; *GI,* gastrointestinal; *gt,* drop; *gtt,* drops; *h,* hour; *IM,* intramuscular; *IOP,* intraocular pressure; *IV,* intravenous; *maint,* maintenance; *max,* maximum; *min,* minute; *NMS,* neuroleptic malignant syndrome; *PB,* protein binding; *PO,* by mouth; *PRN,* as needed; *q4–6h,* every 4 to 6 hours; *qid,* four times a day; *subcut,* subcutaneous; *t½,* half-life; *tid,* three times a day; *UK,* unknown.

TABLE 16.4 Effects of Anticholinergic Drugs

Body Tissues	Responses
Cardiovascular	Heart rate increases with large doses; small doses can decrease heart rate.
Gastrointestinal (GI)	Relaxed smooth muscle tone of GI tract, decreased GI motility and peristalsis; gastric and intestinal secretions are decreased.
Urinary tract	Relaxed bladder detrusor muscle and increased constriction of internal sphincter; urinary retention can result.
Ocular	Dilated pupils (mydriasis) and paralyzed ciliary muscles (cycloplegia) cause a decrease in accommodation.
Glandular	Salivation, perspiration, and bronchial secretions are decreased.
Bronchial	Bronchi are dilated, and bronchial secretions decrease.
Central nervous system	Tremors and rigidity of muscles are decreased; drowsiness, disorientation, and hallucinations can result from large doses.

antagonist—drug. Scopolamine was the second belladonna alkaloid produced. Atropine and scopolamine act on muscarinic receptors, but they have little effect on nicotinic receptors except in high doses. Atropine is useful primarily as a preoperative medication to decrease

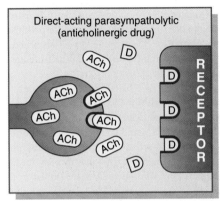

Fig. 16.4 Anticholinergic Response. The anticholinergic drug occupies the receptor sites, blocking acetylcholine. *ACh,* Acetylcholine; *D,* anticholinergic drug.

salivary secretions and as an agent to increase heart rate when bradycardia is present. Atropine can also be used as an antidote for muscarinic agonist poisoning caused by an overdose of a cholinesterase inhibitor or a muscarinic drug such as bethanechol and for neuromuscular blockade reversal. However, if a patient takes atropine or an atropine-like drug (e.g., an antihistamine), side effects can occur. Prototype Drug Chart: Atropine details the pharmacologic behavior of atropine.

Synthetic anticholinergic drugs are also used as antispasmodics to treat peptic ulcers and intestinal spasticity. One example is propantheline bromide, which has been available for several decades. It decreases gastric secretions and GI spasms in duodenal ulcers. Since the introduction of the histamine (H₂) blockers, anticholinergic agents such as propantheline are rarely used to decrease gastric secretions.

Pharmacokinetics. Atropine sulfate is well absorbed orally and parenterally. It crosses the blood-brain barrier and exerts its effect on the central nervous system (CNS). The protein binding is unknown. It crosses the placenta. Atropine has a short half-life of 2 to 4 hours, so there is little cumulative effect. Most of the absorbed atropine is excreted in the urine (75% to 95%).

Pharmacodynamics. Atropine sulfate blocks acetylcholine by occupying the muscarinic receptor. It increases the heart rate by

---

📄 PROTOTYPE DRUG CHART

Atropine

Drug Class	Dosage
Anticholinergic: Parasympatholytic	Bradycardia: A: IV: 0.5–1 mg, repeat q3–5min PRN up to 3 mg

Contraindications	Drug-Lab-Food Interactions
Hypersensitivity *Caution:* Renal, hepatic, or respiratory impairment, COPD, cardiovascular disease, myocardial ischemia, tachycardia, GI obstruction, ileus, ulcerative colitis, GI disease, glaucoma, hyperthyroidism, urinary retention, dysrhythmias, hypertension, diarrhea, myasthenia gravis	Drug: Increases anticholinergic effect with phenothiazines, antihistamines, TCAs, amantadine, quinidine; high-dose anticholinergics may decrease effects of carbidopa/levodopa by delaying GI absorption; anticholinergics may enhance therapeutic effects at therapeutic doses.

Pharmacokinetics	Pharmacodynamics
Absorption: PO/IM: Well absorbed Distribution: PB: 14%–22% Metabolism: t½: 2–4 h Excretion: 75%–95% Excreted in urine	IM: Onset: 10–30 min Peak: 0.5–1 h Duration: 4 h IV: Onset: Immediate Peak: 5 min Duration: UK

Therapeutic Effects/Uses

Preoperative medication to reduce salivation, increase heart rate for bradycardia, for neuromuscular blockade reversal, for cholinergic crisis, and to dilate pupils for ocular diagnostic examinations

Mechanism of Action: Inhibits acetylcholine by occupying the receptors; increases heart rate by blocking vagus stimulation; promotes pupil dilation by blocking iris sphincter muscle

Side Effects	Adverse Reactions
Drowsiness, dizziness, nausea, dry mouth, headache, confusion, insomnia, amnesia, constipation, flushing, restlessness, blurred vision, mydriasis, anxiety, photophobia, palpitations, urinary retention, hyperreflexia, ataxia, weakness, dehydration, injection site reaction	Tachycardia, paradoxical bradycardia, hypertension, hypotension, angina, pulmonary edema, respiratory depression, ileus, seizures *Life-threatening:* Dysrhythmias, laryngospasm, coma

A, Adult; *BPH,* benign prostatic hyperplasia; *COPD,* chronic obstructive pulmonary disease; *GI,* gastrointestinal; *h,* hour; *IM,* intramuscular; *IV,* intravenous; *max,* maximum; *min,* minute; *PB,* protein binding; *PO,* by mouth; *PRN,* as needed; *q5min,* every 5 minutes; *subcut,* subcutaneous; *t½,* half-life; *TCA,* tricyclic antidepressant; *UK,* unknown.

blocking vagus stimulation and promotes dilation of the pupils by paralyzing the iris sphincter. The two most frequent uses of atropine are to decrease salivation and respiratory secretions preoperatively and to treat sinus bradycardia by increasing the heart rate. Atropine also is used ophthalmically for mydriasis and cycloplegia before eye examinations and to treat inflammation of the iris (iritis) and uveal tract.

Its onset of action for the intramuscular (IM) route is 10 to 30 minutes, and it peaks at 30 minutes to 1 hour. The duration is 4 hours. The onset of action for the IV route is immediate, and peak action occurs in 5 minutes.

Side Effects and Adverse Reactions

The common side effects of atropine and atropine-like drugs include xerostomia (dry mouth), nasal dryness, blurred vision, tachycardia, constipation, and urinary retention. Other side effects and adverse reactions are nausea, headache, dehydration, seizures, hypotension or hypertension, photophobia (intolerance of bright light), and coma.

Antiparkinson Anticholinergic Drugs

Studies indicate that anticholinergics affect the CNS as well as the parasympathetic nervous system. Anticholinergics affect the CNS by suppressing the tremors and muscular rigidity of parkinsonism, but they have little effect on mobility and muscle weakness. As a result of these findings, several anticholinergic drugs were developed for the treatment

of parkinsonism (e.g., trihexyphenidyl hydrochloride, biperiden, and benztropine). These drugs can be used alone in the early stages of parkinsonism; they may be used in combination with levodopa/carbidopa to control parkinsonism, or they can be used alone to treat pseudoparkinsonism, which results from the side effects of the phenothiazines in antipsychotic drugs. Drugs used to treat parkinsonism are described in more detail in Chapter 20. Prototype Drug Chart: Benztropine lists the drug data related to benztropine, which is used for parkinsonism.

Pharmacokinetics. Benztropine is well absorbed from the GI tract. Its protein-binding percentage and half-life are unknown. It is excreted in the urine.

Pharmacodynamics. Benztropine decreases involuntary movement and diminishes the signs and symptoms of tremors and muscle rigidity that occur with parkinsonism. It is available as an oral tablet and as parenteral IM and IV injections. Alcohol and other CNS depressants potentiate sedation. Anticholinergics, phenothiazines, and tricyclic antidepressants (TCAs) may increase the anticholinergic effects of benztropine. The side effects are similar to those of other anticholinergic drugs.

Anticholinergics for Treating Motion Sickness

The effects of anticholinergics on the CNS benefit patients who are prone to motion sickness. An example of such an anticholinergic, classified as an antihistamine for motion sickness, is scopolamine. It is available topically as a skin patch placed behind the ear.

🗒 PROTOTYPE DRUG CHART

Benztropine

Drug Class	Dosage
Antiparkinson: anticholinergic agent	Parkinsonism: A: PO/IM: Initially 0.5-1 mg/d at bedtime; *max:* 8 mg/d Drug-induced extrapyramidal symptoms: A: PO/IM/IV: Initially 1–2 mg bid/tid; *maint:* 1–4 mg qd/bid; *max:* 8 mg/d

Contraindications	Drug-Lab-Food Interactions
Hypersensitivity, dementia, children *Caution:* Tachycardia, cardiac disease, autonomic neuropathy, prostatic hypertrophy, psychosis, glaucoma, myasthenia gravis, hyperthermia, alcohol use disorder, urinary retention/obstruction	Drug: Increases anticholinergic effect with phenothiazines, tricyclic antidepressants, and other anticholinergics

Pharmacokinetics	Pharmacodynamics
Absorption: PO: Well absorbed Distribution: PB: UK Metabolism: t½: UK Excretion: In urine	PO: Onset: 1 h Peak: 7 h Duration: 6–10 h

Therapeutic Effects/Uses
To decrease involuntary symptoms of parkinsonism or drug-induced parkinsonism Mechanism of Action: Blocks cholinergic (muscarinic) receptors, thus decreasing acetylcholine to reduce excess cholinergic activity (involuntary movements); also blocks dopamine reuptake to prolong dopamine effects and decrease involuntary movement

Side Effects	Adverse Reactions
Nausea, vomiting, dry mouth, constipation, anhidrosis, dizziness, headache, drowsiness, blurred vision, confusion, depression, hallucinations, weakness, hyperthermia, and paresthesia, mydriasis, urinary retention, photophobia	Tachycardia, ocular hypertension *Life-threatening:* Ileus, coma

A, Adult; *bid,* two times a day; *d,* day; *h,* hour; *IM,* intramuscular; *IV,* intravenous; *max,* maximum; *PB,* protein binding; *PO,* by mouth; *qd,* once daily; *t½,* half-life; *UK,* unknown.

◎ CLINICAL JUDGMENT [NURSING PROCESS]

Anticholinergic Drugs: Atropine

Concept: Perfusion
- The passage of blood flow through arteries and capillaries, which deliver oxygen and nutrients to body cells

Recognize Cues [Assessment]
- Obtain baseline vital signs for future comparisons. Tachycardia is a side effect that occurs with large doses of anticholinergics such as atropine sulfate.
- Assess urine output. Urinary retention may occur.
- Check the patient's medical history. Atropine and atropine-like drugs are contraindicated in patients with narrow-angle glaucoma, obstructive gastrointestinal (GI) disorders, paralytic ileus, ulcerative colitis, benign prostatic hypertrophy, or myasthenia gravis.
- Obtain the patient's drug history. Phenothiazines and antidepressants increase the effect of anticholinergics.

Analyze Cues and Prioritize Hypothesis [Patient Problems]
- Hypertension
- Urinary retention
- Decreased visual acuity
- Constipation

Generate Solutions [Planning]
- Patient secretions will be decreased before surgery.
- Patient's heart rate will be increased.

Take Action [Nursing Interventions]
- Monitor patient vital signs. Report if tachycardia occurs.
- Determine fluid intake and output. Encourage patients to void before taking the medication, and report decreased urine output; anticholinergics can cause urinary retention. Maintain adequate fluid intake.
- Assess bowel sounds. Absence of bowel sounds may indicate paralytic ileus resulting from a decrease in GI motility (peristalsis).
- Examine for constipation caused by a decrease in GI motility. Encourage ingestion of foods that are high in fiber, intake of adequate amounts of fluids, and exercise if possible.
- Use bed alarms for patients who are confused and debilitated. Atropine could cause central nervous system (CNS) stimulation (excitement, confusion) or drowsiness.

- Provide mouth care. Atropine decreases oral secretions and can cause dryness.
- Administer intravenous (IV) atropine undiluted or diluted in 10 mL of sterile water. Rate of administration is 1 mg or some fraction thereof per minute.

Patient Teaching
General
- Direct patients to avoid hot environments and excessive physical exertion. Elevations in body temperature can result from diminished sweat gland activity.
- ⚡ Teach patients with narrow-angle glaucoma to avoid atropine-like drugs. Anticholinergics cause mydriasis and increase intraocular pressure (IOP). Instruct patients to check labels on over-the-counter (OTC) drugs to determine whether they are contraindicated for glaucoma.
- ⚡ Instruct patients not to drive a motor vehicle or participate in activities that require alertness. Drowsiness is common.
- Tell patients with mydriasis after an eye examination to use sunglasses in bright light because of photophobia.

Side Effects
- Advise patients of common side effects such as dry mouth, decreased urination, and constipation that can occur as a result of anticholinergic use.
- Direct patients to increase fluid intake and consumption of high-fiber foods to prevent constipation when taking anticholinergics for a prolonged period.
- Instruct patients to urinate before taking the anticholinergic because urinary retention can be a problem.
- Advise patients to report any marked decrease in urine output.
- Suggest that patients use hard candy, ice chips, or chewing gum. Maintain effective oral hygiene if a patient's mouth is dry. Anticholinergics decrease salivation.
- Encourage patients to use eye drops to moisten dry eyes that result from decreased lacrimation (tearing).

Evaluate Outcomes [Evaluation]
- Evaluate patient response to the anticholinergic.
- Determine whether constipation, urinary retention, or increased pulse rate is a problem.

Prevention of motion sickness is also provided via wristbands and ginger, including ginger gum or candy. Transdermal scopolamine is delivered over 3 days and is frequently prescribed for activities such as flying, cruising on the water, and bus or automobile trips. Other drugs classified as antihistamines for motion sickness are dimenhydrinate, cyclizine, and meclizine hydrochloride. Most of these drugs can be purchased over the counter with the exception of scopolamine.

Examples of anticholinergic drugs and their dosages and common uses are found in Table 16.5. Dosages may vary according to age, sex,

and weight. Because anticholinergic drugs can increase intraocular pressure, they should not be administered to patients diagnosed with glaucoma.

Side Effects and Adverse Reactions

Side effects of antihistamines used as anticholinergics include xerostomia, drowsiness, visual disturbances (especially blurred vision resulting from pupillary dilation), constipation secondary to decreased GI peristalsis, urinary retention related to decreased bladder tone, tachycardia (when taken in large doses), hypotension, dysphagia, anhidrosis, and flushing.

TABLE 16.5 Anticholinergics

Drug	Route and Dosage	Uses and Considerations
Anticholinergics: Gastrointestinal or Cholinergic Blockers		
Atropine sulfate	See Prototype Drug Chart: Atropine	
Dicyclomine hydrochloride	A: PO: Initially 20 mg qid for 7 d; *maint:* 20–40 mg qid for 2 wk; *max:* 160 mg/d A: IM: 10–20 mg q6h for 1–2 d; *max:* 80 mg/d	For IBS. May cause dry mouth, agitation, confusion, dizziness, drowsiness, blurred vision, weakness, and nausea. PB: UK; t½: 9–10 h
Glycopyrrolate	Preoperative: aspiration prophylaxis A: IM: 4 mcg/kg 30 min to 1 h before anesthesia induction	For duodenal ulcer, aspiration prophylaxis. May cause flushing, dry mouth, headache, palpitations, hypotension, tachycardia, blurred vision, sinusitis, nausea, vomiting, constipation, and urinary retention. PB: UK; t½: 0.55–1.25 h
Hyoscyamine SO$_4$	IBS: Immediate release: A: PO/SL: 0.125–0.25 mg q4h PRN; *max:* 1.5 mg/d Extended release: A: 0.375–0.75 mg q12h; *max:* 1.5 mg/d A: subcut/IM/IV: 0.25–0.5 mg bid/qid	Treatment of aspiration prophylaxis and IBS. May cause flushing, confusion, blurred vision, dizziness, drowsiness, photophobia, dysphagia, anhidrosis, constipation, palpitations, tachycardia, urinary retention, and erectile dysfunction. PB: 50%; t½: RR 2–3.5 h, ER 7.5 h
Methscopolamine bromide	A: PO: 2.5 mg tid ac and 2.5–5 mg at bedtime; *max:* 12.5 mg/d	For peptic ulcer. May cause confusion, blurred vision, anhidrosis, dry mouth, constipation, palpitations, tachycardia, urinary retention, and erectile dysfunction. PB: UK; t½: UK
Propantheline bromide	A: PO: 15 mg tid ac; 30 mg at bedtime	For peptic ulcer. May cause dizziness, drowsiness, confusion, anhidrosis, dysphagia, dry mouth, constipation, palpitations, hypotension, weakness, blurred vision, urinary retention, and erectile dysfunction. PB: UK; t½: 1.6 h
Scopolamine	Motion sickness: A: Transdermal: 1 patch behind ear 4 h before antiemetic is needed; *max:* 1 patch q3d	For nausea, vomiting, and motion sickness. May cause dizziness, drowsiness, confusion, blurred vision, tachycardia, bradycardia, dry mouth, anhidrosis, orthostatic hypotension, dysphagia, constipation, photophobia, and urinary retention. PB: 4%; t½: 8 h
Cholinergic Antagonists: Eye		
Cyclopentolate hydrochloride	See Chapter 44	See Chapter 44
Homatropine	See Chapter 44	See Chapter 44
Tropicamide	See Chapter 44	See Chapter 44
Anticholinergic-Antiparkinson Drugs		
Benztropine mesylate	See Prototype Drug Chart: Benztropine	
Trihexyphenidyl hydrochloride	Parkinsonism: Regular tablet or elixir: A: PO: Initially 1 mg, may increase by 2 mg q3–5d; *maint:* 6–10 mg/d, usually tid with meals and at bedtime; *max:* 15 mg/d Extended release: A: PO: 5–10 mg after breakfast; *max:* 15 mg/d	For parkinsonism and drug-induced EPS. May cause dizziness, anxiety, insomnia, nausea, vomiting, constipation, dry mouth, restlessness, and urinary retention. PB: UK; t½: 33 h
Anticholinergic–Antimuscarinic Drugs		
Tolterodine tartrate	See Prototype Drug Chart: Tolterodine Tartrate	
Others		
Ipratropium bromide	A: MDI: 2 inhal tid-qid; *max:* 12 inhal/d	For bronchospasm associated with asthma and COPD, and rhinorrhea associated with allergy and common cold. May cause headache, dyspnea, back pain, epistaxis, nasopharyngitis, sinusitis, dry mouth, nasal dryness, nausea, and chest pain. PB: UK; t½: 2 h

A, Adult; *ac,* before meals; *bid,* two times a day; *COPD,* chronic obstructive pulmonary disease; *d,* day; *EPS,* extrapyramidal syndrome; *ER,* extended release; *GI,* gastrointestinal; *gtt,* drops; *h,* hours; *IBS,* irritable bowel syndrome; *IM,* intramuscular; *inhal,* inhalation; *IOP,* intraocular pressure; *IV,* intravenous; *maint:* maintenance; *max,* maximum; *MDI,* metered-dose inhaler; *min,* minute; *NMS,* neuroleptic malignant syndrome; *PB,* protein binding; *PO,* by mouth; *PRN,* as needed; *q4–6h,* every 4 to 6 hours; *qid,* four times a day; *SL,* sublingual; *sol,* solution; *subcut,* subcutaneous; *t½,* half-life; *tid,* three times a day; *UK,* unknown; *wk,* weeks; *y,* years.

PROTOTYPE DRUG CHART

Tolterodine Tartrate

Drug Class	Dosage
Antimuscarinic agent: anticholinergic	Immediate release: A: PO: 1–2 mg bid; *max:* 4 mg/d Extended release: A: PO: 2–4 mg/d; *max:* 4 mg/d

Contraindications	Drug-Lab-Food Interactions
Hypersensitivity, urinary retention, gastric paresis, GI obstruction, and glaucoma *Caution:* Hypothyroidism, cardiovascular disease, bradycardia, heart failure, GERD, ulcerative colitis, myasthenia gravis, prostatic hypertrophy, renal or hepatic dysfunction, hypokalemia, and hypocalcemia	Drug: Increased effects with amantadine, amoxapine, bupropion, clozapine, cyclobenzaprine, disopyramide, maprotiline, olanzapine, orphenadrine, H_1 blockers, phenothiazines, and TCAs; decreased effects with azole antifungals (e.g., ketoconazole) or macrolide antibiotics (e.g., erythromycin), cyclosporine, and fluoxetine Food: Grapefruit juice may increase drug levels

Pharmacokinetics	Pharmacodynamics
Absorption: GI absorption is decreased with food intake. Distribution: PB: 96% Metabolism: t½: IR, 2–4 h; ER, 7–18 h Excretion: Urine and feces	PO: Onset: UK Peak: IR, 1–2 h; ER, 2–6 h Duration: UK

Therapeutic Effects/Uses
To decrease urinary frequency, urgency, and incontinence Mechanism of Action: Blocks cholinergic (muscarinic) receptors selectively in the urinary bladder

Side Effects	Adverse Reactions
Drowsiness, dizziness, dry mouth and eyes, headache, blurred vision, confusion, diarrhea, abdominal pain, constipation, dyspepsia, dysuria, fatigue, weight gain, arthralgia, hallucinations, and urinary retention	Angioedema, chest pain, tachycardia, peripheral edema *Life-threatening:* Stevens-Johnson syndrome

A, Adult; *bid*, two times a day; *d*, day; *GERD*, gastroesophageal reflux disease; *GI*, gastrointestinal; H_1, histamine 1; *h*, hours; *IR*, immediate release; *max*, maximum; *PB*, protein binding; *PO*, by mouth; *SR*, sustained release; *t½*, half-life; *TCA*, tricyclic antidepressant; *UK*, unknown.

CRITICAL THINKING CASE STUDY

A 70-year-old man is scheduled for surgery to remove gallstones. He has been in fairly good health. His only other clinical problem is a slight tremor in his hands. His health care provider would like him to start on benztropine after surgery for his tremor. Preoperative medications, meperidine 75 mg and atropine sulfate 0.4 mg, were given intramuscularly 1 hour before surgery.

1. What are the advantages of giving atropine sulfate before surgery?
2. What are some contraindications of atropine sulfate?
3. If a patient received an atropine-like drug for several months, what assessments should be made related to its effects?
4. How does atropine sulfate differ from bethanechol chloride?
5. What classification of drug is benztropine and how does it work? Explain your answer.
6. What patient teaching should the nurse include related to the use of benztropine?

REVIEW QUESTIONS

1. A patient is receiving bethanechol. The nurse realizes that the action of this drug is to treat which condition?
   a. Glaucoma
   b. Urinary retention
   c. Delayed gastric emptying
   d. Gastroesophageal reflux disease
   e. Gastroparesis
   f. Parkinsonism
   g. Myasthenia gravis

2. The nurse teaches the patient receiving atropine to expect which side effect?
   a. Diarrhea
   b. Sweating
   c. Blurred vision
   d. Frequent urination

3. When benztropine is ordered for a patient, the nurse acknowledges that this drug is an effective treatment for which condition?
   a. Parkinsonism
   b. Paralytic ileus
   c. Motion sickness
   d. Urinary retention
4. Dicyclomine is an anticholinergic, which the nurse realizes is given to treat which condition?
   a. Mydriasis
   b. Constipation
   c. Urinary retention
   d. Irritable bowel syndrome
5. The nurse realizes that cholinergic agonists mimic which parasympathetic neurotransmitter?
   a. Dopamine
   b. Acetylcholine
   c. Cholinesterase
   d. Monoamine oxidase
6. The nurse is administering bethanechol, a cholinergic agonist, and should know that the expected cholinergic effects include which of the following?
   a. Increased heart rate
   b. Decreased peristalsis
   c. Decreased salivation
   d. Increased pupil constriction
7. When a patient has a cholinergic overdose from excessive dosing of bethanechol, the nurse anticipates administration of which drug as the antidote?
   a. Atropine
   b. Tolterodine
   c. Benztropine
   d. Metoclopramide

Stimulants

http://evolve.elsevier.com/McCuistion/pharmacology

OBJECTIVES

- Explain the effects of stimulants on the central nervous system (CNS).
- Compare attention-deficit/hyperactivity disorder (ADHD) and narcolepsy.
- Differentiate the action of drugs used for ADHD and narcolepsy.

- Contrast the common side effects of amphetamines, anorexiants, analeptics, and caffeine.
- Apply the Clinical Judgment [Nursing Process] for the patient taking CNS stimulants.

OUTLINE

The nervous system is composed of all nerve tissues: brain, spinal cord, nerves, and ganglia. The purpose of the nervous system is to receive stimuli and transmit information to nerve centers for an appropriate response. There are two types of nervous systems: the central nervous system and the peripheral nervous system.

The central nervous system (CNS), composed of the brain and spinal cord, regulates body functions (Fig. 17.1). The CNS interprets information sent by impulses from the peripheral nervous system (PNS) and returns the instruction through the PNS for appropriate cellular actions. Stimulation of the CNS may either increase nerve cell (neuron) activity or block nerve cell activity.

The PNS consists of two divisions: the somatic nervous system (SNS) and the autonomic nervous system (ANS). The SNS is voluntary and acts on skeletal muscles to produce locomotion and respiration. The ANS, also called the *visceral system*, is involuntary; it controls and regulates the functioning of the heart, respiratory system, gastrointestinal (GI) system, and glands. The ANS, a large nervous system that functions without our conscious control, has two subdivisions: the sympathetic and the parasympathetic nervous systems.

The sympathetic nervous system of the ANS is called the *adrenergic system* because its neurotransmitter is norepinephrine. The parasympathetic nervous system is called the *cholinergic system* because its neurotransmitter is acetylcholine. Because organs are innervated by both the sympathetic and the parasympathetic systems, they can produce opposite responses. The sympathetic response is excitability, and the parasympathetic response is inhibition.

The sympathetic and the parasympathetic nerve pathways originate from different locations in the spinal cord. These nervous systems send information by two types of nerve fibers, preganglionic and postganglionic, and by the ganglion between these fibers. The preganglionic nerve fiber carries messages from the CNS to the ganglion, and the postganglionic fiber transmits impulses from the ganglion to body tissues and organs.

Numerous drugs can stimulate the CNS. Medically approved use of CNS stimulants is limited to the treatment of attention-deficit/hyperactivity disorder in children, narcolepsy, and the reversal of respiratory distress. The major groups of CNS stimulants include amphetamines, which stimulate the cerebral cortex of the brain; analeptics, which act on the brain stem and medulla to stimulate respiration; and anorexiants, which are thought to suppress appetite by stimulating the satiety center in the hypothalamic and limbic areas of the brain. Amphetamines and related anorexiants are greatly abused. Long-term use of amphetamines can produce psychological dependence or tolerance, conditions in which larger and larger doses of a drug are needed to reproduce the initial response. These medications are recommended for short-term use only (up to 12 weeks). Gradually increasing a drug dose and then abruptly stopping the drug may result in depression and withdrawal symptoms.

PATHOPHYSIOLOGY

Attention-deficit/hyperactivity disorder (ADHD) might be caused by a dysregulation of the transmitters serotonin, norepinephrine,

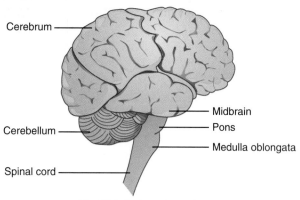

Fig. 17.1 Brain and spinal cord.

and dopamine. ADHD occurs primarily in children, usually before 7 years of age, and may continue through the teenage years. In some cases it may not be identified until early adulthood. The incidence of ADHD is three to seven times more common in boys than in girls. Characteristic behaviors of the various types of ADHD include inattentiveness, inability to concentrate, restlessness (fidgety), hyperactivity (excessive and purposeless activity), inability to complete tasks, and impulsivity.

The child with ADHD may display poor coordination, and there may be abnormal electroencephalograph (EEG) findings. Intelligence is usually not affected, but learning disabilities are often present. This disorder has also been called *minimal brain dysfunction, hyperactivity in children, hyperkinesis,* and *hyperkinetic syndrome with learning disorder.* Some professionals state that ADHD is often incorrectly diagnosed and results in many children receiving unnecessary treatment for months or years.

Narcolepsy is characterized by falling asleep during normal waking activities, such as driving a car or talking with someone. Sleep paralysis, the condition of muscle paralysis that is normal during sleep, usually accompanies narcolepsy and affects the voluntary muscles. The patient with narcolepsy is unable to move and may collapse.

AMPHETAMINES

Amphetamines stimulate the release of the neurotransmitters norepinephrine and dopamine from the brain and sympathetic nervous system (peripheral nerve terminals) and block the reuptake of these transmitters. Amphetamines ordinarily cause euphoria and increased alertness, but they can also cause xerostomia (dry mouth), insomnia, restlessness, tremors, irritability, and weight loss. Cardiovascular problems such as increased heart rate, palpitations, cardiac dysrhythmia, and increased blood pressure can result from cardiac stimulation and vasoconstriction with continuous use of amphetamines. These drugs have a high potential for abuse, tolerance, and dependence. Excessive use may lead to psychosis.

The half-life of amphetamines usually varies from 9 to 15 hours. Amphetamines and dextroamphetamine are prescribed for narcolepsy and ADHD when amphetamine-like drugs are ineffective.

Side Effects and Adverse Reactions

Amphetamines can cause adverse effects in the CNS and the cardiovascular, GI, and endocrine systems. Side effects and adverse reactions include dizziness, headache, euphoria, insomnia, tachycardia, hypertension, palpitations, dry mouth, anorexia, diarrhea, and erectile dysfunction.

Amphetamine-Like Drugs for Attention-Deficit/Hyperactivity Disorder and Narcolepsy

Methylphenidate and dexmethylphenidate, classed as amphetamine-like drugs, are given to increase a child's attention span and cognitive performance (e.g., memory, reading) and to decrease impulsiveness, hyperactivity, and restlessness. Dosage should be minimal in controlling ADHD symptoms. Methylphenidate is also used to treat narcolepsy. Because of the potential for abuse of methylphenidate, it is classified as a Controlled Substance Schedule (CSS) II drug. Prototype Drug Chart: Methylphenidate illustrates the pharmacokinetics, pharmacodynamics, and therapeutic effects of methylphenidate in the treatment of ADHD and narcolepsy. Amphetamine and amphetamine-like drugs should not be taken in the evening or before bedtime because insomnia may result. Drugs should be taken upon awakening.

Modafinil is an amphetamine-like stimulant that increases wakefulness in patients with sleep disorders such as narcolepsy. Its mechanism of action is not fully known.

Methylphenidate is the most frequently prescribed drug used to treat ADHD. Table 17.1 lists the amphetamines and amphetamine-like drugs and their dosages, uses, and considerations, including common side effects and a few serious adverse effects.

Pharmacokinetics. Methylphenidate is well absorbed from the GI mucosa and is usually administered to children twice a day before breakfast and lunch. Because food affects its absorption rate, this drug should be given upon awakening or 30 to 45 minutes before meals. Methylphenidate should be given 6 hours or more before sleep because it can cause insomnia. This drug is excreted in the urine, and 40% of methylphenidate is excreted unchanged.

Pharmacodynamics. Methylphenidate inhibits the reuptake of dopamine and norepinephrine resulting in CNS stimulation and an augmentation of serotonin action. This action helps correct ADHD by decreasing hyperactivity and improving attention span. This drug may also be prescribed for treating narcolepsy. Amphetamine-like drugs are considered generally more effective in treating ADHD than are amphetamines, which are generally avoided because they have a higher potential for abuse, habituation, and tolerance. Sympathomimetics (e.g., pseudoephedrine) and psychostimulants (e.g., caffeine) taken concurrently with methylphenidate increase stimulatory effects of irritability, nervousness, tremors, and insomnia. Concurrent use within 14 days of monoamine oxidase inhibitors (MAOIs) may cause hypertensive crisis. Methylphenidate potentiates the action of CNS stimulants, such as caffeine, and inhibits the metabolism of some barbiturates, such as phenobarbital, which can lead to increased blood levels and potential toxicity.

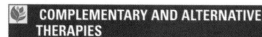

COMPLEMENTARY AND ALTERNATIVE THERAPIES

CNS Stimulants

Korean ginseng may potentiate drug effects of central nervous system (CNS) stimulants.

ANOREXIANTS AND ANALEPTICS

Anorexiants

Anorexiants cause a stimulant effect on the hypothalamic and limbic regions of the brain to suppress appetite. Most of the anorexiants used to suppress appetite (Table 17.2) do not have the serious side effects

📄 PROTOTYPE DRUG CHART

Methylphenidate

Drug Class	Dosage
Amphetamine-like drug: CNS stimulant CSS II	**ADHD:** **Immediate release:** A: PO: 20–30 mg/d in 2–3 divided doses, 30–45 min before breakfast and lunch; *max:* 60 mg/d Adol/C 6–12 y: PO: Initially 5 mg bid before breakfast and lunch; *max:* 60 mg/d **Extended release:** A: PO: Initially 20 mg/d in the morning; *max:* 60 mg/d Adol/C 6–12 y: PO: Initially 20 mg/d in the morning; *max:* 60 mg/d

Contraindications	Drug-Lab-Food Interactions
Anxiety, Tourette syndrome, glaucoma, angina, acute MI, heart failure, dysrhythmias, hyperthyroidism, MAOI therapy, and hereditary fructose intolerance *Caution:* Children <6 y, peripheral vascular disease, psychosis, depression, alcohol abuse, bipolar disorder, hypertension, cardiovascular disease, seizures, GI obstruction, pregnancy	Drug: May increase stimulatory effects of sympathomimetics and psychostimulants; may reduce effect of antihypertensives; increases effects of oral anticoagulants, barbiturates, anticonvulsants, and TCAs; increases hypertensive crisis with MAOIs Food: Caffeine, chocolate, tea, colas may increase effects. Herbs: St. John's wort may decrease drug efficacy

Pharmacokinetics	Pharmacodynamics
Absorption: Well absorbed from GI tract Distribution: PB: 10%–33% Metabolism: t½: 1.3–7.7 h Excretion: 90% excreted unchanged in urine	PO: Onset: 0.5–1 h Regular release: Peak 1.9 h Duration: 3–6 h Extended release: Peak 4.7 h Duration: 8 h

Therapeutic Effects/Uses

To correct hyperactivity caused by ADHD, increase attention span, and control narcolepsy

Mechanism of Action: Research suggests modulation of serotonergic pathways occurs by blocking dopamine transport and increasing sympathomimetic activity

Side Effects	Adverse Reactions
Anorexia, dry mouth, nausea, vomiting, dizziness, insomnia, irritability, restlessness, anxiety, confusion, depression, euphoria, hyperhidrosis, tremors, blurred vision, headache, abdominal pain, weight loss, constipation, diarrhea, paresthesia	Tachycardia, hypertension, bradycardia, growth suppression, palpitations, seizures, psychosis *Life-threatening:* Blood dyscrasias, hepatotoxicity, and ocular hypertension

>, Greater than; <, less than; *A*, adult; *ADHD*, attention-deficit/hyperactivity disorder; *Adol*, adolescent; *bid*, twice a day; *CNS*, central nervous system; *CSS*, Controlled Substances Schedule; *d*, day; *GI*, gastrointestinal; *h*, hour; *MAOI*, monoamine oxidase inhibitor; *max*, maximum; *MI*, myocardial infarction; *min*, minute; *PB*, protein binding; *PO*, by mouth; *t½*, half-life; *TCA*, tricyclic antidepressant; *y*, year.

associated with amphetamines. For weight loss attempts, emphasis should be placed on a nutritious diet, exercise, and behavior modification. Reliance on appetite suppressants should be discouraged. Individuals who take anorexiants should be under the care of a health care provider. Anorexiants are contraindicated in hypertension, hyperthyroidism, glaucoma, and within 14 days of MAOI therapy and should be given with caution in diabetes mellitus, seizures, Tourette syndrome, and bipolar disorder.

Side Effects and Adverse Reactions

Children younger than 12 years should not be given anorexiants, and self-medication with anorexiants should be discouraged. Long-term use of these drugs frequently results in severe side effects such as euphoria, restlessness, insomnia, palpitations, tachycardia, hypertension, and erectile dysfunction.

Analeptics

Analeptics, which are CNS stimulants, mostly affect the brain stem and spinal cord but also affect the cerebral cortex. The primary use of an analeptic is to stimulate respiration. One subgroup of analeptics is the xanthines (methylxanthines). Depending on the dose, caffeine stimulates the CNS, and large doses stimulate respiration. Newborns with respiratory distress might be given caffeine to increase respiration. Table 17.2 lists the analeptics and their dosages, uses, and considerations, including common side effects and a few serious adverse effects.

Side Effects and Adverse Reactions

Side effects from caffeine are similar to those from anorexiants: restlessness, tremors, palpitations, tachycardia, and insomnia. Other side effects include headache, GI irritation (e.g., nausea), and urinary frequency. Excess caffeine affects the CNS and heart and can cause dysrhythmias and seizures. High doses of caffeine in coffee, chocolate, and cold relief medications can cause psychological dependence. The half-life of caffeine is approximately 4 hours; however, the half-life is prolonged in patients with liver disease and in patients who are taking oral contraceptives or are pregnant. Caffeine is contraindicated during pregnancy because its effect on the fetus is unknown.

◎ CLINICAL JUDGMENT [NURSING PROCESS]

Central Nervous System Stimulant: Methylphenidate Hydrochloride

Concept: Cognition
- The process of attaining knowledge through the mental processes of thinking, learning, and memory

Recognize Cues [Assessment]
- Determine whether the patient has a history of heart disease, hypertension, hyperthyroidism, parkinsonism, or glaucoma; in such cases, this drug is usually contraindicated.
- Assess vital signs to be used for future comparisons. Closely monitor patients with cardiac disease because this drug may cause tachycardia, hypertension, and stroke.
- Assess patient mental status, such as mood, affect, and aggressiveness.
- Evaluate height, weight, and growth of children.
- Assess complete blood count (CBC), differential white blood cells (WBCs), and platelets before and during therapy.

Analyze Cues and Prioritize Hypothesis [Patient Problems]
- Hypertension
- Diarrhea
- Reduced functional ability

Generate Solutions [Planning]
- Patient will display less hyperactivity.
- Patient will demonstrate increased attention span.
- Patient's blood pressure and heart rate will be within normal limits.
- Patient will behave in a calm manner.

Take Action [Nursing Interventions]
- Monitor vital signs and report irregularities.
- Evaluate height, weight, and growth of children.
- Observe patients for withdrawal symptoms such as nausea, vomiting, weakness, and headache.
- Monitor patients for side effects such as insomnia, restlessness, nervousness, tremors, irritability, tachycardia, and elevated blood pressure. Report findings.

Patient Teaching
General
- Teach patients to take the drug before meals.
- ⚡ Advise patients to avoid alcohol consumption.
- Encourage use of sugarless gum to relieve dry mouth.
- Teach patients to monitor weight twice a week and report weight loss.
- ⚡ Advise patients to avoid driving and using hazardous equipment when experiencing tremors, nervousness, or increased heart rate.
- ⚡ Teach patients not to abruptly discontinue the drug; the dose must be tapered to avoid withdrawal symptoms. Consult a health care provider before modifying doses.
- ⚡ Encourage patients to read labels on over-the-counter (OTC) products because many contain caffeine. A high plasma caffeine level could be fatal.
- Teach nursing mothers to avoid taking all central nervous system (CNS) stimulants (e.g., caffeine). These drugs are excreted in breast milk and can cause hyperactivity or restlessness in infants.
- Direct families to seek counseling for children with ADHD. Drug therapy alone is not an appropriate therapy program. Notify school nurse of drug therapy regimen.
- Explain to patients and family that long-term use may lead to drug abuse.

Diet
- Advise patients to avoid foods that contain caffeine (e.g., coffee, tea, chocolate, soft drinks, and energy drinks).
- Encourage parents to provide children with a nutritious breakfast because the drug may have anorexic effects.

Side Effects
- Teach patients about drug side effects and the need to report tachycardia and palpitations.
- Monitor children for onset of Tourette syndrome.

Evaluate Outcomes [Evaluation]
- Evaluate effectiveness of drug therapy, level of hyperactivity, and presence of adverse effects.
- Monitor weight, sleep patterns, and mental status.
- Evaluate patient knowledge of methylphenidate therapy.

TABLE 17.1   Amphetamines and Amphetamine-Like Drugs

Drug	Route and Dosage	Uses and Considerations
Amphetamines		
Amphetamine sulfate CSS II	ADHD: Immediate-release tab: A: PO: Initially 5–10 mg/d in morning; *max:* 60 mg/d Adol 6–17 y: PO: Initially 5 mg qd/bid; *max:* 60 mg/d C 3–5 y: PO: Initially 2.5 mg/d; *max:* 40 mg/d Extended release: A: PO: 12.5 mg/d in morning; *max:* 12.5 mg/d Adol/C 6–12 y PO: Initially 6.3 mg/d; *max:* 20 mg/d	For narcolepsy, ADHD, obesity. May cause growth suppression, dizziness, insomnia, headache, blurred vision, euphoria, confusion, anorexia, dry mouth, weight loss, palpitations, tachycardia, anxiety, fatigue, irritability, constipation, diarrhea, and erectile dysfunction. PB: 16%; t½: 10–13 h
Dextroamphetamine sulfate CSS II	ADHD: Immediate release: A: PO: 5 mg qd/bid; *max:* 60 mg/d Adol/C >6 y: PO: 5 mg qd/bid; *max:* 60 mg/d C 3–5 y: PO: 2.5 mg/d; *max:* 40 mg/d Extended release: A/Adol/C >6 y: PO: Initially 5 mg qd/bid; *max:* 60 mg/d	For ADHD and narcolepsy. May cause headache, euphoria, anorexia, abdominal pain, weight loss, growth suppression, insomnia, irritability, palpitations, and blurred vision. PB: UK; t½: 10–12 h

TABLE 17.1 Amphetamines and Amphetamine-Like Drugs—cont'd

Drug	Route and Dosage	Uses and Considerations
Lisdexamfetamine dimesylate CSS II	ADHD: A: PO: Initially 30 mg/d; *max:* 70 mg/d Adol/C >6 y: PO: Initially 20–30 mg/d; *max:* 70 mg/d	For binge-eating disorder and ADHD. May cause insomnia, irritability, anxiety, dizziness, weight loss, nausea, vomiting, constipation, diarrhea, abdominal pain, dry mouth, and bradycardia. PB: UK; t½: <1 h
Combinations of Amphetamines		
Amphetamine and dextroamphetamine	Narcolepsy: A/Adol/C >12 y: PO: Initially 10 mg in the morning; *max:* 60 mg/d C 6–11 y: PO: Initially 5 mg in the morning; *max:* 60 mg/d	For ADHD and narcolepsy. May cause abdominal pain, anorexia, dry mouth, insomnia, headache, weight loss, anxiety, dizziness, nausea, vomiting, and diarrhea. PB: 16% amphetamine, UK dextroamphetamine; t½: 10–13 h amphetamine, 10–12 h dextroamphetamine
Amphetamine-Like Drugs		
Methylphenidate hydrochloride CSS II	See Prototype Drug Chart: Methylphenidate.	
Modafinil CSS IV	A: PO: 200 mg/d in the morning; *max:* 400 mg/d	For narcolepsy, ADHD, shift work sleep disorder, and sleep apnea. May cause headache, dizziness, anxiety, anorexia, nausea, diarrhea, dry mouth, insomnia, rhinitis, back pain. PB: 60%; t½: 15 h
Dexmethylphenidate hydrochloride	Immediate release: A: PO: 2.5 mg bid; *max:* 20 mg/d Extended release: A: PO: 10 mg/d in the morning; *max:* 40 mg/d	For ADHD. May cause headache, dizziness, restlessness, irritability, anxiety, insomnia, anorexia, nausea, vomiting, dry mouth, abdominal pain, nasal congestion, and palpitations. May cause sudden death in patients with structural cardiac abnormalities. PB: UK; t½: 2–4.5 h
Armodafinil	A: PO: 150–250 mg/d in the morning; *max:* 250 mg/d	For narcolepsy, shift work sleep disorder, and sleep apnea. May cause headache, anxiety, dizziness, insomnia, nausea, dry mouth, diarrhea, depression, and suicidal ideation. PB: 60%; t½: 15 h
Selective Norepinephrine Reuptake Inhibitor		
Viloxazine	Adol: PO: 200 mg/d; *max:* 400 mg/d C >6 y: PO: 100 mg/d; *max:* 400 mg/d	For ADHD. May cause drowsiness, headache, fatigue, irritability, insomnia, abdominal pain, anorexia, nausea, vomiting, and infection. PB: 76%–82%; t½: 2–12 h
CNS Stimulant		
Serdexmethylphenidate and dexmethylphenidate	A/Adol/C 6–12 yr: Initially 39.2 mg serdexmethylphenidate, 7.8 mg dexmethylphenidate/d in morning for 1 wk; *max:* 52.3 mg serdexmethylphenidate, 10.4 mg dexmethylphenidate/d	For ADHD. May cause abdominal pain, anorexia, nausea, vomiting, agitation, anxiety, arthralgia, blurred vision, dizziness, headache, insomnia, and irritability. PB: 56% serdexmethylphenidate, 47% dexmethylphenidate; t½: 5.7 h serdexmethylphenidate, 11.7 h dexmethylphenidate
Other Narcolepsy Agents		
Histamine-3 Receptor Antagonists		
Pitolisant	A: PO: Initially 8.9 mg/d upon awakening for 1 wk, then 17.8 mg/d for 1 wk; *max:* 35.6 mg/d	For excessive daytime sleepiness associated with narcolepsy. May cause headache, anxiety, nausea, insomnia, infection, and musculoskeletal pain. PB: 91%–96%; t½: 7.5–24.2 h
Dopamine and Norepinephrine Inhibitors		
Solriamfetol	A: PO: Initially 75 mg/d upon awakening; for 3 days, then may give 150 mg/d; *max:* 150 mg/d	For excessive daytime sleepiness associated with narcolepsy. May cause headache, anxiety, xerostomia, insomnia, hypertension, palpitations, nausea, and diarrhea. PB: <20%; t½: 7.1 h

>, Greater than; <, less than; *A,* adult; *ADHD,* attention-deficit/hyperactivity disorder; *Adol,* adolescent; *bid,* twice a day; *CSS,* Controlled Substances Schedule; *d,* day; *h,* hour; *max,* maximum; *PB,* protein binding; *PO,* by mouth; *t½,* half-life; *UK,* unknown; *y,* year.

TABLE 17.2 Anorexiants and Analeptics

Drug	Route and Dosage	Uses and Considerations
Anorexiants		
Benzphetamine hydrochloride CSS III	A: PO: 25–50 mg daily; *max:* 150 mg/d	Short-term (8–12 wk) treatment for obesity. May cause restlessness, dizziness, headache, insomnia, nausea, dry mouth, dysgeusia, anorexia, diarrhea, anxiety, erectile dysfunction, palpitations, and hypertension. PB: UK, t½: UK
Diethylpropion hydrochloride CSS IV	Immediate release: A: PO: 25 mg tid 1 h before meals; *max:* 75 mg/d Extended release: A: PO: 75 mg/d mid morning; *max:* 75 mg/d	Short-term use for obesity. May cause headache, dizziness, insomnia, dry mouth, abdominal pain, dysgeusia, nausea, constipation, palpitations, restlessness, tremor, and tolerance. PB: UK; t½: 4–8 h
Phentermine hydrochloride CSS IV	A: PO: 15–37.5 mg/d in the morning; *max:* 37.5 mg/d	Short-term use for obesity. May cause restlessness, dizziness, headache, insomnia, euphoria, dysphoria, dry mouth, dysgeusia, constipation, diarrhea, hypertension, tachycardia, palpitations, and tolerance. PB: 17.5 h; t½: 19–24 h
Phentermine-topiramate	Extended release: A: PO: 3.75 mg phentermine/23 mg topiramate/d for 14 d in the morning, then 7.5 mg phentermine/46 mg topiramate/d; *max:* 15 mg phentermine/92 mg topiramate/d	Used short term for obesity. May cause headache, dizziness, pharyngitis, dry mouth, constipation, dysgeusia, tachycardia, hypertension, paresthesia, suicidal ideation, insomnia, infection, and hypokalemia. Evaluate weight loss in 12 weeks. PB: 17.5% phentermine, 15%–41% topiramate; t½: 19–24 h phentermine, 65 h topiramate
Phendimetrazine	Immediate release: A: PO: 35 mg bid/tid, 1 h before meals; *max:* 210 mg/d Extended release: A: PO: 105 mg/d 30–60 min before breakfast; *max:* 105 mg/d	Used short term for obesity. May cause headache, insomnia, dizziness, dry mouth, restlessness, blurred vision, constipation, tachycardia, palpitations, hypertension, erectile dysfunction, tremor, and tolerance. PB: UK; t½: 1.9–9.8 h
Liraglutide	Obesity: A: Subcut: Initially 0.6 mg/d for 1 wk; *max:* 3 mg/d	Used short term for obesity and type 2 diabetes mellitus. May cause headache, anorexia, nausea, vomiting, constipation, diarrhea, tachycardia, palpitations, suicidal ideation, injection site reaction, and hypoglycemia. PB: >98%; t½: 13 h
Naltrexone hydrochloride/ bupropion hydrochloride	Extended release: A: PO: Initially 8 mg naltrexone/90 mg bupropion/d in the morning; *max:* 32 mg naltrexone/360 mg bupropion/d	Used short term for obesity. May cause headache, dizziness, insomnia, nausea, vomiting, constipation, suicidal ideation, hypertension, and erectile dysfunction. PB: 21% naltrexone, 84% bupropion; t½: 4 h naltrexone, 21 h bupropion
Setmelanotide	A: Subcut: Initially 2 mg/d for 2 wk; *max:* 3 mg/d	Short-term use for obesity. May cause abdominal pain, arthralgia, weakness, back pain, fatigue, depression, headache, injection site reaction, nausea, vomiting, diarrhea, and skin hyperpigmentation. PB: 79.1%; t½: 11 h
Analeptics		
Methylxanthines		
Caffeine citrate	Mental alertness: A: PO: 100–200 mg q3–4h PRN; *max:* 1200 mg/d	For neonatal apnea and mental alertness. May cause headache, insomnia, nausea, tachycardia, palpitations, urinary frequency, tremors, and withdrawal. PB: 36%; t½: 3–7 h

>, Greater than; *A,* adult; *bid,* twice a day; *CSS,* Controlled Substances Schedule; *d,* day; *h,* hour; *IV,* intravenous; *max,* maximum; *min,* minute; *PB,* protein binding; *PO,* by mouth; *subcut,* subcutaneous; *t½,* half-life; *tid,* three times a day; *UK,* unknown; *wk,* week; *y,* years.

CRITICAL THINKING CASE STUDY

A 7-year-old child has been diagnosed with attention-deficit/hyperactivity disorder. The physician is considering putting the child on medication.

1. What symptoms does a child with attention-deficit/hyperactivity disorder display?
2. What medication might be prescribed? What class of drugs does the medication fall under?
3. What behavioral improvements might be seen after medication administration?
4. What physical assessment should be completed before medication administration?
5. What teaching should the nurse include related to the use of methylphenidate?

REVIEW QUESTIONS

1. When a 12-year-old child is prescribed methylphenidate, which is most important for the nurse to monitor?
   a. Temperature
   b. Respirations
   c. Intake and output
   d. Height and weight
2. Several children are admitted for diagnosis with possible attention-deficit/hyperactivity disorder. Which is most important for the nurse to observe?
   a. A girl who is lethargic
   b. A girl who lacks impulsivity
   c. A boy with smooth coordination
   d. A boy with an inability to complete tasks
3. The nurse monitoring a patient for methylphenidate withdrawal should observe the patient for which condition?
   a. Tremors
   b. Insomnia
   c. Weakness
   d. Tachycardia
4. The nurse is teaching a patient to self-administer medications. The nurse knows that which drug is used to treat narcolepsy?
   a. Modafinil
   b. Atomoxetine
   c. Lisdexamfetamine
   d. Phendimetrazine
5. The nurse is monitoring a patient who is taking phentermine. Which is important for the nurse to observe? (Select all that apply.)
   a. Euphoria
   b. Dry mouth
   c. Insomnia
   d. Hypotension
   e. Bradycardia
   f. Palpitations

18

Depressants

Jared Robertson III, RN, MN

http://evolve.elsevier.com/McCuistion/pharmacology

Drugs that are central nervous system (CNS) depressants cause varying degrees of depression (reduction in functional activity) within the CNS. The degree of depression depends primarily on the drug and the amount of drug taken. The broad classification of CNS depressants includes sedative-hypnotics, general anesthetics, analgesics, opioid and nonopioid analgesics, anticonvulsants, antipsychotics, and antidepressants. The last five groups of depressant drugs are presented in separate chapters. Sedative-hypnotics and general anesthetics are discussed in this chapter.

TYPES AND STAGES OF SLEEP

Sleep disorders such as insomnia, the inability to fall asleep or remain asleep, occur in 10% to 30% of Americans. Insomnia occurs more frequently in women, and the incidence increases with age.

People spend approximately one-third of their lives, or as much as 25 years, sleeping. Normal sleep is composed of two definite phases: rapid eye movement (REM) and non-rapid eye movement (NREM) sleep. Both REM and NREM sleep occur cyclically at about 90-minute intervals during sleep (Fig. 18.1). The four succeedingly deeper stages of NREM sleep end with an episode of REM sleep, and the cycle begins again. If sleep is interrupted, the cycle begins again with stage 1 of NREM sleep. Individuals perform better during their waking hours if they experience all types and stages of sleep.

During REM sleep, individuals experience most of their recallable dreams. Children have few REM sleep periods and have longer periods of stage 3 and 4 NREM sleep. Older adults experience a decrease in stage 3 and 4 NREM sleep and have frequent waking periods.

It is difficult to rouse a person during REM sleep, and the period of REM sleep episodes becomes longer during the sleep process. Frequently, if a person is roused from REM sleep, a vivid, bizarre dream may be recalled. If these dreams are unpleasant, they may be called *nightmares*. Sleepwalking or nightmares that occur in children take place during NREM sleep.

NONPHARMACOLOGIC METHODS

Before using sedative-hypnotics or over-the-counter (OTC) sleep aids, various nonpharmacologic methods should be used to promote sleep.

Once the nurse discovers why the patient cannot sleep, the following ways to promote sleep may be suggested:

1. Arise at a specific time in the morning.
2. Take few or no daytime naps.
3. Avoid drinks that contain caffeine and alcohol 6 hours before bedtime. Also avoid smoking nicotine products for 6 hours before bedtime.
4. Avoid heavy meals or strenuous exercise before bedtime.
5. Take a warm bath, listen to quiet music, or perform other soothing activities before bedtime.
6. Decrease exposure to loud noises.
7. Avoid drinking copious amounts of fluids before sleep.
8. Drink warm milk before bedtime.

SEDATIVE-HYPNOTICS

Sedative-hypnotics are commonly ordered for treatment of sleep disorders. The mildest form of CNS depression is sedation, which diminishes physical and mental responses at lower dosages of certain CNS depressants but does not affect consciousness. Sedatives are used mostly during the daytime. Increasing the drug dose can produce a hypnotic effect—not hypnosis but a form of "natural" sleep. Sedative-hypnotic drugs are sometimes the same drug; however, certain drugs are used more often for their hypnotic effect. With very high doses of sedative-hypnotic drugs, anesthesia may be achieved.

Sedatives were first prescribed to reduce tension and anxiety. Barbiturates were initially used for their antianxiety effect until the early 1960s, when benzodiazepines were introduced. Because of the many side effects of barbiturates and their potential for physical and mental dependency, they are now less frequently prescribed.

The Centers for Disease Control and Prevention cite that approximately 70 million Americans have chronic sleep problems and suffer from sleep deprivation. The cost is billions of dollars in lost productivity, and millions of dollars are spent each year on OTC sleep aids. The primary ingredient in OTC sleep aids is an antihistamine such as diphenhydramine.

Hypnotics may be short or intermediate acting. Short-acting hypnotics are useful in achieving sleep because they allow the patient to awaken early in the morning without experiencing lingering side effects. Intermediate-acting hypnotics are useful for sustaining sleep; however, after using one, the patient may experience residual drowsiness, or hangover, in the morning. This may be undesirable if the patient is active and requires mental alertness. The ideal hypnotic promotes natural sleep without disrupting normal patterns of sleep and produces no hangover or undesirable effect. Table 18.1 lists the common side effects and adverse reactions associated with sedative-hypnotic use and abuse.

Hypnotic drug therapy should usually be short term to prevent drug dependence and tolerance. Interrupting hypnotic therapy can decrease drug tolerance, but abruptly discontinuing a high dose of hypnotic taken over a long period can cause withdrawal symptoms. In such cases the dose should be tapered to avoid withdrawal symptoms.

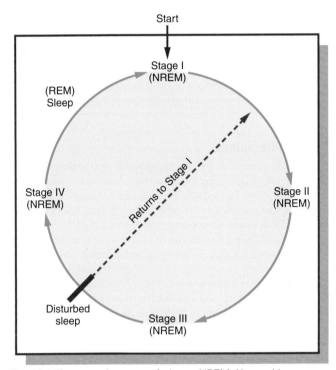

Fig. 18.1 Types and stages of sleep. *NREM,* Non-rapid eye movement (four stages); *REM,* rapid eye movement (dreaming).

TABLE 18.1	Common Side Effects and Adverse Reactions of Sedative-Hypnotics
Side Effects and Adverse Reactions	**Explanation of the Effects**
Hangover	A hangover is residual drowsiness resulting in impaired reaction time. The intermediate- and long-acting hypnotics are frequently the cause of drug hangover. The liver biotransforms these drugs into active metabolites that persist in the body, causing drowsiness.
REM rebound	REM rebound, which results in vivid dreams and nightmares, frequently occurs after taking a hypnotic for a prolonged period then abruptly stopping. However, it may occur after taking only one hypnotic dose.
Dependence	Dependence is the result of chronic hypnotic use. Physical and psychological dependence can result. Physical dependence results in the appearance of specific withdrawal symptoms when a drug is discontinued after prolonged use. The severity of withdrawal symptoms depends on the drug and dosage. Symptoms may include muscular twitching and tremors, dizziness, orthostatic hypotension, delusions, hallucinations, delirium, and seizures. Withdrawal symptoms start within 24 hours and can last for several days.
Tolerance	Tolerance results when there is a need to increase the dosage over time to obtain the desired effect. It is mostly caused by an increase in drug metabolism by liver enzymes. The barbiturate drug category can cause tolerance after prolonged use. Tolerance is reversible when the drug is discontinued.
Excessive depression	Long-term use of a hypnotic may result in CNS depression, which is characterized by lethargy, sleepiness, lack of concentration, confusion, and psychological depression.
Respiratory depression	High doses of sedative-hypnotics can suppress the respiratory center in the medulla.
Hypersensitivity	Skin rashes and urticaria can result when taking barbiturates. Such reactions are rare.

CNS, Central nervous system; *REM,* rapid eye movement.

As a general rule, the lowest dose should be taken to achieve sleep. Patients with severe respiratory disorders should avoid hypnotics, which could cause an increase in respiratory depression. Usually, hypnotics are contraindicated during pregnancy. Ramelteon is the only major sedative-hypnotic approved for long-term use. This drug may be used for treating chronic insomnia.

The category of sedative-hypnotics includes barbiturates, benzodiazepines, and nonbenzodiazepines, among others. Each category is discussed separately. Prototype drug charts are included for benzodiazepines and nonbenzodiazepines.

Barbiturates

Barbiturates were introduced as a sedative in the early 1900s. They are classified as long, intermediate, short, and ultrashort acting.

- The *long-acting* group includes phenobarbital, which is used to control seizures in epilepsy.
- The *intermediate-acting* barbiturates, such as butabarbital, are useful as sleep sustainers for maintaining long periods of sleep. Because these drugs take approximately 1 hour for the onset of sleep, they are not prescribed for those who have trouble getting to sleep. Vital signs should be closely monitored in persons who take intermediate-acting barbiturates.
- The *short-acting* barbiturate secobarbital may be used for procedure sedation. Vital signs should be closely monitored in persons who take short-acting barbiturates.

Barbiturates should be restricted to short-term use (2 weeks or less) because of their numerous side effects, including tolerance to the drug. In the United States barbiturates are classified under the Controlled Substances Act as Schedule II for short-acting, Schedule III for intermediate-acting, and Schedule IV for long-acting hypnotics. In Canada barbiturates are classified as Schedule G. Barbiturates are listed in Table 18.2.

Pharmacokinetics. Pentobarbital has been available for nearly half a century and was the hypnotic of choice until the introduction of benzodiazepines in the 1960s. It has a slow absorption rate and is moderately protein bound. The long half-life is mainly because of the formation of active metabolites resulting from liver metabolism.

Pharmacodynamics. Pentobarbital and secobarbital are used primarily for short-term treatment of insomnia. Other uses include control of seizures, preoperative anxiety, and sedation induction. They have a rapid onset with a short duration of action and are considered short-acting barbiturates.

Many drug interactions are associated with barbiturates. Alcohol, opioids, and other sedative-hypnotics used in combination with barbiturates may further depress the CNS. Pentobarbital increases hepatic enzyme action, causing an increased metabolism and decreased effect of drugs such as oral anticoagulants, glucocorticoids, tricyclic antidepressants, and quinidine. Pentobarbital may cause hepatotoxicity if taken with large doses of acetaminophen.

> ### ⚡ PATIENT SAFETY
>
> **Do Not Confuse:**
> - **Phenobarbital,** a long-acting barbiturate used to control seizures, with **pentobarbital,** an ultra-short-acting barbiturate used as a general anesthetic.

⚠️ Benzodiazepines

Selected benzodiazepines, minor tranquilizers and anxiolytics, were introduced with chlordiazepoxide in the 1960s as antianxiety agents. This drug group is ordered as sedative-hypnotics for inducing sleep. Several benzodiazepines marketed as hypnotics include flurazepam, alprazolam (Prototype Drug Chart: Alprazolam), temazepam, triazolam, estazolam, and quazepam (Table 18.3). Increased anxiety might be the cause of insomnia for some patients, so lorazepam and diazepam can be used to alleviate the anxiety. These drugs are classified as Schedule IV according to the Controlled Substances Act. The benzodiazepines increase the action of the inhibitory neurotransmitter gamma-aminobutyric acid (GABA) to the GABA receptors. Neuron excitability is reduced.

TABLE 18.2   Sedative-Hypnotics: Barbiturates and Other Drugs

Drug	Route and Dosage	Uses and Considerations
Barbiturates: Short-Acting		
Secobarbital sodium CSS II	Sedation induction: A: PO: 200–300 mg 1–2 h before procedure	For sedation induction and insomnia. Use only short term, as effectiveness is lost in about 2 weeks. May cause confusion, drowsiness, constipation, withdrawal, sleep-related behaviors, nightmares, and suicidal ideation. PB: 30%–45%; t½: 15–40 h
Pentobarbital CSS II	Sedation induction: A: IM: 150–200 mg before procedure A: IV: Initially 100 mg; after 1 min assessment, may repeat up to 200–500 mg	For sedation induction, seizures. May cause hypotension, bradycardia, drowsiness, dizziness, ataxia, agitation, confusion, constipation, impaired cognition, erectile dysfunction, and respiratory depression. PB: 35%–45%; t½: 35–50 h
Barbiturates: Intermediate-Acting		
Butabarbital sodium CSS III	Anxiety: A: PO: 15–30 mg tid/qid	To manage anxiety. Use short term (<14 days), and avoid alcohol with all barbiturates. May cause ataxia, drowsiness, sleep-related behaviors, confusion, agitation, bradycardia, hypotension, headache, nightmares, depression, and angioedema. This drug is no longer accepted for use in older adults or debilitated adult patients for insomnia. PB: 50%; t½: 100 h
Barbiturates: Long-Acting		
Phenobarbital CSS IV	Sedation induction: A: IM/IV: 100–200 mg 60–90 min before procedure	Used for seizure control, sedation induction, and insomnia. May cause ataxia, depression, bradycardia, hypotension, dizziness, confusion, drowsiness, headache, impaired judgment, nightmares, constipation, and erectile dysfunction. Monitor for respiratory depression. PB: 20%–45%; t½: 50–120 h for adults, 37–69 h for children, 47–63 h for infants

<, Less than; *A,* adult; *CSS,* Controlled Substances Schedule; *d,* day; *h,* hour; *IM,* intramuscular; *IV,* intravenous; *PB,* protein binding; *PO,* by mouth; *qid,* four times a day; *t½,* half-life; *tid,* three times a day.

⚠ TABLE 18.3 Sedative-Hypnotics: Benzodiazepines, Nonbenzodiazepines, and Opioid Agonists

Drug	Route and Dosage	Uses and Considerations
Benzodiazepines		
Alprazolam CSS IV	See Prototype Drug Chart: Alprazolam	
Estazolam CSS IV	A: PO: 1–2 mg at bedtime; *max:* 2 mg/d Older A: PO: 0.5–1 mg at bedtime; *max:* 2 mg/d	For treatment of insomnia. Should not be used longer than 6 weeks. May cause tolerance, dizziness, drowsiness, anterograde amnesia, confusion, ataxia, edema, dependence, withdrawal, weakness, and sleep-related behaviors. PB: 93%; t½: 10–24 h
Lorazepam CSS IV	Insomnia: A: PO: 2–4 mg at bedtime; *max:* 10 mg/d Older A: PO: Initially 1–2 mg at bedtime; *maint:* 2–4 mg at bedtime; *max:* 10 mg/d	Used for sedation induction and to reduce anxiety, insomnia, and seizures. May cause tolerance, drowsiness, dizziness, hypotension, blurred vision, anterograde amnesia, memory impairment, agitation, nightmares, dependence, injection site reaction, and suicidal ideation. PB: 85%; t½: 12–14 h
Temazepam CSS IV	Insomnia: A: PO: 15–30 mg at bedtime; *max:* 30 mg/d Older A: PO: 7.5 mg at bedtime; *max:* 30 mg/d	To treat insomnia. May cause tolerance, drowsiness, dizziness, confusion, palpitations, hypotension, dependence, withdrawal, anterograde amnesia, and sleep-related behavior. PB: 98%; t½: 8–15 h
Triazolam CSS IV	Insomnia: A: PO: 0.125–0.25 mg at bedtime; *max:* 0.5 mg/d Older A: PO: 0.125 mg at bedtime; *max:* 0.25 mg/d	For management of insomnia. Should not be used longer than 7–10 d at a time to avoid tolerance. Avoid alcohol and smoking when taking triazolam. May cause tolerance, drowsiness, dizziness, nausea, ataxia, confusion, visual impairment, headache, tachycardia, depression, dependence, withdrawal, anterograde amnesia, and sleep-related behaviors. PB: 90%; t½: 1.5–5.5 h
Benzodiazepine Antagonists		
Flumazenil	A: IV: 0.2 mg over 30 s; may repeat after 45 s, then repeat q1min PRN; *max:* 4 doses	For management of benzodiazepine toxicity and sedation reversal. May cause drowsiness, dizziness, blurred vision, ataxia, seizures, hyperacusis, palpitations, vomiting, and dry mouth. PB: 50%; t½: 40–80 min
Nonbenzodiazepines		
Zolpidem tartrate CSS IV	See Prototype Drug Chart: Zolpidem Tartrate	
Eszopiclone CSS IV	Insomnia: A: PO: Initially 1 mg at bedtime; *maint:* 2–3 mg at bedtime; *max:* 3 mg/d Older A: PO: 1–2 mg at bedtime; *max:* 2 mg/d	To treat insomnia. May cause headache, dizziness, drowsiness, unpleasant taste, sleep-related behaviors, infection, depression, and suicidal ideation. PB: 52%–59%; t½: 6 h
Zaleplon CSS IV	Insomnia: A: PO: 10 mg at bedtime; *max:* 20 mg Older A: PO: 5 mg at bedtime; *max:* 10 mg/d	For ultrashort-term treatment of insomnia. May cause headache, dizziness, drowsiness, nausea, abdominal pain, weakness, and sleep-related behaviors. PB: 45%–75%; t½: 1 h
Melatonin Agonist		
Ramelteon	A: PO: 8 mg within 30 min of bedtime; *max:* 8 mg/d	For treatment of insomnia. May cause dizziness, nausea, drowsiness, fatigue, depression, suicidal ideation, and sleep-related behaviors. PB: 82%; t½: 1–2.6 h
Opioid Agonists		
Alfentanil CSS II	A: IV: 130–245 mcg/kg over 3 min as induction; *maint:* 0.5–1.5 mcg/kg/min; *max:* dependent on procedure duration	For general anesthesia induction and maintenance and sedation maintenance. Must be administered by someone trained in general anesthetic administration. May cause dizziness, confusion, dysrhythmias, hypotension or hypertension, respiratory depression, bronchospasm, tachycardia, bradycardia, chest wall rigidity, nausea, and vomiting. Use caution in patients with head trauma and liver dysfunction. PB: 88%–92%; t½: 90–111 min
Sufentanil CSS II	A: IV: 8–30 mcg/kg increments or infusion for induction; *maint:* 0.5–10 mcg/kg intermittent or continuous IV; *max:* dependent on procedure duration	For general anesthesia induction and maintenance, obstetric anesthesia, and severe pain. Must be administered by someone trained in general anesthetic administration. May cause drowsiness, pruritus, bradycardia, hypertension or hypotension, dysrhythmia, chest wall rigidity, bronchospasm, respiratory depression, urinary retention, headache, dizziness, nausea, and vomiting. PB: 93%; t½: 164 min
Remifentanil	A: IV: 0.5–1 mcg/kg/min continuous infusion	For general anesthesia induction and maintenance and moderate to severe pain. Must be administered by someone trained in general anesthetic administration. May cause dizziness, pruritus, confusion, chest wall rigidity, hypotension, bradycardia, dysrhythmias, fever, headache, nausea, and vomiting. PB: 70%; t½: 10–20 min

A, Adult; *CSS,* Controlled Substances Schedule; *d,* day; *h,* hour; *IV,* intravenous; *maint,* maintenance; *max,* maximum; *min,* minute; *PB,* protein binding; *PO,* by mouth; *PRN,* as needed; *q1min,* once per minute; *s,* second; *t½,* half-life.

PROTOTYPE DRUG CHART

! *Alprazolam*

Drug Class	Dosage
Sedative-hypnotic: benzodiazepine CSS IV	Immediate release: A: PO: Initially 0.25–0.5 mg tid, may increase q3–4d; *max:* 4 mg/d Older A: PO: Initially 0.25 mg bid/tid, may increase q3–4d; *max:* 4 mg/d Extended release: A: PO: Initially 0.5–1 mg/d in the morning, may increase q3–4d; *max:* 10 mg/d Older A: PO: Initially 0.5 mg/d, may increase q3–4d; *max:* 10 mg/d

Contraindications	Drug-Lab-Food Interactions
Respiratory depression, acute alcohol intoxication, psychotic reactions, recent respiratory depressants, hypersensitivity *Caution:* Older adults, sleep apnea, renal or liver dysfunction, depression, suicidal ideation, substance abuse, alcohol abuse, psychosis, respiratory depression	Drug: Decreases respiration with alcohol, CNS depressants; azole antifungals (ketoconazole), antibiotics (erythromycin), aprepitant, cimetidine, diltiazem, and verapamil increase blood levels of alprazolam; rifabutin, rifampin, cortisone, and phenytoin decrease blood levels; alprazolam increases digoxin and lithium levels Food: Grapefruit increases alprazolam levels; green tea decreases alprazolam effects

Pharmacokinetics	Pharmacodynamics
Absorption: PO: 90% absorbed from GI tract Distribution: PB: 80% Metabolism: t½: IR, 6.3–26.9 h; ER, 11–16 h Excretion: In urine as metabolites	PO: Onset: 15–30 min Peak: IR, 1–2 h; ER, 9 h Duration: UK

Therapeutic Effects/Uses	
To treat anxiety and panic disorders Mechanism of Action: CNS depression, binds receptors in limbic system and reticular formation, increases GABA to GABA receptors; shift of chloride ions leads to less excitability and stabilizes neuronal membranes	

Side Effects	Adverse Reactions
Lethargy, drowsiness, dizziness, headache, constipation, anterograde amnesia, memory impairment, fatigue, agitation, ataxia, increased appetite, blurred vision, decreased libido, dry mouth, nausea, edema, weight gain/loss, nasal congestion, rash, irritability	Depression, tolerance, dependence, withdrawal, hypotension, tachycardia, seizures *Life-threatening:* Hepatic failure, Stevens-Johnson syndrome

A, Adult; *CNS,* central nervous system; *CSS,* Controlled Substances Schedule; *d,* day; *Dtab,* disintegrating tablet; *ER,* extended release; *GABA,* gamma-aminobutyric acid; *GI,* gastrointestinal; *h,* hour; *IR,* immediate release; *max,* maximum; *min,* minute; *PB,* protein binding; *PO,* by mouth; *t½,* half-life; *tid,* three times a day; *UK,* unknown.

◎ CLINICAL JUDGMENT [NURSING PROCESS]

! *Sedative-Hypnotics: Benzodiazepines*

Concept: Sleep
- A phase of our daily life cycle when the brain and body rest and rejuvenate; the eyes are closed, metabolism slows, and postural muscles are relaxed.

Recognize Cues [Assessment]
- Obtain a drug history of current drugs and complementary and alternative therapies that the patient is taking, especially central nervous system (CNS) depressants, which would potentiate respiratory depression and hypotensive effects.
- Assess baseline vital signs for future comparisons.
- Determine whether the patient has a history of insomnia or anxiety disorders.
- Assess renal function. Urine output should be 1500 mL/day. Renal impairment could prolong drug action by increasing the half-life of the drug.

Analyze Cues and Prioritize Hypothesis [Patient Problems]
- Decreased functional ability
- Reduced stamina
- Decreased level of consciousness
- Decreased ability to cope

Generate Solutions [Planning]
- Patient will receive adequate sleep when taking benzodiazepines.

Take Action [Nursing Interventions]
- Monitor vital signs, especially respirations and blood pressure.
- Use a bed alarm for older adults and for patients receiving a hypnotic for the first time. Confusion can occur, and injury could result.
- Observe the patient for adverse reactions, especially an older adult or a debilitated patient.
- Examine the patient's skin for rashes. Skin eruptions may occur in patients taking benzodiazepines.

Patient Teaching
General
- Teach patients to use nonpharmacologic methods to induce sleep such as taking a warm bath, listening to quiet music, drinking warm fluids, and avoiding drinks with caffeine for 6 hours before bedtime.

CLINICAL JUDGMENT [NURSING PROCESS]—CONT'D

! *Sedative-Hypnotics: Benzodiazepines*

- Encourage patients to avoid alcohol and antidepressant, antipsychotic, and opioid drugs while taking benzodiazepines. Respiratory depression can occur when these drugs are combined.
- Warn patients that certain complementary and alternative therapy products may interact with benzodiazepines (see Complementary and Alternative Therapies). These products may need to be discontinued or the prescription drug dose may need to be modified.
- ⚡ Advise patients not to drive a motor vehicle or operate machinery when using benzodiazepines. Caution is always encouraged.
- Encourage patients to check with a health care provider about over-the-counter (OTC) sleeping aids. Drowsiness may result from taking these drugs; therefore caution while driving is advised.

Side Effects
- Advise patients to report adverse reactions such as cognitive changes and paradoxical reactions to their health care provider. Drug selection or dosage might need to be changed.
- Teach patients that benzodiazepines should be gradually withdrawn, especially if they have been taken for several weeks. Abrupt cessation may result in withdrawal symptoms such as tremors and muscle twitching.

Evaluate Outcomes [Evaluation]
- Assess the effectiveness of benzodiazepines.
- Evaluate respiratory status to ensure that respiratory depression has not occurred.

🌸 COMPLEMENTARY AND ALTERNATIVE THERAPIES

Sedatives

- Kava kava should not be taken in combination with CNS depressants such as barbiturates and opioids. This product may increase the sedative effect.
- Valerian, when taken with alcohol and other CNS depressants such as barbiturates, may increase the sedative effects of the prescribed drug.

⚡ PATIENT SAFETY

Do Not Confuse:
- **Lorazepam,** a benzodiazepine used to reduce anxiety, with **alprazolam,** a benzodiazepine used to treat anxiety and insomnia.

Benzodiazepines (except for temazepam) can suppress stage 4 of NREM sleep, which may result in vivid dreams or nightmares and can delay REM sleep. Benzodiazepines are effective for sleep disorders for several weeks longer than other sedative-hypnotics; to prevent REM rebound, however, they should not be used for longer than 3 to 4 weeks.

Triazolam is a short-acting hypnotic with a half-life of 2 to 5 hours. It does not produce any active metabolites. Adverse effects of anterograde amnesia or memory impairment occur more frequently with triazolam than with other benzodiazepines, and the risk increases with higher doses and with concurrent alcohol or opioid ingestion. Currently, it is seldom prescribed and should not be taken longer than 7 to 10 days.

One adverse effect closely associated with benzodiazepines is anterograde amnesia, an impaired ability to recall events that occur after dosing. Associated with anterograde amnesia are sleep-related behaviors, such as preparing and eating meals, sleep driving, engaging in sex, or making phone calls during sleep without any memory of the event. Alcohol and CNS depressants increase the risk of sleep-related behaviors.

Small doses of benzodiazepines are recommended for patients with renal or hepatic dysfunction. For benzodiazepine overdose, the benzodiazepine antagonist flumazenil may be administered. Benzodiazepines prescribed as antianxiety drugs are discussed in Chapter 22.

Pharmacokinetics. Benzodiazepines are well absorbed through the gastrointestinal (GI) mucosa. They are rapidly metabolized in the liver to active metabolites. Benzodiazepines usually have an intermediate half-life of usually 8 to 24 hours and are highly protein bound. When taken with other highly protein-bound drugs, more free (or unbound) drug is available, resulting in an increased risk for adverse effects.

Pharmacodynamics. Benzodiazepines are used to treat insomnia by inducing and sustaining sleep. They have a rapid onset of action and intermediate- to long-acting effects. The normal recommended dose of a benzodiazepine may be too much for the older adult, so half the dose is recommended initially to prevent overdosing.

Nonbenzodiazepines

Zolpidem is a nonbenzodiazepine that differs in chemical structure from benzodiazepines. It is used for short-term treatment (<10 days) of insomnia. Its duration of action is 6 to 8 hours with a short half-life of 1.4 to 8.4 hours. Zolpidem is metabolized in the liver to three inactive metabolites and is excreted in bile, urine, and feces. When zolpidem is prescribed for older adults, the dose should be decreased. Table 18.3 lists the benzodiazepines and nonbenzodiazepines used as sedative-hypnotics and their dosages, uses, and considerations including common side effects and a few serious adverse effects. Zolpidem is described in the Prototype Drug Chart: Zolpidem Tartrate.

Melatonin Agonists

Ramelteon is in the newest category of sedative-hypnotics called *melatonin agonists*. Ramelteon is the first hypnotic approved by the US Food and Drug Administration (FDA) that is *not* classified as a controlled substance. This drug acts by selectively targeting melatonin receptors to regulate circadian rhythms in the treatment of insomnia. Ramelteon has not been shown to decrease REM sleep. This new drug has a half-life of 1 to 2.6 hours. Adverse effects of ramelteon include drowsiness, dizziness, fatigue, headache, nausea, and suicidal ideation.

Sedatives and Hypnotics for Older Adults

Identifying the cause of insomnia in an older adult should be the first diagnostic consideration, and nonpharmacologic methods should be used before sleep medications are prescribed. Because of physiologic changes in older adults, the use of hypnotics can cause a variety of side effects.

Barbiturates increase CNS depression and confusion in older adults and should *not* be taken for sleep. The short- to intermediate-acting benzodiazepines—such as estazolam, temazepam, and triazolam—are considered to be safer than barbiturates. Long-acting hypnotic benzodiazepines such as flurazepam, quazepam, and diazepam should be avoided. In many cases, older adults should be instructed to take the prescribed benzodiazepine no more than four times a week to avoid side effects and drug dependency. They can choose selected nights to take the hypnotic.

The main sleep problem experienced by older adults is frequent nighttime awakening. Reports have shown that older women experience more troublesome sleep patterns than men. Sleep disturbance

PROTOTYPE DRUG CHART

Zolpidem Tartrate

Drug Class	Dosage
Sedative-hypnotic: Nonbenzodiazepine CSS IV	Immediate release: A males: PO: 5–10 mg at bedtime; *max:* 10 mg/d A females/older A: PO: 5 mg at bedtime; *max:* 10 mg/d for females, 5 mg/d for older adults SL tabs/oral spray: A: PO: 5–10 mg at bedtime; *max:* 10 mg/d Older A: PO: 5 mg at bedtime; *max:* 5 mg/d Extended release: A: PO: 6.25–12.5 mg at bedtime; *max:* 12.5 mg/d Older A: PO: 6.25 mg at bedtime, *max:* 6.25 mg/d
Contraindications	**Drug-Lab-Food Interactions**

Hypersensitivity to benzodiazepine, drug-induced complex
  sleep-related behaviors
Caution: Renal or liver dysfunction; mental depression, suicidal
  ideation; pregnancy; children, older adults, pulmonary disease,
  alcohol/substance abuse, breast feeding
	Drug: Decreases CNS function with alcohol, CNS depressants, anticonvulsants, and
	  phenothiazines; increased levels with azole antifungals; decreased levels with rifampin
	Food: Decreases absorption

Pharmacokinetics	**Pharmacodynamics**
Absorption: PO: well absorbed Distribution: PB: 92% Metabolism: t½: 1.4–8.4 h Excretion: In bile, urine, and feces	PO: Immediate release: Onset: 30 min Peak: 90 min Duration: 6–8 h SL/spray mist: Onset: UK Peak: 35–82 min Duration: UK Extended release: Onset: UK Peak: UK Duration: UK
Therapeutic Effects/Uses	
To treat insomnia Mechanism of Action: CNS depression, neurotransmitter inhibition	
Side Effects	**Adverse Reactions**

Drowsiness, lethargy, headache, hot flashes, hangover (residual sedation),
  irritability, dizziness, ataxia, visual impairment, anxiety, nausea and vomiting,
  edema, erectile dysfunction, anterograde amnesia, memory impairment,
  nightmares, binge eating
	Tolerance, psychological or physical dependence, withdrawal; sleep-related
	  behaviors, hypotension, angioedema, dysrhythmias, depression, suicidal
	  ideation
	Life-threatening: Pulmonary edema, renal failure

A, Adult; *CNS,* central nervous system; *CSS,* Controlled Substances Schedule; *d,* day; *h,* hour; *max,* maximum; *min,* minute; *PB,* protein binding; *PO,* by mouth; *SL,* sublingual; *t½,* half-life; *UK,* unknown.

CLINICAL JUDGMENT [NURSING PROCESS]

Sedative-Hypnotics: Nonbenzodiazepines

Concept: Sleep
- A phase of our daily life cycle when the brain and body rest and rejuvenate; the eyes are closed, metabolism slows, and postural muscles are relaxed.

Recognize Cues [Assessment]
- Assess baseline vital signs and laboratory tests (e.g., aspartate aminotransferase [AST], alanine aminotransferase [ALT], bilirubin) for future comparisons.
- Obtain a drug history. Taking central nervous system (CNS) depressants with nonbenzodiazepine hypnotics can depress respirations.
- Ascertain the patient's problem with sleep disturbance.

Analyze Cues and Prioritize Hypothesis [Patient Problems]
- Decreased functional ability
- Reduced stamina
- Decreased level of consciousness
- Decreased ability to cope

Generate Solutions [Planning]
- Patient will remain asleep for 6 to 8 hours.

Take Action [Nursing Intervention]
- Monitor vital signs. Check for signs of respiratory depression (slow, irregular breathing patterns).

⊚ CLINICAL JUDGMENT [NURSING PROCESS]—CONT'D

Sedative-Hypnotics: Nonbenzodiazepines

- Use bed alarm for older adults or patients receiving nonbenzodiazepines for the first time. Confusion may occur, and injury may result.
- Observe patient for side effects of nonbenzodiazepines such as hangover (residual sedation), lightheadedness, dizziness, or confusion.

Patient Teaching
General

- Teach patients to use nonpharmacologic methods to induce sleep (taking a warm bath, listening to music, drinking warm fluids such as milk, avoiding drinks with caffeine after dinner).
- Encourage patients to avoid alcohol, antidepressants, antipsychotics, and narcotic drugs while taking nonbenzodiazepines. Severe respiratory depression may occur when these drugs are combined.
- Advise patients to take nonbenzodiazepine before bedtime. Alprazolam takes effect within 15 to 30 minutes.

- Suggest that patients urinate before taking nonbenzodiazepines to prevent sleep disruption.
- Encourage patients to check with a health care provider about over-the-counter (OTC) sleeping aids.
- Warn the patient to use caution while driving because drowsiness may occur.

Side Effects

- Advise patients to report adverse reactions such as hangover to a health care provider. Drug selection or dosage may need to be changed if hangover occurs.

Evaluate Outcomes [Evaluation]

- Evaluate effectiveness of sedative-hypnotics in promoting sleep.
- Determine whether side effects such as hangover occur after several days of taking a sedative-hypnotic. Another hypnotic may be prescribed if side effects persist.

---

may be caused by discomfort or pain. Occasionally a nonsteroidal antiinflammatory drug (NSAID) such as ibuprofen may alleviate the discomfort that prevents sleep.

⚠ ANESTHETICS

Anesthetics are classified as *general* and *local*. General anesthetics depress the CNS, alleviate pain, and cause a loss of consciousness. The first anesthetic, nitrous oxide ("laughing gas"), was used for surgery in the early 1800s. It is still an effective anesthetic and is frequently used in dental procedures and surgery.

Pathophysiology

Several theories exist regarding how inhalation anesthetics cause CNS depression and a loss of consciousness. The differing theories suggest the following about inhalation anesthetics:

1. The lipid structure of cell membranes is altered, resulting in impaired physiologic functions.
2. The inhibitory neurotransmitter GABA is activated to the GABA receptor that pushes chloride ions into the neurons. This greatly decreases the action potentials of the neurons.
3. The ascending reticular activating system is altered and the neurons cease to transmit information (stimuli) to the brain.

Balanced Anesthesia

Balanced anesthesia is a combination of drugs frequently used in general anesthesia. Balanced anesthesia may include the following:

1. A hypnotic given the night before
2. Premedication with an opioid analgesic or benzodiazepine (e.g., midazolam) plus an anticholinergic (e.g., atropine) given about 1 hour before surgery to decrease secretions
3. A short-acting nonbarbiturate such as propofol
4. An inhaled gas, often a combination of an inhalation anesthetic, nitrous oxide, and oxygen
5. A muscle relaxant given as needed

Balanced anesthesia minimizes cardiovascular problems, decreases the amount of general anesthetic needed, reduces possible postanesthesia nausea and vomiting, minimizes the disturbance of organ function, and decreases pain. Because the patient does not receive large doses of general anesthetics, fewer adverse reactions occur and recovery is enhanced by allowing quicker mobility.

TABLE 18.4 Stages of Anesthesia

Stage	Name	Description
1	Analgesia	Begins with consciousness and ends with loss of consciousness; speech is difficult, sensations of smell and pain are lost, dreams and auditory and visual hallucinations may occur; this stage may be called the *induction stage*.
2	Excitement or delirium	Produces a loss of consciousness caused by depression of the cerebral cortex; confusion, excitement, or delirium occur, and induction time is short.
3	Surgical	Surgical procedure is performed during this stage. There are four phases: surgery is usually performed in phase 2 and upper phase 3. As anesthesia deepens, respirations become shallower and the respiratory rate is increased.
4	Medullary paralysis	Toxic stage of anesthesia in which respirations are lost and circulatory collapse occurs; ventilatory assistance is necessary.

Stages of General Anesthesia

General anesthesia proceeds through four stages (Table 18.4). The surgical procedure is usually performed during the third stage. If an anesthetic agent is given immediately before inhalation anesthesia, the third stage can occur without the early stages of anesthesia being observed. However, if the drug is given slowly, all stages of anesthesia are usually observed.

Assessment Before Surgery

The patient's response to anesthesia may differ according to variables related to the health status of the individual. These variables include age (young and older adults), a current health disorder (e.g., cardiovascular, pulmonary, renal, liver), pregnancy, history of heavy smoking, and frequent use of alcohol and drugs. These problems must be identified *before* surgery because the type and amount of anesthetic required may need to be adjusted.

❗ TABLE 18.5 Inhalation and Intravenous Anesthetics

Drug	Induction Time	Considerations
Inhalation: Volatile Liquids		
Halothane	Rapid	Highly potent anesthetic; recovery is rapid; could decrease blood pressure, has a bronchodilator effect, and is contraindicated in obstetrics.
Enflurane	Rapid	Can depress respiratory function; ventilatory support may be necessary. This drug should not be used during labor because it could suppress uterine contractions; avoid use in patients with seizure disorders.
Isoflurane	Rapid	Frequently used in inhalation therapy; has a smooth and rapid induction of anesthesia and rapid recovery; could cause hypotension and respiratory depression. This drug should not be used during labor because it suppresses uterine contractions. Cardiovascular effect is minimal.
Desflurane	Rapid	Volatile liquid anesthetic; recovery is rapid after anesthetic administration has ceased; could cause hypotension and respiratory depression.
Sevoflurane	Rapid	For induction and maintenance during surgery; sevoflurane may be given alone or combined with nitrous oxide.
Inhalation: Gas		
Nitrous oxide ("laughing gas")	Very rapid	Must be administered at no less than a mixture of 21% oxygen; potency is low. Recovery is rapid with minimal cardiovascular effect.
Intravenous (Ultra-short-Acting Barbiturates)		
Methohexital sodium	Rapid	Has short duration; frequently used for induction and with other drugs as part of balanced anesthesia; an inhalation anesthesia usually follows.
Thiamylal sodium	Rapid	Used for induction of anesthesia and as anesthesia for electroshock therapy.
Benzodiazepines		
Diazepam	Moderate to rapid	For induction of anesthesia; no analgesic effect.
Midazolam	Rapid	For induction of anesthesia and for endoscopic procedures; IV drug can cause conscious sedation and should be avoided if a cardiopulmonary disorder is present.
Others		
Droperidol and fentanyl	Moderate to rapid	A neuroleptic analgesic when combined with fentanyl (potent opiate narcotic); frequently used with a general anesthetic, can also be used as a preanesthetic drug and is also used for diagnostic procedures; may cause hypotension and respiratory depression.
Etomidate	Rapid	Etomidate is used for short-term surgery, for induction of anesthesia, or with a general anesthetic to maintain the anesthetic state.
Ketamine hydrochloride	Rapid	Used for short-term surgery or for induction of anesthesia; increases salivation, blood pressure, and heart rate; may be used for diagnostic procedures; avoid use in patients with a history of psychiatric disorders.
Propofol	Rapid	For induction of anesthesia; may be used with general anesthesia; duration of action is short; may cause hypotension and respiratory depression. Pain can occur at the injection site, so a local anesthetic (lidocaine) may be administered intravenously before injection of propofol to decrease pain.
Fospropofol	Rapid	For induction and maintenance of anesthesia; may cause hypotension and respiratory depression.

Inhalation Anesthetics

During the third stage of anesthesia, inhalation anesthetics—that is, gas or volatile liquids administered as gas—are used to deliver general anesthesia. Certain gases, notably nitrous oxide, are absorbed quickly, have a rapid action, and are eliminated rapidly. Cyclopropane was a popular inhalation anesthetic from 1930 to 1960, but because of its highly flammable state as ether, it is no longer used. In the late 1950s, halothane was introduced as a nonflammable alternative. Other inhalation drugs used as anesthetics include enflurane, isoflurane, desflurane, and sevoflurane.

Inhalation anesthetics typically provide smooth induction. Upon discontinuing administration of halothane, isoflurane, and enflurane, full recovery of consciousness usually occurs in approximately 1 hour. Recovery from desflurane and sevoflurane is within minutes. Inhalation anesthetics are usually combined with a nonbarbiturate, such as propofol; a strong analgesic, such as morphine; and a muscle relaxant, such as pancuronium, for surgical procedures.

Adverse effects from inhalation anesthetics include respiratory depression, hypotension, dysrhythmias, and hepatic dysfunction. In patients at risk, these drugs may trigger malignant hyperthermia. The newer drugs primarily cause less nausea and vomiting than the older anesthetics.

Intravenous Anesthetics

Intravenous (IV) anesthetics may be used for general anesthesia or for the induction stage of anesthesia. For outpatient surgery of short duration, an IV anesthetic might be the preferred form of anesthesia. Propofol, droperidol, etomidate, and ketamine hydrochloride are commonly used to provide a total intravenous anesthetic (TIVA). IV anesthetics have a rapid onset and short duration of action. Table 18.5 describes the inhalation and IV anesthetics used for general anesthesia.

Midazolam and propofol are commonly administered for the induction and maintenance of anesthesia or for conscious sedation for minor surgery or procedures like intubation and mechanical ventilation.

Patients are sedated and relaxed but, depending on the dose, they are responsive to commands.

Adverse effects from IV anesthetics include respiratory and cardiovascular depression. Propofol supports microbial growth and may increase the risk for bacterial infection. Discarding opened vials within 6 hours is a necessary precaution in the prevention of sepsis.

Topical Anesthetics

Use of topical anesthetic agents is limited to mucous membranes, broken or unbroken skin surfaces, and burns. Topical anesthetics come in different forms: solutions, liquid sprays, ointments, creams, gels, and powders. Topical anesthetics decrease the sensitivity of nerve endings in the affected area.

Local Anesthetics

Local anesthetics block pain at the site where the drug is administered by preventing conduction of nerve impulses. Local anesthetics are useful in dental procedures, suturing skin lacerations, short-term (minor) surgery at a localized area, blocking nerve impulses (nerve block) below the insertion of a spinal anesthetic, and diagnostic procedures such as lumbar puncture and thoracentesis. Local anesthetics may also be used to perform regional blocks—such as brachial plexus, axillary, femoral, or sciatic blocks—to provide analgesia for surgery of the upper or lower extremities.

Most local anesthetics are divided into two groups, the esters and the amides, according to their basic structures. The amides have a very low incidence of allergic reaction.

The first local anesthetic used was cocaine hydrochloride in the late 1800s. Procaine hydrochloride, a synthetic of cocaine, was discovered in the early 1900s. Lidocaine hydrochloride was developed in the mid-1950s to replace procaine except in dental procedures. Lidocaine has a rapid onset and a long duration of action, is more stable in solution, and causes fewer hypersensitivity reactions than procaine. Since the introduction of lidocaine, many local anesthetics have been marketed. Table 18.6 describes the various types of local anesthetics according to short-, moderate-, and long-acting effects.

Orthopedic joint surgeries, mastectomy, cesarean delivery, hysterectomy, hernia repair, and cholecystectomy frequently use the postoperative pain control provided by an anesthetic pump. For example, the patient who has a bilateral hernia repair has a catheter inserted into the deep fascia of the lower abdomen. A continuous flow of bupivacaine, a local anesthetic, is delivered via a Y-connector to both sides. By controlling pain with this delivery method, the patient is allowed increased mobility; reduced opioid use, which reduces associated drowsiness and nausea; and a reduced hospital stay. Yet another use of local the anesthetic, bupivacaine liposome, offers prolonged pain relief of 3 to 5 days when infiltrated in specific approved nerve or field blocks.

Spinal Anesthesia

Spinal anesthesia requires that a local anesthetic be injected into the subarachnoid space below the first lumbar space (L1) in adults and the third lumbar space (L3) in children. If the local anesthetic is given or spreads too high in the spinal column, the respiratory muscles could be affected and respiratory distress or respiratory failure could result. A postdural puncture headache might result after spinal anesthesia (a "spinal"), possibly because of a decrease in cerebrospinal fluid pressure caused by a leak of fluid at the needle insertion point. Encouraging the patient to remain flat after surgery with spinal anesthesia and to take increased fluids usually decreases the likelihood of leaking spinal fluid. Postdural puncture headaches occur most frequently in females and in younger patients, with the highest incidence occurring in obstetric patients. Hypotension also can result after spinal anesthesia due to the ensuing sympathetic blockade and predisposing factors that include sensory block location, history of hypertension, and chronic alcohol intake.

Various sites of the spinal column can be used for a nerve block with a local anesthetic (Fig. 18.2). A spinal block results from the penetration of the anesthetic into the subarachnoid space, which is the space between the pia mater membrane and the arachnoid membrane. An epidural block is the placement of the local anesthetic in the epidural space just posterior to the spinal cord or the dura mater. The epidural space is located between the posterior longitudinal ligament on the anterior side and the ligamentum flavum posteriorly. A caudal block is an epidural block placed by administering a local anesthetic through the sacral hiatus. A saddle block is given at the lower end of the spinal column to block the perineal area. Blood pressure should be monitored

TABLE 18.6 Local Anesthetics

Anesthetics	Type	Uses and Considerations
Short Acting (30 Min to 1 Hour)		
Chloroprocaine hydrochloride	Ester	For infiltration, caudal, and epidural anesthesia; onset of action is 6–12 minutes
Procaine hydrochloride	Ester	For nerve block, infiltration, epidural, and spinal anesthesia; useful in dentistry; use with caution in patients allergic to ester-type anesthetics
Moderate Acting (1–3 Hours)		
Lidocaine hydrochloride	Amide	For nerve block, infiltration, epidural, and spinal anesthesia; allergic reaction is rare. Lidocaine is used to treat cardiac dysrhythmias (see Chapter 37)
Mepivacaine hydrochloride	Amide	For nerve block, infiltration, caudal, and epidural anesthesia; may be used in dentistry
Prilocaine hydrochloride	Amide	For peripheral nerve block, infiltration, caudal, and epidural anesthesia; may be used in dentistry
Long Acting (3–10 Hours)		
Bupivacaine hydrochloride	Amide	For peripheral nerve block, infiltration, caudal, and epidural anesthesia
Dibucaine hydrochloride	Amide	For topical use (creams and ointment) to affected areas
Etidocaine hydrochloride	Amide	For peripheral nerve block, infiltration, caudal, and epidural anesthesia
Tetracaine hydrochloride	Ester	For spinal anesthesia (high and low saddle block); also for topical use to affected areas, such as the eye to anesthetize the cornea, the nose and throat for bronchoscopy, and the skin for relief of pain and pruritus (itching)

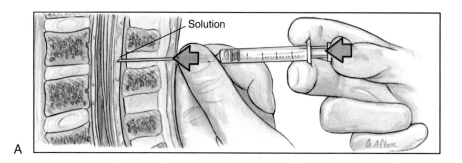

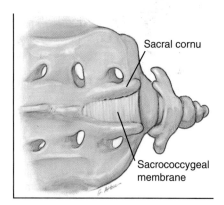

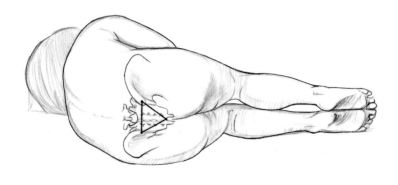

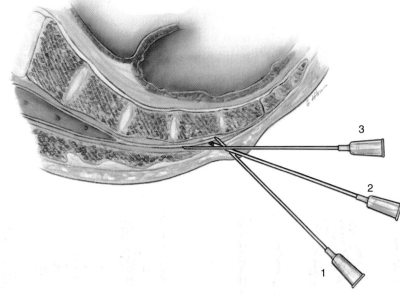

Fig. 18.2 (A) Administration of solution for epidural placement. (B) Caudal anesthesia.

◎ CLINICAL JUDGMENT [NURSING PROCESS]

Anesthetics

Concept: Intraoperative Care
- Monitoring of the patient and the surgical environment throughout a surgical procedure to ensure patient safety

Recognize Cues [Assessment]
- Assess baseline vital signs.
- Obtain a drug and health history, noting drugs that affect the cardiopulmonary system.

Analyze Cues and Prioritize Hypothesis [Patient Problems]
- Airway obstruction
- Acute pain

Generate Solutions [Planning]
- Patient will participate in preoperative preparation and will verbalize understanding of postoperative care.
- Patient's vital signs will remain stable after surgery.

Take Action [Nursing Interventions]
- Monitor the postoperative state of sensorium. Report if a patient remains excessively nonresponsive or confused.
- Observe preoperative and postoperative urine output. Report deficit of hourly or 8-hour urine output.
- ⚡ Monitor vital signs after general and local anesthesia; hypotension and respiratory depression may result.
- Administer an analgesic or a narcotic-analgesic with caution until the patient fully recovers from the anesthetic. To prevent adverse reactions, the dosage might need to be adjusted if the patient is under the influence of an anesthetic.

Patient Teaching
- Explain to patients the preoperative preparation and postoperative nursing assessment and interventions.

Evaluate Outcomes [Evaluation]
- Evaluate the patient's response to the anesthetics. Continue to monitor for adverse reactions.

during administration of these types of anesthesia because a decrease in blood pressure resulting from the drug and procedure might occur. Further discussion of labor and delivery drugs can be found in Chapter 50. Nurses play an important role in patient assessment before and after general and local anesthesia is administered. Preparing the patient for surgery by explaining the preparations and completing the preoperative orders, including premedications, is necessary to enhance the safety and effectiveness of anesthesia and surgery.

■ CRITICAL THINKING CASE STUDY

J.Z., a 72-year-old woman, has difficulty staying asleep. She asks the nurse whether she should take a sleeping medication, such as lorazepam, before bedtime.

1. Before J.Z. takes any sleep aid or hypnotic, what nursing assessments should be made?

2. Describe a nursing plan that may help alleviate J.Z.'s sleep disturbance.
3. Would J.Z. be a candidate for taking a benzodiazepine? Explain your answer.
4. What follow-up plan should the nurse have related to J.Z.'s sleep problem?

■ REVIEW QUESTIONS

1. It is important for the nurse teaching the patient regarding secobarbital to include which information about the drug?
   a. It is a short-acting drug that may cause one to awaken early in the morning.
   b. It is an intermediate-acting drug that frequently causes rapid eye movement rebound.
   c. It is an intermediate-acting drug that frequently causes a hangover effect.
   d. It is a long-acting drug that is frequently associated with dependence.
   e. It is an ultra-short–acting central nervous system depressant that induces hypnosis.
   f. It may cause seizures after prolonged use.
2. A patient taking lorazepam asks the nurse how this drug works. The nurse should respond by stating that it is a benzodiazepine that acts by which mechanism?
   a. Depressing the central nervous system, leading to a loss of consciousness
   b. Depressing the central nervous system, including the motor and sensory activities
   c. Increasing the action of the inhibitory neurotransmitter gamma-aminobutyric acid (GABA) to GABA receptors

   d. Creating an epidural block by placement of the local anesthetic into the epidural space
   e. Increasing melatonin, thus inducing sleep
   f. Increasing cortisol, allowing for natural sleep
3. A patient is taking ramelteon for insomnia. The nurse prepares a care plan that includes monitoring of the patient for side effects/adverse reactions of this drug. Which is a side effect of ramelteon?
   a. Insomnia
   b. Bradycardia
   c. Laryngospasm
   d. Sleep-related behaviors
   e. Increased salivation
   f. Pupillary constriction
4. A patient received spinal anesthesia. Which is most important for the nurse to monitor?
   a. Loss of consciousness
   b. Hangover effects and dependence
   c. Hypotension and headaches
   d. Excitement or delirium
   e. Venous dilation
   f. Increased respiratory rate

5. A nurse is teaching a patient about zolpidem. Which is important for the nurse to include in the teaching of this drug?
   a. The maximum dose is 20 mg/day.
   b. It is used for short-term treatment less than 10 days.
   c. For older adults, the dose is 15 mg at bedtime.
   d. The drug should only be used for 21 days or less.
   e. The drug may cause increased salivation.
   f. The drug may cause excitation.
6. A patient is taking triazolam. Which instructions about this drug are important for the nurse to include?
   a. It may be used as a barbiturate for only 4 weeks.
   b. Use as a nonbenzodiazepine to reduce anxiety.
   c. It may cause agranulocytosis and thrombocytopenia.
   d. Avoid alcohol and smoking while taking this drug.
   e. It is an ultra-short–acting medication.
   f. Long-term use is encouraged.
7. A patient is to receive conscious sedation for a minor surgical procedure. Which drug administration should the nurse expect? (Select all that apply.)
   a. Propofol to reduce anxiety
   b. Lidocaine to provide local anesthesia
   c. Midazolam to promote sedation and following of commands
   d. Ketamine for rapid induction and prolonged duration of action
   e. Phenobarbital for short-acting duration of sleep
   e. Fentanyl for pain control
   f. Intravenous bupivacaine for prolonged analgesia

19

Antiseizure Drugs

OBJECTIVES

- Contrast the two international classifications of seizures with characteristics of each type.
- Differentiate between the types of seizures.
- Summarize the pharmacokinetics, side effects and adverse reactions, therapeutic plasma level, contraindications for use, and drug interactions of phenytoin.

- Compare the actions of hydantoins, long-acting barbiturates, succinimides, benzodiazepines, iminostilbenes, and valproate.
- Apply the Clinical Judgment [Nursing Process] to antiseizure drugs, including patient teaching.

OUTLINE

Approximately 3.4 million people in the United States have active epilepsy, a seizure disorder that results from abnormal electric discharges from the cerebral neurons characterized by a loss or disturbance of consciousness and usually involuntary, uncontrolled movements. Seizures occur when there is a disruption in the electrical functioning of the brain due to an imbalance in the excitation and inhibition of electrical impulses. An excessive amount of excitation discharges could be due to several reasons, such as a defect in the neuronal membrane, the degree of sodium influx, or a decrease in the gamma-aminobutyric acid (GABA) inhibitory action. The electroencephalogram (EEG), computed tomography (CT), and magnetic resonance imaging (MRI) are useful in diagnosing epilepsy. The EEG records abnormal electric discharges of the cerebral cortex. Of all seizure cases, 75% are considered to be primary, or idiopathic (of unknown cause), and the remainder are secondary to brain trauma, brain anoxia (absence of oxygen), infection, or cerebrovascular disorders (e.g., cerebrovascular accident [CVA], stroke). Epilepsy is a chronic, usually lifelong disorder. The majority of persons with seizure disorder had their first seizure before 20 years of age.

Seizures that are not associated with epilepsy could result from fever, stress, hypoglycemic reaction, electrolyte imbalance (hyponatremia), metabolic imbalance (acidosis or alkalosis), and alcohol or drug use disorders. When these conditions are corrected, the seizures cease. Recurrent seizures may result from birth and perinatal injuries, head trauma, congenital malformations, neoplasms (tumors), or idiopathic, or unknown causes.

INTERNATIONAL CLASSIFICATION OF SEIZURES

There are various types of seizures, such as tonic-clonic (formerly known as *grand mal*), absence (formerly known as *petit mal*), and psychomotor. The International Classification of Seizures (Table 19.1) describes two seizure categories: generalized and partial. A person may also have mixed seizures that comprise more than one type.

ANTISEIZURE DRUGS

Drugs used for epileptic seizures are called antiseizure drugs, *anticonvulsants,* or *antiepileptic drugs* (AEDs). Antiseizure drugs stabilize nerve cell membranes and suppress the abnormal electric impulses in the cerebral cortex. These drugs prevent seizures but do not eliminate the cause or provide a cure. Antiseizure drugs are classified as central nervous system (CNS) depressants.

With the use of antiseizure drugs, seizures are controlled in approximately 70% of patients. These drugs are usually taken throughout the person's lifetime; however, the health care provider might discontinue the medication if no seizures have occurred after 3 to 5 years in some cases.

Many types of antiseizure drugs are used to treat seizures, including the hydantoins (phenytoin), long-acting barbiturates (phenobarbital, primidone), succinimides (ethosuximide), benzodiazepines (diazepam, clonazepam), iminostilbanes (carbamazepine), and valproate (valproic acid). Antiseizure drugs are not indicated for all types of seizures. For example, phenytoin is effective in treating tonic-clonic and partial seizures but is not effective in treating absence seizures.

Pharmacophysiology: Action of Antiseizure Drugs

Antiseizure drugs work in one of three ways: (1) by suppressing sodium influx through the drug binding to the sodium channel when it is inactivated, which prolongs the channel inactivation and thereby prevents

TABLE 19.1   International Classification of Seizures

Category	Characteristics
Generalized seizure	Seizures involve both cerebral hemispheres of the brain.
Tonic-clonic seizure	Also called *grand mal seizure,* the most common form; in the *tonic phase,* skeletal muscles contract or tighten in a spasm that lasts 3–5 seconds; in the *clonic phase,* a dysrhythmic muscular contraction occurs with a jerkiness of legs and arms that lasts 2–4 minutes.
Tonic seizure	Sustained muscle contraction
Clonic seizure	Dysrhythmic muscle contraction
Absence seizure	Also called *petit mal seizure;* brief loss of consciousness lasts less than 10 seconds with fewer than three spike waves on the electroencephalogram (EEG) printout. This type usually occurs in children.
Myoclonic seizure	Isolated clonic contraction or jerks that last 3–10 seconds may be limited to one limb (focal myoclonic) or may involve the entire body (massive myoclonic); may be secondary to a neurologic disorder such as encephalitis or Tay-Sachs disease.
Atonic seizure	Head drop, loss of posture, and sudden loss of muscle tone occurs. If lower limbs are involved, the patient could collapse.
Infantile spasms	Muscle spasm
Partial seizure	Involves one hemisphere of the brain; no loss of consciousness occurs in simple partial seizures, but there is a loss of consciousness in complex partial seizures.
Simple seizure	Occurs in motor, sensory, autonomic, and psychic forms; no loss of consciousness occurs.
Motor	Formerly called the *Jacksonian seizure,* this type involves spontaneous movement that spreads; it can develop into a generalized seizure.
Sensory	Visual, auditory, or taste hallucinations
Autonomic response	Paleness, flushing, sweating, or vomiting
Psychological	Personality changes
Complex seizure	Loss of consciousness occurs, and the patient does not recall behavior immediately before, during, and immediately after the seizure.
Psychomotor	Complex symptoms include automatisms (repetitive behavior such as chewing or swallowing motions), behavioral changes, and motor seizures.
Cognitive	Confusion or memory impairment
Affective	Bizarre behavior
Compound	May lead to generalized seizures such as tonic or tonic-clonic

neuron firing; (2) by suppressing the calcium influx, which prevents the electric current generated by the calcium ions to the T-type calcium channel; or (3) by increasing the action of GABA, which inhibits neurotransmitters throughout the brain. The drugs that suppress sodium influx are phenytoin, fosphenytoin, carbamazepine, oxcarbazepine, valproic acid, topiramate, zonisamide, and lamotrigine. Valproic acid and ethosuximide are examples of drugs that suppress calcium influx. Examples of drug groups that enhance the action of GABA are barbiturates, benzodiazepines, and tiagabine. Gabapentin promotes GABA release.

Hydantoins

The first antiseizure drug used to treat seizures was phenytoin, a hydantoin discovered in 1938 and still commonly used for controlling seizures. Hydantoins inhibit sodium influx, stabilize cell membranes, reduce repetitive neuronal firing, and limit seizures. By increasing the electrical stimulation threshold in cardiac tissue, it also acts as an antidysrhythmic. It has a slight effect on general sedation, and it is nonaddicting. However, this drug should *not* be used during pregnancy because it can have a teratogenic effect on the fetus.

⚡ PATIENT SAFETY

Do not confuse:
- **Cerebyx,** a hydantoin antiseizure drug, with **Celebrex,** a nonsteroidal antiinflammatory drug (NSAID). The names of these drugs look and sound alike but are different in their pharmacology.

Drug dosage for phenytoin and other antiseizure drugs is age related. Newborns, persons with liver disease, and older adults require

a lower dosage because of a decrease in metabolism that results in more available drug. Conversely, individuals with an increased metabolic rate, such as children, may require an increased dosage. The drug dosage is adjusted according to the therapeutic plasma or serum level. Phenytoin has a narrow therapeutic range of 10 to 20 mcg/mL, which is generally considered equivalent to 1 to 2 mcg/mL unbound or free phenytoin. The benefits of an antiseizure drug become apparent when the serum drug level is within the therapeutic range. Typically, if the drug level is below the desired range, the patient is not receiving the required drug dosage to control seizure activity. If the drug level is above the desired range, drug toxicity may result. Monitoring the therapeutic serum drug range is of utmost importance to ensure drug effectiveness. Prototype Drug Chart: Phenytoin lists the pharmacologic data associated with phenytoin.

Pharmacokinetics. Phenytoin is slowly absorbed from the small intestine. It is a highly protein-bound (90% to 95%) drug; therefore a decrease in serum protein or albumin can increase the free phenytoin serum level. With a small to average drug dose, the half-life of phenytoin averages approximately 22 hours, but the range can be from 7 to 60 hours. Phenytoin is metabolized to inactive metabolites and excreted in the urine.

Pharmacodynamics. The pharmacodynamics of orally administered phenytoin include onset of action within 30 minutes to 2 hours, peak serum concentration in 1.5 to 3 hours, and a duration of 6 to 12 hours. The onset of action for intravenous (IV) administration is with minutes, peak action is 10 to 30 minutes, and the duration is up to 12 hours.

IV infusion of phenytoin should be administered by direct injection into a large vein via a central line or peripherally inserted central catheter (PICC). The drug may be diluted in saline solution;

PROTOTYPE DRUG CHART

Phenytoin

Drug Class	Dosage
Anticonvulsant: Hydantoin	Status epilepticus: A: IV: LD: 15–20 mg/kg not to exceed 50 mg/min, then in 10 min may give 5–10 mg/kg PRN; *max:* LD: 30 mg/kg Therapeutic serum range: 10–20 mcg/mL Toxic level: >20 mcg/mL
Contraindications	**Drug-Lab-Food Interactions**
Hypersensitivity, AV heart block, bradycardia, Adams-Stokes syndrome *Caution:* Hyponatremia, hypotension, heart failure, vitamin K deficiency, hypoglycemia, psychosis, suicidal ideation, myasthenia gravis, hypothyroidism, alcohol abuse, cardiovascular disease, diabetes mellitus, renal and hepatic impairment, porphyria, older adults, Asian ethnicity, depression, osteoporosis, dysrhythmias, pregnancy, breast feeding	Drug: Increased effects with cimetidine, isoniazid; decreased effects with folic acid, calcium, antacids, sucralfate, cisplatin Decreases effects of anticoagulants, oral contraceptives, antineoplastics, theophylline, cyclosporine, quinidine, dopamine, and rifampin Food: Decreases effects of folic acid, calcium, and vitamin D because absorption is decreased by phenytoin
Pharmacokinetics	**Pharmacodynamics**
Absorption: PO: Slowly absorbed; IM: Erratic rate of absorption Distribution: PB: 90%–95% Metabolism: t½: 7–60 h Excretion: In urine, small amount; in bile and feces, moderate amounts	PO: Onset: 0.5–2 h Peak: 1.5–3 h Duration: 6–12 h IV: Onset: Within minutes to 1 h Peak: 10–30 minutes Duration: >12 h
Therapeutic Effects/Uses	
Treatment of tonic-clonic and partial seizures and status epilepticus Mechanism of Action: Reduces motor cortex activity and alters ion transport by acting on sodium channels on neuronal cell membranes	
Side Effects	**Adverse Reactions**
Headache, confusion, dizziness, drowsiness, tinnitus, insomnia, nystagmus, asthenia, ataxia, paresthesia, hyperreflexia, tremor, gingival hyperplasia, abdominal pain, dysgeusia, nausea, vomiting, constipation,	Hypotension, bradycardia, tachycardia, hyperglycemia, depression, peripheral neuropathy, injection site reaction (purple glove syndrome), cerebral edema *Life-threatening:* Agranulocytosis, leukopenia, thrombocytopenia, hepatic/renal failure, Stevens-Johnson syndrome, ventricular fibrillation, suicidal ideation

>, Greater than; *A*, adult; *d*, day; *h*, hour; *IM*, intramuscular; *IV*, intravenous; *LD*, loading dose; *max*, maximum; *min*, minute; *PB*, protein binding; *PO*, by mouth; *PRN*, as needed; *t½*, half-life.

however, dextrose solution should be avoided because of drug precipitation. The manufacturer recommends use of an in-line filter when the drug is administered as an infusion. IV phenytoin, 50 mg or a fraction thereof, should be administered over 1 minute for adults and at a rate of 25 mg/min for older adults. Infusion rates of more than 50 mg/min may cause severe hypotension or cardiac dysrhythmias, especially for older and debilitated patients. Local irritation at the injection site may be noted, and sloughing—formation of dead tissue that separates from living tissue—may occur. The IV line should always be flushed with saline before and after each dose to reduce venous irritation. Intramuscular (IM) injection of phenytoin irritates tissues and may cause damage. For this reason, and because of its erratic absorption rate, phenytoin is *not* given by the IM route.

Side Effects and Adverse Reactions

The adverse effects of hydantoins include psychiatric effects such as depression, suicidal ideation, Stevens-Johnson syndrome, ventricular fibrillation, and blood dyscrasias such as thrombocytopenia (low

platelet count) and leukopenia (low white blood cell count). Injection site reactions, such as purple glove syndrome (swollen, discolored, and painful extremities that may require amputation), may occur. Patients on hydantoins for long periods might have elevated blood glucose (hyperglycemia) that results from the drug inhibiting the release of insulin. Less severe side effects include nausea, vomiting, gingival hyperplasia (overgrowth of gums or reddened gums that bleed easily), constipation, drowsiness, headaches, slurred speech, confusion, and nystagmus (constant, involuntary, cyclical movement of the eyeball).

Drug-Drug Interactions

Drug interaction is common with hydantoins because they are highly protein bound. Hydantoins compete with other drugs (e.g., anticoagulants, aspirin) for plasma protein-binding sites. The hydantoins displace anticoagulants and aspirin, causing more free-drug availability and increasing their activity. Barbiturates, rifampin, and chronic ingestion of ethanol increase hydantoin metabolism. Drugs like sulfonamides and cimetidine can increase the action of hydantoins by inhibiting liver metabolism, which is necessary for drug excretion. Antacids, calcium preparations, sucralfate, and antineoplastic drugs also decrease the absorption of hydantoins. Antipsychotics and certain herbs can lower the seizure threshold, the level at which seizure may be induced, and they increase seizure activity. The patient should be closely monitored for seizure occurrence.

 COMPLEMENTARY AND ALTERNATIVE THERAPIES

Antiseizure Drugs

- Evening primrose and borage may lower the seizure threshold when taken with antiseizure drugs. The antiseizure dose may need modification.
- Ginkgo may decrease phenytoin, carbamazepine, and valproate effectiveness.

Barbiturates

Phenobarbital, a long-acting barbiturate, is prescribed to treat tonic-clonic, partial, and myoclonic seizures and status epilepticus, a rapid succession of epileptic seizures. Barbiturates reduce seizures by enhancing the activity of GABA, an inhibitory neurotransmitter. Possible teratogenic effects and other side effects related to phenytoin are less pronounced with phenobarbital. The therapeutic serum range of phenobarbital is 15 to 40 mcg/mL. Risks associated with the use of phenobarbital include sedation and tolerance to the drug. High doses may lead to respiratory depression and coma. Discontinuance of phenobarbital should be gradual to avoid recurrence of seizures. Barbiturates may be taken with food to minimize gastrointestinal (GI) irritation.

Succinimides

The succinimide drug group is used to treat absence seizures. Succinimides act by decreasing calcium influx through the T-type calcium channels. The therapeutic serum range of ethosuximide is 40 to 100 mcg/mL. Adverse effects include blood dyscrasias, psychosis, systemic lupus erythematosus, and suicidal ideation.

Benzodiazepines

The benzodiazepines that have antiseizure effects are clonazepam, clorazepate, lorazepam, and diazepam. Clonazepam is effective in controlling absence and myoclonic seizures, but tolerance may occur 6 months after drug therapy starts; consequently, clonazepam dosage must be adjusted. Clorazepate is administered for treating partial seizures.

Diazepam is administered by IV to treat status epilepticus. The drug has a short-term effect; thus other antiseizure drugs, such as phenytoin or phenobarbital, must be given during or immediately after administration of diazepam.

Iminostilbenes

Carbamazepine, an iminostilbene, is used to control tonic-clonic and partial seizures. Carbamazepine is also used for psychiatric disorders (e.g., bipolar disorder), and trigeminal neuralgia (as an analgesic). The therapeutic serum range of carbamazepine is 4 to 12 mcg/mL.

A potentially toxic interaction can occur when grapefruit juice is taken with carbamazepine, and drug concentrations must be carefully monitored.

Valproic Acid

Valproic acid is prescribed for tonic-clonic, absence, and partial seizures, although the safety and efficacy of this drug has not been established for children younger than 2 years of age. Care should be taken when giving this drug to very young children and to patients with liver disorders because hepatotoxicity is one of the possible adverse reactions. Liver enzymes should be monitored. The therapeutic serum range for a patient with seizures is 50 to 100 mcg/mL. Valproic acid may be taken with food to avoid GI distress.

Table 19.2 lists the various antiseizure drugs and their dosages, uses, and considerations, including common side effects and a few serious adverse effects. Table 19.3 lists selected antiseizure drugs frequently prescribed to treat seizure disorders.

Antiseizure drug dosages usually start low and gradually increase over a period of weeks until the serum drug level is within therapeutic range or the seizures cease. Serum antiseizure drug levels should be closely monitored to prevent toxicity.

Antiseizure Drugs and Pregnancy

Approximately one-third of females with a seizure disorder are at greater risk for an increase in seizures during pregnancy. Hypoxia that may occur during seizures places both the pregnant woman and her fetus at risk.

Many antiseizure drugs have teratogenic properties that increase the risk for fetal malformations. Phenytoin and carbamazepine have been linked to fetal anomalies such as cardiac defects and cleft lip and palate. It has been reported that valproic acid is known to cause major congenital malformations in infants in pregnant women who take the drug. As expected, the highest incidence of birth defects occurs when the woman takes combinations of antiseizure drugs.

Antiseizure drugs tend to act as inhibitors of vitamin K, contributing to hemorrhage in infants shortly after birth. Frequently, pregnant women taking antiseizure drugs are given an oral vitamin K supplement during the last week or 10 days of the pregnancy, or vitamin K is administered to the infant soon after birth.

Antiseizure drugs also increase the loss of folate (folic acid) in pregnant women; thus pregnant individuals should take daily folate supplements.

Antiseizure Drugs and Febrile Seizures

Seizures associated with fever usually occur in children between 3 months and 5 years of age. Epilepsy develops in approximately 2.5% of children who have had one or more febrile seizures. Prophylactic antiseizure drug treatment such as phenobarbital or diazepam may be indicated for high-risk patients. Valproic acid should not be given to children younger than 2 years of age because of its possible hepatotoxic effect.

Antiseizure Drugs and Status Epilepticus

Status epilepticus, a continuous seizure state, is considered a medical emergency. If treatment is not begun immediately, death could result. The choices of pharmacologic agents are diazepam administered by IV or lorazepam followed by IV administration of phenytoin. For continued seizures, midazolam or propofol and then high-dose barbiturates are used. These drugs should be administered slowly to avoid respiratory depression.

The pharmacologic behavior of specific anticonvulsants, including a few common side effects and severe adverse effects, is summarized in Table 19.2.

⊙ CLINICAL JUDGMENT [NURSING PROCESS]

Antiseizure Drugs: Phenytoin

Concept: Intracranial Regulation
- The process of regulating function of the brain and nervous system

Recognize Cues [Assessment]
- Obtain a health history that includes current drugs and herbs the patient uses. Report and document any probable drug-drug or herb-drug interactions.
- Assess the patient's knowledge regarding the medication regimen.
- Check urinary output to determine whether it is adequate (>1500 mL/d).
- Determine laboratory values related to renal and liver function. If both blood urea nitrogen (BUN) and creatinine levels are elevated, a renal disorder should be suspected. Elevated serum liver enzymes (alkaline phosphatase, alanine aminotransferase, gamma-glutamyl transferase, 59-nucleotidase) indicate a hepatic disorder.

Analyze Cues and Prioritize Hypothesis [Patient Problems]
- Potential for falls
- Potential for injury
- Need for patient teaching

Generate Solutions [Planning]
- Patient's seizure frequency will diminish.
- Patient will adhere to antiseizure drug therapy.
- Patient's side effects from phenytoin will be minimal.

Take Action [Nursing Interventions]
- Monitor serum drug levels of antiseizure medication to determine therapeutic range (10 to 20 mcg/mL).
- Encourage patient's compliance with medication regimen.
- Monitor patient's complete blood count (CBC) levels for early detection of blood dyscrasias.
- ⚡ Use seizure precautions (environmental protection from sharp objects, such as table corners) for patients at risk for seizures.
- Determine whether the patient is receiving adequate nutrients; phenytoin may cause anorexia, nausea, and vomiting.
- Advise female patients who are taking oral contraceptives and antiseizure drugs to use an additional contraceptive method.

Patient Teaching
General
- Teach patients to shake suspension-form medications thoroughly before use to adequately mix the medication to ensure accurate dosage.
- ⚡ Advise patients not to drive or perform other hazardous activities when initiating antiseizure therapy because drowsiness may occur.
- Counsel female patients contemplating pregnancy to consult with a health care provider because phenytoin and valproic acid may have a teratogenic effect.

- Monitor serum phenytoin levels closely during pregnancy because seizures tend to become more frequent due to increased metabolic rates.
- Warn patients to avoid alcohol and other central nervous system (CNS) depressants because they can cause an added depressive effect on the body.
- Explain to patients that certain herbs can interact with antiseizure drugs (see Complementary and Alternative Therapy), and dose adjustment may be required.
- Encourage patients to obtain a medical alert identification card, medical alert bracelet, or tag that indicates their diagnosis and drug regimen.
- ⚡ Teach patients not to abruptly stop drug therapy but rather to withdraw the prescribed drug gradually under medical supervision to prevent seizure rebound (recurrence of seizures) and status epilepticus.
- Counsel patients about the need for preventive dental checkups.
- Warn patients to take their prescribed antiseizure drug, get laboratory tests as ordered, and keep follow-up visits with health care providers.
- Teach patients not to self-medicate with over-the-counter (OTC) drugs without first consulting a health care provider.
- Advise patients with diabetes to monitor serum glucose levels more closely than usual because phenytoin may inhibit insulin release, causing an increase in glucose level.
- Inform patients of the existence of national, state, and local associations that provide resources, current information, and support for people with epilepsy.

Diet
- Coach patients to take antiseizure drugs at the same time every day with food or milk.

Side Effects
- Tell patients that urine may be a harmless pinkish-red or reddish-brown color.
- Advise patients to maintain good oral hygiene and to use a soft toothbrush to prevent gum irritation and bleeding.
- Teach patients to report symptoms of sore throat, bruising, and nosebleeds, which may indicate a blood dyscrasia.
- Encourage patients to inform health care providers of adverse reactions such as gingivitis, nystagmus, rash, and dizziness. (Stevens-Johnson syndrome begins with a rash.)

Evaluate Outcomes [Evaluation]
- Evaluate effectiveness of drugs in controlling seizures.
- Monitor serum phenytoin levels to determine whether they are within the desired range. High serum levels of phenytoin are frequently indicators of phenytoin toxicity.
- Monitor patients for hydantoin overdose. Initial symptoms are nystagmus and ataxia (impaired coordination). Later symptoms are hypotension, unresponsive pupils, and coma. Respiratory and circulatory support, as well as hemodialysis, are usually used in the treatment of phenytoin overdose.

TABLE 19.2   Anticonvulsants

Drug	Route and Dosage	Uses and Considerations
Barbiturates		
Phenobarbital CSS IV	Status epilepticus: A: IV: 15–18 mg/kg; *max:* 30 mg/kg Seizure prophylaxis: A: PO/IM/IV: 1–3 mg/kg/d in 1–2 divided doses Therapeutic serum range: 15–40 mcg/mL	For tonic-clonic, myoclonic, and partial seizures; status epilepticus; sedation induction and maintenance; anxiety and insomnia. May cause dizziness, drowsiness, weakness, headache, confusion, ataxia, hypotension, bradycardia, nausea, vomiting, constipation, and erectile dysfunction. PB: 20%–45%; t½: 50–120 h
Primidone	Seizure prophylaxis: A: PO: Initially 125–250 mg/d at bedtime; *maint:* 750–1500 mg/d in 3–4 divided doses; *max:* 2 g/d Therapeutic serum range: 5–12 mcg/mL	For tonic-clonic and partial seizures. May cause dizziness, drowsiness, ataxia, confusion, weakness, suicidal ideation, fatigue, nystagmus, anorexia, nausea, vomiting, erectile dysfunction, and respiratory depression. PB: 20%–45%; t½: 10–12 h
Benzodiazepines (Anxiolytics)		
Clonazepam CSS IV	Seizure prophylaxis: A: PO: Initially 1.5 mg/d in 3 divided doses; gradually increase dose q3d until seizures are controlled; *max:* 20 mg/d	For absence and myoclonic seizures and panic disorder. May cause dizziness, drowsiness, anorexia, blurred vision, ataxia, fatigue, dependence, depression, memory impairment, erectile dysfunction, constipation, infection, and dysmenorrhea. PB: 85%; t½: 30–40 h
Clorazepate CSS IV	Partial seizures: A: PO: 7.5 mg bid/tid; *max:* 90 mg/d	May be used for partial seizures, generalized anxiety disorder, and alcohol withdrawal. May cause blurred vision, ataxia, confusion, dizziness, drowsiness, headache, fatigue, dry mouth, tremor, tolerance, dependence, withdrawal, hypotension, and respiratory depression. PB: 97%–98%; t½: 40–50 h
Diazepam CSS IV	Status epilepticus: A: IV: 5–10 mg at 10- to 15-min intervals; *max:* 30 mg	For status epilepticus (drug of choice), partial and tonic-clonic seizures, muscle spasms, anxiety, sedation induction, and alcohol withdrawal. May cause fatigue, dizziness, drowsiness, weight gain/loss, appetite stimulation, headache, urinary retention/incontinence, menstrual irregularity, memory impairment, and respiratory depression. Administer IV slowly to avoid respiratory depression and hypotension; PB: 95%–98%; t½: 48–100 h
Lorazepam CSS IV	Status epilepticus: A: IV: 4 mg at 2 mg/min may repeat in 10–15 min	To control status epilepticus, anxiety, and insomnia and for sedation induction. May cause drowsiness, dizziness, memory impairment, ataxia, confusion, weakness, restlessness, constipation, hypotension, injection site reaction, tolerance, and dependence. PB: 85%; t½: 12–14 h
Midazolam	A: Intranasal: 1 spray (5 mg) into 1 nostril; *max:* 2 doses/single episode	For acute repetitive seizures. May cause headache, hiccups, drowsiness, erythema, throat irritation, hypotension, rhinorrhea, nausea, vomiting, respiratory depression, and apnea. PB: 97%; t½: 2–6 h
Hydantoins		
Fosphenytoin	Status epilepticus: A: IV: Initially 15–20 mg PE/kg; do not exceed 150 mg PE/min; may give additional 5–10 mg PE/kg PRN; *max:* 30 mg PE/kg Therapeutic serum range: 10–20 mcg/mL	For tonic-clonic and partial seizures and status epilepticus. Dilute in D₅W or 0.9% NaCl. May cause dizziness, drowsiness, nystagmus, gingival hyperplasia, ataxia, tinnitus, headache, pruritus, nausea, vomiting, and tremor. PB: 95%–99%; t½: 7–42 h
Phenytoin	See Prototype Drug Chart: Phenytoin	
Iminostilbene		
Carbamazepine	Seizure prophylaxis: A: PO: Initially 200 mg bid; *maint:* 800–1200 mg/d; *max:* 1600 mg/d Therapeutic serum range: 4–12 mcg/mL	For tonic-clonic and partial seizures, trigeminal neuralgia, neuropathic pain, and bipolar disorder. May cause rash, pruritus, dizziness, drowsiness, blurred vision, ataxia, nausea, vomiting, constipation, and weakness. PB: 76%; t½: 25–65 h
Oxcarbazepine	Immediate release: A: PO: Initially 300 mg bid; increase to 2400 mg/d in 2 divided doses; *max:* 2400 mg/d Extended release: A: PO: Initially 600 mg/d; *maint:* 1200–2400 mg/d	For partial seizures. May cause dizziness, drowsiness, confusion, headache, nausea, vomiting, diarrhea, fatigue, weakness, ataxia, rhinitis, infection, anxiety, diplopia, and visual impairment. PB: 40%; t½: 2 h immediate release, 7–11 h extended release
Eslicarbazepine	A: PO: Initially 400 mg/d, may increase weekly; *maint:* 800–1600 mg/d; *max:* 1600 mg/d	For partial seizures. May cause dizziness, drowsiness, ataxia, headache, impaired cognition, fatigue, diplopia, blurred vision, nausea, and vomiting. PB: 40%; t½: 13–20 h
Succinimides		
Ethosuximide	A: PO: Initially 250 mg bid; increase dose gradually; *maint:* 20–40 mg/kg/d; *max:* 1.5 g/d Therapeutic serum range: 40–100 mcg/mL	For absence seizures. May cause dizziness, drowsiness, headache, ataxia, nightmares, impaired cognition, gingival hyperplasia, dyspepsia, nausea, and vomiting. PB: UK; t½: 60 h

TABLE 19.2 Anticonvulsants—cont'd

Drug	Route and Dosage	Uses and Considerations
Valproate		
Valproic acid	Seizure prophylaxis: A: PO: 10–15 mg/kg/d in 2–3 divided doses; *max:* 60 mg/kg/d Therapeutic serum range: 50–100 mcg/mL	For partial, myoclonic, absence, and tonic-clonic seizures; bipolar disorder; and migraine prophylaxis. May cause dizziness, drowsiness, weakness, diplopia, insomnia, anorexia, abdominal pain, dyspepsia, thrombocytopenia, nausea, vomiting, and diarrhea. PB: 90%; t½: 9–16 h
Miscellaneous		
Acetazolamide	Seizure prophylaxis: A: PO/IV: 8–30 mg/kg/d in up to 4 divided doses; *maint:* 375–1000 mg/d; *max:* 1 g/d	For absence, partial, and tonic-clonic seizures; altitude sickness, glaucoma, and edema. Maintain adequate fluid intake to prevent renal impairment. May cause dizziness, drowsiness, confusion, depression, headache, ataxia, fatigue, flushing, dysgeusia, nausea, vomiting, diarrhea, renal failure, and crystalluria. PB: 90%; t½: 10–15 h
Gabapentin	Seizure prophylaxis: A: PO: Initially 300 mg tid; *maint:* 900–1800 mg/d in 3 divided doses; *max:* 3600 mg/d and max time between doses 12 h	For partial, tonic-clonic seizures, restless leg syndrome, and neuropathic pain. May cause dizziness, drowsiness, headache, nystagmus, blurred vision, fatigue, peripheral edema, tremor, ataxia, weakness, hostility, nausea, vomiting, and diarrhea. PB: 3%; t½: 5–7 h
Lamotrigine	Partial seizures: Immediate release: A: PO: Initially 50 mg/d; *maint:* 250 mg bid Extended release: A: PO: Initially 50 mg/d; *maint:* 250–300 mg/d	For partial and tonic-clonic seizures, Lennox-Gastaut syndrome, and bipolar disorder. May cause dizziness, drowsiness, blurred vision, diplopia, fatigue, asthenia, nausea, vomiting, diarrhea, ataxia, tremor, fever, pharyngitis, and rash. PB: 55%; t½: 14–59 h
Levetiracetam	Immediate release: A: PO: Initially 500 mg bid; may increase dose q2wk; *maint:* 1500 mg bid; *max:* 3 g/d Extended release: A: PO: 1 g/d, may increase dose q2wk; *max:* 3 g/d	For partial, tonic-clonic, and myoclonic seizures. May cause drowsiness, dizziness, irritability, headache, cough, fatigue, anorexia, nausea, vomiting, diarrhea, weakness, infection, hallucinations, and hypertension. PB: <10%; t½: 6–8 h
Brivaracetam	A: PO/IV: Initially 50 mg bid; *max:* 200 mg/d	For partial seizures. May cause dizziness, drowsiness, ataxia, fatigue, nausea, vomiting, dysgeusia, euphoria, irritability, and nystagmus. PB: <20%; t½: 9 h
Tiagabine	A: PO: Initially 4 mg/d for 1 wk; *maint:* 32–56 mg/d; *max:* 56 mg/d in 2–4 divided doses	For partial seizures. May cause dizziness, drowsiness, tremor, weakness, ataxia, nausea, vomiting, diarrhea, pharyngitis, and infection. PB: 96%; t½: 7–9 h
Topiramate	Immediate release: A: PO: Initially 25 mg bid; *max:* 400 mg/d Extended release: A: PO: 50 mg/d; *max:* 400 mg/d	For partial and tonic-clonic seizures, Lennox-Gastaut syndrome, and migraine prophylaxis. May cause dizziness, drowsiness, nystagmus, infection, fatigue, dysgeusia, anorexia, nausea, abdominal pain, weight loss, hyperammonemia, and paresthesia. PB: 15%–41%; t½: 21 h
Zonisamide	A: PO: Initially 100 mg/d; may increase after 2 wk; *max:* 600 mg/d	For partial seizures. May cause dizziness, drowsiness, headache, confusion, insomnia, agitation, memory impairment, depression, fatigue, ataxia, diplopia, irritability, anorexia, and nausea. PB: 40%; t½: 63 h
Pregabalin	Partial seizures: A: PO: Initially 150 mg/d in 2–3 divided doses; *max:* 600 mg/d	For partial seizures, neuropathic pain, and fibromyalgia. May cause confusion, drowsiness, dizziness, euphoria, headache, tremor, infection, visual disturbance, peripheral edema, fatigue, xerostomia, appetite stimulation, constipation, weight gain, and ataxia. PB: 0%; t½: 6 h
Lacosamide	A: PO/IV: Initially 100 mg bid; *maint:* 300–400 mg/d in 2 divided doses; *max:* 400 mg/d	For partial and tonic-clonic seizures. May cause dizziness, drowsiness, euphoria, blurred vision, nystagmus, headache, ataxia, tremor, fatigue, nausea, and vomiting. PB: 15%; t½: 13 h
Felbamate	A: PO: Initially 1200 mg/d in 3–4 divided doses; *max:* 3600 mg/d	For partial seizures and Lennox-Gastaut syndrome. May cause drowsiness, dizziness, headache, fatigue, anxiety, paresthesia, dyspepsia, diarrhea, vomiting, and constipation. PB: 25%–35%; t½: 13–23 h
Perampanel	Partial seizures: A: PO: Initially 2 mg/d at bedtime; *maint:* 8–12 mg/d; *max:* 12 mg/d	For partial and tonic-clonic seizures. May cause dizziness, drowsiness, ataxia, headache, fatigue, nausea, vomiting, weight gain, irritability, and hostility. PB: 95%–96%; t½: 105 h
Cenobamate	A: PO: Initially 12.5 mg/d for 2 wk, then 25 mg/d for 2 wk, then 50 mg/d for 2 wk, then 100 mg/d for 2 wk, then 150 mg/d for 2 wk, then 200 mg/d; *max:* 400 mg/d	For partial seizures. May cause dizziness, drowsiness, fatigue, diplopia, headache, blurred vision, nystagmus, ataxia, nausea, vomiting, constipation, dysarthria, and hyperkalemia. PB: 60%; t1/2: 50–60 h

>, Greater than; <, less than; *A,* adult; *bid,* twice a day; *BP,* blood pressure; *CSS,* Controlled Substances Schedule; *d,* day; *EPS,* extrapyramidal symptoms; *GI,* gastrointestinal; *h,* hour; *IM,* intramuscular; *IV,* intravenous; *maint,* maintenance; *max,* maximum; *Mg,* magnesium; *min,* minute; *NaCl,* sodium chloride; *PB,* protein binding; *PE,* phenytoin equivalents; *PO,* by mouth; *PRN,* as needed; *q3d,* every 3 days; *qid,* four times a day; *t½,* half-life; *tid,* three times a day; *UK,* unknown; *wk,* weeks; *URI,* upper respiratory infection; *y,* years.

TABLE 19.3 Selected Anticonvulsants for Seizure Disorders

Seizure Disorder	Drug Therapy
Tonic-clonic	Phenytoin Carbamazepine Fosphenytoin Valproic acid Lamotrigine Primidone Phenobarbital Diazepam Levetiracetam Topiramate
Partial (complex secondarily generalized)	Phenytoin Carbamazepine Oxcarbazepine Levetiracetam Primidone Phenobarbital Tiagabine Topiramate Zonisamide Gabapentin Valproic acid Diazepam Fosphenytoin Lamotrigine Eslicarbazepine Clorazepate Pregabalin Lacosamide Felbamate
Absence (petit mal)	Ethosuximide Valproic acid Clonazepam
Myoclonic, atonic, atypical absence	Valproic acid Levetiracetam Clonazepam
Status epilepticus	Diazepam Fosphenytoin Lorazepam Phenytoin Phenobarbital

CRITICAL THINKING CASE STUDY

A 26-year-old woman takes phenytoin 100 mg three times daily to control tonic-clonic seizures. She and her husband are contemplating starting a family.

1. What action should the nurse take in regard to the patient's family planning?

The patient complains of frequent upset stomach and bleeding gums when brushing her teeth.

2. To decrease gastrointestinal (GI) distress, what can be suggested?
3. To alleviate bleeding gums, what patient teaching for the patient may be included?
4. The nurse checks the patient's serum phenytoin level. What are the indications of an abnormal serum level? What appropriate actions should be taken?

REVIEW QUESTIONS

1. The nurse witnesses a patient's seizure involving generalized contraction of the body followed by jerkiness of the arms and legs. The nurse reports this as which type of seizure?
   a. Myoclonic
   b. Absence
   c. Tonic-clonic
   d. Psychomotor

2. Phenytoin has been prescribed for a patient with seizures. The nurse should include which appropriate nursing intervention in the plan of care?
   a. Report an abnormal phenytoin level of 18 mcg/mL.
   b. Monitor complete blood count levels for early detection of blood dyscrasias.
   c. Encourage the patient to brush teeth vigorously to prevent plaque buildup.
   d. Teach the patient to stop the drug immediately when passing pinkish-red or reddish-brown urine.

3. When administering phenytoin, the nurse realizes more teaching is needed if the patient makes which statement?
   a. "I must shake the oral suspension very well before pouring it in the dose cup."
   b. "I cannot drink alcoholic beverages when taking phenytoin."
   c. "I should take phenytoin 1 hour before meals."
   d. "I will need to get periodic dental checkups."

4. A patient is having absence seizures. Which of the following does the nurse expect to be prescribed for this type of seizure? (Select all that apply.)
   a. Phenytoin
   b. Phenobarbital
   c. Valproic acid
   d. Clonazepam
   e. Ethosuximide

5. A patient is admitted to the emergency department with status epilepticus. Which drug should the nurse most likely prepare to administer to this patient? (Select all that apply.)
   a. Diazepam
   b. Midazolam
   c. Gabapentin
   d. Levetiracetam
   e. Topiramate

6. The nurse should monitor the patient receiving phenytoin for which adverse effect?
   a. Psychosis
   b. Nosebleeds
   c. Hypertension
   d. Gum erosion

7. A nurse administering valproic acid to a patient checks the laboratory values and finds a serum range for valproic acid of 150 mcg/mL. What should the nurse do?
   a. Increase the daily dose to get the patient's level into the therapeutic range.
   b. Hold the morning dose but give the other scheduled dosages for the day.
   c. Ask the patient if he or she is having any adverse effects from the medication.
   d. Hold the medication and notify the health care provider.

20

Drugs for Parkinsonism and Alzheimer Disease

http://evolve.elsevier.com/McCuistion/pharmacology

OBJECTIVES

- Summarize the pathophysiology of Parkinson disease and Alzheimer disease.
- Contrast the actions of anticholinergics, dopaminergics, dopamine agonists, monoamine oxidase B (MAO-B) inhibitors, and catechol-*O*-methyltransferase (COMT) inhibitors in the treatment of Parkinson disease.
- Compare the side effects of various antiparkinson drugs.

- Apply the Clinical Judgment [Nursing Process] to anticholinergics, dopaminergics, and acetylcholinesterase inhibitors.
- Differentiate the various phases of Alzheimer disease with corresponding symptoms.
- Compare the side effects/adverse effects of acetylcholinesterase inhibitors used to treat Alzheimer disease.

OUTLINE

Parkinson disease (PD) is a chronic, progressive neurologic disorder that affects the extrapyramidal motor tract, which controls posture, balance, and locomotion. PD is the most common form of parkinsonism, which is considered a syndrome, or a combination of similar symptoms, because of its major features: rigidity (abnormal increased muscle tone), bradykinesia (slow movement), gait disturbances, and tremors. Rigidity increases with movement. Postural changes caused by rigidity and bradykinesia include the chest and head thrust forward with the knees and hips flexed, a shuffling gait, and the absence of arm swing. Other characteristic symptoms are masked facies (no facial expression), involuntary tremors of the head and neck, and pill-rolling motions of the hands. The tremors may be more prevalent at rest.

Alzheimer disease (AD) is a chronic, progressive, neurodegenerative disorder with marked cognitive dysfunction, such as impairment of memory, reasoning, language, and perception. Various theories exist as to the cause of Alzheimer disease, such as neuritic plaques (also known as senile plaques), degeneration of the cholinergic neurons, and deficiency in acetylcholine (ACh) among them.

PARKINSON DISEASE

PD was first medically described as a neurologic syndrome by James Parkinson in 1817, although fragments of parkinsonism can be found in earlier descriptions. Dr. James Parkinson described PD as having "shaking palsy." Three symptoms were described: (1) involuntary tremors of the limbs, (2) rigidity of muscles, and (3) slowness of movement with a propensity to bend the trunk forward and to pass from a walking to a running pace. In the United States approximately 1 million people have PD, and 60,000 new cases are diagnosed each year. PD generally affects patients 50 to 60 years of age and older, men are more likely to have PD than women, and the number of those diagnosed with PD increases with age, regardless of sex.

PD is a long-term (chronic) condition that gets worse over time (is progressive). PD results from a loss of neurons in a specific part of the brain called the *substantia nigra*. Some chemicals in the substantia nigra make an important brain chemical called dopamine (DA). DA is needed to control movement. As PD worsens, neurons make less DA. This makes it hard to control movement. The cardinal symptoms of PD are rigidity, tremors, gait disturbance, and bradykinesia. Normally the symptoms have a gradual onset and are usually mild and unilateral in the beginning but worsen over time.

Parkinsonism and Extrapyramidal Symptoms

Certain drugs may cause parkinsonism and lead to extrapyramidal symptoms: neuroleptics (antipsychotics and dopamine receptor blockers). The lack of dopamine often mimics idiopathic pathologies of the extrapyramidal system. These include acute dyskinesias (involuntary movement) and dystonic reactions (sustained involuntary contractions of muscles), tardive dyskinesia (repetitive movements), parkinsonism (a condition that causes a combination of the movement abnormalities seen in PD), akinesia (loss of ability to move muscles voluntarily), akathisia (feeling of muscle quivering, restlessness, inability to sit still), and neuroleptic malignant syndrome (an adverse reaction to medications with dopamine receptor-antagonist properties).

Nonpharmacologic Measures

Symptoms of PD can be lessened using nonpharmacologic measures such as patient teaching, exercise, nutrition, and group support. Exercise can improve mobility and flexibility; the patient with PD should enroll in a therapeutic exercise program tailored to this disorder. A balanced diet with fiber and fluids helps prevent constipation and weight loss. Patients with PD and their family members should be encouraged to attend a support group to help cope with and understand this disorder.

Medical marijuana (cannabis) is legalized in many states, and there is strong interest in its therapeutic properties for PD. Despite several clinical studies, it has not been demonstrated that cannabis can directly benefit people with PD. Researchers issue caution for people with PD who use cannabis because of its effect on thinking. PD can impair the executive function—the ability to make plans and limit risky behavior. People with a medical condition that impairs executive function should be cautious about using any medication that can compound this effect.

Pathophysiology

PD is caused by an imbalance of the neurotransmitters DA and ACh, and it is marked by degeneration of neurons of the extrapyramidal (motor) tract in the substantia nigra of the midbrain. The reason for the degeneration of neurons is unknown, but there is some evidence for the role of genetics and environmental factors.

The two neurotransmitters within the neurons of the striatum of the brain are DA, an inhibitory neurotransmitter, and ACh, an excitatory neurotransmitter. DA is released from the dopaminergic neurons, and ACh is released from the cholinergic neurons. DA normally maintains control of ACh and inhibits its excitatory response. In PD, an unexplained degeneration of the dopaminergic neurons occurs, and an imbalance between DA and ACh results. With less DA production, the excitatory response of ACh exceeds the inhibitory response of DA. An excessive amount of ACh stimulates neurons that release gamma-aminobutyric acid (GABA). With increased stimulation of GABA, the symptomatic movement disorders of PD occur. The striatal neurons synthesize DA from levodopa and release DA as needed. Before the next dose of levodopa, symptoms such as slow walking and loss of dexterity return or worsen, but within 30 to 60 minutes of receiving a dose, the patient's functioning is much improved.

Drugs used to treat PD replace the DA deficit and reduce the symptoms. These drugs fall into five categories: (1) anticholinergics, which increase the effects of DA in the brain by reducing the effects of ACh; (2) dopaminergic replacement therapy, which stimulates the production of DA in the brain; (3) dopamine agonists, which mimic the effects of DA in the brain by directly stimulating DA receptors; (4) monoamine oxidase B (MAO-B) inhibitors, which inhibit the inactivation of DA in the brain; (5) catechol-O-methyltransferase (COMT) inhibitors, which inhibit the COMT enzyme that inactivates DA; and (6) dopamine antagonists, which disrupt the activity of DA by blocking DA receptor sites without activating them. Table 20.1 compares the various drugs for PD.

Anticholinergics

Anticholinergic drugs increase the effects of DA in the brain by reducing the effects of ACh. This reduces the rigidity and some of the tremors characteristic of PD but has a minimal effect on bradykinesia. The anticholinergics are parasympatholytics that inhibit the release of ACh. Anticholinergics are still used to treat drug-induced parkinsonism, or pseudoparkinsonism, a side effect of the antipsychotic phenothiazine drug group. Examples of anticholinergics used for PD include trihexyphenidyl and benztropine.

Table 20.2 lists the anticholinergics and their dosages, uses, and considerations. Anticholinergics, also referred to as cholinergic antagonists, are discussed in Chapter 16.

TABLE 20.1	Comparison of Drugs Used to Treat Parkinson Disease
Drug	**Purpose**
Anticholinergics	
Benztropine Trihexyphenidyl	The first group of drugs used to treat PD before levodopa and dopamine agonists were introduced, these were useful in decreasing tremors related to PD. The major use of these agents currently is to treat drug-induced parkinsonism. Treatment starts with a low dosage that is gradually increased. Older adults are more susceptible to the many side effects of anticholinergics, and patients with memory loss or dementia should *not* be on anticholinergic therapy (see Table 20.2).
Dopaminergics	
Levodopa inhalation	Levodopa inhalation is administered via an inhalation pump directly into the lungs. It is used "as needed" for Parkinson disease (PD) patients who are affected by an off period. These periods may come on slowly between regularly scheduled carbidopa/levodopa doses or abruptly at unpredictable times.
Carbidopa-levodopa	To decrease symptoms of PD and parkinsonism; carbidopa, a decarboxylase inhibitor, permits more levodopa to reach the striatum nerve terminals, where levodopa is converted to dopamine. With the use of carbidopa, less levodopa is needed.
Dopamine Agonists (DA)	
Apomorphine	Apomorphine, a nonnarcotic derivative of morphine. Approved as a sublingual film for treatment of acute, intermittent "off" episodes of PD and as a subcutaneous injection in advanced PD. Coadministration with antiemetic is suggested due to high incidence of nausea. Also used as a diagnostic test for dopaminergic responsiveness.

TABLE 20.1 Comparison of Drugs Used to Treat Parkinson Disease—cont'd

Drug	Purpose
Bromocriptine	A synthetic dopamine agonist, an ergot derivative, bromocriptine can be used for early treatment of Parkinson disease. With increasing motor symptoms, it can be given with levodopa therapy. It was the first dopamine agonist marketed for the treatment of PD in adults as monotherapy or as an adjunct to levodopa-based treatment; however, newer dopamine agonists have largely replaced bromocriptine in the treatment of PD.
Cabergoline	A synthetic ergoline-derived dopamine agonist beneficial for motor fluctuations associated with PD. Its advantage over bromocriptine is once-daily dosing due to its longer half-life. Used after other approved treatments have been unsuccessful due to risk of cardiac valvulopathy.
Pramipexole	A DA that differs from other DA in that it is not an ergot alkaloid and is less likely to cause fibrotic and valvular complications.
Ropinirole	An oral, non-ergot, alkaloid dopamine agonist for the treatment of idiopathic PD in adults as early monotherapy and in combinaton with levodopa.
Rotigotine	A transdermal nonergoline dopamine agonist used for the treatment of idiopathic PD and restless leg syndrome (RLS). Effective with and without concomitant levodopa treatment was established in advanced and early stage PD patients.
Monoamine Oxidase B (MAO-B) Inhibitors	
Safinamide	Safinamide is a selective and reversible inhibitor of monoamine oxidase (MAO) Type B. MAO exists as two catabolic isoenzymes, MAO-A and MAO-B. The neurotransmitters serotonin and norepinephrine are primarily catabolized by MAO-A and dopamine is primarily catabolized by MAO-B. Due to its dopaminergic properties, safinamide is effective in the treatment of PD and is FDA approved as an adjunct to levodopa; carbidopa therapy to treat "off" episodes in adults with PD.
Selegiline	Selegiline is a selective monoamine oxidase type-B inhibitor (MAO-B). It works by inhibiting the catabolic enzymes of dopamine and extends its action. Available orally for treatment of PD as an adjunct to levodopa/carbidopa. Recommend decreasing dietary tyramine intake to decrease the risk of hypertensive crisis.
Rasagiline	Rasagiline is a potent, irreversible MAO-B that inhibits the breakdown of dopamine at synapses in the brain and allows neurons to reabsorb more dopamine for use later. It is 5 times more potent an inhibitor than selegiline. If dosing guidelines are followed, tyramine restrictions are not required; however, very high doses of tyramine (aged cheese) may result in hypertensive reaction.
Catechol-*O*-Methyltransferase (COMT) Inhibitors	
Entacapone	A reversible inhibitor of the COMT enzyme that increases the concentration of levodopa and is used in combination with levodopa-carbidopa.
Opicapone	Opicapone is an oral COMT inhibitor used once daily as adjunctive treatment to levodopa-carbidopa in adults with PD experiencing "off" episodes.
Tolcapone	An oral peripherally and centrally acting COMT inhibitor used as an adjunct to levodopa-carbidopa therapy in the treatment of PD. By improving levodopa availability in the CNS, the patient's dose of levodopa can be lowered.
Dopamine Receptor Antagonist (DRA)	
Amantadine	Amantadine decreases the symptoms of PD and drug-induced extrapyramidal reactions. Amantadine is a synthetic antiviral agent that was found to cause symptomatic improvement in PD. It is a weak, uncompetitive antagonist of the N-methyl-D-aspartate (NMDA) receptor. It is used for early treatment of PD, which will delay the necessity of levodopa.
Istradefylline	Istradefylline is a xanthine derivative and an oral adenosine A2A receptor antagonist. It is used as an adjuvant with levodopa-carbidopa therapy in adult PD patients who experience "off" episodes.
Atypical Antipsychotic	
Pimavanserin	Pimavanserin is an atypical antipsychotic, indicated for the treatment of hallucinations and delusions associated with PD psychosis.

◎ CLINICAL JUDGMENT [NURSING PROCESS]

Antiparkinson Anticholinergic Agents

Concept: Mobility
- *Mobility* refers to the ability to move and refers to walking, exercise, and performing self-care. In nursing care, nurses assist the patient in the preservation and rehabilitation of mobility as well as the identification and avoidance of problems with immobility.

Recognize Cues [Assessment]
- Obtain a health history on the patient. Report any history of glaucoma, gastrointestinal (GI) dysfunction, urinary retention, angina, or myasthenia gravis. All anticholinergics are contraindicated if a patient has glaucoma.

- Obtain a drug history on the patient. Report any probable drug-drug interactions, such as with phenothiazines, tricyclic antidepressants (TCAs), and antihistamines, which increase the effect of trihexyphenidyl.
- Assess baseline vital signs for future comparisons. (The pulse rate may increase.)
- Assess the patient's knowledge regarding the medication regimen.
- Assess the patient's ability to ambulate and perform self-care interventions.
- Determine usual urinary output as a baseline for comparison. Urinary retention may occur with continuous use of anticholinergics.

◎ CLINICAL JUDGMENT [NURSING PROCESS]—CONT'D

Antiparkinson Anticholinergic Agents

Analyze Cues and Prioritize Hypothesis [Patient Problems]
- Confusion
- Elimination
- Decreased mobility
- Potential for falls

Generate Solutions [Planning]
- The patient will have decreased involuntary symptoms caused by PD or drug-induced parkinsonism.

Take Action [Nursing Interventions]
- Monitor vital signs, urine output, and bowel sounds. Increased pulse rate, urinary retention, and constipation are side effects of anticholinergic drugs.
- Observe and assess the patient for involuntary movements.
- Assess personal beliefs of patients and family, and modify communications to meet the patient's needs; use an interpreter and community nurse follow-up as needed.

Safety
- Discuss with patient and family the need for "safety always." Depending on the progression of the disease, the patient may need assistance ambulating.
- Discuss bathroom changes such as: A safety bar in the shower, an elevated toilet seat, and a shower chair.
- Discuss with the patient and family a home safety assessment: Remove all throw rugs, add extra lighting, and avoid anything that can block the patient's view when ambulating.

Patient Teaching
General
- Advise patients to avoid alcohol, cigarettes, caffeine, and aspirin to decrease gastric acidity.

Side Effects
- Encourage patients to relieve dry mouth with hard candy, ice chips, or sugarless chewing gum. Anticholinergics may decrease salivation.
- Suggest that patients use sunglasses in direct sunlight because of possible photophobia.
- Advise patients to void before taking the drug to minimize urinary retention.
- ⚡ Counsel patients who take an anticholinergic for control of symptoms of PD to have routine eye examinations because anticholinergics are contraindicated in patients with glaucoma.

Diet
- Encourage patients to ingest foods high in fiber and to increase fluid intake to prevent constipation.
- Instruct patients to avoid alcohol, cigarettes, and caffeine when taking anticholinergic drugs.

Evaluate Outcomes [Evaluation]
- Evaluate the patient's response to trihexyphenidyl or benztropine mesylate to determine whether PD symptoms are controlled and patient can perform self-care.

TABLE 20.2 Antiparkinson Drugs: Anticholinergics

Drug	Route and Dosage	Uses and Considerations
Benztropine	A: PO/IM: Start 0.5–1 mg/d; increase as needed, 0.5 mg at 5- to 6-d intervals; *max:* 8 mg/d Drug-induced extrapyramidal symptoms: A: PO/IM/IV: Initially 1–2 mg bid/tid; *maint:* 1–4 mg qd/bid; *max:* 8 mg/d	To decrease involuntary symptoms of Parkinson disease, tremor, and drug-induced parkinsonism May cause constipation, blurred vision, ocular hypertension, xerostomia (dry mouth), nausea, anhidrosis, and urinary retention Contraindications: Dementia, tachycardia, cardiac disease, autonomic neuropathy, prostatic hypertrophy, psychosis, glaucoma, myasthenia gravis, hyperthermia, alcoholism; contraindicated for use in older adults and children PB: UK; t½: UK
Trihexyphenidyl	A: PO: Initially 1 mg, then increase by 2 mg every 3–5 d; *maint:* 6–10 mg/d, usually tid with meals and at bedtime; *max:* 15 mg/d Extended release: A: PO: 5–10 mg after breakfast in two divided doses 12 h apart; *max:* 15 mg/d	Used for parkinsonism and drug-induced EPS; contraindicated for use in older adults May cause dizziness, anxiety, confusion, insomnia, nausea, vomiting, restlessness, tachycardia, weakness, glaucoma, NMS, and urinary retention Precautions: Abrupt discontinuation, alcoholism, cardiac disease, wide-angle glaucoma, hepatic disease; contraindicated for use in older adults May cause drug interaction: phenothiazine, tricyclic antidepressant, antihistamine PB: UK; t½: 5.6–10.2 h

A, Adult; *bid,* two times a day; *d,* day; *h,* hour; *EPS,* extrapyramidal symptoms; *IM,* intramuscular; *IV,* intravenous; *maint,* maintenance; *max,* maximum; *mg,* milligram; *NMS,* neuroleptic malignant syndrome; *PB,* protein binding; *PO,* by mouth; *t½,* half-life; *tid,* three times day; *UK,* unknown.

Dopaminergics

Levodopa

The first dopaminergic drug was levodopa, which was introduced in 1961. When introduced, levodopa was effective in diminishing symptoms of PD and increasing mobility; this is because the blood-brain barrier admits levodopa but not DA. The enzyme *dopa decarboxylase* converts levodopa to DA in the brain, but this enzyme is also found in the peripheral nervous system and allows 99% of levodopa to be converted to DA *before* it reaches the brain. Therefore only about 1% of levodopa taken is available to be converted to DA once it reaches the brain, and large doses are needed to achieve a pharmacologic response. These high doses may cause many side effects, including nausea, vomiting, dyskinesia, orthostatic hypotension, cardiac dysrhythmias, and psychosis.

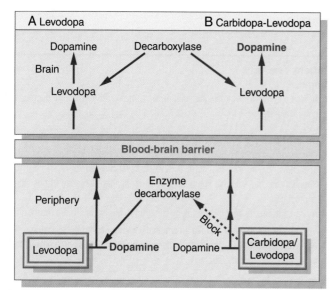

Fig. 20.1 (A) When levodopa is used alone, only 1% reaches the brain because 99% converts to dopamine while in the peripheral nervous system. (B) By combining carbidopa with levodopa, carbidopa can inhibit the enzyme decarboxylase in the periphery, thereby allowing more levodopa to reach the brain.

Levodopa has been unavailable in the United States until recently. In early 2019 the first and only inhaled levodopa used for intermittent treatment of "off episodes" in people with PD taking carbidopa-levodopa was approved by the US Food and Drug Administration (FDA). Off episodes, also known as *off periods*, are defined as the return of Parkinson symptoms that result from low levels of DA between doses of oral carbidopa/levodopa (FDA.gov).

Carbidopa-Levodopa

Due to the side effects of levodopa and the fact that so much levodopa is metabolized before it reaches the brain, an alternative drug, carbidopa, was developed to inhibit the enzyme *dopa decarboxylase*. By inhibiting the enzyme in the peripheral nervous system, more levodopa reaches the brain. The carbidopa is combined with levodopa in a ratio of 1 part carbidopa to 10 parts levodopa. Fig. 20.1 illustrates the comparative action of levodopa and carbidopa-levodopa. By combining levodopa with carbidopa, more DA reaches the basal ganglia and smaller doses of levodopa are required to achieve the desired effect. The disadvantage of the carbidopa-levodopa combination is that with more available levodopa, more side effects may occur, which may include nausea, vomiting, dystonic movement (involuntary abnormal movement), and psychotic behavior. The peripheral side effects of levodopa are not as prevalent; however, angioedema, palpitations, and orthostatic hypotension may occur.

Prototype Drug Chart: Carbidopa-Levodopa lists the pharmacologic behavior of carbidopa-levodopa.

Dopamine Agonists

DA agonists, also called *dopaminergics,* stimulate DA receptor activation and provide relief from PD symptoms such as tremor and rigidity. *Bromocriptine* acts directly on DA receptors in the CNS, cardiovascular system, and GI tract. Bromocriptine is an effective anticholinergic in its class; however, it is not as effective as carbidopa-levodopa in alleviating PD symptoms. Patients who do not tolerate carbidopa-levodopa are frequently given bromocriptine. If bromocriptine is taken with carbidopa-levodopa, usually the drug dosages are reduced, and side effects and drug intolerance decrease.

Apomorphine is a DA agonist and a nonnarcotic derivative of the drug morphine. It contains DA receptor agonist properties and is used for acute, intermittent treatment of off episodes and with advanced PD. Apomorphine has a short duration of action and is inconvenient in the subcutaneous injection form (other forms of administration are being researched); however, the drug has several advantages. These advantages include a quick onset of action, a significant effect on parkinsonian hypomobility (off episodes) unresponsive to oral medications, safety in patients who have a history of psychosis from other DA agonists, and a therapeutic effect comparable to levodopa. Apomorphine is administered under close supervision of the health care provider (HCP) to observe the effect of the drug on the patient's blood pressure and heart rate.

Monoamine Oxidase B Inhibitors

The enzyme MAO-B causes catabolism (breakdown) of DA. *Selegiline* inhibits MAO-B and thus prolongs the action of levodopa. It may be ordered for patients newly diagnosed with PD. The use of selegiline could delay carbidopa-levodopa therapy by 1 year. It decreases "on/off" fluctuations. Large doses of selegiline may inhibit MAO-A, an enzyme that promotes metabolism of tyramine in the GI tract. If not metabolized by MAO-A, ingestion of foods high in tyramine—such as aged cheese, red wine, and bananas—can cause a hypertensive crisis. Severe adverse drug interactions can occur between selegiline and various tricyclic antidepressants (TCAs) or selective serotonin reuptake inhibitors (SSRIs).

Catechol-*O*-Methyltransferase Inhibitors

The enzyme COMT inactivates DA. When taken with a levodopa preparation, COMT inhibitors increase the amount of levodopa concentration in the brain. *Tolcapone* was the first COMT inhibitor to be given with levodopa for advanced PD. This drug can affect liver cell function; therefore serum liver enzymes should be closely monitored.

Entacapone does not affect liver function. The FDA has approved a combination drug of dopaminergics (carbidopa and levodopa) and a COMT inhibitor (entacapone). With various dosage strengths available, this drug combination of carbidopa, levodopa, and entacapone provides greater dosing flexibility and individualization to the patient. This drug combination lessens the "wearing off" effects of levodopa that are sometimes experienced before the next dose. Table 20.3 lists dopaminergics, dopamine agonists, MAO-B inhibitors, COMT inhibitors, dopamine receptor antagonists, and atypical antipsychotics with their dosages, uses, and considerations.

Dopamine Receptor Antagonists

Amantadine

Amantadine, a synthetic antiviral agent, acts on DA receptors. It was introduced as an agent for prophylaxis of seasonal influenza and was later found to cause symptomatic improvement in PD. Although FDA-approved for the prophylaxis and treatment of influenza, the Centers for Disease Control and Prevention (CDC) recommends against using amantadine due to the development of resistant viral strains. The exact mechanism of amantadine in the treatment of PD is unknown. Amantadine may be taken alone or in combination with carbidopa-levodopa or an anticholinergic drug. Initially, it produces improvement in symptoms of PD in approximately two-thirds of patients, but this improvement is usually not sustained because drug tolerance develops. Amantadine can also be used to

📄 **PROTOTYPE DRUG CHART**

Carbidopa-Levodopa

Drug Class	Dosage

Dopaminergic
Antiparkinson: Dopamine replacement
	Immediate release:
	A: PO: Initially 1 tablet containing 25 mg carbidopa/100 mg levodopa tid; *maint:* 70–100 mg
	    of carbidopa per day; *max:* 200 mg/800 mg/dose using 25 mg/100 mg tab
	A: Extended-release tablets: Initially 50 mg carbidopa/200 mg levodopa bid; *max:* 1600 mg/d
	A: Extended-release capsules: Initially 23.75 mg carbidopa/95 mg levodopa tid; *max:* 612.5
	    mg/2450 mg/d
	Enteral suspension: *max:* 2000 mg/d over 16 h

Contraindications	Drug-Lab-Food Interactions

Hypersensitivity to carbidopa-levodopa, narrow-angle glaucoma,
    severe cardiovascular disease, renal impairment, hepatic
    disease, suspicious skin lesions (activates malignant melanoma),
    MAOI therapy, dyskinesia, pulmonary disease
Caution: Peptic ulcer, impulse control syndrome, orthostatic
    hypotension, psychosis, seizure disorder; avoid abrupt
    discontinuation. May cause neuroleptic malignant syndrome (NMS),
    suicidal ideation, open-angle glaucoma (⚡ contraindicated in
    glaucoma patients), phenylalanine-containing forms (PKU).
	Drug: Increased hypertensive crisis with MAOIs, decreased levodopa effect with
	    anticholinergics and antipsychotics; with TCAs, may cause dyskinesia and hypertension;
	    with methyldopa, may cause psychosis.
	Food: High-protein foods decrease levodopa absorption.
	Lab: May increase BUN, AST, ALT, ALP, and LDH

Pharmacokinetics	Pharmacodynamics
Absorption: PO: Well absorbed (99%) Distribution: PB: Widely distributed Metabolism: t½: 1–2 h Excretion: 70%–80% (in urine as metabolites)	PO: Onset: UK Peak: 2 h Duration: 5 h ER: Onset: UK Peak: 3 h Duration: 4–6 h

Therapeutic Effects/Uses

To treat Parkinson disease and parkinsonism; relieves tremor and rigidity.
Mechanism of Action: Transmission of levodopa to brain cells for conversion to dopamine; carbidopa blocks the conversion of levodopa to dopamine in the intestine
    and peripheral tissues. Carbidopa is added to levodopa to inhibit the peripheral destruction of levodopa; thus more levodopa is available for transport to the brain
    cells for conversion to dopamine.

Side Effects	Adverse Reactions

Anorexia, nausea, vomiting, dysphagia, dyskinesia, erythema,
    fatigue, dizziness, headache, dry mouth, constipation, bitter taste,
    twitching, blurred vision, insomnia, excess dark sweating, urine
    discoloration (red, brown, or black)
	Involuntary movements, angioedema, palpitations, orthostatic hypotension, urinary retention,
	    priapism, psychosis, depression with suicidal ideation, hallucinations, sudden sleep onset,
	    impulse control symptoms
	Life-threatening: Agranulocytosis, hemolytic anemia, leucopenia, thrombocytopenia, cardiac
	    dysrhythmias; abrupt discontinuation may cause neuroleptic malignant syndrome

A, Adult; *ALP,* alkaline phosphatase; *ALT,* alanine aminotransferase; *AST,* aspartate aminotransferase; *bid,* two times a day; *BUN,* blood urea nitrogen; *d,* day; *h,* hour; *LDH,* lactic dehydrogenase; *maint,* maintenance; *MAOI,* monoamine oxidase inhibitor; *max,* maximum; *min,* minute; *PB,* protein binding; *PO,* by mouth; *qid,* four times a day; *t½,* half-life; *TCA,* tricyclic antidepressant; *tid,* three times a day; *UK,* unknown.

treat drug-induced parkinsonism. It has few side effects, but the side effects may intensify when the drug is combined with other PD drugs. Amantadine is contraindicated in patients with renal failure, patients undergoing dialysis, and patients with hypersensitivities to amantadine and rimantadine.

Istradefylline

Istradefylline is an adenosine receptor antagonist used to treat PD. It reduces "off" periods resulting from long-term treatment with the antiparkinson drug levodopa. An "off" period is a time when a patient's

medications are not working well, causing an increase in PD symptoms, such as tremors and difficulty walking. It is a selective antagonist.

Atypical Antipsychotic

Pimavanserin is a DA antagonist further classified as an atypical antipsychotic and is the first drug approved by the FDA to treat hallucinations and delusions associated with PD psychosis. Hallucinations or delusions may occur in as many as 50% of patients with PD at some time during their illness. People who experience them see or hear things that are not there (hallucinations) and/or have false beliefs

◎ CLINICAL JUDGMENT [NURSING PROCESS]

Antiparkinson Dopaminergic Agents: Carbidopa-Levodopa

Concept: Mobility

- *Mobility* refers to the ability to move and refers to walking, exercise, and performing self-care. In nursing care, nurses assist the patient in the preservation and rehabilitation of mobility as well as the identification and avoidance of problems with immobility.

Recognize Cues [Assessment]

- Obtain vital signs to use for future comparisons.
- Assess patients for signs and symptoms of PD, including stooped forward posture, shuffling gait, masked facies, and resting tremors.
- Obtain a patient history that includes glaucoma, heart disease, peptic ulcers, kidney or liver disease, and psychosis.
- Obtain a drug history. Report if drug-drug interaction is probable. Drugs that should be avoided or closely monitored are carbidopa-levodopa, bromocriptine, and anticholinergics.

Analyze Cues and Prioritize Hypothesis [Patient Problems]

- Reduced motor function
- Decreased functional ability
- Potential for falls
- Need for health teaching

Generate Solutions [Planning]

- Patient's symptoms of PD will be decreased or absent after 1 to 4 weeks of drug therapy.

Take Action [Nursing Interventions]

- Monitor vital signs and electrocardiogram. Orthostatic hypotension may occur during early use of carbidopa-levodopa and bromocriptine. Instruct patients to rise slowly to avoid faintness.
- Observe for weakness, dizziness, or syncope, which are symptoms of orthostatic hypotension.
- Administer carbidopa-levodopa with low-protein foods. High-protein diets interfere with drug transport to the central nervous system (CNS).
- Observe for symptoms of PD.
- Recognize that elderly patients will need guidance in understanding the disease process of PD.
- Support the patient and their family members who may be dismayed about the diagnosis of PD and lack knowledge of the disease process.
- Secure an interpreter for patients who may have a language barrier.
- Instruct the patient in side effects to report to the health care provider.

Safety

- Ask the doctor for an occupational/physical therapist order to visit the patient's home after discharge. Depending on how the disease progresses, safety changes must be made in the patient's home.

Patient Teaching

General

- ⚡ Urge patients not to abruptly discontinue the medication. Rebound PD (increased symptoms of PD) can occur.
- Inform patients that urine may be discolored and will darken with exposure to air. Perspiration may also be dark. Explain that both are harmless, but clothes may be stained.
- Advise patients to avoid chewing or crushing extended-release tablets.

Side Effects

- Instruct patient in side effects to report to health care provider.
- Encourage patients to report symptoms of dyskinesia.
- Explain that it may take weeks or months before side effects are controlled.

Diet

- Suggest to patients that taking carbidopa-levodopa with food may decrease gastrointestinal (GI) upset, but food will slow the rate of drug absorption.
- Urge patients who take high doses of selegiline to avoid foods high in tyramine such as aged cheese, red wine, cream, yogurt, chocolate, bananas, and raisins to prevent hypertensive crisis.

Amantadine and Bromocriptine

- Urge patients taking amantadine to report any signs of skin lesions, seizures, or depression.
- A history of health problems should have been previously reported to a health care provider; however, it is important for the nurse to review health problems with the patient.
- Advise patients taking bromocriptine to report symptoms of lightheadedness when changing positions, a symptom of orthostatic hypotension.
- Warn patients to avoid alcohol when taking bromocriptine.
- Teach patients to check their heart rate and report rate changes or irregularity.
- Counsel patients not to abruptly stop the drug without first notifying the health care provider.

Evaluate Outcomes [Evaluation]

- Evaluate effectiveness of drug therapy in controlling symptoms of PD.
- Determine whether there is an absence of side effects.
- Determine whether the patient and family have increased knowledge of the drug regimen.

TABLE 20.3   Antiparkinson Medications

Drug	Route and Dosage	Uses and Considerations
Dopaminergics		
Levodopa	Oral inhalation: Inhale contents of 2 capsules (42 mg each), total 84 mg, up to 5 times a day; *max:* 420 mg/d divided into equal doses	Uses: Oral inhalation: Treatment of "off" episodes of PD Absolute contraindications: Closed-angle glaucoma and MAOI therapy. May cause cough, dyskinesia, chest pain, infection, and pharyngitis; t½: 3 h
Carbidopa-levodopa		See Prototype Drug Chart: Carbidopa-Levodopa

TABLE 20.3   Antiparkinson Medications—cont'd

Drug	Route and Dosage	Uses and Considerations
Dopamine Agonists (DA)		
Apomorphine	A: SQ: Initially 2 mg. If tolerable, 1 mg every few days, not to exceed 6 mg; *max:* 6 mg per SQ injection not to exceed 20 mg/d in 5 doses A: SL: Initially 10 mg. If tolerable, 10 mg up to 5 doses daily; increase in 5-mg increments; *max:* 30 mg/day in 5 doses	Apomorphine is administered in a health care setting where the HCP can monitor the patient's BP and pulse. Used as acute, intermittent treatment of "off" episodes and advanced PD. Absolute contraindications: sulfite hypersensitivity. May cause angina, (unspecified) chest pain, dizziness, drowsiness, dyskinesia, ecchymosis, edema, hallucinations, hypotension, injection site reaction, nausea, orthostatic hypertension, peripheral edema, rhinorrhea, vomiting, and yawning. PB: 90%–96%; SQ: t½: 30–60 min; SL: t½: 0.8–3 h
Bromocriptine	A: PO: Initially 1.25 mg bid, gradually increase to usual dose range: 10–30 mg/day PO, in divided doses (with food); *max:* 30 mg/day PO	Used for or treatment of idiopathic or postencephalitic PD. May cause asthenia (weakness), rhinitis, sinusitis, headache, fatigue, nausea, constipation, GI bleeding, hypoglycemia, hypotension. Avoid alcohol use. PB: 90%–96%; t½: 4.8–6 h
Cabergoline	A: Oral: Initially 0.5 mg/d, titrate up as needed; doses range from 1–4 mg/d; *max:* 1 mg 2x/wk	Used for motor fluctuations resulting from PD. May cause constipation, dizziness, headache, and nausea. PB: 40%–42%; t½: 63–69 h ⚡ Caution: Only used if other treatments fail due to risk for cardiac valvulopathy. A full cardiac exam is required before use
Pramipexole	PD: Immediate release: A: PO: Initially: 0.125 mg PO tid; *max:* 4.5 mg/d Extended release: A: PO: Initially 0.375 mg/d; up to 0.75 mg/d	Used for PD and moderate to severe RLS. May cause dizziness, drowsiness, headache, confusion, abnormal dreams, insomnia, asthenia (weakness), orthostatic hypotension, hallucinations, dyskinesia, nausea, and constipation. (Taper off drug gradually.) PB: 15%; t½: 8–12 h ⚡ In patients with cardiac disease or hypotension, close monitoring is required; abrupt discontinuation of drug is prohibited; taper off drug gradually
Ropinirole	PD: Immediate release: A: PO: Initially: 0.25 mg tid; titrate up on weekly basis; *max:* 24 mg/d Extended release: A: PO: Initially 2 mg/d for 1–2 wk, titrate up weekly; *max:* 24 mg/d	Used for PD and restless leg syndrome. May cause dizziness, drowsiness, headache, syncope, dyskinesia, asthenia (weakness), nausea, vomiting, dyspepsia, hypertension, back pain, hallucination, and orthostatic hypotension. PB: 40%; t½: 6–10 h ⚡ Monitor for cardiac adverse effects: hypotension, hypertension, syncope, changes in heart rate; taper before d/c over 7-day period
Rotigotine	Transdermal patch: 2 mg/24 h; titrate up 2 mg/24 h per week Taper before d/c; *max:* 6 mg/24 h	Used for idiopathic PD and RLS. May cause arthralgia, asthenia, dizziness, drowsiness, dyskinesia, fatigue, headache, hyperhidrosis, hypoglycemia, insomnia, nausea, orthostatic hypotension, peripheral edema, pharyngitis, and vomiting. PB: 89.5%; t½ 5–7 h
Monoamine Oxidase B (MAO-B) Inhibitors		
Safinamide	A: 50 mg/PO initially; may increase to 100 mg/d; *max:* 100 mg/d	Used for adjunctive treatment to levodopa-carbidopa therapy in patients with PD experiencing "off" episodes. May cause dyskinesia, elevated hepatic enzymes, and orthostatic hypertension. PB: 76%; t½ 20–26 h
Selegiline	A: PO: 5 mg bid with breakfast and lunch; *max:* 10 mg/d A: PO: ODT tab: 1.25 mg/d for 6 wk, increase to 2.5 mg/d; *max:* 2.5 mg/d; taken without liquid before breakfast	Used for PD and parkinsonism in combination with levodopa or levodopa-carbidopa. May cause dizziness, headache, orthostatic hypotension, nausea (most reported), hallucinations, constipation, depression, confusion, insomnia, and ataxia. PB: 85%–90%; t½: 1.3–2 h ⚡ Contraindicated with any other MAOI, SSRI, or SNRI; titrate off drug; never abruptly d/c; avoid foods high in tyramine, such as aged cheese, red wine, and bananas **Black Box Warning:** Absolute contraindication for use in children; increased risk for suicidal ideation
Rasagiline	A: PO: 1 mg/d due to risk of HTN; *max:* 1 mg/d	Used for PD in early disease and as an adjunct to levodopa in later disease. May cause headache, orthostatic HTN, ataxia, dyskinesia, and GI bleed. PB: 88%–94%; t½: 3 h
Catechol-*O*-Methyltransferase (COMT) Inhibitors		
Entacapone	A: PO: 200 mg with each dose of levodopa-carbidopa (up to 8 doses/d); *max:* 1600 mg/d	Used for PD. Used in combination with levodopa-carbidopa, it prolongs half-life of levodopa and decreases "on/off" fluctuations. Levodopa dose should be decreased when taken with a COMT inhibitor. May cause dizziness, nausea, diarrhea, abdominal pain, dyskinesia, hyperkinesia, orthostatic HTN, dyspnea. PB: 98%; t½: 1–2 h

Continued

TABLE 20.3 Antiparkinson Medications—cont'd

Drug	Route and Dosage	Uses and Considerations
Opicapone	A: PO: 50 mg/d at bedtime (on an empty stomach); *max:* 50 mg/d	Used as a treatment of "off" episodes of PD as an adjunct to carbidopa-levodopa. May cause dyskinesia, constipation, hallucinations, HTN, hypotension, neuroleptic malignant syndrome. PB: 99%, t½: 1–2 h ⚡ Contraindicated with MAOI therapy and pheochromocytoma
Tolcapone	A: PO: Initially 100 mg tid; *max:* 600 mg/d	Used for PD. May cause dizziness, drowsiness, headache, confusion, dystonic reaction, insomnia, anorexia, nausea, constipation, dyskinesia, muscle cramps, hallucinations, vomiting, constipation, and orthostatic hypotension. PB: 99.9%; t½: 2–3 h **Black Box Warning:** Dyskinesia and hepatatoxicity
Dopamine Receptor Antagonist (DRA)		
Amantadine	Immediate release: Young: A: PO: 100 mg bid Geriatric: A: PO: 100 mg daily for several weeks, then increase to 100 mg/bid; *max:* 400 mg/d in divided doses Extended release: A: PO: 129 mg/d in morning (increase at weekly intervals as needed); *max:* 322 mg/d	Used for treatment of PD and drug-induced extrapyramidal reactions. May cause dizziness, headache, anxiety, confusion, insomnia, nausea, blurred vision, ataxia, orthostatic hypotension, and peripheral edema. Do not abruptly stop taking (titrate off drug). PB: 67%; t½: 17 h
Istradefylline	A: Oral: 20 mg/d; max: 40 mg/d	Used as add-on treatment to levodopa and carbidopa in adult PD patients experiencing "off" episodes. May cause dyskinesia, confusion, constipation, delirium, hallucinations, mania, difficulty with impulse control. Use with caution in hepatic disease. PB: 98%; t½: 83 h
Atypical Antipsychotic		
Pimavanserin	A: PO 34 mg/d *without titration; max:* 34 mg/d	Used for the treatment of hallucinations and delusions associated with PD psychosis. May cause confusion, constipation, hallucinations, infection, nausea, peripheral edema, QT prolongation, and stroke **Black Box Warning**: Not approved for dementia-related psychosis unrelated to hallucinations and delusions associated with PD psychosis; increases mortality risk in elderly patients on antipsychotic treatment for dementia-related psychosis

A, Adult; *bid*, twice daily; *BP*, blood pressure; *COMT*, catechol-*O*-methyltransferase; *d*, day; *d/c*, discontinue; *h*, hour; *HCP*, health care provider; *HTN*, hypertension; *incr*, increase; *max*, maximum; *maint*, maintenance; *MAOI*, monoamine oxidase inhibitor; *mg*, milligrams; *min*, minutes; *mL*, milliliters; *NMS*, neuroleptic malignant syndrome; *ODT*, orally disintegrating; *PD*, Parkinson disease; *PB*, protein binding; *PO*, by mouth; *RLS*, restless leg syndrome; *SL*, sublingual; *SSRI*, serotonin reuptake inhibitor; *SNRI*, norepinephrine reuptake inhibitor; *SQ*, subcutaneous; *t½*, half-life; *tid*, three times a day; *tx*, treatment; *w*, with; *wk*, weeks.

(delusions). These are serious symptoms that can lead to thinking and emotions that are so impaired that people experiencing them may not relate to loved ones well or take appropriate care of themselves. In January 2018 the nonprofit Institute for Safe Medication Practices (ISMP) requested that the FDA include stronger warnings on the label for pimavanserin, such as that it may lead to severe adverse effects, including death (https://www.pdlink.org/safety-watchdog-ismp-issues-alert for Parkinson drug).

Precautions for Drugs Used to Treat Parkinson Disease
Side Effects and Adverse Reactions
The common side effects of anticholinergics include dry mouth and dry secretions, urinary retention, constipation, blurred vision, and an increase in heart rate. Mental effects such as restlessness and confusion may occur in older adults.

The side effects of carbidopa-levodopa are numerous. GI disturbances are common because DA stimulates the chemoreceptor trigger zone (CTZ) in the medulla, which stimulates the vomiting center. Taking the drug with food can decrease nausea and vomiting, but food slows the absorption rate. Dyskinesia, impaired voluntary movement, may occur with high levodopa dosages. Cardiovascular side effects include orthostatic hypotension and increased heart rate during early use of levodopa. Nightmares, sudden sleep onset, impulse control symptoms, mental disturbances, and suicidal tendencies may occur.

Pramipexole and *ropinirole* can cause nausea, dizziness, somnolence, weakness, and constipation. These drugs intensify the dyskinesia and hallucinations caused by levodopa. Pramipexole is also FDA approved for treatment of restless legs syndrome.

Tolcapone may cause fatal hepatotoxicity. It is recommended that liver enzymes be drawn frequently. Abrupt discontinuation of tolcapone can cause pyrexia, confusion, and neuroleptic malignant syndrome (NMS). The side effects for tolcapone are GI related (e.g., nausea, anorexia, diarrhea, and vomiting).

Entacapone is not known to affect liver function. With entacapone, the urine can have a brownish orange discoloration. Abrupt discontinuation of entacapone may cause NMS. Both tolcapone and entacapone can intensify the adverse reactions of levodopa (e.g., hallucinations, orthostatic hypotension, constipation, dizziness) because these drugs prolong the effect of levodopa. Both tolcapone and entacapone may lead to intense, uncontrollable urges (sex, gambling, spending money) in addition to suddenly falling asleep. Patients should be warned to avoid driving and other potentially dangerous activities.

Contraindications

Anticholinergics or any drugs that have anticholinergic effects are contraindicated for patients with glaucoma. Those with severe cardiac, renal, or psychiatric health problems should avoid levodopa drugs because of adverse reactions. Patients with chronic obstructive lung diseases such as emphysema can have dry, thick mucus secretions caused by large doses of anticholinergic drugs.

Drug-Drug Interactions

Antipsychotic drugs block the receptors for DA. Carbidopa-levodopa taken with a monoamine oxidase inhibitor (MAOI) antidepressant can cause a hypertensive crisis.

ALZHEIMER DISEASE

Alzheimer disease (AD) is an irreversible neurodegenerative disorder characterized by a decline in a patient's activities of daily living (ADL) and cognitive abilities, as well as changes in behavior.

Pathophysiology

Many physiologic changes contribute to AD. Currently, theories related to the changes that cause AD include the following:

- Degeneration of the cholinergic neuron and deficiency in ACh
- Neuritic plaques that form mainly outside of the neurons and in the cerebral cortex
- Apolipoprotein E_4 (apoE$_4$), which promotes formation of neuritic plaques, which binds beta-amyloid in the plaques
- Beta-amyloid protein accumulation in high levels that may contribute to neuronal injury
- Presence of tau and neurofibrillary tangles that block the neurons and disrupt signals

Fig. 20.2 illustrates a normal healthy neuron and the neuron affected by AD. The etiology of AD is unknown, although factors thought to influence the occurrence of AD are genetic predisposition, virus, infection, or inflammation that attacks brain cells as well as nutritional, environmental, and immunologic factors.

The three phases of AD—(1) preclinical (initial stage), (2) mild cognitive impairment (MCI), and (3) Alzheimer dementia (final stage)—have been modified to assist the clinicians without access to neuropsychological testing, advanced imaging, and cerebrospinal fluid analysis. The modified criteria listed below are reliable for a probable AD diagnosis.

In addition, the patient's deficit must involve at least 2 of the following 5 areas:

1. Impaired ability to acquire and remember new information: repetitive questions or conversations, misplacing personal belongings, forgetting events or appointments, getting lost on a familiar route
2. Impaired reasoning and handling of complex tasks, poor judgment: poor understanding of safety risks, an inability to manage finances, poor decision-making ability, and an inability to plan complex or sequential activities
3. Impaired visuospatial abilities: an inability to recognize faces or common objects or to find objects in direct view despite good acuity, an inability to operate simple implements, and difficulty in orienting clothing to the body

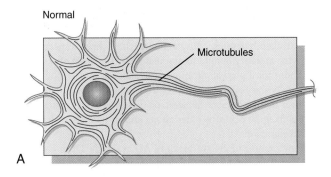

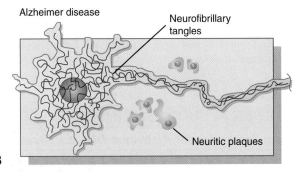

Fig. 20.2 Histologic Changes in Alzheimer Disease. (A) Healthy neuron. (B) Neuron affected by Alzheimer disease shows characteristic neuritic plaques and cellular neurofibrillary tangles.

4. Impaired language functions (speaking, reading, writing): difficulty thinking of common words while speaking, hesitations, and errors in speech, spelling, and writing
5. Changes in personality, behavior, or comportment: uncharacteristic mood fluctuations, such as agitation; impaired motivation and initiative; apathy; loss of drive; social withdrawal; decreased interest in previous activities; loss of empathy; compulsive or obsessive behaviors; and socially unacceptable behaviors

When the diagnosis of AD is unclear, neuropsychological testing is conducted and includes advanced imaging, cerebrospinal fluid analysis, and positron emission tomography (PET).

Acetylcholinesterase/Cholinesterase Inhibitors

The cure for AD is unknown. FDA-approved medications to treat AD symptoms include acetylcholinesterase (AChE) inhibitors. AChE is an enzyme responsible for breaking down ACh and is also known as *cholinesterase*. The AChE inhibitors are donepezil, galantamine, and rivastigmine, a drug that permits more ACh in the neuron receptors. Rivastigmine has effective penetration into the CNS; thus cholinergic transmission is increased. These AChE inhibitors increase cognitive function for patients with mild to moderate AD. A reversible AChE inhibitor used to treat mild to moderate AD is galantamine. Memantine is an N-methyl-D-aspartate (NMDA) receptor antagonist for the management of moderate to severe AD. It can be used alone or along with the AChE inhibitor donepezil.

Rivastigmine

Rivastigmine, an AChE inhibitor, is prescribed to improve cognitive function for patients with mild to moderate AD (see Prototype Drug Chart: Rivastigmine). This drug increases the amount of ACh at the cholinergic synapses. Rivastigmine tends to slow the disease process and has fewer drug interactions than donepezil. Table 20.4 lists the AChE inhibitors used to treat AD.

Pharmacokinetics. Rivastigmine is absorbed faster through the GI tract without food. It has a relatively short half-life and is given twice a day.

The dose is gradually increased. The protein-binding power is average. It readily crosses the blood-brain barrier and is widely distributed.

Pharmacodynamics. Rivastigmine has been successful in improving memory in mild to moderate AD. The onset of action is 0.5 to 1.0 hour for topical application; peak action is 8 to 16 hours. When given orally, the peak is 1 hour. This drug is contraindicated for patients with liver disease because hepatotoxicity may occur. Cumulative drug effect is likely to occur in older adults and in patients with liver and renal dysfunction.

Many organizations are tackling AD research. Drug companies, the US government, and the Alzheimer Association are funding research to learn more about the disease and to find treatments that will reduce symptoms and prevent or cure the disease. Only through clinical research can we gain insights and answers about the safety and effectiveness of new drugs to treat AD. Drug companies are making huge strides in the development and research of Alzheimer medications. The process is long, tedious, and expensive to get drugs approved and ready for marketing. Currently there are several promising drugs in clinical trials.

IgG1 Monoclonal Antibody

Aducanumab is an IV administered amyloid beta-directed antibody indicated for the treatment of adults with AD. It was approved under the FDA's accelerated approval program, which provides patients suffering from a serious disease earlier access to drugs when there is an expectation of clinical benefit as measured by a surrogate endpoint despite some uncertainty about the overall clinical benefit of the drug. The surrogate endpoint that allowed for accelerated approval in 2021 was a reduction of amyloid beta plaque in treated patients. Treatment with aducanumab should be initiated in patients with mild cognitive impairment or mild dementia state of disease (see Table 20.4).

◎ CLINICAL JUDGMENT [NURSING PROCESS]

Drug Treatment for Alzheimer Disease: Rivastigmine

Concept: Cognition

- *Cognition* is the mental action or process of acquiring knowledge and understanding through thought, experience, and the senses. Nurses care for patients with problems in cognition because they may face problems with their physical position or direction, attention span, memories, speaking, and thinking processes.

Recognize Cues [Assessment]

- Assess the patient's mental and physical abilities. Note limitation of cognitive function and self-care.
- Obtain a history that includes any liver or renal disease or dysfunction.
- Assess for memory and judgment losses. Elicit from family members a history of behavioral changes such as memory loss, declining interest in people or home, difficulty in following through with simple activities, and a tendency to wander from home.
- Observe for signs of behavioral disturbances such as hyperactivity, hostility, and wandering.
- Examine the patient for signs of aphasia or difficulty in speech.
- Note patient's physical and motor functions.
- Determine family members' ability to cope with the patient's mental and physical changes.

Analyze Cues and Prioritize Hypothesis [Patient Problems]

- Weight loss
- Decreased self-concept
- Bowel incontinence
- Confusion
- Decreased adherence
- Decreased coping
- Injury

Generate Solutions [Planning]

- Patient's memory will be improved.
- Patient will maintain self-care of body functions with assistance.
- Patient will be provided with assistance for self-care maintenance.

Take Action [Nursing Interventions]

- Maintain consistency in care.
- Assist the patient in ambulation and activity.

- Monitor for side effects related to continuous use of acetylcholinesterase (AChE) inhibitors.
- Record vital signs periodically. Note signs of bradycardia and hypotension.
- Observe any patient behavioral changes, and note any improvement or decline.
- Monitor and assist patient closely to maintain the correct use of the drug dosing plan.
- Provide an interpreter during instruction for the patient and family if a language barrier exists.
- Assist family members in understanding about Alzheimer as a neurologic problem that may be part of the aging process. Explain how symptoms may become more progressive.

Safety

- ⚡ Instruct family in "home safety"; for example, remove area throw rugs, ensure pathways are clear, and keep electrical cords behind furniture to avoid injury when the patient wanders.

Patient Teaching
General

- Explain to the patient and family the purpose for the prescribed drug therapy.
- Clarify times for drug dosing and schedule to the family member responsible for the patient's medications.
- Inform family members of available support groups such as the Alzheimer's Association.

Side Effects

- Inform patients and family members that the patient should rise slowly to avoid dizziness and loss of balance.
- Monitor routine liver function tests because hepatotoxicity is an adverse effect.
- Monitor patient for GI distress.

Diet

- Inform family members about foods that may be prepared for the patient's consumption and tolerance.

Evaluate Outcomes [Evaluation]

- Evaluate effectiveness of the drug regimen by determining whether the patient's mental and physical status shows improvement from drug therapy.

TABLE 20.4 Acetylcholinesterase Inhibitors and Other Drugs for Alzheimer Disease

Drug	Route and Dosage	Uses and Considerations
Donepezil	A: PO: Initially 5 mg/d, upward titration to 10 mg/d should not occur until 4–6 wk; *maint:* 5–10 mg/d; *max:* 23 mg/d	Used for the treatment of mild to moderate Alzheimer disease. May cause GI side effects from mild to severe: diarrhea, headache, infection, vomiting and nausea. Use with caution in older adults. PB: 96%; t½: 70 h
Rivastigmine		See Prototype Drug Chart: Rivastigmine
Memantine	Immediate release: A: PO: Initially 5 mg/d, may increase dose slowly over 3 wk in 5-mg increments; *maint:* 10 mg bid (wk 4); *max:* 20 mg/d Extended release: A: PO: Initially 7 mg/d, increase weekly; *maint:* 28 mg/d; *max:* 28 mg/d Combination memantine and donepezil (extended release): A: 28 mg memantine with 10 mg donepezil once daily in evening; *max:* 228/10 mg/d	Used for moderate to severe Alzheimer disease. May cause serious rash, Stevens-Johnson syndrome, dizziness, headache, drowsiness, confusion, diarrhea, depression, hallucinations, hypertension, hypotension, urinary incontinence and constipation. PB: 45%; t½: 60–80 h
Galantamine	Immediate release: A: PO: Initially 4 mg bid with food; if well tolerated, after 4 wk may increase 8 mg PO bid; if well tolerated, after 4 wk may increase to *maint:* 12 mg bid; *max:* 24 mg/d Extended release: A: PO: Initially 8 mg/d in the morning with food; increase in 4 wk to *maint:* 16 mg PO daily; *max:* 24 mg/d Combination memantine and donepezil (extended release): A: 28 mg memantine with 10 mg donepezil once daily in evening; *max:* 228/10 mg/d	Used for treatment of mild to moderate Alzheimer disease. GI symptoms are most reported: anorexia, abdominal pain, nausea, vomiting, diarrhea, weight loss, and dyspepsia. May cause dizziness, headache, insomnia, fatigue, and suicidal ideation. Use with caution in older adults. PB: 18%; t½: 7 h
Immunoglobulin Gamma Monoclonal Antibody		
Aducanumab	A: IV: titration schedule: (wk 1, wk 2) 1 mg/kg IV; (wk 3, wk 4) 3 mg/kg IV; (wk 5, wk 6) 6 mg/kg IV; *maint:* (wk 7 and beyond) 10 mg/kg IV infusion over 60 min every 4 wk (at least 21 d apart)	Reduces amyloid beta plaques in the brain by binding to forms of beta amyloid protein Side effects include hypersensitivity, headache, confusion, visual impairment, angioedema, cerebral edema, intracranial bleeding. t{½}: 24.8/d

A, Adult; *bid,* twice a day; *d,* day; *h,* hour; *kg,* kilogram; *maint,* maintenance; *max,* maximum; *mg,* milligrams; *PB,* protein binding; *PO,* by mouth; *t½,* half-life; *wk,* week.

📄 PROTOTYPE DRUG CHART

Revastigmine

Drug Class	Dosage
Acetylcholinesterase inhibitor	A: PO: Initially: 1.5 mg bid with food; increase gradually after 4 wk to 3 mg bid Maintenance: 3–6 mg bid; *max:* 12 mg/d Transdermal: Initially 4.6 mg/24 h; may increase after 4 wk to 9.5 mg/d; *max:* 13.3 mg/24 h

Caution	Drug-Lab-Food Interactions
Liver and renal diseases, urinary tract obstruction, orthostatic hypotension, bradycardia, asthma, COPD, seizures, peptic ulcer disease	Drug: Increased effect of theophylline, general anesthetics; TCAs decrease effect; increased effect with cimetidine; NSAIDs increase GI effects; alcohol and tobacco can increase clearance of rivastigmine Lab: Increased ALT, AST

Pharmacokinetics	Pharmacodynamics
Absorption: PO: Food decreases absorption rate Distribution: PB: 40% Metabolism: t½: 1–2 h Excretion: In urine	PO: Onset: UK Peak: 1 h Duration: UK Transdermal: Onset: 30 min–1 h Peak: 8–16 h Duration: 24 h

Therapeutic Effects/Uses

Improves memory loss in mild to moderate Alzheimer disease
Mechanism of Action: Elevates acetylcholine concentration

Continued

📄 PROTOTYPE DRUG CHART—CONT'D

Revastigmine

Side Effects	Adverse Reactions
Anorexia, abdominal pain, GI distress, nausea, vomiting, diarrhea, constipation, weight loss, dizziness, headache, depression, confusion, peripheral edema, dry mouth, dehydration, nystagmus, photophobia	Seizures, bradycardia, orthostatic hypotension, cataracts, myocardial infarction, heart failure *Life-threatening:* Hepatotoxicity, dysrhythmias, suicidal ideation, Stevens-Johnson syndrome

A, Adult; *ALT,* alanine aminotransferase; *AST,* aspartate aminotransferase; *bid,* two times a day; *COPD,* chronic obstructive pulmonary disease; *d,* day; *GI,* gastrointestinal; *h,* hour; *max,* maximum; *min,* minute; *mg,* milligram; *NSAID,* nonsteroidal antiinflammatory drug; *PB,* protein binding; *PO,* by mouth; *t½,* half-life; *TCA,* tricyclic antidepressant; *UK,* unknown; *wk,* weeks.

▌CRITICAL THINKING CASE STUDY

A 79-year-old man was diagnosed with Parkinson disease 10 years ago. During his early treatment, he took selegiline. The drug dosage was increased to alleviate symptoms.

1. How does selegiline alleviate symptoms of Parkinson disease?
2. Which dietary changes are most important to adhere to when a patient is prescribed selegiline?

The patient has developed nausea, depression, and ataxia to selegiline. The HCP stops selegiline and orders carbidopa-levodopa.

3. What are the similarities and differences between selegiline and carbidopa-levodopa?
4. What are the advantages of carbidopa-levodopa?

The family knows of a patient with Parkinson disease who takes the antiviral drug amantadine and does well. They ask whether amantadine is the same as carbidopa-levodopa and, if not, whether their family member can take amantadine instead of carbidopa-levodopa.

5. What is the effect of amantadine on symptoms of Parkinson disease?
6. What would be an appropriate response to the family's question concerning the use of amantadine?
7. What are the uses for dopamine agonists and COMT inhibitors?
8. Certain anticholinergic drugs may be used to control Parkinson disease symptoms. What is the action of these drugs, and what are their side effects? These anticholinergic drugs are usually prescribed for parkinsonism symptoms resulting from what?

▌REVIEW QUESTIONS

1. Which of the following assessment findings would the nurse see in a patient with Parkinson disease? (Select all that apply.)
   a. Abrupt onset of symptoms
   b. Muscle rigidity
   c. Involuntary tremors
   d. Bradykinesia
   e. Bilateral muscle weakness
2. A patient is receiving carbidopa-levodopa for Parkinson disease. What is most important for the nurse know about this drug?
   a. Carbidopa-levodopa may lead to bronchitis.
   b. Carbidopa-levodopa may lead to increased salivation.
   c. Dopaminergics may lead to drowsiness.
   d. Dopaminergics are contraindicated in glaucoma.
3. The nurse has initiated teaching for a family member of a patient with Alzheimer disease. The nurse realizes more teaching is needed when the family member makes which of the following statements?
   a. As the disease progresses, the memory loss will get worse.
   b. There are several theories about the cause of the disease.
   c. Personality changes, wandering, and hostility may occur.
   d. It may take several medications over time to cure the disease.
4. A patient is taking rivastigmine. The nurse should teach the patient and family which information about rivastigmine?
   a. Hepatotoxicity and jaundice are side effects.
   b. The initial dose is 6 mg three times a day.
   c. Gastrointestinal distress is a common side effect.
   d. Increased appetite and weight gain is a side effect.

5. Which is a Take Action [Nursing Intervention] for a patient taking carbidopa-levodopa for Parkinson disease?
   a. Encourage the patient to adhere to a high-protein high sodium diet.
   b. Inform the patient that perspiration may be dark and may stain clothing.
   c. Advise the patient that glucose levels should be checked with urine testing.
   d. Warn the patient that it may take 4 to 5 days before symptoms are controlled.
6. What would the nurse teach a patient who is taking anticholinergic therapy for Parkinson disease? (Select all that apply.)
   a. Avoid alcohol and tobacco.
   b. Relieve dry mouth with hard candy or ice chips.
   c. Use sunglasses to reduce photophobia.
   d. Urinate 2 hours after taking the drug.
   e. Receive routine eye examinations.
7. A patient is taking rivastigmine to improve cognitive function. What should the nurse teach the patient/family member to do? (Select all that apply.)
   a. Rise slowly to avoid dizziness that may cause injury.
   b. Remove obstacles from pathways to avoid injury.
   c. Closely follow the medication dosing schedule.
   d. Have daily blood pressure checks for hypertension.
   e. Receive a monthly glucose panel.

21

Drugs for Neuromuscular Disorders and Muscle Spasms

http://evolve.elsevier.com/McCuistion/pharmacology

OBJECTIVES

- Discuss the pathophysiology of myasthenia gravis and multiple sclerosis.
- Explain the drug group used to treat myasthenia gravis.
- Discuss the drug group used to treat multiple sclerosis.

- Differentiate between the muscle relaxants used for spasticity and those used for muscle spasms.
- Apply the Clinical Judgment [Nursing Process] to drugs used to treat myasthenia gravis and muscle spasms.

OUTLINE

Myasthenia gravis (MG) is an acquired autoimmune disease that impairs the transmission of messages at the neuromuscular junction, resulting in varying degrees of skeletal muscle weakness that increases with muscle use. Although MG can affect any voluntary muscle, those that control eye and eyelid movement (ptosis), facial expression, chewing, and swallowing are most frequently affected due to cranial nerve involvement. MG also affects the muscles of the respiratory system. Respiratory arrest may result from respiratory muscle paralysis. The symptoms of MG are caused by autoimmune destruction of acetylcholine (ACh) sites and a resultant decrease in neuromuscular transmission.

Multiple sclerosis (MS) is a neuromuscular autoimmune disorder that attacks the myelin sheath of nerve fibers, causing lesions known as *plaques*. Although there are no definitive diagnostic tests, the sclerotic plaques are usually detected and measured by magnetic resonance imaging (MRI). Pharmacologic treatment is necessary to control the symptoms of this disorder.

Muscle spasms have various causes, including injury of motor neuron disorders that are associated with conditions such as MS, MG, cerebral palsy, spinal cord injuries (paraplegia [paralysis of the legs]), cerebrovascular accident (CVA [stroke]), or hemiplegia (paralysis of one side of the body). Spasticity of muscles can be reduced with the use of skeletal muscle relaxants.

MYASTHENIA GRAVIS

MG is a chronic autoimmune neuromuscular disease that affects approximately 20 in 100,000 persons. It is estimated that 60,000 Americans are affected. MG can occur in people of any ethnicity and sex; however, more men are affected than women. MG peaks in women around the childbearing years (20 to 30 years of age), whereas the peak onset in men is after 50 years of age. MG can also occur in people outside of this age range. Although it is not a genetic disorder, a familial tendency may be apparent.

Pathophysiology

MG is an autoimmune process in which antibodies attack ACh receptors (AChRs). The result is a decreased amount of AChR sites at the neuromuscular junction. This prevents ACh molecules from attaching to receptors and stimulating normal muscular contraction. The result is ineffective muscle contraction and muscle weakness. About 90% of patients with MG have anti-AChR antibodies that can be detected through serum testing. The other 10% have muscle weakness related to autoantibodies to muscle-specific tyrosine kinase or to other unknown antigens.

Thymic hyperplasia and tumors are common in patients with MG. The thymus gland is involved in systemic immunity that is active during infancy and early childhood, but the gland normally shrinks during adulthood. Approximately 70% of MG patients have thymic hyperplasia. A thymectomy (removal of the thymus gland) is most beneficial because it can cause a reduction of symptoms after the surgery.

MG is characterized primarily by weakness and fatigue of the skeletal muscles. In 90% of cases, eyelid or extraocular muscles are involved. The patients experience ptosis (drooping eyelids) and diplopia (double vision). Other characteristics of MG include dysphagia (difficulty chewing and swallowing), dysarthria (slurred speech), and respiratory muscle weakness.

The group of drugs used to control MG is the acetylcholinesterase (AChE) inhibitors. They inhibit the action of the enzyme AChE. As a result of this action, more ACh is available to activate the cholinergic receptors and promote muscle contraction. The AChE inhibitors are classified as parasympathomimetics.

When muscular weakness in the patient with MG becomes generalized, myasthenic crisis can occur. This complication is a severe, generalized muscle weakness that involves the muscles of respiration, such as the diaphragm and intercostal muscles. Triggers of myasthenic crisis include inadequate dosing of AChE inhibitors, infection, emotional stress, menses, pregnancy, surgery, trauma, hypokalemia, temperature extremes, and alcohol intake. Myasthenic crisis can also occur 3 to 4 hours after taking certain medications (e.g., aminoglycoside and fluoroquinolone antibiotics, beta blockers, phenytoin, and neuromuscular blocking agents; Box 21.1). If muscle weakness remains untreated, death can result from paralysis of the respiratory muscles. Neostigmine, a fast-acting AChE inhibitor, can relieve myasthenic crisis.

Overdosing with AChE inhibitors may cause another complication of MG called cholinergic crisis, which is an acute exacerbation of symptoms. A cholinergic crisis usually occurs within 30 to 60 minutes after taking anticholinergic drugs. This complication is due to continuous depolarization of postsynaptic membranes that create a neuromuscular blockade. The patient with cholinergic crisis often has severe muscle weakness that can lead to respiratory paralysis and arrest. Accompanying symptoms include **miosis** (abnormal pupil constriction), pallor, sweating, vertigo, excessive salivation, nausea, vomiting, abdominal cramping, diarrhea, bradycardia, and **fasciculations** (involuntary muscle twitching).

Acetylcholinesterase Inhibitors

Acetylcholinesterase inhibitors (AChE inhibitors) are also called cholinesterase inhibitors (CHEI). Doses of AChE inhibitors must be individualized to the patient's needs. Patients should always receive the correct dose, at the correct time, to avoid myasthenia crisis and cholinergic crisis.

The first drug used to manage MG is neostigmine methylsulfate, a parasympathomimetic agent (AChE inhibitor). All other AChE drugs should be discontinued 8 hours before administration of neostigmine. Parenteral doses of neostigmine should be accompanied by intravenous (IV) atropine about 30 minutes before administering to counteract the adverse muscarinic effects of neotigmine (Table 21.1).

Pyridostigmine is a reversible AChE inhibitor, preventing the destruction of acetylcholine by cholinesterase and thereby allowing free transmission of nerve impulses across the neuromuscular junction. It has an intermediate action and is given in divided doses. Pyridostigmine is presented in Prototype Drug Chart: Pyridostigmine. Additional uses of pyridostigmine include reversal of neuromuscular

---

BOX 21.1 Medications That May Exacerbate Myasthenia Gravis

- Aminoglycoside antibiotics (gentamicin, neomycin, and tobramycin)
- Beta blockers
- Botulinum toxin
- D-Penicillamine
- [a]Fluoroquinolone antibiotics (moxifloxacin to ciprofloxacin and levofloxacin)
- Chloroquine, hydroxychloroquine
- Immune inhibitors (pembrolizumab, nivolumab, atezolizumab, avelumab, durvalumab, and ipilimumab)
- Iodine radiologic contrast agents
- Macrolides (erythromycin, azithromycin, and clarithromycin)
- Magnesium
- Neuromuscular blocking agents (tubocurarine chloride, pancuronium, succinylcholine)
- Phenytoin
- Quinine, quinidine, procainamide
- Corticosteroids
- Statins (atorvastatin, pravastatin, rosuvastatin, simvastatin)
- [a]Telithromycin
- Zithromax

[a] See http://2019myastheniagravisfoundationofAmerica/cautionarydrugs.

TABLE 21.1 Medications for Myasthenia Gravis

Drug	Route and Dosage	Uses and Considerations
Acetylcholinesterase Inhibitors		
Neostigmine bromide Neostigmine methylsulfate	A: PO: unavailable in United States; treatment of MG A: IM: SC: 0.5 mg; *max:* 0.07 mg/kg Diagnosing MG: IM: 1.5 mg (0.022 mg/kg) single dose (if cholinergic reaction occurs, administer additional IV atropine) Neuromuscular blockade reversal: A: IV: 0.5–2 mg slow IV injection. Repeat as required; *max:* 5 mg total dose	Used for treatment of myasthenia gravis and for neuromuscular blockade reversal and the diagnosis of MG May cause dizziness, headache, nausea, vomiting, bradycardia, hypotension, tachycardia, muscle cramps, seizures, and dyspnea PB: 15%–25%; t½: IM: 51–90 min; t½: IV: 24–113 min
Pyridostigmine		See Prototype Drug Chart: Pyridostigmine
Edrophonium	A: IV: Initially 2 mg over 15–30 s. If cholinergic reaction occurs, discontinue test and administer 0.4–0.5 mg atropine IV. If no response occurs within 45 s, inject another 8 mg. Repeat in 30 min or more to test a positive cholinergic reaction. A: IM: 10 mg; if cholinergic reaction occurs, retest after 30 min with 2 mg to rule out false-negative	Drug of choice for diagnosing MG because of its rapid onset of action and reversibility May cause bradycardia, cardiac arrest, hypotension, laryngospasm, respiratory arrest, and seizures
Immunosuppressant		
Azathioprine	A: PO: 50 mg daily × 1 wk; *gradually increase* to 2–3 mg/kg/d; *max:* 250 mg/d Dosage is based on total body weight	Used for MG poorly controlled with AChE inhibitors May cause infection, leukopenia, nausea and vomiting CBC and platelet required: weekly for the first month; twice monthly for 2–3 months; thereafter, monthly Onset: 6–8 wk Peak: 12 wk Duration: UK PB: 30%; t½: UK ⚡ **Black Box Warning:** Risk for new primary malignancy ❗ High-Alert Drug: Extreme risk of harm if used in error

A, Adult; *AChE,* acetylcholinesterase; *CBC,* complete blood count; *d,* day; *h,* hour; *IM,* intramuscular; *IV,* intravenous; *kg,* kilogram; *max,* maximum dosage; *MG,* myasthenia gravis; *min,* minutes; *PB,* protein binding; *PO,* by mouth; *q,* every; *s,* second; *SC,* subcutaneous; *t½,* half-life; *UK,* unknown; *wk,* weeks.

blockers after surgery and the immediate threat of exposure to the nerve gas Soman by the US military (see Chapter 16).

Pharmacokinetics. Pyridostigmine is poorly absorbed from the gastrointestinal (GI) tract. The half-life of oral pyridostigmine is 3 hours, and the half-life of IV administration is up to 1.5 hours. Because of its short half-life, pyridostigmine should be administered several times a day to avoid muscle weakness and prevent myasthenic crisis. The drug is metabolized by the liver and is excreted in the urine.

Pharmacodynamics. Pyridostigmine increases muscle strength in patients with muscular weakness resulting from MG. Pyridostigmine works to promote transmission of neuromuscular impulses across the myoneural junctions by preventing destruction of ACh. Failure of patients to show clinical improvement may reflect underdosing or overdosing. Overdosing of pyridostigmine can result in cholinergic crisis. This crisis requires emergency medical intervention because of respiratory muscle weakness that can result in respiratory distress. Atropine sulfate injection is the antidote for pyridostigmine overdose to counter the muscarinic effects of ACh. Patients who do not respond to AChE inhibitors may require additional drug treatment such as prednisone, plasma exchange, IV immune globulin, or immunosuppressive drugs.

Prednisone is the drug of choice, but like other immunosuppressants, it reduces the presence of antibodies. Corticosteroids do not produce permanent remission, and the long-term side effects are significant. The immunosuppressive agent azathioprine can be used in conjunction with a lower dose of prednisone. With azathioprine, the complete blood count, including the platelet count, is monitored weekly during the first week of treatment, twice monthly for the second and third months, and monthly, including serum amylase, thereafter. These tests will monitor for leukopenia and hepatatoxicity.

Overdosing and underdosing of AChE inhibitors have similar symptoms: generalized muscle weakness, which can include the muscles of respiration, the diaphragm, and the intercostal muscles, resulting in dyspnea (difficulty breathing) and dysphagia. Additional symptoms that may be present with overdosing are increased salivation (drooling), sweating, and bronchial secretions, along with miosis, bradycardia, and abdominal pain. All doses of AChE inhibitors should be administered on time because late administration of the drug may result in muscle weakness.

Side Effects and Adverse Reactions

Side effects and adverse reactions of AChE inhibitors include GI disturbances (nausea, vomiting, diarrhea, abdominal cramps), increased salivation and tearing, miosis (constricted pupil of the eye), blurred vision, and bradycardia.

Overdosing and underdosing of AChE inhibitors have similar symptoms: muscle weakness, dyspnea, and dysphagia. Underdosing can result in myasthenia crisis, and overdosing can result in cholinergic crisis. The drug edrophonium is a short-acting AChE inhibitor that is used to distinguish between myasthenia crisis and cholinergic crisis. Symptoms are similar for both myasthenia and cholinergic crises; the patient experiences severe muscle weakness. After edrophonium is given, if the symptoms are alleviated because of an increase in AChE, the cause is myasthenia crisis. If the muscle weakness becomes more severe, the cause is cholinergic crisis due to drug overdosing (see Table 21.1).

📄 PROTOTYPE DRUG CHART

Pyridostigmine

Drug Class	Dosage
Acetylcholinesterase (AChE) inhibitors	Myasthenia gravis: RR: A: PO: 600 mg/d in divided doses; Syrup: 60 mg/5 mL in divided doses; average dose is 600 mg/d; *max:* RR: PO 1500 mg/d in divided doses ER: A: PO: 180–540 mg/d bid with at least 6 h between doses. NOTE: *ER is equal to that of a 60-mg regular-release tablet; however, its duration of effectiveness, although varying in individual patients, averages 2.5 times that of a 60-mg dose; max: ER: PO: 180 mg/d* A: IV: 1–2 mg/h (gradually titrate up in increments of 0.5 mg/h to 1 mg/h up to a max rate of 4 mg/h)
Contraindications	**Drug Interactions**
GI and GU obstructions, ileus, bladder obstruction *Caution:* Asthma, bradycardia, seizure disorder, peptic ulcer, cardiac arrhythmias, renal impairment, hyperthyroidism, pregnancy, breastfeeding	Corticosteroids, neuromuscular blockers, aminoglycosides, local anesthetics, magnesium salts; increased toxicity with acetylcholinesterase inhibitors, atropine, tetracyclines, polymyxin B, bacitracin, digoxin, quinidine, and insecticides containing malathion; atropine decreases the effect of pyridostigmine Atropine sulfate injection is an antidote for pyridostigmine
Pharmacokinetics	**Pharmacodynamics**
Absorption: PO: Poorly absorbed ER: 50% absorbed	PO: RR: Onset: 30–45 min PO: ER: Onset: 0.5–1 h IM: Onset: 15 min IV: Onset: Within minutes PB: UK; t½: Oral 3 h; IV up to 1.5 h
Therapeutic Effects/Uses	
Used to control and treat myasthenia gravis, for neuromuscular blockade reversal, and for nerve gas (soman) exposure prophylaxis Mechanism of Action: Promotes transmission of neuromuscular impulses across the myoneural junctions by preventing destruction of acetylcholine	
Side Effects	**Adverse Reactions**
Abdominal pain, confusion, depression, diarrhea, blurred vision, hyperesthesia, fecal and urinary incontinence, seizures	Bradycardia, cardiac dysrhythmias, COPD, hypertension, and seizures

A, Adult; *bid*, twice a day; *C*, child; *COPD*, chronic obstructive pulmonary disease; *d*, day; *ER*, extended release; *GI*, gastrointestinal; *GU*, genitourinary; *h*, hour; *IM*, intramuscular; *IV*, intravenous; *max*, maximum; *mg*, milligram; *min*, minute; *mL*, milliliter; *PB*, protein binding; *PO*, by mouth; *q*, every; *RR*, regular release; *t½*, half-life; *UK*, unknown.

◎ CLINICAL JUDGMENT [NURSING PROCESS]

Drug Treatment for Myasthenia Gravis: Pyridostigmine

Concept: Sensory Perception
- Sensory perception involves interpreting one's surroundings. A good sensory perception depends on normal sensory receptors, an intact reticular activating system, and a functioning nervous system. The nurse is responsible for thorough assessment of the patient to ensure a functioning sensory perception of his or her environment. The nurse is also responsible for implementing patient care or altering the patient's plan of care when malfunction is present.

Recognize Cues [Assessment]
- Obtain a drug history from the patient, which includes all current medications.
- Observe the patient's drug profile for possible drug interactions.
- Record baseline vital signs.
- Assess patient's current laboratory results.
- Assess patient for signs and symptoms of overdosing/underdosing, such as muscle weakness and difficulty breathing and swallowing.
- Instruct patient in signs and symptoms to report to health care provider (HCP).

Analyze Cues and Prioritize Hypothesis [Patient Problems]
- Decreased gas exchange
- Acute respiratory distress
- Decreased functional ability
- Decreased mobility
- Decreased visual acuity
- Decreased ability to cope
- Need for patient teaching

Generate Solutions [Planning]
- Patient's muscle weakness will see improvements with timely administration of pyridostigmine in evenly divided doses as ordered by HCP.
- Patient will identify factors that increase potential for injury.
- Patient will optimize activities of daily living within sensorimotor limitations.

Take Action [Nursing Interventions]
- Monitor effectiveness of drug therapy (AChE inhibitors). Muscle strength should be increased. Both depth and rate of respirations should be assessed and maintained within normal range.

- Administer prescribed AChE inhibitor after dosage recommendations and nursing guidelines.
- Observe patient for signs and symptoms of cholinergic crisis caused by overdosing or underdosing, such as muscle weakness, respiratory failure, increased salivation, sweating, and bronchial secretions along with miosis.
- Involve family members in teaching about prescriptive therapies and disease processes using simple and clear instructions.
- Communicate respect for the patient's cultural beliefs.
- Assess the patient's understanding of adherence to the drug regimen.
- Instruct the patient to notify the HCP before taking any medications other than what the HCP has ordered.
- Stress that medications need to be taken as prescribed.

Patient Teaching
General
- Teach patients to take drugs as ordered to avoid recurrence of symptoms.
- Encourage patients to wear a medical identification bracelet or necklace that indicates health problems.

Safety
- Instruct patient and family in factors that may contribute to injury.

Side Effects
- Teach patients about the side effects of medication and when to notify the HCP.
- Advise patients to report recurrence of symptoms of MG to the HCP.

Diet
- Inform patients to take the drug before meals for best absorption. If gastric irritation occurs, take the drug with food.

Evaluate Outcomes [Evaluation]
- Evaluate effectiveness of drug therapy to maintain muscle strength.
- Determine the absence of respiratory distress.
- Evaluate the correct use of the drug by the patient.
- Evaluate patient's feelings of safety, comfort, and security.

MULTIPLE SCLEROSIS

MS is an autoimmune disorder that attacks the myelin sheath of nerve fibers in the brain and spinal cord, which results in lesions called *plaques*. In the United States, MS affects approximately 1 million people. Most people with MS are diagnosed between 20 and 50 years of age, with at least two to three times more women than men being diagnosed with the disease. Although the cause of MS is unknown, it is thought that the disease develops in a genetically susceptible person because of environmental exposure, like an infection. The onset of MS is usually slow. It is a condition in which there are remissions and exacerbations of multiple symptoms. Common manifestations of MS are motor, sensory, neurologic, cerebellar, and emotional problems. Motor symptoms include weakness or paralysis of the limbs, muscle spasticity, and diplopia. Patients with MS experience sensory abnormalities, including numbness, tingling, blurred vision, vertigo, and tinnitus. Patients may experience neuropathic pain, particularly in the low thoracic and abdominal areas. Cerebellar signs include nystagmus, ataxia, dysarthria, and dysphagia. Many patients experience severe fatigue. If the sclerotic plaque is in the central nervous system (CNS), problems with bowel and bladder function, sexual function, and cognitive dysfunction can occur.

MS is difficult to diagnose. Most physicians use at least one other test besides the medical history and neurologic examination, such as MRI, evoked potential (EP) testing (test that measures the electrical activity of the brain), or analysis of cerebrospinal fluid (CSF), to confirm the diagnosis (see http://www.nationalmssociety.org).

Classifications of Multiple Sclerosis

MS is classified into four primary patterns for treatment purposes:
- *Relapsing-remitting MS (RRMS):* This is the most common pattern. The patient experiences a sudden attack of symptoms and may recover completely until the next attack, or some residual deficits may remain permanently (affects 85%).
- *Primary progressive MS (PPMS):* Slowly worsening neurologic function is evident from the beginning with no relapses or remissions (affects 10%).
- *Secondary progressive MS (SPMS):* The initial course is relapsing-remitting, followed by progression with or without occasional relapses, minor remissions, and plateaus (about 50% of people with RRMS develop SPMS within 10 years).
- *Progressive relapsing MS (PRMS):* This form is progressive from the onset, with clear acute relapses with or without full recovery (affects 5%).
- *Clinically isolated syndrome (CIS):* This form occurs when a patient has only one flareup of MS. CIS does not always develop into MS. The symptoms for CIS are the same as MS.

There is no known cure for MS.

PROTOTYPE DRUG CHART

Beta-Interferon

Drug Class	Dosage
Immunomodulators: Interferon beta-1a Interferon beta-1b Peginterferon beta-1a	**Beta-1a:** A: IM: 30 mcg (6 million International Units) once/wk; *max:* IM 30 mg/wk A: SC: 22 or 44 mcg 3× wk; give doses at least 48 h apart; *max:* 44 mcg SC every 48 h **Beta-1b:** A: SC: 250 mcg every other day. Titrate to required dose every 2 wk, 62.5 mcg SC every other day wk 1 and 2; 125 mcg SC every other day wk 3 and 4; 187.5 mcg SC every other day wk 5 and 6; *max:* 250 mcg SC every other day **Peginterferon beta-1a:** A: Initially 63 mcg SC on Day 1; Day 15, 94 mcg SC once a day; Day 29, 125 mcg SC once; thereafter, continue 125 mcg SC every 14 days; *max:* 125 mcg SC every 14 days

Contraindications	Drug Interactions
Beta-1a: Albumin hypersensitivity, hamster protein hypersensitivity, alcoholism, autoimmune disease, bone marrow suppression, cardiac disease, and children **Beta-1b:** Albumin hypersensitivity, bone marrow suppression, children, depression, *Escherichia coli* protein hypersensitivity, heart failure, hepatitis, seizures, thyroid disease. **Peginterferon beta-1a:** Hypersensitivity to beta interferon, hepatitis, alcoholism, hepatic disease, autoimmune disease, cardiac disease, bone marrow suppression	**Interferon beta-1a and beta-1b:** Antiretroviral NNRTIs; antiretroviral NRTIs; antiretroviral protease inhibitors; ethanol **Peginterferon beta-1a:** Abacavir, dolutegravir, lamivudine, 3TC

Pharmacokinetics	Pharmacodynamics
Interferon beta-1a and beta-1b: SC: 50% absorbed Distribution: UK Metabolism: UK **Peginterferon beta-1a:** Metabolism: Not extensively metabolized in the liver Peak: 1–5 days Excretion: Urine	**Interferon beta-1a:** t½: 19 h **Interferon beta-1b:** t½: 8 min–4.3 h **Peginterferon beta-1a:** t½: 78 h

Therapeutic Effects/Uses

Interferon beta-1a is used for the treatment of RRMS to slow physical disability and to decrease the frequency of clinical exacerbations; also, to prevent or slow the development of CIS in patients who have experienced a first MS episode and have MRI features consistent with MS.
Interferon beta-1b is used for RRMS to decrease the frequency of clinical exacerbations and is used for SPMS to delay neurologic deterioration.
Peginterferon beta-1a is used for treatment of RRMS, including CIS and active SPMS.
Mechanism of Action: Antiviral and immune-regulatory properties are produced by interacting with specific receptor sites on cell surfaces. It is not exactly known how interferon works to treat MS. Beta-interferon is produced by recombinant DNA technology. Beta interferon suppresses the inflammatory response through different mechanisms. It controls the secretions of proinflammatory and antiinflammatory cytokines suppressing T-cell activation.

Side Effects	Adverse Reactions
Depression, dizziness, fatigue, suicidal ideation, vision problems, dyspnea, chest pain, edema, abdominal pain, autoimmune hepatitis, cystitis, neutropenia, injection site reaction, myalgia, arthralgia, muscle spasm, anaphylaxis, flulike symptoms	Increased myelosuppression may occur with other myelosuppressives including antineoplastics; concurrent use of hepatotoxic agents may increase risk of hepatotoxicity Avoid concomitant use with immunomodulating natural products such as astragalus, echinacea, and melatonin

A, Adult; *CIS,* clinically isolated syndrome; *h,* hours; *IM,* intramuscular; *IU,* International Unit; *MS,* multiple sclerosis; mcg, microgram; mg, milligram; *NNRTI,* nonnucleoside reverse transcriptase inhibitor; *NRTI,* nucleoside reverse transcriptase inhibitor; *q,* every; *RRMS,* remitting-relapsing MS; *SC,* subcutaneous; *SPMS,* secondary progressive MS; *t½,* half- life; *UK,* unknown; *wk,* week.

Immunomodulators

Immunomodulators are disease-modifying drugs (DMDs), and they are the first line of treatment for patients with MS. DMDs modulate the course of MS as either an immunosuppressant or immunomodulator. DMDs can slow the progression of the disease and prevent relapses. Immunomodulators include interferon beta-1a, interferon beta-1b, and peginterferon beta-1a, which are popular drugs in the treatment of MS (Prototype Drug Chart: Beta-Interferon). Both interferon beta-1a and interferon beta-1b have been declared orphan status by the US Food and Drug Administration (FDA). Multiple sclerosis affects fewer than 200,000 people in the United States, and the drugs are not expected to recover costs of development and marketing expenses.

Glatiramer acetate is prescribed for relapsing forms of MS. It is available in prefilled syringes, 20 mg/mL or 40 mg/mL, and administered subcutaneously either once daily or three times a week depending on the health care provider's (HCP) orders. It has a favorable safety profile and must be used cautiously in patients with preexisting immunosuppression. Glatiramer modifies the human immune response. Teriflunomide is a pyrimidine synthesis inhibitor immunomodulator used for RRMS, including CIS and active SPMS. It is in oral form and is administered daily. Alemtuzumab, ocrelizumab, and natalizumab are monoclonal antibodies. Ocrelizumab is the first B-cell targeted drug to treat primary progressive MS in adults. Monoclonal antibodies affect the actions of the body's immune system. They target and destroy certain cells while protecting the body's healthy cells from damage. Many have Black Box Warnings along with Institute for Safe Medication Practices (ISMP) safety alerts and are generally reserved for patients who have had an inadequate response to two or more drugs indicated for the treatment of MS. Dimethyl fumarate is a selective immunosuppressant that can lower the patient's immunity, causing an increased risk of infection. It has both neuroprotective and antiinflammatory properties that can help delay disability and disease progression. Mitoxantrone is a potent

immunosuppressant used to reduce the relapse rate in patients with clinically worsening forms of remitting and secondary progressive MS.

Siponimod is a sphingosine-1-phosphate receptor modulator approved by the FDA for the treatment of MS. Before starting treatment with siponimod, an antineoplastic immunomodulator, the patient must have CYP2C9 genotype testing. This drug should not be used by patients who have a CYP2C9 *3/*3 genotype. Ponesimod is a sphingosine-1-phosphate receptor modulator recently approved by the FDA to treat relapsing forms of MS, which includes CIS, RRMS, and active SPMS. Cladribine is a purine antimetabolite. Its drug mechanism of action has not been made clear but is thought to involve lymphocyte depletion through cytotoxic effects on B and T lymphocytes through impairment of the DNA synthesis. Cladribine has Black Box Warnings and ISMP high safety alert status.

No two cases of MS are alike, so the drugs are tailored to the disease pattern and manifestations of the patient. Table 21.2 lists medications used in the treatment of MS. Corticosteroids are used to manage exacerbations of MS. They work by reducing edema and acute inflammation at the site of demyelination.

The study of MS has seen many advances. New pharmacologic methods in medications and treatments are being researched. The

TABLE 21.2   Drugs for Multiple Sclerosis

Drugs	Route and Dosage	Uses and Considerations
Immunomodulators		
Beta-Interferon Interferon beta-1a Interferon beta-1b Peginterferon beta-1a		See Prototype Drug Chart: Beta-Interferon for beta-1a and beta-1b and peginterferon beta-1a
Glatiramer acetate	A: SC 20 mg/mL once daily A: SC 40 mg/mL 3 × wk (administer at least 48 h apart)	Used for treatment of RRMS, CIS, and SPMS May cause chest pain, sinus tachycardia, laryngospasm, candidiasis, dyspnea, erythema, peripheral vasodilation Distribution: Enters lymphatic and systemic circulation Onset/Peak/Duration: UK PB: UK; t½: UK ⚠ Glatiramer 20 mg/mL and 40 mg/mL solutions for injection are NOT interchangeable
Teriflunomide	A: PO: 7 mg or 14 mg once daily; max: 14 mg daily	Used for treatment of RRMS, CIS, and SPMS May cause alopecia, back pain, cystitis, elevated hepatic enzymes, hyperreflexia, hypophosphatemia, lymphopenia, and myasthenia Monitor: ALT and CBC at least monthly for 6 months Absorption: Well absorbed Distribution: UK PB: >99%; t½: 18–19 d **Black Box Warning:** Pregnancy, hepatotoxicity, reproduction risk ⚡ Safety Alert
Immunosuppressants		
Mitoxantrone	A: IV: 12 mg/m² q3mo; max lifetime dose: 140 mg/m² IV ⚠ Requires experienced clinician for administration **Black Box Warning:** Bone marrow suppression, cardiac toxicity, risk of extravasation, and new primary malignancy	Used for the treatment of chronic SPMS or worsening RRMS to reduce neurologic disability and/or frequency of clinical relapses Not indicated for treatment of PPMS May cause anemia, bleeding, constipation, dyspnea, edema, elevated hepatic enzymes, GI bleeding, hematuria, hyperglycemia, hypocalcemia, leukopenia, lymphopenia, neutropenia, stomatitis, and thrombocytopenia Absorption: Complete bioavailability Distribution: Widely distributed Monitor: Liver function labs PB: 78%; t½: 5–8 d
Dimethyl fumarate	A: PO: 120 mg bid for 7 days, then, 240 mg bid; max: 480 mg/d	Used for treatment of RRMS, including CIS and active SPMS May cause leukopenia, nausea, erythema, progressive multifocal leukoencephalopathy, flushing, anaphylactoid reactions, angioedema, and immunosuppression Absorption: Converted to active metabolite (MMF) by enzymes in the GI tract, blood, and tissue Distribution: UK PB: 27%–45%; t½: 1 h

TABLE 21.2 Drugs for Multiple Sclerosis—cont'd

Drugs	Route and Dosage	Uses and Considerations
Sphingosine-1-Phosphate Receptor Modulators		
Fingolimod	A: PO: 0.5 mg once daily	Used for treatment of RRMS, CIS, and active SPMS May cause elevated hepatic enzymes, diarrhea, headache, infection, AV block, bradycardia, stroke, macular edema, seizure, skin cancer, and hepatic failure Monitor: (initially and periodically) CBC, ECG, LFTs, ophthalmologic examination, serum bilirubin, and skin cancer screening examination; cardiac patients should be monitored overnight in hospital for first dose, with careful monitoring thereafter Absorption: 93% after oral administration Distribution: 86% of drug into RBCs PB: >99.7%; t½: 6–9 days
Ozanimod	A: PO: 7-day titration: Days 1–4: 0.23 mg/d; Days 5–7: 0.46 mg/d; Day 8 and after: 0.92 mg/d. If a dose is missed during the first 2 wk, reinitiate titration; *max:* A: PO: 0.92 mg/d	Used for treatment of CIS, RRMS, and active SPMS. Multiple requirements prior to administration: CBC, lymphocyte count, ECG, assess patient's medical profile for drugs that could slow heart rate or AV conduction, test patient's exposure to chickenpox; ALT, AST, and total bilirubin labs; opthalmologic evaluation May cause elevated hepatic enzymes, infection, cystitis, HTN, orthostatic hypotension, AV block, encephalopathy, MS exacerbation, visual impairment, new primary malignancy PB: UK; t½: 21 h, 11 d (active metabolites) Metabolism: liver Excretion: 37% feces, 26% urine
Ponesimod	A: PO: 14-day titration: Days 1 and 2: 2 mg/d; Days 3 and 4: 3 mg/d; Days 5 and 6: 4 mg/d; Day 7: 5 mg/d; Day 8: 6 mg/d; Day 9: 7 mg/d; Day 10: 8 mg/d; Day 11: 9 mg/d; Days 12, 13, and 14: 10 mg/d; on Day 15 and after that, the maintenance dose is 20 mg/d	Used for the treatment of relapsing forms of MS, to include CIS, RRMS, and active SPMS. Before initiation of therapy: CBC, ALT, AST, and lymphocyte counts; ECG; under care of cardiologist; and ophthalmologic exam May cause anemia, bleeding, dyspnea, edema, elevated hepatic enzymes, GI bleeding, neutropenia, hypocalcemia, and hyperglycemia ⚡ **Black Box Warning:** Bone marrow suppression, severe cardiotoxicity, extravasation, new primary malignancy Requires an experienced clinician to administer ❗ ISMP High-Alert Drug and AMB High-Alert Drug
Siponimod (∗1/∗1, ∗2, or ∗2/∗2 CYP2C9 genotypes)	A:PO: Titration regimen: 0.25 mg on Days 1 and 2; 0.5 mg in 2 doses on Day 3; 0.75 mg in 3 doses on Day 4; 1.25 mg in 5 doses on Day 5; begin maintenance dose of 2 mg once daily starting on Day 6; *max:* 2 mg/day	Used for treatment of RRMS, CIS, and active SPMS May cause increased risk of infections (CBC, liver function, and macular eye exam required before beginning treatment), headache, hypertension, increased liver function test PB: Titration regimen: 99.9% Metabolism: CYP2C9 (79.3%), CYP3A4 (18.5%); t½: 30 h ❗ First dose monitoring in patients with cardiac conditions before and during administration; this drug is not recommended for use in patients with CYP2C9 ∗3/∗3 genotypes; genotype must be determined before use
Siponimod (∗1/∗3 or ∗2/∗3 CYP2C9 genotypes)	A:PO: Titration regimen: 0.25 mg Days 1 and 2; 0.5 mg in 2 doses Day 3; 0.75 mg in 3 doses Day 4; begin maintenance dose of 1 mg once daily starting on Day 5; *max:* 2 mg/day	
Synthetic Purine Nucleoside Antimetabolite		
Cladribine	A: PO:1.75 mg/kg divided into 2 cycles and given as divided doses of 1 or 2 tablets once daily over 4 or 5 days for each cycle; second cycle starts 23 to 27 days after last dose of first cycle Administer a second course at least 43 weeks after last dose of first course, second cycle for a cumulative dosage of 3.5 mg/kg *Max:* 20 mg (2 tablets)/cycle day; do not administer additional doses during the next 2 years after 2 treatment courses Safety and efficacy of reinitiating therapy more than 2 years after completing 2 treatment courses has not been studied	Used for RRMS and active SPMS; recommended for patients who cannot tolerate other MS drugs; not recommended for CIS patients because of safety profile May cause anemia, fatigue, fever, lymphopenia, neutropenia, and thrombocytopenia Clinician must avoid contact of drug on skin when administering ❗ **Black Box Warning:** Contraindicated in pregnancy; may cause bone marrow suppression, nephrotoxicity, neurotoxicity, new primary malignancy; reproductive risk ⚡ High-Alert Drug Monitor CBC/diff, hepatitis B serology, LFTs, pregnancy testing, serum creatinine/BUN, TB skin test, skin cancer screening exam

Continued

TABLE 21.2   Drugs for Multiple Sclerosis—cont'd

Drugs	Route and Dosage	Uses and Considerations
Monoclonal Antibody		
⚠ Alemtuzumab	Regimen consists of 2 treatment courses: A: IV: 12 mg over 4 h daily on 5 consecutive days (total dose of 60 mg) for first treatment course; follow 12 mo later with 12 mg IV over 4 h for 3 consecutive days (total dose of 36 mg) for second treatment	Used for the treatment of RRMS and active SPMS May cause abdominal pain, anemia, antibody formation, arthralgia, candidiasis, chills, diarrhea, dyspnea, fever, hypotension, infection, infusion-related reactions, lymphopenia, neutropenia, sinus tachycardia, and thrombocytopenia; may increase risk of thyroid cancer, melanoma, and lymphoproliferative disease Monitor: CBC diff; CD4 and T cell count; serum creatinine, skin cancer screening examination, TFTs, urinalysis, ECG, hepatits B serology, pregnancy testing Onset: UK Peak: UK PB: UK; t½: 2 wk **Black Box Warning:** Autoimmune disease, infection, bone marrow suppression, infusion-related reactions, stroke, new primary malignancy (administration requires a specialized care setting)
⚠ Natalizumab	A: IV: 300 mg over 1 h q4wk	Used for treatment to reduce frequency of exacerbations of RRMS, CIS, active SPMS May cause antibody formation, anaphylactic shock, arthralgia, depression, diarrhea, GI obstruction, infusion-related reactions, constipation, and elevated hepatic enzymes Monitor: anti-JCV antibodies, LFTs, serum bilirubin Distribution: UK PB: UK; t½: 11 d **Black Box Warning:** Leukoencephalopathy ⚠ High-Alert Drug ⚠ Increased risk of PML; consider benefits and risk prior to use.
⚠ Ocrelizumab	A: IV: 300 mg as a single infusion *followed by a second* 300 mg IV infusion 2 wk later *Subsequent infusions of 600 mg IV are administered every 6 months* *Max:* 600 mg/dose IV	Used for treatment of RRMS, CIS, active SPMS, and PPMS May cause infection (upper respiratory and infusion-related reactions), laryngeal edema, new primary malignancy, and sinus tachycardia Patients are premedicated with IV methylprednisolone 100 mg and PO diphenhydramine 30 min before starting infusion Onset/Peak/Duration: UK Monitor: Hepatitis B serology, neurologic functions, IgG serum concentrations PB: UK; t½: 26 days

A, Adult; *AV,* atrioventricular; *AV block,* atrioventricular block; *bid,* twice daily; *BUN,* blood urea nitrogen; *d,* day; *CBC,* complete blood count; *CIS,* clinically isolated syndrome; *diff,* differential; *ECG,* electrocardiogram; *fnx,* function; *GI,* gastrointestinal; *h,* hour; *htn,* hypertension; *JCV,* John Cunningham virus (enzyme-linked immunosorbent assay test for immune compromised); *ISMP,* Institute for Safe Medication Practices; *IV,* intravenous; *LFT,* liver function test; *MMF,* metabolite monomethyl fumarate; *mo,* months; *MS,* multiple sclerosis; *PB,* protein binding; *PML,* progressive multifocal leukoencephalopathy; *PO,* by mouth; *PPMS,* primary progressive MS; *PRMS,* progressive relapsing MS; *RRMS,* relapsing-remitting *MS; SPMS,* secondary progressive MS; *q,* every; *RBC,* red blood cell; *SC,* subcutaneous; *TB,* tuberculosis; *TFT,* thyroid function test; *t½,* half-life; *UK,* unknown; *wk,* weeks.

study on how immune B cells can activate the advancement of MS led to the development of ocrelizumab. Studies to slow brain atrophy in progressive MS are underway. In addition, advancement in stem cell and genetic research are gaining success in the study of MS.

SKELETAL MUSCLE RELAXANTS

Muscle relaxants relieve muscular spasms and pain associated with traumatic injuries and spasticity from chronic debilitating disorders (e.g., MS, stroke [CVA], cerebral palsy, head and spinal cord injuries). Spasticity results from increased muscle tone from hyper excitable neurons; motor neurons transmit nerve signals from your spinal cord to your muscles. Spasticity is a result of demyelination that occurs in nerves that regulate muscle tone. When these nerve signals are disrupted, muscle weakening occurs. The centrally acting muscle relaxants depress neuron activity in the spinal cord or brain and enhance neuronal inhibition of the skeletal muscles.

Centrally Acting Muscle Relaxants

The mechanism of action of centrally acting muscle relaxants is not fully known. Centrally acting muscle relaxants are used in cases of spasticity to suppress hyperactive reflex and for muscle spasms that do not respond to antiinflammatory agents, physical therapy, or other forms of therapy. The centrally acting muscle relaxants are described in Table 21.3.

Prototype Drug Chart: Cyclobenzaprine explains the drug data for the centrally acting muscle relaxant cyclobenzaprine.

Spasticity

Skeletal muscle spasticity is muscular hyperactivity that causes contraction of the muscles, resulting in pain and limited mobility. Centrally acting muscle relaxants act on the spinal cord. Examples of centrally acting muscle relaxants used to treat spasticity are baclofen, dantrolene, and tizanidine. Diazepam, a benzodiazepine, has also been effective for treating spasticity.

🌿 COMPLEMENTARY AND ALTERNATIVE THERAPIES

Diazepam

Kava, valerian, and St. John's wort may potentiate central nervous system depression.

TABLE 21.3   Muscle Relaxants and Related Drugs

Drugs	Route and Dosage	Uses and Considerations
Anxiolytic/Muscle Relaxant		
Cyclobenzaprine	See Prototype Drug Chart: Cyclobenzaprine	
❗ Diazepam *Long-acting benzodiazepine*	A: PO: 2–10 mg bid/qid A: IV/IM: 5–10 mg, q3–4h; *max:* 40 mg/d PO	Diazepam has many uses, one of which is to relieve muscle spasms and spasticity associated with MS and other motor neuron diseases such as CP May cause sedation, memory impairment, urinary incontinence, and urinary retention Contraindicated in MG, glaucoma, respiratory insufficiency, and hepatic disease; not recommended for use in the elderly PB: 98%; t½: A: 30–60 h (up to 100 h for metabolites) Onset: IV: 1–5 min IM: Absorption is slow/erratic Metabolized: Liver Excreted: Urine **Black Box Warning:** Contraindicated in coadministration with other CNS depressants, substance abuse **❗** High-Alert Drug
Muscle Relaxants		
Centrally Acting Muscle Relaxants		
Baclofen	A: PO: Initially 5 mg tid; increase gradually by 5 mg PO tid every 3 d; *max:* 80 mg/d divided over 4 doses *Titrate off baclofen over 2–3 wk to avoid withdrawal side effects*	For muscle spasms caused by MS and spinal cord injury Most common side effects involve CNS (confusion, coma) and GI tract PB: 30%; t½: 2.5–5.7 h Metabolized: 15% liver Excreted: kidneys 70%–85% **Black Box Warning:** Abrupt discontinuation
Tizanidine	A: PO: Starting dose is 2 mg may be repeated q6–8h *Gradually* increase the dose by 2–4 mg, with 1–4 d in between dose increases until satisfactory reduction in muscle tone is achieved *Max:* 36 mg/d	Used to reduce muscle tone associated with spasticity related to cerebral or spinal cord injury, MS, or other spastic disorders May cause bradycardia, cystitis, hypotension, dizziness, drowsiness, and fatigue; abrupt discontinuation is not recommended; use of drug is not recommended in the elderly PB: 30%; t½: 2 h Due to short duration should be reserved for activities when spasticity control is most important
Carisoprodol	A: PO: 18–65 y 250–350 mg/tid A: 66 y and older: Efficacy and safety not established *To reduce abuse potential, the duration of therapy should not exceed 2–3 doses/wk*	Used for relaxation of acute, painful musculoskeletal conditions May cause drowsiness, xerostomia, dizziness, headache, and nausea Use with caution in older adults and in patients with hepatic dysfunction, seizures, and substance abuse This drug has addictive properties and can increase CNS depression PB: UK; t½: 2.4 h
Chlorzoxazone	A: PO: 250–500 mg tid/qid; *max:* 3000 mg/d **❗** Use cautiously in the elderly	Used as a centrally acting skeletal muscle-relaxing agent with sedative properties May cause CNS depression, urine discoloration, dizziness, drowsiness, and malaise; has a sedative effect (not recommended in older adults) PB: UK; t½: 1 h
Methocarbamol	A: PO: Initially 1.5 g qid for 2–3/d; *maint:* 4 g/d in divided doses; *max:* PO: 8 g/d A: IV: IM: 1 g single dose not to exceed 3 mL/min rate IV; do not inject more than 5 mL; *max:* IV: IM: 3 g/d for no more than 3 consecutive days	Used for relief of musculoskeletal pain May cause drowsiness, dizziness, angioedema, bradycardia, and anaphylactoid reactions; patients should not drive or operate machinery when taking this medication; not recommended for use in the elderly PB: UK; t½: 1–2 h
Metaxalone	A: PO: 800 mg tid/qid; *max:* 3200 mg/d	Used for the treatment of musculoskeletal pain associated with MS May cause anaphylactoid reactions, hemolytic anemia, serotonin syndrome, jaundice, dizziness, and drowsiness; not recommended for use in older adults PB: UK; t½: 9+h/-4.8h

Continued

TABLE 21.3 Muscle Relaxants and Related Drugs—cont'd

Drugs	Route and Dosage	Uses and Considerations
Orphenadrine	A: PO: 100 mg bid; *max:* 200 mg/d A: IM/IV: 60 mg q12h; *max:* 120 mg/d	Used for adjunctive therapy for the relief of musculoskeletal pain May cause anaphylactoid reactions, aplastic anemia, ocular hypertension, confusion, dizziness, and drowsiness *Contraindication:* MG and older adults PB: UK; t½: 14 h
Peripherally Acting Muscle Relaxants		
Dantrolene sodium	A: PO: Initially 25 mg/d; increase gradually; *maint:* 100 mg tid *Doses higher than 400 mg/d (100 mg/qid) are not recommended*	Used for chronic neurologic disorders that cause spasms, MS, SCI, stroke, CP Use cautiously in older adults May cause drowsiness, dysphagia, dysphonia, flushing, and headache PB: UK; t½: 8.7 h **Black Box Warning:** Hepatotoxicity
⚠ Succinylcholine	*Muscle relaxation during nonemergent endotracheal intubation:* A: IV: 0.6 mg/kg; *max:* 1.5 mg/kg/dose A: IM: 3–4 mg/kg; *max:* 150 mg/dose *Neuromuscular blockade during surgery:* A: IV: 0.3–1.1 mg/kg once; *max:* 1.1 mg/kg	A parenteral, short-acting, depolarizing neuromuscular blocking agent used during surgical procedures for muscular relaxation and used to allow endotracheal intubation May cause acute quadriplegic myopathy syndrome, anaphylactoid reactions, angioedema, apnea, arrhythmia, asystole, bradycardia, bronchospasm, and cardiac arrest PB: UK; t½: UK Monitor: HR, BP, oxygen saturation, ECG continuously **Black Box Warning**: Contraindicated in children, infants, hyperkalemia, rhabdomyolysis ⚠ Acute-High Alert Drug
Nondepolarizing Neuromuscular Blocking Agent		
⚠ Pancuronium bromide	A: IV: 0.04–0.1 mg/kg; then 0.01 mg/kg at 25- to 60-min intervals *Non-emergent endotrachial intubation:* A: IV: 0.06–0.1 mg/kg/dose *Neuromuscular blockade during surgery:* A: IV: 0.04–0.1 mg/kg; then 0.01 mg/kg at 25- to 60-min intervals	Used for long-acting neuromuscular blockade and paralysis in surgery as an adjunct to general anesthesia May cause bronchospasm, hypotension, edema, and erythema PB: 30%–87%; t½: 89–161 min **Black Box Warning:** Requires experienced clinician ⚠ Acute High-Alert Drug
⚠ Vecuronium bromide	*Non emergent endotrachial intubation:* A: IV: 0.08–0.1 mg/kg/dose *Neuromuscular blockade during surgery:* A: IV: 0.08–0.1 mg/kg once, followed by 0.01–0.015 mg/kg/dose every 12–15 min as needed to maintain blockade	An intermediate-acting nondepolarizing agent used for maintenance of neuromuscular blockade and paralysis as an adjunct to general anesthesia after general anesthesia has been started May cause bronchospasm, erythema, hypotension, and sinus tachycardia PB: UK; t½: 65–75 min **Black Box Warning:** Must be administered by qualified clinician ⚠ Acute High-Alert Drug

A, Adult; *bid,* twice a day; *BP,* blood pressure; *cardio,* cardiovascular; *CNS,* central nervous system; *CP,* cerebral palsy; *CSS,* Controlled Substances Schedule; *d,* day; *ECG,* electrocardiogram; *GI,* gastrointestinal; *h,* hour; *HR,* heart rate; *IM,* intramuscular; *IV,* intravenous; *maint,* maintenance; *max,* maximum; *MG,* myasthenia gravis; *min,* minutes; *mo,* months; *MS,* multiple sclerosis; *PB,* protein binding; *PO,* by mouth; *PRN,* as needed; *q,* every; *qid,* four times a day; *sec,* seconds; *SCI,* spinal cord injury; *t½,* half-life; *tid,* three times a day; *UK,* unknown; *wk,* weeks; *y,* year.

📄 PROTOTYPE DRUG CHART

Cyclobenzaprine

Drug Class	Dosage
Centrally acting muscle relaxant	IR: A: PO 5 mg tid; if needed, may be increased to 7.5–10 mg tid; *max:* 30 mg/d tid
	ER: A: PO: cap: 15 mg/d, may be increased to 30 mg daily if required; *max:* 30 mg/d
	Treatment for both forms is not recommended beyond 3 wk

Contraindications	Drug-Lab-Food Interactions
AV block, acute myocardial infarction, AV block, bundle branch block, cardiac arrhythmias, heart failure, hyperthyroidism, MAOI therapy, and QT prolongation	Drug: Increased CNS depression with alcohol, kava (*Piper methysticum*), valerian, barbiturates, TCAs, and other CNS depressants
Caution: Seizure disorder, alcohol, prostatic hypertrophy, urinary retention, hepatic disease, breastfeeding, driving or operating machinery, morbidity in geriatric patients, sunlight UV exposure; not recommended for use in the elderly	Check drug guide for multiple interactions
	Take with food or milk to decrease GI upset

Pharmacokinetics	Pharmacodynamics
Absorption: PO: Well absorbed	PO: Onset: 1 h
Metabolism: Liver	Peak: 3–8 h
Excretion: primary urine	Duration: 12–24 h
	Distribution: PB: 93%; t½: 8–37 h

Therapeutic Effects/Uses

For short-term treatment of muscle spasms

Mechanism of Action: Cyclobenzaprine relieves muscle spasms through a central action, possibly at the brain stem level, with no direct action on the neuromuscular junction or the muscle involved.

Side Effects	Adverse Reactions
Anticholinergic effects: Blurred vision, constipation, dry mouth, urinary retention, confusion, drowsiness, nausea, nervousness, tachycardia; also, arrhythmias, headache, unpleasant taste	Allergic reactions, angioedema, myocardial infarction, seizure, ileus

A, Adult; *AV*, atrioventricular; *cap*, capsule; *CNS*, central nervous system; *d*, day; *ER*, extended release; *GI*, gastrointestinal; *h*, hour; *IR*, immediate release; *MAOI*, monoamine oxidase inhibitor; *mg*, milligram; *max*, maximum; *MI*, myocardial infarction; *PB*, protein binding; *PO*, by mouth; *SCI*, spinal cord injury; *t½*, half-life; *TCA*, tricyclic antidepressant; *tid*, three times a day; *UV*, ultraviolet; *wk*, week.

Muscle Spasms

Various centrally acting muscle relaxants are used for muscle spasm to decrease pain and increase range of motion. They have a sedative effect and should not be taken concurrently with CNS depressants such as barbiturates, narcotics, and alcohol. These agents, except for cyclobenzaprine, can cause drug dependence. Most muscle relaxants are not recommended for use in older adults. In addition, dizziness and drowsiness are common side effects. Examples of this group of centrally acting muscle relaxants are carisoprodol, chlorzoxazone, cyclobenzaprine, metaxalone, methocarbamol, and orphenadrine citrate.

Pharmacokinetics. Cyclobenzaprine is well absorbed from the GI tract, and its half-life is moderate. Cyclobenzaprine is metabolized in the liver and excreted in urine.

Pharmacodynamics. Cyclobenzaprine alleviates muscle spasm associated with acute painful musculoskeletal conditions. When cyclobenzaprine is taken with alcohol, kava, valerian, sedative-hypnotics, barbiturates, or tricyclic antidepressants (TCAs), increased CNS depression can occur.

Side Effects and Adverse Reactions

The side effects from centrally acting muscle relaxants include drowsiness, dizziness, lightheadedness, headaches, and occasional GI sensitivity (e.g., nausea, vomiting, abdominal distress). Cyclobenzaprine and orphenadrine have anticholinergic effects.

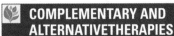

🌿 COMPLEMENTARY AND ALTERNATIVE THERAPIES

Orphenadrine Citrate

Valerian, St. John's wort, and kava may potentiate sedation.

◎ CLINICAL JUDGMENT [NURSING PROCESS]

Muscle Relaxant: Cyclobenzaprine

Concept: Cognition
- *Cognition* is the useful storing and managing of information to focus, acquire, and solve problems. Nurses care for patients who have problems with remembering, attention span, and recall of information. Patients on muscle relaxants may experience cognition problems.

Recognize Cues [Assessment]
- Obtain a medical history. Cyclobenzaprine is contraindicated if the patient has cardiovascular disorders, hyperthyroidism, or hepatic impairment or is taking concurrent monoamine oxidase inhibitors (MAOIs).
- Obtain baseline vital signs.
- Assess the patient's health history to identify the cause of muscle spasm and determine whether it is acute or chronic.
- Observe the patient's drug history for possible drug interactions.
- Assess whether the patient has a history of narrow-angle glaucoma or MG. Cyclobenzaprine and orphenadrine are contraindicated with these health problems.

Analyze Cues and Prioritize Hypothesis [Patient Problems]
- Decreased level of consciousness
- Confusion
- Decreased functional ability

Generate Solutions [Planning]
- The patient will take the muscle relaxants as prescribed by his or her health care provider (HCP).
- The patient will not drive while taking muscle relaxants.
- The patient will not make any major decisions while taking muscle relaxants.

Take Action [Nursing Interventions]
- Monitor serum liver enzyme levels of patients taking dantrolene and carisoprodol. Report to the HCP elevated levels of liver enzymes such as alkaline phosphatase (ALP), aspartate aminotransferase (AST), alanine aminotransferase (ALT), and gamma-glutamyl transferase (GGT).
- Record vital signs. Report abnormal results.

- Observe for central nervous system (CNS) side effects (e.g., dizziness, fatigue, and confusion).
- Instruct patient and family members about the importance of taking prescribed medications as directed by HCP.
- Provide for an interpreter if the patient has a language barrier.

Patient Teaching
General
- Teach patients that the muscle relaxant should not be abruptly stopped. The drug should be tapered over 1 week to avoid rebound spasms.
- Advise patients not to drive, operate dangerous machinery, or make important life-changing decisions when taking muscle relaxants. These drugs have a sedative effect and can cause drowsiness.
- Inform patients that most of the centrally acting muscle relaxants for acute spasms are usually taken for no longer than 3 weeks.
- Teach patients to avoid alcohol and CNS depressants. If muscle relaxants are taken with these drugs, CNS depression may be intensified.
- Advise female patients these drugs must be used cautiously when pregnant or nursing.
- Patients should always check with the HCP before stopping medications.

Side Effects
- Encourage patients to report side effects of the muscle relaxant to their HCP. Common side effects are nausea, vomiting, dizziness, fainting, headache, and diplopia. Dizziness and fainting are most likely caused by orthostatic (postural) hypotension.

Diet
- Advise patients to take muscle relaxants with food to decrease gastrointestinal (GI) upset.

Evaluate Outcomes [Evaluation]
- Evaluate the effectiveness of the muscle relaxant, and determine whether the patient's muscular pain or spasms have decreased or disappeared.

▌ CRITICAL THINKING CASE STUDY

A 29-year-old woman was diagnosed with myasthenia gravis (MG) 2 years ago. She is receiving pyridostigmine 120 mg three times a day. Last evening, the patient was involved in an automobile accident. She was taken to the emergency department unconscious and missed two evening doses of pyridostigmine.

1. How does pyridostigmine alleviate the symptoms of MG?
2. What are the potential side effects and adverse effects of pyridostigmine?

3. What problems are likely to develop after delayed pyridostigmine dosing?
4. What medication is the antidote for pyridostigmine overdose?
5. What problems may develop from pyridostigmine overdosing?
6. What are the similarities between myasthenic crisis and cholinergic crisis?

▌ REVIEW QUESTIONS

1. What is the nurse's best explanation of the pathophysiology of myasthenia gravis?
   a. Degeneration of cholinergic neurons and a deficit in acetylcholine lead to neuritic plaques and neurofibrillary tangles.
   b. A decreased amount of acetylcholine to cholinergic receptors produces weak muscles and reduced nerve impulses.

   c. Myelin sheaths of nerve fibers in the brain and spinal cord develop lesions or plaques affecting the nervous system.
   d. An imbalance of dopamine and acetylcholine leads to degeneration of neurons in midbrain and extrapyramidal motor tracts.

2. The nurse is teaching a patient recently diagnosed with multiple sclerosis about the disease. Which statement is *not* correct concerning multiple sclerosis?
   a. The disease has periods of exacerbations followed by periods of remissions.
   b. Goals of treatment are to decrease the inflammation in the nervous system.
   c. Patients experience muscle weakness, fatigue, and vision and emotional problems.
   d. Multiple sclerosis is an autoimmune disorder that causes plaque to develop.

3. A patient with multiple sclerosis is having muscle spasticity. The nurse anticipates which drug will be prescribed to treat the patient's spasticity?
   a. Neostigmine
   b. Ropinirole
   c. Cyclobenzaprine
   d. Pyridostigmine

4. The nurse anticipates that the health care provider will prescribe which medication to treat a patient with relapsing-remitting multiple sclerosis?
   a. Ambenonium
   b. Pyridostigmine
   c. Mitoxantrone
   d. Glatiramer acetate

5. The nurse is providing medication instructions to a patient with acute muscle spasms who has been prescribed cyclobenzaprine. Which statement indicates to the nurse that the patient understands the instructions?
   a. I plan to take this medication with a glass of milk.
   b. Cyclobenzaprine should be taken once daily at bedtime.
   c. I will only drink one glass of wine a day before taking.
   d. I will be able to take this drug with grapefruit juice.

6. Which instructions will the nurse include in the teaching plan for a patient who is taking pyridostigmine? (Select all that apply.)
   a. Pyridostigmine must always be taken on time.
   b. Take the prescribed dose every other week.
   c. Underdosing can result in myasthenic crisis.
   d. Overdosing can result in cholinergic crisis.
   e. Report the adverse effect of tachycardia to the health care provider (HCP).

7. A patient is beginning to take cyclobenzaprine for treatment of acute back spasms. Which interventions will the nurse include in the care of this patient? (Select all that apply.)
   a. Advise the patient to always take this drug on an empty stomach.
   b. Inform the patient not to abruptly stop taking the muscle relaxant.
   c. Tell the patient to report dizziness and double vision to the health care provider (HCP).
   d. Advise the patient to avoid consuming alcohol beverages.
   e. Taking narcotics at the same time can cause serious side effects.

8. The patient was just prescribed cycobenzaprine for back spasms. The nurse is reviewing the patient's drug profile and plans to contact the HCP about which drug on the patient's daily profile?
   a. Atorvastatin
   b. Conjugated estrogen
   c. Valerian
   d. Penicillin G procaine

9. A patient taking cyclobenzaprine might experience which of the following anticholinergic side effects? (Select all that apply.)
   a. Blurred vision
   b. Dry mouth
   c. Salivation
   d. Constipation
   e. Urinary retention

22

Antipsychotics and Anxiolytics

http://evolve.elsevier.com/McCuistion/pharmacology

OBJECTIVES

- Differentiate between antipsychotic and anxiolytic drug groups.
- Contrast the action, uses, side effects, and adverse effects of traditional typical and atypical antipsychotics.
- Plan nursing interventions, including patient teaching, for the patient taking antipsychotics and anxiolytics.

- Apply the Clinical Judgment [Nursing Process] to the patient taking an atypical antipsychotic, a typical antipsychotic, and an anxiolytic.

OUTLINE

INTRODUCTION

From moods and emotions flow the various thoughts and actions of individuals, which are communicated throughout the central nervous system (CNS) by chemical neurotransmitters. An impulse is communicated by traveling through the presynaptic neuron across the synaptic cleft and binding to a receptor on the postsynaptic neuron, as illustrated in Fig. 22.1.

Neurotransmitters are synthesized in the cytoplasm in the presynaptic neuron and are stored in vesicles, which safeguard neurotransmitters from being destroyed by enzymes. When an impulse arrives by way of an action potential at a presynaptic neuron, vesicles are triggered to move to the cell membrane wall and release the transmitter into the synaptic cleft.

Neurotransmitters function with the help of receptors, which are embedded in the membrane of the postsynaptic neuron. Receptors are configured in size and shape to interlock with specific transmitters. Immediately upon connection of neurotransmitters to receptors, an action is exerted and the transmitter is removed. Once released, transmitters can be broken down into inactive substances by enzymes, diffused away from the synapse into intracellular fluid, or returned to the presynaptic neuron in a process called *reuptake*.

The major neurotransmitters that affect psychopathology include gamma-aminobutyric acid (GABA), serotonin, dopamine,

norepinephrine, and acetylcholine. The GABA neurotransmitter is associated with the regulation of anxiety. When the level of GABA neurotransmitters is reduced, anxiety disorders may result. Benzodiazepines (antianxiety drugs) act by binding to a GABA receptor site, making the postsynaptic receptor more sensitive to GABA and its neurotransmission. This connection decreases the signs and symptoms of anxiety.

Dopamine-containing neurons are thought to be involved in the regulation of cognition, emotional responses, and motivation, and dopamine neurotransmitters are associated with schizophrenia and other psychoses. Antipsychotic drugs block dopamine receptors in the postsynaptic neuron.

Faulty release, reuptake, or elimination of neurotransmitters may lead to an imbalance of neurotransmission and subsequent pathology. Disorders can then develop that can affect an individual's thoughts, feelings, and behaviors.

CNS depressants used to manage symptoms of psychosis and anxiety disorders include antipsychotics and anxiolytics, which may cause psychosis. Antipsychotics are also known as *neuroleptics* or *psychotropics,* but the preferred name for this group is either *antipsychotics* or *neuroleptics*. The term neuroleptic refers to any drug that modifies psychotic behavior and exerts an antipsychotic effect. Anxiolytics are also called *antianxiety drugs* or *sedative-hypnotics*. Certain anxiolytics are used to treat sleep disorders,

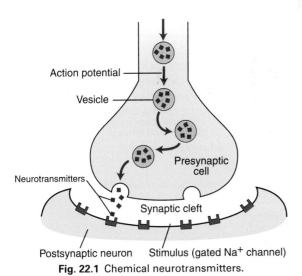

Action potential

Vesicle

Presynaptic cell

Neurotransmitters

Postsynaptic neuron   Stimulus (gated Na$^+$ channel)

Synaptic cleft

Fig. 22.1 Chemical neurotransmitters.

seizures, and withdrawal symptoms from alcohol or other abuse substances. Some of these drugs are also used for conscious sedation and anesthesia supplementation. However, the anxiolytics described in this chapter are used specifically to treat anxiety and psychotic behaviors.

PSYCHOSIS

Psychosis, or loss of contact with reality, is manifested in a variety of mental or psychiatric disorders. Psychosis is usually characterized by more than one symptom, such as difficulty in processing information, disorganized thoughts, distortion of reality, delusions, hallucinations, incoherence, catatonia, and aggressive or violent behavior. Schizophrenia, a chronic psychotic disorder, is the major category of psychosis in which many of these symptoms are manifested.

The symptoms of schizophrenia usually develop in adolescence or early adulthood and are divided into three groups: (1) cognitive symptoms, (2) positive symptoms, and (3) negative symptoms. *Cognitive symptoms* are characterized by disorganized thinking, memory difficulty, and decreased ability to focus attention. *Positive symptoms* may be characterized by exaggeration of normal function (e.g., agitation), incoherent speech, hallucinations, delusions, and paranoia. *Negative symptoms* are characterized by a decrease or loss in function and motivation. A poverty or simplicity of speech, blunted affect, inertia, poor self-care, and social withdrawal are apparent. Negative symptoms tend to be more chronic and persistent. The typical, conventional, or traditional group of antipsychotics (first-generation antipsychotics) is more helpful for managing positive symptoms. A group of antipsychotics called *atypical* (second-generation antipsychotics) has been found to be the newest treatment for both positive and negative symptoms of schizophrenia.

Antipsychotics compose the largest group of drugs used to treat mental illness. Specifically, these drugs improve the thought processes and behavior of patients with psychotic symptoms, especially those with schizophrenia and other psychotic disorders. They are not used as a primary treatment for anxiety or depression. The theory is that psychotic symptoms result from an imbalance in the neurotransmitter dopamine in the brain. Sometimes these antipsychotics are called *dopamine antagonists*. Antipsychotics block D$_2$ dopamine receptors in the brain and thus reduce psychotic symptoms. Many antipsychotics block the chemoreceptor trigger zone (CTZ) and vomiting (emetic) center in the brain, producing an antiemetic (prevents or relieves nausea and vomiting) effect. However, when dopamine is blocked, symptoms of extrapyramidal syndrome (EPS) or parkinsonism (a chronic neurologic disorder that affects the extrapyramidal motor tract) such as tremors, masklike facies, rigidity, and shuffling gait may develop.

Many patients who take high-potency antipsychotic drugs may require long-term medication for symptoms of parkinsonism.

ANTIPSYCHOTIC AGENTS

Antipsychotics are divided into two major categories: *typical* and *atypical*. The typical antipsychotics, introduced in 1952, are subdivided into phenothiazines and nonphenothiazines. *Nonphenothiazines* include butyrophenones, dibenzoxazepines, dihydroindolones, and thioxanthenes. The butyrophenones block only the neurotransmitter dopamine. The *phenothiazines* and the thioxanthenes block norepinephrine, causing sedative and hypotensive effects early in treatment.

Atypical antipsychotics make up the second category of antipsychotics. Clozapine, discovered in the 1960s and made available in Europe in 1971, was the first atypical antipsychotic agent. It was not marketed in the United States until 1990 because of adverse hematologic reactions. Atypical antipsychotics are effective for treating schizophrenia and other psychotic disorders in patients who do not respond to or are intolerant of typical antipsychotics. Because of their decreased side effects, atypical antipsychotics are often used instead of traditional typical antipsychotics as first-line therapy.

Pharmacophysiologic Mechanisms of Action

Antipsychotics block the actions of dopamine and thus may be classified as dopaminergic antagonists. There are five subtypes of dopamine receptors numbered D$_1$ through D$_5$. All antipsychotics block the D$_2$ (dopaminergic) receptor, which in turn promotes the presence of EPS, resulting in drug-induced pseudoparkinsonism in varying degrees. Atypical antipsychotics have a weak affinity to D$_2$ receptors and a stronger affinity to D$_4$ receptors, and they block the serotonin receptor. These agents cause fewer EPS than the typical (phenothiazine) antipsychotic agents, which have a strong affinity to D$_2$ receptors.

Adverse Reactions
Extrapyramidal Syndrome

Pseudoparkinsonism, which resembles symptoms of parkinsonism, is a major side effect of typical antipsychotic drugs. Symptoms of pseudoparkinsonism or EPS include stooped posture, masklike facies, rigidity, tremors at rest, shuffling gait, pill-rolling motions of the hands, and bradykinesia. When patients take high-potency typical antipsychotic drugs for extended periods, EPS is more pronounced. Patients who take low-strength antipsychotics such as chlorpromazine are not as likely to have symptoms of pseudoparkinsonism as those who take fluphenazine.

During early treatment with typical antipsychotic agents for schizophrenia and other psychotic disorders, two adverse extrapyramidal reactions that may occur are acute dystonia and akathisia. Tardive dyskinesia is a later phase of extrapyramidal reaction to antipsychotics. Use of anticholinergic drugs helps decrease pseudoparkinsonism symptoms, acute dystonia, and akathisia but has little effect on alleviating tardive dyskinesia. Complementary and Alternative Therapies: Antipsychotic Agents details interactions with antipsychotic agents.

> ### 🌿 COMPLEMENTARY AND ALTERNATIVE THERAPIES
> #### *Antipsychotic Agents*
>
> - Kava kava may increase the risk and severity of dystonic reactions when taken with phenothiazines.
> - Kava kava may increase the risk and severity of dystonia when taken concurrently with fluphenazine.
> - Ginkgo may potentiate drug effects in patients with schizophrenia who are taking antipsychotics such as haloperidol, olanzapine, and clozapine.
> - St. John's wort may decrease drug levels of clozapine.

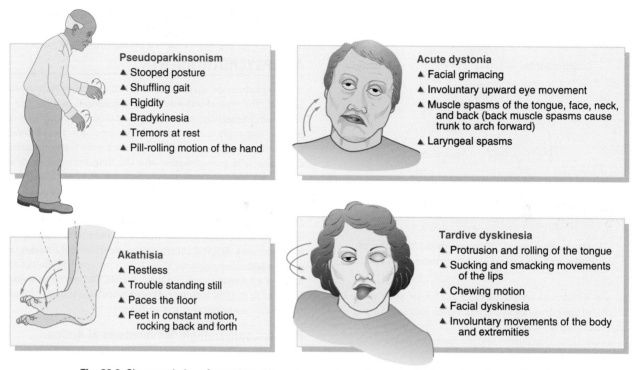

Fig. 22.2 Characteristics of pseudoparkinsonism, acute dystonia, akathisia, and tardive dyskinesia.

The symptoms of acute dystonia usually occur in 5% of patients within days of taking typical antipsychotics. Characteristics of the reaction include muscle spasms of the face, tongue, neck, and back; facial grimacing; abnormal or involuntary upward eye movement; and laryngeal spasms that can impair respiration. This condition is treated with an anticholinergic antiparkinson drug such as benztropine. The benzodiazepine lorazepam may also be prescribed.

Akathisia occurs in approximately 20% of patients who take a typical antipsychotic drug. With this reaction, the patient has trouble standing still, is restless, paces the floor, and is in constant motion (e.g., rocks back and forth). Akathisia is best treated with a benzodiazepine such as lorazepam or a beta blocker such as propranolol.

Tardive dyskinesia is a serious adverse reaction that occurs in approximately 20% to 30% of patients who have taken a typical antipsychotic drug for more than 1 year. The prevalence is higher in cigarette smokers. The likelihood of developing tardive dyskinesia depends on the dose and duration of the antipsychotic factor. Characteristics of tardive dyskinesia include protrusion and rolling of the tongue, sucking and smacking movements of the lips, chewing motion, and involuntary movement of the body and extremities. In older adults, these reactions are more frequent and severe. The antipsychotic drug should be stopped in all who experience tardive dyskinesia, and another antipsychotic agent should be substituted. Benzodiazepines, calcium channel blockers, and beta blockers are sometimes helpful in decreasing tardive dyskinesia, although no one agent is effective for all patients. High doses of vitamin E may be helpful, and its use to treat tardive dyskinesia is currently under investigation. Clozapine has also been effective for treating tardive dyskinesia. Tetrabenazine, used to improve symptoms of Huntington disease, seems to be effective in treating tardive dyskinesia. Tetrabenazine reduces dopamine, norepinephrine, and serotonin levels. Amantadine has also been helpful in reducing drug-induced involuntary movements. Fig. 22.2 shows the characteristics of pseudoparkinsonism, acute dystonia, akathisia, and tardive dyskinesia.

Neuroleptic Malignant Syndrome

Neuroleptic malignant syndrome (NMS) is a rare but potentially fatal condition associated with antipsychotic drugs. Predisposing factors include excess agitation, exhaustion, and dehydration. NMS symptoms involve muscle rigidity, hyperthermia, altered mental status, profuse diaphoresis, blood pressure fluctuations, tachycardia, dysrhythmias, seizures, rhabdomyolysis, acute renal failure, respiratory failure, and coma. Treatment of NMS involves immediate withdrawal of antipsychotics, adequate hydration, hypothermic blankets, and administration of antipyretics, benzodiazepines, and muscle relaxants such as dantrolene.

Phenothiazines

Chlorpromazine hydrochloride was the first phenothiazine introduced for treating psychotic behavior in patients in psychiatric hospitals. The phenothiazines are subdivided into three groups: aliphatic, piperazine, and piperidine, which differ mostly in their side effects.

The *aliphatic phenothiazines* produce a strong sedative effect and decreased blood pressure and may cause moderate EPS (pseudoparkinsonism). Chlorpromazine hydrochloride is in the aliphatic group and may produce pronounced orthostatic hypotension, low blood pressure that occurs when an individual assumes an upright position from a supine position.

The *piperazine phenothiazines* produce more EPS than other phenothiazines. They also cause dry mouth, blurred vision, weight gain, and agranulocytosis. Examples of piperazine phenothiazines are fluphenazine and perphenazine.

The *piperidine phenothiazines* have a strong sedative effect, cause few EPS, have a low to moderate effect on blood pressure, and have no antiemetic effect. Thioridazine is an example of piperidine phenothiazines. Table 22.1 summarizes the effects of the phenothiazines.

Most antipsychotics can be given orally (tablet or liquid), intramuscularly (IM), or intravenously (IV). For oral use, the liquid form might be preferred because some patients may hide tablets in their

TABLE 22.1 Effects of Phenothiazines (Varies Within Class)

Group	Sedation	Hypotension	EPS	Antiemetic
Aliphatic	+++	+++	++	++
Chlorpromazine and triflupromazine				+++
Piperazine	++	+	+++	+++
Piperidine	+++	+++	+	—
Nonphenothiazines				
Haloperidol	+	+	+++	+++
Loxapine	++	++	+++	—
Molindone	+/++	+	+++	—
Thiothixene	+	+	+++	—
Atypical Antipsychotics				
Risperidone	+	+	+/0	—

—, No effect; +, mild effect; ++, moderate effect; +++, severe effect; *EPS*, symptoms of extrapyramidal syndrome.

cheek or under their tongue to avoid taking them. Mouth checks are necessary for noncompliant patients. In addition, the absorption rate is faster with the liquid form, and a peak serum drug level occurs in 2 to 3 hours. The antipsychotics are highly protein bound (>90%), and excretion of the drugs and their metabolites is slow. Phenothiazines are metabolized by liver enzymes into phenothiazine metabolites. Metabolites can be detected in the urine several months after the medication has been discontinued. Phenothiazine metabolites may cause a harmless pinkish to red-brown urine color. The *full* therapeutic effects of oral antipsychotics may not be evident for 3 to 6 weeks after initiation of therapy, but an observable therapeutic response may be apparent after 7 to 10 days.

Noncompliance with antipsychotics is common. Medication teaching in the following areas is of utmost importance: (1) encourage the patient to take the medication as prescribed, (2) explain and emphasize essential information to compensate for the patient's knowledge deficit, and (3) provide an interpreter for patients whose first language is not English.

Prototype Drug Chart: Fluphenazine shows the drug characteristics of fluphenazine, a phenothiazine antipsychotic used to manage psychosis. Box 22.1 shows the symptoms and suggested treatment for overdose of phenothiazines.

📄 PROTOTYPE DRUG CHART

Fluphenazine

Drug Class	Dosage
Antipsychotic: Neuroleptic piperazine phenothiazine	Schizophrenia: A: PO: Initially 2.5–10 mg/d in single or 2–3 divided doses, increase gradually; *max:* 20 mg/d Older A: PO: 1–2.5 mg/d in 2–3 divided doses; *max:* 20 mg/d A: IM/subcut: 12.5–25 mg single dose; *max:* 10 mg/d of immediate release injection, 100 mg/dose of decanoate depot injection
Contraindications	**Drug-Lab-Food Interactions**
Hypersensitivity, CNS depression, coma, blood dyscrasias, children *Caution:* Dysrhythmias, GI obstruction, ileus, cardiovascular disease, bradycardia, urinary retention, BPH, leukopenia, neutropenia, agranulocytosis, diabetes mellitus, hepatic and renal damage, glaucoma, parkinsonism, seizure disorder, older adults, suicidal ideation, tardive dyskinesia, alcohol use disorder	Drug: Increased depressive effects when taken with alcohol or other CNS depressants; MgSO₄, lithium, and beta blockers increase effects; antacids and antiparkinson drugs decrease effects Complementary and alternative therapies: Kava kava may increase dystonia
Pharmacokinetics	**Pharmacodynamics**
Absorption: Rapidly absorbed Distribution: PB 91%–99% Metabolism: t½: HCl, 14.4–16.4 h Excretion: In urine	PO: Onset: UK Peak: 2.8 h Duration: UK IM decanoate: Onset: 24 h Peak: 48–96 h Duration: 4–6 wk
Therapeutic Effects/Uses	
To manage symptoms of psychosis including schizophrenia Mechanism of Action: Blocks dopamine receptors in the brain and controls psychotic symptoms	
Side Effects	**Adverse Reactions**
Drowsiness, dizziness, headache, dry mouth, blurred vision, hyperhidrosis, weight gain, constipation, erectile/ejaculatory dysfunction, urinary retention, peripheral edema, skin hyperpigmentation	Hyper/hypotension, tachycardia, ileus, EPS, seizures, psychosis, hyper/hypoglycemia, hyponatremia, cerebral edema, pseudoparkinsonism *Life-threatening:* Agranulocytosis, aplastic anemia, hemolytic anemia, leukopenia, eosinophilia, neutropenia, thrombocytopenia, angioedema, bronchospasm, NMS

>, Greater than; *A,* adult; *BPH,* benign prostatic hyperplasia; *CNS,* central nervous system; *d,* day; *ER,* extended release; *EPS,* symptoms of extrapyramidal syndrome; *h,* hours; *HCl,* hydrochloride; *IM,* intramuscular; *maint,* maintenance; *max,* maximum; *MgSO₄,* magnesium sulfate; *NMS,* neuroleptic malignant syndrome; *PB,* protein binding; *PO,* by mouth; *q6–8h,* every 6 to 8 hours; *subcut,* subcutaneous; *t½,* half-life; *wk,* weeks; *y,* years.

BOX 22.1   Symptoms and Suggested Treatment for Overdose of Phenothiazines

Symptoms
- Unable to arouse; blood pressure fluctuations; tachycardia; agitation; delirium; convulsions; dysrhythmias; neuroleptic malignant syndrome; extrapyramidal symptoms; and renal, cardiac, and respiratory failure

Treatment
- Maintain airway, gastric lavage, activated charcoal administration, adequate hydration, anticholinergics, and norepinephrine

Pharmacokinetics. Oral absorption of fluphenazine is rapid and unaffected by food. This drug is strongly protein bound and has a long half-life; therefore the drug may accumulate in the body. Fluphenazine is metabolized by the liver, crosses the blood-brain barrier and placenta, and is excreted as metabolites primarily in the urine. With hepatic dysfunction, the phenothiazine dose may need to be decreased. Lack of drug metabolism in the liver will cause an elevation in serum drug level.

Pharmacodynamics. Fluphenazine blocks postsynaptic dopamine receptors increasing dopamine turnovers and is prescribed primarily for psychotic disorders. This drug has anticholinergic properties and should be cautiously administered to patients with glaucoma, especially narrow-angle glaucoma. Because hypotension is a side effect of these phenothiazines, any antihypertensives simultaneously administered can cause an additive hypotensive effect. Narcotics and sedative-hypnotics administered simultaneously with these phenothiazines can cause an additive CNS depression. Antacids decrease the absorption rate of both drugs and all phenothiazines, so they should be given 1 hour before or 2 hours after an oral phenothiazine.

The peak action of fluphenazine is 2.8 hours. Fluphenazine decanoate has delayed absorption, with an onset of action of 24 hours and a duration of 4 to 6 weeks.

Nonphenothiazines

The many groups of nonphenothiazine antipsychotics include butyrophenones, dibenzoxazepines, dihydroindolones, and thioxanthenes.

In the *butyrophenone* group, a frequently prescribed nonphenothiazine is haloperidol. Haloperidol's pharmacologic behavior is similar to that of the phenothiazines. It is a potent antipsychotic drug in which the equivalent prescribed dose is smaller than that of drugs of lower potency, such as chlorpromazine. The initial oral drug dose for haloperidol is 0.5 to 2 mg, whereas the drug dose for chlorpromazine is 10 to 25 mg. Long-acting preparations of haloperidol decanoate and fluphenazine decanoate are given for slow release via injection every 2 to 4 weeks. Administration precautions should be taken to prevent soreness and inflammation at the injection site. Because the medication is a viscous liquid, a large-gauge needle (e.g., 21 gauge) should be used with the Z-track method for administration in a deep muscle; Chapter 10 provides further explanation of the Z-track method of injection. The injection site should not be massaged, and sites should be rotated. These medications should not remain in a plastic syringe longer than 15 minutes. Prototype Drug Chart: Haloperidol provides the drug data related to haloperidol.

Pharmacokinetics. Haloperidol is absorbed well through the gastrointestinal (GI) mucosa. It has a long half-life and is highly protein bound, so the drug may accumulate. Haloperidol is metabolized in the liver and is excreted in urine and feces.

Pharmacodynamics. Haloperidol alters the effects of dopamine by blocking dopamine receptors; thus sedation and EPS may occur. The drug is used to control psychosis and to decrease agitation in adults and children. Dosages need to be decreased in older adults because of decreased liver function and potential side effects. Haloperidol may be prescribed for children with hyperactive behavior. Because it has anticholinergic activity, care should be taken when administering it to patients with a history of glaucoma.

Haloperidol has a similar onset of action, peak time of concentration, and duration of action as the phenothiazines. It has strong EPS effects. Skin and sun protection is necessary for prolonged use because of the possible side effect of photosensitivity.

From the *dibenzoxazepine* group, loxapine is a moderately potent agent. It has moderate sedative and orthostatic hypotensive effects and strong EPS effects.

The typical antipsychotic molindone hydrochloride from the *dihydroindolone* group is a moderately potent agent. It has low sedative and orthostatic hypotensive effects and strong EPS effects.

In the nonphenothiazine group known as *thioxanthenes* is thiothixene, a highly potent typical antipsychotic drug. It has side effects similar to those of molindone with low sedative and orthostatic hypotensive effects and strong EPS effects.

Side Effects and Adverse Reactions

Several side effects are associated with antipsychotics. The most common side effect for all antipsychotics is drowsiness. Many of the antipsychotics have some anticholinergic effects: dry mouth, increased heart rate, urinary retention, and constipation can occur. Blood pressure decreases with the use of antipsychotics; aliphatics and piperidines cause a greater decrease in blood pressure than the others.

EPS can begin within 5 to 30 days after initiation of antipsychotic therapy and are most prevalent with the phenothiazines, butyrophenones, and thioxanthenes. These symptoms include pseudoparkinsonism, akathisia, dystonia (prolonged muscle contractions with twisting, repetitive movements), and tardive dyskinesia. Tardive dyskinesia may develop in 20% of patients taking antipsychotics for long-term therapy. Antiparkinson anticholinergic drugs may be given to control EPS, but they are not always effective in treating tardive dyskinesia.

High dosing or long-term use of some antipsychotics can cause blood dyscrasias (blood cell disorders) such as agranulocytosis. The white blood cell (WBC) count should be closely monitored and reported to the health care provider if an extreme decrease in leukocytes is observed.

Dermatologic side effects seen early in drug therapy are pruritus and marked photosensitivity. Patients are urged to use sunscreen, hats, and protective clothing, and to stay out of the sun.

Drug Interactions

Because phenothiazines lower the seizure threshold, dosage adjustment of an anticonvulsant may be necessary. If either aliphatic phenothiazine or the thioxanthene group is administered, a higher dose of anticonvulsant might be necessary to prevent seizures.

Antipsychotics interact with alcohol, hypnotics, sedatives, narcotics, and benzodiazepines to potentiate the sedative effects of antipsychotics. Atropine counteracts EPS and potentiates antipsychotic effects. Use of antihypertensives can cause an additive hypotensive effect.

Antipsychotics should *not* be given with other antipsychotic or antidepressant drugs except to control psychotic behavior for selected individuals who are refractory to drug therapy. Under ordinary circumstances, if one antipsychotic drug is ineffective, a different one is prescribed. Individuals should *not* take alcohol or other CNS depressants (e.g., narcotic analgesics, barbiturates) with antipsychotics because additive depression is likely to occur.

PROTOTYPE DRUG CHART

Haloperidol and Haloperidol Decanoate

Drug Class	Dosage
Antipsychotic: Neuroleptic (nonphenothiazine)	Schizophrenia: A: PO: Initially 0.5–2 mg bid/tid; *max:* 100 mg/d Decanoate depot: A: IM: Initially 10–15 times previous PO dose of haloperidol equivalents *max:* 450 mg/month

Contraindications	Drug-Lab-Food Interaction
Parkinsonism, CNS depression, coma *Caution:* Alcohol use disorder, dementia, glaucoma, dehydration, CAD, liver damage, urinary retention, narrow-angle glaucoma, cardiovascular disease, neutropenia, leukopenia, agranulocytosis, seizures	Effects of haloperidol may be increased by amiodarone, kava kava, magnesium sulfate, metoclopramide, promethazine, antidepressants, antidysrhythmics; haloperidol may increase effects of anticholinergics, CNS depressants, glucagon, opioid agonists, oxycodone, potassium chloride, thiazide diuretics; effects of haloperidol may be decreased by acetylcholinesterase inhibitors, glycopyrrolate; haloperidol may decrease the effects of amphetamines, systemic epinephrine, nitroglycerine

Pharmacokinetics	Pharmacodynamics
Absorption: PO: 60% absorbed Distribution: PB: 92% Metabolism: t½: 12–37 h PO, 3 weeks decanoate depot IM Excretion: In urine and feces	PO: Onset: 60–90 min Peak: 4–6 h Duration: 24–72 h IM: Onset: 15–30 min Peak: 20–40 min Duration: 4–8 h IM: Decanoate: Onset: UK Peak: 6 d Duration: 3–4 wk

Therapeutic Effects/Uses

To treat acute psychoses, schizophrenia, Tourette syndrome
Mechanism of Action: Alters the effect of dopamine on the CNS; the mechanism for antipsychotic effects is unknown

Side Effects	Adverse Reactions
Drowsiness, edema, headache, blurred vision, depression, confusion, euphoria, cataracts, lethargy, tremor, dry mouth, constipation, weight gain/loss, restlessness, hyperhidrosis, erectile dysfunction, urinary retention	Tachycardia, orthostatic hypotension, EPS, hyper/hypoglycemia, hyponatremia, seizures, retinopathy, osteopenia *Life-threatening:* Laryngeal edema, bronchospasm, dysrhythmias, eosinophilia, aplastic anemia, hemolytic anemia, agranulocytosis, leukopenia, neutropenia, thrombocytopenia, pancytopenia, hepatic failure, NMS, rhabdomyolysis

A, Adult; *ADHD,* attention-deficit/hyperactivity disorder; *bid,* twice a day; *CAD,* coronary artery disease; *CNS,* central nervous system; *d,* day; *EPS,* symptoms of extrapyramidal syndrome; *h,* hour; *IM,* intramuscularly; *maint,* maintenance; *max,* maximum; *min,* minute; *NMS,* neuroleptic malignant syndrome; *PB,* protein binding; *PO,* by mouth; *t½,* half-life; *tid,* three times a day; *UK,* unknown; *wk,* week; *y,* year.

When discontinuing antipsychotics, the drug dosage should be reduced gradually to avoid sudden recurrence of psychotic symptoms and seizures. Table 22.2 lists common antipsychotic drugs—phenothiazines and nonphenothiazines—and their dosages, uses, and considerations, including common side effects and a few serious adverse effects.

Antipsychotic Dosage for Older Adults

Older adults usually require smaller doses of antipsychotics—from 25% to 50% less than young and middle-aged adults. Regular to high doses of antipsychotics increase the risk of severe side effects. Dosage amounts need to be individualized according to the patient's age and physical status. In addition, dosage changes may be necessary during antipsychotic therapy. Antipsychotics have a black box warning that states mortality is increased in elderly patients with dementia-related psychosis.

Atypical Antipsychotics (Serotonin/Dopamine Antagonists)

Atypical antipsychotics differ from typical traditional antipsychotics in that the atypical agents are effective in treating both positive and negative symptoms of schizophrenia. The typical antipsychotics

have not been effective in the treatment of negative symptoms. Two advantages of the atypical agents are that they are effective in treating negative symptoms and that they are unlikely to cause symptoms of EPS, including tardive dyskinesia. Atypical drugs available include clozapine, risperidone, olanzapine, ziprasidone, and aripiprazole. These agents have a greater affinity for blocking serotonin and dopaminergic D_4 receptors than primarily blocking the dopaminergic D_2 receptor responsible for mild and severe EPS. Weight gain, drowsiness, unsteady gait, headache, insomnia, depression, diabetes mellitus, and dyslipidemia are common side effects of atypical antipsychotics.

Clozapine was the first atypical antipsychotic agent used to treat schizophrenia and other psychoses. It is not as likely to cause symptoms of EPS, although they may occur. Tremors and occasional rigidity have been reported. Serious adverse reactions of clozapine are seizures and agranulocytosis, a decrease in the production of granulocytes that involves the body's immune defenses. Currently, clozapine is only indicated for the treatment of severely ill schizophrenic patients who have not responded to traditional antipsychotic drugs. The WBC (leukocyte) count needs to be closely monitored for leukopenia; if the level

CLINICAL JUDGMENT [NURSING PROCESS]

Phenothiazines and Nonphenothiazines

Concept: Cognition
- Mental activities used to process and apply information

Recognize Cues [Assessment]
- Assess baseline vital signs for use in future comparisons.
- Obtain a patient health history that includes present drug therapy. If the patient is taking an anticonvulsant, the drug dose might need to be increased because antipsychotics tend to lower the seizure threshold.
- Assess mental status and cardiac, eye, and respiratory disorders before starting drug therapy, and continue daily assessment.

Analyze Cues and Prioritize Hypothesis [Patient Problems]
- Confusion
- Anxiety
- Decreased functional ability
- Decreased ability to cope

Generate Solutions [Planning]
- Patient will appear calmer.
- Patient will communicate coherently.
- Patient will carry out personal activities of daily living.
- Patient will demonstrate organized thoughts.
- Patient will communicate understanding of reality.

Take Action [Nursing Interventions]
- Monitor vital signs. Orthostatic hypotension is likely to occur.
- Remain with patients while medication is taken and swallowed; some patients hide antipsychotics in the mouth to avoid taking them.
- Avoid skin contact with liquid concentrates to prevent contact dermatitis. Liquid must be protected from light and should be diluted with fruit juice.
- Administer oral doses with food or milk to decrease gastric irritation.
- Dilute oral solution of fluphenazine in fruit juice, water, or milk. Avoid apple juice and caffeinated drinks.
- Administer deep into muscle because drug irritates fatty tissue. Do *not* administer intravenously.
- Check blood pressure for marked decrease or increase 30 minutes after drug is injected.
- Do *not* mix in same syringe with heparin, pentobarbital, cimetidine, or dimenhydrinate.
- Chill suppository in refrigerator for 30 minutes before removing foil wrapper.
- Observe for extrapyramidal syndrome (EPS) symptoms such as acute dystonia, akathisia, pseudoparkinsonism, and tardive dyskinesia (see Fig. 22.2) and report these promptly to the health care provider.
- ⚡ Assess for symptoms of neuroleptic malignant syndrome (NMS): increased fever, pulse, and blood pressure; muscle rigidity; increased creatine phosphokinase and white blood cell (WBC) count; altered mental status; acute renal failure; varying levels of consciousness; pallor; diaphoresis; tachycardia; and dysrhythmias.
- Record urine output; urinary retention may result.
- Monitor serum glucose level.
- Engage patient in interactions with staff, other patients, and attending therapies.

Patient Teaching
General
- Encourage patients to take the drug exactly as ordered. In schizophrenia and other psychotic disorders, antipsychotics do not cure the mental illness but do alleviate symptoms. Many patients on medication can function outside of an institutional setting. Adherence to a drug regimen is extremely important.

- Inform patients that medication may take 6 weeks or longer to achieve full clinical effect.
- ⚡ Caution patients not to consume alcohol or other central nervous system (CNS) depressants such as narcotics; these drugs intensify the depressant effect on the body.
- Recommend that patients not abruptly discontinue the drug. Seek advice from a health care provider before making any changes in dosage.
- Encourage patients to read labels on over-the-counter (OTC) preparations. Some are contraindicated when taking antipsychotics.
- Teach smoking cessation because smoking increases the metabolism of some antipsychotics.
- Guide patients to maintain good oral hygiene by frequently brushing and flossing teeth.
- Encourage patients to talk with a health care provider regarding family planning. The effect of antipsychotics on the fetus is not fully known; however, there may be teratogenic effects.
- Explain to the breastfeeding patient that phenothiazine passes into breast milk, possibly causing drowsiness and unusual muscle movement in the infant.
- Warn patients about the importance of routine follow-up examinations.
- ⚡ Encourage patients to obtain laboratory tests on schedule. WBCs are monitored for 3 months, especially during the start of drug therapy. Leukopenia, or decreased WBCs, may occur. Be alert to symptoms of malaise, fever, and sore throat, which may be an indication of agranulocytosis, a serious blood dyscrasia.
- Teach patients, especially those taking clozapine, to report symptoms of infection promptly to the health care provider.
- Advise patients to wear an identification bracelet indicating the medication taken.
- Inform patients that tolerance to the sedative effect develops over a period of days or weeks.

Side Effects
- ⚡ Direct patients to avoid potentially dangerous situations, such as driving, until drug dosing has been stabilized.
- Inform patients about EPS and instruct them to promptly report symptoms to a health care provider.
- Encourage patients to wear sunglasses for photosensitivity, to limit exposure to direct sunlight, and to use sunscreen and protective clothing to prevent a skin rash.
- Warn patients about orthostatic hypotension and possible dizziness.
- Teach patients who are taking aliphatic phenothiazines such as chlorpromazine that the urine might be pink or red-brown; this discoloration is harmless.
- Inform patients that changes may occur related to sexual functioning and menstruation. Women could have irregular menstrual periods or amenorrhea, and men might experience impotence and gynecomastia (enlargement of breast tissue).
- Suggest lozenges or hard candy if mouth dryness occurs. Advise patients to consult a health care provider if dry mouth persists for more than 2 weeks.
- Encourage patients to avoid extremes in environmental temperatures and exercise.
- Advise patients to rise slowly from sitting or lying to standing to prevent a sudden decrease in blood pressure.

Evaluate Outcomes [Evaluation]
- Evaluate the effectiveness of the drug and whether the patient has acceptably reduced psychotic symptoms at the *lowest* dose possible.
- Ascertain whether the patient can cope with everyday living situations and attend to activities of daily living.
- Determine whether any side effects or adverse reactions to the drug have occurred.

TABLE 22.2 Phenothiazines and Nonphenothiazines

Drug	Route and Dosage	Uses and Considerations
Chlorpromazine hydrochloride	Schizophrenia: A: PO: Initially 10–25 mg 2–4 times/d; *maint:* 200–400 mg/d; *max:* 1000 mg/d (2000 mg/d for short periods)	For acute psychosis, schizophrenia, intractable hiccups, nausea, and vomiting. May cause drowsiness, dizziness, weight gain, dry mouth, blurred vision, photosensitivity, orthostatic hypotension, peripheral edema, constipation, erectile/ejaculation dysfunction, and EPS. PB: 90%–99%; t½: 2–30 h
Fluphenazine hydrochloride	See Prototype Drug Chart: Fluphenazine	
Perphenazine	Schizophrenia: A: PO: Initially 4–16 mg bid/qid; after obtaining maximum response, gradually reduce dose; *max:* 24 mg/d (64 mg/d for short periods)	For schizophrenia, severe nausea and vomiting. May cause headache, dry mouth, drowsiness, dizziness, appetite stimulation, constipation, insomnia, weight gain, akathisia, urinary retention, and EPS. PB: 91%–99%; t½: 9–12 h
Thioridazine hydrochloride	A: PO: Initially 50–100 mg tid; *maint:* 200–800 mg/d; *max:* 800 mg/d	For schizophrenia. May cause dizziness, drowsiness, dry mouth, weight gain, appetite stimulation, nausea, vomiting, constipation, akathisia, hypotension, and EPS. PB: 96%–99%; t½: 21–24 h
Haloperidol	See Prototype Drug Chart: Haloperidol	
Loxapine	Schizophrenia: A: PO: Initially 10 mg bid (50 mg in severely disturbed patients); *maint:* 60–100 mg/d; *max:* 250 mg/d for severe symptoms, 100 mg/d for outpatients	For schizophrenia and bipolar disorder. May cause dizziness, drowsiness, dry mouth, insomnia, dysgeusia, constipation, hypotension, and bronchospasm. PB: 96.6%; t½: 5–19 h
Molindone hydrochloride	A: PO: Initially: 50–75 mg/d in 3–4 divided doses; *max:* 225 mg/d	For schizophrenia. May cause blurred vision, dry mouth, hypersalivation, drowsiness, urinary retention, nausea, constipation, and EPS. PB: UK; t½: 1.5 h
Thiothixene hydrochloride	A: PO: Initially 2 mg tid; *maint:* 20–30 mg/d; *max:* 60 mg/d	For schizophrenia. May cause blurred vision, appetite stimulation, dry mouth, weight gain, akathisia, constipation, erectile/ejaculation dysfunction, hypotension, peripheral edema, and EPS. PB: 90%; t½: 3.4–34 h
Clozapine	A: PO: Initially: 12.5 mg/qd or bid; gradually increase to *maint:* 300–450 mg/d in 3 divided doses; *max:* 900 mg/d	For schizophrenia. May cause dizziness, drowsiness, insomnia, dyspepsia, hypersalivation, nausea, vomiting, constipation, tachycardia, and EPS. PB: 97%; t½: 4–12 h
Olanzapine	Schizophrenia: A: PO: Initially 5–10 mg/d; *max:* 20 mg/d Older A: PO: Initially 5 mg/d; *max:* 20 mg/d	For schizophrenia, bipolar disorder, depression. May cause headache, dizziness, drowsiness, weakness, dry mouth, weight gain, constipation, akathisia, depression, hyperglycemia, hypercholesterolemia, hypertriglyceridemia, appetite stimulation, and EPS. PB: 93%; t½: 21–54 h
Quetiapine	Schizophrenia: Immediate release: A: PO: Initially 25 mg/bid; *maint:* 400–800 mg/d in divided doses; *max:* 800 mg/d Extended release: A: PO: 300 mg at bedtime; *max:* 800 mg/d Older A: PO: Initially 50 mg/d, *max:* 800 mg/d	For schizophrenia, bipolar disorder, and depression. May cause dizziness, drowsiness, headache, agitation, dry mouth, hypercholesterolemia, weight gain, hypertriglyceridemia, fatigue, hyper/hypotension, and EPS. PB: 83%; t½: 6 h immediate release, 7 h extended release
Asenapine	Schizophrenia: A: SL: Initially 5 mg bid; may increase after 1 wk; *max:* 20 mg/d A: Transdermal: Initially 3.8 mg patch/d; *max:* 7.6 mg patch/d	For schizophrenia and bipolar disorder. May cause dizziness, drowsiness, insomnia, headache, paresthesia, fatigue, hypertriglyceridemia, weight gain, akathisia, hyperglycemia, and EPS. PB: 95%; t½: 24 h
Risperidone	Schizophrenia: A: PO: Initially 2 mg/d; *maint:* 4–8 mg/d; *max:* 16 mg/d Older A: PO: Initially 0.5 mg bid; *maint:* 4–8 mg/d; *max:* 16 mg/d	For management of schizophrenia and bipolar disorder. May cause dizziness, drowsiness, headache, weight gain, akathisia, anxiety, agitation, dry mouth, tachycardia, orthostatic hypotension, insomnia, fatigue, appetite stimulation, nausea, vomiting, constipation, and EPS. PB: 90%; t½: 3 h
Ziprasidone	Schizophrenia: A: PO: 20 mg bid with food; may increase q2d; *max:* 160 mg/d	For schizophrenia and bipolar disorder. May cause dizziness, drowsiness, headache, insomnia, nausea, constipation, hypercholesterolemia, weight gain, urinary retention, and EPS. PB: 99%; t½: 7 h
Iloperidone	A: PO: Initially 1 mg bid; *maint:* 6–12 mg bid; *max:* 24 mg/d	For schizophrenia. May cause dizziness, drowsiness, nasal congestion, diarrhea, hyperlipidemia, hyperprolactinemia, dry mouth, hypertriglyceridemia, weight gain, nausea, and tachycardia. PB: 95%; t½: 18–33 h
Aripiprazole	See Prototype Drug Chart: Aripiprazole	
Cariprazine	Schizophrenia: A: PO: Initially 1.5 mg/d; *max:* 6 mg/d	For schizophrenia and bipolar disorder. May cause insomnia, drowsiness, dizziness, headache, restlessness, weight gain, nausea, vomiting, constipation, akathisia, and EPS. PB: 91%–97%; t½: 2–4 d
Brexpiprazole	Schizophrenia: A: PO: Initially 1 mg/d; *maint:* 2–4 mg/d; *max:* 4 mg/d	For schizophrenia and depression. May cause headache, drowsiness, dizziness, blurred vision, weight gain, pharyngitis, orthostatic hypotension, tachycardia, akathisia, and EPS. PB: 99%; t½: 91 h

Continued

TABLE 22.2   Phenothiazines and Nonphenothiazines—cont'd

Drug	Route and Dosage	Uses and Considerations
Paliperidone	Extended-release tablet: A: PO: Initially 6 mg/d; may increase dose q5d; *max:* 12 mg/d A: IM: Initially 234 mg, then 1 wk later 156 mg; *maint:* 5 wk after first dose begin 117 mg/month; *max:* 234 mg q1month	For schizophrenia. May cause anxiety, drowsiness, headache, agitation, tachycardia, hypercholesterolemia, hypertriglyceridemia, hyperlipidemia, hyperkinesis, vomiting, weight gain, tremor, akathisia, and EPS. PB: 74%; t½: 23 h
Lumateperone	A: PO: 42 mg/d; *max:* 42 mg/d	For schizophrenia. May cause drowsiness, dizziness, fatigue, dry mouth, nausea, vomiting, hypercholesterolemia, hyperglycemia, hyperlipidemia, and hypertriglyceridemia. PB: 97.4%; t½: 18 h
Olanzapine and samidorphan	A: PO: Initially 5 mg olanzapine/10 mg samidorphan/d or 10 mg olanzapine/10 mg samidorphan/d; *max:* 20 olanzapine/10 mg samidorphan/d	For schizophrenia and bipolar disorder. May cause dizziness, drowsiness, headache, dry mouth, appetite stimulation, weight gain, hyperglycemia, hypertriglyceridemia, hyperprolactinemia, and orthostatic hypotension. PB: olanzapine 93%, samidorphan 23%–33%; t½: olanzapine 35–52 h, samidorphan 7–11 h

>, Greater than; *A,* adult; *bid,* twice a day; *d,* day; *EPS,* symptoms of extrapyramidal syndrome; *h,* hour; *IM,* intramuscular; *maint,* maintenance; *max,* maximum; *NMS,* neuroleptic malignant syndrome; *PB,* protein binding; *PO,* by mouth; *q2d,* every 2 days; *SL,* sublingual; *t½,* half-life; *tid,* three times a day; *UK,* unknown; *wk,* weeks; *y,* years.

falls below 3000 mm³, clozapine should be discontinued. Seizures have been reported in 3% of patients taking the drug. Dizziness, sedation, tachycardia, orthostatic hypotension, and constipation are common side effects.

Another atypical agent used to treat the positive and negative symptoms of schizophrenia is risperidone. Its action is similar to that of clozapine, and the occurrence of EPS and tardive dyskinesia is low. It does not cause agranulocytosis. Paliperidone is the major active metabolite of risperidone and is an extended-release tablet with once-a-day dosing. Paliperidone should be swallowed whole and not chewed, divided, or crushed. The most common adverse effects include EPS, insomnia, headache, and akathisia.

Like clozapine and risperidone, the atypical antipsychotic olanzapine is effective for treating the positive and negative symptoms of schizophrenia.

Like all the other atypical antipsychotics, quetiapine is less likely to cause EPS. Severe tardive dyskinesia may occur, but it is rare.

For individuals with cardiac dysrhythmias, ziprasidone must be prescribed with caution because its use may lead to a prolonged QT interval; electrocardiograms (ECGs) should be monitored. Ziprasidone is contraindicated in patients with a history of prolonged QT interval or with other concurrent drugs known to prolong QT interval. Patients taking quetiapine, clozapine, risperidone, olanzapine, ziprasidone, and aripiprazole should be monitored for hyperglycemia and other symptoms of diabetes mellitus.

Prototype Drug Chart: Aripiprazole illustrates drug characteristics of aripiprazole, an atypical antipsychotic. When anxiety, hallucinations, agitation, mania, confusion, or depression and other symptoms are noted, the health care provider should check the medications that the patient is taking.

ANXIOLYTICS

Anxiolytics, or *antianxiety drugs,* are primarily used to treat excessive anxiety. The major anxiolytic group is benzodiazepines, a minor tranquilizer group. Long before benzodiazepines were prescribed for anxiety and insomnia, barbiturates were used. Benzodiazepines are considered more effective than barbiturates because they enhance the action of GABA, an inhibitory neurotransmitter within the CNS. Benzodiazepines have fewer side effects and may

be less dangerous in overdosing. Long-term use of barbiturates causes drug tolerance and dependence and may cause respiratory distress. Currently, barbiturates are not drugs of choice for treating anxiety. Benzodiazepine-like drugs are used to treat insomnia. Selective serotonin reuptake inhibitors (SSRIs), serotonin norepinephrine reuptake inhibitors (SNRIs), tricyclic antidepressants (TCAs), and monoamine oxidase inhibitors (MAOIs) are used to treat various anxiety disorders. These drugs are discussed in Chapter 23.

Table 22.3 lists approved uses for benzodiazepines. Drugs used to treat insomnia, including benzodiazepines, are discussed in Chapter 18.

A certain amount of anxiety may make a person more alert and energetic, but when anxiety is excessive, it can be disabling, and anxiolytics may be prescribed. The action of anxiolytics resembles that of the sedative-hypnotics but *not* that of the antipsychotics.

An estimated 264 million people have an anxiety disorder. Excessive anxiety may be characterized by sweating palms, pacing, palpitations, tachycardia, restlessness, irritability, difficulty concentrating, disturbed sleep, nausea, diarrhea, urinary frequency, and dyspnea. Common anxiety disorders include general anxiety disorder, social anxiety disorder, obsessive-compulsive disorder, panic disorder, and posttraumatic stress disorder. These agents treat the symptoms but do not cure them. Long-term use of anxiolytics is discouraged because tolerance develops within weeks or months, depending on the agent. Drug tolerance can occur in less than 2 to 3 months in patients who take phenobarbital.

Nonpharmacologic Measures

Some of the symptoms of a severe attack of anxiety, or panic attack, include dyspnea (difficulty in breathing), choking sensation, chest pain, heart palpitations, dizziness, faintness, sweating, trembling and shaking, and fear of losing control. Before giving anxiolytics, nonpharmacologic measures should be used for decreasing anxiety. These measures might include using a relaxation technique, psychotherapy, or support groups.

! Benzodiazepines

Benzodiazepines have multiple uses as anticonvulsants, sedative-hypnotics, preoperative drugs, substance abuse withdrawal agents, and anxiolytics. Most of the benzodiazepines are used mainly for severe or prolonged anxiety. Examples include

PROTOTYPE DRUG CHART

Aripiprazole

Drug Class	Dosage
Nonphenothiazine: Atypical antipsychotic	Schizophrenia: Immediate-release tablets: A: PO: 10–15 mg/d, may increase q2wk; *maint:* 10–30 mg/d; *max:* 30 mg/d Extended release (Abilify Maintena): A: IM: Initially 400 mg/month; *max:* 400 mg/month

Contraindications	Drug-Lab-Food Interactions
Hypersensitivity *Caution:* Dysrhythmias, dehydration, CNS depression, dementia, hypovolemia, heart failure, suicidal ideation, myocardial infarction, hyperglycemia, hypotension, parkinsonism, seizures, agranulocytosis, neutropenia, leukopenia, bradycardia, cerebrovascular disease, diabetes mellitus, hypertriglyceridemia, alcohol use disorder	Drug: Antidiabetic agents decrease drug levels and increase risk of hyperglycemia; alpha blockers and antihypertensives increase risk of hypotension; other antipsychotics enhance risk of NMS, EPS, anticholinergic effects, hypotension, and seizures; CNS depressants may increase sedation and orthostatic hypotension; SSRIs may increase risk of serotonin syndrome; calcium channel blockers may increase blood levels Food: Grapefruit juice may increase blood levels Herbal: St. John's wort may decrease blood levels Lab: Increased blood glucose

Pharmacokinetics	Pharmacodynamics
Absorption: Well absorbed, not affected by food Distribution: PB: 99% Metabolism: t½: 75 h; extended release 30–47 d Excretion: In urine and feces	PO: Onset: UK Peak: 3–5 h Duration: UK IM: Immediate release: Onset: UK Peak: 1–3 h Duration: UK IM: ER: Peak: 5–7 d Duration: UK

Therapeutic Effects/Uses

To manage schizophrenia, bipolar disorder, autism, depression, Tourette syndrome
Mechanism of Action: Interferes with the binding of dopamine to dopamine (D_2) and serotonin 5-hydroxytryptamine (5-HT$_2$) receptors

Side Effects	Adverse Reactions
Drowsiness, memory impairment, weight gain/loss, headache, fatigue, blurred vision, peripheral edema, insomnia, anxiety, agitation, dizziness, fever, dry mouth, nausea, vomiting, constipation, rash, tremor, urinary retention, impulse control symptoms, appetite stimulation, hyperhidrosis, akathisia, erectile dysfunction	Hyper/hypotension, tachycardia, palpitations, bradycardia, hypokalemia, diabetes mellitus, rhabdomyolysis, hypertriglyceridemia, hypercholesterolemia, dysrhythmias, seizures, EPS, hyper/hypoglycemia, hyponatremia *Life-threatening:* Suicidal ideation, NMS, angioedema, agranulocytosis, neutropenia, leukopenia, laryngospasm

>, Greater than; *A,* adult; *CNS,* central nervous system; *d,* day; *EPS,* symptoms of extrapyramidal syndrome; *ER,* extended release; *h,* hour; *IM,* intramuscularly; *maint,* maintenance; *max,* maximum; *NMS,* neuroleptic malignant syndrome; *PB,* protein binding; *PO,* by mouth; *q2d,* every 2 days; *SSRI,* selective serotonin reuptake inhibitor; *t½,* half-life; *UK,* unknown; *wk,* week.

chlordiazepoxide, diazepam, clorazepate dipotassium, lorazepam, and alprazolam. The most frequently prescribed benzodiazepine is lorazepam. Many of the benzodiazepines are used for more than one purpose.

Benzodiazepines are lipid soluble and are absorbed readily from the GI tract. They are highly protein bound (80% to 98%). Benzodiazepines are primarily metabolized by the liver and are excreted in urine, so the drug dosage for patients with liver or renal disease should be lowered accordingly to avoid possible cumulative effects. Traces of benzodiazepine metabolites could

be present in the urine for weeks or months after the person has stopped taking the drug. These are Controlled Substance Schedule IV (CSS IV) drugs.

The first benzodiazepine, chlordiazepoxide, became widely used for its sedative effect in 1962. Diazepam was the most frequently prescribed drug in the early 1970s. Lorazepam is the prototype drug of benzodiazepine and is described in Prototype Drug Chart: Benzodiazepine.

Pharmacokinetics. Lorazepam is highly lipid soluble, and the drug is rapidly absorbed from the GI tract. The drug is highly protein bound,

TABLE 22.3 Approved Uses for Benzodiazepines

Prescribed Uses	Drugs
Anxiety	Alprazolam Chlordiazepoxide Chlorazepate Diazepam Lorazepam
Anxiety associated with depression	Alprazolam Clonazepam Lorazepam
Insomnia, short-term use	Estazolam Flurazepam Quazepam Temazepam Triazolam
Seizures and status epilepticus	Clonazepam Clorazepate Diazepam Lorazepam
Alcohol withdrawal	Clorazepate Chlordiazepoxide Diazepam Lorazepam
Skeletal muscle spasms	Diazepam
Preoperative medications	Chlordiazepoxide Diazepam Lorazepam Midazolam

COMPLEMENTARY AND ALTERNATIVE THERAPIES

Benzodiazepines

Kava kava should not be combined with benzodiazepines because it increases the sedative effect.

and the half-life is 12 hours. Lorazepam is excreted primarily in the urine.

Pharmacodynamics. Lorazepam acts on the limbic, thalamic, and hypothalamic levels of the CNS. The onset of action is 20 to 30 minutes for IM administration and 2 to 3 minutes IV. The serum level of oral lorazepam peaks in 2 hours.

It is recommended that benzodiazepines be prescribed for no longer than 3 to 4 months. Beyond 4 months, the effectiveness of the drug lessens. Table 22.4 lists the anxiolytics and their dosages, uses, and considerations, including common side effects and a few serious adverse effects.

Side Effects and Adverse Reactions

The side effects associated with benzodiazepines are sedation, dizziness, headaches, dry mouth, blurred vision, rare urinary incontinence, and constipation. Adverse reactions include leukopenia (decreased WBC count) with symptoms of fever, malaise, and sore throat; tolerance to the drug dosage with continuous use; and physical dependency. Box 22.2 lists guidelines for treating benzodiazepine overdose.

Benzodiazepines should not be abruptly discontinued because withdrawal symptoms are likely to occur. Withdrawal symptoms caused by short-term benzodiazepine use are similar to those from the sedative-hypnotics: agitation, nervousness, insomnia, tremor, anorexia, muscular cramps, and sweating; however, they are slow to develop, taking 2 to 10 days, and can last several weeks, depending on the benzodiazepine's half-life. When discontinuing a benzodiazepine, the drug dosage should be gradually decreased over a period of days, depending on dose or length of time on the drug. Withdrawal symptoms from long-term, high-dose benzodiazepine therapy include paranoia, delirium, panic, hypertension, and status epilepticus. Convulsions during withdrawal may be prevented with simultaneous substitution of an anticonvulsant. Alcohol and other CNS depressants should *not* be taken with benzodiazepines because respiratory depression can result. Tobacco, caffeine, and sympathomimetics decrease the effectiveness of benzodiazepines. Benzodiazepines are contraindicated during pregnancy because of possible teratogenic effects.

Miscellaneous Anxiolytics

The anxiolytic buspirone hydrochloride binds to serotonin and dopamine receptors. It may not be effective until 1 to 2 weeks after continuous use. It has fewer of the side effects of sedation and physical and psychological dependency associated with many benzodiazepines. The most common side effects of buspirone include drowsiness, dizziness, headache, nausea, nervousness, and excitement. It is important to note that buspirone has an interaction with grapefruit juice that can lead to toxicity. To avoid this interaction, buspirone users should be advised to limit intake of grapefruit juice to 8 ounces daily or half of a grapefruit.

PROTOTYPE DRUG CHART

! Lorazepam

Drug Class	Dosage
Anxiolytic: Benzodiazepine	Anxiety: A: PO: initially 2–3 mg/d in divided doses; increase gradually PRN; *maint:* 1–10 mg/d in divided doses; *max:* 10 mg/d Older A: PO: Initially 1–2 mg/d in divided doses; *maint:* 2–6 mg/d; *max:* 10 mg/d

Contraindications	Drug-Lab-Food Interactions
Hypersensitivity, glaucoma *Caution:* Hepatic or renal dysfunction, COPD, alcohol and substance use disorder, depression, seizures, CNS depression, parkinsonism, psychosis, pregnancy, suicidal ideation	Drug: Increases CNS depression when taken with alcohol, CNS depressants, and anticonvulsants; cimetidine increases lorazepam plasma levels, increases phenytoin levels, decreases levodopa effects; smoking and caffeine decrease antianxiety effects; oral contraceptives decrease effects

Pharmacokinetics	Pharmacodynamics
Absorption: Rapid from GI tract Distribution: PB: 85% Metabolism: t½: 12–14 h Excretion: In urine	PO: Onset: UK Peak: 2 h Duration: UK IM: Onset: 20–30 min Peak: 3 h Duration: 6–8 h IV: Onset: 2–3 min Peak: UK Duration: 6–8 h

Therapeutic Effects/Uses

To control anxiety, and to treat status epilepticus; for sedation induction; for insomnia
Mechanism of Action: Potentiates GABA effects by binding to specific benzodiazepine receptors and inhibiting GABA neurotransmission

Side Effects	Adverse Reactions
Drowsiness, dizziness, weakness, headache, confusion, depression, euphoria, amnesia, ataxia, blurred vision, restlessness, constipation, erectile dysfunction, injection site reaction	Hyper/hypotension, bradycardia, tachycardia, hearing loss, tolerance, dependence, seizures, hyponatremia, heart failure *Life-threatening:* Suicidal ideation, NMS, agranulocytosis, thrombocytopenia, pancytopenia, respiratory depression

>, Greater than; *A,* adult; *CNS,* central nervous system; *COPD,* chronic obstructive pulmonary disease; *d,* day; *GABA,* gamma-aminobutyric acid; *GI,* gastrointestinal; *h,* hour; *IM,* intramuscularly; *IV,* intravenously; *maint,* maintenance; *max,* maximum; *min,* minute; *NMS,* neuroleptic malignant syndrome; *PB,* protein binding; *PO,* by mouth; *PRN,* as needed; *t½,* half-life; *UK,* unknown; *y,* years.

! TABLE 22.4 Anxiolytics

Drug	Route and Dosage	Uses and Considerations
Benzodiazepines		
Alprazolam CSS IV	Panic disorders: Immediate release: A: PO: Initially 0.5 mg tid, may increase q3–4d; *max:* 10 mg/d Older A: PO: Initially 0.25 bid/tid, may increase q3–4d; *max:* 10 mg/d Extended release: A: PO: Initially 0.5–1 mg/d in the morning, may increase q3–4d; *max:* 10 mg/d Older A: PO: Initially 0.5 mg/d, may increase q3–4d; *max:* 10 mg/d	For anxiety, panic disorders, and generalized anxiety disorder. May cause dizziness, drowsiness, anxiety, impaired memory/cognition, nausea, dysarthria, fatigue, depression, weight gain/loss, constipation, withdrawal, and appetite stimulation. PB: 80%; t½: 6.3–26.9 h immediate release, 11–16 h extended release
Chlordiazepoxide hydrochloride CSS IV	Anxiety disorders: A: PO: 5–10 mg bid/qid; for severe anxiety: 20–25 mg tid/qid; *max:* 100 mg/d Older A: PO: 5 mg bid/qid; *max:* 20 mg/d	For anxiety, alcohol withdrawal syndrome (DTs). May cause nausea, drowsiness, confusion, ataxia, tolerance, dependence, and withdrawal. PB: 96%; t½: 5–30 h
Clorazepate dipotassium CSS IV	Anxiety: A: PO: Initially 7.5–15 mg bid or 15 mg at bedtime; *maint:* 15–60 mg/d; *max:* 60 mg/d Older A: PO: 3.75–7.5 mg bid or 7.5 mg at bedtime; *maint:* 15–60 mg/d; *max:* 60 mg/d	For anxiety, alcohol withdrawal syndrome, and partial seizures. May cause drowsiness, dizziness, blurred vision, hypotension, ataxia, amnesia, depression, suicidal ideation, tolerance, dependence, and withdrawal. PB: 97%–98%; t½: 40–50 h

Continued

TABLE 22.4   Anxiolytics—cont'd

Drug	Route and Dosage	Uses and Considerations
Diazepam CSS IV	Anxiety: A: PO: 2–10 mg bid/qid; *max:* 40 mg/d Older A: PO: 2–2.5 mg qd/bid; *max:* 40 mg/d A: IM/IV: 2–10 mg; repeat in 3–4 h PRN	For anxiety, muscle spasms, alcohol withdrawal, seizures, status epilepticus, and sedation induction. May cause drowsiness, memory impairment, respiratory depression, dysarthria, fatigue, appetite stimulation, weight gain/loss, menstrual irregularity, and urinary retention/incontinence. PB: 95%–98%; t½: 48–100 h
Lorazepam CSS IV	See Prototype Drug Chart: Lorazepam	
Oxazepam CSS IV	Anxiety: A: PO: Initially 10–15 mg tid/qid; for severe symptoms, 15–30 mg tid/qid; *max:* A 120 mg/d Older A: PO: Initially 10 mg tid; *max:* 60 mg/d	For anxiety and acute alcohol withdrawal. May cause dizziness, rash, drowsiness, headache, hypotension, dependence, tolerance, and withdrawal. PB: 85%–95%; t½: 5–15 h
Azapirones		
Buspirone hydrochloride	A: PO: Initially: 7.5 mg bid; *maint:* 15–30 mg/d in divided doses; *max:* 60 mg/d Older A: PO: 5 mg bid; *maint:* 15–30 mg/d in divided doses; *max:* 60 mg/d	For anxiety and generalized anxiety disorder. May cause drowsiness, ataxia, dizziness, blurred vision, headache, nausea, edema, erectile/ejaculatory dysfunction, and EPS. PB: 86%; t½: 2–3 h
Benzodiazepine Antagonists		
Flumazenil	Benzodiazepine toxicity: A: IV: Initially 0.2 mg; may give 0.3 mg in 30 s, then may give 0.5 mg at 1-min intervals; *max:* 5 mg	For sedation reversal and benzodiazepine toxicity. May cause dizziness, dyspnea, blurred vision, headache, anxiety, ataxia, agitation, insomnia, hyperhidrosis, vomiting, dry mouth, palpitations, and tremor. PB: 50%; t½: 40–80 min

>, Greater than; *A,* adult; *bid,* twice a day; *CNS,* central nervous system; *CSS,* Controlled Substances Schedule; *d,* day; *DTs,* delirium tremens; *EPS,* symptoms of extrapyramidal symptoms; *h,* hour; *IM,* intramuscularly; *IV,* intravenously; *maint,* maintenance; *max,* maximum; *min,* minute; *PB,* protein binding; *PO,* by mouth; *PRN,* as needed; *q,* every; *q4–6h,* every 4 to 6 hours; *qd,* every day; *qid,* four times a day; *s,* seconds; *t½,* half-life; *tid,* three times a day; *y,* years.

◎ CLINICAL JUDGMENT [NURSING PROCESS]

Benzodiazepines

Concept: Anxiety
- More intense worry about everyday issues than situation demands

Recognize Cues [Assessment]
- Assess for suicidal ideation.
- Obtain a history of the patient's anxiety reaction.
- Determine the patient's support system (family, friends, groups).
- Obtain a drug history. Report possible drug-drug interactions.

Analyze Cues and Prioritize Hypothesis [Patient Problems]
- Anxiety
- Insomnia
- Decreased ability to cope
- Decreased functional ability

Generate Solutions [Planning]
- Patient will appear calmer after nonpharmacologic methods, anxiolytic drugs, or support/group therapy.
- Patient will sleep better.
- Patient will appear to cope better with everyday situations.
- Patient will carry out own activities of daily living.

Take Action [Nursing Interventions]
- Observe patient for side effects of anxiolytics. Recognize that drug tolerance and physical and psychological dependency can occur with most anxiolytics.
- Recognize that anxiolytic dosages should be lower for older adults, children, and debilitated persons than for middle-aged adults.

- Monitor vital signs, especially blood pressure and pulse; orthostatic hypotension may occur.
- Encourage family to be supportive of the patient.

Patient Teaching
General
- ⚡ Advise patients not to drive a motor vehicle or operate dangerous equipment when taking anxiolytics because sedation is a common side effect.
- ⚡ Warn patients not to consume alcohol or central nervous system (CNS) depressants such as narcotics while taking an anxiolytic.
- Teach patients ways to control excess stress and anxiety with relaxation techniques such as long walks.
- Inform patients that an effective response may take 1 to 2 weeks.
- Encourage patients to follow drug regimens and not to abruptly stop taking a drug after prolonged use because withdrawal symptoms can occur. The drug dose is usually tapered when a drug is discontinued.

Side Effects
- Encourage patients to rise slowly from sitting to standing positions to avoid dizziness from orthostatic hypotension.

Evaluate Outcomes [Evaluation]
- Evaluate the effectiveness of drug therapy by determining whether the patient is less anxious and more able to cope with stresses and anxieties.
- Determine whether the patient is taking the anxiolytic drug as prescribed and is adhering to patient teaching instructions.

BOX 22.2 Suggested Treatment for Overdose of Benzodiazepines

1. Administer an emetic and follow with activated charcoal if the patient is conscious; use gastric lavage if the patient is unconscious.
2. Administer the benzodiazepine antagonist flumazenil intravenously if required.
3. Maintain an airway, give oxygen as needed for decreased respirations, and monitor vital signs.
4. Give intravenous vasopressors for severe hypotension.
5. Request a mental health consultation for the patient.

CRITICAL THINKING SINGLE EPISODE CASE STUDY

Cognitive Skill: Enhanced Hot Spot
Objective: Knowledge of medication side effects.
A 35-year-old woman with a diagnosis of schizophrenia has stopped taking her medication. After experiencing agitation, delusions, and hallucinations, she was admitted to the hospital for evaluation. The physician prescribed risperidone 2 mg per day. After several days, the patient is stabilized and ready for discharge. The nurse teaches the patient about the side effects of risperidone.

Place a check mark next to the side effect of risperidone that is most important for the patient to report to the physician.

_____ A. Dizziness
_____ B. Weight loss
_____ C. Drowsiness
_____ D. Blurred vision
_____ E. Appetite stimulation
_____ F. Diarrhea
_____ G. Akathisia

Answers
✓ A. Dizziness
_____ B. Weight loss
✓ C. Drowsiness
_____ D. Blurred vision
✓ E. Appetite stimulation
_____ F. Diarrhea
✓ G. Akathisia

Rationale:
Risperidone is an atypical antipsychotic drug and is the first line of treatment options for the management of schizophrenia. Risperidone exhibits strong antagonist activity at alpha-1 receptors, which likely contributes to adverse cardiovascular effects such as orthostatic hypotension, which may cause dizziness, syncope, drowsiness, and akathisia (muscle quivering and restlessness). It has a high affinity at H-1 histamine receptor sites and has been demonstrated to partially account for adverse effects such as sedation, drowsiness, appetite stimulation, and weight gain. It does not cause weight loss, blurred vision, or diarrhea.

Reference:
Pharmacology: A patient centered pharmacology approach. 10th ed. McCuistion, L., et al (2021) Elsevier; www.clinicalkey.com/pharmacology; Lehne's pharmacology for nursing care (10th ed). Rosenack, J, etal (2019) Elsevier.

▌ REVIEW QUESTIONS

1. The nurse suspects that a patient who is experiencing facial grimacing, involuntary upward eye movement, and muscle spasms of the tongue and face may have which condition?
   a. Akathisia
   b. Acute dystonia
   c. Tardive dyskinesia
   d. Pseudoparkinsonism
2. A patient asks the nurse to explain how antipsychotic drugs work to make him feel better. The nurse understands that antipsychotics act in which way?
   a. Blocking actions of dopamine
   b. Blocking actions of epinephrine
   c. Promoting prostaglandin synthesis
   d. Enhancing the action of gamma-aminobutyric acid
3. An antipsychotic agent, fluphenazine, is ordered for a patient with psychosis. The nurse understands that this agent can lead to symptoms of extrapyramidal syndrome (EPS). What are the symptoms of EPS?
   a. Hypertension
   b. Nausea and vomiting
   c. Hyperthermia and dysrhythmias
   d. Tremors, rigidity, and shuffling gait
4. An atypical antipsychotic is prescribed for a patient with psychosis. The nurse understands that this category of medications includes which drugs? (Select all that apply.)
   a. Clozapine
   b. Fluphenazine
   c. Haloperidol
   d. Olanzapine
   e. Aripiprazole

5. A patient is prescribed lorazepam. What does the nurse know to be true regarding lorazepam?
   a. It is used to treat anxiety, status epilepticus, insomnia, and sedation induction.
   b. It has a maximum adult dose of 25 mg/day.
   c. It causes plasma levels to be decreased when combined with cimetidine.
   d. It interferes with the binding of dopamine receptors.
6. A patient is receiving aripiprazole. Which nursing intervention(s) will the nurse include in the patient's care plan? (Select all that apply.)
   a. Administer before meals on an empty stomach to facilitate absorption.
   b. Remain with the patient until medication is swallowed.
   c. Monitor vital signs to detect orthostatic hypotension.
   d. Assess the patient for evidence of neuroleptic malignant syndrome.
   e. Observe the patient for acute dystonia, akathisia, and tardive dyskinesia.
7. A patient appears to have had an overdose of phenothiazines. The nurse anticipates that which intervention(s) may be used to treat phenothiazine overdose? (Select all that apply.)
   a. Gastric lavage
   b. Adequate hydration
   c. Maintaining an airway
   d. Fluphenazine
   e. Risperidone
   f. Activated charcoal administration

Antidepressants and Mood Stabilizers

http://evolve.elsevier.com/McCuistion/pharmacology

OBJECTIVES

- Contrast the various categories of different antidepressants and give an example of one drug for each category.
- Describe the side effects and adverse reactions of antidepressants.
- Plan nursing interventions, including patient teaching, for antidepressants (tricyclic antidepressants [TCAs], monoamine oxidase inhibitors [MAOIs], selective serotonin reuptake inhibitors [SSRIs], serotonin norepinephrine reuptake inhibitors [SNRIs], and atypical antidepressants).
- Explain the uses of lithium and its serum/plasma therapeutic ranges, side effects and adverse reactions, and nursing interventions.
- Apply the Clinical Judgment [Nursing Process] to the patient taking lithium, carbamazepine, and valproic acid.

OUTLINE

Antidepressants are used for depressive episodes accompanied by feelings of hopelessness and helplessness. They can be prescribed for 1 month to 12 months or perhaps longer.

Mood-stabilizing agents such as lithium are effective for bipolar disorder. Drug therapy for treating bipolar disorder is discussed in this chapter.

DEPRESSION

Depression is the most common mental illness, affecting approximately 14.8 million Americans. Fewer than 50% of individuals with depression seek treatment despite the fact that about 70% of individuals with depression have a full remission with effective treatment. Women between the ages of 25 and 45 years are two to three times more likely than men to experience major depression. Depression is characterized primarily by mood changes and loss of interest in normal activities and is second only to hypertension as the most common chronic clinical condition.

Contributing causes of depression include genetic predisposition, social and environmental factors, and biologic conditions. Some signs of major depression include loss of interest in most activities, depressed mood, weight loss or gain, insomnia or hypersomnia, loss of energy, fatigue, feelings of despair, decreased ability to think or concentrate, and suicidal thoughts. Approximately 66% of all suicides are related to depression. Depressed men, especially older Caucasian men, are more likely to commit suicide successfully than depressed women. Antidepressants can mask suicidal ideation.

The three types of depression are (1) *reactive*, (2) *major*, and (3) *bipolar disorder*, previously referred to as *manic depression*. Reactive depression usually has a sudden onset after a precipitating event (e.g., depression resulting from a loss, such as death of a loved one). The patient knows why he or she is depressed and may call this "the blues." Usually, this type of depression lasts for months, and a benzodiazepine agent may be prescribed. *Major depression* is characterized by loss of interest in work and home, inability to concentrate and complete tasks, difficulty sleeping or excessive sleeping, feelings of fatigue and worthlessness, and deep depression, also known as dysphoria. Major depression can be either *primary* (unrelated to other health problems) or *secondary* to a health problem such as a physical or psychiatric disorder or drug use. Antidepressants have been effective in treating major depression. Bipolar disorder involves swings between two moods: manic (euphoric) and depressive (dysphoric). Lithium was originally the drug of choice for treating this type of disorder. Other mood stabilizers such as carbamazepine, valproic acid or divalproex, and lamotrigine are also currently first-line drugs of choice for bipolar disorder.

Pathophysiology

Many theories exist as to the cause of major depression. A common one suggests an insufficient amount of brain monoamine neurotransmitters (norepinephrine, serotonin, perhaps dopamine). It is thought that decreased levels of serotonin permit depression to occur, and decreased levels of norepinephrine cause depression. However, there can be other physiologic causes of depression, and social and environmental factors play a role.

Serotonin neurotransmission is associated with arousal and general activity levels of the central nervous system (CNS). Serotonin functions to regulate sleep, wakefulness, and mood as well as the delusions, hallucinations, and withdrawal of schizophrenia. Antidepressants block the reuptake of serotonin into the presynaptic neuron. A structurally specific drug is more likely to affect only the specific receptors for which it is intended and not the receptors specific for other neurochemicals, which would produce unintended effects. Selective serotonin reuptake inhibitor (SSRI) drugs are specific and generally produce fewer side effects in the treatment of depression than older antidepressants such as monoamine oxidase inhibitors (MAOIs).

Norepinephrine is associated with control of arousal, attention, vigilance, mood, affect, and anxiety. This neurotransmitter is involved with thinking, planning, and interpreting. Tricyclic antidepressants (TCAs) block the reuptake of norepinephrine into the presynaptic neuron and effectively treat depressive disorders. MAOIs inactivate norepinephrine, dopamine, and serotonin by inhibiting the monoamine oxidase enzyme to relieve signs and symptoms of depression.

Faulty release, reuptake, or elimination of neurotransmitters may lead to an imbalance of neurotransmission and subsequent pathology. Disorders can then develop that can affect an individual's thoughts, feelings, and behaviors.

Complementary and Alternative Therapy for Depression

St. John's wort and ginkgo biloba have been suggested for the management of mild depression, but these should not be taken along with prescription antidepression medications. St. John's wort can decrease reuptake of the neurotransmitters serotonin, norepinephrine, and dopamine. The use of these and many complementary and alternative products should be discontinued 1 to 2 weeks before surgery. The patient should check with a health care provider regarding complementary and alternative therapies.

 COMPLEMENTARY AND ALTERNATIVE THERAPIES

Selective Serotonin Reuptake Inhibitors

- Feverfew may interfere with SSRI antidepressants such as fluoxetine.
- St. John's wort interacts with SSRIs, which may cause serotonin syndrome (dizziness, headache, sweating, and agitation).

ANTIDEPRESSANT AGENTS

Antidepressants are divided into five groups: (1) tricyclic antidepressants (TCAs), or tricyclics; (2) selective serotonin reuptake inhibitors (SSRIs); (3) serotonin norepinephrine reuptake inhibitors (SNRIs); (4) atypical antidepressants that affect various neurotransmitters; and (5) monoamine oxidase inhibitors (MAOIs). TCAs and MAOIs were marketed in the late 1950s, and many of the SSRIs and atypical antidepressants were available in the 1980s. The SSRIs and SNRIs are popular antidepressants because they do not cause sedation, hypotension, anticholinergic effects, or cardiotoxicity as do many of the TCAs. However, users of SSRIs can experience sexual dysfunction, but this can be managed. With unpleasant side effects or lack of improvement, the patient is usually changed to another category of drug.

Tricyclic Antidepressants

Tricyclic antidepressants (TCAs) are used to treat major depression because they are effective and less expensive than SSRIs and other drugs. Imipramine was the first TCA marketed in the 1950s.

The action of TCAs is to block the uptake of the neurotransmitters norepinephrine and serotonin in the brain. The clinical response of TCAs occurs after 2 to 4 weeks of drug therapy. If there is no improvement after 2 to 4 weeks, the antidepressant is slowly withdrawn and another antidepressant is prescribed. *Polydrug therapy,* the practice of giving several antidepressants or antipsychotics together, should be avoided if possible because of potential serious side effects.

The effectiveness of TCAs in treating major depression is well documented. This group of drugs elevates mood, increases interest in daily living and activity, and decreases insomnia. For agitated depressed persons, amitriptyline, doxepin, or trimipramine may be prescribed because of their highly sedative effect. TCAs are often given at night to minimize problems caused by their sedative action. When discontinuing TCAs, the drugs should be gradually decreased to avoid withdrawal symptoms such as nausea, vomiting, anxiety, and akathisia. Imipramine hydrochloride is used for the treatment of enuresis (involuntary discharge of urine during sleep in children).

The TCA drugs include amitriptyline, imipramine, trimipramine, doxepin, desipramine, nortriptyline, and protriptyline. The TCA drugs desipramine and nortriptyline are major metabolites of imipramine and amitriptyline.

Pharmacokinetics. Amitriptyline is strongly protein bound. The half-life is 10 to 50 hours, and a cumulative drug effect may result. Amitriptyline is primarily excreted in urine.

Pharmacodynamics. Amitriptyline is well absorbed, but antidepressant effects develop slowly over several weeks. The onset of the antidepressant effect of amitriptyline is 1 to 3 weeks, and the peak concentration is 2 to 5 hours. Drug doses are decreased for older patients to reduce side effects.

Side Effects and Adverse Reactions

The TCAs have many side effects: orthostatic hypotension, sedation, anticholinergic effects, cardiotoxicity, and seizures. Rising from a sitting position too rapidly can cause dizziness and lightheadedness (*orthostatic hypotension*), so the patient should be instructed to rise slowly to an upright position. The TCAs block the histamine receptors; thus sedation is likely to occur initially but decreases with continuous use of the drug. Because TCAs block the cholinergic receptors, they can cause anticholinergic effects such as tachycardia, urinary retention, constipation, dry mouth, and blurred vision. Other side effects of TCAs include allergic reactions (skin rash, pruritus, and weight gain), sexual dysfunction (erectile dysfunction, ejaculatory dysfunction), and suicidal ideation. Most TCAs can cause blood dyscrasias (leukopenia, thrombocytopenia, and agranulocytosis) that require close monitoring of blood cell counts. Amitriptyline may lead to symptoms of extrapyramidal syndrome (EPS). Clomipramine can cause neuroleptic malignant syndrome (NMS). Because the seizure threshold is decreased by TCAs, patients with seizure disorders may need TCA dose adjustment. The most serious adverse reaction to TCAs is cardiotoxicity, such as dysrhythmias that may result from high doses of the drug. The therapeutic serum range of TCAs should be monitored.

Drug Interactions

Alcohol, hypnotics, sedatives, and barbiturates potentiate CNS depression when taken with TCAs. Concurrent use of MAOIs with amitriptyline may lead to cardiovascular instability and toxic psychosis. Antithyroid medications taken with amitriptyline may increase the risk of dysrhythmias.

Selective Serotonin Reuptake Inhibitors

Selective serotonin reuptake inhibitors (SSRIs) block the reuptake of serotonin into the nerve terminal of the CNS, thereby enhancing its transmission at the serotonergic synapse. These drugs do *not* block the uptake of dopamine or norepinephrine, and they do *not* block cholinergic and alpha$_1$-adrenergic receptors. SSRIs are more commonly used to treat depression than TCAs, and they have fewer side effects than TCAs.

The primary use of SSRIs is for major depressive disorders. They are also effective for treating anxiety disorders such as obsessive-compulsive disorder (OCD), panic disorders, phobias, posttraumatic stress disorder (PTSD), and other forms of anxiety. Fluvoxamine is useful for treating OCD in children and adults. SSRIs have also been used to treat eating disorders and selected drug abuses. Miscellaneous uses for SSRIs include decreasing premenstrual tension syndrome, preventing migraine headaches, and preventing or minimizing aggressive behavior in patients with borderline personality disorder.

The SSRIs include fluoxetine, fluvoxamine, sertraline, paroxetine, citalopram, and escitalopram. Fluoxetine has been effective in 50% to 60% of patients who fail to respond to TCA therapy (*TCA-refractory depression*). The US Food and Drug Administration (FDA) approved a weekly delayed-release fluoxetine dose of 90 mg. However, before taking the weekly dose, the patient should respond to a daily maintenance dose of 20 mg/day without serious effects.

Many SSRIs have an interaction with grapefruit juice that can lead to possible toxicity. It is recommended that daily intake be limited to 8 ounces of grapefruit juice or one half of a grapefruit.

Prototype Drug Chart: Fluoxetine describes the drug characteristics of the SSRI fluoxetine.

Pharmacokinetics. Fluoxetine is strongly protein bound, and the half-life is 4 to 6 days; therefore a cumulative drug effect may result from long-term use. Fluoxetine is metabolized and excreted by the kidneys.

Pharmacodynamics. Fluoxetine is well absorbed; however, its antidepressant effect develops slowly over several weeks. The onset of fluoxetine's initial antidepressant effect is between 3 and 4 weeks, and peak concentration with consistent therapy is at 6 to 8 hours after ingestion. The drug dose for older adults should be decreased to reduce side effects.

Side Effects and Adverse Reactions

Fluoxetine produces common side effects such as dry mouth, blurred vision, insomnia, headache, anorexia, nausea, diarrhea, and suicidal ideation. Fluoxetine has fewer side effects than amitriptyline.

📄 PROTOTYPE DRUG CHART

Fluoxetine

Drug Class	Dosage
Antidepressant: Selective serotonin reuptake inhibitor	Depression: Immediate release: A: PO: Initially 20 mg/d in the morning; *max:* 80 mg/d Delayed release: A: PO: 90 once weekly; *max:* 90 mg/wk
Contraindications	**Drug-Lab-Food Interactions**
Hypersensitivity, MAOI therapy *Caution:* Dehydration, cardiac disease, thyroid disease, dysrhythmias, hepatic disease, seizures, diabetes mellitus, anticoagulant therapy, diarrhea, hypokalemia, hypocalcemia, suicidal ideation, older adults	Drug: Increased effects of CNS and respiratory depression, hypotensive effect with alcohol and CNS depressants; increased bleeding potential with aspirin, NSAIDs, anticoagulants; MAOIs and SSRIs increase risk of serotonin syndrome. Complementary and alternative therapy: St. John's wort increases risk for serotonin syndrome; increased effect of hypoglycemics
Pharmacokinetics	**Pharmacodynamics**
Absorption: PO: well absorbed Distribution: PB: 94.5% Metabolism: Fluoxetine: t½: 4–6 d Excretion: Excreted primarily in urine	PO: Onset: 3–4 wk initially Peak: 6–8 h Duration: UK

Therapeutic Effects/Uses

To treat depression, bipolar disorder, bulimia disorder, obsessive-compulsive disorder, panic disorder, and premenstrual dysphoric disorder
Mechanism of Action: Serotonin action is enhanced in nerve cells because of selective serotonin reuptake blockade at neuronal membranes.

Side Effects	Adverse Reactions
Headache, dizziness, drowsiness, insomnia, anxiety, weakness, confusion, abnormal dreams, tremors, hyperhidrosis, pharyngitis, dry mouth, anorexia, nausea, diarrhea, constipation, peripheral edema, akathisia, urinary retention, erectile/ejaculatory dysfunction	Seizures, angioedema, hypo/hyperkalemia, hyponatremia, hypocalcemia, dehydration, GI bleeding/obstruction, osteoporosis, bone fractures, tachycardia, orthostatic hypotension, dysrhythmias, hearing loss *Life-threatening:* Stevens-Johnson syndrome, hepatic/renal failure, thrombocytopenia, leukopenia, serotonin syndrome, stroke, suicidal ideation

A, Adult; *CNS,* central nervous system; *d,* day; *MAOI,* monoamine oxidase inhibitor; *max,* maximum; *NSAID,* nonsteroidal antiinflammatory drug; *PB,* protein binding; *PO,* by mouth; *SSRI,* selective serotonin reuptake inhibitor; *t½,* half-life; *UK,* unknown; *wk,* week.

Some patients may experience sexual dysfunction when taking SSRIs. Men have discontinued taking fluoxetine after experiencing a decrease in sexual arousal. Some women have become anorgasmic, whereas males reported erectile dysfunction and delayed ejaculation when taking paroxetine HCl. The side effects often decrease or cease over the 1- to 4-week period of waiting for the therapeutic effect to emerge.

Serotonin Norepinephrine Reuptake Inhibitors

SNRIs inhibit the reuptake of serotonin and norepinephrine, increasing availability in the synapse. SNRIs are used for major depression. Other approved uses are for generalized anxiety disorder and social anxiety disorder. Other SNRIs include duloxetine, levomilnacipran, and desvenlafaxine.

Side Effects and Adverse Effects

Side effects for this classification include drowsiness, dizziness, insomnia, headache, amnesia, blurred vision, and erectile/ejaculation dysfunction. Adverse effects of this drug are hypertension, orthostatic hypotension, tachycardia, seizures, NMS, and suicidal ideation.

Atypical Antidepressants

Atypical antidepressants, or *second-generation antidepressants*, became available in the 1980s and have been used for major depression, reactive depression, and anxiety. They affect one or two of the three neurotransmitters: serotonin, norepinephrine, and dopamine. One of the first atypical antidepressants marketed was amoxapine; another atypical antidepressant drug is maprotiline.

Maprotiline is sometimes considered to be aTCA because of their pharmacologic similarities. Atypical antidepressants should *not* be taken with MAOIs and should not be used within 14 days after discontinuing MAOIs.

Side Effects and Adverse Effects

Side effects for atypical antidepressants include dizziness, drowsiness, dry mouth, constipation, orthostatic hypotension, tachycardia, palpitations, and erectile/ejaculatory dysfunction. Adverse effects include seizures.

Monoamine Oxidase Inhibitors

Another group of antidepressants is the monoamine oxidase inhibitors (MAOIs). The enzyme monoamine oxidase (MAO) inactivates norepinephrine, dopamine, epinephrine, and serotonin. By inhibiting MAO, the levels of these neurotransmitters rise. Two forms of MAO enzyme exist in the body: MAO-A and MAO-B. These enzymes are found primarily in the liver and brain. MAO-A inactivates dopamine in the brain, whereas MAO-B inactivates norepinephrine and serotonin. The MAOIs are nonselective and inhibit both MAO-A and MAO-B. Inhibition of MAO by MAOIs is thought to relieve the symptoms of depression. Four MAOIs are currently prescribed: (1) tranylcypromine sulfate, (2) isocarboxazid, (3) selegiline HCl, and (4) phenelzine sulfate. These MAOIs are detailed in Table 23.1.

For the treatment of depression, MAOIs are as effective as TCAs; however, because of adverse reactions, such as the risk of hypertensive crisis resulting from food and drug interactions, only 1% of patients who take antidepressants take an MAOI. Currently, MAOIs are not the antidepressants of choice and are usually prescribed when the patient does not respond to TCAs or second-generation antidepressants. However, MAOIs are still used for mild, reactive, and atypical depression (chronic anxiety, hypersomnia, fear). MAOIs and TCAs should not be taken together when treating depression.

Drug and Food Interactions

Certain drug and food interactions with MAOIs can be fatal. Any drugs that are CNS stimulants or sympathomimetics, such as vasoconstrictors and cold medications that contain phenylephrine and pseudoephedrine, can cause a hypertensive crisis when taken with an MAOI. In addition, foods that contain tyramine—aged cheese (cheddar, Swiss, bleu), cream, yogurt, coffee, chocolate, bananas, raisins, Italian green beans, liver, pickled foods, sausage, soy sauce, yeast, beer, and red wines—have sympathomimetic-like effects and can cause a hypertensive crisis. MAOI users *must avoid* these types of food and drugs. Frequent blood pressure monitoring is essential, and patient teaching regarding foods and over-the-counter (OTC) drugs to avoid is an important nursing responsibility. Because of the danger associated with hypertensive crisis, many psychiatrists will not prescribe MAOIs for depression unless other drugs have failed to be effective for the patient. However, this group of drugs is effective for treating depression if taken properly.

 COMPLEMENTARY AND ALTERNATIVE THERAPIES

Monoamine Oxidase Inhibitors

- Ginseng, ephedra (ma-huang), and St. John's wort may lead to palpitations, heart attack, and hypertensive crisis when taken with antidepressant MAOIs.
- Ginseng may lead to manic episodes when taken in combination with MAOIs such as tranylcypromine sulfate.
- An excessive dose of anise may interfere with MAOIs.
- An increased use of brewer's yeast with MAOIs can increase blood pressure.

In teaching patients about the foods and drugs to avoid when taking MAOIs, some individuals respond better to verbal instructions and education with reinforcement from videos than to printed communications. Complementary and Alternative Therapies: Monoamine Oxidase Inhibitors details complementary and alternative therapy interactions with MAOIs.

Side Effects and Adverse Reactions

Side effects of MAOIs include CNS stimulation (insomnia), orthostatic hypotension, and anticholinergic effects.

MOOD STABILIZERS

Mood stabilizers are used to treat bipolar affective disorder. Lithium was the first drug used to manage this disorder. Some refer to lithium as an *antimania drug* effective in controlling manic behavior that arises from underlying bipolar disorder. Lithium has a calming effect but may cause some memory loss and confusion. It controls any evidence of flight of ideas and hyperactivity. If the person stops taking lithium, manic behavior may return. Lithium, carbamazepine, valproic acid or divalproex, lamotrigine, cariprazine, and aripiprazole are currently first-line drugs for bipolar disorder.

Lithium is an inexpensive drug that must be closely monitored, and it has a narrow therapeutic serum range of 0.8 to 1.2 mEq/L. Serum lithium levels greater than 1.5 mEq/L may produce early signs of toxicity. The serum lithium level should be monitored biweekly until the therapeutic level has been obtained, and then it must be monitored at least every 1 to 2 months on the maintenance dose. Serum sodium levels also need to be monitored because lithium tends to deplete sodium.

◎ CLINICAL JUDGMENT [NURSING PROCESS]

Antidepressants

Concept: Mood and Affect
- A conscious state of mind or feeling

Recognize Cues [Assessment]
- Assess the patient's baseline vital signs and weight for future comparisons. Tricyclic antidepressants (TCAs) should be avoided in patients with cardiovascular disease and hypertension and should be used cautiously in patients with seizure disorders.
- Note the patient's hepatic and renal function by assessing urine output (>1500 mL/day), blood urea nitrogen (BUN), and serum creatinine and hepatic enzyme levels.
- Obtain a health history of episodes of depression; assess mental status, and assess for suicidal tendencies.
- Secure a drug history of the current drugs, alcohol, and herbs the patient is taking. Central nervous system (CNS) depressants can cause an additive effect. Antidepressants that cause anticholinergic-like symptoms are contraindicated if a patient has glaucoma.
- Assess for tardive dyskinesia and neuroleptic malignant syndrome (NMS), including hyperpyrexia, muscle rigidity, tachycardia, and cardiac dysrhythmias.

Analyze Cues and Prioritize Hypothesis [Patient Problems]
- Confusion
- Anxiety
- Hopelessness
- Decreased ability to cope
- Social isolation

Generate Solutions [Planning]
- Patient will display a calmer attitude.
- Patient will cope with at least one current issue.
- Patient will interact with others.

Take Action [Nursing Interventions]
- Observe patients for signs and symptoms of depression: mood changes, insomnia, apathy, or lack of interest in activities.
- Monitor vital signs. Orthostatic hypotension is common. Check for anticholinergic-like symptoms such as dry mouth, increased heart rate, urinary retention, and constipation. Check weight two to three times per week.
- ⚡ Monitor patients for suicidal tendencies when marked depression is present.

- Observe patients for seizures when anticonvulsants are taken; antidepressants lower the seizure threshold, and the anticonvulsant dose might need to be increased.
- ⚡ Monitor for drug-drug and food-drug interactions. Sympathomimetic-like drugs and foods that contain tyramine may cause a hypertensive crisis if taken with monoamine oxidase inhibitors (MAOIs).
- Check patients for extremely high blood pressure when taking MAOIs.
- Provide patients with a list of foods to avoid when taking MAOIs to avoid hypertensive crisis. These foods include cheese, red wine, beer, liver, bananas, yogurt, and sausage.

Patient Teaching
General
- Teach patients to take the medication as prescribed. Compliance is important.
- Inform patients that full effectiveness of a drug may not be evident until 1 to 2 weeks after the start of therapy.
- Encourage patients to keep medical appointments.
- Caution patients not to consume alcohol or any CNS depressants because of their addictive effect.
- ⚡ Inform patients that many complementary and alternative therapy products interact with antidepressants, especially MAOIs and selective serotonin reuptake inhibitors (SSRIs). Complementary and alternative therapies may need to be discontinued, or the antidepressant drug dosage may need to be modified (see Complementary and Alternative Therapies: Selective Serotonin Reuptake Inhibitors and Monoamine Oxidase Inhibitors).
- ⚡ Warn patients not to drive or be involved in potentially dangerous mechanical activity until stabilization of the drug dose has been established.
- Advise patients not to abruptly stop taking the drug. A health care provider should gradually decrease the drug dose.
- Encourage patients planning pregnancy to consult with a health care provider about possible teratogenic effects of the drug on the fetus.
- Advise patients to take the drug with food if gastrointestinal (GI) distress occurs.

Side Effects
- Advise patients that antidepressants may be taken at bedtime to decrease dangers from the sedative effect, and suggest they check with a health care provider. Transient side effects include nausea, drowsiness, headaches, and nervousness.

Evaluate Outcomes [Evaluation]
- Evaluate the effectiveness of the drug therapy regarding whether a patient's depression is controlled or has ceased.

TABLE 23.1 Antidepressants

Drug	Route and Dosage	Uses and Considerations
Tricyclic Antidepressants (TCAs)		
Amitriptyline hydrochloride	A: PO: Initially 75 mg/d in divided doses; *maint:* 50–100 mg/d at hs; *max:* 300 mg/d for inpatients, 150 mg/d for outpatients Older A: PO: Initially 10–25 mg at bedtime; *maint:* 50–100 mg/d; *max:* 150 mg/d Therapeutic serum range: 120–150 ng/mL	For depression. May cause drowsiness, dizziness, orthostatic hypotension, blurred vision, memory impairment, insomnia, ataxia, dry mouth, hyperhidrosis, constipation, nausea, weight gain, lethargy, tremor, and EPS. PB: 95%; t½: 10–50 h
Clomipramine hydrochloride	A: PO: Initially 25 mg/d, may increase to 100 mg/d in divided doses with meals; after titration, entire dose may be given at bedtime; *max:* 250 mg/d	For OCD and depression. May cause tremor, dizziness, drowsiness, headache, insomnia, fatigue, dry mouth, nausea, constipation, orthostatic hypotension, hyperhidrosis, and erectile/ejaculatory dysfunction. PB: 97%; t½: 19–37 h
Desipramine hydrochloride	A: PO: Initially 50–75 mg/d in 2–4 divided doses, increased gradually; *maint:* 100–200 mg/d; *max:* 300 mg/d for inpatients, 200 mg/d for outpatients Older A: Initially 25 mg/d at bedtime; *maint:* 100 mg/d in divided doses; *max:* 150 mg/d for inpatients, 100 mg/d for outpatients Therapeutic serum range: 125–300 ng/mL	For depression. May cause dizziness, drowsiness, headache, blurred vision, tremor, dry mouth, nausea, constipation, orthostatic hypotension, weight gain, erectile dysfunction, and EPS. PB: 90%; t½: 7–60 h
Doxepin hydrochloride	A: PO: Initially 75 mg/d at bedtime; or in 2–3 divided doses; *maint:* 75–150 mg/d; *max:* 300 mg/d Therapeutic serum range: 50–150 ng/mL	For depression and anxiety. May cause dizziness, drowsiness, blurred vision, orthostatic hypotension, dry mouth, constipation, erectile/ejaculatory dysfunction, weight gain, and skin irritation. PB: 80%; t½: 6–8 h
Imipramine hydrochloride	A: PO: Initially 75 mg/d; *maint:* 50–150 mg/d; *max:* 200 mg/d for outpatients, 300 mg/d for inpatients Older A: Initially 30–40 mg/d at bedtime; *maint:* 75–100 mg/d; *max:* 100 mg/d Therapeutic serum range: 125–250 ng/mL	For depression. May cause dizziness, drowsiness, headache, ataxia, blurred vision, fatigue, dysarthria, dry mouth, nausea, constipation, orthostatic hypotension, tremor, urinary retention, weight gain, and erectile/ejaculatory dysfunction. PB: 85%–95%; t½: 8–16 h
Mirtazapine	A: PO: Initially 15 mg at bedtime; *maint:* 15–45 mg/d; *max:* 45 mg/d	For depression. May cause dizziness, drowsiness, weakness, abnormal dreams, appetite stimulation, dry mouth, constipation, hypercholesterolemia, weight gain, hypertriglyceridemia, and erectile/ejaculatory dysfunction. PB: 85%; t½: 20–40 h
Nortriptyline hydrochloride	A: PO: Initially 25–50 mg at hs or in divided doses; *max:* 150 mg/d Older A: PO: Initially 10–25 mg/d at bedtime; *maint:* 30–50 mg/d; *max:* 50 mg/d Therapeutic serum range: 50–150 ng/mL	For depression. May cause dizziness, drowsiness, headache, blurred vision, weight gain, dry mouth, nausea, vomiting, constipation, appetite stimulation, erectile/ejaculatory dysfunction, and tremor. PB: 93%–95%; t½: 16–90 h
Protriptyline hydrochloride	A: PO: Initially 5–10 mg tid/qid; *max:* 60 mg/d Older A: PO: Initially 5 mg tid; *max:* 30 mg/d Therapeutic serum range: 70–250 ng/mL	For depression. May cause dizziness, drowsiness, headache, blurred vision, insomnia, tremor, dysarthria, dry mouth, erectile/ejaculatory dysfunction, nausea, vomiting, and constipation. PB: 90%; t½: 54–92 h
Trimipramine maleate	A: Initially 75 mg/d in divided doses for outpatients, 100 mg for inpatients; *max:* 200 mg/d for outpatients, 300 mg/d for inpatients Older A: Initially 50 mg/d in divided doses; *max:* 100 mg/d Therapeutic serum range: 150–300 ng/mL	For depression. May cause dizziness, drowsiness, fatigue, tremor, headache, dry mouth, nausea, constipation, weight gain, erectile/ejaculatory dysfunction, and appetite stimulation. PB: 95%; t½: 20–26 h
Selective Serotonin Reuptake Inhibitors (SSRIs)		
Citalopram	A:<60 y: PO: Initially 20 mg/d, may increase after 1 wk; *max:* 40 mg/d A >60 y: PO: 20 mg/d; *max:* 20 mg/d	For depression. May cause drowsiness, insomnia, dry mouth, hyperhidrosis, nausea, diarrhea, tremor, ejaculation dysfunction, and seizures. PB: 80%; t½: 35 h
Fluoxetine hydrochloride	See Prototype Drug Chart: Fluoxetine	
Paroxetine hydrochloride	Depression: Immediate-release tablets: A: PO: Initially 20 mg/d in a.m.; *max:* 50 mg/d Older A: PO: Initially 10 mg/d; *max:* 40 mg/d Controlled-release tablets: A: PO: Initially 25 mg/d in a.m.; *max:* 62.5 mg/d Older A: PO: Initially 12.5 mg/d; *max:* 50 mg/d	For depression, general anxiety disorder, social anxiety disorder, panic disorder, PTSD, and OCD. May cause dizziness, drowsiness, insomnia, headache, asthenia, hyperhidrosis, dry mouth, nausea, constipation, diarrhea, tremors, and erectile/ejaculatory dysfunction. PB: 93%–95%; t½: 21 h for immediate release, 15–20 h for controlled release

Continued

TABLE 23.1 Antidepressants—cont'd

Drug	Route and Dosage	Uses and Considerations
Sertraline hydrochloride	Depression: A: PO: 25–50 mg/d; *max:* 200 mg/d	For depression, OCD, PTSD, panic disorder, social anxiety disorder. May cause dizziness, drowsiness, agitation, insomnia, fatigue, tremor, dry mouth, erectile/ejaculatory dysfunction, nausea, and diarrhea. PB: 98%; t½: 26 h
Fluvoxamine	Depression: Immediate release: A: PO: Initially 50 mg/d at bedtime; *maint:* 50–300 mg/d; *max:* 300 mg/d	For OCD and depression. May cause dizziness, drowsiness, headache, insomnia, anxiety, asthenia, dry mouth, anorexia, nausea, diarrhea, constipation, and erectile/ejaculatory dysfunction. PB: 80%; t½: 15.6 h immediate release
Escitalopram	Depression: A: PO: 10 mg/d, may increase to 20 mg/d after 1 wk; *max:* 20 mg/d Older A: PO: 10 mg/d; *max:* 10 mg/d	For depression and generalized anxiety disorder. May cause drowsiness, fatigue, headache, insomnia, dry mouth, nausea, diarrhea, orthostatic hypotension, and erectile/ejaculation dysfunction. PB: 56%; t½: 27–32 h

Atypical (Second-Generation) Antidepressants

Drug	Route and Dosage	Uses and Considerations
Amoxapine	A: PO: Initially 50 mg bid/tid; *max:* 400 mg/d for outpatients, 600 mg/d for inpatients Older A: PO: 25 mg bid/tid; *max:* 300 mg/d Therapeutic serum range is 200–400 ng/mL	For depression. May cause drowsiness, blurred vision, dry mouth, constipation, orthostatic hypotension, palpitations, tachycardia, edema, EPS, and erectile/ejaculatory dysfunction. PB: >90%; t½: 8 h
Maprotiline hydrochloride	A <60 y: PO: Initially 25–75 mg/d in divided doses for outpatients, 100–150 mg/d for inpatients; *max:* 225 mg/d Older A: Initially 25 mg/d; *maint:* 50–75 mg/d; *max:* 150 mg/d	For depression. May cause dizziness, drowsiness, blurred vision, confusion, dry mouth, constipation, tachycardia, palpitations, seizures, urinary retention, ataxia, and erectile dysfunction. PB: 88%; t½: 51 h

Aminoketone Antidepressants

Drug	Route and Dosage	Uses and Considerations
Bupropion hydrochloride	Depression: Immediate release: A: PO: Initially 100 mg bid; *max:* 450 mg/d, 150 mg/dose Sustained release: A: PO: Initially 150 mg/d in the morning; *maint:* 200 mg bid; *max:* 400 mg/d, 200 mg single dose Extended release: A: PO: 150 mg/d in the morning; *max:* 450 mg/d	For depression, seasonal affective disorder, and tobacco cessation. May cause dizziness, insomnia, headache, dry mouth, anorexia, nausea, vomiting, constipation, hyperhidrosis, agitation, tachycardia, weight gain/loss, tremor, and erectile/ejaculatory dysfunction. PB: 84%; t½: 8–24 h immediate release, 20–37 h sustained and extended release

Miscellaneous Antidepressants

Drug	Route and Dosage	Uses and Considerations
Mirtazapine	Initially 15 mg at bedtime; *maint:* 15–45 mg/d; *max:* 45 mg/d	For depression. May cause dizziness, drowsiness, weakness, abnormal dreams, appetite stimulation, dry mouth, constipation, hypercholesterolemia, weight gain, hypertriglyceridemia, and erectile/ejaculatory dysfunction. PB: 85%; t½: 20–40 h
Esketamine	A: Nasal spray: 56 mg Day 1; 56 or 84 mg 2 times/wk during wk 1–4; 56 or 84 mg/once a week during wk 5–8; thereafter 56 or 84 mg q1wk or q2wk	For treatment-resistant depression in addition to an oral antidepressant. May cause dizziness, drowsiness, dissociation, headache, nausea, and dysgeusia. PB: insignificant; t½: 7–12 h
Vilazodone	A: PO: Initially 10 mg/d for 1 wk; *maint:* 20–40 mg/d with food; *max:* 40 mg/d	For depression. May cause dizziness, blurred vision, insomnia, headache, nausea, dry mouth, vomiting, diarrhea, and erectile/ejaculatory dysfunction. PB: 96%–99%; t½: 25 h
Nefazodone	A: PO: Initially 50–100 mg bid; *maint:* 300–600 mg/d; *max:* 600 mg/d Older A: Initially 50 mg bid; *maint:* 300–600 mg/d in 2 divided doses; *max:* 600 mg/d	For depression. May cause headache, drowsiness, dizziness, insomnia, blurred vision, dry mouth, weakness, infection, nausea, diarrhea, and constipation. PB: 99%; t½: 2–4 h
Trazodone hydrochloride	Immediate release: A: PO: Initially 150 mg/d in divided doses; *max:* 400 mg/d for outpatients, 600 mg/d for inpatients Extended release: A: PO: Initially 150 mg/d at bedtime, *max:* 375 mg/d	For depression. May cause drowsiness, dizziness, blurred vision, headache, fatigue, tachycardia, palpitations, dry mouth, nausea, vomiting, constipation, diarrhea, erectile/ejaculatory dysfunction, and hearing loss. PB: 89%–95%; t½: 10 h
Vortioxetine	A: PO: Initially 5–10 mg/d; *maint:* 5–20 mg/d; *max:* 20 mg/d	For depression. May cause dizziness, dry mouth, nausea, vomiting, diarrhea, constipation, and orgasm and erectile/ejaculatory dysfunction. PB: 98%; t½: 66 h

Serotonin Norepinephrine Reuptake Inhibitors (SNRIs)

Drug	Route and Dosage	Uses and Considerations
Desvenlafaxine	A: PO: Initially 50 mg/d; *max:* 400 mg/d	For depression. May cause dizziness, drowsiness, fatigue, insomnia, hyperhidrosis, dry mouth, anorexia, nausea, vomiting, constipation, hypercholesterolemia, orthostatic hypotension, tremor, withdrawal, and erectile/ejaculatory dysfunction. PB: 30%; t½: 11 h

TABLE 23.1 Antidepressants—cont'd

Drug	Route and Dosage	Uses and Considerations
Duloxetine	Depression: A: PO: Initially 20 mg/bid; *maint:* 60 mg/d; *max:* 120 mg/d	For major depression, diabetic neuropathy, fibromyalgia, generalized anxiety disorder, and chronic musculoskeletal pain. May cause dizziness, drowsiness, headache, insomnia, fatigue, weakness, dry mouth, anorexia, abdominal pain, nausea, constipation, weight loss, and erectile/ejaculatory dysfunction. PB: 90%; t½: 8–17 h
Levomilnacipran	A: PO: Initially 20 mg/d for 2 d, then 40 mg/d; *maint:* 40–120 mg/d; *max:* 120 mg/d	For depression. May cause orthostatic hypotension, hyperhidrosis, nausea, vomiting, constipation, tachycardia, erectile/ejaculatory dysfunction, urinary retention, and palpitations. PB: 22%; t½: 12 h

Monoamine Oxidase Inhibitors (MAOIs)

Drug	Route and Dosage	Uses and Considerations
Isocarboxazid	A: PO: Initially 10 mg bid; *maint:* 40 mg/d in divided doses; *max:* 60 mg/d	For treatment-resistant depression. May cause dizziness, headache, insomnia, dry mouth, nausea, constipation, weight gain, withdrawal, erectile/ejaculatory dysfunction. PB: UK; t½: 2.5 h
Phenelzine sulfate	A: PO: Initially 15 mg tid; *maint:* 15–90 mg/d; *max:* 90 mg/d	For treatment-resistant depression. May cause dizziness, drowsiness, headache, insomnia, blurred vision, hyperhidrosis, dry mouth, constipation, weight gain, hyperreflexia, paresthesia, peripheral edema, erectile/ejaculation dysfunction. PB: UK; t½: 12 h
Tranylcypromine sulfate	A: PO: Initially 15 mg bid; *max:* 60 mg/d	For treatment-resistant depression. May cause dizziness, drowsiness, insomnia, constipation, orthostatic hypotension, peripheral edema, dry mouth, diarrhea, weight gain, erectile/ejaculatory dysfunction. PB: UK; t½: 2.5 h
Selegiline hydrochloride	Depression: A: Transdermal: 6 mg patch/d; *max:* 12 mg patch/d	For depression and parkinsonism. May cause dizziness, headache, insomnia, dry mouth, abdominal pain, nausea, diarrhea, orthostatic hypotension, impulse control disorder, hallucinations, and erectile dysfunction. PB: 85%–90%; t½: 1.3–2 h

Mood Stabilizers

Drug	Route and Dosage	Uses and Considerations
Lithium citrate	See Prototype Drug Chart: Lithium	
Carbamazepine	Bipolar disorder: Immediate release: A: PO: Initially 200 mg bid; *maint:* 600–1600 mg/d in divided doses; *max:* 1600 mg/d Extended-release capsule: A: PO: Initially 200 mg bid; *max:* 1600 mg/d Therapeutic serum level: 4–12 mcg/mL	For bipolar disorder, seizures, neuropathic pain, trigeminal neuralgia. May cause dizziness, drowsiness, blurred vision, weakness, ataxia, dry mouth, nausea, vomiting, and constipation. PB: 76%; t½: 25–65 h
Valproic acid, divalproex	Bipolar disorder: Delayed release: A: PO: Initially 750 mg/d in divided doses; *max:* 60 mg/kg/d Extended release: A: PO: Initially 25 mg/kg/d; *max:* 60 mg/kg/d Therapeutic range: 50–125 mcg/mL	For bipolar disorder, seizures, and migraine prophylaxis. May cause dizziness, drowsiness, headache, insomnia, weakness, blurred vision, diplopia, abdominal pain, nausea, vomiting, diarrhea, and tremor. PB: 90%; t½: 9–16 h
Lamotrigine	Bipolar disorder: A: PO: Initially 25 mg/d for 2 wk, then 50 mg/d for 2 wk, then 100 mg/d for 1 wk; thereafter give 200 mg/d	For bipolar disorder, seizures, Lennox-Gastaut syndrome. May cause dizziness, drowsiness, blurred vision, diplopia, fever, rash, nausea and vomiting. PB: 55%; t½: 14–59 h
Cariprazine	Bipolar disorder: A: PO: Initially 1.5 mg/d; Day 2 give 3 mg/d; *maint:* 3–6 mg/d; *max:* 6 mg/d	For bipolar disorder and schizophrenia. May cause dizziness, drowsiness, headache, insomnia, vomiting, weight gain, nausea, constipation, akathisia, and EPS. PB: 91%–97%; t½: 2–4 d
Aripiprazole	Bipolar disorder: Immediate release: A: PO: Initially 10–15 mg/d; *max:* 30 mg/d	For bipolar disorder, schizophrenia, autism, depression, Tourette syndrome. May cause drowsiness, headache, anxiety, agitation, insomnia, nausea, fatigue, hyperglycemia, and blurred vision. PB: 99%; t½: 75 h
Olanzapine and samidorphan	A: PO: 10 mg olanzapine/10 mg samidorphan/d or 15 mg olanzapine/10 mg samidorphan/d; *maint:* 5–20 mg olanzapine/10 mg samidorphan/d; *max:* 20 mg olanzapine/10 mg samidorphan/d	For bipolar disorder and schizophrenia. May cause hyperprolactinemia, weight gain, hyperglycemia, dizziness, drowsiness, hypertriglyceridemia, dry mouth, appetite stimulation, headache, and orthostatic hypotension.

>, Greater than; *A,* adult; *bid,* twice a day; *CNS,* central nervous system; *d,* day; *EPS,* extrapyramidal syndrome symptoms; *GI,* gastrointestinal; *h,* hour; *maint,* maintenance; *MAOI,* monoamine oxidase inhibitor; *max,* maximum; *OCD,* obsessive-compulsive disorder; *PB,* protein binding; *PO,* by mouth; *PTSD,* posttraumatic stress disorder; *qid,* four times a day; *t½,* half-life; *tid,* three times a day; *TCA,* tricyclic antidepressant; *UK,* unknown; *wk,* week(s); *y,* year.

Lithium must be used with caution, if at all, by patients taking diuretics. Prototype Drug Chart: Lithium lists the pharmacologic behavior of lithium.

Pharmacokinetics. More than 95% of lithium is absorbed through the gastrointestinal (GI) tract. The protein-binding capacity of lithium is 15%. The half-life of lithium ranges from 18 to 36 hours. Because of its long half-life, cumulative drug action may result. The liver metabolizes lithium, and most of the drug is excreted unchanged in the urine.

Pharmacodynamics. Lithium is prescribed mostly for the stabilization of bipolar affective disorder. The onset of action is fast, but the patient may not achieve the desired effect for 5 to 6 days. Increased sodium intake increases renal excretion, so the sodium intake needs to be closely monitored. Increased urine output can result in body fluid loss and dehydration; therefore adequate fluid intake of 1 to 2 L should be maintained daily.

Antiseizure drugs such as carbamazepine, lamotrigine, and valproic acid/valproate/divalproex have been used in place of lithium for some patients. These antiseizure agents are further discussed in Chapter 19. The antipsychotic drugs olanzapine, ziprasidone, and aripiprazole are approved to treat acute mania and mixed episodes of bipolar disorder. Antipsychotic drugs are discussed in Chapter 22.

📄 PROTOTYPE DRUG CHART

Lithium

Drug Class	Dosage
Mood stabilizer	Immediate release: A: PO: Initially 300 mg tid; *maint:* 300–600 mg/bid–tid Extended release: A: PO: Initially 900 mg bid; *maint:* 900–1200 mg/d Therapeutic drug range: 0.8–1.2 mEq/L

Contraindications	Drug-Lab-Food Interactions
Hypersensitivity *Caution:* Hepatic and renal disease, pregnancy, breastfeeding, cardiac disease, dehydration, hyponatremia, hypercalcemia, hypokalemia, diarrhea, children, older adults, infection, parkinsonism, thyroid disease, seizure disorder, suicidal ideation	Drug: May increase lithium level with thiazide diuretics, methyldopa, haloperidol, NSAIDs, antidepressants, carbamazepine, calcium channel blockers, spironolactone, ACE inhibitors, sodium bicarbonate, phenothiazines; may increase lithium excretion with theophylline, aminophylline; may increase risk of serotonin syndrome with SSRIs and SNRIs; may increase hyperglycemia with antidiabetics; caffeine may decrease lithium levels; CNS stimulants and direct renin inhibitors may increase risk of mania Lab: Increased urine and blood glucose, protein; decreased serum sodium level Food: Increase sodium intake; lithium may cause sodium depletion Complementary and alternative therapy: Use of St. John's wort, kava kava, and valerian may lead to neurotoxicity

Pharmacokinetics	Pharmacodynamics
Absorption: PO: Well absorbed Distribution: PB: 15% Metabolism: t½: 18–36 h Excretion: 98% in urine, mostly unchanged	PO: Onset: UK Peak: 0.25–3 h Duration: 24 h Extended release: Onset: UK Peak: 4–6 h Duration: UK

Therapeutic Effects/Uses
To treat bipolar disorder, manic episodes Mechanism of Action: Alteration of ion transport in muscle and nerve cells; increased receptor sensitivity to serotonin

Side Effects	Adverse Reactions
Headache, memory impairment, blurred vision, metallic taste, thirst, dry mouth, dental caries, drowsiness, dizziness, fatigue, ataxia, tremor, anorexia, nausea, vomiting, diarrhea, polyuria, dehydration, hypotension, abdominal pain, restlessness, erectile dysfunction, weight gain/loss, peripheral edema	Urinary and fecal incontinence, thyroid disease, hyperglycemia, proteinuria, leukocytosis, nephrotoxicity *Life-threatening:* Dysrhythmias, seizures, angioedema, cardiac arrest, diabetes insipidus, serotonin syndrome, neuroleptic malignant syndrome

A, Adult; *ACE,* angiotensin-converting enzyme; *bid,* twice a day; *CNS,* central nervous system; *d,* day; *h,* hour; *maint,* maintenance; *NSAID,* nonsteroidal antiinflammatory drug; *PB,* protein binding; *PO,* by mouth; *SNRI,* serotonin norepinephrine reuptake inhibitor; *SSRI,* selective serotonin reuptake inhibitor; *t½,* half-life; *tid,* three times a day; *UK,* unknown; *y,* year; *>,* greater than.

⊚ CLINICAL JUDGMENT [NURSING PROCESS]

Mood Stabilizer: Lithium

Concept: Mood and Affect
- A conscious state of mind or feeling

Recognize Cues [Assessment]
- Assess for suicidal ideation.
- Assess baseline vital signs for future comparisons.
- Evaluate neurologic status, including gait, level of consciousness, reflexes, and tremors.
- Note hepatic and renal function by assessing urine output (>600 mL/day) and whether blood urea nitrogen (BUN) and serum creatinine and liver enzyme levels are within normal range. Assess for toxicity. Draw weekly blood levels initially and then every 1 to 2 months. Therapeutic serum levels for lithium are 0.8 to 1.2 mEq/L. Signs and symptoms of serum levels above 1.5 mEq/L are nausea and vomiting, diarrhea, ataxia, blurred vision, confusion, and tremors. Above 2.5 mEq/L, signs and symptoms of toxicity progress to include seizures, cardiac dysrhythmias, coma, and permanent neurologic impairment. At 3.5 mEq/L or higher, signs of toxicity are potentially lethal. Withhold medication and notify a health care provider immediately if any of these occur.
- Obtain a health history of episodes of depression or manic depressive behavior.
- Obtain a drug history. Diuretics, tetracyclines, methyldopa, probenecid, and nonsteroidal antiinflammatory drugs (NSAIDs) such as ibuprofen decrease renal clearance of lithium, causing drug accumulation.

Analyze Cues and Prioritize Hypothesis [Patient Problems]
- Diarrhea
- Confusion
- Anxiety
- Decreased visual acuity
- Hopelessness
- Decreased ability to cope
- Social isolation

Generate Solutions [Planning]
- Patient will display a calmer attitude.
- Patient will cope with at least one current issue.
- Patient will interact with others.

Take Action [Nursing Interventions]
- Observe patients for signs and symptoms of depression: mood changes, insomnia, apathy, or lack of interest in activities.
- Monitor vital signs. Hypotension is common.
- Draw blood samples for lithium levels immediately before the next dose (8 to 12 hours after the previous dose).
- ⚡ Monitor for signs of lithium toxicity. Report high (>1.5 mEq/L) serum lithium levels immediately to a health care provider.
- ⚡ Monitor patients for suicidal tendencies when marked depression is present.
- Evaluate urine output and body weight. Fluid volume deficit may occur as a result of polyuria.

- Observe patients for fine and gross motor tremors and presence of slurred speech, which are signs of adverse reaction.
- Assist patients in conserving energy when in a manic phase.
- Check cardiac monitor, blood pressure, and heart rate. Loss of fluids and electrolytes may cause electrolyte imbalance and cardiac dysrhythmias.
- Monitor serum electrolytes and report abnormal findings.

Patient Teaching
General
- Teach patients to take lithium as prescribed. Emphasize the importance of adherence to the therapy, laboratory tests, and follow-up visits with a health care provider. If lithium is stopped, manic symptoms will reappear.
- Encourage patients to keep medical appointments. Have patients check with a health care provider before taking over-the-counter (OTC) preparations.
- Warn patients not to drive a motor vehicle or engage in potentially dangerous mechanical activity until a stable lithium level is established.
- Advise patients to maintain adequate fluid intake (2 to 3 L/day initially and 1 to 2 L/day maintenance). Fluid intake should increase in hot weather.
- Teach patients to take lithium with meals to decrease gastric irritation.
- Inform patients that effectiveness of the drug may not be evident until 1 to 2 weeks after the start of therapy. Compliance in taking the prescribed lithium doses on a daily basis is a major problem with bipolar patients. Sometimes, when a patient has a period of emotional stability, he or she does not believe that the drug is needed and may stop taking the lithium.
- Advise patients planning pregnancy to consult with a health care provider about possible teratogenic effects of the drug on the fetus, especially during the first 3 months.
- Encourage patients to wear or carry an identification tag or bracelet indicating the drug taken.

Diet
- Advise patients to avoid caffeine products (coffee, tea, cola) because they can aggravate the manic phase of bipolar disorder by decreasing lithium levels.
- Advise patients to maintain adequate sodium intake and to avoid crash diets that affect physical and mental health.

Side Effects
- Advise patients to contact a health care provider if they experience symptoms of toxicity. Early symptoms include diarrhea, drowsiness, loss of appetite, muscle weakness, nausea, vomiting, slurred speech, and trembling. Late symptoms include blurred vision, confusion, increased urination, convulsions, severe trembling, and unsteadiness.

Evaluate Outcomes [Evaluation]
- Evaluate the effectiveness of the drug therapy and determine if patient is free of bipolar behavior.
- Allow patients to verbalize their understanding of symptoms of toxicity.
- Determine whether the patient demonstrates a subsiding or resolution of symptoms.

Side Effects and Adverse Reactions

The many side effects of lithium—dry mouth, thirst, polyuria (loss of water and sodium in increased urination), weight gain, metallic taste, and peripheral edema of the hands and ankles—can be annoying to the patient. If taken during pregnancy, lithium may have teratogenic effects.

Lithium and nonsteroidal antiinflammatory drugs (NSAIDs) should *not* be given together, because NSAIDs may increase lithium levels. Caffeine and loop diuretics may decrease lithium levels. Lithium should be prescribed with extreme caution for patients who have a cardiovascular disease due to an increased risk of lithium toxicity. Frequent monitoring of lithium levels is necessary. Caution must also be used in patients with thyroid disease, as hypothyroidism may occur.

■ CRITICAL THINKING CASE STUDY

A 37-year-old woman is receiving fluoxetine 20 mg in the morning for depression. The patient complains of insomnia and GI upset.

1. What could you suggest to help her avoid insomnia? Explain your answer.
2. How might the patient avoid GI upset when taking fluoxetine? What food should be avoided?

   The patient states that she does not think the fluoxetine is helping. She states that she has heard about complementary and alternative therapies that may be taken for depression. She has also heard that fluoxetine can be taken weekly.

3. Is the patient's fluoxetine dose within normal dosage range? Explain your answer.
4. How would you respond to the patient about the use of certain complementary and alternative therapies for depression?
5. What would your response be concerning the use of fluoxetine in a weekly dose?

■ REVIEW QUESTIONS

1. A patient is admitted with bipolar affective disorder. The nurse acknowledges which medication as one used to treat this disorder for some patients in place of lithium?
   a. Thiopental
   b. Ginkgo biloba
   c. Fluvoxamine
   d. Divalproex
2. The nurse realizes that some complementary and alternative therapies interact with selective serotonin reuptake inhibitors. Which complementary and alternative therapy interactions may cause serotonin syndrome? (Select all that apply.)
   a. Feverfew
   b. Ma huang
   c. St. John's wort
   d. Ginkgo biloba
3. A selective serotonin reuptake inhibitor is prescribed for a patient. The nurse knows that which drug is a selective serotonin reuptake inhibitor?
   a. Paroxetine
   b. Amitriptyline
   c. Divalproex sodium
   d. Bupropion hydrochloride
4. A patient is taking tranylcypromine sulfate for depression. What advice should the nurse include in the teaching plan for this medication?
   a. Warn the patient about weight loss.
   b. Instruct the patient to avoid beer and cheddar cheese.

   c. Encourage the patient to take ginseng and ephedra.
   d. Encourage the patient to eat fruit such as bananas.
5. Which statement is true concerning lithium?
   a. The maximum dose is 3.4 g/day.
   b. The therapeutic drug range is 2.5 to 3.5 mEq/L.
   c. Lithium increases receptor sensitivity to gamma-aminobutyric acid.
   d. Concurrent nonsteroidal antiinflammatory drugs (NSAIDs) may increase lithium levels.
6. When a patient is taking an antidepressant, what should the nurse do? (Select all that apply.)
   a. Monitor the patient for suicidal tendencies.
   b. Observe the patient for orthostatic hypotension.
   c. Teach the patient to take the drug with food if gastrointestinal distress occurs.
   d. Tell the patient that the drug may not have full effectiveness for 1 to 2 weeks.
   e. Advise the patient to maintain adequate fluid intake of 2 L/day.
7. A patient is taking lithium. The nurse should be aware of the importance of which nursing intervention(s)? (Select all that apply.)
   a. Observe the patient for motor tremors.
   b. Monitor the patient for hypotension.
   c. Draw lithium blood levels immediately after a dose.
   d. Advise the patient to drink 750 mL/day of fluid in hot weather.
   e. Advise the patient to avoid caffeinated foods and beverages.
   f. Teach the patient to take lithium with meals to decrease gastric irritation.

24

Antiinflammatories

http://evolve.elsevier.com/McCuistion/pharmacology

OBJECTIVES

- Explain the pathophysiologic basis of the five cardinal signs of inflammation.
- Compare the action of various nonsteroidal antiinflammatory drugs (NSAIDs).
- Explain the use of disease-modifying antirheumatic drugs (DMARDs).

- Differentiate between the side effects and adverse reactions of NSAIDs and DMARDs.
- Correlate the Clinical Judgment [Nursing Process] associated with NSAIDs and corticosteroids, including patient teaching.
- Apply the Clinical Judgment [Nursing Process] to the patient taking DMARDs.
- Compare the action of various antigout medications.

OUTLINE

INTRODUCTION

Inflammation is a response to tissue injury caused by the release of chemical mediators that trigger both a vascular response and the migration of fluid and cells—leukocytes, or white blood cells—to the injured site. The chemical mediators are histamines, kinins, and prostaglandins. The process of inflammation is a protective mechanism in which the body attempts to neutralize and destroy harmful agents at the site of injury and to establish conditions for tissue repair.

Although a relationship exists between inflammation and infection, these terms should *not* be used interchangeably. **Infection** is caused by microorganisms and *results* in inflammation, but not all inflammations are caused by infections. Only a small percentage of inflammations are caused by infection. Other causes of inflammation include trauma, surgical interventions, extreme heat or cold, and caustic chemical agents.

Antiinflammatory drugs reduce fluid migration and pain, lessening loss of function and increasing the patient's mobility and comfort.

PATHOPHYSIOLOGY

The five characteristics of inflammation, called *the cardinal signs of inflammation,* are (1) redness, (2) swelling (edema), (3) heat, (4) pain, and (5) loss of function. Table 24.1 gives the description and explanation of the cardinal signs of inflammation. Inflammation also has two phases: the *vascular phase,* which occurs 10 to 15 minutes after an injury; and the *delayed phase.* The vascular phase is associated with vasodilation and increased capillary permeability, during which blood substances and fluid leave the plasma and go to the injured site. The delayed phase occurs when leukocytes infiltrate the inflamed tissue.

Various chemical mediators are released during the inflammation process (Fig. 24.1). *Histamine,* the first mediator in the inflammatory process, causes dilation of the arterioles and increases capillary permeability, allowing fluid to leave the capillaries and flow into the injured area. *Kinins,* such as bradykinin, also increase capillary permeability and the sensation of pain.

TABLE 24.1	**Cardinal Signs of Inflammation**
Signs	**Description and Explanation**
Erythema (redness)	Redness occurs in the first phase of inflammation. Blood accumulates in the area of tissue injury because of the release of the body's chemical mediators (kinins, prostaglandins, and histamine). These chemical mediators dilate the arterioles.
Edema (swelling)	Swelling is the second phase of inflammation. Plasma leaks into the interstitial tissue at the injury site. Kinins and histamine increase capillary permeability.
Heat	Heat at the inflammatory site can be caused by increased blood accumulation and may result from pyrogens, substances that produce fever, which interfere with the temperature-regulating center in the hypothalamus.
Pain	Pain is caused by tissue swelling and release of chemical mediators.
Loss of function	Function is lost because of the accumulation of fluid at the tissue injury site and because of pain, which decreases mobility at the affected area.

Among these are prostaglandins, chemical mediators that have been isolated from the exudate at inflammatory sites. Prostaglandins have many effects, which include vasodilation, relaxation of smooth muscle, increased capillary permeability, and sensitization of nerve cells to pain.

Cyclooxygenase (COX) is the enzyme responsible for converting arachidonic acid into prostaglandins and their products. This synthesis of prostaglandins causes inflammation and pain at a tissue injury site. COX has two enzyme forms, COX-1 and COX-2. *COX-1* protects the stomach lining and regulates blood platelets, and *COX-2* triggers inflammation and pain.

ANTIINFLAMMATORY AGENTS

Drugs such as aspirin inhibit the biosynthesis of prostaglandin and are therefore called *prostaglandin inhibitors.* Because prostaglandin inhibitors affect the inflammatory process, they are more commonly called *antiinflammatories or antiinflammatory drugs.*

Antiinflammatories also relieve pain (analgesic), reduce elevated body temperature (antipyretic), and inhibit platelet aggregation (anticoagulant). Aspirin is the oldest antiinflammatory drug, but it was first used for its analgesic and antipyretic properties. As a result of searching for a more effective drug with fewer side effects, many other antiinflammatories or prostaglandin inhibitors have been discovered. Although these drugs have potent antiinflammatory effects that mimic the effects of corticosteroids (cortisone), they are *not* chemically related to corticosteroids and therefore are called nonsteroidal antiinflammatory drugs (NSAIDs). Most NSAIDs are used to decrease inflammation and pain for patients who have some type of musculoskeletal condition.

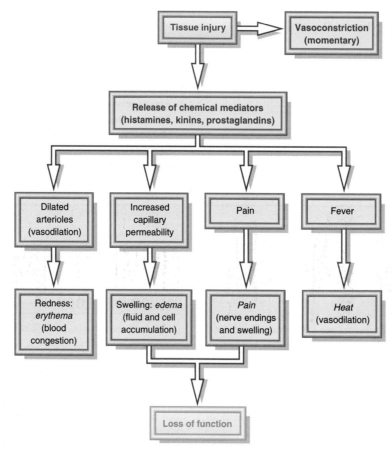

Fig. 24.1 Chemical mediator response to tissue injury.

NONSTEROIDAL ANTIINFLAMMATORY DRUGS

NSAIDs include aspirin and aspirin-like drugs that inhibit the enzyme COX, which is needed for the biosynthesis of prostaglandins. Chapters 25 and 40 present expanded discussions of NSAIDs in their roles as analgesics and anticoagulants, respectively. These drugs may be called *prostaglandin inhibitors* with varying degrees of analgesic and antipyretic effects, but they are used primarily as antiinflammatories to relieve inflammation and pain. Their antipyretic effect is less than their antiinflammatory effect. With several exceptions, NSAID preparations are not suggested for use in alleviating mild headaches and mildly elevated temperature. Preferred drugs for headaches and fever are aspirin (adults only for fever), acetaminophen, and ibuprofen. NSAIDs are more appropriate for reducing swelling, pain, and stiffness in joints.

Most NSAIDs cost more than aspirin. Other than aspirin, the only NSAIDs that can be purchased over the counter (OTC) are ibuprofen and naproxen. All other NSAIDs require a prescription. Examples of prescription products on the market that contain NSAID contents alone or in combination include celecoxib, meloxicam, oxaprozin, nabumetone, sulindac, and ketorolac. If a patient can take aspirin for the inflammatory process without gastrointestinal (GI) upset, salicylate products are usually recommended.

There are six groups of NSAIDs:

1. Salicylates
2. *Para*-chlorobenzoic acid derivatives, or indoles
3. Propionic acid derivatives
4. Fenamates
5. Oxicams
6. Selective COX-2 inhibitors

The first five NSAID groups on the list are known as *first-generation NSAIDs*, and the COX-2 inhibitors are called *second-generation NSAIDs*.

TABLE 24.2 Antiinflammatory Agents: Nonsteroidal

Drug	Route and Dosage	Uses and Considerations
First-Generation NSAIDs		
Salicylates		
Aspirin	See Prototype Drug Chart: Aspirin	
Diflunisal	Osteoarthritis: A: PO: 250–500 mg bid; *max:* 1500 mg/d	For mild to moderate pain, osteoarthritis, and rheumatoid arthritis. Avoid if hypersensitive to aspirin. May cause rash, headache, nausea, diarrhea, dyspepsia, GI bleeding/perforation, abdominal pain, elevated hepatic enzymes, and hearing loss. PB: 99%; t½: 8–12 h
Salicylate Derivatives		
Olsalazine sodium	A: PO: 500 mg q12h; *max:* 1 g/d	For ulcerative colitis. May cause headache, arthralgia, nausea, diarrhea, dyspepsia, and abdominal pain. PB: 99%; t½: 1 h
Sulfasalazine	Rheumatoid arthritis: A: PO: Initially 0.5–1 g/d; *maint:* 2 g/d in 2–3 divided doses; *max:* 3 g/d	For ulcerative colitis and rheumatoid arthritis. Avoid if allergic to sulfonamides or aspirin. May cause headache, dizziness, rash, anorexia, nausea, abdominal pain, vomiting, dyspepsia, and oligospermia. PB: 99%; t½: 5–7 h
Para-Chlorobenzoic Acid (Indoles)		
Indomethacin	Rheumatoid arthritis: Regular release: A: PO: 25 mg bid/tid with food; *max:* 200 mg/d Sustained release: A: PO: 75 mg/d; *max:* 150 mg/d	For mild to severe pain, acute gout, tendinitis, arthralgia, ankylosing spondylitis, and arthritis. May cause dizziness, headache, nausea, vomiting, constipation, dyspepsia, hyperkalemia, and hyponatremia. Take with food. Avoid if allergic to aspirin. PB: 99%; t½: 2.6–11.2 h
Sulindac	Rheumatoid arthritis: A: PO: 150–200 mg bid; *max:* 400 mg/d	For arthritis, bursitis, ankylosing spondylitis, gout, and tendinitis. May cause dizziness, headache, rash, dyspepsia, nausea, vomiting, diarrhea, abdominal pain, constipation, and elevated hepatic enzymes. Take with food or milk. PB: 93%; t½: 8 h
Etodolac	Arthritis: Regular release: A: PO: Initially 300 mg bid/tid; *maint:* 600–1200 mg/d; *max:* 1200 mg/d Extended release: A: PO: 400–1000 mg/d; *max:* 1200 mg/d	For mild to moderate pain, rheumatoid arthritis, and osteoarthritis. May cause dizziness, weakness, dyspepsia, nausea, diarrhea, abdominal pain, flatulence, and pyrosis. Take with food. PB: 99%; t½: 6–7 h
Propionic Acid		
Fenoprofen calcium	Rheumatoid arthritis: A: PO: Initially 400–600 mg tid/qid; *max:* 3200 mg/d	For mild to moderate pain, osteoarthritis, and rheumatoid arthritis. May cause drowsiness, dizziness, rash, headache, weakness, pruritus, dyspepsia, nausea, constipation, palpitations, tinnitus, and peripheral edema. Take with food. PB: 99%; t½: 2.5–3 h
Flurbiprofen sodium	Arthritis: A: PO: 200–300 mg/d in 2–4 divided doses; *max:* 300 mg/d, 100 mg/dose	For mild to moderate pain, osteoarthritis, and rheumatoid arthritis. May cause dizziness, blurred vision, insomnia, flatulence, abdominal pain, dyspepsia, nausea, diarrhea, constipation, and GI bleeding. Take with food. PB: 99%; t½: 3–9 h
Ibuprofen	See Prototype Drug Chart: Ibuprofen	

Continued

TABLE 24.2   Antiinflammatory Agents: Nonsteroidal—cont'd

Drug	Route and Dosage	Uses and Considerations
Ketoprofen	Arthritis: Immediate release: A: PO: Initially 50 mg qid or 75 mg tid (older A, initially 50 mg tid or 75 mg bid); *max:* 300 mg/d Extended release: A: PO: 200 mg/d; *max:* 200 mg/d Older A: PO: 100–150 mg/d; *max:* 200 mg/d	For mild to moderate pain, osteoarthritis, and rheumatoid arthritis. May cause headache, insomnia, nausea, dyspepsia, diarrhea, flatulence, abdominal pain, and constipation. PB: 99%; t½: immediate release, 0.9–3.3 h; extended release, 5.4 h
Naproxen	Rheumatoid arthritis: A: PO: 250–500 mg bid; *max:* 1500 mg/d Delayed release: A: PO: 375–500 mg bid; *max:* 1500 mg/d Controlled release: A: PO: Initially 750–1000 mg/d; *max:* 1500 mg/d	For mild to moderate pain, osteoarthritis, rheumatoid arthritis, ankylosing spondylitis, and gout. May cause dizziness, drowsiness, pharyngitis, dyspepsia, influenza, elevated hepatic enzymes, dyspnea, headache, nausea, vomiting, diarrhea, abdominal pain, constipation, flatulence, tinnitus, edema, and GI bleeding/perforation/ulcer. Take with food or with a full glass of water. PB: 99%; t½: 12–17 h
Oxaprozin	A: PO: 600–1200 mg/d based upon weight; *max:* 1800 mg/d	For osteoarthritis and rheumatoid arthritis. May cause edema, dizziness, drowsiness, confusion, headache, tinnitus, abdominal pain, dyspepsia, nausea, vomiting, constipation, diarrhea, or GI bleeding/perforation/ulcer. PB: 99%; t½: 41.4 h
Anthranilic Acids (Fenamates)		
Meclofenamate	Arthritis: A: PO: Initially 200–400 mg/d in 3–4 divided doses; *max:* 400 mg/d	For mild to moderate pain, dysmenorrhea, osteoarthritis, and rheumatoid arthritis. May cause dizziness, headache, rash, nausea, vomiting, diarrhea, abdominal pain, flatulence, and pyrosis. PB: 99%; t½: 2 h
Mefenamic acid	Pain: A: PO: Initially: 500 mg, then 250 mg q6h PRN for 7 d or less; *max:* 1250 mg/d	For mild to moderate pain and dysmenorrhea. May cause dizziness, headache, nausea, vomiting, abdominal pain, constipation, flatulence, diarrhea, dyspepsia, edema, tinnitus, and GI bleeding/perforation. PB: 90%; t½: 2 h
Oxicams		
Piroxicam	A: PO: 20 mg/d; *max:* 20 mg/d	For osteoarthritis and rheumatoid arthritis. May cause edema, dizziness, headache, rash, pruritus, anorexia, nausea, vomiting, diarrhea, constipation, flatulence, abdominal pain, tinnitus, and GI bleeding/perforation/ulcer. PB: 99%; t½: 50 h
Meloxicam	A: PO: 7.5–15 mg/d; *max:* 15 mg/d	For osteoarthritis and rheumatoid arthritis. May cause dizziness, headache, edema, dyspepsia, nausea, diarrhea, abdominal pain, eructation, arthralgia, and GI bleeding/perforation. PB: 99.4%; t½: 15–20 h
Naphthylalkanones		
Nabumetone	A: PO: 1000 mg/d or 500 mg bid; *max:* 2000 mg/d	For osteoarthritis and rheumatoid arthritis. May cause headache, dizziness, dyspepsia, nausea, vomiting, diarrhea, abdominal pain, constipation, tinnitus, flatulence, pruritus, rash, and edema. PB: 99%; t½: 24 h
Second-Generation NSAIDs		
COX-2 inhibitors		
Celecoxib	See Prototype Drug Chart: Celecoxib	
Miscellaneous		
Tolmetin	A: PO: Initially: 400 mg tid; *maint:* 600–1800 mg/d in divided doses; *max:* 1800 mg/d	For osteoarthritis, rheumatoid arthritis, and juvenile rheumatoid arthritis. May cause dizziness, headache, weakness, peripheral edema, weight loss/gain, hypertension, abdominal pain, nausea, vomiting, diarrhea, flatulence, and dyspepsia. Take with food. PB: 99%; t½: 1–2 h
Diclofenac sodium	Osteoarthritis: Immediate release: A: PO: 35–50 mg bid/tid; *max:* 150 mg/d Extended release: A: PO: 50–100 mg/d; *max:* 150 mg/d	For mild to severe pain, rheumatoid arthritis, osteoarthritis, migraine, and ankylosing spondylitis. May cause anemia, lacrimation, ocular hypertension/pain, xerophthalmia, blurred vision, keratitis, dermatitis, dyspepsia, vomiting, edema, and GI bleeding/perforation. Take with food. PB: 99%; t½: 2 h

TABLE 24.2   Antiinflammatory Agents: Nonsteroidal—cont'd

Drug	Route and Dosage	Uses and Considerations
Ketorolac tromethamine	Short-term pain: A >50 kg: PO: Initially 20 mg dose, then 10 mg q4–6h; *max:* 40 mg/d A <50 kg and Older A: PO: Initially 10 mg dose, then 10 mg q4–6h; *max:* 40 mg/d A >50 kg: IM/IV: 30 mg IV or 60 mg IM; *max:* 120 mg/d A <50 kg and Older A: IM/IV: 15 mg IV or 30 mg IM; *max:* 60 mg/d Nasal spray: A >50 kg: Intranasal: 1 spray (15.75 mg/spray) q6–8h each nostril; *max:* 4 doses/d A <50 kg and Older A: Intranasal: 1 spray q6–8h 1 nostril; *max:* 4 doses/d	For short-term moderate to severe pain management of 5 days or less and for ocular inflammation. First injectable NSAID. May cause drowsiness, dizziness, dyspepsia, nausea, vomiting, diarrhea, abdominal pain, flatulence, constipation, hypertension, diaphoresis, corneal edema, injection site reaction, GI bleeding/perforation, and ocular inflammation/pain. PB: 99%; t½: PO, 2.4–9 h; IM, 3.5–9.2 h

A, Adult; *bid,* twice a day; *COX,* cyclooxygenase; *d,* day; *GI,* gastrointestinal; *h,* hour; *IM,* intramuscular; *IV,* intravenous; *maint,* maintenance; *max,* maximum; *NSAID,* nonsteroidal antiinflammatory drug; *PB,* protein binding; *PO,* by mouth; *PRN,* as needed; *q12h,* every 12 hours; *qd,* every day; *qid,* four times a day; *t½,* half-life; *tid,* three times a day; *y,* year; *>,* greater than; *<,* less than.

Table 24.2 provides dosage information and considerations for use for the most commonly used NSAIDs. The half-lives of NSAIDs differ greatly; some have a short half-life of 2 hours, and others have a moderate to long half-life of 6 to 24 hours. Aspirin should not be taken with an NSAID because of the potentiation of side effects. In addition, combined therapy does not increase effectiveness.

Salicylates

Aspirin comes from the family of salicylates derived from salicylic acid. Aspirin is also called *acetylsalicylic acid (ASA)* after the acetyl group used in its composition.

Adolph Bayer developed aspirin in 1899, making it the oldest antiinflammatory agent. It was the most frequently used antiinflammatory agent before the introduction of ibuprofen. Aspirin is a prostaglandin inhibitor that decreases the inflammatory process. It is also considered an antiplatelet drug for patients with cardiac or cerebrovascular disorders; aspirin decreases platelet aggregation, and thus blood clotting is decreased. Because high doses of aspirin are usually needed to relieve inflammation, gastric distress—which includes anorexia, dyspepsia, nausea, vomiting, diarrhea, constipation, abdominal pain, heartburn, and flatulence—is a common problem. In such cases, enteric-coated (EC) tablets may be used. Aspirin should *not* be taken with other NSAIDs because it decreases the blood level and effectiveness of NSAIDs.

Aspirin and other NSAIDs relieve pain by inhibiting the COX enzyme, which is needed for the biosynthesis of prostaglandins. As mentioned earlier, the two enzyme forms of COX, COX-1 and COX-2 (Fig. 24.2), serve different purposes: COX-1 protects the stomach lining and regulates blood platelets, promoting blood clotting, whereas COX-2 triggers pain and inflammation at the injured site. NSAIDs usually inhibit or block *both* COX-1 and COX-2. Inhibition of COX-1 produces the desirable effect of decreasing platelet aggregation, but it has the undesirable effect of decreasing protection to the stomach lining; therefore stomach bleeding and ulcers may occur with aspirin and NSAID agents. When COX-2 is inhibited, pain and fever are reduced and inflammation is suppressed, but COX-2 inhibitors do *not* cause gastric ulceration, and they have no effect on platelet function.

Newer NSAIDs, called COX-2 inhibitors, block only COX-2 and not COX-1. These drugs leave protection for the stomach lining intact, so no gastric bleeding or ulcers result, but they still deliver relief for pain and inflammation.

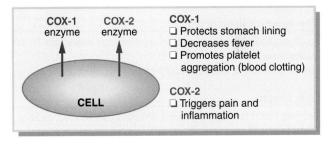

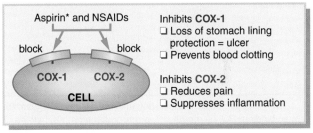

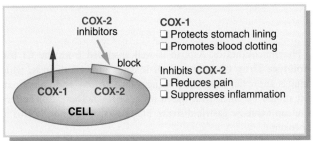

*Aspirin is only one of the NSAIDs.

Fig. 24.2 Uses of COX-1 and COX-2 inhibitors.

A COX-2 inhibitor approved by the US Food and Drug Administration (FDA) is celecoxib. Drugs similar to COX-2 inhibitors include meloxicam and nabumetone, which allow some stomach protection. Patients at risk for stroke or heart attack who take aspirin to prevent blood clotting (decreased platelet aggregation) would not benefit from COX-2 inhibitors. If the COX-1 enzyme were not blocked, increased blood clotting would remain even though the stomach lining is protected.

Many researchers believe that COX-2 inhibitors may prevent some types of cancer, such as colon cancer. Fruits and vegetables block the COX-2 enzyme naturally, protecting the colon from malignant growths.

PROTOTYPE DRUG CHART

Aspirin

Drug Class	Dosage
Analgesic: Antiinflammatory drug	Arthritis: A: PO: 325 or 650 mg q4h PRN; *max:* 3900 mg/d Toxic serum salicylate level: >300 mcg/mL

Contraindications	Drug-Lab-Food Interactions
Hypersensitivity to salicylates or NSAIDs *Caution:* Renal or hepatic disorders, gout, alcohol abuse, anticoagulant therapy, GI bleeding history, bone marrow suppression, head trauma, immunosuppression, pregnancy	Drug: Increased risk of bleeding with anticoagulants and other NSAIDs; increased risk of hypoglycemia with oral hypoglycemic drugs; increased ulcerogenic effect with glucocorticoids; decreased effects of ACE inhibitors, loop diuretics, and probenecid; effects are decreased by corticosteroids. Lab: Decreased cholesterol, potassium, T_3, and T_4 levels; increased uric acid, PT, and bleeding time

Pharmacokinetics	Pharmacodynamics
Absorption: PO: 80%–100% Distribution: PB: 20%–95%, crosses placenta Metabolism: t½: 15–20 min Excretion: 50% in urine	PO: Onset: 15–30 min Peak: 1–2 h Duration: 4–6 h

Therapeutic Effects/Uses

To reduce pain, inflammatory symptoms, fever; decrease inflammation for osteoarthritis and rheumatoid arthritis; and arterial thromboembolism, MI, TIA, stroke prophylaxis

Mechanism of Action: Inhibits prostaglandin synthesis, hypothalamic heat regulator center, and platelet aggregation

Side Effects	Adverse Reactions
Dizziness, headache, dyspepsia, nausea, abdominal pain, anorexia, confusion, diaphoresis, agitation, lethargy, gastritis, vomiting, pruritus, rash, and dehydration	Tinnitus, hearing loss, hypokalemia, hypernatremia, elevated hepatic enzymes, hypo/hyperglycemia, proteinuria, metabolic acidosis, cerebral edema, hyperuricemia, GI bleeding/ulceration/perforation, visual impairment, seizures, intracranial bleeding *Life-threatening:* Reye syndrome, angioedema, bronchospasm, agranulocytosis, hemolytic anemia, aplastic anemia, leukopenia, thrombocytopenia, pancytopenia, respiratory alkalosis, renal/hepatic failure, pulmonary edema, Stevens-Johnson syndrome

A, Adult; *ACE*, angiotensin-converting enzyme; *d*, day; *GI*, gastrointestinal; *h*, hour; *min*, minute; *NSAID*, nonsteroidal antiinflammatory drug; *PB*, protein binding; *PO*, by mouth; *PT*, prothrombin time; *t½*, half-life; T_3, triiodothyronine; T_4, thyroxine.

Pharmacokinetics. Aspirin is well absorbed from the GI tract (Prototype Drug Chart: Aspirin). It can cause GI distress, which includes anorexia, nausea, vomiting, diarrhea, and abdominal pain, so it should be taken with water, milk, or food. The EC or buffered form can decrease gastric distress. EC tablets should not be crushed or broken.

Aspirin has a short half-life. It should not be taken during the last trimester of pregnancy because it could cause premature closure of the ductus arteriosus in the fetus. Children with flu symptoms should not take aspirin because it may cause the potentially fatal Reye syndrome.

Pharmacodynamics. Like other NSAIDs, aspirin inhibits prostaglandin synthesis by inhibiting COX-1 and COX-2; thus it decreases inflammation and pain. The onset of action for aspirin is within 30 minutes. It peaks in 1 to 2 hours, and the duration of action is an average of 4 to 6 hours. The action for the rectal preparation of aspirin can be erratic because of blood supply and fecal material in the rectum; it may take a week or longer for a therapeutic antiinflammatory effect.

Hypersensitivity to Salicylate Products

Patients may be hypersensitive to aspirin. Tinnitus (ringing in the ears), vertigo (dizziness), and bronchospasm—especially in asthmatic patients—are symptoms of aspirin overdose or hypersensitivity to aspirin.

Salicylates are present in numerous foods such as prunes, raisins, and licorice, and in spices such as curry and paprika.

Para-Chlorobenzoic Acid

One of the first NSAIDs introduced was indomethacin, a *para*-chlorobenzoic acid. It is used for rheumatoid arthritis (RA), gouty arthritis, and osteoarthritis, and it is a potent prostaglandin inhibitor. It is highly protein bound (99%) and displaces other protein-bound drugs, resulting in potential toxicity. It has a moderate half-life (2.6 to

◎ CLINICAL JUDGMENT [NURSING PROCESS]

Salicylate: Aspirin

Concept: Inflammation
- An immunologic response of the body to injury or infection involving redness, swelling, warmth, and pain

Recognize Cues [Assessment]
- Determine a medical history. Ask the patient about previous gastric distress, gastric bleeding, or liver disease. Aspirin can cause gastric irritation, and it prolongs bleeding time by inhibiting platelet aggregation.
- Obtain a drug history. Report if a drug-drug interaction is probable.

Analyze Cues and Prioritize Hypothesis [Patient Problems]
- Acute pain
- Injury
- Nausea
- Reduced functional ability

Generate Solutions [Planning]
- The patient will report a pain level has decreased within 1 hour of medication administration.
- The patient's swelling and redness will be reduced.

Take Action [Nursing Interventions]
- Monitor serum salicylate (aspirin) level when a patient takes high doses of aspirin for chronic conditions such as arthritis. The normal therapeutic range is 15 to 30 mg/dL. Mild toxicity occurs at a serum level greater than 30 mg/dL, and severe toxicity occurs above 50 mg/dL.
- Observe the patient for signs of bleeding such as dark, tarry stools; bleeding gums; petechiae (round red spots); ecchymosis (excessive bruising); and purpura (large red spots) when the patient takes high doses of aspirin.

Patient Teaching
General

- Advise patients not to take aspirin with alcohol or with drugs that are highly protein bound, such as the anticoagulant warfarin. Aspirin displaces drugs like warfarin from the protein-binding site, causing increased anticoagulant levels.
- Suggest that patients inform their dentist before a dental visit if they are taking high doses of aspirin.
- Instruct patients to discontinue aspirin approximately 7 days before surgery to reduce risk of bleeding (with the health care provider's approval).
- Advise patients to keep aspirin bottles out of reach of children.
- ⚡ Educate parents to call the poison control center immediately if a child has taken a large or unknown amount of aspirin or acetaminophen.
- Instruct patient not to cut or break an enteric-coated (EC) aspirin tablet.
- ⚡ Warn patients not to administer aspirin for virus or flu symptoms in children. Reye syndrome (vomiting, lethargy, delirium, and coma) has been linked with aspirin and viral infections. Acetaminophen is usually prescribed for cold and flu symptoms.
- Inform patients that aspirin tablets can cause gastrointestinal (GI) distress.
- Inform patients with dysmenorrhea to take acetaminophen instead of aspirin 2 days before and during the first 2 days of the menstrual period.

Side Effects
- Direct patients to report side effects such as drowsiness, tinnitus (ringing in the ears), headaches, flushing, dizziness, GI distress, GI bleeding, visual changes, and seizures.

Diet
- Instruct patients to take aspirin and ibuprofen with food, at mealtime, or with plenty of fluids. EC aspirin helps prevent GI distress.

Evaluate Outcomes [Evaluation]
- Evaluate the effectiveness of aspirin in relieving pain. If pain persists, another analgesic such as ibuprofen may be prescribed.
- Determine whether the patient shows any of the side effects of aspirin.

11.2 hours). Indomethacin is very irritating to the stomach and should be taken with food.

Two other *para*-chlorobenzoic acid derivatives—sulindac and tolmetin—produce less severe adverse reactions than indomethacin. Tolmetin is also highly protein bound at 99% and has a short half-life of 1 to 2 hours. This group of NSAIDs may cause sodium and water retention and increased blood pressure.

Propionic Acid Derivatives

The propionic acid group is a relatively new group of NSAIDs. These drugs are aspirin-like but have stronger effects and create less GI irritation. Drugs in this group are highly protein bound, so drug interactions might occur, especially when given with another highly protein-bound drug. Propionic acid derivatives are better tolerated than other NSAIDs. Gastric upset occurs, but it is not as severe as with aspirin and indomethacin. Severe adverse reactions such as blood dyscrasias are not frequently seen. Ibuprofen is the most widely used propionic acid NSAID, and it may be purchased OTC in lower doses (200 mg). Prototype Drug Chart: Ibuprofen details the pharmacologic behavior of ibuprofen. Five other propionic acid agents are fenoprofen calcium, naproxen, ketoprofen, flurbiprofen, and oxaprozin.

Pharmacokinetics. Ibuprofens are well absorbed from the GI tract. These drugs have a short half-life but are highly protein bound. If ibuprofen is taken with another highly protein-bound drug, severe side effects may occur. The drug is metabolized in the liver to inactivate metabolites and is excreted as inactive metabolites in the urine.

Pharmacodynamics. Ibuprofen inhibits prostaglandin synthesis and is therefore effective in alleviating inflammation and pain. It has a short onset of action, peak concentration time, and duration of action. It may take several days for the antiinflammatory effect to be evident.

Many drug interactions are associated with ibuprofen. Because ibuprofen can increase the effects of warfarin, sulfonamides, many of the cephalosporins, and phenytoin, it should be avoided with these drugs. However, when taken with aspirin, its effect can be decreased. Hypoglycemia may result when ibuprofen is taken with insulin or an oral hypoglycemic drug, and risk of toxicity is high when ibuprofen is taken concurrently with calcium channel blockers.

Fenamates

The fenamate group includes potent NSAIDs used for acute and chronic arthritic conditions. Fenamates decrease prostaglandin synthesis by inhibition of COX-1 and COX-2. As with most NSAIDs, gastric

PROTOTYPE DRUG CHART

Ibuprofen

Drug Class	Dosage
NSAID: Propionic acid derivative	Rheumatoid arthritis: A: PO: 400–800 mg tid/qid; *max:* 3200 mg/d

Contraindications	Drug-Lab-Food Interactions
Hypersensitivity, coronary artery bypass graft surgery *Caution:* Bleeding disorders, cardiac disease, dysrhythmias, pregnancy, lactation, systemic lupus erythematosus, asthma, peptic ulcer, anticoagulant therapy, dehydration, Crohn disease, renal or hepatic disease, alcohol use disorder, GI bleeding/perforation, bone marrow suppression, ulcerative colitis, older adults	Drug: Increased bleeding time with oral anticoagulants; increased effects of phenytoin, sulfonamides, warfarin; decreased effect with aspirin; may increase severe side effects of lithium

Pharmacokinetics	Pharmacodynamics
Absorption: PO: Well absorbed Distribution: PB: 99% Metabolism: t½: 1.7–2.5 h Excretion: In urine, mostly as inactive metabolites; some in bile	PO: Onset: 30 min–1 h Peak: 2–4 h Duration: 6–8 h

Therapeutic Effects/Uses

To reduce inflammatory process; to relieve pain; antiinflammatory effect for arthritic conditions; to reduce fever, dysmenorrhea, headache
Mechanism of Action: Inhibits COX-1 and COX-2 by blocking arachidonate binding, thus relieving pain and inflammation

Side Effects	Adverse Reactions
Headache, dizziness, blurred vision, drowsiness, dyspepsia, pyrosis, nausea, vomiting, constipation, diarrhea, abdominal pain, flatulence, edema, rash, pruritus, fluid retention	Hearing loss, GI bleeding/perforation/ulcer, tinnitus, seizure *Life-threatening:* Anaphylaxis, angioedema, anemia, neutropenia, hemolytic anemia, aplastic anemia, agranulocytosis, thrombocytopenia, pancytopenia, renal failure, Stevens-Johnson syndrome

A, Adult; *d,* day; *h,* hour; *max,* maximum; *min,* minute; *NSAID,* nonsteroidal antiinflammatory drug; *PB,* protein binding; *PO,* by mouth; *qid,* four times a day; *t½,* half-life; *tid,* three times a day.

irritation is a common side effect; patients with a history of peptic ulcer should avoid taking fenamates. Other side effects include edema, dizziness, tinnitus, and pruritus. Two fenamates are meclofenamate sodium monohydrate and mefenamic acid.

Oxicams

Piroxicam and meloxicam, oxicams, are indicated for long-term arthritic conditions such as RA and osteoarthritis. Oxicams decrease prostaglandin synthesis by inhibition of COX-1 and COX-2. They too can cause gastric problems such as ulceration and epigastric distress, but the incidence is lower than for some other NSAIDs. Oxicams are well tolerated, and their major advantage over other NSAIDs is their long half-life, which allows them to be taken only once daily.

Full clinical response to piroxicam may take 1 to 2 weeks. This drug is also highly protein bound and may interact with another highly protein-bound drug when taken together. Piroxicam should *not* be taken with aspirin or other NSAIDs.

General Side Effects and Adverse Reactions With First-Generation NSAIDs

Most NSAIDs tend to have fewer side effects than aspirin when taken at antiinflammatory doses, but gastric irritation is still a common problem when NSAIDs are taken without food. In addition,

sodium and water retention may occur. Alcoholic beverages consumed with NSAIDs may increase gastric irritation and should be avoided.

 COMPLEMENTARY AND ALTERNATIVE THERAPIES

Nonsteroidal Antiinflammatory Drugs

Dong quai, feverfew, garlic, ginger, and ginkgo may cause bleeding when taken with nonsteroidal antiinflammatory drugs (NSAIDs).

Selective COX-2 Inhibitors

Cyclooxygenase-2 (COX-2) inhibitors, second-generation NSAIDs, became available in the past several years to decrease inflammation and pain. Most NSAIDs are nonselective inhibitors that inhibit COX-1 and COX-2. By inhibiting COX-1, protection of the stomach lining is decreased, and clotting time is also decreased, which may benefit the patient with cardiovascular or coronary artery disease (CAD). Selective COX-2 inhibitors are the drugs of choice for patients with severe arthritic conditions who need high doses of an antiinflammatory drug, because large doses of NSAIDs may cause peptic ulcer and gastric bleeding.

◎ CLINICAL JUDGMENT [NURSING PROCESS]

Nonsteroidal Antiinflammatory Drug (NSAID): Ibuprofen

Concept: Inflammation
- An immunologic response of the body to injury or infection involving redness, swelling, warmth, and pain

Recognize Cues [Assessment]
- Check the patient's history for allergy to NSAIDs such as ibuprofen. If an allergy is present, notify the health care provider.
- Obtain a drug and herbal history, and report any possible drug-drug or herb-drug interactions. NSAIDs can increase the effects of phenytoin, sulfonamides, and warfarin. Most NSAIDs are highly protein bound and can displace other highly protein-bound drugs like warfarin.
- Determine the medical history. NSAIDs are contraindicated if a patient has severe renal or liver disease, peptic ulcer, or bleeding disorder.
- Assess for gastrointestinal (GI) distress and peripheral edema, which are common side effects of NSAIDs.

Analyze Cues and Prioritize Hypothesis [Patient Problems]
- Acute pain
- Injury
- Nausea
- Reduced functional ability
- Decreased mobility

Generate Solutions [Planning]
- The patient will report a pain level has decreased within 1 hour of medication administration.
- The patient's swelling and redness will be reduced within 1 week.

Take Action [Nursing Interventions]
- Observe the patient for bleeding gums, petechiae, ecchymoses, or black, tarry stools. Bleeding time can be prolonged when NSAIDs are taken, especially with a highly protein-bound drug such as warfarin (anticoagulant).
- Report if a patient has GI discomfort. Administer NSAIDs at mealtime or with food to prevent GI upset.
- Monitor vital signs and check for peripheral edema, especially in the morning.

- Do not give directions such as "take one blue pill" at a specified time. Instead, provide the name and the dosage of medications.

Patient Teaching
General
- ⚡ Advise patients not to take aspirin and acetaminophen with NSAIDs. Taking an NSAID with aspirin could cause GI upset and possibly GI bleeding.
- Advise patients to avoid alcohol when taking NSAIDs. GI distress or gastric ulcer may result.
- Alert patients that many complementary and alternative therapy products may interact with NSAIDs and could cause bleeding. Doses of NSAIDs and/or herbs may need to be modified to avoid possible bleeding.
- Direct patients to inform the dentist or surgeon before a procedure if they are taking ibuprofen or other NSAIDs for a continuous period.
- Warn female patients not to take NSAIDs 1 to 2 days before menstruation to avoid heavy menstrual flow. If discomfort occurs, acetaminophen is usually prescribed.
- ⚡ Advise pregnant patients to avoid NSAIDs. Congenital abnormalities may occur when NSAIDS are taken during early pregnancy, and excess bleeding might occur during delivery.
- Inform patients that it may take several weeks to experience the desired drug effect of some NSAIDs and disease-modifying antirheumatic drugs (DMARDs).

Side Effects
- Educate patients about the common side effects of NSAIDs. GI distress, peripheral edema, purpura or petechiae, and dizziness can occur. Report occurrences of side effects.

Diet
- Advise patients to take NSAIDs with meals or snacks to reduce GI distress.

Evaluate Outcomes [Evaluation]
- Evaluate the effectiveness of the drug therapy, such as a decrease in pain and in swollen joints and an increase in mobility.

Currently, only one drug, celecoxib, is classified as a COX-2 inhibitor. Nabumetone and meloxicam are similar drugs that can be used; however, they are not considered true COX-2 inhibitors, although they do inhibit COX-2 more than COX-1. Celecoxib is described in Prototype Drug Chart: Celecoxib.

Use of NSAIDs in Older Adults

Older adults frequently use NSAIDs to treat pain associated with inflammation caused by osteoarthritis, RA, and neuromuscular-skeletal disorders. As older adults age, the number of drugs taken daily increases; therefore drug interactions are more common, especially when numerous drugs are taken with NSAIDs. With the use of NSAIDs, GI distress—including ulceration—is four times more common in older adults, and hospitalization is often necessary.

The introduction of COX-2 inhibitors (second-generation NSAIDs) has decreased the incidence of GI problems associated with NSAID use; however, edema is likely to occur. Renal function should be evaluated, and older adults should increase their fluid intake for adequate hydration. To decrease possible complications, the NSAID dose should be lowered.

CORTICOSTEROIDS

Corticosteroids such as prednisone, prednisolone, and dexamethasone are frequently used as antiinflammatory agents. This group of drugs controls inflammation by suppressing or preventing many of the components of the inflammatory process at the injured site. Corticosteroids have been widely prescribed for arthritic conditions, and although they are not the drug of choice for arthritis because of their numerous side effects, they are frequently used to control arthritic flare-ups.

The half-life of a corticosteroid is long (>24 hours), and it is administered once a day in a large prescribed dose. When discontinuing long-term steroid therapy, the dosage should be tapered over a period of 5 to 10 days. Steroids are discussed in more detail in Chapter 46.

DISEASE-MODIFYING ANTIRHEUMATIC DRUGS

When NSAIDs do not control immune-mediated arthritic disease sufficiently, other drugs, although more toxic, can be prescribed to alter the disease process. The disease-modifying antirheumatic drugs (DMARDs) include immunosuppressive agents, immunomodulators, and antimalarials. DMARDs help alleviate the symptoms of RA

📄 PROTOTYPE DRUG CHART

Celecoxib

Drug Class	Dosage
Nonsteroidal antiinflammatory: COX-2 inhibitor	Arthritis: A: PO: 100 mg bid or 200 mg qd; *max:* 800 mg/d, older adult 400 mg/d

Contraindications	Drug-Lab-Food Interactions
Hypersensitivity, coronary artery bypass surgery *Caution:* Renal or hepatic dysfunction, angina, hypertension, dysrhythmias, heart failure, cardiac disease, dehydration, peptic ulcer disease, GI bleeding/perforation, anticoagulant therapy, alcohol abuse, peripheral vascular disease, older adults	Drug: Decreased effect of ACE inhibitors; increased INR and GI bleeding with warfarin and SNRIs; may increase toxicity with lithium; fluoroquinolones may increase the risk of seizures; fluconazole and ketoconazole increase celecoxib levels Complementary and alternative therapies: Ginkgo biloba may increase bleeding risk

Pharmacokinetics	Pharmacodynamics
Absorption: Well absorbed in GI tract Distribution: PB: 97% Metabolism: t½: 11.2 h Excretion: Primarily in feces	PO: Onset: UK Peak: 3 h Duration: UK

Therapeutic Effects/Uses	
To treat osteoarthritis and rheumatoid arthritis; to relieve dysmenorrhea and moderate to severe pain; for ankylosing spondylitis, migraine Mechanism of Action: Inhibits COX-2, which normally promotes prostaglandin synthesis and inflammatory response, but does not inhibit COX-1	

Side Effects	Adverse Reactions
Headache, dizziness, drowsiness, sinusitis, pharyngitis, cough, anorexia, abdominal pain, nausea, dyspepsia, flatulence, vomiting, diarrhea, constipation, infection, arthralgia, peripheral edema, rash	GI bleeding/obstruction/ulcer/perforation, hypertension, hearing loss, dyspnea, tendon rupture, hypo-hypernatremia, tinnitus, thromboembolism *Life-threatening:* Anaphylaxis, angioedema, bronchospasm, renal/hepatic failure, aplastic anemia, agranulocytosis, leukopenia, pancytopenia, thrombocytopenia, Stevens-Johnson syndrome

A, Adult; *ACE,* angiotensin-converting enzyme; *bid,* twice a day; *COX,* cyclooxygenase; *d,* day; *GI,* gastrointestinal; *h,* hour; *INR,* international normalized ratio; *max,* maximum; *PB,* protein binding; *PO,* by mouth; *qd,* every day; *SNRI,* serotonin norepinephrine reuptake inhibitor; *t½,* half-life; *UK,* unknown.

for the 2 million persons in the United States affected by the disorder. DMARDs are described in Table 24.3. Other indications for use of DMARDs include osteoarthritis, psoriatic arthritis, severe psoriasis, ankylosing spondylitis, Crohn disease, and ulcerative colitis.

Immunosuppressive Agents

Immunosuppressives are used to treat refractory RA, arthritis that does not respond to antiinflammatory drugs. In low doses, selected immunosuppressive agents have been effective in the treatment of RA. Drugs such as azathioprine, cyclophosphamide, and methotrexate—primarily used to suppress cancer growth and proliferation—might be used to suppress the inflammatory process of RA when other treatments fail. In one study of patients receiving cyclophosphamide, few new erosions of joint cartilage were present, suggesting that the disease process was not active.

Immunomodulators

Immunomodulators treat moderate to severe RA by disrupting the inflammatory process and delaying disease progression. Interleukin 1 (IL-1) receptor antagonists and tumor necrosis factor (TNF) blockers are two groups of drugs classified as immunomodulators.

Anakinra, an IL-1 receptor antagonist, blocks activity of IL-1 by inhibiting it from binding to interleukin receptors located in cartilage and bone. IL-1 is a proinflammatory cytokine that contributes to synovial inflammation and joint destruction. Anakinra is administered subcutaneously. The peak is 3 to 7 hours, and the half-life is 4 to 6 hours.

TNF blockers bind to TNF and block it from attaching to TNF receptors on synovial cell surfaces. By neutralizing TNF, a contributor to synovitis, the inflammatory disease process is delayed. Etanercept was the first TNF blocker developed. It is administered subcutaneously, and the half-life ranges from 72 to 132 hours. Signs and symptoms of RA are suppressed rapidly with etanercept therapy but reappear if the drug is discontinued. Other TNF blockers include infliximab, adalimumab, and leflunomide. Infliximab is administered intravenously over at least 2 hours, adalimumab is administered subcutaneously, and leflunomide is administered orally. Infliximab is described in Prototype Drug Chart: Infliximab.

Both IL-1 receptor antagonists and TNF blockers predispose the patient to severe infections; they are contraindicated in active infection and should be discontinued when an infection occurs. Immunomodulators are usually very expensive.

TABLE 24.3 Antiinflammatory Drugs: Disease-Modifying Antirheumatic Drugs

Drug	Route and Dosage	Uses and Considerations
Golimumab	Rheumatoid arthritis: A: Subcut: 50 mg every month A: IV: 2 mg/kg over 30 min, repeat after 4 wk, then q8wk	For RA, psoriatic arthritis, ankylosing spondylitis, and ulcerative colitis. May cause injection site reaction, antibody development, hypertension, elevated hepatic enzymes, influenza, and infection. PB: UK; t½: 2 wk
Anakinra	Rheumatoid arthritis: A: Subcut: 100 mg/d; *max:* 100 mg/d	For RA and COVID-19. May cause injection-site reaction, headache, fever, nausea, vomiting, diarrhea, abdominal pain, arthralgia, pharyngitis, sinusitis, antibody formation, and infection. PB: UK; t½: 4–6 h
Etanercept	Psoriasis: A: Subcut: 50 mg twice weekly for 3 months, then 50 mg/wk; *max:* 100 mg/wk	For RA, psoriatic arthritis, psoriasis, and ankylosing spondylitis. May cause injection site reaction, antibody formation, diarrhea, pharyngitis, rash, sinusitis, influenza, and infection. PB: UK; t½: 72–132 h
Infliximab	See Prototype Drug Chart: Infliximab	
Rituximab	Rheumatoid arthritis: A: IV: 1000 mg on day 1 and day 15, then q24wk	For RA, lymphocytic leukemia, and non-Hodgkin lymphoma. May cause antibody formation, headache, depression, fever, chills, peripheral edema, anemia, nausea, diarrhea, abdominal pain, alopecia, dizziness, angioedema, peripheral neuropathy, infection, and weakness. PB: UK; t½: 5.17–77.5 d
Adalimumab	Rheumatoid arthritis: A: Subcut: 40 mg q2wk; *max:* 40 mg/wk or 80 mg q2wk	For RA, psoriatic arthritis, Crohn disease, ulcerative colitis, psoriasis, and ankylosing spondylitis. May cause injection site reaction, headache, nausea, abdominal pain, infection, rash, sinusitis, and antibody formation. PB: UK; t½: 10–20 d
Leflunomide	A: PO: LD:100 mg/d for 3 d; *maint:* 10–20 mg/d	For RA. May cause hypertension, dizziness, headache, alopecia, rash, abdominal pain, weakness, back pain, elevated hepatic enzymes, dyspepsia, nausea, diarrhea and infection. PB: 99%; t½: 18–19 d
Abatacept	Rheumatoid arthritis: A >100 kg: IV: 1 g over 30 min q2wk for 3 doses, then 1 g q4wk A 60–100 kg: IV: 750 mg over 30 min q2wk for 3 doses, then q4wk A <60 kg: IV: 500 mg over 30 min q2wk for 3 doses, then q4wk A: Subcut: 125 mg/wk	For RA and psoriatic arthritis. May cause dizziness, headache, diarrhea, pharyngitis, sinusitis, antibody formation, infection, hypo/hypertension, influenza, and infusion-related reaction. PB: UK; t½: 14.3 d
Tofacitinib	Immediate release: A: PO: 5 mg bid; *max:* 10 mg bid Extended release: A: PO: 11 mg/d; *max:* 11 mg/d	For RA, psoriatic arthritis, and ulcerative colitis. May cause headache, nausea, diarrhea, gastritis, pharyngitis, infection, anemia, and rash. PB: 40%; t½: 3 h immediate release, 6–8 h extended release
Tocilizumab	A: IV: Initially 4 mg/kg over 1 h q4wk; *max:* 800 mg/dose A <100 kg: Subcut: 162 mg q2wk A >100 kg: Subcut: 162 mg/wk	For RA and juvenile idiopathic arthritis. May cause infusion/injection-related reaction, headache, hyperlipidemia, elevated hepatic enzymes, neutropenia, infection, pharyngitis, constipation, and hypertension. PB: UK; t½: subcut 5–13 d; IV, 11–13 d
Secukinumab	Psoriasis: A: Subcut: 300 mg wk 0–4, followed by 300 mg q4wk; *max:* 300 mg/dose	For psoriasis, psoriatic arthritis, and ankylosing spondylitis. May cause oral ulceration, neutropenia, infection, pharyngitis, rhinitis, and antibody formation. PB: UK; t½: 22–31 d
Apremilast	Psoriatic arthritis: A: PO: Initially 10 mg in the morning; day 2, 10 mg bid; day 3, 10 mg in morning and 20 mg in evening; day 4, 20 mg bid; day 5, 20 mg in morning and 30 mg in evening; *maint:* 30 mg bid starting on day 6; *max:* 60 mg/d	For psoriatic arthritis and psoriasis. May cause headache, abdominal pain, nausea, vomiting, diarrhea, weight loss, and infection. PB: 68%; t½: 6–9 h
Canakinumab	Adol/C >2 y >7.5 kg: Subcut: 4 mg/kg q4wk; *max:* 300 mg/dose A: Subcut: 4 mg/kg q4wk; *max:* 300 mg/dose	For systemic juvenile idiopathic arthritis. May cause headache, injection-site reaction, nausea, abdominal pain, diarrhea, weight gain, musculoskeletal pain, pharyngitis, rhinitis, influenza, and infection. PB: UK; t½: 26 d
Sarilumab	A: Subcut: 200 mg q2wk; reduce dose to 150 mg q2wk to manage elevated hepatic enzymes, neutropenia, and thrombocytopenia	For moderate to severe rheumatoid arthritis and COVID-19. May cause elevated hepatic enzymes, antibody formation, erythema, infection, pruritus, neutropenia, thrombocytopenia, injection site reaction, and hypercholesterolemia. PB: UK; t½: 8–43 d depending upon concentration

Continued

TABLE 24.3   Antiinflammatory Drugs: Disease-Modifying Antirheumatic Drugs—cont'd

Drug	Route and Dosage	Uses and Considerations
Ixekizumab	Psoriatic arthritis: A: Subcut: LD: 160 mg/wk, then 80 mg q4wk	For psoriatic arthritis and plaque psoriasis. May cause antibody formation, infection, injection site reaction, neutropenia, influenza, ocular infection, conjunctivitis, and nausea. PB: UK; t½: 13 d
Certolizumab pegol	Rheumatoid arthritis: A: Subcut: Two 200 mg on wk 0, 2, 4; then 200 mg q2wk or 400 mg q4wk	For Crohn disease, rheumatoid arthritis, psoriatic arthritis, ankylosing spondylitis, and plaque psoriasis. Should be given as monotherapy or concomitantly with nonbiological disease-modifying antirheumatic drugs. May cause antibody formation, infection, arthralgia, back pain, headache, hypertension, rash, pharyngitis, fatigue, and cough. PB: UK; t½: 14 d
Baricitinib	Rheumatoid arthritis: A: PO: 2 mg/d	For RA and COVID-19. May cause infection, nausea, and elevated hepatic enzymes. PB: 45%; t½: 12 h
Upadacitinib	A: PO: 15 mg/d	For RA. May cause infection, cough, nausea, lymphopenia, neutropenia, and elevated hepatic enzymes. PB: 52%; t½: 8–14 h

A, Adult; *bid*, twice daily; *d*, day; *GI*, gastrointestinal; *h*, hour; *IV*, intravenous; *maint*, maintenance; *max*, maximum; *min*, minute; *PB*, protein binding; *PO*, by mouth; *q2*, every two; *RA*, rheumatoid arthritis; *Subcut*, subcutaneous; *t½*, half-life; *UK*, unknown; *wk*, week; *y*, year; *>*, greater than.

📄 PROTOTYPE DRUG CHART

Infliximab

Drug Class	Dosage
Immunomodulator: Tumor necrosis factor blocker	Rheumatoid arthritis: A: IV: Initially 3 mg/kg over 2 h on wk 0, 2, and 6; *maint:* 3 mg/kg q8wk; *max:* 10 mg/kg/dose q4wk Crohn disease: A: IV: Initially 5 mg/kg over 2 h on wk 0, 2, and 6; *maint:* 5–10 mg/kg q8wk; *max:* 10 mg/kg/dose

Contraindications	Drug-Lab-Food Interactions
Hypersensitivity *Caution:* Hepatic dysfunction, bone marrow suppression, diabetes mellitus, COPD, heart failure, immunosuppression, multiple sclerosis, seizures, corticosteroid therapy, infection, leukopenia	Drug: May decrease effectiveness of vaccines; concurrent immunosuppressives may increase risk for infection or adverse effects

Pharmacokinetics	Pharmacodynamics
Absorption: UK Distribution: UK Metabolism: t½: 8–9.5 d Excretion: UK	IV: Onset: RA: 3–7 d; Crohn disease: 1–2 wk Peak: UK Duration: RA: 6–12 wk; Crohn disease 8–48 wk

Therapeutic Effects/Uses

To treat psoriasis, rheumatoid arthritis, psoriatic arthritis, ankylosing spondylitis, ulcerative colitis, and Crohn disease
Mechanism of Action: Binds to TNF and blocks it from attaching to TNF receptors on synovial cell surfaces; reduces infiltration of inflammatory cells and delays inflammatory process

Side Effects	Adverse Reactions
Headache, dizziness, cough, fatigue, chills, flushing, fever, nausea, dyspepsia, diarrhea, constipation, abdominal pain, hyperhidrosis, weight loss, edema, dehydration, rash, pharyngitis, visual impairment, arthralgia, myalgia, sinusitis, candidiasis, infusion related reaction, phlebitis	Severe infections, hypo/hypertension, chest pain, dyspnea, seizures, bone fractures, anemia, pulmonary edema, bradycardia, GI obstruction, antibody formation, elevated hepatic enzymes *Life-threatening:* Bronchospasm, leukopenia, neutropenia, pancytopenia, hemolytic anemia, thrombocytopenia, hepatotoxicity, Stevens-Johnson syndrome

A, Adult; *COPD*, chronic obstructive pulmonary disease; *d*, day; *h*, hour; *IV*, intravenous; *maint*, maintenance; *max*, maximum; *RA*, rheumatoid arthritis; *q8*, every 8; *t½*, half-life; *TNF*, tumor necrosis factor; *UK*, unknown; *wk*, week.

CLINICAL JUDGMENT [NURSING PROCESS]

Disease-Modifying Antirheumatic Drug: Infliximab

Concept: Inflammation
- An immunologic response of the body to injury or infection involving redness, swelling, warmth, and pain

Recognize Cues [Assessment]
- Determine a medical history. Ask patient if there is any history of seizures, diabetes mellitus, multiple sclerosis, or kidney or liver disease. Infliximab may increase the risk of bleeding time.
- Obtain baseline complete blood count (CBC) and renal and liver function tests.

Analyze Cues and Prioritize Hypothesis [Patient Planning]
- Acute pain
- Injury
- Nausea
- Reduced functional ability
- Decreased mobility

Generate Solutions [Planning]
- The patient will report that pain level has decreased within 1 hour of medication administration.
- The patient's swelling and redness will be reduced within 1 week.

Take Action [Nursing Interventions]
- Obtain a negative tuberculosis skin test before initiating infliximab therapy.
- Monitor patients for signs and symptoms of infection. If a serious infection occurs while a patient is receiving infliximab therapy, antibiotic therapy should be initiated, and infliximab should be discontinued.
- Monitor laboratory tests for blood dyscrasias (CBC) and renal and liver function (blood urea nitrogen [BUN], serum creatinine, alkaline phosphatase [ALP], aspartate aminotransferase [AST], alanine aminotransferase [ALT]).
- Flush intravenous (IV) tubing with normal saline before and after administration. Deliver IV medication through a 1.2-micron or smaller filter.
- Administer each dose over a minimum of 2 hours.
- Discontinue IV dose of infliximab if the patient develops acute infusion reaction (e.g., chest pain, fever, chills, dyspnea, pruritus, urticaria, hypotension, or hypertension).
- Monitor patients up to 2 hours after infusion for acute infusion reaction.

Patient Teaching
General
- Encourage patients to keep medical appointments and to have regularly scheduled laboratory tests that include CBC and renal and liver function tests for early detection of blood dyscrasias and renal and liver damage.
- Advise patients to avoid live vaccines while taking infliximab.

Side Effects
- Teach patients to report dizziness, chills, depression, dyspnea, severe infections, seizures, fatigue, or rash immediately.
- Teach patients to report severe infections immediately.

Evaluate Outcomes [Evaluation]
- Evaluate patient response to the disease-modifying antirheumatic drug (DMARD). If pain persists, the drug regimen may need modification.
- Determine the presence of adverse reactions. Drug therapy for pain may need to be changed.

Antimalarials

Antimalarial drugs may be used to treat RA when other methods of treatment fail. The mechanism of action of antimalarials in suppressing RA is unclear. The effect may take 4 to 12 weeks to become apparent. Antimalarials are usually used in combination with NSAIDs in patients whose arthritis is not under control.

ANTIGOUT DRUGS

Gout is an inflammatory condition that attacks joints, tendons, and other tissues. It may be called *gouty arthritis*. The most common site of acute gouty inflammation is at the joint of the hallux (big toe). Gout is characterized by a uric acid metabolism disorder and a defect in purine (products of certain proteins) metabolism, which results in an increase in urates (uric acid salts) and an accumulation of uric acid (hyperuricemia) or an ineffective clearance of uric acid by the kidneys. Uric acid solubility is poor in acid urine, and urate crystals may form, causing urate calculi. Gout may appear as bumps, or *tophi*, in the subcutaneous tissue of earlobes, elbows, hands, and at the base of the great toe. In addition to tophi, the complications of untreated or prolonged periods of gout include gouty arthritis, urinary calculi, and gouty nephropathy.

To promote uric acid excretion and to prevent renal calculi, fluid intake should be increased while taking antigout drugs. Foods high in purine—such as organ meats, sardines, salmon, gravy, herring, liver, and meat soups—and alcohol, especially beer, should be avoided. Alcohol causes both an overproduction and underexcretion of uric acid. To reduce acidity, acetaminophen should be taken for discomfort instead of aspirin (salicylic acid).

Antiinflammatory Gout Drug: Colchicine

The first drug used to treat gout was colchicine, introduced in 1936. This antiinflammatory gout drug inhibits the migration of leukocytes to the inflamed site. It is effective in alleviating acute symptoms of gout, but it is not effective for decreasing inflammation that occurs in other inflammatory disorders. Colchicine does not inhibit uric acid synthesis and does not promote uric acid excretion. It should not be used if the patient has a severe renal, cardiac, or GI problem. Gastric irritation is a common problem, so colchicine should be taken with food. With high doses, nausea, vomiting, diarrhea, or abdominal pain occurs in approximately 75% of patients taking the drug.

Colchicine is well absorbed in the GI tract, and its peak concentration time is within 2 hours. Most of the drug is excreted in the feces, but 10% to 20% is excreted in the urine.

Xanthine Oxidase Inhibitors

Allopurinol, first marketed in 1963, is *not* an antiinflammatory drug; instead, it increases uric acid excretion in the urine by inhibiting the xanthine oxidase enzyme, which blocks metabolism of xanthine to uric acid. It also reduces uric acid production, preventing the precipitation of an attack. This drug is frequently used as a prophylactic to prevent gout, and it is a drug of choice for patients with chronic tophaceous gout. Allopurinol is also indicated for gout patients with renal impairment. It is useful for patients who have renal obstructions caused by uric acid stones and for patients with blood disorders such as leukemia and polycythemia vera. It is also given to patients who do not respond well to uricosuric drugs such as probenecid.

Increased fluid intake is recommended to promote diuresis and alkalinization of the urine.

Febuxostat was FDA approved in 2009 for the treatment of hyperuricemia associated with gout. This drug is more selective for xanthine oxidase than allopurinol. Febuxostat may cause gout exacerbations as allopurinol does. It has a greater risk of promoting cardiovascular adverse events. Febuxostat is eliminated by both hepatic and renal pathways.

Prototype Drug Chart: Febuxostat presents the pharmacologic behavior of febuxostat, another uric acid biosynthesis inhibitor.

Pharmacokinetics. The half-life of febuxostat is 5 to 8 hours. The protein-binding percentage is 99.2%. Approximately 49% is excreted in urine and 45% in feces.

Pharmacodynamics. Febuxostat inhibits the production of uric acid by inhibiting the enzyme xanthine oxidase, which is needed in the synthesis of uric acid. Its onset of action is unknown; its peak time averages 1 to 1.5 hours. The duration of action of febuxostat is unknown.

Uricosurics

Uricosurics increase the rate of uric acid excretion by inhibiting its reabsorption. These drugs are effective in alleviating chronic gout, but they should not be used during acute attacks. Probenecid is a uricosuric that has been available since 1945. It blocks the reabsorption of uric acid and promotes its excretion. Probenecid can be taken with colchicine. To begin initial therapy for relieving symptoms of gout and inhibiting uric acid reabsorption, small doses of colchicine should be given before adding probenecid. If gastric irritation occurs, probenecid should be taken with meals. It has an average half-life of 3 to 12 hours and is 75% to 95% protein bound. Table 24.4 gives dosages and considerations for the commonly used antigout drugs.

📋 PROTOTYPE DRUG CHART

Febuxostat

Drug Class	Dosage
Antigout: Xanthine oxidase inhibitor	A: PO: Initially 40 mg/d; 40–80 mg/d; *max:* 120 mg/d

Contraindications	Drug-Lab-Food Interactions
Hypersensitivity *Caution:* Hepatic/renal disorder, cardiac disease, stroke, chemotherapy	Drug: Increased effect of theophylline, azathioprine, didanosine, mercaptopurine, pegloticase Lab: Increased AST, ALT, BUN

Pharmacokinetics	Pharmacodynamics
Absorption: PO: 49% absorbed Distribution: PB: 99.2% Metabolism: t½: 5–8 h Excretion: 49% in urine and 45% in feces	PO: Onset: UK Peak: 1–1.5 h Duration: UK

Therapeutic Effects/Uses

To treat gout and hyperuricemia

Mechanism of Action: Blocks hypoxanthine and xanthine metabolism to reduce uric acid synthesis to decrease uric acid blood and urine concentrations

Side Effects	Adverse Reactions
Dizziness, headache, blurred vision, anorexia, dry mouth, dysgeusia, abdominal pain, nausea, dyspepsia, vomiting, diarrhea, constipation, arthralgia, myalgia, weakness, edema, dehydration, rash, pruritus, erectile dysfunction	Bradycardia, gout exacerbations, Guillain-Barre syndrome, dyspnea, chest pain, diabetes mellitus, hyperglycemia, anemia, elevated hepatic enzymes, hyperlipidemia, hypertriglyceridemia, hypercholesterolemia, cholecystitis, rhabdomyolysis *Life-threatening:* Thrombocytopenia, neutropenia, leukopenia, pancytopenia, angioedema, hepatic/renal impairment, dysrhythmias, Stevens-Johnson syndrome

A, Adult; *ALT,* alanine aminotransferase; *AST,* aspartate aminotransferase; *BUN,* blood urea nitrogen; *d,* day; *h,* hour; *max,* maximum; *PB,* protein binding; *PO,* by mouth; *t½,* half-life; *UK,* unknown.

TABLE 24.4 Antigout Drugs

Drug	Route and Dosage	Uses and Considerations
Antiinflammatory Gout Drugs		
Colchicine	Acute gout attack: A: PO: Initially 1.2 mg; then 0.6 mg in 1 h; *max:* 1.8 mg over 1-h period Prophylaxis: A: PO: 0.6 mg qd/bid; *max:* 1.2 mg/d	For gout. Not for patients with renal or gastric disorders. May cause headache, nausea, vomiting, diarrhea, fatigue, and peripheral neuropathy. Take with food. PB: 34%–44%; t½: 1.7–31.2 h

TABLE 24.4 Antigout Drugs—cont'd

Drug	Route and Dosage	Uses and Considerations
Xanthine Oxidase Inhibitors		
Allopurinol	Gout: A: PO: Initially 100 mg/d; *max:* 800 mg/d	For gout, hyperuricemia, and renal calculi. May cause nausea, vomiting, diarrhea, and GI bleeding/obstruction. PB: UK; t½: 1–2 h
Febuxostat	See Prototype Drug Chart: Febuxostat	
Uricosurics		
Probenecid	A: PO: Initially 250 mg bid for 1 wk; *maint:* 500 mg bid; *max:* 2 g/d	For hyperuricemia and gout. May cause dizziness, flushing, headache, fever, nausea, vomiting, and anemia. Increase fluid intake. PB: 75%–95%; t½: 3–12 h
Combinations		
Lesinurad-allopurinol	A: PO: 1 tab/d (lesinurad 200 mg, allopurinol 200–300 mg)	For hyperuricemia associated with gout. May cause headache, dizziness, dysgeusia, dyspepsia, nausea, diarrhea, abdominal pain, vomiting, and influenza. PB: lesinurad 98%, allopurinol UK; t½: lesinurad 5 h, allopurinol 1–2 h

A, Adult; *bid,* twice a day; *d,* day; *GI,* gastrointestinal; *h,* hour; *maint,* maintenance; *max,* maximum; *PB,* protein binding; *PO,* by mouth; *qd,* every day; *t½,* half-life; *UK,* unknown; *wk,* week; *y,* year; *>,* greater than.

◉ CLINICAL JUDGMENT [NURSING PROCESS]

Antigout Drug: Allopurinol

Concept: Inflammation
- An immunologic response of the body to injury or infection involving redness, swelling, warmth, and pain

Recognize Cues [Assessment]
- Obtain a medical history of any gastric, renal, cardiac, or liver disorders. Antigout drugs are excreted via kidneys, so sufficient renal function is needed. Drug dosage and drug selection might need to be changed.
- Obtain a drug history. Report possible drug-drug interactions.
- Assess serum uric acid value for future comparisons.
- Record urine output. Use initial urine output for future comparisons.
- Check laboratory tests such as blood urea nitrogen (BUN), serum creatinine, alkaline phosphatase (ALP), aspartate aminotransferase (AST), alanine aminotransferase (ALT), and lactate dehydrogenase (LDH), and compare with future laboratory test results.

Analyze Cues and Prioritize Hypothesis [Patient Problems]
- Acute pain
- Injury
- Nausea
- Reduced functional ability
- Decreased mobility

Generate Solutions [Planning]
- The patient will report that pain level has decreased within 1 hour of medication administration.
- The patient's swelling and redness will be reduced within 1 week.

Take Action [Nursing Interventions]
- Report gastrointestinal (GI) symptoms, gastric pain, nausea, vomiting, or diarrhea for patients taking antigout drugs. Administer these drugs with food to alleviate gastric distress.
- Record urine output. Because the drugs and uric acid are excreted through the urine, kidney stones might occur, so both water intake and urine output should be increased.

- ⚡ Monitor laboratory tests for renal and liver function (BUN, serum creatinine, ALP, AST, ALT).

Patient Teaching
General
- ⚡ Encourage patients to keep medical appointments and to have regularly scheduled laboratory tests for renal and liver function and complete blood count (CBC). Some antigout drugs may cause blood dyscrasias, so blood tests should be monitored.
- Instruct patients to increase fluid intake; it will increase drug and uric acid excretion.

Side Effects
- Advise patients to report to a health care provider any side effects of antigout drugs such as anorexia, nausea, vomiting, diarrhea, stomatitis, dizziness, rash, pruritus, and metallic taste.
- Advise patients to have a yearly eye examination because visual changes can result from prolonged use of allopurinol.

Diet
- Warn patients to avoid alcohol and caffeine because they can increase uric acid levels.
- Suggest that patients not take large doses of vitamin C while taking allopurinol; kidney stones may occur.
- Tell patients not to ingest foods high in purine content such as organ meats, salmon, sardines, gravy, and legumes. Foods with purine increase uric acid levels.
- Direct patients to report any gastric distress. Encourage them to take antigout drugs with food or at mealtime.

Evaluate Outcomes [Evaluation]
- Evaluate response to the antigout drug. If pain persists, the drug regimen may need modification.
- Determine the presence of adverse reactions. Drug therapy for gout pain may need to be changed.

Side Effects and Adverse Reactions

Side effects of uricosurics may include flushed skin, fever, dizziness, and headache. Kidney stones resulting from the uric acid could be prevented by increasing water intake and maintaining a urine pH above 6. Blood dyscrasias may occur. Aspirin use should be avoided with probenecid because it inhibits the action of probenecid.

CRITICAL THINKING CASE STUDY

A 72-year-old woman had taken 650 mg of aspirin four times a day for 8 months to alleviate her chronic symptoms of pain and inflammation associated with arthritis. Four weeks ago, a peptic ulcer developed.

1. Explain the process by which the patient could have a peptic ulcer. How could this have been prevented?

2. Compare the similarities and differences in the side effects of salicylates with those of acetic acid agents, propionic acid agents, COX-2 inhibitors, and phenylacetic acid.

3. What teaching points should the patient receive before and during the time she takes aspirin?

4. How would COX-2 inhibitors prevent the development of a peptic ulcer?

REVIEW QUESTIONS

1. A patient is taking ibuprofen. The nurse understands that COX-1 and COX-2 inhibitors are different in that ibuprofen is more likely than celecoxib to cause which adverse effect?
   a. Fever
   b. Constipation
   c. Peptic ulcer disease
   d. Metallic taste when eating

2. When teaching a patient who is receiving allopurinol, what should the nurse encourage the patient to do?
   a. Eat more meat.
   b. Increase vitamin C intake.
   c. Have annual eye examinations.
   d. Take medication 2 hours before meals.

3. A patient is admitted to the hospital with an acute gout attack. The nurse expects that which medication will be ordered to treat acute gout?
   a. Colchicine
   b. Allopurinol
   c. Probenecid
   d. Sulfinpyrazone

4. A patient is taking aspirin for arthritis. Which adverse reaction should the nurse teach the patient to report to the health care provider?
   a. Tinnitus

   b. Weight loss
   c. Sinusitis
   d. Palpitations

5. The nurse is teaching a patient about taking aspirin. Which are important points to include? (Select all that apply.)
   a. Advise the patient to avoid alcohol while taking aspirin.
   b. Instruct the patient to take aspirin before meals on an empty stomach.
   c. Instruct the patient to inform the dentist of the aspirin dosage before having dental work.
   d. Instruct the patient to inform the surgeon of the aspirin dosage before having surgery.
   e. Suggest that aspirin may be given to children for flu symptoms.
   f. Advise patient that urine may be a harmless pinkish-red or reddish-brown color.

6. A patient is taking infliximab and asks the nurse what side effects/adverse reactions to expect from this drug. The nurse lists which side effects? (Select all that apply.)
   a. Fatigue
   b. Headache
   c. Chest pain
   d. Renal damage
   e. Severe infections

25

Analgesics

http://evolve.elsevier.com/McCuistion/pharmacology

OBJECTIVES

- Differentiate between acute and chronic pain.
- Compare indications for nonopioid and opioid analgesics.
- Describe the serum therapeutic ranges of aspirin and acetaminophen.
- Contrast the side effects of aspirin and opioids.

- Explain the methadone treatment program.
- Discuss nursing interventions and patient teaching related to nonopioid and opioid analgesics.
- Formulate a Clinical Judgment [Nursing Process] for a patient with morphine patient-controlled analgesia.

OUTLINE

Pain is an unpleasant sensory and emotional experience related to tissue injury. Due to the subjective nature of pain, the nurse must be knowledgeable and skillful in the assessment and measurement of pain to achieve optimal pain management.

Pain management is regarded as such a significant component of nursing care that pain has become known as the "fifth vital sign." The Joint Commission (TJC) has incorporated the assessment, documentation, and management of pain into its standards, which reflect the importance of this vital sign. The nurse's role is to assess the patient's pain level, alleviate the patient's pain through nonpharmacologic and pharmacologic treatments, thoroughly document the patient's response to treatment, and teach patients and their significant others to manage pain control when appropriate.

An individual's pain threshold reflects the level of stimulus needed to create a painful sensation, and individual genetic makeup contributes to the variations in pain threshold from person to person. The mu (μ) opioid receptor gene controls the number of μ-receptors present. When an individual has a large number of μ-receptors, the pain threshold is high, and pain sensitivity is reduced.

The amount of pain a person can endure without having it interfere with normal functioning is called pain tolerance. This psychological aspect of pain varies greatly in individuals because it is subjective and because pain tolerance is influenced by factors such as age, sex, culture, ethnicity, previous experience, anxiety level, and specific circumstances, such as a traumatic event.

Analgesics, both nonopioid and opioid, are prescribed for the relief of pain. The choice of analgesic depends on the severity of the pain. Mild to moderate pain is frequently relieved with the use of nonopioid, also known as *nonnarcotic,* analgesics. Moderate to severe pain usually requires an opioid, or *narcotic,* analgesic.

Drugs used for pain relief are presented in this chapter. Many of the same nonopioid analgesics that are taken for pain, such as the nonsteroidal antiinflammatory drugs (NSAIDs), are also taken for antiinflammatory purposes. This application for these drugs is covered in Chapter 24.

The most common classification of pain is by duration. Acute pain can be mild, moderate, or severe, and it is usually associated with a specific tissue injury. The onset of acute pain is usually sudden and of short duration lasting less than 3 months. Chronic pain usually has a vague origin and gradual onset with a prolonged duration (more than 3 months) of long-lasting discomfort.

Pain may also be classified by its origin. Nociceptors, sensory receptors for pain, are activated by noxious stimuli—mechanical, thermal, and chemical—in peripheral tissues. When tissue damage occurs, injured cells release chemical mediators that affect the exposed nerve endings of the nociceptors. Pain that originates from tissue injury is nociceptor pain, which includes somatic pain—that is, pain from structural tissues such as bones and muscles—and visceral (organ) pain. Neuropathic pain is an unusual sensory disturbance that often involves neural supersensitivity. This pain is due to injury or disease of the peripheral nervous system (PNS) or central nervous system (CNS). The patient with neuropathic

TABLE 25.1   Types of Pain

Type of Pain	Definition	Drug Treatment
Acute	Pain occurs suddenly, is of short duration (less than 3 months), and responds to treatment; it can result from trauma, tissue injury, inflammation, or surgery.	Mild pain: Nonopioid drugs, such as acetaminophen and NSAIDs Moderate pain: Combination of nonopioid and opioid drugs, such as oxycodone and acetaminophen Severe pain: Potent opioids, such as morphine or hydrocodone
Chronic	Pain persists for more than 3 months and is difficult to treat or control.	Nonopioid drugs are suggested. Opioids, if used, should meet these criteria: • Oral or transdermal • Long duration of action • Include adjunct therapy • Cause minimal respiratory depression
Cancer	Pain occurs from pressure on nerves and organs, blockage to blood supply, or metastasis to bone.	NSAIDs and opioid drugs administered PO, transdermally, via IM or IV routes, intrathecally, or with PCA
Somatic	Pain is in skeletal muscle, ligaments, and joints.	Nonopioids: NSAIDs; also act as antiinflammatories and muscle relaxants
Superficial	Pain is from surface areas such as skin and mucous membranes.	Mild pain: Nonopioid Moderate pain: Combination of opioid and nonopioid analgesic drugs
Vascular	Pain occurs from vascular or perivascular tissues contributing to headaches or migraines.	Nonopioid drugs
Visceral	Pain is from smooth muscle and organs.	Opioid drugs

IM, Intramuscular; *IV,* intravenous; *NSAIDs,* nonsteroidal antiinflammatory drugs; *PCA,* patient-controlled analgesia; *PO,* by mouth.

pain usually complains of burning, tingling, or electric shock sensations in the affected area, often triggered by light touch. Diabetic neuropathy associated with diabetes mellitus is an example of peripheral neuropathic pain. Severe, intractable pain from a herniated disk or spinal cord injury is evidence of neuropathic pain from the CNS.

PATHOPHYSIOLOGY

The most common pain theory is called the *gate theory,* proposed by Melzack and Wall in 1965. According to this theory, tissue injury activates nociceptors and causes the release of chemical mediators, such as substance P, prostaglandins, bradykinin, histamine, serotonin, acetylcholine, glutamate, adenosine triphosphate, leukotrienes, and potassium. These substances initiate an action potential along a sensory nerve fiber and sensitize pain receptors. Nociceptive action potentials are transmitted via afferent nerve fibers. One type of pain fiber that primarily transmits impulses from the periphery is the A-delta (A-δ) fiber. Because A-δ pain fibers are wrapped in a myelin sheath, they transmit impulses rapidly in acute pain. The C-fiber is a type of pain fiber that is small and unmyelinated, and because C-fibers are unmyelinated, they transmit impulses slowly. C-fibers are more often associated with chronic, dull pain.

A pain signal begins at the nociceptors in the periphery and proceeds throughout the CNS. Knowing how and where pharmacologic agents work is essential to controlling pain. The body produces neurohormones called endorphins (peptides) that naturally suppress pain conduction, although the method is not completely understood. Opioids such as morphine activate the same receptors as endorphins to reduce pain. NSAIDs control pain at the peripheral level by blocking the action of cyclooxygenase, a pain-sensitizing chemical, and interfering with the production of prostaglandins. Cortisone decreases pain by blocking the action of phospholipase, reducing the production of both prostaglandins and leukotrienes. In neuropathic pain, anticonvulsant drugs inhibit the transmission of nerve impulses by stabilizing the neuronal membrane and inactivating peripheral sodium channels.

To ascertain severity of pain, the health care provider should ask the patient to rate the degree of pain on a scale of 0 to 10, with 10 being the worst or most severe pain. For example, a patient who indicates a pain level of 9 may verbalize a decrease in pain to a level of 7 within 30 to 45 minutes after receiving pain medication. Many scales and instruments are available to the nurse for assessment and measurement of the patient's pain level. Table 25.1 lists the types of pain and the drug groups that may be effective in relieving each type.

Undertreatment of Pain

Undertreatment of pain is a major issue in health care today. Postoperative pain is inadequately managed in 80% or more of patients in the United States. When acute postoperative pain is poorly controlled, associated factors include delayed recovery time, extended duration of opioid use, functional ability, impaired quality of life, higher health care costs, and increased morbidity. Some reasons for undertreatment are sociocultural variables that mediate a patient's willingness to acknowledge being in pain, the patient's inability to describe pain, the patient's fear of substance use disorder, the nurse's inability to measure pain, lack of regular pain assessment rounds, attitudes of the health care team, an unwillingness to believe the patient's report of pain, inaccurate knowledge on the part of the health care provider concerning substance use disorder and tolerance, and prescription of an inadequate analgesic dose.

Unrelieved pain leads to a multitude of harmful effects that involve almost all organs of the body. As a result of unrelieved pain, the patient may develop increased respiratory and heart rates, hypertension, increased stress response, urinary retention, fluid overload, electrolyte imbalance, glucose intolerance, hyperglycemia, pneumonia, atelectasis, anorexia, paralytic ileus, constipation, weakness, confusion, infection, or psychological and physical suffering.

Inadequate pain management leads to high health care costs. It is estimated that the cost of extended hospital stays, readmissions to the hospital, and outpatient visits due to inadequate pain management exceeds $200 billion per year.

NONOPIOID ANALGESICS

Nonopioid analgesics such as aspirin, acetaminophen, ibuprofen, and naproxen are less potent than opioid analgesics and are used to treat mild to moderate pain. Nonopioids are usually purchased over the counter, but cyclooxygenase 2 (COX-2) inhibitors require a prescription. Nonopioids are effective for the dull, throbbing pain of headaches; dysmenorrhea (menstrual pain); inflammation; minor abrasions; muscular aches and pain; and mild to moderate arthritis. Most analgesics also have an antipyretic effect and will lower an elevated body temperature. Some, such as aspirin, have antiinflammatory and antiplatelet effects as well.

Nonsteroidal Antiinflammatory Drugs

All NSAIDs have an analgesic effect as well as an antipyretic and antiinflammatory action. NSAIDs such as aspirin, ibuprofen, and naproxen can be purchased as over-the-counter (OTC) drugs. Aspirin, a salicylate NSAID, is the oldest nonopioid analgesic drug still in use. Adolf Bayer marketed the original formulation in 1899, and currently aspirin can be purchased under many names and with added ingredients.

The American Academy of Pediatrics, Centers for Disease Control and Prevention (CDC), US Food and Drug Administration (FDA), National Reye's Syndrome Foundation, US Surgeon General, and World Health Organization (WHO) recommend aspirin products not be given to children and adolescents younger than 19 years of age during episodes of fever or viral illnesses because of the danger of Reye syndrome. Reye syndrome is a rare but serious condition associated with viral infections treated with salicylates that causes swelling of the brain and liver. In these circumstances, acetaminophen is recommended instead of aspirin.

In addition to its analgesic, antipyretic, and antiinflammatory properties, aspirin decreases platelet aggregation (clotting). Some health care providers may therefore prescribe one 81-mg, 162-mg, or 325-mg aspirin tablet every day or one 325-mg tablet every other day as a preventive measure against transient ischemic attacks (TIAs, or ministrokes), heart attacks, or any thromboembolic episode. Aspirin is discussed in depth in Chapter 24 along with other NSAIDs.

Aspirin and other NSAIDs relieve pain by inhibiting biosynthesis of prostaglandin by different forms of the COX enzyme. As explained in Chapter 24, NSAIDs inhibit or block both COX-1 and COX-2 enzymes, whereas COX-2 inhibitors are selective and only inhibit COX-2 enzyme. Inhibition of COX-1 decreases protection of the stomach lining, whereas inhibition of COX-2 decreases inflammation and pain. As a result of an NSAID's inhibition of COX-1, gastric irritation and bleeding may occur. Aspirin is the drug of choice for alleviating pain and inflammation in arthritic conditions, but when given in high doses, severe gastrointestinal (GI) irritation and possible ulceration develop in approximately 20% of patients. Some pharmaceutical companies have developed antiinflammatory and analgesic drugs that inhibit only COX-2. The COX-2 inhibitors were developed to eliminate the GI side effects associated with aspirin and other NSAIDs. COX-2 inhibitors are discussed in depth in Chapter 24.

Side Effects and Adverse Reactions

A common side effect of NSAIDs is gastric distress, including anorexia, nausea, vomiting, and diarrhea. These drugs should be taken with food, at mealtime, or with a full glass of fluid to help reduce this problem. Excessive bleeding might occur as a side effect if an NSAID is taken for dysmenorrhea during the first 2 days of menstruation. Adverse effects of salicylate toxicity include tinnitus, vertigo, hyperventilation, and potential metabolic acidosis.

Some patients are hypersensitive to aspirin. Dyspnea, bronchospasm, and urticaria are some of the symptoms that indicate anaphylaxis to salicylate products. Certain foods also contain salicylates: prunes, raisins, paprika, and licorice. Those with a hypersensitivity to aspirin and salicylate products may be sensitive to other NSAIDs. This hypersensitivity may be related to inhibition of the COX enzyme by the salicylate. It is recommended that aspirin not be given to children or adolescents unless specifically directed by a health care provider because of the danger of Reye syndrome.

Acetaminophen

The analgesic acetaminophen, a para-aminophenol derivative, was first marketed in the mid-1950s as an analgesic and antipyretic drug used for muscular aches and pains, and for fever caused by viral infections in infants, children, adults, and older adults. It is a popular nonprescription drug; it constitutes 25% of all OTC drugs sold. Acetaminophen is a nonopioid drug, but it is *not* an NSAID. Because acetaminophen does not have the antiinflammatory properties of aspirin, it is not the drug of choice for any inflammatory process. Acetaminophen is a safe, effective drug when used at therapeutic doses, causes little to no gastric distress, and does not interfere with platelet aggregation. Complementary and Alternative Therapies: Capsaicin describes the use of these products in pain relief. An intravenous (IV) formulation of acetaminophen was approved by the FDA for treating pain and fever. It should be administered undiluted over 15 minutes. There is no link between acetaminophen and Reye syndrome, and unlike aspirin and NSAIDs, it does not increase the potential for excessive bleeding if taken for dysmenorrhea (Prototype Drug Chart: Acetaminophen).

🌸 COMPLEMENTARY AND ALTERNATIVE THERAPIES

Capsaicin

Capsaicin, which is found naturally in cayenne pepper, is selective for C-fiber nociceptors and relieves some arthritis pain in topical cream or gel form.

Pharmacokinetics. Acetaminophen is well absorbed from the GI tract. Rectal absorption may be erratic because of the presence of fecal material or a decrease in blood flow to the colon. Because of acetaminophen's short half-life, it can be administered every 4 hours as needed with a maximum dose of 4 g/day for adults. However, it is suggested that a patient who frequently takes acetaminophen limit the dose to 2000 mg/day (2 g/day) to avoid the possibility of hepatic or renal dysfunction. More than 85% of acetaminophen is metabolized to drug metabolites by the liver.

Large doses or overdoses can be toxic to the hepatic cells, so when large doses are administered over a long period, the serum level of acetaminophen should be monitored. The therapeutic serum range is 10 to 20 mcg/mL. Hepatic enzyme levels (aspartate aminotransferase [AST], alanine aminotransferase [ALT], alkaline phosphatase [ALP]) and serum bilirubin should also be monitored. Ingesting alcohol concurrently with acetaminophen may lead to hepatic injury, hepatic failure, and death. When acetaminophen toxicity occurs, acetylcysteine is the antidote, which reduces liver injury by converting toxic metabolites to a nontoxic form.

Pharmacodynamics. Acetaminophen weakly inhibits prostaglandin synthesis, which decreases pain sensation. It is effective in eliminating mild to moderate pain and headaches and is useful for its antipyretic effect. Acetaminophen does not possess antiinflammatory action. When given orally, its onset of action is within 10 to 30 minutes, and the peak concentration occurs within 30 to 60 minutes. Severe adverse reactions may occur with an overdose, so acetaminophen in liquid or chewable form should be kept out of children's reach.

PROTOTYPE DRUG CHART

Acetaminophen

Drug Class	Dosage
Analgesic	Pain: Immediate release: A: PO/PR: 325–650 mg q4–6h PRN; *max:* 4 g/d Extended release: A: PO: 650–1300 mg q8h PRN; *max:* 3900 mg/d
Contraindications	**Drug-Lab-Food Interactions**
Hypersensitivity *Caution:* Renal/hepatic disease, hypertension, diabetes mellitus, alcohol use disorder, hypovolemia, malnutrition, older adults	Increased effect with caffeine, diflunisal Decreased effect with oral contraceptives, antacids, anticholinergics, cholestyramine, charcoal, barbiturates, carbamazepine, and phenytoin
Pharmacokinetics	**Pharmacodynamics**
Absorption: Rapidly absorbed PO; rectal absorption is erratic. Distribution: PB: 10%–25%; crosses the placenta, excreted in breast milk Metabolism: t½: 2–3 h Excretion: In urine as metabolites	PO: Onset: 10–30 min Peak: 30–60 min Duration: 4–6 h Rectal: Onset: UK Peak: UK Duration: UK
Therapeutic Effects/Uses	
To decrease pain and fever Mechanism of Action: Inhibition (weak) of prostaglandin synthesis, inhibition of hypothalamic heat regulator center	
Side Effects	**Adverse Reactions**
Headache, insomnia, anxiety, fatigue, anorexia, nausea, vomiting, constipation, peripheral edema	Oliguria, hearing loss, hypomagnesemia, elevated hepatic enzymes *Life-threatening:* Hepatic/renal failure, hypokalemia, rhabdomyolysis, anemia, hemolytic anemia, agranulocytosis, neutropenia, thrombocytopenia, pancytopenia

A, Adult; *d,* day; *h,* hour; *max,* maximum dosage; *min,* minute; *PB,* protein binding; *PO,* by mouth; *PR,* per rectum; *PRN,* as needed; *q,* every; *qid,* four times a day; *supp,* suppository; *t½,* half-life; *TDM,* therapeutic drug monitoring; *UK,* unknown; *y,* year; *>,* greater than; *<,* less than.

Side Effects and Adverse Reactions

An overdose of acetaminophen can be extremely toxic to liver cells; death could occur in 1 to 4 days from hepatic necrosis. If a child or adult ingests excessive amounts of acetaminophen tablets or liquid, a poison control center should be contacted immediately, and the child or adult should be taken to the emergency department. Early symptoms of hepatic damage include nausea, vomiting, diarrhea, and abdominal pain.

Table 25.2 lists the commonly used nonopioid analgesics and their dosages, uses, and considerations.

! OPIOID ANALGESICS

Opioid analgesics, called opioid agonists, are prescribed for moderate and severe pain. In the United States the Harrison Opioid Act of 1914 required that all forms of opium be sold with a prescription and that it no longer be used as a nonprescription drug. The Controlled Substances Act of 1970 classified drugs with high abuse potential, opioids among them, in five schedule categories according to their potential for drug abuse (see Chapter 8). Addiction, or substance use disorder, is defined as a psychological and physical dependence upon a substance beyond normal voluntary control, usually after prolonged use of a substance.

Morphine, a prototype opioid, is obtained from the sap of seedpods of the opium poppy plant. Codeine is another drug obtained from opium. In the past decades, many synthetic and semisynthetic opioids have been developed; for example, meperidine.

Although nonopioid analgesics act on the PNS at the pain receptor sites, opioid analgesics act mostly on the CNS. Opioids act primarily by activating the μ-receptors, but they also exert a weak activation of the kappa (κ) receptors. Analgesia, respiratory depression, euphoria, and sedation are effects of μ-receptor activation. Activation of κ-receptors leads to analgesia and sedation but has no effect on respiratory depression and euphoria.

Opioids not only suppress pain impulses but also suppress respiration and coughing by acting on the respiratory and cough centers in the medulla of the brain stem. One example of such an opioid is morphine, a potent analgesic that can readily depress respirations. Codeine is not as potent as morphine (1/15 to 1/20 as potent), but it also relieves mild to moderate pain and suppresses cough, which allows it also to be classified as an antitussive. Most opioids, with the exception of meperidine, have an antitussive (cough suppression) effect. The opioids have two isomers, levo and dextro. The levo-isomers of opioids produce an analgesic effect only; however, both levo- and dextro-isomers possess an antitussive response. The dextro-isomers do not cause physical dependence, but the levo-isomers do. Synthetic cough suppressants are discussed in Chapter 35.

In addition to pain relief and antitussive effects, many opioids possess antidiarrheal effects. Common side effects with high doses

⊚ CLINICAL JUDGMENT [NURSING PROCESS]

Analgesic: Acetaminophen

Concept: Pain
- An unpleasant feeling of discomfort usually associated with tissue damage

Recognize Cues [Assessment]
- Obtain a medical history of liver dysfunction. Overdosing or extremely high doses of acetaminophen can cause hepatotoxicity, hepatic failure, and death.
- Ascertain the severity of pain. Nonopioid nonsteroidal antiinflammatory drugs (NSAIDs), such as ibuprofen, or an opioid may be necessary to relieve pain.

Analyze Cues and Prioritize Hypothesis [Patient Problems]
- Injury
- Acute pain
- Nausea
- Diarrhea
- Discomfort
- Decreased mobility

Generate Solutions [Planning]
- The patient will report pain has decreased within 1 hour after medication administration.

Take Action [Nursing Interventions]
- Check hepatic enzyme tests such as alanine aminotransferase (ALT), alkaline phosphatase (ALP), gamma-glutamyl transferase (GGT), 5′-nucleotidase, and bilirubin for elevations in patients who take high doses of acetaminophen or overdoses.

Patient Teaching
General
- Teach patients to keep acetaminophen out of children's reach. Acetaminophen for children is available in flavored tablets and liquid, and high doses can cause hepatotoxicity, hepatic failure, and death.

- Advise patients not to self-medicate with acetaminophen for more than 10 days. Teach adult caregivers not to medicate children for more than 5 days without a health care provider's approval.
- ⚡ Direct parents to call a poison control center immediately if a child has taken a large or unknown amount of acetaminophen.
- ⚡ Teach patients to check acetaminophen dosages on the label of over-the-counter (OTC) drugs. Do not exceed the recommended dosage. The suggested safe maximum adult acetaminophen dosage is 4 g/day to avoid hepatic damage (see Prototype Drug Chart: Acetaminophen).
- Teach patient to avoid alcohol ingestion while taking acetaminophen.

Side Effects
- Encourage patients to report side effects. Overdosing can cause severe hepatic damage, hepatic failure, and death.
- ⚡ Check the serum acetaminophen level if toxicity is suspected. The therapeutic serum level is 10 to 20 mcg/mL; the toxic level is greater than 200 mcg/mL 4 hours after ingestion and is usually associated with hepatotoxicity. The antidote for acetaminophen is acetylcysteine. Dosage is based on the serum acetaminophen level.

Evaluate Outcomes [Evaluation]
- Evaluate the effectiveness of acetaminophen in relieving pain using consistent pain scale. If pain persists, another analgesic may be needed.
- Determine whether the patient is taking the recommended dosage. Observe and report any side effects.

TABLE 25.2 Analgesics

Generic	Route and Dosage	Uses and Considerations
Para-Aminophenol		
Acetaminophen	See Prototype Drug Chart: Acetaminophen	
Nonsteroidal Antiinflammatory Drugs (NSAIDs)		
Aspirin	Minor pain: A: PO: 325–650 mg q4h PRN	For relief of headaches, pain, fever, and inflammation, and thromboembolism prevention. May cause nausea, vomiting, anorexia, dyspepsia, abdominal pain, gastritis, dizziness, hearing loss, tinnitus, elevated hepatic enzymes, and bleeding. Aspirin should be taken with food. Avoid with alcohol. Avoid in children and teenagers younger than 19 years during episodes of fever or viral illnesses. PB: 20%–95%; t½: 15–20 min
Diflunisal	Pain: A: PO: Initial LD 500 mg–1 g; *maint:* 250–500 mg q8–12h PRN; *max:* 1500 mg/d	For mild to moderate pain, osteoarthritis, and RA. May cause headache, tinnitus, hearing loss, nausea, vomiting, diarrhea, abdominal pain, dyspepsia, rash, GI ulcer/bleeding/perforation, and elevated hepatic enzymes. PB: 99%, t½: 8–12 h
Ibuprofen	Severe Pain: A: PO: 400–800 mg q6h PRN; *max:* 3200 mg/d	For reducing fever, mild to severe pain, osteoarthritis, RA, and dysmenorrhea. May cause headache, dizziness, tinnitus, edema, anemia, nausea, dyspepsia, vomiting, diarrhea, flatulence, rash, abdominal pain, and constipation. Should be taken with food, at mealtime, or with plenty of fluids. PB: 99%; t½: 1.7–2.5 h

Continued

TABLE 25.2   Analgesics—cont'd

Generic	Route and Dosage	Uses and Considerations
Propionic Acids		
Naproxen	Mild to moderate pain: A: PO: Initially 500 mg, then 250 mg q6–8h; *max:* 1250 mg/d	For mild to moderate pain, fever, osteoarthritis, RA, bursitis, ankylosing spondylitis, gout, and dysmenorrhea. May cause dizziness, drowsiness, pharyngitis, headache, abdominal pain, flatulence, nausea, vomiting, diarrhea, constipation, rash, edema, influenza, dyspepsia, elevated hepatic enzymes, tinnitus, and GI bleeding/ulcer/perforation. PB: 99%; t½: 12–17 h
Acetic Acids (Indoles)		
Indomethacin	Moderate to severe pain: Regular-release capsules: A: PO: 20 mg tid or 40 mg bid/tid; *max:* 200 mg/d, not recommended for older A Extended release: A: PO: 75 mg qd/bid; *max:* 150 mg/d, not recommended for older A	For mild to severe pain, gout, tendinitis, osteoarthritis, RA, and ankylosing spondylitis. May cause dizziness, headache, nausea, vomiting, dyspepsia, constipation, hyperkalemia, and hyponatremia. Take with food. Avoid if allergic to aspirin. PB: 99%; t½: 2.6–11.2 h
Ketorolac	A ≥50 kg: Intranasal: 1 spray each nostril, q6–8h; *max:* 4 doses/d Older A <50 kg: Intranasal: 1 spray 1 nostril q6–8h; *max:* 4 doses/d	For short-term pain management (5 days or less). May cause drowsiness, dizziness, nausea, vomiting, diarrhea, dyspepsia, abdominal pain, constipation, flatulence, diaphoresis, injection site reaction, and ocular edema. PB: 99%; t½: PO, 2.4–9 h; IM, 3.5–9.2 h
Nabumetone	A: PO: 1000 mg/d or 500 mg bid; *max:* 2000 mg/d	For pain from osteoarthritis and RA. May cause dizziness, headache, tinnitus, pruritus, dyspepsia, vomiting, nausea, abdominal pain, diarrhea, constipation, flatulence, rash, and edema. PB: 99%; t½: 24 h
Oxicams		
Meloxicam	A: PO: 7.5–15 mg/d; *max:* 15 mg/d	For pain from osteoarthritis and RA. May cause dizziness, headache, edema, dyspepsia, arthralgia, nausea, eructation, diarrhea, abdominal pain, constipation, cystitis, and GI bleeding/perforation. PB: 99.4%; t½: 15–20 h
Cyclooxygenase 2 (COX-2) Inhibitors		
Celecoxib	Moderate to severe pain: A: PO: initially 400 mg followed by additional 200 mg on day 1 if needed; *maint:* 200 mg bid; *max:* 800 mg/d, older A 400 mg/d	For moderate to severe pain, osteoarthritis, and RA. May cause headache, hypertension, peripheral edema, dyspepsia, nausea, vomiting, diarrhea, abdominal pain, pharyngitis, infection, and arthralgia. Use caution in patients with severe renal or liver disorders and for those allergic to salicylates or sulfonamides. PB: 97%; t½: 11.2 h
Miscellaneous		
Baricitinib	A: PO: 2 mg/d	For moderate to severe RA in adults with inadequate response to 1 or more TNF antagonists. Hgb must be 8 g/dL or more, ANC must be 1000 cells/mm^3 or more, and ALC must be 500 cells/mm^3 or more. May cause infection, elevated hepatic enzymes, and nausea. PB: 45%; t½: 12 h
Norepinephrine and Serotonin Reuptake Inhibitors		
Tramadol	Severe pain: Immediate release: A: PO: Initially: 25 mg/d; *maint:* 50–100 mg q4–6h PRN; *max:* 400 mg/d, 300 mg/d for A >75 y Extended release: A: PO: 100 mg/d; *max:* 300 mg/d	For moderate to severe pain. May cause drowsiness, dizziness, weakness, headache, anxiety, agitation, euphoria, flushing, dry mouth, nausea, dyspepsia, vomiting, diarrhea, constipation, and tremor. PB: 20%; t½: 6.3–7.4 h for immediate release, 7.9–8.8 h for extended release
Milnacipran	A: PO: Initially 12.5 mg qd on day 1, 12.5 bid on days 2–3, 25 mg bid days 4–7, then 50 mg bid	For management of fibromyalgia. May cause nausea, headache, constipation, hot flashes, insomnia, and dizziness. PB: 13%; t½: 4–10 h

A, Adult; *alc,* absolute lymphocyte count; *anc,* absolute neutrophil count; *bid,* twice a day; *CNS,* central nervous system; *d,* day; *GI,* gastrointestinal; *hgb,* hemoglobin; *h,* hour; *IM,* intramuscular; *IV,* intravenous; *maint,* maintenance; *max,* maximum dosage; *min,* minute; *PB,* protein binding; *PO,* by mouth; *PR,* per rectum; *PRN,* as needed; *q,* every; *RA,* rheumatoid arthritis; *t½,* half-life; *y,* year; *>,* greater than; *<,* less than.

of most opioids include nausea and vomiting, particularly in ambulatory patients; constipation; a moderate decrease in blood pressure; and orthostatic hypotension. High doses of opioids may also cause respiratory depression; urinary retention, usually in older adults; and antitussive effects. See Complementary and Alternative Therapies: Sedatives for interactions with opioids.

COMPLEMENTARY AND ALTERNATIVE THERAPIES

Sedatives

Opioids taken with kava, valerian, and St. John's wort may increase sedation.

Morphine

Morphine, an extraction from opium, is a potent opioid analgesic (Prototype Drug Chart: Morphine Sulfate). Morphine is effective against acute pain resulting from acute myocardial infarction (AMI) and cancer, relieves dyspnea resulting from pulmonary edema, and may be used as a preoperative medication to relieve anxiety. Although it is effective in relieving severe pain, it can cause respiratory depression, orthostatic hypotension, miosis, urinary retention, constipation resulting from reduced bowel motility, and cough suppression. An antidote for morphine excess or overdose is the opioid antagonist naloxone.

Pharmacokinetics. Morphine may be taken orally, although GI absorption can be somewhat erratic. For quick relief of severe pain, such as with AMI, or for fast relief of anxiety and to reduce hypertension, it is given intravenously. Morphine is 20% to 35% protein bound and may also be administered rectally and epidurally. Oral morphine undergoes first-pass hepatic metabolism, meaning the liver metabolizes the drug before morphine is available to the rest of the body. Only a small amount of morphine crosses the blood-brain barrier to produce an analgesic effect. It has a short half-life of 2 to 4 hours, and 90% is excreted in the urine. Morphine crosses the placenta and is excreted in breast milk.

Pharmacodynamics. Morphine binds with the opiate receptor in the CNS. Parenterally, the onset of action is rapid, especially when

PROTOTYPE DRUG CHART

⚠ *Morphine Sulfate*

Drug Class	Dosage
Opioid CSS II	Immediate release: A: PO: Initially 15–30 mg q4h PRN Extended release: A: PO: 15 mg q8–12h PRN or 30 mg/d A: IV/IM/subcut: 2–10 mg/70 kg q3–4h PRN
Contraindications	**Drug-Lab-Food Interactions**
Hypersensitivity, CNS or respiratory depression, status asthmaticus, increased intracranial pressure, shock, alcohol use disorder, ileus, hypovolemia, dysrhythmias, shock *Caution:* Respiratory insufficiency, seizures, renal or hepatic disorders, urinary retention, sleep apnea, older adults	Drug: Increased effects of alcohol, sedative-hypnotics, antipsychotic drugs, muscle relaxants Complementary and Alternative Therapies: St. John's wort may decrease drug effect (see Complementary and Alternative Therapies: Sedatives). Lab: Increased AST, ALT
Pharmacokinetics	**Pharmacodynamics**
Absorption: PO, varies; IV, rapid Distribution: PB: 20%–35%; crosses placenta, excreted in breast milk Metabolism: t½: 2–4 h Excretion: 90% in urine	PO: Onset: 30 min Peak: IR 1 h, ER 3–4 h Duration: IR 3–5 h; ER 8–24 h Subcut: Onset: 15–30 min Peak: 50–90 min Duration: 3–6 h IM: Onset: 15–30 min Peak: 30–60 min Duration: 3–6 h IV: Onset: 5–10 min Peak: 20 min Duration: 3–6 h

Therapeutic Effects/Uses

To relieve moderate to severe pain
Mechanism of Action: Depression of the CNS; depression of pain impulses by binding with opiate receptors in the CNS

Side Effects	Adverse Reactions
Anorexia, dry mouth, nausea, abdominal pain, diarrhea, constipation, flatulence, fever, drowsiness, dizziness, agitation, anxiety, dysgeusia, confusion, depression, urinary retention, rash, blurred vision, miosis, weakness, flushing, euphoria, peripheral edema, paresthesia, diaphoresis, pruritus, infection, back pain, insomnia, erectile dysfunction	Orthostatic hypotension, bradycardia, tachycardia, palpitations, seizures, ileus, psychological dependence, dyspnea *Life-threatening:* Respiratory depression, anemia, leukopenia, thrombocytopenia, pulmonary edema, GI obstruction, dysrhythmias

A, Adult; *ALT,* alanine aminotransferase; *AST,* aspartate aminotransferase; *CNS,* central nervous system; *CSS,* Controlled Substances Schedule; *d,* day; *h,* hour; *IM,* intramuscular; *IV,* intravenous; *min,* minute; *mo,* month; *PB,* protein binding; *PO,* by mouth; *PRN,* as necessary; *q,* every; *subcut,* subcutaneous; *SR,* sustained release; *t½,* half-life; *UK,* unknown.

administered intravenously. Onset of action is 15 to 30 minutes for subcutaneous (subcut) and intramuscular (IM) injections. The duration of action with most types of drug administration is 3 to 6 hours; with controlled-release morphine sulfate tablets, duration is 8 to 24 hours.

COMPLEMENTARY AND ALTERNATIVE THERAPIES

St. John's Wort

> St. John's wort may potentiate drug effects of oral morphine and decrease drug levels of oxycodone.

Meperidine

One of the first synthetic opioids, meperidine became available in the mid-1950s. It is classified as a Schedule II drug according to the Controlled Substances Act. Meperidine has a shorter duration of action than morphine, and its potency varies according to the dosage. Meperidine can be given orally or via IM and IV routes, and it is primarily effective in GI procedures. It does not have the antitussive property of opium preparations.

During pregnancy, meperidine is preferred to morphine because it does not diminish uterine contractions and causes less neonatal respiratory depression. Meperidine causes less constipation and urinary retention than morphine. Meperidine is not indicated for patients with chronic pain, severe liver dysfunction, sickle cell disease, a history of seizures, severe coronary artery disease (CAD), or cardiac dysrhythmias. When older adults and patients with advanced cancer receive large doses of meperidine, neurotoxicity (e.g., nervousness, tremors, agitation, irritability, seizures) is reported. Meperidine should *not* be prescribed for long-term use; the dosage is frequently limited to 150 mg/dose for a period no longer than 48 to 72 hours.

Meperidine is metabolized in the liver to an active metabolite; therefore the dose should be decreased for patients with hepatic or renal insufficiency. It is excreted in the urine in a metabolite form called *normeperidine*. Meperidine should not be taken with alcohol or sedative-hypnotics because combination of these drugs causes an additive CNS depression. A major side effect of meperidine is a decrease in blood pressure, which should be monitored, especially if the patient is an older adult.

Table 25.3 lists opioids and their dosages, uses, and considerations.

◎ CLINICAL JUDGMENT [NURSING PROCESS}

⚠ Opioid Analgesic: Morphine Sulfate

Concept: Pain
- An unpleasant feeling of discomfort usually associated with tissue damage

Recognize Cues [Assessment]
- Obtain a medical history. Contraindications for morphine include severe respiratory disorders, increased intracranial pressure, and severe renal disease. Morphine may cause seizures.
- Determine a drug history and check for drug allergies. Report if a drug-drug interaction is probable. Morphine increases the effects of alcohol, sedatives and hypnotics, antipsychotic drugs, and muscle relaxants, and it can cause respiratory depression.
- Assess vital signs, noting the rate and depth of respirations, as well as pupil size for future comparisons; opioids commonly decrease respirations and systolic blood pressure and may cause miosis.
- Monitor urinary output; morphine can cause urinary retention.
- Assess the type of pain, location, and duration before giving opioids.

Analyze Cues and Prioritize Hypothesis [Patient Problems]
- Decreased gas exchange
- Injury
- Acute pain
- Hypotension
- Falls
- Urinary retention
- Constipation
- Discomfort

Generate Solutions [Planning]
- The patient will report pain is decreased within 1 hour after medication administration.

Take Action [Nursing Interventions]
- Administer morphine before pain reaches its peak to maximize effectiveness of the drug.
- Monitor vital signs at frequent intervals to detect respiratory changes and hypotension. Fewer than 10 respirations per minute can indicate respiratory distress.

- Record the patient's urine output because urinary retention is a side effect of morphine. Urine output should be at least 600 mL/day.
- Check bowel sounds for decreased peristalsis; constipation is a side effect of morphine. A dietary change or mild laxative might be needed.
- ⚡ Check for pupil changes and reaction. Pinpoint pupils can indicate morphine overdose.
- ⚡ Have naloxone available as an antidote to reverse respiratory depression if morphine overdose occurs.
- Validate the dose of morphine before administration. Check older adults for alertness and orientation because confusion is a side effect of morphine. Use side rails and take other safety precautions as necessary.

Patient Teaching
General
- Encourage patients not to use alcohol or central nervous system (CNS) depressants with any opioid analgesics such as morphine. Respiratory depression can result, as well as dizziness and the potential fall risk.
- Suggest nonpharmacologic measures to relieve pain as the patient recuperates from surgery. As recovery progresses, a nonopioid analgesic may be prescribed.

Side Effects
- Alert patients that with continuous use, opioids such as morphine can become a substance use disorder. If this occurs, inform patients about methadone treatment programs and other resources in the area.
- Encourage patients to report dizziness while taking morphine. Dizziness could be due to orthostatic hypotension. Advise patients to ambulate with caution or only with assistance.
- ⚡ Teach patients to report difficulty in breathing, blurred vision, and headaches.

Evaluate Outcomes [Evaluation]
- Evaluate the effectiveness of morphine in lessening or alleviating pain using a consistent pain scale. If pain persists after several days, the dose should be increased or the opioid should be changed.
- Determine the stability of vital signs. Any decrease in respiration or blood pressure should be reported.

⚠ TABLE 25.3 Opioids: Opium and Synthetics

Generic	Route and Dosage	Uses and Considerations
Codeine sulfate, codeine phosphate CSS II	A: PO: 15–60 mg q4h PRN; *max:* 360 mg/d	For mild to moderate pain and as an antitussive. May cause drowsiness, dizziness, euphoria, miosis, weakness, orthostatic hypotension, constipation, and dependence. PB: 7%–25%, t½: 3 h
Hydrocodone bitartrate CSS II	Pain: A: PO: Initially 10 mg q12h	For moderate to severe pain. May cause headache, anxiety, dyspepsia, nausea, vomiting, abdominal pain, constipation, arthralgia, dyspnea, dehydration, peripheral edema, flushing, and infection. Taper off upon discontinuation. PB: 36%; t½: 7–12 h
Hydromorphone hydrochloride CSS II	A: PO: Initially 2.5–10 mg q3-6h or 2–4 mg q4–6h PRN A: IM/subcut: 1–2 mg q2–3h PRN A: IV: 0.2–1 mg over 2–3 min q2–3h PRN Rectal: 3 mg q6–8h PRN	For moderate to severe pain. May cause dizziness, drowsiness, fatigue, headache, abdominal pain, nausea, vomiting, constipation, diarrhea, weakness, peripheral edema, hyperhidrosis, and arthralgia. PB: 8%–19%; t½: 2–3 h
Meperidine CSS II	Severe Pain: A: PO/subcut/IM/IV: 50–150 mg q3–4h PRN, give IV over 4–5 min; *max:* 150 mg/dose	For severe pain and sedation induction and maintenance. May cause dizziness, drowsiness, confusion, euphoria, weakness, visual impairment, dry mouth, nausea, vomiting, constipation, orthostatic hypotension, urinary retention, dependence, and respiratory depression. PB: 65%–75%; t½: 3–5 h
Morphine sulfate CSS II	See Prototype Drug Chart: Morphine Sulfate	
Oxycodone hydrochloride CSS II	Severe pain: Immediate release: A: PO: 5–15 mg q4–6h PRN Extended release: A: PO: 10 mg q12h PRN	For moderate to severe pain. Avoid taking drug over an extended period of time. May cause drowsiness, blurred vision, dry mouth, nausea, vomiting, constipation, diarrhea, weakness, euphoria, edema, and urinary retention. Take with food to avoid GI distress. PB: 45%; t½: 3–5 h
Oxycodone with acetaminophen and oxycodone with aspirin CSS II	Immediate release: A: PO: 1–2 tabs (2.5–10 mg oxycodone/325 mg acetaminophen) q6h PRN Extended release: A: PO: 2 tabs q12h With aspirin: A: PO: 1 tab (4.8355 mg oxycodone/325 mg aspirin) q6h PRN; *max:* 12 tabs/d	For moderate to severe pain. May cause dizziness, drowsiness, headache, confusion, nausea, vomiting, constipation, and urticaria. Take with food or liquid. PB: oxycodone 45%, acetaminophen 10%–25%, ASA 20%–90%; t½: oxycodone 3–5 h, acetaminophen 4 h, ASA 15–20 min
Fentanyl CSS II	Pain: A: IM/IV: 50–100 mcg 30–60 min before surgery (slow IV over 1–2 min); may repeat in 1–2 h for postoperative pain	For moderate to severe pain and anesthesia induction and maintenance. May cause drowsiness, dizziness, euphoria, headache, confusion, fatigue, weakness, hypokalemia, vomiting, nausea, constipation, rash, and tolerance. PB: 80%–85%; t½: IV, 2–4 h; transdermal, 20–27 h; transmucosal, 3–14 h
Methadone CSS II	Pain: A: PO: Initially 2.5 mg q8–12h PRN A: IV/subcut/IM: 2.5–10 mg q8–12h	For moderate to severe pain, opiate agonist dependence and withdrawal. May cause dizziness, drowsiness, blurred vision, confusion, euphoria, orthostatic hypotension, edema, constipation, urinary retention, dependence, and respiratory depression. PB: 85%–90%; t½: 8–59 h
Oxycodone-naloxone	A: PO: oxycodone 10 mg, naloxone 5 mg q12h; *max:* oxycodone 80 mg, naloxone 40 mg	For severe pain. May cause abdominal pain, constipation, dry mouth, diarrhea, anxiety, weakness, confusion, hyperhidrosis, orthostatic hypotension, and withdrawal. PB: oxycodone 45%, naloxone 60%; t½: oxycodone 3–5 h, naloxone 0.5–2 h
Oxycodone-naltrexone	A: PO: oxycodone 10 mg, naltrexone 1.2 mg q12h	For severe pain. May cause abdominal pain, weakness, abnormal dreams, anxiety, dry mouth, dyspepsia, diarrhea, euphoria, hyperhidrosis, confusion, and blurred vision. PB: oxycodone 45%, naltrexone 21%–28%; t½: oxycodone 3–5 h, naltrexone 4 h

A, Adult; *CSS,* Controlled Substances Schedule; *d,* day; *ER,* extended release; *GI,* gastrointestinal; *h,* hour; *IM,* intramuscular; *IV,* intravenous; *max,* maximum; *min,* minute; *PB,* protein binding; *PO,* by mouth; *PRN,* as necessary; *q,* every; *subcut,* subcutaneous; *t½,* half-life; *tab,* tablet; *y,* year.

⚡ **PATIENT SAFETY**

Do not confuse…

- **Meperidine** (opioid analgesic) with **morphine** (opioid analgesic), **meprobamate** (antianxiety), or **hydromorphone** (opioid analgesic).
- **Demerol** (opioid analgesic) with **Desyrel** (antidepressant) or **Dilaudid** (opioid analgesic).

Hydromorphone

Hydromorphone is a semisynthetic opioid similar to morphine. The analgesic effect is approximately six times more potent than that of morphine with fewer hypnotic effects and less GI distress. This opioid has a faster onset and shorter duration of action than morphine. Hydromorphone is classified as a Schedule II drug according to the Controlled Substances Act. Tolerance to hydromorphone increases gradually.

This drug is given orally, rectally, or via subcut, IM, and IV routes for the relief of moderate to severe pain. When given intravenously, dilution of each dose with 5 mL of sterile water or normal saline is preferred. Direct IV administration of 2 mg or less should be given over 2 to 3 minutes. Hydromorphone is readily absorbed in the body and is excreted in the urine. Respirations should be monitored closely, and adequate hydration should be provided.

Side Effects and Adverse Reactions

Many side effects are known to accompany the use of opioids. Of particular importance are signs of respiratory depression (respiration <10 breaths/min). Other side effects include orthostatic hypotension (decrease in blood pressure when rising from a sitting or lying position), drowsiness, dizziness, weakness, confusion, constipation, and urinary retention. In addition, pupillary constriction (a sign of toxicity), tolerance, and psychological and physical dependence may occur with prolonged use.

Increased metabolism of opioids contributes to tolerance, which causes an increased need for higher doses of the opioid. If chronic use of the opioid is discontinued, symptoms of withdrawal that result from cessation of drug administration usually occur within 24 to 48 hours after the last opioid dose. Withdrawal syndrome is caused by physical dependence. Symptoms of withdrawal syndrome include irritability, diaphoresis (sweating), restlessness, muscle twitching, tachycardia, and increased blood pressure. Withdrawal symptoms from opioids are unpleasant but not as severe or life-threatening as those that accompany withdrawal from sedative-hypnotics, a process that may lead to seizures.

Contraindications

Use of opioid analgesics is contraindicated for patients with head injuries. Opioids decrease respiration, which promotes carbon dioxide (CO_2) retention leading to increased intracranial pressure.

Opioid analgesics given to a patient with a respiratory disorder only intensify the respiratory distress. In a patient with asthma, opiates decrease respiratory drive while simultaneously increasing airway resistance.

Opioids may cause hypotension and are not indicated for patients in shock or for those who have very low blood pressure. If an opioid is necessary, the dosage needs to be adjusted accordingly; otherwise, the hypotensive state may worsen. For an older adult or a person who is debilitated, the opioid dose usually needs to be decreased.

Morphine is the opioid analgesic prototype; all other opioids are measured in comparison to morphine.

Combination Drugs

To treat moderate to severe pain, combination drugs that comprise an NSAID and an opioid analgesic may be used. Examples are ibuprofen and hydrocodone, a combination of an NSAID and an opioid. Another combination for the treatment of mild to moderate pain is acetaminophen and codeine. When using a combination of drugs, smaller doses of each drug are required, thereby decreasing side effects. Also, using a combination of drugs for pain helps to decrease drug dependency that may result from possible long-term use of an opioid agent.

Patient-Controlled Analgesia

Patient-controlled analgesia (PCA) is an alternative route for opioid administration for self-administered pain relief as needed. Usually a loading dose (e.g., 2 to 10 mg of morphine) is given initially to achieve pain relief. Within predetermined safety limits, the patient controls administration of the opioid analgesic based on the amount of pain. To receive the opioid, the patient pushes a button on the PCA device, which releases a specific dose of analgesic (e.g., 1 mg morphine) into the IV line. The nurse sets the PCA pump with the opioid analgesic dose prescribed by the health care provider by regulating the time intervals (every several minutes) at which the drug can be received. A lockout mechanism on the electronically controlled infusion pump prevents the patient from constantly pushing the button and causing a drug overdose. The PCA device maintains a near-constant analgesic level, avoiding episodes of severe pain or oversedation. It is imperative that the patient, not the family or the nurse, control the PCA device to avoid overdosing. Morphine is used most often for PCA, but fentanyl and hydromorphone may also be given.

Transdermal Opioid Analgesics

Transdermal opioid analgesics provide continuous, around-the-clock pain control that is helpful to patients who suffer from chronic pain. The transdermal method is not useful for acute or postoperative pain. An example of a transdermal opioid analgesic is fentanyl, which is administered via a transdermal patch. This patch comes in various strengths—12.5, 25, 50, 75, and 100 mcg/h. Maximum serum fentanyl levels occur within 24 hours of when the patch is first applied. Fentanyl is also available for IM and IV use. Fentanyl is more potent than morphine. For older adults, the use of a lower fentanyl transdermal dose is usually suggested. The health care provider must exercise caution when prescribing fentanyl for patients who weigh less than 110 pounds.

Analgesic Titration

Analgesics may be titrated to increase or decrease the dosage. Usually postoperative pain will decrease over time, and analgesics will be titrated downward. However, the patient with cancer-related pain usually has a continual increase in pain and will require an upward titration. Titration can be accomplished by changing the dose, the interval between doses, the route of administration, or the drug. When titrating analgesics, the dosage is decided after assessing the patient's respiratory rate and pain level.

Opioid Use in Special Populations
Children

Pain management in children is complex because it is more difficult to assess their pain. Some children will not verbalize discomfort when they are in severe pain, and some are fearful of treatments like injections that relieve pain. Nurses should use age-appropriate communication skills to ascertain a child's need for pain relief. The "ouch scale"

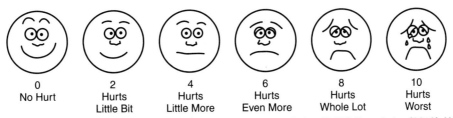

Fig. 25.1 Wong-Baker FACES® Pain Rating Scale. (From Wong-Baker FACES Foundation [2019]. Wong-Baker FACES® Pain Rating Scale. Published with permission from http://www.WongBakerFACES.org. Originally published in *Whaley & Wong's Nursing Care of Infants and Children.* © Elsevier Inc.)

illustrated in Fig. 25.1 can be helpful in determining a child's level of pain. Also, the parent may help identify the presence and degree of the child's pain. Crying and whining may be indicators of a need for pain relief or may represent other needs.

A child, like an adult, should be given medication before the pain becomes severe. The use of oral liquid medication for pain relief, if appropriate, is generally more acceptable to the child. The nurse may alleviate the child's fear and help with drug compliance by using drawings and pictures related to areas of pain in the body and pain relief with smiling faces.

Older Adults

Usually, adults who are 65 years of age or older require adjustment to drug doses to avoid severe side effects. Merely decreasing the usual adult dosage of opioid analgesic is not always the answer for older adults. Many take an array of medications for their health problems, increasing the possibility of drug interactions and drug side effects. In older adults, side effects from the use of opioids are more pronounced; therefore, the nurse must closely monitor for adverse reactions in older adults who take opioid analgesics. As a person ages, liver and renal functions decrease, causing the rate of metabolism and excretion of the drug to decrease. As a result, drug accumulation may occur.

Older adults tend to have different beliefs and fears than younger generations regarding opioids. They may believe that pain is inevitable due to aging, or they may fear addiction. Older adults may not want to report pain because they do not want to be a burden. The nurse must perform pain assessment with a supportive approach in an unhurried manner and should give the patient accurate drug information.

Pain assessment may be more difficult with older adults due to the decrease in cognitive and sensory perceptual abilities. Dementia or hearing and visual deficits may interfere with communication. The nurse may need to rely on a more thorough physical assessment to discover the presence of pain, because self-reporting may not be reliable.

In the presence of decreased renal and hepatic function, drugs that tend to be more toxic in older adults include meperidine and pentazocine. Analgesics are usually metabolized in the liver and are excreted in the urine. Usual doses of analgesics in older adults may result in excessive sedation and prolonged duration of action. Chronologic age is one of several factors that influence medication use and dosage. Comorbidity must also be considered.

Cognitively Impaired Individuals

Any cognitively impaired individual may be unable to report pain adequately. The nurse should use a measurement scale that is appropriate for the patient. Some physical signs of pain include moans, grimacing, clenched teeth, noisy respirations, and restlessness.

Oncology Patients

Cancer pain is managed according to three levels of analgesia based on the WHO "ladder" as follows:

Step 1—Mild Pain: Nonopioids with or without an adjuvant medication

Step 2—Moderate Pain: Nonopioids and mild opioids with or without an adjuvant medication

Step 3—Severe Pain: Stronger opioids at higher dosage levels with or without an adjuvant medication

Opioids are titrated for oncology patients until pain relief is achieved or the side effects become intolerable. For effective pain management in patients with cancer, extremely high doses may be required. There are no set dosage limits for oncology patients.

Individuals With a History of Substance Use Disorder

Often patients with a history of substance use disorder require pain medication. A thorough pain assessment is necessary to find out the cause of pain. The nurse needs to know that opioids are effective and safe in this population, even though larger doses in greater frequency may be required. Studies have shown that withholding opioids in this population has not increased recovery from addiction. However, opioid agonist-antagonists such as pentazocine should be avoided in chemically dependent patients because these drugs may precipitate withdrawal syndrome.

ADJUVANT THERAPY

Medications used as adjuvant analgesics have been developed for other purposes and were later found to be effective for pain relief in neuropathy. Adjuvant therapy is usually used along with a nonopioid and opioid analgesic. Examples of adjuvant analgesics include anticonvulsants, antidepressants, corticosteroids, antidysrhythmics, and local anesthetics.

Antiseizure medications such as gabapentin act on the peripheral nerves and CNS by inhibiting spontaneous neuronal firing. They are used for neuropathic pain and for prevention of migraine headaches. Tricyclic antidepressants (TCAs) such as amitriptyline prevent the reuptake of serotonin and norepinephrine in the cells. Lower doses of TCAs than those usually prescribed for depression are effective in treating peripheral neuropathy. Corticosteroids serve as effective analgesics by reducing nociceptive stimuli. Antidysrhythmics such as mexiletine block sodium channels to reduce pain. Local anesthetics—for example, a lidocaine patch—can provide effective analgesia by interrupting the transmission of pain signals to the brain.

Adjuvant medications potentiate opioid analgesia for severe persistent pain in diabetic neuropathy, cancer, migraine headaches, and rheumatoid arthritis. When any of the adjuvant medications are used in conjunction with an NSAID and an opioid, dosages may be kept lower to reduce adverse effects.

TREATMENT FOR SUBSTANCE USE DISORDER

Refer to Chapter 8 for a discussion of therapies for substance use disorder.

OPIOID AGONIST-ANTAGONISTS

Opioid agonist-antagonists, medications in which an opioid antagonist is added to an opioid agonist, may be used to decrease substance use disorder. Pentazocine, an opioid agonist-antagonist analgesic, can be given by injection (subcut, IM, and IV). Pentazocine is classified as a Schedule IV drug. Butorphanol tartrate, buprenorphine, and nalbuphine hydrochloride are examples of other opioid agonist-antagonist analgesics. Reports say that pentazocine and butorphanol can cause dependence. Opioid agonist-antagonist drugs are not given for cancer pain because of the risk of potential CNS toxicity from the high doses required. These analgesics are considered safe for use during labor, but their safety during early pregnancy has not been established.

Prototype Drug Chart: Nalbuphine details the pharmacologic behavior of nalbuphine, and Table 25.4 lists the various opioid agonist-antagonists.

Pharmacokinetics. Nalbuphine can be administered orally or via IM, subcut, or IV routes. It is rapidly absorbed parenterally. Its protein binding capacity is less than 30%. Nalbuphine has a short half-life of 3 to 6 hours. It is metabolized in the liver and excreted in the urine.

Pharmacodynamics. Nalbuphine is effective in alleviating moderate to severe pain. The onset of action is rapid, and peak time occurs within 30 minutes with IV administration. The duration of action is 3 to 4 hours for IV administration and 3 to 6 hours for intramuscular/subcutaneous administration.

OPIOID ANTAGONISTS

Opioid antagonists are antidotes for drug toxicity of natural and synthetic opioid analgesics. The opioid antagonists have a higher affinity to the opiate receptor site than the opioid being taken. An opioid antagonist blocks the receptor and displaces any opioid that would normally be at the receptor, which inhibits the opioid action. Indications for opioid antagonists include reversal of postoperative opioid depression and opioid overdose.

Naloxone is administered via an IM or IV route, and naltrexone hydrochloride is administered orally by tablet or liquid. These drugs are perfect examples of pharmacologic antagonists because they reverse the respiratory and CNS depression (sedation and hypotension) caused by opioids. Table 25.5 lists the opioid antagonists.

When receiving opioid antagonists, the patient should be monitored continuously. The opioid action may exceed that of opioid antagonists, and further analgesia may be needed. For example, fentanyl and a combination of drugs given during surgery may lead to excessive respiratory depression. Naloxone may be given as an opioid antidote. The patient's respiratory and CNS status should be monitored closely for indications of analgesic reversal (tachycardia, nausea, vomiting, and sweating) and the possible need for further analgesia. The patient receiving naloxone should also be observed for bleeding because this drug may cause an elevated partial thromboplastin time.

HEADACHES: MIGRAINE AND CLUSTER

Migraine headaches are characterized by a unilateral throbbing head pain accompanied by nausea, vomiting, and photophobia. These symptoms frequently persist for 4 to 24 hours and for several days in some cases. Two-thirds of migraine headaches are experienced by women

---

📄 PROTOTYPE DRUG CHART

Nalbuphine

Drug Class	Dosage
Opioid agonist-antagonist	Pain: A: IV/IM/subcut: 10 mg q3–6h PRN; *max:* 20 mg/dose, 160 mg/d

Contraindications	Drug-Lab-Food Interactions
Hypersensitivity *Caution:* Alcohol or drug use disorder, respiratory insufficiency, head injury, increased ICP, biliary tract disease, renal or hepatic dysfunction, older adults	Drug: CNS depression is potentiated with alcohol or other CNS depressants.

Pharmacokinetics	Pharmacodynamics
Absorption: Readily occurs parenterally Distribution: PB: 50%; crosses placenta, excreted in breast milk Metabolism: t½: 3–6 h Excretion: In urine, bile, and feces	Onset: 2–3 min IV; <15 min IM/subcut Peak: 30 min IV; 30 min IM Duration: 3–4 h IV; 3–6 h IM/subcut

Therapeutic Effects/Uses

To relieve moderate to severe pain and for anesthesia induction and maintenance
Mechanism of Action: Inhibits pain impulses transmitted in the CNS by binding with opiate receptors and increasing pain threshold

Side Effects	Adverse Reactions
Dizziness, drowsiness, headache, dry mouth, nausea, vomiting, diaphoresis, erectile dysfunction	Bradycardia, hypo/hypertension, dyspnea *Life-threatening:* Respiratory depression, seizures, dependence

A, Adult; *CNS,* central nervous system; *d,* day; *h,* hour; *ICP,* intracranial pressure; *IM,* intramuscular; *IV,* intravenous; *max,* maximum; *min,* minute; *PB,* protein binding; *q,* every; *subcut,* subcutaneous; *t½,* half-life; <, less than.

TABLE 25.4 Opioid Agonist-Antagonists and Opioid Agonist

Generic	Route and Dosage	Uses and Considerations
Buprenorphine hydrochloride CSS V	Pain: A: IM/IV: Initially, 0.3 mg (older adults 0.15 mg); may repeat in 30–60 min, then q6–8h PRN; *max:* 0.6 mg/dose IM, 0.3 mg/dose IV A: Transdermal: 5 mcg/h patch q7d; *max:* 20 mcg/h A: Transmucosal: 75 mcg/d or q12h; *max:* 900 mcg q12h	For moderate to severe pain, opiate dependence, and withdrawal. May cause dizziness, drowsiness, headache, anxiety, insomnia, back and abdominal pain, nausea, constipation, diaphoresis, and weakness. PB: 96%; t½: IV 1.2–7.2 h, transdermal 26 h
Butorphanol tartrate CSS IV	A: IM: 1–4 mg q3–4h PRN A: IV: 0.5–2 mg q3–4h PRN A: Nasal spray: 1 mg (1 spray into 1 nostril), may apply additional spray in 60–90 min in other nostril, then q3–4h PRN	For moderate to severe pain and anesthesia induction and maintenance. May cause dizziness, drowsiness, insomnia, nasal congestion, nausea, vomiting, withdrawal, and tolerance. PB: 80%; t½: 2–9 h
Nalbuphine hydrochloride CSS IV	See Prototype Drug Chart: Nalbuphine	
Pentazocine lactate CSS IV	A: Subcut/IM/IV: 30 mg q3–4 h PRN; *max:* 360 mg/d	For moderate to severe pain and anesthesia induction and maintenance. May cause dizziness, drowsiness, confusion, nausea, vomiting, and tolerance. PB: UK; t½: 1.5–10 h
Sufentanil	A: SL: 30 mcg q1h PRN up to 72 h; *max:* 12 tabs/d (30 mcg tab)	For acute pain when alternative treatment options are inadequate, and anesthesia induction. May cause nausea, vomiting, headache, chest wall rigidity, dizziness, and hypo/hypertension. PB: 93%; t½: 13.4 h
Oliceridine	A: IV: 1.5 mg, then 0.75 mg q1h PRN; *max:* 3 mg/dose, 27 mg/d	For acute severe pain. May cause dizziness, drowsiness, headache, nausea, vomiting, constipation, back pain, pruritus, and hypoxia.

A, Adult; *CNS*, central nervous system; *CSS*, Controlled Substances Schedule; *d*, day; *GI*, gastrointestinal; *h*, hour; *IM*, intramuscular; *IV*, intravenous; *IVP*, intravenous push; *max*, maximum; *min*, minutes; *PB*, protein binding; *PRN*, as needed; *q*, every; *subcut*, subcutaneous; *sl*, sublingual; *t½*, half-life; *UK*, unknown; *>*, greater than.

⚡ PATIENT SAFETY

Do not confuse...
- **Nubain,** a narcotic agonist-antagonist analgesic for moderate to severe pain, with **Nebcin,** an aminoglycoside antibiotic, or **Nuprin,** an OTC analgesic, antipyretic NSAID.

◎ CLINICAL JUDGMENT [NURSING PROCESS]

Opioid Agonist-Antagonist Analgesic: Nalbuphine

Concept: Pain
- An unpleasant feeling of discomfort associated usually with tissue damage

Recognize Cues [Assessment]
- Obtain a drug history from the patient. Report if a drug-drug interaction is probable. When taken with nalbuphine, central nervous system (CNS) depressants can cause respiratory depression.
- Note baseline vital signs for future comparisons.
- Assess the type of pain, duration, and location before giving the drug.

Analyze Cues and Prioritize Hypothesis [Patient Problems]
- Decreased gas exchange
- Acute pain
- Discomfort
- Constipation

Generate Solutions [Planning]
- The patient will report that pain has decreased within 1 hour after medication administration.

Take Action [Nursing Interventions]
- Monitor vital signs. Note any changes in respirations.
- Check bowel sounds and the date of the last bowel movement to identify constipation. Decreased peristalsis may result in constipation. A mild laxative may be necessary.

- Determine urine output. Report if urine output is less than 30 mL/h or less than 600 mL/day.
- Administer intravenous (IV) nalbuphine undiluted. Do not mix with barbiturates.

Patient Teaching
General
- ⚡ Warn patients not to use alcohol or CNS depressants while taking nalbuphine. Respiratory depression can occur.
- Suggest nonpharmacologic methods for lessening pain, such as changing position or ambulation.

Side Effects
- Advise patients to report side effects of nalbuphine: dizziness, headaches, constipation, dysuria, rash, or blurred vision. Hallucinations, tachycardia, and respiratory depression are adverse reactions that might occur.

Evaluate Outcomes [Evaluation]
- Evaluate the effectiveness of nalbuphine in relieving pain. If ineffective, another opioid analgesic may need to be ordered.
- Determine stability of vital signs. Note whether a change in respirations, pulse rate, or blood pressure occurs. Report abnormal findings.

TABLE 25.5 Opioid Antagonists

Generic	Route and Dosage	Uses and Considerations
Naloxone hydrochloride	Opiate agonist overdose: A: IV/IM/Subcut: 0.4–2 mg; may repeat q2–3 min; *max:* 2 mg/dose A: Intranasal: 1 spray (2 or 4 mg) may repeat dose in alternate nostrils q2–3min PRN	For opioid overdose and opioid-induced respiratory depression. May cause flushing, agitation, hypo/hypertension, confusion, dizziness, tachycardia, headache, hyperhidrosis, nausea, vomiting, and dyspnea. PB: 60%; t½: 0.5–2 h
Naltrexone hydrochloride	A: PO: 25–50 mg/d with food for 12 wk; *max:* 150 mg/d A: IM: 380 mg/dose q4wk; *max:* 380 mg/dose	For opioid agonist and alcohol dependence. May cause dizziness, headache, insomnia, anxiety, anorexia, nausea, diarrhea, abdominal pain, constipation, bleeding, weakness, and injection site reaction. PB: 21%; t½: 21%–28%
Lofexidine	A: PO: Initially 0.54 mg qid for 5–7 d; *max:* 2.88 mg/d	For opioid withdrawal. May cause dizziness, drowsiness, bradycardia, orthostatic hypotension, insomnia, dry mouth, tinnitus, and withdrawal. PB: 55%; t½: 17–22 h

A, Adult; *d*, day; *GI*, gastrointestinal; *IM*, intramuscular; *IV*, intravenous; *max*, maximum; *min*, minute; *PB*, protein binding; *PO*, by mouth; *q*, every; *subcut*, subcutaneous; *t½*, half-life; *UK*, unknown; *wk*, weeks; *y*, years; >, greater than; <, less than.

in their 20s and 30s. Symptoms usually decrease or are absent during pregnancy and menopause. The intensity of migraine pain can disrupt daily activities.

Pathophysiology

The exact etiology of migraine headaches is unknown, although many theories exist. A common theory suggests a series of neurovascular events initiates a migraine headache. Neuronal hyperexcitability occurs in the cerebral cortex, especially in the occipital cortex. Specific factors that trigger a migraine headache include foods, monosodium glutamate, aspartame, fatigue, stress, too much or too little sleep, missed meals, odors, light, hormone changes, drugs, and weather. Foods such as cheese, chocolate, and red wine can trigger an attack.

The two types of migraine are *migraines associated with an aura*, which occurs minutes to 1 hour before onset, and *migraines without aura*.

Cluster headaches are characterized by a severe, unilateral, non-throbbing pain usually located around the eye. They occur in a series of cluster attacks in which one or more attacks occur every day for several weeks. Cluster headaches are not associated with an aura and do not cause nausea and vomiting. Men are more commonly affected by cluster headaches than women.

Treatment of Migraine Headaches

Preventive treatment for migraines includes (1) beta-adrenergic blockers, such as propranolol and atenolol; (2) anticonvulsants, such as valproic acid and gabapentin; and (3) TCAs, such as amitriptyline and imipramine.

Treatment of a migraine attack depends on the intensity of pain. Drugs used to treat migraines include analgesics, opioid analgesics, ergot alkaloids, and selective serotonin (5-HT) receptor agonists, also known as *triptans*. For mild migraine attacks, aspirin, acetaminophen, or NSAIDs such as ibuprofen or naproxen may be prescribed. Aspirin may be used in combination with caffeine. Meperidine and butorphanol nasal spray are opioid analgesics that are occasionally used.

Antimigraine medication should be taken early during a migraine attack. Nausea and vomiting might occur, and antiemetics decrease these symptoms. Dihydroergotamine, an ergot alkaloid, can be administered subcutaneously, intramuscularly, intravenously, and by means of a nasal spray.

The triptans, 5-HT receptor agonists, are the most recently developed group of drugs for the treatment of migraine headaches. Sumatriptan, a selective serotonin receptor agonist with a short duration of action, was the first triptan drug. It is considered more effective than ergot alkaloids in treating acute migraine attacks. Table 25.6 lists the ergot alkaloids and the 5-HT receptor agonists and their dosages, uses, and considerations.

> ⚡ **PATIENT SAFETY**
>
> **Do not confuse...**
> - **Sumatriptan** with **zolmitriptan.** Both drugs are triptans but have different dosages.
> - **Amerge,** a triptan used for migraines, with **Amaryl,** a sulfonylurea used for diabetes mellitus, or **Altace,** an angiotensin-converting enzyme (ACE) inhibitor used for hypertension and heart failure.

Prototype Drug Chart: Sumatriptan provides further information on the pharmacology of sumatriptan.

TABLE 25.6 Drugs Used to Treat Severe Migraine Headaches

Drug	Route and Dosage	Uses and Considerations
Ergot Alkaloids		
Dihydroergotamine mesylate	A: Intranasal: 1 spray (0.5 mg) in each nostril; may repeat in 15 min; *max:* 4 sprays (2 mg total dose), 3 mg/d, 4 mg/wk A: IM/subcut/IV: 1 mg; may repeat q1h until resolved; *max:* Subcut/IM 3 mg/d, IV 2 mg/d	For migraine and cluster headaches. May cause drowsiness, dizziness, rhinitis, pharyngitis, paresthesia, dysgeusia, nausea, vomiting, and diarrhea. PB: 90%–93%; t½: 9–10 h
Selective Serotonin Receptor Agonists (Triptans)		
Sumatriptan	See Prototype Drug Chart: Sumatriptan	
Naratriptan	A: PO: 1–2.5 mg; may repeat in 4 h; *max:* 5 mg/d	For migraines. May cause dizziness, drowsiness, nausea, vomiting, fatigue, and paresthesia. PB: 28%–31%; t½: 6 h
Rizatriptan benzoate	A: PO: 5–10 mg; may repeat q2h; *max:* 30 mg/d	For migraines. May cause dizziness, drowsiness, dry mouth, nausea, weakness, paresthesia, and fatigue. PB: 14%; t½: 2–3 h
Zolmitriptan	A: PO: 1.25–2.5 mg; may repeat in 2 h; *max:* 5 mg/dose; 10 mg/d A: Oral disintegrating tab: 2.5 mg; *max:* 5 mg/dose, 10 mg/d Nasal inhalation: A: 2.5–5 mg in 1 nostril; may repeat in 2 h; *max:* 10 mg/d	For migraines. May cause dizziness, drowsiness, dysgeusia, dry mouth, nausea, paresthesia, hyperesthesia, and weakness. PB: 25%; t½: 3 h
Almotriptan	A: PO: 6.25–12.5 mg; may repeat in 2 h; *max:* 25 mg/d	For migraines. May cause drowsiness, dizziness, paresthesia, headache, nausea, and vomiting. PB: 35%; t½: 3–4 h
Frovatriptan	A: PO: 2.5 mg; may repeat in 2 h; *max:* 7.5 mg/d	For migraines. May cause dizziness, flushing, headache, dry mouth, nausea, vomiting, diarrhea, paresthesia, and fatigue. PB: 15%; t½: 26 h
Eletriptan	A: PO: 20–40 mg; may repeat in 2 h; *max:* 40 mg/dose, 80 mg/d	For migraines. May cause dizziness, drowsiness, flushing, headache, hyperhidrosis, dry mouth, nausea, weakness, and paresthesia. PB: 85%; t½: 13 h
Lasmiditan	A: PO: 50, 100, or 200 mg as single dose; *max:* 1 dose/24 h or 200 mg/d	For migraines. May cause dizziness, drowsiness, fatigue, weakness, hypoesthesia, paresthesias, nausea, and vomiting. PB: 55%–60%; t½: 5.7 h
Gene-Related Peptide		
Erenumab	A: Subcut: 70–140 mg/mo	For migraine prophylaxis. May cause antibody formation, injection site reaction, constipation, alopecia, muscle cramps, erythema, and pruritus. PB: UK; t½: 28 d
Fremanezumab	A: Subcut: 225 mg/mo or 675 mg q3mo	For migraine prophylaxis. May cause antibody formation, injection site reaction, erythema, rash, urticaria, and pruritus. PB: UK; t½: 31 d
Galcanezumab	A: Subcut: LD 240 mg, then 120 mg q1mo	For migraine prophylaxis and cluster headaches. May cause antibody formation, injection site reaction, erythema, rash, and pruritus. PB: UK; t½: 27 d
Rimegepant	A: PO: 75 mg as single dose; *max:* 75 mg/d	For migraines. May cause nausea, dyspnea, abdominal pain, dyspepsia, and rash. PB: 96%; t½: 11 h
Ubrogepant	A: PO: 50 or 100 mg as single dose, may give second dose in 2 h PRN; *max:* 200 mg/d	For migraines. May cause dry mouth, fatigue, and nausea. PB: 87%; t½: 5–7 h
Eptinezumab	A: IV: 100 mg q3months with 30 min infusion; *max:* 300 mg q3mo	For migraine prophylaxis. May cause flushing, pharyngitis, rash, urticaria, angioedema, and antibody formation. PB: UK; t½: 27 d
Atogepant	A: PO: 10, 30, or 60 mg/d; *max:* 60 mg/d	For episodic migraine prophylaxis. May cause anorexia, nausea, constipation, weight loss, drowsiness, and fatigue. PB: UK; t½: 11 h

A, Adult; *CAD*, coronary artery disease; *d*, day; *GI*, gastrointestinal; *h*, hour; *IHD*, ischemic heart disease; *IM*, intramuscular; *IV*, intravenous; *LD*, loading dose; *max*, maximum; *MI*, myocardial infarction; *min*, minute; *PB*, protein binding; *PO*, by mouth; *q*, every; *subcut*, subcutaneous; *t½*, half-life; *tab*, tablet; *wk*, week; *y*, years; *>*, greater than.

📄 PROTOTYPE DRUG CHART

Sumatriptan

Drug Class	Dosage
Selective serotonin receptor agonist: Antimigraine	A: PO: Initially 25–100 mg, may repeat in 2 h; *max:* 200 mg/d A: Subcut: 3–6 mg, may repeat after 1 h; *max:* 12 mg/d A: Intranasal: 5–20 mg in 1 nostril, may repeat after 2 h; *max:* 40 mg/d

Contraindications	Drug-Lab-Food Interactions
Hypersensitivity, CAD, peripheral vascular disease, hypertension, cerebrovascular disease *Caution:* Renal or hepatic dysfunction, dysrhythmias, intracranial bleeding, obesity, DM, smoking, seizures, older adults	Drug: Risk of vasospasm and blood pressure elevation with dihydroergotamine and other ergot alkaloids; increased levels and toxicity within 2 weeks of MAOIs; increased risk of serotonin syndrome or neuroleptic malignant syndrome with SSRIs

Continued

PROTOTYPE DRUG CHART—CONT'D

Pharmacokinetics

Absorption: Rapidly absorbed after subcut injection
Distribution: PB: 14%–21%
Metabolism: t½: 2 h
Excretion: Urine and feces

Pharmacodynamics

PO: Onset: 60 min
Peak: 2 h; duration: 24–48 h
Subcut: Onset: 10 min
Peak: 5–20 min; duration: 24–48 h
Intranasal: Onset: 15 min
Peak: 1–1.5 h; duration: 24–48 h

Therapeutic Effects/Uses

To treat migraine and cluster headaches
Mechanism of Action: Causes vasoconstriction of cranial arteries to relieve migraine attacks

Side Effects

Dizziness, headache, blurred vision, paresthesia, fatigue, flushing, drowsiness, dysgeusia, myalgia, hyperhidrosis, nausea, vomiting, injection site reaction, pruritus, skin irritation

Adverse Reactions

Hypotension, hypertensive crisis, angina, dysrhythmias, bradycardia, tachycardia, thrombosis, seizures, hearing loss, ocular hemorrhage, GI bleeding/obstruction

Life-threatening: Coronary artery vasospasm, renal failure, angioedema, hemolytic anemia, pancytopenia, thrombocytopenia, intracranial hemorrhage, stroke, MI, cardiac arrest, suicidal ideation

5-HT, Serotonin; *A,* adult; *AV,* atrioventricular; *CAD,* coronary artery disease; *d,* day; *DM,* diabetes mellitus; *h,* hour; *MAOI,* monoamine oxidase inhibitor; *max,* maximum; *MI,* myocardial infarction; *min,* minute; *PB,* protein binding; *PO,* by mouth; *SSRI,* selective serotonin reuptake inhibitor; *subcut,* subcutaneous; *t½,* half-life.

CRITICAL THINKING SINGLE EPISODE CASE STUDY

Cognitive Skill: Prioritize Hypotheses
Objective: Prioritize nursing care for a postoperative patient receiving a prescribed analgesic.

A 79-year-old male client on the medical surgical unit is complaining of abdominal pain. This patient has a history of ulcerative colitis and 24 hours prior received emergent resection of the colon. During the morning assessment the nurse notes his last dose of 2 mg IV morphine was administered on the previous shift 6 hours prior. It is ordered every 4 hours. The nurse administers the patient's prescribed dose of 2 mg IV morphine after the morning assessment and vital signs check.

Which nursing actions are required related to the client's condition and prescribed pain medication? Choose the most likely options for the information missing from the statements below by selecting from the lists of options provided.

The nurse will continue to monitor the patient's _____(A)_____ and assess the depth and rate of the patient's _____(A)_____. Instruct the patient to report signs and symptoms of _____(A)_____, _____(A)_____, and _____(A)_____. Monitor and observe for changes in the patient's _____(B)_____. The nurse will withhold pain medication for any difficulty in the patient's _____(B)_____ and respirations below _____(B)_____. Instruct the patient to notify the nurse immediately upon return or increase of the patient's _____(B)_____.

Option A	Option B
tinnitus	dry skin
dizziness	breathing
vital signs	pedal edema
sore throat	mental status
respirations	abdominal pain

constipation	episodes of sneezing
hypotension	12 breaths per minute
feeling of fullness	20 breaths per minute

Answers:

The nurse will continue to monitor the patient's vital signs and asses the depth and rate of the patient's respirations. Instruct the patient to report signs and symptoms of dizziness, constipation, and hypotension. Monitor and observe for changes in the patient's mental status. The nurse will withhold pain medication for any difficulty in the patient's breathing and respirations below 12 breaths per minute. Instruct the patient to notify the nurse immediately upon return or increase of the patient's abdominal pain.

Rationale:

Morphine binds with the opiate receptors in the central nervous system, producing analgesia and sedation. The onset of action when administered parenterally is 15–20 min. Morphine injection has high risk for low respiratory rate, which can result in respiratory depression. If the patient is experiencing breathing difficulty and their respirations are below 12 breaths per minute, the nurse should withhold the medication and notify the provider because the patient may be developing respiratory distress. Also, it is known to cause sedation, hypotension, constipation, and changes in mental status. It is important to administer the morphine before pain reaches its peak to maximize the effectiveness of the drug, so instruct the patient to report any periods of increased abdominal pain.

Reference:
McCuistion, et al.: Pharmacology, Chapter 25 (see Prototype Drug Chart). In Burchum J, Rosenthal L, editors: *Lehne's Pharmacology for Nursing Care*, 10th ed, 2019.

REVIEW QUESTIONS

1. A patient requires a nonopioid medication. The nurse knows that which medication will cause the least gastrointestinal distress?
   a. Aspirin
   b. Ketorolac
   c. Celecoxib
   d. Ibuprofen

2. A patient states during a medical history that he takes several acetaminophen tablets throughout the day for acute pain. The nurse teaches the patient that the dosage should not exceed which amount?
   a. 1 g/day
   b. 3 g/day
   c. 4 g/day
   d. 6 g/day

3. For the patient receiving periodic morphine via intravenous push, which of the following findings would be of utmost concern to the nurse?
   a. Increased temperature
   b. Decreased bowel sounds
   c. Decreased respirations
   d. Increased red blood cell count

4. A patient is admitted to the emergency department with signs of respiratory depression after self-injection with hydromorphone. The admitting nurse knows that which drug will reverse respiratory depression caused by opioid overdose?
   a. Fentanyl
   b. Naloxone
   c. Butorphanol
   d. Sufenta

5. Assessing a patient after intravenous morphine administration, the nurse notes cold, clammy skin; a pulse of 40 beats/min; respirations of 10 breaths/min; and constricted pupils. Which medication will the patient likely need next?
   a. Naloxone
   b. Meloxicam
   c. Pentazocine
   d. Propoxyphene

6. For the patient taking acetaminophen, what should the nurse do? (Select all that apply.)
   a. Monitor routine liver enzyme tests.
   b. Encourage the patient to check package labels of over-the-counter drugs to avoid overdosing.
   c. Report side effects immediately, as toxicity can cause severe hepatic damage.
   d. Teach the female patient that oral contraceptives can increase the effect of acetaminophen.
   e. Teach the patient that caffeine decreases the effects of acetaminophen.

7. For the patient who is taking nalbuphine, what should the nurse do? (Select all that apply.)
   a. Monitor any changes in respirations.
   b. Instruct the patient to report hypohidrosis.
   c. Administer intravenous nalbuphine undiluted.
   d. Explain to the patient to expect an excessive amount of urine output.
   e. Instruct the patient to avoid alcohol when taking nalbuphine to avoid respiratory depression.

8. A patient is having a migraine attack. The nurse should know that which drugs are used to treat migraine attacks?
   a. Triptans
   b. Anticonvulsants
   c. Tricyclic antidepressants
   d. Beta-adrenergic blockers

26

Penicillins, Other Beta-Lactams, and Cephalosporins

http://evolve.elsevier.com/McCuistion/pharmacology

OBJECTIVES

- Explain the mechanisms of action of antibacterial drugs.
- Differentiate between bacteria that are naturally resistant and those that have acquired resistance to an antibiotic.
- Summarize the three general adverse effects associated with antibacterial drugs.
- Differentiate between narrow-spectrum and broad-spectrum antibiotics.

- Compare the effects of the natural, broad-spectrum (extended), penicillinase-resistant, and antipseudomonal penicillins.
- Contrast the effects of first-, second-, third-, fourth-, and fifth-generation cephalosporins.
- Apply the Clinical Judgment [Nursing Process] for patients receiving penicillins and cephalosporins.

OUTLINE

INTRODUCTION

Disease-producing microorganisms may be gram-positive or gram-negative bacteria, viruses, protozoans, or fungi. The degree to which they are pathogenic depends on the microorganism and its virulence.

This chapter discusses penicillins, other beta-lactam antibacterials, and cephalosporins and their effects. It includes mechanisms of antibacterial action, body defenses, resistance to antibacterials, use of antibacterial combinations, general adverse reactions to antibacterials, and narrow- and broad-spectrum antibiotics.

The penicillins are primarily bacteriostatic drugs, those that inhibit bacterial growth, but they may also be bactericidal (bacteria killing), depending on the drug dose, serum level, and pathogen (the

disease-producing microorganism). Cephalosporins and other beta-lactams are bactericidal drugs.

PATHOPHYSIOLOGY

Bacteria, known as *prokaryotes,* are single-celled organisms that lack a true nucleus and nuclear membrane. Most bacteria have a rigid cell wall, and the structure of the cell wall determines the shape of the bacteria. One classification of bacteria involves the appearance or shape under a microscope. A *bacillus* is a rod-shaped organism, and *cocci* are spherical. When cocci appear in clusters, they are called *staphylococci*; when they are arranged in chains, they are called *streptococci*. Bacteria reproduce by cell division about every 20 minutes.

Another classification of bacteria involves staining properties of the cell. The Gram staining method was devised in 1882 by Hans Christian Gram, a Danish bacteriologist. Gram staining determines the ability of the bacterial cell wall to retain a purple stain by a basic dye. Crystal violet is normally used in the staining process but may be substituted with methylene blue. If bacteria retain a purple stain, they are classified as gram-positive microorganisms. Those bacteria not stained are known as gram-negative microorganisms. Examples of gram-positive bacteria include *Staphylococcus aureus*, *Streptococcus pneumoniae*, group B *Streptococcus* (GBS), and *Clostridium perfringens*. Examples of gram-negative bacteria include *Neisseria meningitides*, *Escherichia coli*, and *Haemophilus influenzae*.

Bacteria produce toxins that cause cell lysis (cell breakdown). Many bacteria produce the enzyme beta-lactamase, which destroys beta-lactam antibiotics such as penicillins and cephalosporins.

ANTIBACTERIAL DRUGS

ANTIBACTERIALS/ANTIBIOTICS

Although the terms *antibacterial*, *antimicrobial*, and *antibiotic* are frequently used interchangeably, there are some subtle differences in meaning. Antibacterials and antimicrobials are substances that inhibit bacterial growth or kill bacteria and other microorganisms—microscopic organisms that include viruses, fungi, protozoa, and rickettsiae. Technically, the term *antibiotic* refers to chemicals produced by one kind of microorganism that inhibit the growth of or kill another. For practical purposes, however, these terms may be used interchangeably. Several drugs, including antiinfective and chemotherapeutic agents, have actions similar to those of antibacterial and antimicrobial agents. Antibacterial drugs do not act alone in destroying bacteria. Natural body defenses, surgical procedures to excise infected tissues, and dressing changes may be needed along with antibacterial drugs to eliminate the infecting bacteria.

Antibacterial drugs are either obtained from natural sources or manufactured. The use of moldy bread on wounds to fight infection dates back 3500 years. In 1928 British bacteriologist Alexander Fleming noted that a mold that had contaminated his bacterial cultures was inhibiting bacterial growth. The mold was *Penicillium notatum*; thus Fleming called the substance *penicillin*. In 1939 Howard Florey expanded on Fleming's findings and purified penicillin so it could be used commercially. Penicillin was used during World War II and was marketed in 1945.

Mechanisms of Antibacterial Action

Five mechanisms of antibacterial action are responsible for the inhibition of growth or destruction of microorganisms: (1) inhibition of bacterial cell wall synthesis, (2) alteration of membrane permeability, (3) inhibition of protein synthesis, (4) inhibition of the synthesis of bacterial ribonucleic acid (RNA) and deoxyribonucleic acid (DNA), and (5) interference with metabolism within the cell (Table 26.1).

Pharmacokinetics. Antibacterial drugs must not only penetrate the bacterial cell wall in sufficient concentrations but also have an affinity for (attraction to) the binding sites on the bacterial cell. The length of time the drug remains at the binding sites increases the effect of the antibacterial action. This time factor is controlled by the pharmacokinetics—the distribution, half-life, and elimination—of the drug.

Antibacterials that have a longer half-life usually maintain a greater concentration at the binding site; therefore frequent dosing is not required. Most antibacterials are not highly protein bound, with a few exceptions (e.g., oxacillin, ceftriaxone, cefprozil, cloxacillin, nafcillin, clindamycin). Protein binding does not have a major influence on the effectiveness of most antibacterial drugs. The steady state of the antibacterial drug occurs after the fourth to fifth half-lives, and after the seventh half-life, the drug is eliminated from the body, mainly through urine.

Pharmacodynamics. The drug concentration at the site and the exposure time for the drug play important roles in bacterial eradication. Antibacterial drugs are used to achieve the minimum effective

TABLE 26.1 Mechanisms of Action of Antibacterial Drugs

Action	Effect	Drugs
Inhibition of cell wall synthesis	Bactericidal effect Enzyme breakdown of cell wall Inhibition of enzyme in synthesis of cell wall	Penicillin Cephalosporins Bacitracin Vancomycin
Alteration of membrane permeability	Bacteriostatic or bactericidal effect Increases membrane permeability Cell lysis caused by loss of cellular substances	Amphotericin B Nystatin Polymyxin Colistin
Inhibition of protein synthesis	Bacteriostatic or bactericidal effect Interferes with protein synthesis without affecting normal cell Inhibits steps of protein synthesis	Aminoglycosides Tetracyclines Erythromycin Lincomycin
Inhibition of synthesis of bacterial RNA and DNA	Inhibits synthesis of RNA and DNA in bacteria Binds to nucleic acid and enzymes needed for nucleic acid synthesis	Fluoroquinolones
Interference with cellular metabolism	Bacteriostatic effect Interferes with steps of metabolism within cells	Sulfonamides Trimethoprim Isoniazid Nalidixic acid Rifampin

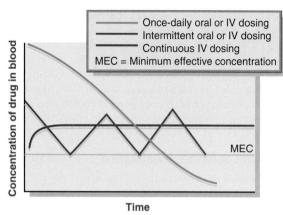

Fig. 26.1 Effects of concentrated drug dosing.

concentration (MEC) necessary to halt the growth of a microorganism. Many antibacterials have a bactericidal effect against the pathogen when the drug concentration remains constantly above the MEC during the dosing interval. Duration of use of the antibacterial varies according to the type of pathogen, site of infection, and immunocompetence of the host. With some severe infections, a continuous infusion regimen is more effective than intermittent dosing because of constant drug concentration and time exposure. Once-daily antibacterial dosing—such as with aminoglycosides, macrolides, and fluoroquinolones—has been effective in eradicating pathogens and has not caused severe adverse reactions (ototoxicity, nephrotoxicity) in most cases. The ease of compliance with once- or twice-daily drug dosing also increases the patient's adherence to the drug regimen.

Fig. 26.1 illustrates the effect of three methods of drug dosing. The drug dose is effective when it remains above the MEC.

Body Defenses

Body defenses and antibacterial drugs work together to stop the infectious process. The effect that antibacterial drugs have on an infection depends not only on the drug but also on the host's defense mechanisms. Factors such as age, nutrition, immunoglobulins, white blood cells (WBCs), organ function, and circulation influence the body's ability to fight infection. Older adults and undernourished individuals have less resistance to infection than younger, well-nourished populations. If the host's natural body defense mechanisms are inadequate, drug therapy might not be as effective. As a result, drug therapy may need to be closely monitored or revised. When circulation is impeded, an antibacterial drug may not be distributed properly to the infected area. In addition, immunoglobulins—antibody proteins such as IgG and IgM—and other elements of the immune response system, such as WBCs needed to combat infections, may be depleted in individuals with poor nutritional status.

Resistance to Antibacterials

Bacteria can be either sensitive or resistant to certain antibacterials. When bacteria are *sensitive* to a drug, the pathogen is inhibited or destroyed; however, if bacteria are *resistant,* the pathogen continues to grow despite administration of that antibacterial drug.

Bacterial resistance can result naturally, called inherent resistance, or it may be acquired. A natural, or inherent, resistance occurs without previous exposure to the antibacterial drug. For example, the gram-negative bacterium *Pseudomonas aeruginosa* is inherently resistant to penicillin G. An acquired resistance is caused by prior exposure to the antibacterial. Although *S. aureus* was once sensitive to penicillin G, repeated exposures have caused this organism to evolve and become resistant to that drug. Penicillinase, an enzyme produced by the

microorganism, is responsible for causing its penicillin resistance. Penicillinase metabolizes penicillin G, causing the drug to be ineffective; however, penicillinase-resistant penicillins that are effective against *S. aureus* are now available.

Antibiotic resistance is a major problem. In the early 1980s pharmaceutical companies thought that enough antibiotics were on the market, so they concentrated on developing antiviral and antifungal drugs. As a result, fewer new antibiotics were developed during the 1980s. Now pharmaceutical companies have developed many new antibiotics, but antibiotic resistance continues to develop, especially when antibiotics are used frequently. As bacteria reproduce, some mutation occurs, and eventually the mutant bacteria survive the effects of the drug. One explanation is that the mutant bacterial strain may have grown a thicker cell wall.

In large health care institutions, there is a tendency toward drug resistance in bacteria. Mutant strains of organisms have developed, thus increasing their resistance to antibiotics that were once effective against them. Infections acquired while patients are hospitalized are called health care–acquired infections (previously known as nosocomial infections). Many of these infections are caused by drug-resistant bacteria, and this can prolong hospitalization, which is costly to both the patient and third-party health care insurers.

Another problem related to antibiotic resistance is that bacteria can transfer their genetic instructions to another bacterial species, and the other bacterial species then becomes resistant to that antibiotic as well. Bacteria can also pass along high resistance to a more virulent and aggressive bacterium (e.g., *S. aureus,* enterococci).

Methicillin was the first penicillinase-resistant penicillin; it was developed in 1959 in response to the resistance of *S. aureus*. In 1968 strains of *S. aureus* were beginning to become resistant to methicillin. Highly resistant bacteria, so-called methicillin-resistant *S. aureus* (MRSA), became resistant not only to methicillin but to all penicillins and cephalosporins as well. Resistance that was once found only in hospitals began to emerge in 1981 in the community. Methicillin is now off the market, and the treatment of choice for MRSA is vancomycin. Other effective drugs used to treat MRSA include linezolid, tedizolid, daptomycin, TMP-SMZ, doxycycline, clindamycin, and telavancin, a glycopeptide antiinfective.

Many enterococcal strains are resistant to penicillin, ampicillin, gentamicin, streptomycin, and vancomycin. Another big resistance problem is vancomycin-resistant *Enterococcus faecium* (VREF), which can cause death in persons with weakened immune systems. The incidence of VREF in hospitals has increased, and a strain of MRSA has also been reported to be resistant to vancomycin (vancomycin-resistant *S. aureus,* or VRSA). One antibiotic after another is ineffective against new resistant strains of bacteria, and major medical problems result. As new drugs are developed, drug resistance will probably also develop.

Pharmaceutical companies and biotech firms are working on new classes of drugs to overcome the problem of bacterial resistance to antibiotics. A class of antibiotics known as *oxazolidinones* was discovered by a pharmaceutical company in 1988, but the company could not overcome the toxicity problems with this class of drug; however, another pharmaceutical company has taken the compound and made it less toxic. This antibiotic, linezolid, is effective against MRSA, VREF, and penicillin-resistant streptococci. Quinupristin-dalfopristin, which consists of two streptogramin antibacterials, is marketed in a 30:70 combination for intravenous (IV) use against life-threatening infection caused by VREF and for treatment of bacteremia, *S. aureus,* and *Streptococcus pyogenes.*

Another way to attack antimicrobial resistance is to develop drugs that disable the antibiotic-resistant mechanism in the bacteria. Patients would take the antibiotic-resistance disabler along with the antibiotic already on the market, making the drug effective again. Developing a

TABLE 26.2 General Adverse Reactions to Antibacterial Drugs

Type	Considerations
Allergy or hypersensitivity	Allergic reactions to drugs may be mild or severe. Examples of mild reactions are rash, pruritus, and hives. An example of a severe response is anaphylactic shock, which results in vascular collapse, laryngeal edema, bronchospasm, and cardiac arrest. Severe allergic reaction generally occurs within 20 minutes, and shortness of breath is often the first symptom of anaphylaxis. Mild allergic reaction is treated with an antihistamine, whereas anaphylaxis requires treatment with epinephrine, bronchodilators, and antihistamines.
Superinfection	Superinfection is a secondary infection that occurs when the normal microbial flora of the body are disturbed during antibiotic therapy. Superinfections can occur in the mouth, respiratory tract, intestine, genitourinary tract, and skin. Fungal infections frequently result in superinfections, although bacterial organisms (e.g., *Proteus, Pseudomonas, Staphylococcus*) may be the offending microorganisms. Superinfections rarely develop when drug is administered for less than 1 week, and they occur more commonly with the use of broad-spectrum antibiotics. For fungal infection of the mouth, nystatin is frequently used.
Organ toxicity	The liver and kidneys are involved in drug metabolism and excretion, and antibacterials may result in damage to these organs. For example, aminoglycosides can be nephrotoxic and ototoxic.

bacterial vaccine is another way to combat bacteria and lessen the need for antibiotics. The bacterial vaccine against pneumococcus has been effective in decreasing the occurrence of pneumonia and meningitis among various age groups.

Antibiotic misuse, a major problem today, increases antibiotic resistance. Studies reveal that 23% to 37.8% of patients in hospitals receive antibiotics, and 50% of this population is receiving antibiotics inappropriately. When antibiotics are taken unnecessarily—such as for viral infections when no bacterial infection is present—or incorrectly (e.g., skipping doses, not taking the full antibiotic regimen), resistance to antibacterials may develop. Consumer education is important because many patients demand antibiotics for viral conditions, even though antibiotics are ineffective against viruses; however, viral infections that persist could compromise the body's immune system and thus promote a secondary bacterial infection. The nurse should teach patients about the proper use of antibiotics to prevent situations that promote drug resistance to bacteria.

Cross-resistance can also occur among antibacterial drugs that have similar actions, such as the penicillins and cephalosporins. To ascertain the effect antibacterial drugs have on a specific microorganism, culture and sensitivity (C&S) or antibiotic susceptibility laboratory testing is performed. C&S can detect the infective microorganism present in a sample (e.g., blood, sputum, swab) and the best drug to kill it. The organism causing the infection is determined by culture, and antibiotics the organism is sensitive to are determined by sensitivity. The susceptibility or resistance of one microorganism to several antibacterials can be determined by the C&S test. Multiantibiotic therapy, or daily use of several antibacterials, delays the development of microorganism resistance.

Use of Antibiotic Combinations

Combination antibiotics should not be routinely prescribed or administered except for specific uncontrollable infections. Usually a single antibiotic will successfully treat a bacterial infection; however, when severe infection persists and is of an unknown origin or has been unsuccessfully treated with several single antibiotics, a combination of two or three antibiotics may be suggested. Before beginning antibiotic therapy, a culture or cultures should be taken to identify the bacteria.

When two antibiotics are combined, the result may be additive, potentiative, or antagonistic. The *additive* effect is equal to the sum of the effects of two antibiotics. The *potentiative* effect occurs when one antibiotic potentiates the effect of the second antibiotic, *increasing* its effectiveness. The *antagonistic* result is achieved with combination of a drug that is bactericidal, such as penicillin, and a drug that is bacteriostatic, such as tetracycline; when these two drugs are used together, the desired effect may be greatly *reduced*.

General Adverse Reactions to Antibacterials

Three major adverse reactions associated with the administration of antibacterial drugs are (1) allergic (hypersensitivity, anaphylaxis) reactions, (2) superinfection, and (3) organ toxicity. Table 26.2 describes these adverse reactions, all of which require close monitoring of the patient.

Narrow-Spectrum and Broad-Spectrum Antibiotics

Antibacterial drugs can be classified as either narrow spectrum or broad spectrum. The narrow-spectrum antibiotics are primarily effective against one type of organism. For example, penicillin and erythromycin are used to treat infections caused by gram-positive bacteria. Certain broad-spectrum antibiotics, such as tetracycline and third- and fifth-generation cephalosporins, can be effective against both gram-positive and gram-negative organisms. Because narrow-spectrum antibiotics are selective, they are more active against those single organisms than the broad-spectrum antibiotics. Broad-spectrum antibiotics are frequently used to treat infections when the offending microorganism has not been identified by the C&S test.

PENICILLINS AND CEPHALOSPORINS

PENICILLINS

Penicillin, a natural antibacterial agent obtained from the mold genus *Penicillium*, was introduced to the military during World War II and is considered to have saved many soldiers' lives. It became widely used in 1945 and was considered a "miracle drug." With the advent of penicillin, many patients survived who would have normally died from wound and severe respiratory infections.

Penicillin's beta-lactam ring structure interferes with bacterial cell wall synthesis by inhibiting the bacterial enzyme necessary for cell division and cellular synthesis. The bacteria die of cell lysis (cell breakdown). The penicillins can be both bacteriostatic and bactericidal, depending on the drug and dosage. Penicillin G is primarily bactericidal.

Penicillins are mainly referred to as *beta-lactam antibiotics*. Bacteria can produce a variety of enzymes, such as beta-lactamases, that can inactivate penicillin and other beta-lactam antibiotics such as the cephalosporins. The beta-lactamases, which attack penicillins, are called *penicillinases*.

Penicillin G was the first penicillin administered orally and by injection. With oral administration, only about one-third of the dose is absorbed. Because of its poor absorption, penicillin G given by injection (IV and intramuscular [IM]) is more effective in achieving a therapeutic serum penicillin level. Because it is an aqueous drug solution, aqueous penicillin G has a short duration of action, and the IM injection is very painful. As a result, a longer-acting form of penicillin, procaine penicillin (milky color), was produced to extend the activity of the drug. Procaine (an anesthetic) in the penicillin decreases the pain related to injection.

Penicillin V was the next type of penicillin produced. Although two-thirds of the oral dose is absorbed by the gastrointestinal (GI) tract, it is a less potent antibacterial drug than penicillin G. Penicillin V is effective against mild to moderate infections, including anthrax as a weapon of bioterrorism.

Initially, penicillin was overused. It was first introduced for the treatment of staphylococcal infections, but after a few years, mutant strains of *Staphylococcus* developed that were resistant to penicillins G and V because of the bacterial enzyme penicillinase, which destroys penicillin. This led to the development of new broad-spectrum antibiotics with structures similar to penicillin to combat infections resistant to penicillins G and V.

Food in the stomach does not significantly alter absorption of penicillin V, so it should be taken after meals. Amoxicillins are penicillins that are unaffected by food.

Broad-Spectrum Penicillins (Aminopenicillins)

Broad-spectrum penicillins are used to treat both gram-positive and gram-negative bacteria. They are not, however, as broadly effective against all microorganisms as they were once considered to be. This group of drugs is costlier than penicillin and therefore should not be used when ordinary penicillins, such as penicillin G, are effective. The broad-spectrum penicillins are effective against some gram-negative organisms such as *E. coli*, *H. influenzae*, *Shigella dysenteriae*, *Proteus mirabilis*, and *Salmonella* species. However, these drugs are not penicillinase resistant; because they are readily inactivated by beta-lactamases, they are ineffective against *S. aureus*. Examples of this group are ampicillin and amoxicillin (Table 26.3). Amoxicillin is the most prescribed penicillin derivative for adults and children.

Penicillinase-Resistant Penicillins (Antistaphylococcal Penicillins)

Penicillinase-resistant penicillins (antistaphylococcal penicillins) are used to treat penicillinase-producing *S. aureus*. Dicloxacillin is an oral preparation of these antibiotics, whereas nafcillin and oxacillin are IM and IV preparations. This group of drugs is *not* effective against gram-negative organisms and is less effective than penicillin G against gram-positive organisms. See Prototype Drug Chart: Amoxicillin and Table 26.3 to compare the similarities and differences in the broad-spectrum penicillin amoxicillin and the penicillinase-resistant penicillin dicloxacillin.

Extended-Spectrum Penicillins (Antipseudomonal Penicillins)

The antipseudomonal penicillins are a group of broad-spectrum antibiotics effective against *P. aeruginosa*, a gram-negative bacillus that is difficult to eradicate. These drugs are also useful against many gram-negative organisms such as *Proteus*, *Serratia*, *Enterobacter*, and *Acinetobacter* species, and also *Klebsiella pneumoniae*. The antipseudomonal penicillins are *not* penicillinase resistant. Their pharmacologic action is similar to that of aminoglycosides, but they are less toxic.

Table 26.3 lists the drugs in the four categories of penicillin-type antibacterials. The administration routes (oral, IM, or IV) of various types of penicillins, along with the cephalosporins, are available on the Evolve website.

Beta-Lactamase Inhibitors

When a broad-spectrum antibiotic such as amoxicillin is combined with a beta-lactamase enzyme inhibitor such as clavulanic acid, the resulting antibiotic combination inhibits the bacterial beta-lactamases, making the antibiotic effective and extending its antimicrobial effect. There are three beta-lactamase inhibitors: (1) clavulanic acid, (2) sulbactam, and (3) tazobactam. These inhibitors are not given alone but are combined with a penicillinase-sensitive penicillin such as amoxicillin, ampicillin, or piperacillin. The combination drugs currently marketed include amoxicillin-clavulanic acid (for oral use), and ampicillin-sulbactam and piperacillin-tazobactam (for use parenterally).

📄 PROTOTYPE DRUG CHART

Amoxicillin

Drug Class	Dosage
Amoxicillin: Broad-spectrum penicillin	Lower respiratory infections: A: PO: 875 mg q12h or 500 mg q8h; *max:* 1750 mg/d

Contraindications	Drug-Lab-Food Interactions
Allergy to penicillin, hypersensitivity *Caution:* Hypersensitivity to cephalosporins, renal impairment, asthma, inflammatory bowel disease, ulcerative colitis, older adults, pseudomembranous colitis, mononucleosis, GI disease, breastfeeding	Drug: Increased effect with aspirin, allopurinol, probenecid; increased bleeding with oral anticoagulants; increased effect of methotrexate; decreased effect with tetracycline, erythromycin Lab: Increased serum AST, ALT, BUN, and creatinine; increased PT, INR Food: Decreased effect with acidic fruits and juices

Pharmacokinetics	Pharmacodynamics
Absorption: PO: >80% in the GI tract Distribution: PB: 20%–25% Metabolism: t½: 1–1.5 h Excretion: 70% in urine	PO: Onset, duration: UK Peak: 1–2 h

Therapeutic Effects/Uses

For treating otitis media, tonsillitis, sinusitis, and skin, respiratory, and urinary tract infections. Amoxicillin is effective against *Helicobacter pylori* and *Escherichia coli and* species of *Haemophilus*, *Enterococcus*, *Proteus*, *Staphylococcus*, and *Streptococcus*

Mechanism of Action: Amoxicillin inhibits the enzyme in cell wall synthesis and has a bactericidal effect

Side Effects	Adverse Reactions
Nausea, vomiting, diarrhea, abdominal pain, dysphagia, rash, dysgeusia, tongue and tooth discoloration, headache, dizziness, anxiety, confusion, candidiasis, insomnia, crystalluria, dermatitis	Superinfection, prolonged bleeding time *Life-threatening:* Anaphylaxis, angioedema, eosinophilia, leukopenia, thrombocytopenia, CDAD, seizures

A, Adult; *ALT,* alanine aminotransferase; *AST,* aspartate aminotransferase; *BUN,* blood urea nitrogen; *CDAD, Clostridium difficile*–associated diarrhea; *d,* day; *GI,* gastrointestinal; *h,* hour; *INR,* international normalized ratio; *max,* maximum dosage; *mo,* months; *PB,* protein binding; *PO,* by mouth; *PT,* prothrombin time; *q,* every; *t½,* half-life; *UK,* unknown; *>,* greater than; *<,* less than.

TABLE 26.3 Antibacterials: Penicillins

Generic	Route and Dosage	Uses and Considerations
Basic Penicillins		
Penicillin G procaine	Pneumococcal pneumonia: A: IM: 600,000–1.2 million units/d for at least 10 d; *max:* 2.4 million units/d	For treating diphtheria, skin infections, staphylococcal/streptococcal, syphilis, endocarditis, scarlet fever, and respiratory infections. May cause arthralgia, edema, nausea, vomiting, diarrhea, rash, superinfection, CDAD, and tongue discoloration. PB: 60%; t½: UK
Penicillin G benzathine	Upper respiratory infection: A: IM: 1.2 million units as a single dose; *max:* 2.4 million units/d	For streptococcal, syphilis, and respiratory infections and for rheumatic fever prophylaxis. May cause arthralgia, edema, nausea, vomiting, diarrhea, rash, tongue discoloration, superinfection, and CDAD. PB: 60%; t½: UK
Penicillin G	Streptococcal infection: A: IM/IV: 12–24 million units/d divided q4–6h; *max:* 80 million units/d	For anthrax, meningitis, diphtheria, skin and clostridial infections, gonorrhea, syphilis, pericarditis, endocarditis, and serious respiratory infections. May cause arthralgia, nausea, vomiting, diarrhea, rash, tongue discoloration, myalgia, superinfection, and CDAD. PB: 45%–68%; t½: 20–30 min
Penicillin V potassium	Otitis media: A: PO: 250–500 mg q6h for at least 2 d; *max:* 2 g/d	For streptococcal infections, ulcerative gingivitis, otitis media, skin infections, and endocarditis prophylaxis. May cause rash, nausea, vomiting, diarrhea, contact dermatitis, peripheral neuropathy, tongue discoloration, superinfection, candidiasis, and CDAD. Not recommended in renal failure. PB: 75%–89%; t½: UK
Broad-Spectrum Penicillins		
Amoxicillin	See Prototype Drug Chart: Amoxicillin	
Amoxicillin-clavulanate	Lower respiratory infection: Immediate release: A: PO: 500–875 mg amoxicillin and 125 mg clavulanate q8h for at least 5 d Extended release: A: PO: 2000 mg amoxicillin and 125 mg clavulanate q12h for at least 5 d	For treating otitis media, sinusitis, and respiratory, skin, and urinary tract infections. May cause dermatitis, nausea, vomiting, diarrhea, rash, urticaria, tooth/tongue discoloration, superinfection, candidiasis, and CDAD. PB: amoxicillin 18%, clavulanate 25%; t½: amoxicillin 1–1.5 h, clavulanate 1 h
Ampicillin	Respiratory infection: A: PO: 250 mg qid; *max:* 2 g/d A>40kg: IM/IV: 250–500 mg q6h; *max:* 200 mg/kg/d A<40kg: IM/IV: 25–50 mg/kg/d IV q6–8h; *max:* 200 mg/kg/d	For meningitis, endocarditis, bacteremia, anthrax, and gastrointestinal, skin, respiratory, intraabdominal, urinary tract, and severe infections. May cause dysphagia, glossitis, nausea, vomiting, diarrhea, rash, stomatitis, tongue discoloration, superinfection, and CDAD. PB: 15%–25%; t½: 1–1.5 h
Ampicillin-sulbactam	Skin infections: A: IM/IV: 1 g ampicillin/0.5 g sulbactam q6h for 1–4 wk or 2 g ampicillin 1 g sulbactam q6h for 1–4 wk; *max:* 8 g ampicillin 4 g sulbactam	For skin, respiratory, intraabdominal, and gynecologic infections. May cause headache, phlebitis, injection site reaction, rash, glossitis, nausea, vomiting, diarrhea, tongue discoloration, CDAD, edema, candidiasis, and superinfection. PB: sulbactam 38%, ampicillin 15%–25%; t½: both 1–1.5 h
Penicillinase-Resistant Penicillins		
Dicloxacillin sodium	Skin infections: A: PO: 250–500 qid for 5–7 d	For mastitis, skin structure, and respiratory infections. May cause abdominal pain, arthralgia, myalgia, rash, stomatitis, nausea, vomiting, diarrhea, tongue discoloration, CDAD, and superinfection. PB: 95%–99%; t½: 30–42 min
Nafcillin	Endocarditis: A: IV: 12 g/d in divided doses q4–6h for 6 wk; *max:* 6 g/d	For treating endocarditis, meningitis, bacteremia, mastitis, and skin, respiratory, and bone/joint infections. May cause abdominal pain, arthralgia, stomatitis, nausea, vomiting, diarrhea, tongue discoloration, rash, CDAD, superinfection, phlebitis, and injection site reaction. PB: 70%–90%; t½: 0.5–1.5 h
Oxacillin sodium	Meningitis: A: IV: 2 g q4h; *max:* 6 g/d	For endocarditis, meningitis, bacteremia, mastitis, and skin, respiratory, and bone/joint infections. May cause abdominal pain, rash, tongue discoloration, stomatitis, arthralgia, myalgia, nausea, vomiting, diarrhea, CDAD, superinfection, and injection site reaction. PB: 89%–94%; t½: 30 minutes
Extended-Spectrum Penicillins		
Piperacillin tazobactam	Community-acquired pneumonia: A: IV: 4 g piperacillin/0.5 g tazobactam over 30 min q6h at least 7 d; *max:* 16 g piperacillin/2 g tazobactam/d	For intraabdominal, skin, urinary tract, and respiratory infections. May cause headache, pruritus, candidiasis, abdominal pain, dyspepsia, nausea, vomiting, diarrhea, constipation, CDAD, rash, insomnia, and superinfection. PB: 30%; t½: 0.7–1.5 h

A, Adult; *CDAD, Clostridium difficile*–associated diarrhea; *d,* day; *GI,* gastrointestinal; *h,* hour; *IM,* intramuscular; *IV,* intravenous; *max,* maximum; *min,* minutes; *PB,* protein binding; *PID,* pelvic inflammatory disease; *PO,* by mouth; *q,* every; *STI,* sexually transmitted infection; *t½,* half-life; *UK,* unknown; *UTI,* urinary tract infection; *wk,* weeks; *y,* years; *>,* greater than; *<,* less than.

Pharmacokinetics. Amoxicillin is well absorbed from the GI tract, whereas dicloxacillin is only partially absorbed. Protein-binding power differs between the two drugs—amoxicillin is 20% to 25% protein bound, but dicloxacillin is highly protein bound (95% to 99%). Drug toxicity may result when other highly protein-bound drugs are used with dicloxacillin. Both drugs have short half-lives. Sixty percent of amoxicillin is excreted in the urine; dicloxacillin is excreted in bile and urine.

Pharmacodynamics. Both amoxicillin and dicloxacillin are penicillin derivatives and are bactericidal. These drugs interfere with bacterial cell wall synthesis, causing cell lysis. Amoxicillin may be produced with or without clavulanic acid, an agent that prevents the breakdown of amoxicillin by decreasing resistance to the antibacterial drug. The addition of clavulanic acid intensifies the effect of amoxicillin. The amoxicillin–clavulanic acid preparation and amoxicillin trihydrate have similar pharmacokinetics and pharmacodynamics as well as similar side effects and adverse reactions. When probenecid is taken with amoxicillin or dicloxacillin, the serum antibacterial levels may be increased.

The effects of amoxicillin are decreased when taken with erythromycin and tetracycline. The onset of action, serum peak concentration time, and duration of action for amoxicillin and dicloxacillin are very similar.

Geriatrics

Most beta-lactam antibiotics are excreted via the kidneys. With older adults, assessment of renal function is most important. Serum blood urea nitrogen (BUN) and serum creatinine should be monitored. With a decrease in renal function, the antibiotic dose should be decreased.

Side Effects and Adverse Reactions

Common adverse reactions to penicillin administration are hypersensitivity and superinfection, the occurrence of a secondary infection when the flora of the body are disturbed (see Table 26.2). Anorexia, nausea, vomiting, and diarrhea are common GI disturbances, often referred to as *GI distress*. This may be alleviated some by taking penicillin with food. Rash is an indicator of a mild to moderate allergic reaction; severe allergic reaction leads to anaphylactic shock. Clinical manifestations of a severe allergic reaction include laryngeal edema, severe bronchoconstriction with stridor, and hypotension. Allergic effects occur in 5% to 10% of persons receiving penicillin compounds; therefore close monitoring during the first and subsequent doses of penicillin is essential.

Drug Interactions

The broad-spectrum penicillins, amoxicillin and ampicillin, may decrease the effectiveness of oral contraceptives. Potassium supplements can increase serum potassium levels when taken with potassium penicillin G or V. When penicillin is mixed with an aminoglycoside in IV solution, the actions of both drugs are inactivated.

◎ CLINICAL JUDGMENT [NURSING PROCESS]

Antibacterials: Penicillins

Concept: Infection
- A condition in which microorganisms enter the body and release toxins

Recognize Cues [Assessment]
- Assess for allergy to penicillin or cephalosporins. The patient who is hypersensitive to amoxicillin should not take *any* type of penicillin products because severe allergic reaction could occur. A small percentage of patients who are allergic to penicillin could also be allergic to a cephalosporin product.
- Evaluate laboratory results, especially liver enzymes. Report elevated alkaline phosphatase (ALP), alanine aminotransferase (ALT), and aspartate aminotransferase (AST).
- Record urine output. If amount is inadequate (<30 mL/h or <600 mL/day), the drug or drug dosage may need to be changed.

Analyze Cues and Prioritize Hypothesis [Patient Problems]
- Tissue injury
- Vomiting
- Nausea

Generate Solutions [Planning]
- The patient's white blood cells (WBCs) will be within normal limits.

Take Action [Nursing Interventions]
- Obtain a sample (e.g., swab, blood, sputum) for laboratory culture and antibiotic sensitivity testing (C&S test) to discern the infective organism before antibiotic therapy is started.
- Monitor for signs and symptoms of superinfection, especially in patients taking high doses of an antibiotic for a prolonged time. Signs and symptoms include stomatitis (mouth ulcers), genital discharge (vaginitis), and anal or genital itching.
- ⚡ Examine the patient for allergic reaction to the penicillin product, especially after the first and second doses. This may be a mild reaction, such as a rash, or a severe reaction, such as respiratory distress or anaphylaxis.
- ⚡ Have epinephrine available to counteract a severe allergic reaction.

- Do not mix aminoglycosides with a high-dose or extended-spectrum penicillin G because this combination may inactivate the aminoglycoside.
- Assess the patient for bleeding if high doses of penicillin are being given; a decrease in platelet aggregation (clotting) may result.
- Monitor body temperature and the infected area.
- Dilute antibiotic for IV use in an appropriate amount of solution as indicated in the package insert.

Patient Teaching
General
- Teach patients to always take the *entire* prescribed penicillin product, such as amoxicillin, until the bottle is empty. If only a portion of the penicillin is taken, drug resistance to that antibacterial agent may develop in the future.
- Advise patients allergic to penicillin to wear a medical alert bracelet or necklace and to carry a card that indicates the allergy. Patients should notify their health care providers of any allergy to penicillin when reporting their health history.
- Keep drugs out of reach of small children. Request childproof containers.
- Tell patients to report any side effects or adverse reactions that may occur while taking the drug.
- Encourage patients to increase fluid intake; fluids can aid in regulating body temperature and in excreting the drug.
- Warn patients or the parents of children taking antibiotics that chewable tablets must be chewed or crushed before swallowing.
- Advise female patients of childbearing years to use an additional form of birth control while taking penicillins.

Diet
- Advise patients to take medication with food to avoid gastric irritation.

Evaluate Outcomes [Evaluation]
- Evaluate the effectiveness of antibacterial agents by determining whether the infection has resolved and whether any side effects, including superinfection, have occurred.

TABLE 26.4 Other Beta-Lactam Antibiotics

Generic	Route and Dosage	Uses and Considerations
Aztreonam	Skin infections: A: IM/IV: 1–2 g q8–12h; *max:* 8 g/d	For bacteremia and intraabdominal, skin, respiratory, gynecologic, and urinary tract infections. May cause fever, rash, nasal congestion, cough, wheezing, vomiting, abdominal pain, CDAD, neutropenia, injection site reaction, elevated hepatic enzymes, and superinfection. PB: 56%–65%; t½: 1.7 h
Ertapenem	Skin infections: A: IM/IV: 1 g/d for 7–14 d; *max:* 1 g/d	For bacteremia, community-acquired pneumonia, and complicated urinary tract, skin, pelvic, and intraabdominal infections. May cause drowsiness, confusion, agitation, elevated hepatic enzymes, abdominal pain, nausea, diarrhea, vomiting, headache, CDAD, injection site reaction, superinfection, and anemia. PB: 95%; t½: 4.5 h
Imipenem and cilastatin	Urinary tract infection: A: IV: 500 mg q6h; *max:* 4 g/d	For sepsis, endocarditis, and gynecologic, intraabdominal, respiratory, urinary tract, skin, and bone/joint infections. May cause rash, nausea, vomiting, diarrhea, urine discoloration, injection site reaction, phlebitis, CDAD, seizures, and superinfection. PB: imipenem 20%, cilastatin 40%; t½: both 1 h
Meropenem	Skin infections: A: IV: 500 mg–1 g q8h; *max:* 1 g q8h	For treating meningitis and intraabdominal, respiratory, and skin infections. May cause headache, rash, nausea, vomiting, diarrhea, constipation, CDAD, anemia, injection site reaction, hyperbilirubinemia, and superinfection. PB: 2%; t½: 1 h
Meropenem, vaborbactam	A: IV: 2 g meropenem and 2 g vaborbactam q8h up to 14 d; administer over 3 h; *max:* 6 g meropenem and 6 g vaborbactam/d	For complicated UTIs, including pyelonephritis. May cause headache, injection site reaction, phlebitis, fever, nausea, diarrhea, hypokalemia, and elevated hepatic enzymes. PB: meropenem 2%, vaborbactam 33%; t½: meropenem 1.22 h, vaborbactam 1.68 h
Imipenem, cilastatin, relebactam	Intraabdominal infections: A: IV: 500 mg imipenem, 500 mg cilastatin, 250 mg rebebactam q6h for 4–14 d; *max:* 2 g imipenem, 2 g cilastatin, 1 g relebactam/d	For UTIs, nosocomial pneumonia, and complicated intraabdominal infections. May cause headache, anemia, elevated hepatic enzymes, constipation, hypokalemia, hyponatremia, fever, erythema, nausea, vomiting, diarrhea, and hypertension. PB: imipenem 20%, cilastatin 40%, relebactam 22%; t½: imipenem 1 h, cilastatin 1 h, relebactam 1.2 h

A, Adult; *CDAD, Clostridium difficile*–associated diarrhea; *d,* day; *GI,* gastrointestinal; *h,* hour; *IM,* intramuscular; *IV,* intravenous; *max,* maximum; *mo,* months; *PB,* protein binding; *PO,* by mouth; *q,* every; *t½,* half-life; *>,* greater than.

OTHER BETA-LACTAM ANTIBACTERIALS

Like penicillins, these beta-lactam antibacterials preferentially bind to specific penicillin-binding proteins located inside the bacterial cell wall and are bactericidal. This group includes aztrenam, imipenem/cilastatin, and meropenem. Aztreonam's effectiveness is limited to aerobic gram-positive infections. Imipenem/cilastatin and meropenem are effective against a broader spectrum of activity than many other beta-lactam antibacterials. These three antibacterials are less nephrotoxic than many other antibacterials. Table 26.4 describes these other beta-lactam antibacterials and their dosages, uses, and considerations.

Side Effects and Adverse Reactions

Side effects and adverse reactions to aztrenam, imipenem/cilastatin, and meropenem include headache, nausea, vomiting, diarrhea, anemia, eosinophilia, and neutropenia. Rash may also occur. Severe adverse reactions include anaphylaxis, angioedema, seizures, and *Clostridium difficile*–associated diarrhea.

CEPHALOSPORINS

In 1948 a fungus called *Emericellopsis minimum* (*Cephalosporium acremonium*) was discovered in seawater at a sewer outlet off the coast of Sardinia. This fungus was found to be active against gram-positive and gram-negative bacteria and resistant to beta-lactamase, an enzyme that acts against the beta-lactam structure of penicillin. In the early 1960s cephalosporins were used with clinical effectiveness. For cephalosporins to be effective against numerous organisms, their molecules were chemically altered, and semisynthetic cephalosporins were produced. Like penicillin, the cephalosporins

have a beta-lactam structure and act by inhibiting the bacterial enzyme necessary for cell wall synthesis. Lysis to the cell occurs, and the bacterial cell dies.

First-, Second-, Third-, Fourth-, and Fifth-Generation Cephalosporins

Cephalosporins are a major antibiotic group used in hospitals and in health care offices. These drugs are bactericidal with actions similar to those of penicillin. For antibacterial activity, the beta-lactam ring of cephalosporins is necessary.

Five groups of cephalosporins have been developed, identified as *generations*. Each generation is effective against a broader spectrum of bacteria, an increased resistance to destruction by beta-lactamases, and an increased ability to reach cerebrospinal fluid (Table 26.5).

Not all cephalosporins are affected by the beta-lactamases. First-generation cephalosporins are effective against most gram-positive bacteria and are destroyed by beta-lactamases, but not all second-generation cephalosporins are affected by beta-lactamases. Second-generation cephalosporins are effective against gram-positive and some gram-negative bacteria. Third-generation cephalosporins are resistant to beta-lactamases. They have broad-spectrum antibacterial activity and are effective against *P. aeruginosa.* The fourth-generation cephalosporin, cefepime, has broad-spectrum activity, is highly resistant to beta-lactamases, and has good penetration to cerebrospinal fluid. The fifth-generation cephalosporins are broad-spectrum drugs effective against MRSA.

Approximately 10% of persons allergic to penicillin are also allergic to cephalosporins because both groups of antibacterials have similar molecular structures. If a patient is allergic to penicillin and taking a cephalosporin, the nurse should watch for a possible allergic reaction to the cephalosporin, although the likelihood of a reaction is small.

TABLE 26.5 Activity of the Five Generations of Cephalosporins

Generation	Activity
First	Effective mostly against gram-positive bacteria (streptococci and most staphylococci) and some gram-negative bacteria (*Escherichia coli* and species of *Klebsiella, Proteus, Salmonella,* and *Shigella*)
Second	Same effectiveness as first generation but with a broader spectrum against other gram-negative bacteria such as *Haemophilus influenzae, Neisseria gonorrhoeae* and *N. meningitidis, Enterobacter* species, and several anaerobic organisms
Third	Same effectiveness as first and second generations and also effective against gram-negative bacteria (*Pseudomonas aeruginosa* and *Serratia* and *Acinetobacter* species) but with increased resistance to destruction by beta-lactamases
Fourth	Similar to third-generation drugs and highly resistant to most beta-lactamase bacteria with broad-spectrum antibacterial activity and good penetration to cerebrospinal fluid; effective against *E. coli; P. aeruginosa; Klebsiella, Proteus,* and *Streptococcus* species; and certain staphylococci
Fifth	Similar characteristics of third and fourth generations, also broad spectrum, and the only cephalosporins effective against methicillin-resistant *Staphylococcus aureus* (MRSA)

📄 PROTOTYPE DRUG CHART

Ceftriaxone

Drug Class	**Dosage**
Ceftriaxone: Third-generation cephalosporin	Intraabdominal A: IM/IV: 1–2 g q12–24h for 4–7 d; *max:* 4 g/d

Contraindications	**Drug-Lab-Food Interactions**
Hypersensitivity to cephalosporins *Caution:* Calcium IVs, hypersensitivity to penicillins, vitamin K deficiency, anticoagulants, hepatic/renal dysfunction, pseudomembranous colitis, urinary tract obstruction, older adults	Drug: Increased nephrotoxicity with loop diuretics, aminoglycosides, calcium salts, and vancomycin; increased bleeding with anticoagulants Lab: May increase AST, ALT, ALP, LDH, PT, and INR

Pharmacokinetics	**Pharmacodynamics**
Absorption: IM, IV Distribution: PB: 85%–95% Metabolism: t½: 6–9 h Excretion: In urine	IM: Onset, duration: UK Peak: 1.5–4 h IV: Onset: Immediate; duration: UK Peak: 30 min

Therapeutic Effects/Uses

For treating otitis media, meningitis, gonorrhea, bacteremia, and skin, respiratory, bone/joint, intraabdominal, and urinary tract infections.
Ceftriaxone is effective against *Klebsiella, Haemophilus, Clostridium, Citrobacter, Bacteroides, Acinetobacter, Neisseria, Proteus, Salmonella, Serratia, Shigella, Staphylococcus, Staphylococcus,* and *Escherichia coli.*
Mechanism of Action: Inhibits bacterial cell wall synthesis causing cell lysis; bactericidal effect

Side Effects	**Adverse Reactions**
Nausea, dyspepsia, dysgeusia, stomatitis, glossitis, vomiting, diarrhea, abdominal cramps, flatulence, rash, flushing, diaphoresis, fever, pruritus, headaches, dizziness, edema, injection site reaction, epistaxis, chills, vaginitis, azotemia, candidiasis, elevated hepatic enzymes	Superinfection, bleeding, palpitations, biliary obstruction, cholelithiasis, nephrolithiasis, jaundice, hyperbilirubinemia, anemia, hematuria, hypothrombinemia *Lifethreatening:* Seizures, anaphylaxis, angioedema, bronchospasm, agranulocytosis, aplastic anemia, hemolytic anemia, leukopenia, thrombocytopenia, neutropenia, eosinophilia, renal failure, CDAD, Stevens-Johnson syndrome, thrombocytosis

A, Adult; *ALP,* alkaline phosphatase; *ALT,* alanine aminotransferase; *AST,* aspartate aminotransferase; *CDAD, Clostridium difficile*–associated diarrhea; *d,* day; *h,* hour; *IM,* intramuscular; *INR,* international normalized ratio; *IV,* intravenous; *LDH,* lactic dehydrogenase; *max,* maximum; *min,* minute; *PB,* protein binding; *PT,* prothrombin time; *q,* every; *t½,* half-life; *UK,* unknown.

Only a few cephalosporins are administered orally. These include cephalexin, cefadroxil, cefaclor, cefuroxime, cefdinir, cefprozil, cefixime, cefpodoxime, cefditoren, and ceftibuten. The rest of the cephalosporins are administered IM and IV. Prototype Drug Chart: Ceftriaxone describes the drug data related to ceftriaxone.

Pharmacokinetics. Cefazolin is administered IM and IV, and cefaclor is given orally. The protein-binding power of cefazolin is greater than that of cefaclor. The half-life of each drug is short, and the drugs are excreted 60% to 80% unchanged in the urine.

Pharmacodynamics. Cefazolin and cefaclor inhibit bacterial cell wall synthesis and produce a bactericidal action. For IM and IV use of cefazolin, the onset of action is almost immediate, and peak concentration time is 5 to 15 minutes with IV use. The peak concentration time for an oral dose of cefaclor is 30 to 60 minutes.

TABLE 26.6 Antibacterials: Cephalosporins

Generic	Route and Dosage	Uses and Considerations
First Generation		
Cefadroxil	UTI: A: PO: 1–2 g/d in 1–2 divided doses for 3–7 d; *max:* 2 g/d	For treating pharyngitis, tonsillitis, and urinary tract and skin infections. May cause rash, pruritus, nausea, vomiting, diarrhea, CDAD, angioedema, elevated hepatic enzymes, and superinfection. Well absorbed by the GI tract and not affected by food. PB: UK; t½: 1–2 h
Cefazolin sodium	UTI: A: IM/IV: 1 g q6–12h; *max:* 12 g/d	For endocarditis, bacteremia, mastitis, prostatitis, epididymitis, and skin, bone/joint, biliary, respiratory, and urinary tract infections. May cause rash, pruritus, CDAD, superinfection, nausea, vomiting, diarrhea, injection site reaction, elevated hepatic enzymes, eosinophilia, and thrombocytopenia. PB: 75%–85%; t½: 1.8–2 h
Cephalexin	URI: A: PO: 250–500 mg q12h for 7–14 d; *max:* 4 g/d	For treating mastitis, otitis media and skin, bone/joint, respiratory, and genitourinary infections. May cause CDAD, rash, urticaria, nausea, vomiting, diarrhea, elevated hepatic enzymes, eosinophilia, thrombocytopenia, and superinfection. PB: 10%–15%; t½: 1 h
Second Generation		
Cefaclor	Lower respiratory infection: Immediate release: A: PO: 250–500 mg q8h; *max:* 1.5 g/d Extended release: A: PO: 500 mg q12h for 7 d; *max:* 1 g/d	For pharyngitis, tonsillitis, otitis media, and skin, respiratory, and urinary tract infections. May cause headache, pharyngitis, rhinitis, rash, nausea, diarrhea, CDAD, pruritus, cough, abdominal pain, candidiasis, vaginitis, eosinophilia, elevated hepatic enzymes, and superinfection. PB: 25%; t½: 1 h
Cefotetan	UTI: A: IM/IV: 500 mg q12h or 1–2 g q24h; *max:* 6 g/d IV, 4 g/d IM	For gynecologic, intraabdominal, respiratory, urinary tract, skin, and bone/joint infections. May cause CDAD, nausea, diarrhea, phlebitis, rash, pruritus, elevated hepatic enzymes, seizures, eosinophilia, and superinfection. PB: 78%–91%; t½: 3–4.6 h
Cefoxitin sodium	Respiratory infection: A: IM/IV: 1–2 g q6–8h; *max:* 12 g/d	For bacteremia, intraabdominal, gynecologic, skin, respiratory, bone/joint, and urinary tract infections. May cause rash, pruritus, urticaria, elevated hepatic enzymes, thrombocytopenia, diarrhea, CDAD, and superinfection. PB: 73%; t½: 40–60 min
Cefprozil	Skin infection: A: PO: 250–500 mg q12h for 10 d or 500 mg/d for 10 d; *max:* 1 g/d	For treating sinusitis, tonsillitis, pharyngitis, otitis media, and respiratory and skin infections. May cause rash, pruritus, nausea, diarrhea, CDAD, elevated hepatic enzymes, vaginitis, eosinophilia, and superinfection. PB: 36%; t½: 1.3 h
Cefuroxime	Chronic bronchitis: A: PO: 250–500 mg q12h for 5–7 d; *max:* 1 g/d	For meningitis, otitis media, gonorrhea, bacteremia, pharyngitis, tonsillitis, sinusitis, and skin, respiratory, urinary tract, and bone/joint infections. May cause rash, CDAD, phlebitis, vaginitis, nausea, vomiting, diarrhea, dermatitis, elevated hepatic enzymes, eosinophilia, and superinfection. PB: 50%; t½: 1–2 h
Third Generation		
Cefdinir	Skin infection: A: PO: 300 mg q12h for 10 d; *max:* 600 mg/d	For treating otitis media, acute sinusitis, tonsillitis, and respiratory, and skin infections. May cause headache, rash, nausea, diarrhea, CDAD, elevated hepatic enzymes, proteinuria, candidiasis, and superinfection. PB: 60%–70%; t½: 1.7 h
Cefixime	Bronchitis: A: PO: 400 mg/d in divided doses q12–24h for at least 5–7 d; *max:* 400 mg/d	For treating otitis media, tonsillitis, gonorrhea, pharyngitis, bronchitis, and urinary tract infections. May cause headache, dizziness, vomiting, diarrhea, flatulence, rash, nausea, dyspepsia, abdominal pain, CDAD, and superinfection. PB: 65%–70%; t½: 3–4 h
Cefotaxime	UTI: A: IM/IV: 1–2 g q8h for moderate to severe and 2 g IV q6–8h for severe; *max:* 12 g/d	For treating bacteremia, sepsis, meningitis, and gynecologic, skin, bone/joint, intraabdominal, respiratory, and urinary tract infections. May cause rash, pruritus, fever, nausea, vomiting, diarrhea, colitis, CDAD, injection site reaction, eosinophilia, and superinfection. PB: 13%–38%; t½: 1–1.5 h
Cefpodoxime	Respiratory infection: A: PO: 200 mg q12h for 5–14 d; *max:* 800 mg/d	For treating otitis media, tonsillitis, sinusitis, gonorrhea, pharyngitis, and skin, respiratory, and urinary tract infections. May cause headache, abdominal pain, nausea, vomiting, diarrhea, CDAD, and superinfection. Food enhances drug absorption. PB: 22%–33%; t½: 3 h
Ceftazidime	Intraabdominal infection: A: IM/IV: 2 g q8h for 4–7 d; *max:* 6 g/d	For treating bacteremia, meningitis, and gynecologic, intraabdominal, skin, respiratory, bone/joint, and urinary tract infections. May cause injection site reaction, diarrhea, fever, rash, pruritus, phlebitis, CDAD, eosinophilia, thrombocytosis, and superinfection. PB: 10%; t½: 1.4–2 h
Ceftriaxone	See Prototype Drug Chart: Ceftriaxone	
Ceftibuten	Bronchitis: A: PO: 400 mg/d for 5–10 d; *max:* 400 mg/d	For treating otitis media, tonsillitis, pharyngitis, bronchitis, and respiratory infections. May cause headache, CDAD, dyspepsia, dizziness, eosinophilia, superinfection, abdominal pain, nausea, vomiting, and diarrhea. PB: 65%; t½: 2–2.5 h
Cefditoren	Chronic bronchitis: A: PO: 400 mg bid for 5–10 d; *max:* 800 mg/d	For treating pharyngitis, tonsillitis, and respiratory and skin infections. May cause CDAD, dyspepsia, diarrhea, nausea, abdominal pain, headache, and superinfection. Avoid in patients with milk protein hypersensitivity. PB: 88%; t½: 1.6 h
Ceftazidime and avibactam	UTI: A: IV: 2 g ceftazidime/0.5 g avibactam over 2 h q8h for 7–14 d; *max:* 6 g ceftazidime/1.5 g avibactam/d	For treating intraabdominal, respiratory, and urinary tract infections. May cause headache, dizziness, pruritus, nausea, vomiting, diarrhea, constipation, CDAD, and superinfection. PB: 5%–8% avibactam, 10% ceftazidime; t½: 2 h avibactam, 1.5–2 h ceftazidime

Continued

TABLE 26.6 Antibacterials: Cephalosporins—cont'd

Generic	Route and Dosage	Uses and Considerations
Fourth Generation		
Cefepime	Pneumonia: A: IV: 1–2 g q8–12h for 10 d; *max:* 6 g/d	For treating febrile neutropenia, bacteremia, and respiratory, skin, intraabdominal, and urinary tract infections. May cause headache, nausea, diarrhea, CDAD, injection site reaction, elevated hepatic enzymes, eosinophilia, hypoprothrombinemia, hypophosphatemia, and superinfection. PB: 20%; t½: 2 h
Fifth Generation		
Ceftaroline fosamil	Skin infections: A: IV: 600 mg q12h for 5–14 d; *max:* 1200 mg/d	For treating skin and respiratory infections. May cause headache, fever, rash, nausea, vomiting, diarrhea, pruritus, elevated hepatic enzymes, superinfection, and CDAD. PB: 20%; t½: 1.6 h
Ceftolozane and tazobactam	Intraabdominal infection: A: IV: 1 g ceftolozane/0.5 g tazobactam q8h for 4–14 d; *max:* 6 g ceftolozane, 3 g tazobactam/d	For treating intraabdominal, respiratory, and urinary tract infections. May cause headache, insomnia, nausea, vomiting, diarrhea, constipation, CDAD, fever, superinfection, elevated hepatic enzymes, intracranial bleeding, renal failure, and hypokalemia. PB: ceftolozane 16%–21%, tazobactam 30%; t½: ceftolozane 3–4 h, tazobactam 2–3 h

A, Adult; *bid,* two times a day; *CDAD, Clostridium difficile*–associated diarrhea; *d,* day; *GI,* gastrointestinal; *h,* hour; *IM,* intramuscularly; *IV,* intravenously; *max,* maximum; *min,* minutes; *mo,* month; *PB,* protein binding; *PID,* pelvic inflammatory disease; *PO,* by mouth; *q,* every; *t½,* half-life; *UK,* unknown; *URI,* upper respiratory infection; *UTI,* urinary tract infection; *y,* years; <, less than; >, greater than.

◎ CLINICAL JUDGMENT [NURSING PROCESS]

Antibacterials: Cephalosporins

Concept: Infection
- A condition in which microorganisms enter the body and release toxins

Recognize Cues [Assessment]
- Assess for allergy to cephalosporins or penicillins. If a patient is allergic to one type or class of cephalosporin, that patient should not receive any other type of cephalosporin or penicillin.
- Record vital signs and urine output. Report abnormal findings, which may include elevated temperature or decreased urine output.
- Evaluate laboratory results, especially those that indicate renal and liver function (blood urea nitrogen [BUN], serum creatinine, aspartate aminotransferase [AST], alanine aminotransferase [ALT], alkaline phosphatase [ALP], and bilirubin). Use these laboratory results for baseline values, and report any abnormal findings.

Analyze Cues and Prioritize Hypothesis [Patient Problems]
- Tissue injury
- Vomiting
- Nausea

Generate Solutions [Planning]
- The patient's white blood cells (WBCs) will be within normal limits.

Take Action [Nursing Interventions]
- Culture the infected area before cephalosporin therapy is started. The organism causing the infection can be determined by culture, and the antibiotics the organism is sensitive to are determined by sensitivity. If antibiotic therapy is started before culture result is reported, the antibiotic may need to be changed after culture and sensitivity (C&S) test results are received.

Patient Teaching
General
- Keep drugs out of reach of children. Request childproof containers.
- Tell patients to report signs of superinfection, such as mouth ulcers or discharge from the anal or genital area.
- Advise patients to ingest buttermilk, yogurt, or an acidophilus supplement to prevent superinfection of the intestinal flora.
- Instruct patients to take the complete course of medication, even when symptoms of infection have ceased.
- Infuse all IV cephalosporins over 30 minutes or as ordered to prevent pain and irritation.
- Observe for hypersensitivity reactions.

Side Effects
- Warn patients to report any side effects from use of oral cephalosporin drugs; these may include anorexia, nausea, vomiting, headache, dizziness, itching, and rash.

Diet
- Advise patients to take medication with food if gastric irritation occurs.
- Encourage patients to take an adequate amount of fluids to avoid dehydration from diarrhea.

Evaluate Outcomes [Evaluation]
- Evaluate the effectiveness of the cephalosporin by determining whether the infection has ceased and that no side effects, including superinfection, have occurred.

When probenecid is administered with either of these drugs, urine excretion of cefazolin and cefaclor is decreased, which increases the action of the drug. The effects of cefazolin and cefaclor can be decreased if the drug is given with tetracyclines or erythromycin. These drugs can cause false-positive laboratory results for proteinuria and glucosuria, especially when they are taken in large doses.

Table 26.6 lists the cephalosporins by their designated generation and also gives dosages, uses, and considerations.

Side Effects and Adverse Reactions

The side effects and adverse reactions to cephalosporins include GI disturbances (nausea, vomiting, diarrhea), alteration in blood clotting time (increased bleeding) with administration of large doses, and nephrotoxicity (toxicity to the kidney) in individuals with a preexisting renal disorder.

Drug Interactions

Drug interactions can occur with certain cephalosporins and alcohol. For example, alcohol consumption may cause a disulfiram-like reaction (flushing, dizziness, headache, nausea, vomiting, and muscular cramps) while taking cefotetan. Alcohol should be avoided while taking cefotetan and for 2 to 3 days after discontinuation. Cefotetan may increase the effects of warfarin, salicylates, and aminoglycosides.

CRITICAL THINKING CASE STUDY

A child 6 years of age has otitis media. The health care provider ordered amoxicillin 250 mg every 8 hours. The nurse asks the child's parent if he is allergic to any drugs, and the parent says that he is allergic to penicillin.

1. What are the similarities and differences in penicillin and amoxicillin? Explain your answer.
2. What nursing action should the nurse take? Why?
   The health care provider changed the amoxicillin order to cefaclor 250 mg every 8 hours. The therapeutic dosage for children is 20–40 mg/kg/d in three divided doses. The child weighs 40 pounds.

3. What are the similarities and differences in amoxicillin and cefaclor? Explain your answer.
4. Is the prescribed cefaclor dosage for the child within safe parameters? Explain your answer.
5. What should the nurse include in patient teaching for the child and his parent?

REVIEW QUESTIONS

1. Amoxicillin is prescribed for a patient who has a respiratory infection. The nurse is teaching the patient about this medication and realizes that more teaching is needed when the patient makes which statement?
   a. This medication should not be taken with food.
   b. I will take my entire prescription of medication.
   c. I should report to the physician any genital itching.
   d. If I experience any excess bleeding, I will contact the health care provider.
2. A patient is taking a cephalosporin. The nurse anticipates which appropriate nursing intervention(s) for this medication? (Select all that apply.)
   a. Monitoring renal function studies
   b. Monitoring liver function studies
   c. Infusing intravenous medication over 30 minutes
   d. Monitoring the patient for mouth ulcers
   e. Advising the patient to stop the medication when he or she feels better
3. Penicillin G has been prescribed for a patient. Which nursing intervention(s) should the nurse perform for this patient? (Select all that apply.)
   a. Collect culture and sensitivity before the first dose.
   b. Monitor the patient for mouth ulcers.
   c. Instruct the patient to limit fluid intake to 1000 mL/day.
   d. Have epinephrine on hand for a potential severe allergic reaction.
   e. No particular interventions are required for this patient.

4. A patient is receiving amoxicillin. The nurse understands that the action of this drug is by which process?
   a. Inhibition of protein synthesis
   b. Alteration of membrane permeability
   c. Inhibition of bacterial cell wall synthesis
   d. Alteration of bacterial ribonucleic acid synthesis
5. A patient is prescribed dicloxacillin. For which adverse effect should the nurse monitor the patient?
   a. Constipation
   b. Tongue discoloration
   c. Hypertension
   d. Hemolytic anemia
6. A patient has been prescribed amoxicillin. What does the nurse know is true about this medication?
   a. It has a normal adult dose of 2 grams q6h.
   b. It has a common side effect of hypotension.
   c. It has an intramuscular administration route.
   d. It is used to treat respiratory infections.

27

Macrolides, Oxazolidinones, Lincosamides, Glycopeptides, Ketolides, and Lipopeptides

http://evolve.elsevier.com/McCuistion/pharmacology

OBJECTIVES

- Describe the side effects/adverse effects of erythromycin.
- Apply the Clinical Judgment [Nursing Process] for azithromycin, including patient teaching.
- Compare the side effects/adverse effects of oxazolidinones, lincosamides, ketolides, and lipopeptides.

- Summarize the nurse's role in detecting ototoxicity and nephrotoxicity associated with the administration of vancomycin.

OUTLINE

INTRODUCTION

Disease-producing microorganisms may be gram-positive or gram-negative bacteria, viruses, protozoans, or fungi. The degree to which they are pathogenic depends on the microorganism and its virulence. This chapter discusses drugs prescribed to combat disease-producing microorganisms.

The groups of antibacterials discussed in this chapter include macrolides (erythromycin, clarithromycin, and azithromycin), lincosamides, glycopeptides, ketolides, lipopeptides, and oxazolidinones.

The macrolides, oxazolidinones, lincosamides, and ketolides are primarily bacteriostatic drugs, those that inhibit bacterial growth, but they may also be bactericidal (bacteria killing), depending on the drug dose, serum level, and pathogen (the disease-producing microorganism). Glycopeptides and lipopeptides are bactericidal drugs.

Macrolides, oxazolidinones, lincosamides, glycopeptides, and ketolides are discussed together because they have spectrums of antibiotic effectiveness similar to that of penicillin, although they differ in structure. Drugs from these groups are used as penicillin substitutes, especially in individuals who are allergic to penicillin. Erythromycin is the drug frequently prescribed if the patient has a hypersensitivity to penicillin.

MACROLIDES

Macrolide antibiotics—which include azithromycin, clarithromycin, and erythromycin—are called *broad-spectrum antibiotics*. Erythromycin, the first macrolide, was derived from the fungus-like bacteria *Streptomyces erythreus* and was first introduced in the early 1950s. Macrolides bind to the 50S ribosomal subunits and inhibit protein synthesis. At low to moderate drug doses, macrolides have a bacteriostatic effect, and with high drug doses, their effect is bactericidal. Macrolides can be administered orally or by IV but not intramuscularly because it is too painful. IV macrolides should be infused slowly to avoid unnecessary pain (phlebitis).

Gastric acid destroys erythromycin in the stomach; therefore acid-resistant salts are added (e.g., ethylsuccinate, stearate, estolate) to decrease breakdown into small particles (dissolution) in the stomach. This allows the drug to be absorbed in the intestine. Normally, food does not hamper the absorption of acid-resistant macrolides. Table 27.1 lists the dosages, uses, and considerations of macrolides.

Macrolides are active against most gram-positive bacteria and are moderately active against some gram-negative bacteria, although resistant organisms may emerge during treatment. Macrolides are used to treat mild to moderate infections of the respiratory tract, sinuses, GI tract, and skin and soft tissue in addition to treating diphtheria, impetigo contagiosa, and sexually transmitted infections (STIs).

TABLE 27.1 Antibacterials: Macrolides, Oxazolidinones, Lincosamides, Glycopeptides, Ketolides, and Lipopeptides

Generic	Route and Dosage	Uses and Considerations
Macrolides		
Azithromycin	See Prototype Drug Chart: Azithromycin	
Clarithromycin	Skin infections: Regular release: A: PO: 250 mg q12h for 7–14 d; *max:* 1.5 g/d	For treating otitis media, tonsillitis, sinusitis, pharyngitis, and *Helicobacter pylori*, skin, and respiratory infections. May cause headache, rash, dysgeusia, dyspepsia, nausea, vomiting, diarrhea, flatulence, CDAD, abdominal pain, elevated hepatic enzymes, and superinfection. PB: 42%–70%; t½: 3–7 h
Erythromycin base	Respiratory infections: A: PO: 25 mg q6h or 500 mg q12h; *max:* 4 g/d A: IV: 15–20 mg/kg/d in divided doses q6h; *max:* 4 g/d	For treating acne, impetigo, tonsillitis, urethritis, STIs, Legionnaires' disease, PID, diphtheria, listeriosis, pertussis, and respiratory, GI, and skin infections. May cause dry, irritated skin; superinfection; CDAD; anorexia; pruritus; erythema; phlebitis; jaundice; elevated hepatic enzymes; nausea; vomiting; diarrhea; and abdominal pain. PB: 75%–90%; t½: 1.5 h
Fidaxomicin	A: PO: 200 mg bid for 10 d; *max:* 400 mg/d	For treating CDAD. May cause nausea, vomiting, diarrhea, abdominal pain, GI bleeding/constipation, fever, rash, pruritus, and elevated hepatic enzymes. PB: UK; t½: 6.9–16.5 h
Oxazolidinones		
Linezolid	Nosocomial pneumonia: A: PO/IV: 600 mg q12h for at least 7 d; *max:* 1200 mg/d	For treating bacteremia, sepsis, MRSA, VREF, tuberculosis, and respiratory and skin infections. May cause headache, pruritus, tongue/tooth discoloration, nausea, vomiting, diarrhea, abdominal pain, dizziness, anemia, thrombocytopenia, serotonin syndrome, CDAD, and superinfection. PB: 31%; t½: 4.26–5.4 h
Tedizolid	A: PO/IV: 200 mg/d for 6 d; *max:* 200 mg/d	For treating skin infections. May cause headache, nausea, vomiting, diarrhea, infusion-related/injection site reactions, phlebitis, erythema, serotonin syndrome, CDAD, and superinfection. PB: 70%–90%; t½: 12 h
Lincosamides		
Clindamycin	Lower respiratory infection: A: PO: 150–450 mg q6h for 7–21 days; *max:* 1800 mg/d A: IM/IV: 300–600 mg q6–12h; *max:* 2700 mg/d IV, 2400 mg/d IM	For treating PID, acne, bacteremia, mastitis, MRSA, and respiratory, intraabdominal, skin, gynecologic, and bone/joint infections. May cause dry skin, nausea, vomiting, diarrhea, CDAD, erythema, pruritus, superinfection, headache, candidiasis, and back pain. Should be taken with full glass of water. PB: 80%–95%; t½: 2–3 h
Lincomycin	A: IM: 600 mg q12–24h; *max:* 1.2 g/d A: IV: 600 mg-1 g q8–12h; *max:* 8 g/d	For treating severe infections. May cause glossitis, stomatitis, headache, candidiasis, dizziness, nausea, vomiting, diarrhea, CDAD, superinfection, injection site reaction, and rash. PB: 77%–82%; t½: 4.4–6.4 h
Glycopeptides		
Vancomycin hydrochloride	Clostridium difficile infection: A: PO: 125 mg qid for 10–14 d, then 125 mg bid for 1 wk, then 125 mg qd for 1 wk, then 125 mg q2–3d for 2–8 wk; *max:* 2 g/d Therapeutic range: Trough: 5–20 mcg/mL Peak: 30–40 mcg/mL	For treating bacteremia, mastitis, endocarditis, enterocolitis due to *Staphylococcus aureus*, MRSA, CDAD, and respiratory, skin, and bone/joint infections. May cause fever, headache, fatigue, back pain, peripheral edema, nausea, vomiting, flatulence, diarrhea, abdominal pain, hypokalemia, tinnitus, CDAD, vancomycin infusion reaction (red man syndrome), neutropenia, ototoxicity, nephrotoxicity, and superinfection. PB: 55%; t½: 4–6 h
Oritavancin	Skin infection: A: IV: 1200 mg as a single dose over 3 h; *max:* 1200 mg	For treating skin infections. May cause erythema, nausea, vomiting, diarrhea, dizziness, headache, peripheral edema, infusion site reaction, elevated hepatic enzymes, phlebitis, tachycardia, vancomycin infusion reaction (red man syndrome), superinfection, and CDAD. PB: 85%; t½: 245 h
Telavancin	Respiratory infections: A: IV: 10 mg/kg/d over 60 min for 7–21 d; *max:* 10 mg/kg/d	For treating MRSA and respiratory and skin infections. May cause erythema, chills, dizziness, pruritus, rash, renal failure, metallic taste, nausea, vomiting, diarrhea, infusion site reaction, CDAD, and superinfection. PB: 93%; t½: 8–9 h
Ketolides		
Telithromycin	A: PO: 800 mg/d for 7–10 d; *max:* 800 mg/d	For treating community-acquired pneumonia. May cause visual disturbances, dizziness, abdominal pain, nausea, vomiting, diarrhea, CDAD, myasthenia gravis exacerbation, hepatotoxicity, and superinfection. PB: 60%–70%; t½: 10 h
Lipopeptides		
Daptomycin	Skin infection: A: IV: 4 mg/kg/d for 7–14 d; *max:* 6 mg/kg/d	For treating endocarditis, bacteremia, and skin infections. May cause rash, pruritus, insomnia, edema, dizziness, hypo/hypertension, chest pain, headache, hyperhidrosis, nausea, vomiting, diarrhea, abdominal pain, CDAD, and superinfection. PB: 90%–93%; t½: 8–9 h

A, Adult; *bid,* twice daily; *CDAD, Clostridium difficile*–associated diarrhea; *d,* day; *GI,* gastrointestinal; *h,* hour; *IM,* intramuscular; *IV,* intravenous; *max,* maximum; *min,* minutes; *mo,* month; *MRSA,* methicillin-resistant *Staphylococcus aureus; PB,* protein binding; *PID,* pelvic inflammatory disease; *PO,* by mouth; *q,* every; *STI,* sexually transmitted infection; *t½,* half-life; *UK,* unknown; *VREF,* vancomycin-resistant *Enterococcus faecium; wk,* weeks; *y,* years; <, less than; >, greater than.

Erythromycin is the drug of choice for the treatment of mycoplasmal pneumonia and Legionnaires' disease. Clarithromycin is also available in a once-a-day extended-release tablet to be taken for 7 days. Azithromycin is frequently prescribed for upper and lower respiratory infections, STIs, and uncomplicated skin infections. Table 27.1 lists the drugs developed from the derivatives of erythromycin, and Prototype Drug Chart: Azithromycin details the pharmacologic behavior of azithromycin.

Pharmacokinetics. Clarithromycin and erythromycin are readily absorbed from the GI tract, mainly by the duodenum. Azithromycin is incompletely absorbed from the GI tract, and only 37% reaches systemic circulation. Azithromycin and erythromycin can be administered intravenously, but intermittent infusions should be diluted in normal saline (NS) or in 5% dextrose in water (D_5W) to prevent phlebitis or burning sensations at the injection site. Azithromycin 500 mg should be diluted in 250 to 500 mL of fluid, and erythromycin lactobionate 1 g should be diluted in 200 to 1000 mL. Macrolides are excreted in bile, feces, and urine. Because only a small amount is excreted in urine, renal insufficiency is not a contraindication for macrolide use.

Pharmacodynamics. Macrolides suppress bacterial protein synthesis. The onset of action of oral preparations of erythromycin is 1 hour, peak concentration time is 4 hours, and duration of action is 6 hours. Newer macrolides have a longer half-life and are administered less frequently. Clarithromycin is administered twice a day for immediate release, and the extended-release formulation is administered once a day. Azithromycin has a 68-hour half-life.

Side Effects and Adverse Reactions

Side effects and adverse reactions to macrolides include GI disturbances such as nausea, vomiting, diarrhea, and abdominal cramping. Severe diarrhea occurs when antibacterials kill normal flora, allowing an overgrowth of *Clostridium difficile*. This superinfection is called *Clostridium difficile*–associated diarrhea (CDAD), also known as pseudomembranous colitis. A release of bacterial toxins causes injury, inflammation, and bleeding in the colon lining. This condition causes abdominal cramping, 5 to 10 watery diarrheal stools per day, and bloody stools. Frequency of stools may increase to 20 per day in severe cases. Conjunctivitis may develop as a side effect of azithromycin, and the patient should avoid wearing contact lenses if this occurs. Allergic reactions to erythromycin are rare. Hepatotoxicity (liver toxicity) can occur when erythromycin and azithromycin are taken in high doses with other hepatotoxic drugs, such as acetaminophen (high doses), phenothiazines, and sulfonamides. Liver damage is usually reversible when the drug is discontinued. Erythromycin should not be taken with clindamycin or lincomycin because they compete for receptor sites.

Drug Interactions

Macrolides can increase serum levels of theophylline (a bronchodilator), carbamazepine (an anticonvulsant), and warfarin (an anticoagulant). If these drugs are given with macrolides, their drug serum levels should be closely monitored. To avoid severe toxic effects, erythromycin should not be used with other macrolides. Antacids may reduce azithromycin peak levels when taken at the same time.

Extended Macrolide Group

Derivatives of erythromycin have been effective in the treatment of numerous organisms. Like erythromycin, they also inhibit protein synthesis. Many of these macrolides have a longer half-life and are administered once a day. After the introduction of erythromycin, the first extended macrolide drug developed was clarithromycin, which has been effective against many bacterial infections. Clarithromycin is administered twice a day for immediate-release form, and the

---

📄 PROTOTYPE DRUG CHART

Azithromycin

Drug Class	Dosage
Antibacterial macrolide	Chronic bronchitis exacerbation: Immediate release: A: PO: 500 mg for 1 d, or 500 mg/d for 3 d, then follow with 250 mg/d for 4 days; *max:* 500 mg/d

Contraindications	Drug-Lab-Food Interactions
Hypersensitivity to macrolides, hepatitis, jaundice *Caution:* Bradycardia, hypokalemia, hypomagnesemia, dysrhythmias, hepatic/renal dysfunction, diarrhea, CDAD, hypocalcemia, rheumatoid arthritis, cardiac disease, myasthenia gravis, thyroid disorder, breastfeeding, older adults	Drug: Increases effects of digoxin, cyclosporine, and warfarin; decreases effects of penicillins and clindamycin

Pharmacokinetics	Pharmacodynamics
Absorption: PO: 38% absorbed Distribution: PB: 51% Metabolism: t½: 40–68 h Excretion: In bile, a small amount in urine	PO: Onset, duration: UK Peak: 2–3 h Extended release: Peak: 3–5 h IV: Onset, duration, peak: UK

Therapeutic Effects/Uses

For treating bacterial conjunctivitis, otitis media, tonsillitis, sinusitis, PID, STIs, and skin and respiratory infections. For patients who are allergic to penicillin. Azithromycin is effective against species of *Clostridium, Haemophilus, Chlamydia, Mycobacterium, Neisseria, Staphylococcus,* and *Streptococcus*

Mechanism of Action: Inhibits the steps of protein synthesis; bacteriostatic or bactericidal effect

Side Effects	Adverse Reactions
Blurred vision, ocular irritation/pain, photosensitivity, headache, tinnitus, edema, drowsiness, dizziness, fever, fatigue, tongue discoloration, dysgeusia, anorexia, nausea, vomiting, diarrhea, flatulence, abdominal cramps, pruritus, rash, injection site reaction, weakness, agitation, vaginitis, constipation	Superinfection, hearing loss, angioedema, seizures, hyperbilirubinemia, hypotension, azotemia, cholestasis, myasthenia gravis exacerbation, hypo/hyperkalemia, hyponatremia *Life-threatening:* Hepatotoxicity, anemia, eosinophilia, anaphylaxis, bronchospasm, CDAD, leukopenia, thrombocytopenia, Stevens-Johnson syndrome

A, Adult; *CDAD, Clostridium difficile*–associated diarrhea; *d,* day; *h,* hour; *IV,* intravenous; *max,* maximum; *PB,* protein binding; *PID,* pelvic inflammatory disease; *PO,* by mouth; *STI,* sexually transmitted infection; *t½,* half-life; *UK,* unknown.

⊙ CLINICAL JUDGMENT [NURSING PROCESS]

Antibacterials: Macrolides

Concept: Infection
- A condition in which microorganisms enter the body and release toxins

Recognize Cues [Assessment]
- Assess vital signs and urine output. Report abnormal findings.
- Check laboratory tests (liver enzyme values) to determine liver function. Order liver enzyme tests periodically for patients taking large doses of azithromycin for a continuous period.
- Obtain a history of drugs the patient currently takes. The peak level of azithromycin may be decreased by antacids.

Analyze Cues and Prioritize Hypothesis [Patient Problems]
- Tissue injury
- Nausea
- Vomiting

Generate Solutions [Planning]
- The patient's white blood cells (WBCs) will be within normal limits.

Take Action [Nursing Interventions]
- Obtain a sample from the infected area and send it to the laboratory for culture and sensitivity (C&S) testing before starting azithromycin therapy. Antibiotic therapy can be initiated after obtaining the culture sample.
- Monitor vital signs, urine output, and laboratory values, especially liver enzymes (alkaline phosphatase [ALP], alanine aminotransferase [ALT], aspartate aminotransferase [AST], and bilirubin).

- Monitor the patient for liver damage resulting from prolonged use and high dosage of macrolides such as azithromycin. Signs of liver dysfunction include elevated liver enzyme levels and jaundice.
- Administer oral azithromycin 1 hour before or 2 hours after meals. Give with a full glass of water, *not* fruit juice. Give the drug with food if gastrointestinal (GI) upset occurs. Chewable tablets should be chewed, *not* swallowed whole.
- Dilute in an appropriate amount of solution as indicated in the drug circular for intravenous (IV) azithromycin.
- Administer antacids either 2 hours before or 2 hours after azithromycin.

Patient Teaching
General
- Instruct patients to take the full course of the antibacterial agent as prescribed. Drug compliance is most important for all antibacterials (antibiotics).

Side Effects
- Encourage patients to report side effects, including adverse reactions (nausea, vomiting, diarrhea, abdominal cramps, itching).
- Teach patients to report any evidence of superinfection, secondary infection resulting from drug therapy; for some patients, stomatitis or vaginitis may occur.
- ⚡ Tell patients to report the onset of loose stools or diarrhea. *Clostridium difficile*–associated diarrhea (CDAD) should be ruled out.

Evaluate Outcomes [Evaluation]
- Evaluate the effectiveness of azithromycin by determining whether the infection has been controlled or has ceased and that no side effects, including superinfection, have occurred.

---

extended-release formulation is given once a day. Another extended macrolide is azithromycin. This drug has a long half-life of up to 68 hours.

Elimination of these drugs is via bile and feces. Azithromycin is frequently prescribed for upper and lower respiratory tract infections, STIs, and uncomplicated skin infections.

When erythromycin is given concurrently with verapamil, diltiazem, clarithromycin, fluconazole, ketoconazole, and itraconazole, erythromycin blood concentration and the risk of sudden cardiac death increase. Table 27.1 lists the drugs developed from the derivatives of erythromycin.

Common side effects of clarithromycin are nausea, diarrhea, and abdominal discomfort. With azithromycin, the side effects of nausea, diarrhea, and abdominal pain are common.

OXAZOLIDINONES

Like macrolides, oxazolidinones inhibit protein synthesis on the 50S ribosomal subunit of bacteria. This action prevents formation of 70S initiation complex, which is necessary for bacterial reproduction. Linezolid and tedizolid are examples of oxazolidinones. Drugs in this antibacterial classification are bacteriostatic or bactericidal and are effective against gram-positive infections. Table 27.1 lists the oxazolidinones.

Side Effects and Adverse Reactions

Side effects and adverse reactions to linezolid and tedizolid include headache, nausea, vomiting, diarrhea, anemia, and thrombocytopenia. Severe adverse reactions include CDAD and serotonin syndrome.

LINCOSAMIDES

Like erythromycin, lincosamides inhibit bacterial protein synthesis and have both bacteriostatic and bactericidal actions, depending on drug dosage. Clindamycin and lincomycin are examples of lincosamides. Clindamycin is more widely prescribed than lincomycin because it is active against most gram-positive organisms, including *S. aureus* and anaerobic organisms. It is not effective against gram-negative bacteria (e.g., *E. coli* and *Proteus* and *Pseudomonas* species). Clindamycin is absorbed better than lincomycin through the GI tract and maintains a higher serum drug concentration. Clindamycin is considered more effective than lincomycin and has fewer toxic effects. Table 27.1 lists the lincosamides.

Side Effects and Adverse Reactions

Side effects and adverse reactions to clindamycin and lincomycin include GI irritation, which may manifest as nausea, vomiting, and stomatitis. Rash may also occur. Severe adverse reactions include colitis and anaphylactic shock.

Drug Interactions

Clindamycin and lincomycin are incompatible with aminophylline, phenytoin, barbiturates, and ampicillin.

GLYCOPEPTIDES

Vancomycin, a glycopeptide bactericidal antibiotic, was widely used in the 1950s to treat staphylococcal infections. Vancomycin is used against drug-resistant *S. aureus* and in cardiac surgical prophylaxis for individuals with penicillin allergies. Serum vancomycin levels should be monitored.

Vancomycin has become ineffective for treating enterococci. Antibiotic-resistant enterococci can cause staphylococcal endocarditis.

Telavancin, a glycopeptide, treats selected gram-positive bacteria and skin infections. This drug is a semisynthetic derivative of vancomycin with bactericidal action against MRSA. Telavancin has an advantage of once-daily dosing. Oritavancin has the further advantage of being administered in a single dose.

Pharmacokinetics. Vancomycin is given orally for treatment of staphylococcal enterocolitis and antibiotic-associated pseudomembranous colitis due to *C. difficile*. When vancomycin is given orally, it is not absorbed systemically and is excreted in the feces. Vancomycin is also given intravenously for septicemia; for severe infections due to MRSA; and for bone, skin, and lower respiratory tract infections that do not respond or are resistant to other antibiotics. Intermittent vancomycin doses should be diluted in 100 mL for 500 mg and 200 mL for 1 g of D_5W, NS, or lactated Ringer's (LR), and should be administered over 60 to 90 minutes. Vancomycin is excreted in the urine when given by IV route. It is 55% protein bound, and the half-life is 4 to 6 hours.

Pharmacodynamics. Vancomycin inhibits bacterial cell wall synthesis and is active against several gram-positive microorganisms. The peak action is 30 minutes after the end of the infusion.

Side Effects and Adverse Reactions

Vancomycin may cause nephrotoxicity and ototoxicity. Ototoxicity results in damage to the auditory or vestibular branch of cranial nerve VIII. Such damage can result in permanent hearing loss (auditory branch) or temporary or permanent loss of balance (vestibular branch). Side effects may include headache, dizziness, fatigue, fever, nausea, vomiting, flatulence, abdominal pain, diarrhea, back pain, peripheral edema, and injection site reaction. Too-rapid injection of IV vancomycin can cause a condition known as vancomycin infusion reaction, previously known as *red man syndrome* or *red neck syndrome*. Characterized by red blotching of the face, neck, arms, upper body, and back, this is a toxic effect rather than an allergic reaction. Other effects include hypotension, tachycardia, wheezing, dyspnea, paresthesias, erythema, pruritus, and urticaria, and may lead to cardiac arrest. Adverse effects include eosinophilia, neutropenia, phlebitis, CDAD, hypokalemia, renal failure, and Stevens-Johnson syndrome.

Drug Interactions

Dimenhydrinate can mask ototoxicity when taken with vancomycin. The risk of nephrotoxicity and ototoxicity may be potentiated when vancomycin is taken with furosemide, aminoglycosides, amphotericin B, colistin, cisplatin, and cyclosporine. Vancomycin may inhibit methotrexate excretion and can increase methotrexate toxicity. The absorption of oral vancomycin may be decreased when given with cholestyramine and colestipol.

KETOLIDES

Ketolides are structurally related to macrolides but have greater bactericidal ability. The first drug in this class, telithromycin, is used for adults 18 years of age and older to treat mild to moderate community-acquired pneumonia. This disorder is usually caused by *S. pneumoniae* and *H. influenzae*.

Pharmacokinetics. Telithromycin is given orally and is well absorbed by the GI tract; it is unaffected by food intake. Telithromycin is excreted in the feces and urine. It is 60% to 70% protein bound, and the half-life is 10 hours.

Pharmacodynamics. Telithromycin inhibits protein synthesis in microorganisms by binding to the bacterial ribosomal RNA site of the 50S subunit, resulting in bacterial cell death. The peak action is 1 hour.

Side Effects and Adverse Reactions

Side effects and adverse reactions to telithromycin include visual disturbances (blurred vision and diplopia), dizziness, altered taste, nausea, vomiting, diarrhea, anaphylaxis, and liver failure. Telithromycin may also lead to an exacerbation of myasthenia gravis.

Drug Interactions

Telithromycin levels are increased when taken concurrently with antilipidemics (simvastatin, lovastatin, and atorvastatin), itraconazole, ketoconazole, and benzodiazepines. Class 1A or class III antidysrhythmics may lead to life-threatening dysrhythmias. Blood levels of telithromycin are decreased when taken with rifampin, phenytoin, carbamazepine, or phenobarbital, producing a subtherapeutic drug level. Telithromycin can increase levels of cisapride and pimozide, which can lead to toxicity; these two drugs are therefore contraindicated for the patient taking telithromycin. Digoxin, metoprolol, midazolam, ritonavir, sirolimus, and tacrolimus levels are increased when taken concurrently with telithromycin. Concurrent use of telithromycin with ergot alkaloid derivatives leads to ergot toxicity (severe peripheral vasospasm and impaired sensation).

LIPOPEPTIDES

Daptomycin is a US Food and Drug Administration (FDA)-approved antibiotic in the category of *lipopeptides*. Daptomycin acts by binding to the bacterial membrane and causing rapid depolarization of its membrane potential, inhibiting protein, DNA, and RNA synthesis. This action results in bacterial cell death.

Indications for daptomycin include complicated skin infections due to gram-positive microorganisms, septicemia due to *S. aureus* infection, and infective endocarditis due to MRSA infection.

Pharmacokinetics. Daptomycin is administered by IV at a dose of 4 mg/kg daily. Each 500-mg vial of the medication is diluted in 10 mL of NS 0.9% and allowed to stand for 10 minutes. After gentle rotation of the vial to ensure dilution, further dilute in 50 to 100 mL of NS and administer over 30 minutes. Drug should *not* be mixed with dextrose-containing diluents. The protein-binding capacity is 90% to 93%, and half-life averages 8 to 9 hours. Daptomycin is primarily excreted by the kidneys.

Pharmacodynamics. Daptomycin binds to the bacterial membrane and causes cell death. An effective trough concentration of 5.9 mcg/mL is usually achieved by the third dose.

Side Effects and Adverse Reactions

Side effects that may occur when taking daptomycin include hypertension, hypotension, dizziness, insomnia, nausea, vomiting, and diarrhea. More serious adverse effects that have occurred with daptomycin are chest pain, anemia, peripheral neuropathy, anaphylaxis, rhabdomyolysis, angioedema, *Clostridium difficile*–associated diarrhea, Stevens-Johnson syndrome, and renal failure.

Drug Interactions

When daptomycin is given with 3-hydroxy-3-methylglutaryl coenzyme A (HMG-CoA) reductase inhibitors (statins, such as simvastatin or atorvastatin), the risk of rhabdomyolysis and elevated levels of creatine phosphokinase (CPK) is increased. Daptomycin toxicity may be increased when given concurrently with tobramycin, and warfarin may lead to increased bleeding when taken with daptomycin.

CRITICAL THINKING CASE STUDY

A 54-year-old male is ordered clarithromycin 250 mg every 12 hours for his newly developed chronic bronchitis.

1. Is the dose within normal dosage range? Explain your answer.

2. What side effects should the nurse teach the patient about?

3. What are some adverse effects that the patient should report to the health care provider?

REVIEW QUESTIONS

1. A patient is prescribed daptomycin. Which action(s) should the nurse implement? (Select all that apply.)
   a. Monitor blood values for toxicity.
   b. Dilute in 50 to 100 mL of normal saline and administer intravenously over 30 minutes.
   c. Monitor the patient for allergic reactions such as rhabdomyolysis.
   d. Advise the patient to take the medication on an empty stomach, even if gastrointestinal distress occurs.
   e. Culture the infected area before administering the first dose.

2. A patient is taking azithromycin. Which nursing intervention(s) would the nurse plan to implement for this patient? (Select all that apply.)
   a. Monitor periodic liver function tests.
   b. Dilute with 50 mL of 5% dextrose in water for intravenous administration.
   c. Instruct the patient to report any loose stools or diarrhea.
   d. Instruct the patient to report evidence of superinfection.
   e. Teach the patient to take oral drug 1 hour before or 2 hours after meals.
   f. Advise the patient to avoid antacids from 2 hours before 2 hours after administration.

3. For which serious adverse effect should the nurse closely monitor a patient who is taking lincosamides?
   a. Seizures
   b. Ototoxicity
   c. Hepatotoxicity
   d. *Clostridium difficile*–associated diarrhea

4. The nurse enters a patient's room to find that his heart rate is 120, his blood pressure is 70/50, and he has red blotching of his face and neck. Vancomycin is running intravenous piggyback. The nurse believes that this patient is experiencing a severe adverse effect called *red man syndrome*. What action will the nurse take?
   a. Stop the infusion and call the health care provider.
   b. Reduce the infusion to 10 mg/minute.
   c. Encourage the patient to drink more fluids, up to 2 L/day.
   d. Report onset of Stevens-Johnson syndrome to the health care provider.

28

Tetracyclines, Glycylcyclines, Aminoglycosides, and Fluoroquinolones

OBJECTIVES

- Apply the Clinical Judgment [Nursing Process] for tetracyclines, including patient teaching.
- Compare the similarities and differences between tetracyclines and glycylcyclines.
- Summarize the nurse's role in detecting ototoxicity and nephrotoxicity associated with the administration of aminoglycosides.
- Explain the importance for ordering peak and trough concentration levels for aminoglycosides.

- Develop a teaching plan for a patient prescribed a fluoroquinolone (quinolone).
- Contrast the nursing interventions for each of the drug categories: tetracyclines, glycylcyclines, aminoglycosides, and fluoroquinolones.
- Apply the Clinical Judgment [Nursing Process] to the patient taking fluoroquinolones.

OUTLINE

INTRODUCTION

The groups of antibacterials discussed in this chapter include tetracyclines, glycylcyclines, aminoglycosides, and fluoroquinolones (quinolones).

TETRACYCLINES

Tetracyclines, isolated from *Streptomyces aureofaciens* in 1948, were the first broad-spectrum antibiotics effective against gram-positive and gram-negative bacteria, and many other organisms—mycobacteria, rickettsiae, spirochetes, and chlamydiae, to name a few. Tetracyclines act by inhibiting bacterial protein synthesis and have a bacteriostatic effect.

Tetracyclines are not effective against *S. aureus* (except for the newer tetracyclines), nor are they effective against *Pseudomonas* or *Proteus* species, but they can be used against *Mycoplasma pneumoniae*. Tetracycline in combination with metronidazole and bismuth subsalicylate is useful in treating *Helicobacter pylori,* a bacterium in the stomach that can cause peptic ulcer. For years, oral and topical tetracyclines have been used to treat severe acne vulgaris, and low doses are usually prescribed to minimize the toxic effect of the drug.

The tetracyclines are frequently prescribed for oral use, although they are also available for intravenous (IV) use to treat severe infections (Prototype Drug Chart: Doxycycline). The newer oral preparations of tetracyclines (i.e., doxycycline, minocycline) are more rapidly and completely absorbed. Tetracyclines should not be taken with magnesium and aluminum antacid preparations, milk products containing calcium, or iron-containing drugs because these substances bind with tetracycline and prevent absorption of the drug. It is suggested that tetracyclines, except for doxycycline and minocycline, be taken on an empty stomach 1 hour before or 2 hours after mealtime; the absorption of doxycycline and minocycline is improved with food ingestion. Table 28.1 describes the tetracycline preparations and their dosages, uses, and considerations. The tetracyclines are listed according to whether they are short-, intermediate-, or long-acting drugs.

Continuous use of tetracyclines has resulted in bacterial resistance to the drugs. Tetracycline resistance has increased in the treatment of pneumococcal and gonococcal infections; therefore, tetracyclines are not as useful in treating these infections. Although tetracyclines are widely used, they have numerous side effects, adverse reactions, toxicities, and drug interactions.

📄 PROTOTYPE DRUG CHART

Doxycycline

Drug Class	Dosage
Antibacterial: Tetracycline	Urinary tract infection: Delayed release: A: PO: 100 mg q12h on day 1, then 100 mg/d A: IV: 200 mg on day 1, then 100–200 mg/d

Contraindications	Drug-Lab-Food Interactions
Hypersensitivity *Caution:* Renal and hepatic dysfunction, asthma, diabetes mellitus, obesity, chemotherapy, sulfite hypersensitivity, diarrhea, CDAD, immunosuppression, STI, sunlight exposure, breastfeeding, pregnancy, older adults	Drug: May increase effects of digoxin and warfarin; doxycycline absorption decreases with sucralfate, antacids, iron, calcium, magnesium, zinc, barbiturates, phenytoin, quinapril, and rifampin; decreases effects of oral contraceptives, ciprofloxacin, and penicillin; may alter lithium levels Lab: Decreases serum potassium level Food: Dairy products decrease effect

Pharmacokinetics	Pharmacodynamics
Absorption: PO: 100% absorbed Distribution: PB: 80%–90% Metabolism: t½: 12–25 h Excretion: Urine and feces	PO: Onset, duration: UK Peak: 3 h IV: Onset: Rapid Peak, duration: UK

Therapeutic Effects/Uses
For treating acne, anthrax, amebiasis, cholera, brucellosis, psittacosis, epididymitis, malaria, tularemia, plague, STIs, rickettsia, and respiratory, urinary tract, and skin infections. Doxycycline is effective against *Escherichia coli* and MRSA, and species of *Clostridium, Haemophilus, Enterococcus, Chlamydia, Neisseria, Klebsiella, Staphylococcus, Streptococcus,* and *Shigella* Mechanism of Action: Inhibits the steps of protein synthesis; bacteriostatic or bactericidal

Side Effects	Adverse Reactions
Abdominal pain, glossitis, dysphagia, dry mouth, tooth/nail discoloration, nausea, vomiting, diarrhea, headache, blurred vision, diplopia, photosensitivity, rash, cough, injection site reaction, nasopharyngitis, skin hyperpigmentation, anxiety, sinusitis, throat irritation, nasal congestion, dyspepsia, back pain, influenza, musculoskeletal pain, elevated hepatic enzymes, candidiasis, Jarisch-Harxheimer reaction	Superinfection, angioedema, hypertension, enterocolitis, hyperglycemia, pancreatitis, esophageal ulceration *Life-threatening:* Anaphylaxis, eosinophilia, thrombocytopenia, hemolytic anemia, neutropenia, hepatotoxicity, increased intracranial pressure, CDAD, Stevens-Johnson syndrome

A, Adult; *CDAD, Clostridium difficile*–associated diarrhea; *d,* day; *h,* hour; *IV,* intravenous; *MRSA,* methicillin-resistant *Staphylococcus aureus*; *PB,* protein binding; *PO,* by mouth; *q,* every; *STI,* sexually transmitted infection; *t½,* half-life; *UK,* unknown; *UTI,* urinary tract infection; *y,* year; <, less than; >, greater than.

Side Effects and Adverse Reactions

GI disturbances such as nausea, vomiting, and diarrhea are side effects of tetracyclines. Photosensitivity (sunburn reaction) may occur in persons taking tetracyclines, especially demeclocycline. Pregnant patients should *not* take tetracycline during the first trimester of pregnancy because of possible teratogenic effects. Women in the last trimester of pregnancy and children younger than 8 years of age should also *not* take tetracycline because it irreversibly discolors the permanent teeth. Minocycline can cause damage to the vestibular part of the inner ear, which may result in difficulty maintaining balance. Outdated tetracyclines should always be discarded because the drug breaks down into a toxic by-product. Renal failure results with some tetracyclines, especially when given in high doses with other nephrotoxic drugs. Because tetracycline can disrupt the microbial flora of the body, superinfection (secondary infection resulting from drug therapy) is another adverse reaction that might result. Blood dyscrasias may occur with tetracyclines.

Drug Interactions

Antacids and iron-containing drugs can prevent absorption of tetracycline from the GI tract. Milk and foods high in calcium can inhibit tetracycline absorption. To avoid drug interaction, these should be taken at least 2 hours apart from tetracycline. Be aware that lipid-soluble tetracyclines, such as doxycycline and minocycline, are actually better absorbed from the GI tract when taken *with* milk products and food.

The desired action of oral contraceptives can be lessened when taken with tetracyclines. The activity of penicillins given with a tetracycline can be decreased because the tetracyclines could cause a bacterial resistance to the action of penicillin. Administering tetracycline with an aminoglycoside may increase the risk of nephrotoxicity.

GLYCYLCYCLINES

Tigecycline is an antibiotic in a category called *glycylcyclines,* synthetic analogues of the tetracyclines (see Table 28.1). Tigecycline acts by

TABLE 28.1   Antibacterials: Tetracyclines and Glycylcyclines

Generic	Route and Dosage	Uses and Considerations
Short-Acting Tetracycline		
Tetracycline	URI: A: PO: 500 mg bid or 250 mg q6h; *max:* 2 g/d	For treating acne, tularemia, shigellosis, intestinal amebiasis, psittacosis, anthrax, plague, gingivitis, cholera, MRSA, STIs, and *Helicobacter pylori*, skin, urinary tract, and respiratory infections. May cause headache, dermatitis, glossitis, tooth/tongue/nail discoloration, nausea, vomiting, diarrhea, blood dyscrasias, and superinfection. PB: 65%; t½: 6–12 h
Intermediate-Acting Tetracycline		
Demeclocycline hydrochloride	Respiratory infection: A: PO: 150 mg q6h or 300 mg q12h; *max:* 1.2 g/d	For treating acne, gingivitis, anthrax, amebiasis, cholera, plague, STIs, and skin, respiratory, and urinary tract infections. May cause headache, tooth discoloration, glossitis, nausea, vomiting, diarrhea, CDAD, blood dyscrasias, renal failure, and superinfection. PB: 65%–90%; t½: 10–17 h
Miscellaneous Tetracyclines		
Doxycycline hyclate	See Prototype Drug Chart: Doxycycline	
Minocycline hydrochloride	Respiratory infection: A: PO/IV: Initially: 200 mg; *maint:* 100 mg q12h; *max:* 200 mg/d PO; 400 mg/d IV	For treating anthrax, cholera, plague, meningitis, MRSA, STIs, acne, and respiratory, urinary tract, and skin infections. May cause dizziness, fatigue, headache, stomatitis, dental caries/pain, nausea, vomiting, flushing, erythema, dry mouth, anorexia, gingivitis, tooth/tongue discoloration, oral ulceration, pruritus, CDAD, blood dyscrasias, renal failure, and superinfection. Take drug with food. PB: 76%; t½: 11–24 h
Omadacycline	Pneumonia: A: IV: LD 200 mg once or 100 mg bid on day 1, then 100 mg/d for 7–14 d A: PO: After IV LD, 300 mg/d for 7–14 d	For community-acquired pneumonia and skin infections. May cause injection site reaction, headache, hypertension, nausea, vomiting, diarrhea, constipation, tooth discoloration, elevated hepatic enzymes, CDAD, superinfection, and insomnia. PB: 20%; t½: 15.5–16.83 h
Eravacycline	A: IV: 1 mg/kg q12h for 4–14 d; *max:* 2 mg/kg/d	For complicated intraabdominal infections. May cause tooth discoloration, injection site reaction, hypotension, nausea, vomiting, diarrhea, CDAD, and wound dehiscence. PB: 79%–90%; t½: 20 h
Glycylcyclines		
Tigecycline	Skin infections: A: IV: Initially: 100 mg over 30–60 min; *maint:* 50 mg q12h for 7–14 d; *max:* 100 mg/d	For treating community-acquired pneumonia, MRSA, and skin and intraabdominal infections. May cause dizziness, headache, weakness, anemia, superinfection, nausea, vomiting, diarrhea, abdominal pain, rash, tooth discoloration, azotemia, elevated hepatic enzymes, photosensitivity, anaphylaxis, and CDAD. PB: 71%–89%; t½: 27–42 h

A, Adult; *CDAD, Clostridium difficile*–associated diarrhea; *d,* day; *GI,* gastrointestinal; *h,* hour; *IV,* intravenous; *maint,* maintenance; *max,* maximum; *min,* minutes; *MRSA,* methicillin-resistant *Staphylococcus aureus; PB,* protein binding; *PO,* by mouth; *q,* every; *STI,* sexually transmitted infection; *t½,* half-life; *URI,* upper respiratory infection; *y,* year; *>,* greater than.

⊚ CLINICAL JUDGMENT [NURSING PROCESS]

Antibacterials: Tetracyclines

Concept: Infection
- A condition in which microorganisms enter the body and release toxins

Recognize Cues [Assessment]
- Assess vital signs and urine output. Report abnormal findings.
- Check laboratory results, especially those that indicate renal and liver function (blood urea nitrogen [BUN], serum creatinine, aspartate aminotransferase [AST], alanine aminotransferase [ALT], bilirubin).
- Obtain a history of dietary intake and drugs the patient currently takes. Dairy products, antacids, iron, calcium, and magnesium decrease drug absorption. Digoxin absorption is increased, which may lead to digitalis toxicity.

Analyze Cues and Prioritize Hypothesis [Patient Problems]
- Tissue injury
- Vomiting
- Nausea

Generate Solutions [Planning]
- The patient's white blood cells (WBCs) will be within normal limits.

Take Action [Nursing Interventions]
- Obtain a sample for culture from the infected area and send it to the laboratory for culture and sensitivity (C&S). Antibiotic therapy can be started after the culture sample has been taken.
- Administer tetracycline 1 hour before or 2 hours after meals for optimum absorption.
- Monitor laboratory values to assess liver and kidney function (in particular, liver enzymes, BUN, and serum creatinine).
- Record vital signs and urine output.

Patient Teaching
General
- Instruct patients to store tetracycline away from light and extreme heat. Tetracycline decomposes in light and heat and causes the drug to become toxic.
- Advise patients to check expiration dates on bottles of tetracycline; out-of-date tetracycline can be toxic.
- ⚡ Inform female patients who are contemplating pregnancy to avoid taking tetracycline because of possible teratogenic effects.

CLINICAL JUDGMENT [NURSING PROCESS]—CONT'D

Antibacterials: Tetracyclines

- Warn parents that children younger than 8 years of age should not take tetracycline because it can cause discoloration of permanent teeth.
- Encourage patients to take the complete course of tetracycline as prescribed.

Side Effects

- Advise patients to use a sun block and protective clothing during sun exposure. Photosensitivity is associated with tetracycline.
- Encourage patients to report signs of a superinfection (mouth ulcers, anal or genital discharge).
- Advise patients to use additional contraceptive techniques and *not* to rely on oral contraceptives when taking the drug because contraceptive effectiveness may decrease.

- Teach patients to use effective oral hygiene several times a day to prevent or alleviate mouth ulcers (stomatitis).

Diet

- Educate patients to avoid milk products, iron, and antacids. Tetracycline should be taken 1 hour before or 2 hours after meals with a full glass of water. If gastrointestinal (GI) upset occurs, the drug can be taken with nondairy foods.

Evaluate Outcomes [Evaluation]

- Evaluate the effectiveness of tetracycline by determining whether the infection has been controlled or has ceased and that there are no side effects.

PROTOTYPE DRUG CHART

Gentamicin Sulfate

Drug Class	Dosage
Antibacterial: Aminoglycoside	Respiratory infection: A: IM/IV: 3–5 mg/kg/d in 3–4 divided doses TDM: Peak: 5–8 mcg/mL Trough: <1–2 mcg/mL

Contraindications	Drug-Lab-Food Interactions
Hypersensitivity *Caution:* Renal disease, neuromuscular disorders (myasthenia gravis, parkinsonism), electrolyte imbalance, dehydration, hearing impairment, CDAD, ulcerative colitis, ototoxicity, respiratory depression, older adults	Drug: Increases risk of ototoxicity with loop diuretics and methoxyflurane; increases risk of nephrotoxicity with NSAIDs, amphotericin B, cephalosporins, cisplatin, furosemide, and vancomycin Lab: Increases BUN, serum AST, ALT, LDH, bilirubin, and creatinine; decreases serum potassium and magnesium

Pharmacokinetics	Pharmacodynamics
Absorption: IM, IV Distribution: PB: 0%–30% Metabolism: t½: 2 h Excretion: Unchanged in urine	IM/IV: Onset: rapid Peak: IM 30–60 min, IV 30 min Duration: UK

Therapeutic Effects/Uses

For treating endocarditis, meningitis, bacteremia, sepsis, and respiratory, intraabdominal, bone/joint, skin, and urinary tract infections. Aminoglycosides are effective against *Pseudomonas aeruginosa, Escherichia coli,* and species of *Proteus, Enterococcus, Haemophilus, Klebsiella, Salmonella, Serratia, Staphylococcus,* and *Streptococcus*

Mechanism of Action: Inhibits bacterial protein synthesis; bactericidal effect

Side Effects	Adverse Reactions
Stomatitis, nausea, vomiting, alopecia, rash, pruritus, skin/ocular irritation, photosensitivity, headache, dizziness, confusion, depression, tinnitus, weakness, arthralgia, conjunctivitis, phlebitis, injection site reaction, paresthesias, vitamin B_6 and B_{12} deficiency	Peripheral neuropathy, laryngeal edema, hearing loss, ototoxicity, hypokalemia, hypomagnesemia, hyponatremia, neurotoxicity, hyperbilirubinemia *Life-threatening:* Anaphylaxis, nephrotoxicity, thrombocytopenia, anemia, agranulocytosis, eosinophilia, leukopenia, hepatic dysfunction, increased intracranial pressure

A, Adult; *ALT,* alanine aminotransferase; *AST,* aspartate aminotransferase; *BUN,* blood urea nitrogen; *CDAD, Clostridium difficile*-associated diarrhea; *d,* day; *h,* hour; *IM,* intramuscular; *IV,* intravenous; *LDH,* lactic dehydrogenase; *min,* minutes; *MRSA,* methicillin-resistant *Staphylococcus aureus; NSAID,* nonsteroidal antiinflammatory drug; *PB,* protein binding; *q,* every; *t½,* half-life; *TDM,* therapeutic drug monitoring; *UK,* unknown; *<,* less than.

blocking protein synthesis in bacterial cells, resulting in a bacteriostatic action. Indications for use are community-acquired pneumonia, complicated skin infections, and intraabdominal infections, including *S. aureus, E. coli, S. pyogenes, K. pneumoniae,* and *C. perfringens.*

Pharmacokinetics. Tigecycline is administered IV at an initial loading dose of 100 mg over 30 to 60 minutes, followed by 50 mg every 12 hours. The protein-binding capacity of tigecycline ranges from 71% to 89%, and the half-life is 27 to 42 hours. The drug is eliminated from the body in bile, feces, and urine, but biliary excretion is the primary route.

Pharmacodynamics. Tigecycline binds to the 30S ribosomal subunit and causes cell death. It has broad-spectrum activity against gram-positive and gram-negative bacterial pathogens.

Side Effects and Adverse Reactions

Because of their related structural formulas, many side effects of tigecycline are similar to those of tetracycline. The most common side effects of tigecycline involve the GI tract and include nausea, vomiting, abdominal pain, and diarrhea. *Clostridium difficile*–associated diarrhea (CDAD) may occur but is rare. Other side effects are photosensitivity, tooth discoloration, weakness, headache, dizziness, anemia, and thrombocythemia. Elevated hepatic enzymes, hepatic failure, and Stevens-Johnson syndrome may also occur.

Drug Interactions

Oral contraceptives may be less effective when given concurrently with tigecycline. Warfarin levels may be increased and may lead to bleeding when taken with tigecycline.

AMINOGLYCOSIDES

Aminoglycosides act by inhibiting bacterial protein synthesis. The aminoglycoside antibiotics are used against gram-negative bacteria such as *E. coli* and *Proteus* and *Pseudomonas* species. Some gram-positive cocci are resistant to aminoglycosides, so penicillins or cephalosporins may be used.

Streptomycin sulfate, derived from the bacterium *Streptomyces griseus* in 1944, was the first aminoglycoside available for clinical use and was used to treat tuberculosis. Because of its ototoxicity and the bacterial resistance that can develop, it is infrequently used today. Despite its toxicity, streptomycin is the drug of choice to treat tularemia and plague.

Aminoglycosides are for serious infections, and they cannot be absorbed from the GI tract, nor can they cross into the cerebrospinal fluid; they cross the blood-brain barrier in children but not in adults. These agents are primarily administered IM and IV, except for a few aminoglycosides (e.g., neomycin) that may be given orally to decrease bacteria and other organisms in the bowel. Neomycin is frequently used as a preoperative bowel antiseptic.

The aminoglycosides currently used to treat *P. aeruginosa* infection include gentamicin, tobramycin, and amikacin. *P. aeruginosa* is sensitive to gentamicin. Amikacin may be used when there is bacterial resistance to gentamicin and tobramycin. Prototype Drug Chart: Gentamicin Sulfate lists the drug data related to the aminoglycoside gentamicin.

Pharmacokinetics. Gentamicin is administered IM and IV. This drug has a short half-life, and the drug dose can be given three to four times a day. Excretion of this drug is primarily unchanged in the urine.

Pharmacodynamics. Gentamicin inhibits bacterial protein synthesis and has a bactericidal effect. The onset of action is rapid or immediate, and the peak action for gentamicin is 30 minutes to 1 hour for IM and 30 minutes for IV administration.

To ensure a desired blood level, aminoglycosides are usually administered IV. The patient's blood levels are drawn periodically to determine the drug's peak (highest concentration) and trough (lowest concentration) blood levels. A therapeutic drug level can be

TABLE 28.2	Antibacterials: Aminoglycosides	
Generic	**Route and Dosage**	**Uses and Considerations**
Amikacin sulfate	Respiratory infections: A: IM/IV: 15 mg/kg/d in divided doses q8–12h; *max:* 1.5 g/d TDM: Peak: 25–40 mcg/mL; *trough:* <5 mg/mL	For treating meningitis, sepsis, bacteremia, and respiratory, urinary, bone/joint, skin, and intraabdominal infections. May cause cough, fatigue, throat irritation, nausea, diarrhea, wheezing, hemoptysis, dysphonia, aphonia, laryngitis, myalgia, arthralgia, weakness, back pain, ototoxicity, dyspnea, CDAD, nephrotoxicity, and bronchospasm. PB: 0%–11%; t½: 2 h
Gentamicin sulfate	See Prototype Drug Chart: Gentamicin Sulfate	
Neomycin sulfate	Skin infections: A: Topical: Apply a thin film of 0.5% cream or ointment to infected area up to four times daily	For treating hepatic encephalopathy, skin infections, and bowel preparation. May cause vitamin D, B_6, and B_{12} deficiency, nausea, vomiting, diarrhea, rash, pruritus, and superinfection. PB: 0%–30%; t½: UK
Streptomycin sulfate	Respiratory infection: A: IM: 1–2 g/d in divided doses q6–12h TDM: Peak: 40–50 mcg/mL; *trough:* <5 mcg/mL	For treating meningitis, endocarditis, bacteremia, tuberculosis, plague, and respiratory and urinary tract infections. May cause weakness, vitamin B_6 and B_{12} deficiency, fever, injection site reaction, rash, tinnitus, paresthesia, nephrotoxicity, and hearing loss. PB: 34%; t½: 2–3 h
Tobramycin sulfate	Bone/joint infection: A: IM/IV: 3–5 mg/kg/d in 3–4 divided doses; give IV over 30–60 min; *max:* 10 mg/kg/d; older A 7.5 mg/kg/d TDM: Peak: 5–8 mcg/mL, Trough: 1–2 mcg/mL	For treating bacteremia, sepsis, meningitis, and respiratory, urinary tract, intraabdominal, skin, external eye, and bone/joint infections. May cause headache, anorexia, abdominal pain, nausea, vomiting, dysphonia, weakness, chest pain, cough, dyspnea, fever, pharyngitis, rhinitis, hemoptysis, ototoxicity, nephrotoxicity, CDAD, and superinfection. PB: 30%; t½: 2–3 h

A, Adult; *CDAD, Clostridium difficile*–associated diarrhea; *d,* day; *GI,* gastrointestinal; *h,* hour; *IM,* intramuscular; *IV,* intravenous; *max,* maximum; *min,* minutes; *PB,* protein binding; *PID,* pelvic inflammatory disease; *PO,* by mouth; *q,* every; *t½,* half-life; *TDM,* therapeutic drug monitoring; *UK,* unknown; <, less than.

◎ CLINICAL JUDGMENT [NURSING PROCESS]

Antibacterials: Aminoglycosides

Concept: Infection
- A condition in which microorganisms enter the body and release toxins

Recognize Cues [Assessment]
- Record vital signs and urine output. Compare these results with future vital signs and urine output. Nephrotoxicity is an adverse reaction to most aminoglycosides.
- Assess laboratory results to determine renal and liver function, including blood urea nitrogen (BUN), serum creatinine, alkaline phosphatase (ALP), alanine aminotransferase (ALT), aspartate aminotransferase (AST), and bilirubin. Serum electrolytes should also be checked. Aminoglycosides may decrease serum potassium and magnesium levels.
- Obtain a medical history related to renal or hearing disorders. Large doses of aminoglycosides could cause nephrotoxicity or ototoxicity.

Analyze Cues and Prioritize Hypothesis [Patient Problems]
- Tissue injury
- Vomiting
- Nausea

Generate Solutions [Planning]
- The patient's white blood cells (WBCs) will be within normal limits.

Take Action [Nursing Interventions]
- Send a sample from the infected area to the laboratory for culture to determine the organism and its antibiotic sensitivity before the aminoglycoside is started.
- Monitor intake and output. Urine output should be at least 600 mL/day. Immediately report any decrease in urine output. Urinalysis may be ordered daily, and results should be checked for proteinuria, casts, blood cells, and appearance.
- ⚡ Check for hearing loss. Aminoglycosides can cause ototoxicity.
- Evaluate laboratory results and compare with baseline values. Report abnormal results.
- Monitor vital signs. Note whether body temperature has decreased.
- Dilute gentamicin in 50 to 200 mL of normal saline (NS) or 5% dextrose in water (D_5W) solution and administer intravenously (IV) over 30 to 60 minutes.
- ⚡ Check that therapeutic drug monitoring (TDM) has been ordered for peak and trough drug levels. Blood should be drawn 45 to 60 minutes after drug has been administered for peak levels and minutes before next drug dosing for trough levels. Gentamicin peak values should be 5 to 8 mcg/mL, and trough values should be less than 1 to 2 mcg/mL.
- Monitor for signs and symptoms of superinfection; these include stomatitis (mouth ulcers), genital discharge (vaginitis), and anal or genital itching.

Patient Teaching

General
- Encourage patients to increase fluid intake unless fluids are restricted.

Side Effects
- Advise patients to report aminoglycoside side effects, which include nausea, vomiting, tremors, tinnitus, pruritus, and muscle cramps.
- Direct patients to use a sun block and protective clothing during sun exposure because aminoglycosides can cause photosensitivity.

Evaluate Outcomes [Evaluation]
- Evaluate the effectiveness of the aminoglycoside by determining whether the infection has ceased and whether any side effects have occurred.

TABLE 28.3 Antibacterials: Fluoroquinolones (Quinolones)

Generic	Route and Dosage	Uses and Considerations
Fluoroquinolones		
Ciprofloxacin hydrochloride	See Prototype Drug Chart: Ciprofloxacin	
Levofloxacin	Chronic bronchitis: A: PO/IV: 500 mg/d for 5–7 d; *max:* 750 mg/d	For acute bacterial sinusitis, UTI, exacerbation of chronic bronchitis, community-acquired pneumonia, skin infections, tuberculosis, conjunctivitis, plaque, and anthrax prophylaxis. May cause dysgeusia, headache, insomnia, nausea, vomiting, diarrhea, abdominal pain, constipation, dizziness, CDAD, visual impairment, tendon rupture, and Stevens-Johnson syndrome. PB: 24%–38%; t½: 6–8 h
Moxifloxacin	Sinusitis: A: PO/IV: 400 mg/d for 10 d; *max:* 400 mg/d	For treating sinusitis, conjunctivitis, plaque, and respiratory, intraabdominal, and skin infections. May cause cough, fever, pharyngitis, rhinitis, rash, ocular irritation/bleeding/pain/lacrimation, headache, dizziness, nausea, diarrhea, CDAD, tendon rupture, and superinfection. PB: 30%–50%; t½: 12 h
Ofloxacin	UTI: A: PO: 200 mg q12h for 3–7 d; *max:* 800 mg/d	For treating otitis media/externa, PID, STIs, prostatitis, and respiratory, urinary tract, ophthalmic, and skin infections. May cause dry mouth, nausea, vomiting, diarrhea, vaginitis, headache, dizziness, rash, pruritus, dysgeusia, insomnia, CDAD, superinfection, candidiasis, polyuria, and tendon rupture. PB: 20%–32%; t½: 4–8 h
Delafloxacin	Skin infection: A: PO: 450 mg q12h for 5–14 d; *max:* 900 mg/d A: IV: 300 mg q12h for 5–14 d; *max:* 600 mg/d	For respiratory and skin infections. May cause headache, dizziness, anxiety, dysgeusia, nausea, diarrhea, abdominal pain, tendon rupture, CDAD, elevated hepatic enzymes, and superinfection. PB: 84%; t½: 4.2–8.5 h PO, 3.7 h IV

A, Adult; *CDAD*, *Clostridium difficile*–associated diarrhea; *d*, day; *GI*, gastrointestinal; *h*, hour; *IV*, intravenous; *max*, maximum; *PB*, protein binding; *PID*, pelvic inflammatory disease; *PO*, by mouth; *q*, every; *STI*, sexually transmitted infection; *t½*, half-life; *TDM*, therapeutic drug monitoring; *UK*, unknown; *URI*, upper respiratory infection; *UTI*, urinary tract infection; *VREF*, vancomycin-resistant *Enterococcus faecium*; *y*, year; >, greater than; <, less than.

PROTOTYPE DRUG CHART

Ciprofloxacin

Drug Class	Dosage
Antibacterials: Quinolone, fluoroquinolone	UTI: Regular release: A: PO: 250 mg q12h for 3 d; *max:* 1.5 g/d Extended release: A: PO: 500 mg/d for 3 d; *max:* 1 g/d A: IV: 200–400 mg q12h for 7–14 d; *max:* 1.2 g/d

Contraindications	Drug-Lab-Food Interactions
Hypersensitivity to other quinolones *Caution:* Renal/hepatic dysfunction, children, severe renal disease, stroke, neurotoxicity, dehydration, rheumatoid arthritis, seizures, dysrhythmias, myasthenia gravis, tendon rupture, diarrhea, diabetes mellitus, cardiovascular/cerebrovascular disease, colitis, tendinitis, older adults	Drug: Increases effects of theophylline, and caffeine; increases levels of ciprofloxacin with NSAIDs, and probenecid; decreases drug absorption with iron, and calcium; may increase warfarin effects Lab: Increased AST, ALT; prolonged bleeding time

Pharmacokinetics	Pharmacodynamics
Absorption: PO: rapidly absorbed Distribution: PB: 20%–40% Metabolism: t½: 4 h Excretion: 35%–50% excreted in urine, 20%–35% excreted in feces	IR: PO: Onset: 0.5–1 h Peak: 1–2 h Duration: UK ER: PO: Onset: UK Peak: 1–4 h Duration: UK

Therapeutic Effects/Uses
For treating sinusitis, plague, anthrax prophylaxis, typhoid fever, STIs, prostatitis, and respiratory, enteric, intraabdominal, bone/joint, urinary tract, and skin infections, as well as corneal ulcers, bacterial conjunctivitis, and otitis media/externa. Ciprofloxacin is effective against *Escherichia coli* and species of *Enterobacter, Haemophilus, Klebsiella, Neisseria, Proteus, Pseudomonas, Serratia, Chlamydia, Enterococcus, Staphylococcus,* and *Streptococcus* Mechanism of Action: Inhibits the enzyme DNA gyrase, which is needed for bacterial DNA synthesis; bactericidal effect

Side Effects	Adverse Reactions
Dizziness, syncope, anxiety, irritability, flushing, dry mouth , dyspepsia, anorexia, dysgeusia, nausea, vomiting, diarrhea, abdominal cramps, constipation, headache, ocular irritation/pain/ulceration, nystagmus, corneal deposits, blurred vision, myalgia, arthralgia, restlessness, confusion, pharyngitis, rhinorrhea, insomnia, weakness, nightmares, tremor, ocular pruritus, conjunctival hyperemia, injection site reaction, peripheral neuropathy, paresthesia, tinnitus, phlebitis, photosensitivity	Neurotoxicity, crystalluria, myasthenia, ileus, GI bleeding, hypercholesterolemia, tendon rupture, superinfection, hearing loss, bradycardia, tachycardia, hypo/hyperglycemia, hypertriglyceridemia, hypo/hypertension, bradycardia *Life-threatening:* Anaphylaxis, angioedema, anemia, leukopenia, agranulocytosis, thrombocytopenia, aplastic anemia, eosinophilia, hemolytic anemia, pancytopenia, increased intracranial pressure, Stevens-Johnson syndrome, seizures, CDAD, hepatic/renal failure, dysrhythmias, suicidal ideation

A, Adult; *ALT,* alanine aminotransferase; *AST,* aspartate aminotransferase; *CDAD, Clostridium difficile*–associated diarrhea; *d,* day; *DNA,* deoxyribonucleic acid; *h,* hour; *IV,* intravenous; *NSAID,* nonsteroidal antiinflammatory drug; *PB,* protein binding; *PO,* by mouth; *t½,* half-life; *UK,* unknown.

maintained by monitoring the trough level, and peak levels are useful to monitor for toxicity. Many other antibiotics should be monitored as well to maintain effective blood levels.

IV aminoglycosides can be given concurrently with penicillins and cephalosporins but should not be mixed together in the same container. When combinations of antibiotics are given by IV, the IV line is flushed after each antibiotic has been administered to ensure that the antibiotic was completely delivered.

Side Effects and Adverse Reactions

Serious adverse reactions to aminoglycosides include ototoxicity and nephrotoxicity. Renal function, drug dose, and age are all factors that determine whether a patient will develop nephrotoxicity from aminoglycoside therapy. Careful drug dosing is especially important with younger and older patients. The nurse must assess changes in patients' hearing, balance, and urinary output. Prolonged use of aminoglycosides could result in a superinfection, and specific serum aminoglycoside levels should be closely monitored to avoid adverse reactions. Table 28.2 lists the aminoglycosides and their dosages, uses, and considerations.

Drug Interactions

When aminoglycosides are administered concurrently with penicillins, the desired effects of the aminoglycosides are greatly decreased;

preferably, these drugs should be given several hours apart. The drug action of oral anticoagulants such as warfarin can increase when taken simultaneously with aminoglycoside administration, and the risk of ototoxicity increases when ethacrynic acid and an aminoglycoside are given.

FLUOROQUINOLONES (QUINOLONES)

The mechanism of action of fluoroquinolones is to interfere with the enzyme DNA gyrase, which is needed to synthesize bacterial DNA. Their antibacterial spectrum includes bactericidal action on both gram-positive and gram-negative organisms. The fluoroquinolones are effective against some gram-positive organisms, such as *S. pneumoniae*, and also against *H. influenzae*, *P. aeruginosa*, and *Salmonella* and *Shigella* species. This group of antibiotics is useful in the treatment of urinary tract, bone, and joint infections; bronchitis; pneumonia; gastroenteritis; and gonorrhea. Table 28.3 lists the various fluoroquinolones.

Ciprofloxacin is a synthetic antibacterial related to nalidixic acid. This fluoroquinolone has a broad spectrum of action on gram-positive and gram-negative organisms, including *P. aeruginosa*. Ciprofloxacin is approved for use for urinary tract and lower respiratory tract infections and for skin, soft tissue, bone, and joint infections.

The use of fluoroquinolones as urinary antibiotics is discussed in Chapter 48. Prototype Drug Chart: Ciprofloxacin lists the drug data related to levofloxacin. Levofloxacin is used primarily to treat respiratory problems such as community-acquired pneumonia, chronic bronchitis, acute sinusitis, and uncomplicated skin infections in addition to urinary tract infections.

Moxifloxacin is available for once-a-day oral and parenteral dosing. This drug is prescribed to treat the same infections other fluoroquinolones are effective against. Moxifloxacin is more active than levofloxacin against *S. pneumoniae*. It is also effective against some strains of *S. aureus* and enterococci but is not effective against vancomycin-resistant *Enterococcus faecium*. The fluoroquinolones are included in Table 28.3.

⚡ PATIENT SAFETY

Fluoroquinolones, especially levofloxacin, should be reserved for patients who have no other alternative treatment options for uncomplicated urinary tract infection (UTI), acute bacterial exacerbation of chronic bronchitis, or acute bacterial sinusitis due to disabling and potentially irreversible serious adverse reactions. These adverse reactions include tendon rupture, tendinitis, peripheral neuropathy, central nervous system (CNS) effects, and exacerbation of myasthenia gravis. (Black Box Warning.)

◎ CLINICAL JUDGMENT [NURSING PROCESS]

Antibacterials: Fluoroquinolones

Concept: Infection
- A condition in which microorganisms enter the body and release toxins

Recognize Cues [Assessment]
- Record vital signs along with intake and urine output. Compare these results with future vital signs and urine output. Fluid intake should be at least 2000 mL/day.
- Assess laboratory results (blood urea nitrogen [BUN] and serum creatinine) to determine renal function.
- Obtain a drug and diet history. Antacids and iron preparations decrease absorption of fluoroquinolones such as levofloxacin, and levofloxacin can increase the effects of theophylline and caffeine and can also increase the effects of oral hypoglycemics. When levofloxacin is taken with nonsteroidal antiinflammatory drugs (NSAIDs), central nervous system (CNS) reactions may occur, which includes seizures.

Analyze Cues and Prioritize Hypothesis [Patient Problems]
- Tissue injury
- Vomiting
- Nausea

Generate Solutions [Planning]
- The patient's white blood cells (WBCs) will be within normal limits.

Take Action [Nursing Interventions]
- Obtain a specimen from the infected site, and send it to the laboratory for culture and sensitivity (C&S) before initiating antibacterial drug therapy.
- Monitor intake and output. Urine output should be at least 750 mL per day. The patient should be well hydrated, and fluid intake should be greater than 2000 mL daily to prevent crystalluria (crystals in the urine). Urine pH should be below 6.7.
- Record vital signs and report any abnormal findings.
- Check laboratory results, especially BUN and serum creatinine. Elevated values may indicate renal dysfunction.

- Administer levofloxacin 2 hours before or after antacids and iron products for best absorption. Give with a full glass of water. If gastrointestinal (GI) distress occurs, the drug may be taken with food.
- Dilute intravenous (IV) levofloxacin in recommended amount of solution (NS, D_5W, D_5NS). Infuse over 60–90 minutes.
- Check for signs and symptoms of superinfection: stomatitis (mouth ulcers), furry black tongue, and anal or genital discharge or itching.
- ⚡ Monitor serum theophylline levels when taken concurrently with levofloxacin, which can increase theophylline levels. Check for symptoms of CNS stimulation such as nervousness, insomnia, anxiety, and tachycardia.
- ⚡ Monitor blood glucose. Levofloxacin can increase the effects of oral hypoglycemics.

Patient Teaching
General
- Teach patients to drink at least 6 to 8 glasses (8 oz) of fluid daily.
- Encourage patients to avoid caffeinated products.

Side Effects
- Direct patients to avoid operating motor vehicles or hazardous machinery while taking the drug, at least until drug stability has occurred, because of possible drug-related dizziness.
- Inform patients that photosensitivity is a side effect of most fluoroquinolones. Patients should wear sunglasses, sun block, and protective clothing when in the sun.
- Encourage patients to report side effects such as dizziness, nausea, vomiting, diarrhea, flatulence, abdominal cramps, tinnitus, rash, and tendon rupture (very rare). Older adults are more likely to develop side effects.

Evaluate Outcomes [Evaluation]
- Evaluate the effectiveness of the fluoroquinolone by determining whether the infection has resolved and the body temperature has returned within normal range.

Pharmacokinetics. Ciprofloxacin is rapidly absorbed from the GI tract. It has a low protein-binding effect of 20% to 40% and a moderately short half-life of 4 hours. Ciprofloxacin is excreted in the urine feces.

Pharmacodynamics. Ciprofloxacin inhibits bacterial DNA synthesis by inhibiting the enzyme DNA gyrase. The drug has a high tissue distribution. If possible, it should be taken before meals because food slows the absorption rate; antacids also decrease the absorption rate. Ciprofloxacin increases the effect of theophylline and caffeine.

Ciprofloxacin has an average onset of action of 30 minutes to 1 hour, and the peak concentration time is 1 to 2 hours. The duration of action is unknown.

CRITICAL THINKING CASE STUDY

A 46-year-old female patient has a wound infection. The culture report states that the infection is due to *Pseudomonas aeruginosa,* and the patient's temperature has risen to 104°F (40°C). Amikacin sulfate is to be administered intravenously in 100 mL of 5% dextrose in water (D₅W solution) over 45 minutes every 8 hours. The dosage is 15 mg/kg/day in three divided doses. The patient weighs 165 pounds.

1. What is the drug classification of amikacin? How many milligrams of amikacin should the patient receive every 8 hours?
2. What type of intravenous (IV) infusion should be used? What would be the IV flow rate?
3. When would a wound culture be obtained to determine the appropriate antibacterial agent? Explain your answer.

4. What are the similarities of amikacin to other aminoglycosides such as gentamicin? Would one aminoglycoside be preferred over another? Explain your answer.

The nurse assesses the patient for hearing and urinary function before and during amikacin therapy.

5. Why should a hearing assessment be included?
6. The patient's urine output in the last 8 hours was 125 mL. Explain the possible cause for the amount of urine output. What nursing action should be taken?
7. What laboratory tests monitor renal function?
8. The health care provider requests peak and trough serum amikacin levels. When should the blood samples to determine peak serum level and trough serum level be drawn?

REVIEW QUESTIONS

1. A patient is receiving tetracycline. Which advice should the nurse include when teaching this patient about tetracycline?
   a. Take sunscreen precautions when at the beach.
   b. Take an antacid with the drug to prevent severe gastrointestinal distress.
   c. Obtain frequent hearing tests for early detection of hearing loss.
   d. Obtain frequent eye checkups for early detection of retinal damage.
2. A patient is taking levofloxacin. What does the nurse know to be true regarding this drug?
   a. It is administered by intravenous only.
   b. Levofloxacin may cause hypertension.
   c. This drug is classified as an aminoglycoside.
   d. An adverse effect is tendon rupture.

3. Which instruction(s) will the nurse include when teaching patients about gentamicin? (Select all that apply.)
   a. Patients should report any hearing loss.
   b. Patients should use sunscreen when taking gentamicin.
   c. Intravenous gentamicin will be given over 20 minutes.
   d. Patients are monitored for mouth ulcers and vaginitis.
   e. Peak levels will be drawn 30 minutes before the intravenous dose.
   f. Patients should increase fluid intake.
4. Which nursing intervention(s) should the nurse consider for the patient taking ciprofloxacin? (Select all that apply.)
   a. Obtain culture before drug administration.
   b. Tell the patient to avoid taking ciprofloxacin with antacids.
   c. Monitor the patient for tinnitus.
   d. Encourage fluids to prevent crystalluria.
   e. Infuse intravenous ciprofloxacin over 60 minutes.
   f. Monitor blood glucose because ciprofloxacin can decrease effects of oral hypoglycemics.

29

Sulfonamides and Nitroimidazoles Antibiotics

http://evolve.elsevier.com/McCuistion/pharmacology

OBJECTIVES

- Explain the action of sulfonamides.
- Explain the pharmacokinetics of the sulfonamides.
- Formulate the Clinical Judgment [Nursing Process] to the patient taking trimethoprim-sulfamethoxazole.

- Develop a teaching plan for a patient prescribed metronidazole.
- Describe side effects/adverse effects for a patient taking quinupristin-dalfopristin.

OUTLINE

INTRODUCTION

Sulfonamide, a synthetic antibacterial, was introduced in 1935. Sulfonamides are one of the oldest antibacterial agents used to combat infection. When penicillin was initially marketed, the sulfonamide drugs were not widely prescribed because penicillin was considered a "miracle drug." However, use of sulfonamides has increased as a result of newer sulfonamides and drugs that combine a sulfonamide with an antibacterial agent in preparations such as trimethoprim-sulfamethoxazole (TMP-SMZ). This chapter discusses sulfonamides and nitroimidazoles.

SULFONAMIDES

Sulfonamides were first isolated from a coal tar derivative compound in the early 1900s and were produced for clinical use against coccal infections in 1935. Sulfonamides were the first group of drugs used against bacteria, although they are not classified as antibiotics because they were not obtained from biologic substances. The sulfonamides are bacteriostatic because they inhibit bacterial synthesis of folic acid, which is essential for bacterial growth. Humans do not synthesize folic acid; rather, they acquire it through the diet; therefore sulfonamides selectively inhibit bacterial growth without affecting normal cells. Folic acid (folate) is required by cells for biosynthesis of RNA, DNA, and proteins.

The clinical usefulness of sulfonamides alone, not in combination, has decreased for several reasons. The availability and effectiveness of penicillin and other antibiotics have increased, and bacterial resistance to some sulfonamides can develop. Sulfonamides may be used as an alternative drug for patients who are allergic to penicillin. They are still used to treat urinary tract and ear infections and may be used for newborn eye prophylaxis. Sulfonamides are approximately 90% effective against *E. coli*; therefore they are frequently a preferred treatment for urinary tract infections, which are often caused by *E. coli*. They are also useful in the treatment of meningococcal meningitis and against *Chlamydia* species and *Toxoplasma gondii*. Sulfonamides are *not* effective against viruses and fungi.

Pharmacokinetics. Sulfonamide drugs are well absorbed by the gastrointestinal (GI) tract, and they are well distributed to body tissues and the brain. The liver metabolizes the sulfonamide drug, and the kidneys excrete it.

Pharmacodynamics. Many sulfonamides are for oral administration because they are absorbed readily by the GI tract. They are also available in solution and as ointments for ophthalmic use and in cream form (silver sulfadiazine and mafenide acetate) for burns. Most of the early sulfonamides were highly protein bound and displaced other drugs by competing for protein sites. The two categories of sulfonamides, classified according to their duration of action, are *short-acting sulfonamides* that have a rapid absorption and excretion rate and *intermediate-acting sulfonamides* with moderate to slow absorption and a slow excretion rate.

Sulfadiazine is useful in prophylactic treatment of streptococcal infections in patients with rheumatic fever who are hypersensitive to penicillin. Older sulfonamides such as sulfadiazine are poorly soluble in urine and can cause crystallization, which could damage the kidneys if fluid and water intake are insufficient; however, newer sulfonamides have greater water solubility. Therefore crystal formations in the urine and renal damage are unlikely. Table 29.1 describes the sulfonamides.

Side Effects and Adverse Reactions

Side effects of sulfonamides may include an allergic response such as skin rash and itching. Anaphylaxis is uncommon. Blood disorders such as hemolytic anemia, aplastic anemia, and low white blood cell (WBC) and platelet counts could result from prolonged use and high dosages. GI disturbances such as anorexia, nausea, and vomiting may also occur. The early sulfonamides were insoluble in acid urine, and crystalluria (crystals in the urine) and hematuria (blood in the urine) were common problems. Increasing fluid intake dilutes the drug, which helps prevent crystalluria. Photosensitivity, an excessive reaction to direct sunlight or ultraviolet (UV) light that leads to redness and burning of the skin, can also occur; therefore the patient should avoid sunbathing and excess ultraviolet light. **Cross-sensitivity**, a sensitivity or allergy to one sulfonamide that leads to sensitivity to another sulfonamide, might occur with the different sulfonamides but does not occur with other antibacterial drugs. Sulfonamides should be avoided during pregnancy to avoid congenital malformations, neural tube defects, and kernicterus.

Trimethoprim-Sulfamethoxazole

TMP-SMZ contains one part trimethoprim and five parts sulfamethoxazole to produce a synergistic effect that increases the desired drug response. Trimethoprim is an antibacterial agent that interferes with bacterial folic acid synthesis just as sulfonamides do; it is classified as a urinary tract antiinfective that may be used alone for uncomplicated urinary tract infections, and it is also effective against the gram-negative bacteria *E. coli* and also *Proteus* and *Klebsiella* species. In the 1970s trimethoprim was combined with sulfamethoxazole, an intermediate-acting sulfonamide, to prevent bacterial resistance to sulfonamide drugs and to obtain a better response against many organisms. Giving both drugs together in one compounded form causes bacterial resistance to develop much more slowly than if only one of the drugs were to be used alone.

TMP-SMZ is effective in treating urinary, intestinal, lower respiratory tract, and middle ear (otitis media) infections; prostatitis; and gonorrhea. It is also used to prevent *Pneumocystis carinii* in patients with acquired immunodeficiency syndrome (AIDS). Increased fluid intake is strongly recommended to avoid complications such as crystalluria. Prototype Drug Chart: Trimethoprim-Sulfamethoxazole describes the pharmacologic behavior of TMP-SMZ.

Pharmacokinetics. TMP-SMZ is well absorbed from the GI tract and is moderately protein bound. Its half-life is 6 to 12 hours; thus it is administered twice a day. It is excreted as unchanged metabolites in the urine.

Pharmacodynamics. Trimethoprim, a nonsulfonamide antibiotic, enhances the activity of the drug combination. TMP-SMZ blocks steps in the bacterial synthesis of protein and nucleic acid, producing a bactericidal effect.

TMP-SMZ can be administered orally or intravenously (IV). Orally the drug has a moderately rapid onset of action; drug action is immediate via the IV route. Serum peak concentration time for oral use is 1 to 4 hours and 30 minutes to 1 hour for IV use. TMP-SMZ increases the hypoglycemic response when taken with sulfonylureas (oral hypoglycemic agents). It can also increase the activity of oral anticoagulants.

Side Effects and Adverse Reactions

Side effects of TMP-SMZ may include mild to moderate rashes, anorexia, nausea, vomiting, diarrhea, stomatitis, crystalluria, and photosensitivity. Serious adverse reactions are rare; however, agranulocytosis, aplastic anemia, and myocarditis have been reported as possible life-threatening conditions.

Topical and Ophthalmic Sulfonamides

Sulfonamides can be administered for topical and ophthalmic uses, but because topical use of sulfonamides can cause hypersensitivity reactions, they are used infrequently. Mafenide acetate is a sulfonamide derivative prescribed to prevent sepsis in cases of second- and

TABLE 29.1	**Antibacterials: Sulfonamides**	
Generic	**Route and Dosage**	**Uses and Considerations**
Sulfadiazine	Urinary tract infection: A: PO: LD 2–4 g, then 2–4 g/d in 3–6 divided doses; *max:* 4 g/d	For treating otitis media, meningitis, malaria, nocardiosis, toxoplasmosis, chancroid, chlamydial conjunctivitis, and UTIs and for rheumatic fever prophylaxis. May cause headache, insomnia, crystalluria, stomatitis, edema, abdominal pain, arthralgia, anorexia, nausea, vomiting, and diarrhea. Increase fluid intake to >2000 mL/d. PB: 38%–48%; t½: 17 h
Sulfasalazine	Ulcerative colitis: Uncoated tablets: A: PO: Initially 1 g q6–8h; *maint:* 500 mg q6–12h; *max:* 4 g/d Enteric coated tablets: A: PO: Initially 3–4 g/d in divided doses; *maint:* 2 g/d	For treating ulcerative colitis and rheumatoid arthritis. May cause headache, dizziness, stomatitis, fever, dyspepsia, abdominal pain, anorexia, nausea, vomiting, oligospermia, elevated hepatic enzymes, rash, and pruritus. Take drug after eating. PB: 99%; t½: 5.7–7.6 h
Trimethoprim-sulfamethoxazole	See Prototype Drug Chart: Trimethoprim-Sulfamethoxazole	

A, Adult; *d,* day; *GI,* gastrointestinal; *h,* hour; *IV,* intravenous; *maint,* maintenance; *max,* maximum; *mo,* month; *PB,* protein binding; *PO,* by mouth; *q,* every; *t½,* half-life; *UTI,* urinary tract infection; *y,* year; *>,* greater than.

third-degree burns. Silver sulfadiazine is another topical sulfonamide used to treat burns. Both of these drugs are discussed in more detail in Chapter 45.

Sulfacetamide sodium is a sulfonamide for ophthalmic and topical uses. In ophthalmic preparations (liquid drops and ointments), sulfacetamide sodium is used to treat ocular infections. It is often used as prophylactic treatment after an eye injury or after removal of a foreign body. Do *not* use ointment for the eye unless it has *ophthalmic* printed on the drug label. Sulfacetamide sodium is discussed in more detail in Chapter 44.

Topical sulfacetamide sodium *for the skin* is a cream, gel, lotion, or cleanser and is used to treat seborrheic dermatitis and acne. This dermatologic form is *not* used for the eye.

NITROIMIDAZOLES

Nitroimidazoles act by disrupting DNA and protein synthesis in susceptible bacteria and protozoa. The nitroimidazoles are effective against *H. pylori* and bacterial species (such as *Bacteroides*, *Clostridium*, *Gardnerella*, *Prevotella*, *Peptococcus*, *Giardia*), and protozoa (such as *Trichomonas vaginalis*). Nitroimidazoles are used for prophylaxis for surgical infections and to treat *Clostridium difficile*–associated diarrhea

(CDAD), anaerobic infections, amebiasis, giardiasis, trichomoniasis, bacterial vaginosis, and acne rosacea. Metronidazole and tinidazole are two of the most effective drugs available to treat anaerobic bacterial infections. Both nitroimidazoles are used with other agents to treat *H. pylori* infections associated with peptic and duodenal ulcers. Metronidazole was FDA approved in 1963, and tinidazole was approved in 2004.

Nitroimidazoles are primarily administered orally, parenterally, and topically. When metronidazole is given IV intermittently, it should be administered slowly over 30 to 60 minutes. Avoid contact with the eyes when using topical product. Table 29.2 lists nitroimidazoles and their dosages, uses, and considerations.

⚡ PATIENT SAFETY

Preventing Medication Errors

Do not confuse...
- **Septra**, an antibacterial sulfonamide, with **Sectral**, a beta-adrenergic antagonist used to manage dysrhythmias.
- **Sulfadiazine**, a short-acting antibacterial sulfonamide, with **sulfasalazine**, an intermediate-acting antibacterial sulfonamide.

📋 PROTOTYPE DRUG CHART

Trimethoprim-Sulfamethoxazole (TMP-SMZ)

Drug Class	Dosage
Antibacterial: Sulfonamide	Acute exacerbation of chronic bronchitis: A: PO: TMP 160 mg, SMZ 800 mg q12h for 5–14 d

Contraindications	Drug-Lab-Food Interactions
Severe renal/hepatic disease, hypersensitivity to sulfonamides, infants *Caution:* Diabetes mellitus, thyroid disorder, electrolyte imbalance, folate deficiency, bradycardia, hypertension, dysrhythmias, colitis, diarrhea, cardiac disease, alcohol use disorder, older adults, pregnancy, breastfeeding	Drug: Increased anticoagulant effect with warfarin; increased hypoglycemic effect with oral hypoglycemic drugs, increased potassium levels with ACE inhibitors and spironolactone, increased digoxin and sulfonylurea levels, increased phenytoin and methotrexate toxicity Lab: May increase BUN, serum creatinine, AST, ALT, and ALP

Pharmacokinetics	Pharmacodynamics
Absorption: PO: Well absorbed Distribution: PB: 44% for TMP; 70% for SMZ; crosses placenta Metabolism: t½: 8–10 h for TMP, 6–12 h for SMZ Excretion: In urine as metabolites	PO: Onset: 2 h Peak: 1–4 h Duration: 12 h

Therapeutic Effects/Uses	
For treating otitis media, traveler's diarrhea, shigellosis, MRSA, and respiratory and urinary tract infections. TMP-SMZ is effective against *Salmonella* and species of *Haemophilus*, *Staphylococcus,* and *Klebsiella* Mechanism of Action: Inhibits folic acid synthesis and protein synthesis of nucleic acids; bactericidal effect	

Side Effects	Adverse Reactions
Anorexia, stomatitis, glossitis, nausea, vomiting, diarrhea, abdominal pain, weakness, ataxia, rash, depression, headache, insomnia, photosensitivity, tinnitus, arthralgia, myalgia	Rhabdomyolysis, systemic lupus erythematosus, crystalluria *Life-threatening:* Anaphylaxis, angioedema, seizures, myocarditis, leukopenia, thrombocytopenia, hemolytic anemia, aplastic anemia, agranulocytosis, eosinophilia, neutropenia, hyperkalemia, hyponatremia, hypoglycemia, CDAD, Stevens-Johnson syndrome, renal/hepatic impairment

A, Adult; *ACE*, angiotensin-converting enzyme; *ALP*, alkaline phosphatase; *ALT*, alanine aminotransferase; *AST*, aspartate aminotransferase; *BUN*, blood urea nitrogen; *CDAD*, Clostridium difficile–associated diarrhea; *d*, day; *h*, hour; *IV*, intravenous; *MRSA*, methicillin-resistant *Staphylococcus aureus*; *PB*, protein binding; *PO*, by mouth; *q*, every; *SMZ*, sulfamethoxazole; *TMP*, trimethoprim; *t½*, half-life; *UK*, unknown.

TABLE 29.2   Antibacterials: Nitroimidazoles

Generic	Route and Dosage	Uses and Considerations
Metronidazole	Amebiasis: A: PO: 500 or 750 mg q8h for 5–10 d; *max:* 4 g/d A: IV: 750 mg q8h for 7–10 d; *max:* 4 g/d	For treating acne, amebiasis, bacterial vaginosis, endocarditis, meningitis, skin, bacteremia, trichomoniasis, and bone/joint, gynecologic, skin, intraabdominal, and respiratory infections and for surgical infection prophylaxis. May cause headache, rash, dizziness, weakness, dry mouth, metallic taste, candidiasis, nausea, vomiting, diarrhea, abdominal pain, pruritus, vaginitis, vaginal discharge, and superinfection. PB: <20%; t½: 8 h
Tinidazole	Intestinal amebiasis: A: PO: 2 g/d with food for 3 d; *max:* 2 g/d	For treating amebiasis, giardiasis, trichomoniasis, and bacterial vaginosis. May cause candidiasis, metallic taste, nausea, vomiting, anorexia, vaginitis, weakness, tongue/urine discoloration, and superinfection. PB: 12%; t½: 12–14 h
Secnidazole	Bacterial vaginosis: A: PO: 2 g single dose; *max:* 2 g	For trichomoniasis and bacterial vaginosis. May cause headache, candidiasis, abdominal pain, dysgeusia, nausea, vomiting, diarrhea, and vaginitis. PB: <5%; t½: 17 h

A, Adult; *CDAD, Clostridium difficile*–associated diarrhea; *d,* day; *GI,* gastrointestinal; *h,* hour; *IV,* intravenous; *max,* maximum; *PB,* protein binding; *PO,* by mouth; *q,* every; *t½,* half-life; *y,* year; *>,* greater than.

⊚ CLINICAL JUDGMENT [NURSING PROCESS]

Antibacterials: Sulfonamides

Concept: Infection
- A condition in which microorganisms enter the body and release toxins

Recognize Cues [Assessment]
- Assess the patient's renal function by checking urinary output (>600 mL/day), blood urea nitrogen (BUN; normal, 8 to 25 mg/dL), and serum creatinine (normal, 0.5 to 1.5 mg/dL).
- Obtain a medical history from the patient. Sulfonamides such as trimethoprim-sulfamethoxazole (TMP-SMZ) are contraindicated for patients with severe renal or liver disease.
- Determine whether the patient is hypersensitive to sulfonamides. An allergic reaction can include rash, skin eruptions, and itching. A severe hypersensitivity reaction includes erythema multiforme—an erythematous macular, papular, or vesicular eruption that can cover the entire body—or exfoliative dermatitis, characterized by desquamation, scaling, and itching of the skin.
- Obtain a history of drugs the patient currently takes. Oral antidiabetic drugs (sulfonylureas) given with sulfonamides increase the hypoglycemic effect; use of warfarin with sulfonamides increases the anticoagulant effect.
- Assess baseline laboratory results, especially complete blood count (CBC). Blood dyscrasias may occur as a result of high doses of sulfonamides over a continuous period, causing life-threatening conditions.

Analyze Cues and Prioritize Hypothesis [Patient Problems]
- Tissue injury
- Vomiting
- Nausea

Generate Solutions [Planning]
- The patient's white blood cells (WBCs) will be within normal limits.

Take Action [Nursing Interventions]
- Administer sulfonamides with a full glass of water. Extra fluid intake can prevent crystalluria and kidney stone formation.
- Record intake and output. To decrease the risk of crystalluria, fluid intake should be at least 2000 mL/day, and urine output should be at least 1200 mL/day. Sulfonamide sulfadiazine is more likely to cause crystalluria than combination drugs.
- Monitor vital signs. Note whether the patient's temperature has gone down.
- Observe the patient for hematologic reactions that may lead to life-threatening anemias. Early signs are sore throat, purpura, and decreasing WBC and platelet counts. Check CBC, and compare values with baseline findings.
- Check for signs and symptoms of superinfection. Symptoms include stomatitis (mouth ulcers), furry black tongue, anal or genital discharge, and itching.

Patient Teaching
General
- Encourage patients to drink several quarts of fluid daily while taking sulfonamides to avoid crystalluria.
- Advise pregnant patients to avoid sulfonamides during the last 3 months of pregnancy.
- Counsel patients not to take antacids with sulfonamides because antacids decrease the absorption rate of sulfonamide drugs.
- ⚡ Warn patients with an allergy to one sulfonamide that all sulfonamide preparations should be avoided, with health care provider's approval, because of the possibility of cross-sensitivity. Observe the patient for rash or any skin eruptions.

Self-Administration
- Teach patients to take sulfonamides 1 hour before or 2 hours after meals with a full glass of water.

Side Effects
- ⚡ Direct patients to report bruising or bleeding that could be a result of a drug-induced blood disorder. Advise patients to have their blood cell count monitored on a regular basis.
- Warn patients to wear sunglasses, avoid direct sunlight, and use sun block and protective clothing to decrease the risk of photosensitive reactions.

Evaluate Outcomes [Evaluation]
- Evaluate the effectiveness of sulfonamide therapy by determining whether the infection has been alleviated and the blood cell count is within normal range.

TABLE 29.3   Miscellaneous Antibacterial Drugs

Generic	Route and Dosage	Uses and Considerations
Unclassified Drugs		
Chloramphenicol	Salmonella: A: IV: 50–100 mg/kg/d in 4 divided doses for 14–21 d; *max:* 100 mg/kg/d TDM: Peak: 10–20 mcg/mL Trough: 5–10 mcg/mL	For treating only serious infections, such as bacteremia, salmonella, rickettsial infection, typhoid fever, and meningitis. May cause headache, glossitis, confusion, depression, anemia, rash, nausea, vomiting, diarrhea, peripheral neuropathy, vitamin B_{12} deficiency, angioedema, and nephritis. PB: 60%; t½: 4.1 h
Quinupristin-dalfopristin	Skin infections: A: IV: 7.5 mg/kg given over 1 h, q12h for at least 7 d; *max:* 15 mg/kg/d	For treating skin infections. May cause infusion site reaction, rash, arthralgia, myalgia, CDAD, nausea, vomiting, diarrhea, hyperbilirubinemia, edema, and superinfection. PB: 11%–19%; t½: 0.7–0.85 h
Obiltoxaximab	A >40 kg: IV: 16 mg/kg as single dose A: <40 kg: IV: 24 mg/kg as single dose	For prophylaxis and treatment of anthrax. May cause headache, cough, nasal congestion, vomiting, hematoma, superinfection, rash, pruritus, and injection site reaction. PB: UK; t½: UK
Lefamulin	A: PO: 600 mg q12h for 5 d; *max:* 1200 mg/d A: IV: 150 mg q12h for 5–7 d; *max:* 300 mg/d	For community-acquired pneumonia. May cause headache, injection site reaction, nausea, vomiting, diarrhea, hypokalemia, CDAD, superinfection, and elevated hepatic enzymes. PB: 94.8%–97.1%; t½: 3–20 h

A, Adult; *CDAD, Clostridium difficile*–associated diarrhea; *d,* day; *GI,* gastrointestinal; *h,* hour; *IV,* intravenous; *max,* maximum; *PB,* protein binding; *PID,* pelvic inflammatory disease; *PO,* by mouth; *q,* every; *STI,* sexually transmitted infection; *t½,* half-life; *TDM,* therapeutic drug monitoring; *UK,* unknown; *URI,* upper respiratory infection; *UTI,* urinary tract infection; *VREF,* vancomycin-resistant *Enterococcus faecium; y,* year; *>,* greater than; *<,* less than.

 COMPLEMENTARY AND ALTERNATIVE THERAPIES

Milk thistle may decrease absorption of metronidazole.

Pharmacokinetics. Both metronidazole and tinidazole are well absorbed from the GI tract and are usually not given parenterally unless the patient cannot tolerate oral medications. The protein-binding capacity of nitroimidazoles ranges from 5% to 12%, and the half-life is 8 to 14 hours. These drugs are eliminated from the body via urine and feces.

Pharmacodynamics. Nitroimidazoles disrupt DNA and protein synthesis becoming bactericidal, amebicidal, and trichomonacidal. It is recommended that tinidazole be taken with food, but metronidazole can be given without regard to food. When metronidazole is used in the extended release form, it should be taken on an empty stomach. The topical form is only minimally absorbed. The peak action for both agents is 1 to 3 hours.

Side Effects and Adverse Reactions

Common side effects that may occur when taking nitroimidazoles include headache, dizziness, insomnia, weakness, dry mouth, dysgeusia, anorexia, nausea, vomiting, diarrhea, tongue/urine discoloration, and superinfection. More serious adverse reactions that have occurred with metronidazole and tinidazole are leukopenia, peripheral neuropathy, seizures, and Stevens-Johnson syndrome. A disulfiram-like reaction may occur when metronidazole is taken with excessive amounts of alcohol. Symptoms of disulfiram-like reaction include flushing, throbbing headache, visual disturbance, confusion, dyspnea, nausea, vomiting, tachycardia, syncope, and circulatory collapse.

MISCELLANEOUS ANTIBACTERIAL DRUGS (TABLE 29.3)

Chloramphenicol does not belong to any major drug group. Chloramphenicol was discovered in 1947 and exerts its bacteriostatic action by inhibiting bacterial protein synthesis. Because of the toxic effects of chloramphenicol, including blood dyscrasias related to bone marrow suppression, it is used only to treat serious infections. It is effective against gram-negative and gram-positive bacteria, and many other microorganisms, such as rickettsiae, *Mycoplasma,* and *H. influenzae.*

Quinupristin-dalfopristin is in a class of drugs called streptogramin antibiotics. It is effective for treating vancomycin-resistant *Enterococcus* faecium bacteremia and skin infected by *S. aureus* and *S. pyogenes.* It acts by disrupting the protein synthesis of the organism. When administering the drug through a peripheral IV line, pain, edema, and phlebitis may occur.

Obiltoxaximab is a monoclonal antibody and was FDA approved in 2016 for prophylaxis and treatment of anthrax. It prevents the lethal factor of anthrax from intracellular entry by inhibiting the binding of the protective antigen of *Bacillus anthracis* toxin to cellular receptors. This drug is administered IV as a single dose over 90 minutes.

Lefamulin is first in its class of pleuromutilin antibiotic, which is used for the treatment of community-acquired pneumonia. It can be bacteriostatic or bactericidal. Lefamulin inhibits bacterial protein synthesis. The most common side effects are diarrhea, injection site reaction, nausea, and vomiting.

CRITICAL THINKING CASE STUDY

A 46-year-old female has a severe urinary tract infection. She takes trimethoprim-sulfamethoxazole 160 mg/800 mg every 6 hours.

1. What are the similarities and differences between trimethoprim-sulfamethoxazole and sulfadiazine?
2. Is the dose within the recommended drug dose and dosing interval?

Patient teaching is an important part of nursing interventions. Explain the nurse's role regarding patient teaching concerning the following:

3. What is the required amount of daily fluid intake?
4. What time of day should sulfonamides be taken?
5. Why should bruising and bleeding be reported?
6. What effect does trimethoprim-sulfamethoxazole have on warfarin?

REVIEW QUESTIONS

1. A patient is taking sulfasalazine. What should the nurse teach the patient to do?
   a. Drink at least 10 glasses of fluid per day.
   b. Monitor blood glucose carefully to avoid hyperglycemia.
   c. Avoid operating a motor vehicle because this drug may cause drowsiness.
   d. Take this drug with an antacid to decrease the risk of gastrointestinal distress.
2. The nurse is teaching a patient about sulfadiazine. Which instructions will the nurse include in the teaching?
   a. Avoid caffeine during sulfonamide treatment.
   b. Administer in 50 mL of fluid over 30 minutes.
   c. Avoid sulfonamides during the third trimester of pregnancy.
   d. Use an ultraviolet light to enhance drug effectiveness.
3. A patient is ordered to take trimethoprim-sulfamethoxazole. The nurse knows to be aware of which adverse effect?
   a. Bronchospasm
   b. Tendon rupture
   c. Red man syndrome
   d. *Clostridium difficile*–associated diarrhea

4. The nurse is teaching a patient about trimethoprim-sulfamethoxazole. Which instructions will the nurse plan to include? (Select all that apply.)
   a. Report any bruising or bleeding.
   b. Report any diarrhea or bloody stools.
   c. Report any fever, rash, or sore throat.
   d. Avoid unprotected exposure to sunlight.
   e. Report thirst and polyuria.
5. A patient is taking a sulfonamide for an acute urinary tract infection. Which medication does the nurse realize is a short-acting sulfonamide?
   a. Sulfadiazine
   b. Sulfasalazine
   c. Seconidazole
   d. Trimethoprim-sulfamethoxazole

30

Antituberculars, Antifungals, and Antivirals

http://evolve.elsevier.com/McCuistion/pharmacology

OBJECTIVES

- Compare first-line and second-line antitubercular drugs and give examples of each.
- Differentiate between the groups of antifungal drugs.
- Explain the uses of polyenes.

- Differentiate the adverse reactions of antitubercular, antifungal, and antiviral drugs.
- Apply the Clinical Judgment [Nursing Process] for patients taking antitubercular, antifungal, and antiviral drugs.

OUTLINE

This chapter covers antituberculars, antifungals, and antivirals. Although these drug categories differ from one another, they each contain drugs that inhibit or kill organisms that cause disease.

TUBERCULOSIS

Tuberculosis (TB) is caused by the acid-fast bacillus *Mycobacterium tuberculosis*. The number of TB cases had declined until the mid-1980s, when the number of cases started to increase. The increase in cases of TB was attributed to multiple factors, such as human immunodeficiency virus (HIV), increased immigration, and the spread of multidrug-resistant TB (MDR TB). According to the US Department of Health and Human Services (DHHS), TB is one of the world's leading causes of death due to infectious diseases in persons older than 5 years of age. The Centers for Disease Control and Prevention (CDC) reported in 2017 that 10 million people worldwide developed TB, and about 1.3 million die because of it. In 2018 the United States reported a total of 9029 TB cases. MDR TB continues to be a serious health concern. Patients started on therapy for TB who do not finish the prescribed therapy can develop and spread resistant strains of *M. tuberculosis*.

PATHOPHYSIOLOGY

TB is transmitted from one person to another by droplets dispersed in the air through coughing, sneezing, and speaking. TB microorganisms can be inhaled into the lungs; therefore persons in close contact with the infected patient are at highest risk of becoming infected. Others at high risk for contracting the disease include the immunocompromised (e.g., patients with HIV, diabetes, and renal failure, and those taking certain medications, such as cortisol), people living or working in high-risk residential settings (e.g., nursing homes, shelters, correctional facilities), those who inject illegal drugs, and health care workers who serve high-risk patients.

Not everyone infected with TB will develop clinical manifestations; rather, some will harbor the microorganisms and will have what is called latent tuberculosis infection; these persons are at risk of developing TB disease later, and only those with active TB disease can infect others. Symptoms of active TB include anorexia, cough with blood-tinged sputum, chest pain, fever, night sweats, weight loss, and positive acid-fast bacilli in the sputum. Isolating infectious persons and initiating treatment for TB disease as soon as possible is the best way to decrease transmission.

Nurses should be aware that persons coming to the United States from high-risk countries where TB disease is common may have been vaccinated with bacille Calmette-Guérin (BCG) as a child. This vaccine is seldom used in the United States. Previous vaccination with BCG may cause a positive reaction to skin testing; however, it does not affect interferon-gamma release assay (IGRA) blood testing, and the person does not have TB disease.

ANTITUBERCULAR DRUGS

Antitubercular drugs (Table 30.1), which include antimycobacterials, are prescribed to people with active TB and those exposed to TB. Streptomycin was the first drug used in the treatment of TB disease in 1943. However, it was noted that patients began to deteriorate after 3 months of therapy due to drug resistance. In 1952 isoniazid (INH) began to see widespread use in the treatment of TB disease and was felt to be a "wonder drug." To this day, INH remains the first-line treatment for TB disease. INH is a bactericidal drug that inhibits tubercle cell wall synthesis and blocks pyridoxine (vitamin B$_6$), which is used for intracellular enzyme production. When INH is prescribed, pyridoxine may also be prescribed to avoid vitamin B deficiency and to minimize peripheral neuropathy. INH is administered orally. Prototype Drug Chart: Isoniazid lists the data for INH.

Prophylactic antituberculars are drugs to prevent TB disease in individuals with latent TB infection. Prophylaxis is recommended for those who have a clinically significant result on tuberculin skin testing (≥5 mm for immunocompromised individuals or ≥10 mm for high-risk groups; Box 30.1) or a positive IGRA result. Patients who have converted from a negative to a positive TB skin test (TST) or from a negative to positive IGRA should be considered candidates for prophylactic therapy as well. Prototype Drug Chart: Isoniazid shows guidelines for latent TB infection treatment with INH.

Prophylactic therapy is contraindicated for persons with liver disease because INH is the primary antitubercular drug used, and it may cause INH-induced liver damage. Other antitubercular drugs may also cause liver damage if given in high doses over an extended period.

Single-drug therapy is ineffective in the treatment of TB disease due to drug resistance. Using a combination of antitubercular drugs has been shown to decrease bacterial resistance. Additionally, using combination therapy has decreased the duration of treatment from 2 years to 6 to 9 months. Different combinations of drugs can be used with INH, rifampin, ethambutol, and pyrazinamide.

Antitubercular drugs are divided into two categories: first-line drugs that form the core of treatment regimens and drugs used in the treatment of drug-resistant TB. First-line drugs—those drugs chosen first, such as INH, rifampin, pyrazinamide, and ethambutol—are considered more effective and less toxic than drugs used in the treatment of drug-resistant TB. Drugs used in the treatment of drug-resistant TB, in which *M. tuberculosis* is resistant to at least one first-line drug, or MDR TB, in which *M. tuberculosis* is resistant to INH and rifampin plus one other first-line drug, are used in combination with first-line drugs to treat drug-resistant *M. tuberculosis*. See Table 30.1 for drugs used in the treatment of drug-resistant TB.

Combination therapy against active TB is more effective in eradicating infection than any single drug. The treatment regimen is divided into two phases: the initial phase lasts 2 months, and the continuation phase consists of the next 4 or 7 months. The total treatment plan can be up to 9 months or longer, depending on response to drug therapy. If drug resistance develops, other antibacterial drugs such as aminoglycosides (streptomycin, kanamycin, amikacin) or fluoroquinolones (levofloxacin, ciprofloxacin, or ofloxacin) may be given as part of combination therapy. Combination therapy for drug-resistant TB disease consists of a minimum of three drugs, but preferably four to five drugs, administered as part of directly observed therapy to ensure adherence. Drug therapy should be managed by an expert in the disease, and susceptibility testing to determine drug resistance should be performed before drug therapy; however, treatment with first-line therapy should not be delayed if active TB is suspected. Aminoglycoside antibiotics should not be taken if kidney dysfunction is present. When antibacterial agents are used continuously or at high doses, serum drug levels should be closely monitored to avoid drug toxicity.

Many drug-drug interactions and side effects occur with antituberculars. To increase adherence to drug therapy, direct observation therapy (DOT) is recommended.

Side Effects and Adverse Reactions

Side effects and adverse reactions to antituberculars differ according to the drug prescribed. For INH, peripheral neuropathy can be a problem, especially for those who are malnourished, have diabetes mellitus, or are alcoholics. This condition can be prevented if pyridoxine (vitamin B$_6$) is administered. Hepatotoxicity (liver toxicity) is an adverse reaction to many antituberculars. Patients with moderate to severe liver dysfunction should *not* take these drugs. Patients with liver disease should have hepatic transaminases monitored closely. Patients may also develop headaches, blood dyscrasias, paresthesias, gastrointestinal (GI) distress (e.g., nausea, vomiting, diarrhea, dyspepsia), and ocular toxicity. An ophthalmic examination before and during treatment is warranted. INH may cause hyperglycemia, hyperkalemia, hypophosphatemia, and hypocalcemia. Rifampin turns body fluids orange, and soft contact lenses may be permanently discolored. It may also cause thrombocytopenia and GI intolerance. The patient taking ethambutol may develop dizziness, confusion, hallucinations, and joint pain. Streptomycin may lead to many adverse effects such as ototoxicity, optic nerve toxicity, encephalopathy, angioedema, central nervous system (CNS) and respiratory depression, nephrotoxicity, and hepatotoxicity.

> ⚡ **PATIENT SAFETY**
>
> **Do not confuse…**
> - **Rifampin** with other antituberculars such as **rifabutin** and **rifapentine**.

SPECIAL POPULATIONS

Tuberculosis and Pregnancy

The benefits of treating a pregnant woman with TB disease outweigh the risks of treatment. Women with untreated TB disease are at risk for passing the infection to the fetus and delivering a newborn with low birthweight. The drugs used in initial treatment of TB do cross the placenta but do not appear to harm the fetus.

Treatment of latent TB infection in the pregnant woman includes INH daily or twice weekly for 9 months with pyridoxine supplementation. Three-month combination therapy of INH with rifapentinem, referred to as *3HP*, is not recommended for pregnant women or those planning to become pregnant within 3 months.

The pregnant woman with active TB should be treated with INH, rifampin, and ethambutol daily for 2 months followed by INH and rifampin daily or twice weekly for 7 months for a total of 9 months. Streptomycin should *not* be used due to potential harmful effects on the fetus. Pyrazinamide is also *not* recommended due to unknown effects on the fetus.

Tuberculosis and HIV Coinfection

HIV is a risk factor for the development of TB, and TB disease is one of the leading causes of death for people coinfected with HIV. Left untreated, latent TB infection can quickly develop into TB disease. The recommended treatment for an adult with latent TB infection and HIV is INH daily for 9 months.

Adults with HIV and TB disease should be treated for 6 months with INH, rifabutin, pyrazinamide, and ethambutol during the initial

TABLE 30.1 Antitubercular Drugs

Generic	Route and Dosage	Uses and Considerations
First-Line Treatment for Tuberculosis Disease		
Ethambutol	A: PO: 15–25 mg/kg/d or 25–30 mg/kg 3 × wk	Used in combination with other antitubercular drugs. A common adverse effect is eye damage that causes blurred or changed vision, including color vision. May also cause toxic epidermal necrolysis, thrombocytopenia, and anaphylaxis. Give with food to decrease GI disturbance. Monitor LFTs. PB: 20%–30%; t½: 3–4 h
Isoniazid (INH)	See Prototype Drug Chart: Isoniazid	
Pyrazinamide	A: PO: Based on lean body weight: 40–55 kg: 1000 mg/d or 1500 mg 3 × wk 56–75 kg: 1500 mg/d or 2500 mg 3 × wk 76–90 kg: 2000 mg/d or 3000 mg 3 × wk	Used in combination with other antitubercular drugs. Common adverse effects include arthralgia and myalgia. May also cause hepatotoxicity and thrombocytopenia. Monitor LFTs and serum uric acid. PB: 50%; t½: 9–10 h
Rifabutin	A: PO: 300 mg/d; *max:* 600 mg/d	Used in combination with other antitubercular drugs. May divide dose to 150 mg twice daily with GI concerns (e.g., nausea, vomiting). PB: 85%; t½: Average 45 h; decrease dose by 50% for creatinine clearance less than 30 mL/min Monitor LFTs
Rifampin[a]	A: PO: 10 mg/kg/d; *max:* 600 mg/d	Used in combination with other antitubercular drugs. Take one hour before or two hours after eating. Contents of capsules may be mixed with applesauce or jelly. PB: 80%; t½: 3–5 h
Rifapentine	Active: A: PO: 600 mg twice weekly for two months Latent: A: Single weight-based dose weekly ≥12 years and 32.1–50 kg: 750 mg × 12 wk ≥12 years and >50 kg: 900 mg × 12 wk	Rifapentine *must* be used in combination with other antitubercular drugs in patients with TB disease who are HIV negative or for latent TB infection to prevent progression to TB disease. Rifapentine has a longer half-life than rifampin; the interval between doses should be at least 72 h. Monitor for toxicity if drug is taken with an anticoagulant or anticonvulsant or with digoxin. Monitor for thrombocytopenia, ecchymosis, and indigestion. Do not use concurrently with oral contraceptives. PB: 98%; t½: 13 h
Drugs for Multidrug-Resistant Tuberculosis		
(Used in combination with first-line drugs based on sensitivity)		
Aminosalicylate	A: PO: 3.3–4 g every 8 h or 5–6 g every 12 h	Used in combination with other antitubercular drugs as a second-line therapy. Do not take within 6 hours of rifampin. May be taken with or after meals or with antacid if stomach upset occurs. Monitor LFTs. GI disturbances (e.g., nausea, vomiting, diarrhea, abdominal pain) are the most common complaints. PB: 50%–60%; t½: 26 min
Capreomycin	A ≤59 y: IV/IM: 15 mg/kg/d; *max:* 1 g/d A >59 y: IV/IM: 10 mg/kg/d; *max:* 750 mg/d	Used in combination with other antitubercular drugs. Inject into a large muscle mass. Because of possible nephrotoxicity, use caution when administering to patients with renal impairment. Other toxicity includes ototoxicity. PB: UK; t½: 4–6 h
Cycloserine	A: PO: 10–15 mg/kg/d in divided doses; *max:* 1000 mg/d	Used in combination with other antitubercular drugs. May be taken without regard to food. Pyridoxine 200 mg to 300 mg/d taken concurrently can relieve or prevent neurotoxic effects. Contraindicated in patients with a history of ETOH abuse, severe anxiety, major depression, psychosis, severe renal disease, and seizure disorders. Monitor cycloserine concentrations (toxic level >30 mcg/mL). PB: UK; t½: 10 h
Ethionamide	A: PO: 15–20 mg/kg/d as a single dose or in 2–3 divided doses; *max:* 1 g/d	Used in combination with other antitubercular drugs. Not first-line treatment. Contraindicated in severe hepatic impairment. Dosage adjustment required for kidney dysfunction. An ophthalmologic examination should be done and blood glucose and hepatic function should be monitored before and periodically during treatment. Drug may be taken without regard to food. PB: 30%; t½: 2 h
Streptomycin	A: IM: <59 yo: 15 mg/kg/d IM; *max:* 1 g/d >59 yo: 10 mg/kg/d IM; 51 g/d	Used in combination with other antitubercular drugs. Inject into a large muscle mass. Contraindicated in people with aminoglycoside hypersensitivity. Monitor for ototoxicity, nephrotoxicity, and neurotoxicity. PB: 35%; t½: 2–3 h

A, Adult; *d,* day; *ETOH,* ethanol (alcohol); *GI,* gastrointestinal; *h,* hour; *HIV,* human immunodeficiency virus; *IM,* intramuscular; *IV,* intravenous; *LFT,* liver function test; *max,* maximum; *min,* minutes; *PB,* protein binding; *PO,* by mouth; *t½,* half-life; *TB,* tuberculosis; *UK,* unknown; *wk,* week; *y,* year; *>,* greater than; *≥,* greater than or equal to; *≤,* less than or equal to.
[a]Rifampin is the preferred agent from the class of rifamycins (rifabutin, rifampin, and rifapentine).

📋 PROTOTYPE DRUG CHART

Isoniazid

Drug Class	Dosage
Antimycobacterial (antitubercular)	Latent TB infection: A: PO/IM: 5 mg/kg/d up to 300 mg/d or 15 mg/kg 2–3 × wk; max: 900 mg 2–3 × wk. See the CDC website at www.cdc.gov for complete dosing regimens.

Contraindications	Drug-Lab-Food Interactions
Severe renal or hepatic disease, alcoholism, diabetic retinopathy; severe hypersensitivity to pyrazinamide or ethionamide; concurrent use with MAOI therapy. Crosses placenta; enters breast milk. Use with caution if benefit outweighs risks.	Drug: Potent inhibitor of CYP450 enzyme system; many drug-drug interactions can occur (see the package insert for a complete list). Increased effect with alcohol, rifampin, and cycloserine; decreased GI absorption while taking aluminum antacids; inhibits the metabolism of benzodiazepines, phenytoin, fosphenytoin, SSRIs, SNRIs, and valproic acid. MAOIs could potentiate the effects of INH. Food: Avoid tyramine-containing foods. Give with meal to decrease GI upset; drug absorption is better 1 h before or 2 h after meals. Herb: Green tea, guarana, and ginseng could potentiate the effects of INH. Lab: Increases LFTs, bilirubin, and glucose; decreases platelets and granulocytes

Pharmacokinetics	Pharmacodynamics
Absorption: Rapidly absorbed in the GI tract when given PO; absorption slowed with food Distribution: PB: 10%–15% Metabolism: t½: 1–4 h Excretion: 75% in urine; remainder in feces, saliva, and sputum	PO/IM: Onset: Rapid Peak: 1–2 h Duration: 6–8 h

Therapeutic Effects/Uses
To treat active tuberculosis and as a prophylactic measure against tuberculosis Mechanism of Action: Bactericidal; inhibits bacterial cell wall synthesis by interfering with lipid and DNA synthesis. No cross-resistance with other antitubercular drugs occurs except with ethionamide. Pyridoxine supplementation reduces neurotoxic side effects.

Side Effects	Adverse Reactions
Drowsiness, tremors, rash, blurred vision, photosensitivity, tinnitus, dizziness, nausea, vomiting, dry mouth, constipation, diarrhea with oral solution, injection site reaction with IM administration	Vitamin B6 deficiency, optic neuritis, seizures, agranulocytosis, hemolytic anemia, aplastic anemia, thrombocytopenia, eosinophilia, and methemoglobinemia *Life-threatening:* Toxic encephalopathy, fatal hepatitis

A, Adult; *CDC,* Centers for Disease Control and Prevention; *CYP450,* cytochrome P450; *d,* day; *GI,* gastrointestinal; *h,* hour; *IM,* intramuscular; *INH,* isoniazid; *MAOI,* monoamine oxidase inhibitor; *max,* maximum; *PB,* protein binding; *PO,* by mouth; *SNRI,* serotonin norepinephrine reuptake inhibitor; *SSRI,* selective serotonin reuptake inhibitor; *t½,* half-life; *TB,* tuberculosis; *UK,* unknown; *wk,* week; *y,* year.

phase. The 4-month continuation phase should consist of INH and rifabutin. A pregnant woman with HIV and TB disease should be treated the same as a nonpregnant woman but with concern for the fetus when choosing drug therapy.

Tuberculosis and Pediatrics

Children are more likely than adults to become sick more quickly by TB. Because of this, children with latent TB infection should be treated to prevent development of TB disease. The recommended treatment is INH for 9 months. Treatment of TB disease should be managed by a pediatric TB expert in conjunction with drug susceptibility studies. It is very important for the nurse to make sure parents understand that if a child stops taking the drugs before therapy is finished, the child can become sick again. Additionally, nurses should stress to parents that if drugs are not taken correctly, the bacteria may become resistant to the drug. Drug-resistant TB is harder and more expensive to treat.

Tuberculosis and Other Special Populations

Consideration of other special populations for TB includes the homeless and foreign-born, including Hispanics/Latinos and Asians. According to the CDC, 1% of the US population experiences homelessness in a given year. Of the foreign-born people with TB, 32% were Hispanics/Latinos. Lack of resources and reduced public health capacity increase the challenges faced in treating people with TB. There are many barriers in properly treating these vulnerable populations in eradicating TB. Socioeconomic, cultural, and language barriers are just a few that increase the risk for latent TB infection.

▍FUNGUS

PATHOPHYSIOLOGY

An infection caused by a fungus may also be called *mycosis, tinea,* or *candidiasis.* A fungal infection may be local or systemic. Local fungal infections can be acquired by contact with an infected person. Fungi known as *dermatophytes* can cause local fungal infections involving the integumentary system, which includes mucous membranes, hair, nails, and moist skin areas. When *Candida albicans* affects the mouth, it is called *oral candidiasis* or *thrush.* Vaginal candidiasis is common in

BOX 30.1 Determining When to Treat Latent Tuberculosis Infection

People with a positive tuberculin skin test (TST) reaction of ≥5 mm if they are:
- HIV positive
- Recent contacts of someone with active tuberculosis (TB disease)
- Persons with fibrotic changes on chest radiography consistent with old TB
- Organ transplant recipients
- Persons who are immunosuppressed for other reasons (e.g., those taking the equivalent of >15 mg/day of prednisone for 1 month or longer, those taking tumor necrosis factor alpha [TNF-α] antagonists)

People with a positive TST reaction of ≥10 mm if they are:
- Recent immigrants (<5 years) from high-prevalence countries
- Injection drug users
- Residents and employees of high-risk congregate settings (e.g., correctional facilities, nursing homes, homeless shelters, hospitals, and other health care facilities)
- Mycobacteriology laboratory personnel
- Children under 4 years of age or children or adolescents exposed to adults in high-risk categories

From http://www.cdc.gov/tb/topic/treatment/decideltbi.htm.

women who are pregnant, diabetic, immunocompromised, or taking certain medications (e.g., antibiotics, oral contraceptives, and dapagliflozin). Systemic fungal infections may involve the lungs, CNS, or abdomen and are usually transmitted to an individual through inhalation into the lungs. Fungal infections may be mild, such as tinea pedis (athlete's foot), or severe, such as fungal disease of the lungs or fungal meningitis.

Fungal infections are also classified as *opportunistic* or *primary*. Opportunistic infections usually occur in the immunocompromised or debilitated population (e.g., patients who have cancer or AIDS) or in those taking antibiotics, corticosteroids, chemotherapy, or other immunosuppressive drugs. Fungi such as *Candida* species (yeast) are part of the normal flora of the mouth, skin, intestine, and vagina. An opportunistic infection, such as systemic candidiasis, may occur when the body's defense mechanisms are impaired such that they allow overgrowth of the fungus. Other opportunistic infections are aspergillosis, mucormycosis, *Pneumocystis* pneumonia, and fusariosis. Primary infections typically occur in immunocompetent persons and result from inhaled spores. Primary infections include coccidioidomycosis, blastomycosis, paracoccidioidomycosis, cryptococcosis, and histoplasmosis, including progressive disseminated histoplasmosis.

⊚ CLINICAL JUDGMENT [NURSING PROCESS]

Antitubercular Drugs

Concept: Drug Adherence
- The ability or lack of the ability to take drugs as prescribed

Concept: Safety
- Protection of the patient from potential or actual harm; is a basic human need

Recognize Cues [Assessment]
- Assess for financial means to obtain drugs for tuberculosis (TB).
- Assess the means to follow up with appropriate person.
- Determine any past instances of TB in the patient's health history—including the last purified protein derivative (PPD) tuberculin test and the reaction or the serum interferon-gamma release assay (IGRA) result, the last chest radiograph and result, and the last ophthalmic examination—along with any allergies.
- Obtain a general medical history from the patient. Most antitubercular drugs are contraindicated if the patient has severe hepatic disease.
- Check laboratory results for liver function studies, bilirubin, blood urea nitrogen (BUN), and serum creatinine. These baseline values can be compared with future laboratory test results.
- Evaluate the patient for signs and symptoms of paresthesia (tingling, numbness, or burning).
- Assess for hearing changes if the antitubercular drug regimen includes streptomycin. Drug-induced ototoxicity is the major irreversible toxicity of aminoglycosides.

Analyze Cues and Prioritize Hypothesis [Patient Problems]
- Pulmonary infection

Generate Solutions [Planning]
- Patient will verbalize understanding for strict adherence to drug treatments.
- Patient will be free of symptoms of new infections.
- Patient will have a negative sputum test for acid-fast bacilli 2 to 3 months postantitubercular treatment.

Take Action [Nursing Interventions]
- Consult case management for financial help with drug treatment.
- Obtain initial follow-up appointment before discharge.

- If isoniazid (INH) is ordered, administer the drug 1 hour before or 2 hours after meals because food decreases the absorption rate. Other antitubercular drugs are given without regard to meals.
- Give pyridoxine (vitamin B_6) as prescribed with INH to prevent peripheral neuropathy.
- Monitor serum liver enzyme levels. Elevated levels may indicate liver toxicity.
- Collect sputum specimens for acid-fast bacilli early in the morning. Usually three consecutive morning sputum specimens are sent to the laboratory.
- Encourage eye examinations for patients taking INH and ethambutol because these antitubercular drugs may cause visual disturbances.
- Emphasize the importance of complying with the drug regimen.
- Tell patients who take INH to take the drug 1 hour before meals or 2 hours after meals for better absorption.
- ⚡ Direct patients to take antitubercular drugs as prescribed. Ineffective treatment and development of drug resistance might occur if drugs are taken intermittently or discontinued when symptoms are decreased or when the patient is feeling better. *Adherence to the drug regimen is essential to prevent the spread of drug-resistant* M. tuberculosis.
- Advise patients to keep medical appointments and to participate in sputum testing, which is important in evaluating the effectiveness of drug regimens.
- Warn patients contemplating pregnancy to first check with their health care provider about taking the antitubercular drugs ethambutol and rifampin.
- Increase access to health care. Community involvement and culturally sensitive patient education are important. Explain to patients who have active TB that family members should get a TB skin test (TST) and may receive a prophylactic drug for 6 months to 1 year. Emphasize the importance of family members seeking medical care.
- Provide a written sheet for drug and treatment regimens in the language the patient speaks or reads most easily. Explain the importance of good hygiene (e.g., discarding tissues that contain sputum, separating dishes, using a dishwasher to clean dishes if possible).
- Understand the significance of community if multiple individuals in the same community are treated for latent TB infection. Make all attempts to place community members on a treatment plan to increase compliance through social support.

◎ CLINICAL JUDGMENT [NURSING PROCESS]—CONT'D

Antitubercular Drugs

- Instruct patients not to take antacids while taking antitubercular drugs because they decrease drug absorption. Patients should also avoid alcohol because it increases the risk of hepatotoxicity.
- Alert patients receiving ethambutol to take daily single doses to avoid visual problems. Divided doses of ethambutol may cause visual disturbances.
- Inform patients taking rifampin that urine, feces, saliva, sputum, sweat, and tears may turn a harmless red-orange color. Soft contact lenses may be permanently stained.
- Guide patients to report any numbness, tingling, or burning of hands and feet. Peripheral neuropathy is a common side effect of INH. Vitamin B₆ prevents peripheral neuropathy.

- Encourage patients to avoid direct sunlight to decrease the risk of photosensitivity. Patients should use a sunscreen with a minimum sun protection factor (SPF) of 30 and ultraviolet A and B (UVA/UVB) protection while in the sun.

Evaluate Outcomes [Evaluation]
- Evaluate the effectiveness of the antitubercular drugs. Sputum specimens for acid-fast bacilli should be negative after taking antitubercular drugs for several weeks or months.

ANTIFUNGAL DRUGS

Antifungal drugs, also called antimycotic drugs, are used to treat fungal infections. Typically, antifungals are fungistatic or fungicidal depending on the susceptibility of the fungus and the dosage. The antifungal drugs are classified into the following groups (Table 30.2):

- Polyenes (amphotericin B, nystatin)
- Azoles (fluconazole)
- Antimetabolites (flucytosine)
- Echinocandins (caspofungin)
- Miscellaneous antifungals (griseofulvin)

Polyenes

Amphotericin B

The polyene antifungal drug of choice for severe, life-threatening systemic fungal infection is amphotericin B, which is effective against numerous fungal diseases that include histoplasmosis, cryptococcosis, coccidioidomycosis, aspergillosis, blastomycosis, zygomycosis, including mucormycosis, and systemic candidiasis. Polyene antifungals act by binding to the fungal cell membrane to form open channels that increase cell permeability and leakage of intracellular components, especially potassium. Because of its toxicity, amphotericin B is administered with close supervision.

Pharmacokinetics. Amphotericin B is highly protein bound (>90%) and has a long half-life of approximately 15 days. Only 5% of the drug is excreted in the urine. Renal disease does not affect the excretion of amphotericin B.

Pharmacodynamics. Amphotericin B is not absorbed from the GI tract; therefore it is administered intravenously in low doses for treating systemic fungal infections. Peak effect occurs 1 to 2 hours after intravenous (IV) infusion, and the duration is 24 hours.

Side Effects and Adverse Reactions. Side effects and adverse reactions for amphotericin B include fever, shaking, chills, flushing, loss of appetite, dizziness, nausea, vomiting, headache, shortness of breath, and tachypnea. These symptoms may occur 1 to 3 hours after the infusion has started. Pretreatment with acetaminophen, diphenhydramine, or hydrocortisone administered 30 to 60 minutes before infusion may alleviate these symptoms. Additionally, patients may experience hypotension, paresthesia, and thrombophlebitis. Amphotericin B is *highly toxic* and can cause nephrotoxicity and electrolyte imbalance, especially hypokalemia and hypomagnesemia (low serum potassium and magnesium levels). Urinary output, BUN, and serum creatinine levels must be closely monitored. Amphotericin

B is also toxic to bone marrow; therefore complete blood counts (CBCs) should be monitored periodically.

Nystatin

Nystatin is another polyene antifungal drug that is administered orally or topically to treat *Candida* infection. It is available in suspension, cream, and ointment forms. Nystatin is poorly absorbed by the GI tract. The more common use of nystatin is as an oral suspension for *Candida* infection of the mouth (oral thrush). The suspension is swished in the mouth for several minutes to ensure contact with the mucous membranes and then is either disposed of or swallowed. If the throat area is involved, the patient should also gargle with nystatin before swishing and swallowing or spitting. Prototype Drug Chart: Nystatin lists the data for nystatin.

Azole Antifungals

The azole group is effective against candidiasis (local and systemic), coccidioidomycosis, cryptococcosis, histoplasmosis, and paracoccidioidomycosis. Ketoconazole was the first effective antifungal drug that was orally absorbed. Fluconazole, itraconazole, posaconazole, and voriconazole are other azole drugs used to treat systemic fungal infections. These antifungals can be taken orally, unlike amphotericin B and caspofungin, which are administered by the IV route only. Fluconazole, a systemic azole antifungal agent, is described in Prototype Drug Chart: Fluconazole.

Azoles inhibit cytochrome P450 (CYP450) in fungal cells, interfering with the formation of ergosterol. Because ergosterol is a major sterol in the fungal cell membrane, cell permeability and leakage are increased. Numerous azoles are used in topical preparations (e.g., creams, ointments, powders, shampoos, sprays, and solutions) to treat candidiasis and tinea infections. Azoles and other topical antifungal agents are presented in Table 30.2.

Antimetabolites

The antimetabolite flucytosine acts by selectively penetrating the fungal cell, which converts the drug into fluorouracil, an antimetabolite that disrupts fungal DNA and RNA synthesis. Flucytosine is well absorbed from the GI tract, and it is used in combination with other antifungal drugs, such as amphotericin B. Antimetabolites are discussed further in Chapter 32.

Echinocandins

Echinocandins are the newest class of antifungals. Three echinocandins are available in the United States: anidulafungin, caspofungin, and micafungin. The action of echinocandins is to inhibit

TABLE 30.2 Antifungal Drugs

Generic	Route and Dosage	Uses and Considerations
Polyenes		
Amphotericin B deoxycholate	A: IV: Test dose: 1 mg IV over 20–30 min Load: 0.25–0.5 g/kg IV over 2–6 h Maintenance: 0.25–1.5 mg/kg IV/d	For patients with potentially life-threatening fungal infections. May require pretreatment with an analgesic, antihistamine, antipyretic, and corticosteroid for pain, fever, chills, or rigor. Electrolyte loss and nephrotoxicity can occur. Protect drug against light and infuse slowly via an in-line filter. PB: 90%–95%; t½: Initial plasma half-life 24 h with elimination half-life of 15 days
Nystatin	See Prototype Drug Chart: Nystatin	
Azole Antifungals		
Fluconazole	See Prototype Drug Chart: Fluconazole	
Itraconazole	A: PO: 200–400 mg/d Other dosing regimens are available for severe infection or for patients who are immunocompromised.	For a variety of fungal infections. Targets CYP450 enzymatic pathway. Avoid concurrent use with PPIs, H₂ blockers, or antacids. Take on an empty stomach. Pregnancy considerations: contraindicated in pregnancy and in those contemplating pregnancy; PB: 99%; t½: 34–42 h
Ketoconazole	Systemic: A: PO: 200–400 mg/d as a single dose Topical: A: Apply a sufficient amount to affected and surrounding areas once daily for 2 wk.	For a variety of fungal infections. Treatment may last 1–6 months for systemic infections. Take with food to avoid GI discomfort. Oral administration may cause hepatotoxicity; may cause QT prolongation. Higher doses can inhibit adrenal cortisol synthesis. PB: 93%–96%; t½: 2–8 h
Posaconazole	Oral candidiasis: A: PO: 100 mg/d up to 200 mg tid for 14–21 d Prophylactic: A: PO: 200–300 mg bid/tid A: IV: 300 mg bid initially, then 300 mg/d	For oral candidiasis and prophylactic treatment of invasive *Aspergillus* and *Candida* infections in immunosuppressed patients. Different formulations are not interchangeable. Ensure proper dosage formulation, strength, and frequency. Do not chew, divide, or crush delayed-release tablets. Administer with food or as an IV infusion via a central line with an in-line filter. PB: >98%; t½: 26–35 h depending on formulation
Voriconazole	A: PO: Weight-based dosing: 200–400 mg q12h A: IV: 6 mg/kg q12h on day 1, then 3–4 mg/kg q12h	For aspergillosis, candidiasis, fusariosis, and scedosporiosis. Patients with HIV coinfection may need a higher dose. Grapefruit juice should be avoided. Take PO dose on an empty stomach. PB: 58%; t½: variable; dose dependent
Antimetabolites		
Flucytosine	A: PO: 50–150 mg/kg/d in divided doses q6h for 7–10 d; *max:* 150 mg/kg/d TDM: 50–100 mcg/mL; toxic levels >100 mcg/mL	Usually given in conjunction with amphotericin B for treatment of systemic candidiasis and cryptococcosis, to decrease the development of resistance to flucytosine. Fungal resistance occurs if drug is given alone. Monitor LFTs. PB: 2%–4%; t½: 3–8 h
Echinocandins		
Anidulafungin	A: IV: 100–200 mg loading dose on day 1, then 50–100 mg/d	For *Candida* infections. Infusion time is dose dependent. Monitor liver function tests. PB: 99%; t½: 30–60 min
Caspofungin	A: IV: 70 mg on day 1, then 50 mg/d	For *Aspergillus* and *Candida* infections. Give IV as an infusion over 1 h. Monitor CBC and liver transaminases. PB: 97%; t½: 9–50 h
Micafungin	A: IV: 100–150 mg/d	For *Candida* infection. Patients with HIV coinfection may require a higher dose. Does not have significant effect on the CYP450 enzyme system. To minimize excessive foaming, do not vigorously shake the vial. Infuse slowly over 1 h. Rapid infusion can cause histamine-mediated reactions. PB: 99%; t½: 11–21 h
Miscellaneous Antifungals		
Griseofulvin	A: PO: 375–750 mg/d; can be given in 2–4 divided doses/d; *max:* 1000 mg/d	For tinea infection, including onychomycosis. Available in microsize and ultramicrosize; dosage depends on formulation. Give with a fatty meal to increase absorption. Tablets can be crushed and mixed with food; swallow without chewing. Avoid during pregnancy and caution is advised while breastfeeding. PB: UK; t½: 9–22 h

A, Adult; *bid,* twice daily; *CBC,* complete blood count; *CYP450,* cytochrome P450; *d,* day; *GI,* gastrointestinal; *h,* hour; *H₂,* histamine 2; *HIV,* human immunodeficiency virus; *IV,* intravenous; *max,* maximum; *min,* minute; *mo,* month; *PB,* protein binding; *PO,* by mouth; *PPI,* proton pump inhibitor; *q,* every; *t½,* half-life; *TDM,* therapeutic drug monitoring; *tid,* three times daily; *UK,* unknown; *wk,* weeks; *y,* year; *>,* greater than; *≥,* greater than or equal to.

📋 PROTOTYPE DRUG CHART

Nystatin

Drug Class	Dosage
Polyene antifungal	A: PO susp: 400,000 to 600,000 units swished in the mouth then swallowed 4 ×/d for 7–14 d A: Top: Apply to affected area bid until healed. A: PO cap: 500,000–1 million units tid for at least 48 h

Contraindications	Drug-Lab-Food Interactions
Caution: Pregnancy, diabetes mellitus, paraben hypersensitivity, breastfeeding. Not for use in systemic mycoses.	Drug: Azole antifungals inhibit the synthesis of the fungal sterol ergosterol, which decreases the effectiveness of nystatin.

Pharmacokinetics	Pharmacodynamics
Absorption: Poorly absorbed in the GI the tract when given PO Absorption: Susp/top: Not absorbed from intact skin or mucous membranes Distribution: PB: Not subject to plasma PB Metabolism: t½: Not metabolized Excretion: PO: In feces, unchanged	PO: Onset symptom relief: 24–72 h; peak and duration: UK Susp/top: Onset, peak, and duration: UK

Therapeutic Effects/Uses
To treat cutaneous and mucocutaneous mycotic infections Mechanism of Action: Binds to sterols (ergosterol) causing the loss of intracellular potassium and other cellular contents

Side Effects	Adverse Reactions
PO: Diarrhea, nausea, vomiting, abdominal pain Top: Contact dermatitis	Top/susp: Hypersensitivity reaction *Life-threatening:* PO/top/susp: Stevens-Johnson syndrome

A, Adult; *bid*, twice daily; *cap*, capsule; *d*, day; *GI*, gastrointestinal; *h*, hour; *PB*, protein binding; *PO*, by mouth; *susp*, suspension; *t½*, half-life; *tid*, three times daily; *top*, topical; *UK*, unknown.

biosynthesis of essential components of the fungal cell wall, which interferes with growth and reproduction of *Candida* and *Aspergillus* species. Echinocandins are administered intravenously because they are not absorbed in the GI tract. Phlebitis at the IV site and increased aspartate aminotransferase (AST) and alanine aminotransferase (ALT) are common adverse effects. Rapid infusion can cause histamine-mediated reactions.

⚡ PATIENT SAFETY

Amphotericin B
The two formulations of amphotericin B are amphotericin B deoxycholate and liposomal amphotericin B. Dosing for each formulation is different; therefore caution is advised.

❘ VIRUSES

A virus is an obligate intracellular organism that must reside within a living host cell to survive and reproduce. Viruses enter healthy cells, live and reproduce within living cells, and use their DNA and RNA to generate more viruses. The growth cycle of viruses depends on host cell enzymes and cell substrates for viral replication. With the exception of HIV and certain kinds of viral hepatitis, viruses are self-limiting illnesses that usually do *not* require treatment with a specific antiviral. Current antivirals target influenza, herpes, and hepatitis.

PATHOPHYSIOLOGY

Influenza, commonly called *the flu*, is a highly contagious viral infection that causes mild to severe illness that can result in hospitalization or even death. Influenza is usually seasonal and is more prevalent from fall to spring. There are three main types of influenza: A, B, and C. *Influenza A* causes a moderate to severe infection. There are two subtypes found in humans, designated by the hemagglutinin (H) and neuraminidase (N) proteins, H1N1 and H3N2, found on the viral surface. *Influenza B* usually causes mild illness in children. Two strains are currently found in humans: B/Yamagata and B/Victoria. *Influenza C* infection is a mild respiratory illness not thought to cause epidemics. Influenza is transmitted easily via contaminated droplets during coughing, sneezing, or talking. Droplets enter into the respiratory tract of the unaffected person and begin replication 24 hours before the appearance of symptoms. Usually influenza has an abrupt onset, with the first symptoms being high fever, headache, fatigue, and myalgia (muscle aches). Chills; sore throat; nonproductive cough; watery nasal discharge; weakness; red, watery eyes; and photophobia can also occur.

Herpesviruses are large viruses that cause infections. Among the most familiar are herpes simplex virus type 1 (HSV-1) and type 2 (HSV-2); varicella-zoster viruses (HSV-3, or VZV), more commonly known as *chickenpox* and *shingles*; Epstein-Barr virus (EBV, or human herpesvirus 4 [HHV-4]); and cytomegalovirus (CMV, or human herpesvirus 5 [HHV-5]). HSV-1 is usually associated with cold sores (vesicular lesions) and is capable of latency, the establishment and maintenance of latent infection in nerve cell ganglia proximal to the site of infection.

PROTOTYPE DRUG CHART

Fluconazole

Drug Class	Dosage
Azole antifungal	Cryptococcal meningitis: A: PO/IV: 400 mg on day 1, then 200–400 mg/d Systemic candidiasis (candidemia): A: PO/IV: 800 mg on day 1, then 400 mg/kg/d Candiduria (UTI due to candiasis, esophageal): A: PO/IV: 200–400 mg/d Most other candidiasis, oropharyngeal: A: PO/IV: 200 mg on day 1, then 100 mg/d Candidiasis, vulvovaginal (uncomplicated) 150 mg × 1 Candidasis, vulvovaginal (severe) 150 mg × 72 hours × 2

Contraindications	Drug-Lab-Food Interactions
Caution: Hypersensitivity, first trimester pregnancy; secreted in breast milk, QT prolongation, renal or hepatic disease	Drug: Because this drug inhibits the CYP450 isoenzyme, many drug-drug interactions are possible. See package insert for complete detail. Increases PT in patients taking warfarin; increases hypoglycemia when taken with oral sulfonylureas; increases phenytoin, cyclosporine, and haloperidol levels; decreases fluconazole level with cimetidine and rifampin; decreases the effect of clopidogrel; increases incidences of QT prolongation with cisapride, terfenadine, thioridazine, ondansetron, and other CYP3A4 substrates Food: May be administered without regard to food Herb: None significant

Pharmacokinetics	Pharmacodynamics
Absorption: PO: Oral administration with 90% bioavailability Distribution: PB: 11%–12% Metabolism: t½: 20–50 h; does not undergo first-pass metabolism Excretion: 80% in urine unchanged, 11% as metabolites	Lab: May increase LFTs PO: Onset: Rapid Peak: 1–2 h Duration: UK IV: Onset, peak, and duration: UK

Therapeutic Effects/Uses

To treat *Candida* infections and cryptococcal meningitis; as prophylaxis for patients undergoing BMT or radiation therapy
Mechanism of Action: Increases permeability of the fungal cell membrane by inhibiting ergosterol synthesis

Side Effects	Adverse Reactions
PO: GI upset (e.g., nausea, vomiting, diarrhea, abdominal pain, dyspepsia), rash, headache, hypokalemia	Hepatotoxicity, seizures, leukopenia, agranulocytosis, thrombocytopenia, Stevens-Johnson syndrome, QT prolongation, renal failure, fatal cardiac arrhythmias, toxic epidermal necrolysis

A, Adult; *BMT*, bone marrow transplant; *CYP*, cytochrome P; *d*, day; *GI*, gastrointestinal; *h*, hour; *IV*, intravenous; *PB*, protein binding; *PO*, by mouth; *PT*, prothrombin time; *t½*, half-life; *UK*, unknown; *UTI*, urinary tract infection.

HSV-2 is usually associated with vesicular lesions and small ulcerations on the genitalia (genital herpes). The HSV-2 virus remains dormant by traveling through the peripheral nerves to the sacral dorsal nerve root ganglia. The reactivation and replication of latent HSV always occurs in the area supplied by the ganglia in which latency was established. Reactivation can be induced by various factors that include fever, trauma, emotional stress, sunlight, and menstruation. Both HSV-1 and HSV-2 are capable of causing recurrent infections, and both can replicate in the mucous membranes and skin of the oropharynx or genitalia. Virus is transmitted by contact with infectious lesions or secretions. Signs and symptoms usually include eruption of small pustules and vesicles, fever, headache, malaise, myalgia, and tingling, itching, and pain in the affected area.

VZV causes chickenpox and shingles. Chickenpox is a highly contagious viral infection that causes generalized pruritic vesicles and fever. Serious illness, hospitalizations, and deaths from VZV have decreased by 90% since vaccination began in 1995; however, some outbreaks still occur. When a person who has previously been infected with chickenpox becomes older or develops a weakened immune system, VZV that has lain dormant in nerve root ganglia can reactivate. The reactivation, called shingles, is a painful vesicular rash along the region of skin innervated by the nerve root ganglia, or dermatome, where the virus had lain dormant. In addition to the rash, the patient may also develop fever, malaise, myalgia, and pain along the involved dermatome.

EBV most commonly causes infectious mononucleosis, a condition manifested by fever, tonsillitis, and enlarged lymph nodes in the neck. EBV resides in lymphocytes, epithelial cells, and muscle cells and has a latency period.

CMV is a common viral infection that affects people of all ages. Most people infected with CMV do not exhibit symptoms and are unaware they have the virus. However, people with weakened immune systems (such as those with HIV, transplant recipients, and those

◎ CLINICAL JUDGMENT [NURSING PROCESS]
Antifungals

Concept: Drug Adherence
- The ability or lack of the ability to take drugs as prescribed

Concept: Safety
- Protection of the patient from potential or actual harm; is a basic human need

Recognize Cues [Assessment]
- Obtain a medical history that includes any serious renal or hepatic disorders. Antifungal agents such as amphotericin B, fluconazole, flucytosine, and ketoconazole are contraindicated if the patient has a serious renal or liver disease.
- Assess the ability to swallow. Oral candidiasis can impede swallowing, which can decrease appropriate nutritional intake.
- Check laboratory tests for liver function (alkaline phosphatase [ALP], alanine aminotransferase [ALT], aspartate aminotransferase [AST], gamma-glutamyl transferase [GGT]), blood urea nitrogen (BUN), bilirubin, and serum creatinine because elevated levels can indicate liver or renal dysfunction. Use these test results for future comparisons.
- Assess any prior use of antifungals.

Analyze Cues and Prioritize Hypothesis [Patient Problems]
- Potential for nonadherence
- Potential for decreased tissue integrity
- Potential for decreased nutrition

Generate Solutions [Planning]
- Patient will list potential complications and when to call the medical provider.
- Patient will verbalize appropriate means to protect self from further injury.
- Patient will identify proper nutrition while on antifungals to prevent further injury and improve healing.

Take Action [Nursing Interventions]
- Obtain a culture to determine the fungus type (e.g., *Candida*).

- Monitor the patient's urinary output; many antifungal drugs can cause nephrotoxicity.
- Check laboratory results for BUN, serum creatinine, ALP, ALT, AST, bilirubin, and electrolytes and compare these with baseline findings. Certain antifungals can cause hepatotoxicity and nephrotoxicity when high doses are taken for an extended period.
- Record vital signs and compare these with baseline findings.
- Observe for side effects and adverse reactions to antifungal drugs, which may include nausea, vomiting, headache, phlebitis, and signs and symptoms of electrolyte imbalance.
- Advise patients to take drugs as prescribed. Compliance is of the utmost importance because discontinuing a drug too soon may result in relapse.
- Instruct patients to keep appointments to monitor laboratory testing of serum liver enzymes, BUN, creatinine, and electrolytes.
- Advise patients not to consume alcohol.
- Educate patients on proper administration of topical preparations.
- Respect the patient's apprehension and fear concerning the use of topical antifungal drugs and the desire to use alternative methods. Evaluate the patient's method of topical administration in regard to safe practice. If the method is considered unsafe, explain why and suggest modifications. If appropriate, involve other persons for clarification.
- Teach patients to avoid operating hazardous equipment or motor vehicles when taking antifungals that may cause visual changes, sleepiness, dizziness, or lethargy (e.g., amphotericin B, ketoconazole, or flucytosine).
- Encourage patients to report side effects such as nausea, vomiting, diarrhea, dermatitis, rash, dizziness, tinnitus, edema, and flatulence. These symptoms may occur when taking certain antifungal drugs.

Evaluate Outcomes [Evaluation]
- Evaluate the effectiveness of the antifungal drug by noting the diminishing or absence of the fungal infection.

taking immunosuppressant drugs), along with pregnant women, unborn babies, and neonates, are at risk for developing signs and symptoms (e.g., lymphadenopathy and splenomegaly). In susceptible individuals, CMV infection can lead to blindness (CMV retinitis) or fatal pneumonia.

Viral hepatitis infections, such as with hepatitis B and C viruses (HBV and HCV, respectively), are serious liver infections. Many people with HBV and HCV are unaware they have the virus. These viruses can persist undetected for years, increasing the likelihood of transmitting the disease to others. HBV and HCV are blood-borne pathogens spread through blood and body fluids. They are leading causes of hepatic cancer and the most common reason for hepatic failure and subsequent liver transplant. Signs and symptoms of viral hepatitis include fatigue, jaundice, abdominal pain, malaise, and nausea.

NON-HIV ANTIVIRALS

Antiviral drugs are used to prevent or delay the spread of viral infections. They inhibit viral replication by interfering with viral nucleic acid synthesis in the cell. Some groups of antiviral drugs are effective against various viruses, such as influenzas A and B, herpesviruses, HBV and HCV, and HIV. The non-HIV antiviral drugs are listed in Table 30.3. Interferon alfa-2a and -2b used to treat HBV and HCV are discussed in Chapter 34. Drugs for HIV are discussed in Chapter 29.

Influenza Antivirals

Current recommendations for the treatment of influenza type A and B are oseltamivir or zanamivir. These are neuraminidase inhibitors, a group of drugs that decrease the release of the virus from infected cells by inhibiting the activity of neuraminidase, a viral glycoprotein, thus decreasing viral spread and shortening the duration of flu symptoms. Zanamivir and oseltamivir should be taken within 48 hours of flu symptoms, but they are *not* substitutes for the influenza vaccines.

Side Effects and Adverse Reactions

The side effects and adverse reactions of these two neuraminidase inhibitors include dizziness, headache, insomnia, vertigo, fatigue, and GI disturbances such as nausea, vomiting, and diarrhea. ⚡ Nurses must be aware of a US Food and Drug Administration (FDA) advisory that persons receiving oral oseltamivir should be monitored closely for abnormal behavior. Incidence of self-injury and delirium have been reported in postmarketing surveillance.

Herpes Antivirals

The synthetic purine nucleoside antiviral group is effective in interfering with the steps of viral nucleic acid (DNA) synthesis. Drugs in this group of nucleoside analogues include ribavirin, acyclovir, famciclovir, ganciclovir sodium, valacyclovir, and valganciclovir. These drugs are effective in managing herpes simplex viruses (HSV-1, HSV-2) and VZV (chickenpox and shingles).

TABLE 30.3   Non-HIV Antivirals

Generic	Route and Dosage	Uses and Considerations
Antivirals: Influenza		
Amantadine	Influenza A: A: PO: 200 mg/d in 1–2 divided doses	Primary use is as prophylaxis against influenza A. Because of resistance in circulating influenza A, amantadine is no longer recommended; influenza A is sensitive to oseltamivir and zanamivir. If used, amantadine should be started within 24–48 h of onset of signs/symptoms and continued for 24–48 h after resolution. Avoid aspirin-containing products in children with influenza virus. Can be taken without regard to food. Contraindicated in kidney failure. PB: 67%; t½: 16 h
Cidofovir	A: IV: Induction treatment: 5 mg/kg IV over 1 h, once/week × 2 weeks Maintenance treatment: 5 mg/kg IV q2weeks	For CMV retinitis in HIV-infected patients. Give concomitantly with hydration (1 liter NS before treatment and 1 liter NS after treatment) and 2 g probenecid 3 h before each dose and 1 g at 2 h and 8 h after dose completion to minimize renal toxicity. Use chemotherapeutic precautions, including preparing the drug under laminar flow and using protective gloves and gowns. *Contraindications:* Sulfonamide hypersensitivity, renal impairment PB: <6%; t½: 2.6 h
Foscarnet	Acyclovir-resistant herpesvirus: A: IV: 40 mg/kg q8h CMV retinitis: A: IV: 90 mg/kg q12h or 60 mg/kg/d q8h	For CMV retinitis and acyclovir-resistant mucocutaneous HSV. Administer via slow IV infusion. Patient must be hydrated with 750 to 1000 mL minimize renal toxicity. Monitor renal function. PB: 14%–17%; t½: 3.3–4 h
Oseltamivir	Influenza A & B treatment (start within 48 h of symptom onset): A: PO: 75 mg bid for 5 d Prophylaxis (start within 48 h of exposure) 75 mg daily × 10 d	Treatment should begin within 48 h of flu symptoms. May be taken without regard to food. Monitor renal function. PB: 3%, t½: 1–3 h
Rimantadine	A: PO: 100 mg bid; *max:* 200 mg/d	Formerly used for prophylaxis and treatment against influenza A virus. If used, monitor renal and hepatic functions; dosing may need to be adjusted. Because of resistance in circulating influenza A, rimantadine is not recommended; influenza A is sensitive to oseltamivir and zanamivir. Avoid aspirin-containing products in children with influenza. PB: 40%; t½: 25.4 h
Zanamivir	Inhaler: A: 2 oral inhalations bid for 5 d Prophylaxis: A: 2 oral inhalations once daily for 10 d	Effective against influenzas A and B. Treatment should begin within 36 h of exposure or 48 h of onset of symptoms. Take bronchodilators before zanamivir. PB: <10%; t½: 2.5–5 h
Antivirals: Herpes Species		
Acyclovir	See Prototype Drug Chart: Acyclovir	Also available as a topical
Famciclovir	Herpes zoster: A: PO: 500 mg q8h for 7 d Herpes simplex: A: PO: 250 mg tid for 7–10 d Herpes genitalis: recurrent A: PO: 1000 mg bid for 1 d Herpes genitalis: suppressive A: PO: 250 mg sq 12 h × 12 months Herpes labialis: initial A: PO: 250 mg q 8 h × 7–10 d Herpes labialis: suppressive A: PO: 250 mg q 12 h × 12 months	For herpes zoster, herpes genitalis, herpes labialis, and HSV. Start treatment within 48 h of rash onset. Dose adjustment is necessary in patients coinfected with HIV. Monitor renal function; dose adjustment may be necessary with impaired renal function. Can be taken without regard to food. PB: <20%; t½: 2–4 h
Ganciclovir	CMV retinitis: A: 5 mg/kg IV q 12 h × 14–21 d Maintenance: 5 mg/kg IV qd CMV prevention transplant recipient: A: 5 mg/kg IV q12h × 7–14 d A: Ophthal: 1 drop to each affected eye 5 ×/d until healed, then 1 drop tid for 7 d	For CMV infection in immunocompromised patients and for herpes simplex keratitis. Monitor for hematologic toxicity. Handle drugs according to guidelines for chemotherapeutics. *Contraindicated in patients with severe thrombocytopenia.* Monitor renal function; dose may need to be adjusted. PB: 1%–2%; t½: 2.5–3.6 h
Penciclovir	A: Topical: Apply q2h while awake for 4 d	For recurrent herpes labialis (cold sores). Start within 1 h of onset of symptoms. Do not administer to mucous membranes. PB: 20%; t½: 2 h

Continued

TABLE 30.3 Non-HIV Antivirals—cont'd

Generic	Route and Dosage	Uses and Considerations
Trifluridine	A: Ophthal: 1 gtt q2h to each affected eye while awake; *max:* Not to exceed 21 d treatment	Used primarily for keratoconjunctivitis due to HSV. Remove contact lenses before use. If more than one ophthalmic drug is used, separate instillations by at least 5–10 min. Store under refrigeration. PB: UK; t½: 12–18 min
Valacyclovir	Herpes labialis A: PO: 2 g q 12 hr × 2 doses Genital herpes Initial: A: PO: 1 g every 12 h × 10 d Recurrent: A: PO: 500 mg q 12 h × 3 d Suppressive A: PO 1 g/d Herpes zoster: A: PO: 1 g tid for 7 d	Effective against varicella and HSV. May be taken without regard to food. Monitor kidney function; dose reduction is required. PB: 14%–18%; t½: 2.5–3.3 h
Valganciclovir	CMV retinitis: A: PO: 900 mg bid CMV prophylaxis: A: PO: 900 mg once daily	For CMV disease prophylaxis in transplant recipients and CMV retinitis in AIDS patients. Monitor kidney function; may need dose adjustment. Monitor CBC; do not give if ANC <500 cells/mm³. Do not crush or break tablets. Oral solution is not recommended for adults and should not be mixed with other liquids. PB: 1%–2% as ganciclovir; t½: 4.08 h
Antivirals: Hepatitis		
Adefovir	A: PO: 10 mg/d	For chronic HBV, used in combination with lamivudine. Can be taken without regard to food. Monitor renal function. Renal impairment and LFTs require dose adjustment. Monitor HBV DNA. PB: <4%; t½: 7.5 h
Convenience drug pack with ombitasvir/ paritaprevir/ritonavir and dasabuvir	A: PO: 1-day convenience pack with fixed dosage: ombitasvir 12.5 mg, paritaprevir 75 mg, ritonavir 50 mg × 2 tabs and dasabuvir 250 mg × 2 tabs	For HCV with or without cirrhosis. Monitor liver function and HCV RNA concentration. May take with food. Duration of treatment depends on genotype. Combination drug; see individual drugs for PB and t½ information
Entecavir	A: PO: 0.5–1 mg/d	For chronic HBV. Take on an empty stomach. Monitor liver function and HBV DNA viral load. Patients with renal impairment may need dose adjustment. PB: 13%; t½: 128–149 h
Lamivudine	See Chapter 29	Synthetic nucleoside analogue for HBV and HIV
Ledipasvir/sofosbuvir	A: PO: ledipasvir 90 mg/sofosbuvir 400 mg fixed dose tab; 1 tab daily	For chronic HCV; includes patients with other comorbid conditions (e.g., decompensated liver disease, HIV, liver transplant) as combination therapy with sofosbuvir. Monitor liver function, HCV RNA concentration, and renal function. Must be taken with food if coadministering with ribavirin. Duration of treatment depends on genotype; dependent on genotype, ribavirin may be added. Combination drug; see individual drugs for PB and t½ information
Peginterferon alfa-2a	HBV: A: Subcut or IM: 30–35 million units/wk in divided doses × 16 wk HCV: 180 mcg SQ/wk	For HBV and HCV with compensated liver disease. See Chapter 34 for other uses and considerations. If severe reactions occur, reduce dose. For HCV, may be used in combination with ribavirin. Dosage modification required for neutropenia, thrombocytopenia, and kidney dysfunction. PB: UK; t½: 160 h
Ribavirin	Hepatitis C, in combination therapy: A ≥75 kg: PO: 1200 mg/d in 2 divided doses A <75 kg: PO: 1000 mg/d in 2 divided doses Other dosing regimens are available.	Effective for HCV when used as combination therapy with other antivirals. Aerosolized ribavirin therapy requires an experienced clinician. Health care workers should protect eyes when administering aerosol to prevent ocular irritation. Contraindicated during pregnancy. Dosage and duration, as well as coadministration of peginterferon alfa-2a dependent on genotype. Do not open, crush, or chew capsules; give with food. PB: NA; t½: 120–170 h
Sofosbuvir	A: PO: 400 mg once daily	For chronic HCV as combination therapy with ribavirin or peginterferon alfa. Drug combination and treatment duration are dependent on genotype. Monitor HCV RNA concentration and renal function. May be taken without regard to food. PB: 61%–65%; t½: 0.4 h (sofosbuvir) and 27 h (metabolite GS-41203)

TABLE 30.3   Non-HIV Antivirals—cont'd

Generic	Route and Dosage	Uses and Considerations
Tenofovir disoproxil	A: PO: 300 mg once daily.	For chronic HBV. Has an additive or synergistic activity when combined with other antiretroviral agents. PB: Minimally bound; t½: 32 h

A, Adult; *AIDS*, acquired immunodeficiency syndrome; *bid*, twice daily; *CBC*, complete blood count; *CMV*, cytomegalovirus; *gtt*, drops; *h*, hour; *HBV*, hepatitis B virus; *HCV*, hepatitis C virus; *HIV*, human immunodeficiency virus; *HSV*, herpes simplex virus; *IM*, intramuscular; *IV*, intravenous; *max*, maximum; *min*, minutes; *mo*, month; *NA*, not applicable; *Ophthal*, ophthalmic solution; *PB*, protein binding; *PO*, by mouth; *q*, every; *RSV*, respiratory syncytial virus; *subcut*, subcutaneous; *t½*, half-life; *tab*, tablet; *tid*, three times daily; *UK*, unknown; *wk*, weeks; *y*, year; *>*, greater than; *≥*, greater than or equal to; *<*, less than.

📄 PROTOTYPE DRUG CHART

⚡ *Acyclovir*

Drug Class	Dosage
Nucleotide analog antiviral	Herpes genitalis: Initial infection 200 mg 5 times daily for a total of 1 g daily for 10 days. Therapy should be initiated as early as possible following onset of signs and symptoms Herpes zoster: 800 mg 5 times daily for 7 to 10 days. Treatment should be initiated within 72 h of the onset of lesions Chickenpox: 20 mg/kg (not to exceed 800 mg) orally, 4 times daily for 5 days. Therapy should be initiated within 24 h of the appearance of rash

Contraindications	Drug-Lab-Food Interactions
Known hypersensitivity to acyclovir and its components, milk protein hypersensitivity *Caution:* Renal impairment, electrolyte imbalance, dehydration, seizure disorder, crosses placenta; distributed in breast milk, young children	Drug: Increased nephrotoxicity and neurotoxicity with aminoglycosides, probenecid, interferon, and ibuprofen; decreases effect of phenytoin; increases serum concentrations of other antivirals (e.g., tenofovir, entecavir) Lab: May increase AST, ALT, serum creatinine, BUN Food: Food does not affect absorption. Herb: None significant

Pharmacokinetics	Pharmacodynamics
Absorption: PO: Poorly absorbed, 10%–20% Distribution: PB: 9%–33% Metabolism: t½: PO: 2.5–3 h Excretion: Unchanged in urine (90%–92%)	PO: Onset: UK; peak: 2.5–3.3 h; duration: UK IV: Onset: UK; peak: 1 h; duration: UK

Therapeutic Effects/Uses

To treat herpes simplex and varicella-zoster viruses
Mechanism of Action: Inhibits viral DNA synthesis and inhibits viral DNA polymerase and viral DNA chain; inactivates viral DNA polymerase

Side Effects	Adverse Reactions
Nausea, anorexia, vomiting, diarrhea, headache, lethargy, rash	Leukopenia, hepatitis, kidney dysfunction, agitation, hemolytic uremic syndrome, and TTP *Life-threatening:* Coma, seizures, Steven-Johnsons syndrome, toxic epidermal necrolysis, and erythema multiform

A, Adult; *ALT*, alanine aminotransferase; *AST*, aspartate aminotransferase; *BUN*, blood urea nitrogen; *d*, day; *h*, hour; *HSV*, herpes simplex virus; *IV*, intravenous; *mo*, months; *PB*, protein binding; *PO*, by mouth; *q*, every; *t½*, half-life; *UK*, unknown.

Acyclovir, famciclovir, and valacyclovir appear equally effective in the treatment of initial episodes and recurrent episodes of genital herpes, but famciclovir appears somewhat less effective for suppression of viral shedding. Topical antivirals for herpes simplex viruses include acyclovir, penciclovir, and trifluridine.

Cytomegalovirus Antivirals

Four antivirals are effective in treating CMV retinitis in persons with acquired immunodeficiency syndrome (AIDS): ganciclovir, valganciclovir, cidofovir, and foscarnet. Ganciclovir and valganciclovir are synthetic purine nucleoside analogues. Ganciclovir was the first

CLINICAL JUDGMENT [NURSING PROCESS]

Antiviral: Acyclovir

Concept: Infection
- The introduction of pathogen eliciting an immune response.

Concept: Safety
- Protection of the patient from potential or actual harm; is a basic human need

Recognize Cues [Assessment]
- Obtain a medical history from the patient that includes any serious renal or hepatic diseases.
- Determine baseline vital signs and obtain a complete blood count (CBC). Use these findings for comparisons with future results.
- Assess baseline laboratory results, particularly blood urea nitrogen (BUN), serum creatinine, liver function studies, bilirubin, and electrolytes. Use these results for future comparisons.
- Evaluate baseline vital signs and urine output. Report abnormal findings.

Analyze Cues and Prioritize Hypothesis [Patient Problems]
- Decreased immunity

Generate Solutions [Planning]
- Patient will exhibit decreased symptoms of viral infections.

Take Action [Nursing Interventions]
- Check the patient's CBC. Report abnormal results (leukopenia, thrombocytopenia, low hemoglobin and hematocrit).
- Monitor other laboratory tests (BUN, serum creatinine, liver function studies); compare with baseline values.
- Record the patient's urinary output. An antiviral drug such as acyclovir can affect renal function.
- Monitor vital signs, especially blood pressure. Acyclovir and amantadine may cause orthostatic hypotension.
- Observe for signs and symptoms of side effects. Most antiviral drugs have many side effects.

- Check for superimposed infection (superinfection) caused by high doses and prolonged use of an antiviral drug such as acyclovir.
- Administer oral acyclovir as prescribed. Oral doses can be taken at mealtime.
- Dilute the antiviral drug in an appropriate amount of solution as indicated in the drug circular when giving intravenously. Administer intravenous (IV) drug over 60 minutes. Never give acyclovir as a bolus (IV push).
- Advise patients to maintain adequate fluid intake to ensure sufficient hydration for drug therapy and to increase urine output.
- Instruct patients with genital herpes to avoid spreading infection by practicing sexual abstinence or by using condoms correctly and consistently. Patients must be aware that although condoms reduce the transmission of disease, they may not eliminate it. Advise women with genital herpes to have a Pap test done as indicated by their health care provider. Cervical cancer is more prevalent in women with genital herpes simplex.
- Teach non-English-speaking patients and family members how to properly use antivirals by providing materials in the patient's first language. Pictures may be helpful.
- Guide patients to report adverse reactions, including a decrease in urine output and central nervous system (CNS) changes such as dizziness, anxiety, or confusion.
- Warn patients with dizziness resulting from orthostatic hypotension to arise slowly from a sitting to a standing position.
- Tell patients to report any side effects associated with the antiviral drug; this may include nausea and vomiting, diarrhea, increased bleeding time, rash, urticaria, and menstrual abnormalities.

Evaluate Outcomes [Evaluation]
- Evaluate the effectiveness of the antiviral drug in eliminating the virus or in decreasing symptoms.
- Determine whether any side effects are present.

---

drug approved for treatment of CMV retinitis. Cidofovir is a nucleotide analogue that suppresses viral replication by inhibiting DNA polymerase. Foscarnet selectively inhibits viral-specific DNA polymerases and reverse transcriptases. Due to the emergence of drug resistance, many times it is necessary to use a combination of agents to effectively manage CMV retinitis (Prototype Drug Chart: Acyclovir Sodium).

Side Effects and Adverse Reactions

A limiting factor in all antiviral therapy for CMV and herpes is hematologic toxicity. All patients should be closely monitored for signs of bone marrow suppression and toxicity, including thrombocytopenia, granulocytopenia, and leukopenia. Additionally, all antivirals should be dose adjusted in the setting of kidney dysfunction. Kidney function should be closely monitored during drug therapy because acute kidney failure can occur.

Side effects and adverse reactions to antiviral drugs include nausea, vomiting, and diarrhea; headache; dizziness; rash and pruritus; and hematuria. Additionally, when antiviral drugs are administered IV, extravasation may lead to sloughing of the skin. Topical preparations can cause local irritations, and contact lenses should be removed before instilling ophthalmic antivirals.

Hepatitis Antivirals

Viral hepatitis can be caused by at least five distinct viruses that affect the liver: hepatitis A virus (HAV), HBV, HCV, hepatitis D (delta hepatitis, HDV), and hepatitis E. Hepatitis A and E are self-limiting

illnesses and do not usually require antiviral therapy. HBV and HCV can develop into chronic hepatitis; those with HBV can be coinfected with HDV. The CDC and the World Health Organization (WHO) have developed guidelines for screening, treatment, and surveillance of persons with HBV and HCV. Currently, HAV and HBV are vaccine preventable. Vaccines are discussed in Chapter 31.

No specific therapy exists for people with acute HBV. Instead, treatment is mostly supportive. Antivirals are given for people with chronic HBV and signs of liver disease progression to attempt to suppress viral replication and potentially halt liver disease and liver-related deaths. Treatment with antivirals is recommended for all people with chronic HBV who are at high risk of disease progression regardless of age. Currently, five antiviral drugs are approved for this indication: lamivudine, adefovir, entecavir, tenofovir, and peginterferon alfa-2a. Except for peginterferon alfa-2a, all of these are nucleoside analogues, and all have been shown to delay the progression of liver disease (e.g., cirrhosis, hepatic carcinoma). Adefovir inhibits reverse transcription, entecavir inhibits several major stages of viral replication, and lamivudine and tenofovir inhibit the synthesis of viral DNA; however, no antiviral therapy cures HBV. Lamivudine and adefovir are no longer the preferred agents in the treatment of HBV.

Hepatitis C is more prevalent among people who inject drugs. HCV is an RNA virus, whereas HBV is a DNA virus. As with HBV, HCV can cause chronic infection that leads to liver cirrhosis, liver failure, and hepatic carcinoma. No vaccine against HCV is currently available. In addition to peginterferon alfa-2a, NS5A inhibitors (e.g., ledipasvir) and polymerase inhibitors (e.g., sofosbuvir) can treat HCV. Many of these antivirals are prepackaged as combination therapy.

Persons with HCV should have genotype testing; HCV has 6 genotypes and more than 50 subtypes, and genotyping can help predict treatment response and duration of treatment. For example, genotypes 2 and 3 respond better to peginterferon alfa-2a or a combination of peginterferon alfa-2a and ribavirin than does genotype 1. Genotypes 2 and 3 only need 24 months of treatment, whereas genotype 1 requires 48 months. Genotype 1 is the most common genotype in the United States. The Infectious Diseases Society of America (IDSA) and the American Association for the Study of Liver Diseases (AASLD) have published treatment guidelines based on genotype (see https://www.hcvguidelines.org).

Table 30.3 lists the antivirals, uses, and considerations for viral hepatitis. Chapter 29 further illustrates nucleoside analogues.

Side Effects and Adverse Effects

Side effects range from mild to life threatening. Transient exacerbations of viral hepatitis can occur if antivirals are suddenly stopped. HBV and HCV can become resistant to antivirals; therefore routine monitoring of renal and hepatic functions are warranted in addition to monitoring viral load. Nucleoside analogues can cause hepatotoxicity or lactic acidosis, and dose adjustments are recommended in patients with renal impairment. Side effects for peginterferon include depression, fatigue, flulike symptoms, pancytopenia, alopecia, arthralgia, myalgia, anorexia, dysgeusia, thyroid dysfunction, and infection. Ophthalmic dysfunction can also occur (e.g., papilledema, vasculature obstruction). Ribavirin is teratogenic and can also cause hemolytic anemia, and protease inhibitors can cause skin reactions, dysgeusia, and photosensitivity.

CRITICAL THINKING CASE STUDY

A 41-year-old homeless man has had a constant cough and night sweats for several months. He consumes about a fifth of liquor over 2 days. Acid-fast bacilli (AFB) smear on the sputum is positive. The health care provider orders a 6- to 9-month antitubercular drug regimen, with the time of therapy to be determined according to sputum and radiograph test results. For 2 months, the patient takes isoniazid (INH), rifampin, and pyrazinamide daily. For the next 4 to 7 months, he takes INH and rifampin biweekly.

1. What are some of the patient's risk factors for contracting tuberculosis (TB)? Give other risk factors for contracting TB.
2. The patient received first-line antitubercular drugs for treatment of TB. How can the health professional determine whether the drugs are effective in eradicating the bacillus *Mycobacterium tuberculosis*? Explain your answer.
3. What is the nurse's role in patient teaching concerning the drug regimen?
4. Name at least two serious adverse reactions that can occur when antitubercular drugs are given over an extended period.
5. What laboratory tests should be monitored while the patient takes isoniazid and rifampin? Why?
6. The health care provider orders pyridoxine to be given daily. Give the rationale for the use of pyridoxine.

REVIEW QUESTIONS

1. A patient is beginning isoniazid and rifampin treatment for tuberculosis. The nurse gives the patient which instruction?
   a. Do not skip doses.
   b. Take both drugs three times daily.
   c. Take an antacid with the drugs.
   d. Take rifampin initially.
2. A patient taking isoniazid is worried about the negative effects of the drug. The nurse provides information knowing that which is an adverse effect of the drug?
   a. Ototoxicity
   b. Hepatotoxicity
   c. Nephrotoxicity
   d. Optic nerve toxicity
3. The nurse teaches a patient taking amphotericin B to report which signs and symptoms to the health care provider?
   a. Change in sight
   b. Decrease in hearing
   c. Decrease in urine
   d. Painful red rash and blisters
4. A patient has been diagnosed with tuberculosis and is to begin antitubercular therapy with isoniazid, rifampin, and ethambutol. Which actions are appropriate for the nurse to do? (Select all that apply.)
   a. Encourage periodic eye examinations.
   b. Instruct the patient to take medications with meals.
   c. Suggest that the patient take antacids with medications to prevent gastrointestinal distress.
   d. Advise the patient to report numbness and tingling of the hands or feet.
   e. Alert the patient that body fluids may develop a red-orange color.
   f. Teach the patient to avoid direct sunlight and to use sunblock.

5. Zanamivir is ordered for a patient with which disorder?
   a. Herpes simplex virus type 2
   b. Herpes simplex virus type 1
   c. Varicella-zoster virus
   d. Hepatitis B virus
6. Acyclovir has been ordered for a patient with genital herpes. Which nursing interventions are appropriate for this patient? (Select all that apply.)
   a. Monitor the patient's blood urea nitrogen and creatinine.
   b. Monitor the patient's blood pressure for hypertension.
   c. Administer intravenous acyclovir over 30 minutes.
   d. Advise maintenance of adequate fluid intake.
   e. Monitor complete blood count for blood dyscrasias.
7. A mother of two children was just diagnosed with hepatitis C virus. Which of the following is *incorrect* about hepatitis C virus?
   a. A vaccine has been available for 5 years.
   b. Hepatitis C virus can be transmitted by blood and body fluids.
   c. Hepatitis C virus can cause hepatic carcinoma.
   d. Persons with hepatitis C virus can become chronic carriers.

31

Antimalarials, Anthelmintics, and Peptides

OBJECTIVES

- Explain the two-phase parasitic process in transmission of the action of antimalarial drugs in people with malaria.
- Identify side effects and adverse reactions of people responding to antimalarial drugs.
- Correlate preventive measures with a safe and protective environment for people at risk for malaria.
- Apply the Clinical Judgment [Nursing Process], including patient teaching of route and side effects for people receiving antimalarial drugs.
- Describe the transmission of helminths in people infected with cestodes and nematodes.
- Identify the side effects and adverse reactions of anthelmintic drugs.

- Correlate transmission with prevention in people with helminthic infections.
- Apply the Clinical Judgment [Nursing Process] for people receiving anthelmintic drugs including patient teaching on protective measures during self-management.
- Discuss effects of peptides in antibiotic-resistant bacteria.
- Summarize the side effects and adverse reactions of peptides used as microbials including colistimethate, polymyxins, bacitracin, and metronidazole.
- Apply the Clinical Judgment [Nursing Process] for people taking antimicrobial peptides.

OUTLINE

ANTIMALARIAL DRUGS

Malaria is a life-threatening disease that was eliminated from the U.S. in the early 1950s. Since that time, about 2,000 cases of malaria have been diagnosed each year in the U.S. In 2018 an estimated 228 million cases of malaria occurred worldwide and 405,000 people died, mostly children in the sub-Saharan African region. Malaria is caused by multiple species of protozoan parasites of the genus *Plasmodium* that are carried by infected *Anopheles* mosquitoes, and it remains one of the most prevalent protozoan diseases. After the mosquito infects the human, the protozoan parasite passes through two phases: the tissue phase and the erythrocytic phase. The tissue phase (invasion of body tissue) produces no clinical symptoms in the human, but the erythrocytic phase (invasion of the red blood cells) causes symptoms of chills, fever, and sweating. The incubation period is 10 to 35 days, followed by flulike symptoms. Preventing transmission of malaria can be done by controlling the mosquito first through insecticide-treated mosquito nets and second with spraying.

There are approximately 50 species of *Plasmodium,* four of which cause malaria: *P. malariae, P. ovale, P. vivax,* and *P. falciparum. P. vivax* is the most prevalent, whereas *P. falciparum* is the most severe. In spite of having more than 200 million cases of malaria globally, in the United States malaria is confined mainly to persons who enter the country after having

traveled abroad, primarily because of travel to regions in the world where malaria is endemic and drug-resistant malaria parasites have evolved.

Treatment of malaria depends on the type of *Plasmodium* and the organism's life cycle. Quinine was the only antimalarial drug available from 1820 until the early 1940s. Antimalarial drugs provide treatment and prophylaxis, and synthetic antimalarial drugs have since been developed that are as effective as quinine and cause fewer toxic effects. When drug-resistant malaria occurs, combinations of antimalarials are used to facilitate effective treatment. Chloroquine is a commonly prescribed drug for malaria. Antimicrobial resistance to chloroquine therapy is widespread, so it is critical to determine whether chloroquine is appropriate for use. If drug resistance occurs to chloroquine, another antimalarial such as mefloquine hydrochloride (HCl) or combinations of antimalarials with or without antibiotics (e.g., tetracycline, doxycycline, clindamycin) may be prescribed.

Three methods used to eradicate malaria are prophylaxis (prevention), treatment for the acute attack, and prevention of relapse. Many synthetic antimalarials, chloroquine and primaquine among them, are used prophylactically. Chloroquine and mefloquine are frequently used to treat an acute malarial attack. Mefloquine HCl and the combination drug atovaquone-proguanil are used to treat chloroquine-resistant *P.*

PROTOTYPE DRUG CHART

Chloroquine Phosphate

Drug Class	Dosage
Antimalarial	Malaria treatment (uncomplicated): A: PO: 16.6 mg (10 mg base)/kg/dose PO once (*max:* 1000 mg/dose [600 mg base/dose]), then 8.3 mg (5 mg/base)/kg/dose PO in 6 to 8h (*max:* 500 mg/dose [300 mg base/dose]), then 8.3 mg (5 mg base)/kg/dose PO once daily for 2 days (*max:* 500 mg/dose [300 mg base/dose]). For *P. vivax* or *P. ovale*, give in combination with primaquine phosphate. Malaria prophylaxis: A: PO: 500 mg (300 mg base)/wk on same day of each wk, starting 2 wk before entering the endemic area and continuing for 8 wk after leaving the area. *max:* A: PO: 1000 mg/d (600 mg base/d)

Contraindications	Drug-Lab-Food Interactions
Chloroquine hypersensitivity and ocular disease (retinal and visual field changes) *Caution:* Cardiac disease, renal disease, psoriasis, alcoholism, G6PD deficiency, hepatic disease, GI disease, neurologic disorders (seizures, hearing impairment), and hypoglycemia	Use appropriately to avoid chloroquine antimicrobial resistance Multiple drug-drug interactions; please refer to drug reference Drug: Increases effects of digoxin, neuromuscular blockers; decreased absorption with antacids and laxatives Monitor Labs: Blood glucose, CBC, and ECG Food: Take with food to avoid GI upset

Pharmacokinetics	Pharmacodynamics
Absorption: Well absorbed from GI tract Distribution: Widely distributed into body tissue PB: 55% Metabolism: Partially in the liver Half-life:1–2 mo Excretion: Excreted slowly in urine, feces, breast milk; crosses placenta	Onset: Rapid Peak: 1–2 h Duration: Days to weeks

Therapeutic Effects/Uses

Treatment and prophylaxis of uncomplicated malaria due to susceptible strains of *P. falciparum, P. knowlesi, P. ovale, P. malariae,* and *P. vivax.* Chloroquine phosphate is under investigation and is not recommended for treatment of severe acute respiratory syndrome coronavirus 2 (SARS-CoV-2), the virus that causes coronavirus disease 2019 (COVID-19).

Mechanism of Action: Inhibits parasite replication, transcription of DNA to RNA by forming complexes with DNA of parasite

Side Effects	Adverse Reactions
Anorexia, nausea, vomiting, diarrhea, abdominal cramps, fatigue, pruritus, headache, nervousness, visual impairment, insomnia, photosensitivity, hair discoloration, skin and eyes may appear yellowish	Heart block and cardiac arrhythmia, ECG changes, hypotension, psychosis, dermatologic reactions (pruritus, urticaria), seizures; may cause dizziness, so use caution driving a vehicle; avoid sun exposure Extrapyramidal reaction, Stevens-Johnson syndrome, toxic epidermal necrolysis, DRESS syndrome *Life-threatening:* Loss of consciousness, agranulocytosis, aplastic anemia, corneal opacity, macular degeneration, thrombocytopenia, ototoxicity, cardiovascular collapse, anaphylactic shock

A, Adult; *CBC,* complete blood count; *DNA,* deoxyribonucleic acid; *ECG,* electrocardiogram; *G6PD,* glucose-6-phosphate dehydrogenase; *GI,* gastrointestinal; *h,* hour; *mo,* month; *PB,* protein binding; *PO,* by mouth; *RBC,* red blood cell; *RNA,* ribonucleic acid; *wk,* week.

falciparum. Both chloroquine and hydroxychloroquine may also have activity against severe acute respiratory syndrome conronavirus 2 (SARS-CoV-2). Both are under investigational use for SARS-CoV-2, the virus that causes coronavirus disease 2019 (COVID-19). Data are limited and efficacy has not been established. The National Institute of Health (NIH) COVID-19 treatment guidelines recommend against the use of both chloroquine and hydroxychloroquine for treatment of COVID-19. The Federal Drug Administration (FDA) has revoked the Emergency Use Authorization (EUA) of both chloroquine and hydroxychloroquine. The Prototype Drug Chart: Chloroquine Phosphate lists the drug data for chloroquine phosphate.

Pharmacokinetics. Chloroquine phosphate is well absorbed from the gastrointestinal (GI) tract. It is moderately protein binding, and the drug has a long half-life. Because of the drug's long half-life, the first two doses have a loading dose effect. After the initial loading dose is administered, the next dose is followed at 6 to 8 h after the first dose. The third and fourth doses are given at 24 h, respectively. Chloroquine is metabolized in the liver to active metabolites and is largely excreted in the urine, with small amounts in the feces. The elimination half-life is 108–291 h. This drug has two absolute contraindications: chloroquine hypersensitivity and ocular disease. Antimalarial drugs concentrate first in the liver; if the patient drinks large amounts of alcohol or has a liver disorder, the liver enzymes will require closer monitoring. Renal impairment may also occur as an adverse effect of antimalarials.

Pharmacodynamics. Chloroquine phosphate inhibits the malaria parasite's growth by interfering with its protein synthesis. Whether the drug is given orally or intramuscularly (IM), the onset of action is rapid. The peak effect is slower when given orally. The duration of effect of the drug is very long, from days to weeks.

Side Effects and Adverse Reactions

General side effects and adverse reactions to antimalarials include GI upset, retinal damage, cranial nerve VIII involvement (quinine and chloroquine), renal impairment (quinine), and cardiovascular effects (quinine).

Table 31.1 lists commonly ordered antimalarial drugs and their dosage, uses, and considerations. Note that *quinine* is an antimalarial

TABLE 31.1 **Antimalarials**

Generic	Route and Dosage	Uses and Considerations
Artesunate	A: IV: 2.4 mg/kg/dose administered at 0, 12, and 24 h, and thereafter, once daily until able to switch to oral therapy. For patients who cannot tolerate oral therapy, continue for a total of 7 days or switch to IV doxycycline or clindamycin for 7 days; *max:* A: IV: 2.4 mg/kg/dose IV.	Used to treat severe malaria and active against microorganism strains of *P. falciparium, P. malariae, P. ovale, P. sp,* and *P. vivax.* Caution: Breastfeeding and pregnancy; contraindicated in hypersensitivity to drug. Monitor: CBC during treatment and × 4 wk after d/c PB: 93%; t½: 0.3 h
Chloroquine phosphate	See Prototype Drug Chart: Chloroquine Phosphate	
Hydroxychloroquine sulfate	Malaria: A: PO: 800 mg (620 mg base), then 400 mg (310 mg base) dose at 6, 24, 48 h after initial dose for a total dose of 2,000 mg (1,550 mg base). *max:* A: PO: 80 mg/dose (620 mg base dose) for malaria up to a total of 2,000 mg (1,500 mg base) in 48 h. Malaria prophylaxis: A: PO: 400 mg (310 mg base) dose wk on the same day of each wk, starting 1 to 2 wk before entering the endemic area and continuing for 4 wk after leaving the area. *max:* A: PO: 400 mg/wk (310 mg base/wk).	Used to treat and prevent malaria due to susceptible strains of *P. falciparum, P. vivax, P. malariae, P. ovale,* and *P. knowlesi;* also an alternative to chloroquine sensitivity. Dosage varies for treating malaria. Recommend concomitant use with primaquine. Give with meals or milk to reduce GI distress *Caution:* During pregnancy, in patients with psoriasis, renal impairment, or ocular disturbances, and with history of alcoholism or hepatic impairment. Can cause sensorimotor disorder including neuropathy, GI upset, cardiomyopathy, hypoglycemia, and suicidal ideation Consider monitoring complete blood count (CBC), electrocardiogram (ECG), and ophthalmologic examination PB: 45%; t½: 32–50 d
Mefloquine hydrochloride	A: PO: 1250 mg as a single dose or, alternately, 750 mg as initial dose, then 500 mg 6–12 hours after initial dose Malaria prophylaxis: A: PO: 250 mg PO weekly on the same day of each week for 1–2 wk before travel, then weekly during travel, and 4 wk after leaving endemic area. *Max:* A: PO: 1250 mg once for treatment or 250 mg once/wk for prophylaxis.	Used for treatment of malaria prophylaxis or for treatment of susceptible strains of malaria. It is the treatment of choice for malaria in the United States Contraindicated in people with cardiac conditions, seizures, psychosis, and hepatic disease 〔!〕 Psychiatric Event Absolute contraindications: Anxiety, depression, melfloquine, quinidine, or quinine hypersensitivities, psychosis, schizophrenia, and seizures Safety/Monitoring: Ophthalmic exam; LFTs, neurologic exams if long-term use Is secreted in breast milk. PB: 98%; t½: 13–33 d Not recommended in travel to Southeast Asia.
Primaquine phosphate	Malaria: A: PO: 52.6 mg (30 mg base) × 14 days in combination with chloroquine Malaria prophylaxis: A: PO: 52.6 mg (30 mg base) × 2 days before entering malaria-risk area continue during travel then 7 days after leaving the endemic area. *Max:* A: PO: 15 mg base daily; however, higher doses of 30 mg base daily have been used	Used to treat malaria caused by *Plasmodium vivax, P. ovale,* and *P. falciparum.* Also, for Malaria Prevention of Relapse Adverse reactions: GI distress, rash WBC production (granulocytopenia), cardiac arrhythmias, acute hemolytic anemia in patients with G6PD deficiency Pregnancy test at baseline, CBC, ECG if risk of prolonged QT interval Contraindications: Cardiac disease, rheumatoid arthritis, pregnancy, systemic lupus erythematosus (SLE) PB: UK; t½: 6 h

TABLE 31.1 Antimalarials—cont'd

Generic	Route and Dosage	Uses and Considerations
Quinine sulfate	Severe malaria (prior to the start of IV artesunate): A: PO: 650 mg every 8 h. Discontinue when IV artesunate is started. Uncomplicated malaria: A: PO: 648–650 mg every 8 h for 3 d *Max:* A: PO: 1944 mg/d for uncomplicated and severe malaria	Used to treat malaria caused by *P. falciparum* including chloroquine-resistant strains and chloroquine-resistant strains of *P. vivax* Combination drug therapy includes tetracycline, clindamycin, or doxycycline. **!** **Black Box Warning:** Muscular cramps Absolute Contraindications: Blackwater fever, hemolytic-uremic syndrome, long QT syndrome, mefloquine, quinine, and quinidine hypersentivities, myasthenia gravis, optic neuritis, QT prologation, thrombocytopenia, and thrombotic thrombocytopenic purpura PB: 70%; t½: 8–21 h
Combination Antimalarial Drugs		
Atovaquone; Proguanil	Malaria: A: PO: 4 tabs (250 mg atovaquone; 100 mg proguanil per tablet) once d for 3 consecutive days Malaria prophylaxis: A: PO: 1 tab (250 mg atovaquone; 100 mg proguanil per tab) for a day. Begin 1–2 d before entering endemic area. Continue daily during the stay and for 7 days after leaving the area *Max:* A: PO: total of atovaquone 250 mg/100 mg (1 tablet) proguanil per day PO for prophylaxis; 1 g/400 mg proguanil (4 tablets) per day PO for treatment (3 days only) C: PO: 21–30 kg 2 tablets/d; begin 2 days before entering; continue daily during the stay and for 7 days after leaving the area	For acute and uncomplicated prophylaxis and treatment of malaria due to *P. falciparum* or *P. vivax;* effective for chloroquine-resistant strains Not administered with known hypersensitivity to atovaquone or proguanil Adverse reactions: GI distress, elevated hepatic enzymes, headache, insomnia, visual disturbances Take with food or milk at same time each day *Caution:* Renal and hepatic impairment PB: 75%–99%; t½: 2–3 d/12–21 h
Artemether; Lumefantrine	Acute, uncomplicated malaria: A: PO: 4 tablets (20 mg artemether; 120 mg lumefantrine per tablet) as initial dose and 4 tablets at 8 h after initial dose, then 4 tablets twice daily (morning and evening) for 2 d for a total course of 24 tablets. *Max:* A: PO: 3 g or more: 8 tabs/d	Used to treat malaria in patients with acute, uncomplicated infections due to *P. falciparum* Adverse Effects: Abdominal pain, arthralgia, chills, fever, peptic ulcer disease, proteinuria, ataxia, wheezing, anorexia, palpitations, and hepatomegaly. Caution in breastfeeding PB: 95.4%/99.7%; t½: 2–3 h/3–6 d

A, Adult; *Adol,*adolescent; *C*, child; *CBC*, complete blood count; *d*, day; *d/c*, discharge; *G-6-PD*, glucose-6-phosphate dehydrogenase; *GI*, gastrointestinal; *h*, hour; *IV*, intravenous; *LFT*, Liver function test; *max*, maximum; *P*, plasmodium; *PB*, protein binding; *PO*, by mouth; *q*, every; *t½*, half-life; *tabs*, tablets; *UK*, unknown; *WBC*, white blood cell; *wk*, week; *y*, year; *>*, greater than; *<*, less than.

drug and *quinidine* is an antidysrhythmic drug. A medication guideline developed by the US Food and Drug Administration (FDA) accompanies mefloquine each time it is dispensed. This type of guideline is used only for drugs that require monitoring for serious adverse effects. Adverse effects of mefloquine include severe anxiety, restlessness, disorientation, depression, hallucinations, paranoia, and suicidal thoughts, which may continue after the drug is discontinued. The manufacturer of malarial drugs indicates these drugs have been shown active against most strains of microorganisms either in vitro and/or in clinical infections. However, the safety and effectiveness in treating clinical infections due to organisms in vitro data have not been established in adequate and well-controlled clinical trials.

> ⚡ **PATIENT SAFETY**
>
> **Do not Confuse...**
> * **Quinine** (antimalarial) with **quinidine** (antidysrhythmic).
> * **Hydroxychloroquine** (antimalarial drug) and **hydroxyurea** (chemotherapy drug).

ANTHELMINTIC DRUGS

Helminths are parasitic worms that cause disease worldwide. Transmission occurs in areas of poor sanitation and hygiene from infected soil to the person, whereupon the helminth then feeds on host tissue (Centers for Disease Control and Prevention [CDC], 2020). Helminth infection affects the host's immunity resulting in disability in the host and, if left untreated, causes developmental delays in children. The most common site for helminthiasis (worm infection) is the intestine. Other sites for parasitic infection are the lymphatic system, blood vessels, and liver.

Classification of helminths includes (1) cestodes (tapeworms), (2) trematodes (flukes), (3) intestinal nematodes (roundworms), and (4) extraintestinal tissue-invading nematodes (trichinosis, onchocerciasis, and filariae). They enter the human host via contaminated food, bites of carrier insects, or direct penetration of the skin.

The cestodes (tapeworms) enter the intestine via contaminated food and attach to the intestinal wall. There are four types of cestodes: *Taenia solium* (pork tapeworm), *T. saginata* (beef tapeworm), *Diphyllobothrium latum* (fish tapeworm), and *Hymenolepis nana* (dwarf tapeworm). Cestodes have heads and hooks or suckers that attach to the tissue.

The trematodes (flukes) are flat parasites that feed on the host and include *Fasciola hepatica* (liver fluke), which inhabits the biliary track; *Fasciolopsis buski* (intestinal fluke) common in Southeast Asia; *Paragonimus westermani* (lung fluke); and *Schistosoma* species (blood flukes), which are acquired outside the US.

Intestinal nematodes infect and feed on intestinal tissue: *Ascaris lumbricoides* (giant roundworm) are prevalent worldwide, *Necator americanus* (hookworm) are common in rural areas, *Enterobius vermicularis* (pinworm) are most common in the US, *Strongyloides stercoralis* (threadworm) are common in the southern US, and *Trichuris trichiura* (whipworm) are common worldwide.

Extraintestinal nematodes are tissue-invading: *Trichinella spiralis* (pork roundworm) can cause trichinosis, a disease caused by ingestion of raw or inadequately cooked pork that contains larvae of the *T. spiralis* parasite, which can be diagnosed by muscle biopsy. By thoroughly cooking pork, the roundworm is destroyed. *Onchocerciasis volvulus* (river blindness) is transmitted by an infected fly causing worm-filled skin lesions and ocular lesions leading to blindness.

Side Effects and Adverse Reactions

The common side effects of anthelmintics (agents that destroy worms) include various manifestations of GI distress, such as anorexia, nausea, vomiting, and occasionally diarrhea and stomach cramps. The neurologic problems associated with anthelmintics are dizziness, weakness, headache, and drowsiness. Adverse reactions do not occur frequently because the drugs usually are given for a short period (1 to 3 days). Prototype Drug Chart: Ivermectin lists dosages and drug data for ivermectin, and Table 31.2 lists anthelmintic drugs prescribed to treat various types of parasitic worms.

PEPTIDES

Antimicrobial peptides (AMPs) are broad-spectrum, powerful defenses that kill parasites, fungi, and viruses. The Center for

---

⊚ CLINICAL JUDGMENT [NURSING PROCESS]

Antimalarials

Concept: Infection
- Invasion and growth of malaria parasitic microorganism in body tissues resulting in cellular infection and destruction

Concept: Nutrition
- Optimal cellular metabolism during antimalarial prophylaxis and treatment

Concept: Immunity
- Protective physiologic response to the malarial protozoa

Recognize Cues [Assessment]
- Assess patient's hearing by establishing an auditory baseline and hearing tests at scheduled intervals. Drugs such as quinine or chloroquine may affect cranial nerve VIII.
- Assess patient for visual changes including establishing a baseline and then checking vision at scheduled intervals.
- Note patient's level of consciousness.
- Secure a history of whether the patient has traveled out of the country to a malaria-endemic area.
- Obtain a patient history of malaria and whether antimalarial drugs were taken.
- Note renal function by assessing urinary color, output (>600 mL/day), and blood urea nitrogen (BUN).
- Assess patient for presence of allergies including skin rash, tissue swelling, and altered ventilation.
- Monitor electrocardiogram (ECG).

Analyze Cues and Prioritize Hypothesis [Patient Problems]
- Decreased visual acuity
- Decreased level of consciousness
- Decreased immunity
- Need for health teaching
- Skin rash with pruritus
- Diarrhea
- Nausea and vomiting

Generate Solutions [Planning]
- Patient will exhibit vital signs at baseline level showing absence of malarial symptoms.
- Patient will take antimalarial drugs at the times and dosages prescribed.

- Patient will use preventive measures when in the outside environment.

Take Action [Nursing Interventions]
- ⚡ Monitor renal and liver function by checking urine output (>600 mL/d) and liver enzymes.
- ⚡ Report if the patient's serum liver enzymes are elevated and if renal function tests are abnormal.
- Observe the patient for side effects and adverse reactions from antimalarial drugs such as chloroquine and quinine; impaired consciousness, headache, or seizures; ventricular fibrillation monitored by ECG; and skeletal muscle weakness.
- Identify home-based safety measures to avoid injuries during periods of weakness, decreased vision, and difficulty hearing.

Patient Teaching
- Advise patient traveling to malaria-endemic countries to receive prophylactic doses of an antimalarial drug before leaving, during the visit, and upon their return.
- Teach patient to take oral antimalarial drugs with food or at mealtime if gastrointestinal (GI) upset occurs.
- Monitor patient returning from malaria-endemic areas for malarial symptoms of nausea, vomiting, diarrhea, abdominal cramps, pruritus, visual changes, and dizziness.
- Inform patient who takes chloroquine or hydroxychloroquine to report vision changes immediately, such as blurred and low vision, redness, and irritation.
- Provide patients with information on herbal supplements that may be harmful when taking prescribed medications.

Side Effects
- Direct patients to report signs and symptoms of anorexia, nausea, vomiting, diarrhea, abdominal cramps, pruritus, visual disturbances, hearing loss, and dizziness.

Evaluate Outcomes [Evaluation]
- Evaluate the effectiveness of the antimalarial drug by determining that the patient is free of symptoms.
- Evaluate the patient's self-management in prophylaxis and medication regimen.

PROTOTYPE DRUG CHART

Ivermectin

Drug Class	Dosage
Broad-spectrum anthelmintic (antiparasitic)	Administered topically and orally Onchocerciasis: A: PO: Doses are prescribed to provide approx 150 mcg/kg as a single dose Repeated doses may be necessary Dosage based on weight. Strongyloidiasis: A: PO: 200 mcg/kg single dose Doses are based on weight Follow up treatment is required Pediculosis capitis: A: Topical: 1 tube Follow instructions on tube Pediculosis corporis: A :PO: 20 to 40 mcg/kg/dose for 2 doses, administer 7 days apart
Contraindications	**Drug-Lab-Food Interactions**
Contraindicated for those hypersensitive to the drug's components. *Caution:* Asthma, hepatic impairment, and immunosuppression; not recommended with breastfeeding	Drug: Use with caution with aprepitant or fosaprepitant. Do not use with ceritinib, idelalisib, and mirabegron. Mitotane decreases effectiveness; boceprevir, posaconazole, and telaprevir increases risk of toxicity; may increase INR when used concurrently with warfarin Food: Take on an empty stomach with water Lab: Monitor ophthalmic examinations; obtain and monitor stool examinations, ALT, AST, and pregnancy testing
Pharmacokinetics	**Pharmacodynamics**
Absorption: Well absorbed Distribution: Widely distributed within the body; does not cross blood-brain barrier Half-life: 16–28 h Metabolism: Liver; PB: 93%; t½ 16–28 h Excretion: In feces (over 12 d) and urine (<1%)	Peak: 4 h Onset: UK Duration: UK
Therapeutic Effects/Uses	
An antiparasitic agent, drug of choice for strongloidiasis and onchoerciasis. Used topically for pediculosis capitis. Mechanism of Action: Binds with chloride ions, increases cell permeability to kill parasite	
Side Effects	**Adverse Reactions**
Pruritus, urticaria, fever, arthralgia, dizziness, diarrhea, nausea, skin irritation, xerosis, ocular irritation, back pain, lethargy, rash, asthenia, fatigue, vomiting, anorexia, abdominal pain, vertigo, tremor, drowsiness	Angioedema, Stevens-Johnson syndrome, toxic epidermal necrolysis, seizures, ocular hemorrhage, coma, keratitis, uveitis, visual impairment

A, adult; *ALT,* alanine aminotransferase;*AST,* aspartate aminotransferase; *d,* day; *h,* hour; *PB,* protein binding; *PO,* by mouth; <, less than; >, greater than.

Communicable Disease, a governmental health agency that prevents and reduces communicable diseases in the United States and globally, has launched an initiative for health care providers and patients to prevent drug-resistant infection. There is ongoing research in combining antibiotics as multidrug regimens, which in turn can reduce antibiotic resistance. Mismanagement of antibiotics has created an increased antibiotic resistance whereby a drug is no longer able to treat a disease. Examples include methicillin-resistant *Staphylococcus aureus* (MRSA) and carbapenem-resistant *Enterobacteriaceae* (CRE), *Clostridium difficile* (C. Diff), and *vancomycin-resistant entercocci* (VRE).

Peptide classifications include antiviral, antimicrobial, antifungal, and antiparasitic. The two groups of peptides used as antibiotics are the polymyxins and bacitracin. Peptides are derived from cultures of *Bacillus subtilis,* and this group appears to weaken the bacterial cell membrane function causing cell death.

Colistimethate

Colistimethate is a polypeptide antibiotic that targets aerobic gram-negative bacteria. It is used to treat *Pseudomonas aeruginosa,* CRE, and *Klebsiella* and *Shigella* species. This antibiotic has the capacity to penetrate and disrupt the bacterial cell. Colistimethate is available in forms administered IM, intravenously (IV), and by inhalation. Common reactions include dyspepsia, tingling, slurred speech, dizziness, paresthesia, pruritus, rash, and fever. Serious reactions include nephrotoxicity,

⊚ CLINICAL JUDGMENT [NURSING PROCESS]

Anthelmintics

Concept: Nutrition
- Deficient nutrients needed for cellular metabolism resulting from intestinal parasites leading to nutritional deficiencies

Concept: Infection
- Presence of tissue inflammation from invading helminths causing gastrointestinal (GI) distress and neurologic effects.

Recognize Cues [Assessment]
- Note whether the patient has traveled to countries outside the US or has been in areas that are overcrowded with poor sanitation.
- Identify close contacts with patients infected by helminths.
- Assess the patient's health behavior when at home; also assess handwashing facilities, disposal of waste, access to safe drinking water, and whether the patient walks barefoot in soil.
- Secure a history of foods (especially beef and pork) the patient has eaten and how the food was prepared to determine if it was raw, undercooked, or contaminated.
- Document whether any other person in the household has been checked for helminths.
- Determine presence and intensity of anal itching, diarrhea, and abdominal discomfort in the patient before and during treatment and medication management.
- Assess the patient's baseline vital signs and then monitor changes at prescribed intervals while patient is responding to anthelmintic medications.
- Note type of helminthiasis to ensure the anthelmintic drug is specific to the organisms.

Analyze Cues and Prioritize Hypothesis [Patient Problems]
- Coping
- Decreased adherence to medication regimen
- Decreased functional ability when performing self-care management
- Decreased immunity
- Need for health teaching
- Reduced sensory perception (vision)
- Diarrhea, nausea, and vomiting

Generate Solutions [Planning]
- The patient will demonstrate handwashing before eating.
- The patient will explain how to prepare foods properly to avoid recurrence.
- The patient will identify changes needed at home to ensure sanitation in food preparation.
- The patient will describe methods of infection control within the home.

Take Action [Nursing Interventions]
- ⚡ Discuss benefits of handwashing before eating and after working in the soil or with animals.
- Monitor patient's fluid and urinary output during anthelmintic medication use, checking for fluid loss from vomiting, diarrhea, and inadequate fluid intake.
- Collect the stool specimen in a clean container. Avoid having stool come in contact with water, urine, or chemicals, which could destroy parasitic worms.
- ⚡ Administer the prescribed anthelmintic after meals to prevent or minimize occurrence of GI distress.
- ⚡ Monitor adverse reactions, which can include wheezing, abdominal pain, abdominal distention, and high fever.
- Check laboratory values of iron, iodine, and vitamin A to monitor nutritional status.
- Obtain an interpreter when necessary. Avoid relying on family members who may not fully disclose or understand medical terminology.
- Provide community-based resources for patients discharged to areas at high risk for poor sanitation.

Patient Teaching
- Explain to the patient the importance of handwashing before meals and after going to the toilet. The parasite can be transferred within the family if proper hygiene is not used.
- Advise the patient to take daily showers and not baths.
- Encourage the patient to change sheets, bedclothes, towels, and underwear daily.
- Advise the patient that a second course of anthelmintic may be necessary if helminthiasis persists after therapy.
- Emphasize the importance of taking the prescribed drug at the designated times and keeping health care appointments.
- Teach the patient to read all directions regarding over-the-counter (OTC) drugs before use and avoid self-medication.
- Warn the patient that drowsiness may occur and that operating a car or machinery should be avoided if this should happen.
- Encourage collaboration between family, patient, and health care provider when reporting side effects or adverse reactions.

Evaluate Outcomes [Evaluation]
- Evaluate effectiveness of anthelmintic therapy and absence of side effects.
- Determine the patient's self-management ability in proper hygiene, handwashing, and cleaning bed linen to avoid the spread of parasitic worms.
- Evaluate the patient's knowledge of maintaining adequate food and fluid intake to provide strength and healing.

---

neurotoxicity, neuromuscular blockade, respiratory distress, apnea, superinfection, and *C. difficile*–associated diarrhea. Acute respiratory distress syndrome can occur when the antibiotic is administered by inhalation.

Polymyxins

Polymyxins were one of the early groups of antimicrobials, but many of the early drugs were discontinued because of severe toxic reactions such as neurotoxicity and nephrotoxicity. Polymyxins are polypeptide antibiotics that consist of five different chemical compounds, polymyxins A through E. Currently, polymyxin B and polymyxin E (also

known as *colistin*) are used in clinical practice. Polymyxins produce a bactericidal effect by interfering with the cell membrane of the bacterium, thereby causing cell death. They affect most gram-negative bacteria, such as *P. aeruginosa*, *Escherichia coli*, and *Klebsiella* and *Shigella* species.

The polymyxins are not absorbed through the oral route except for colistin, which exerts action on the colon and is excreted in the feces. Intramuscular injection of polymyxins produces intense pain at the injection site. Consequently, parenteral polymyxins are administered at a slow IV infusion rate. Table 31.3 lists antiinfective peptides with dosage and uses.

TABLE 31.2 Anthelmintics

Generic	Route and Dosage	Uses and Considerations
Ivermectin	See Prototype Drug Chart: Ivermectin	
Praziquantel	Liver flukes (clonorchiasis and opisthorchiasis): A: PO: 25 mg/kg/dose tid q 4–6/h × 1 d Schistosomiasis: A: PO 20 mg/kg/dose tid (q 4–6/h) × 1 day Cysticercosis (tapeworms): A: PO: 50 mg/kg/d × given in 3 divided doses Taeniasis (tapeworms): A: PO: 5–10 mg/kg as single dose Neurocysticercosis (pork tapeworm infection): 50 mg/kg/d given in 3 divided doses, usually in combination with other medications *Max:* A: PO: 75 mg/kg/d	Used for schistosomiasis, clonorchiasis, and opisthorchiasis; also effective for certain cestode (tapeworm) infections Contraindicated in hypersensitivity to drug class; ocular schistosomiasis and cysticercosis, CNS lesions, and seizures. Caution in hepatic impairment and arrhythmias Adverse reactions: urticaria, drowsiness, abdominal pain, vertigo, anorexia, asthenia, pruritus, vomiting, diarrhea, myalgia, fatigue, dizziness, nausea, weakness, headache, rash, fever, arrhythmia, AV block, bradycardia, and malaise ⚡ In neurocysticercosis, anticonvulsive therapy is recommended for those with seizure disorders PB: 80%–85%; t½: 0.8–1.5 h
Pyrantel pamoate	Enterobiasis and trichostrongyliasis (pinworms): A: PO: 11 mg/kg base (*max:* 1 g) as single dose. Uncinariasis (hookworm): A: PO: 11 mg/kg base (*max:* 1 g) daily × 3 days Ascariasis (intestinal human parasite): A: PO: 11 mg/kg base (*max:* 1 g) daily × 3 days as an alternative to other treatments; *max:* A: PO: 11 mg/kg/dose, not to exceed 1 g/dose	Antihelminthic for treating pinworm infection Caution: hypersensitivity to drug class; use with caution in hepatic impairment Adverse reactions: abdominal cramps and distention, nausea, vomiting, diarrhea, anorexia, rectal tenesmus, headache, and dizziness Use with caution in pregnancy and breastfeeding PB: UK; t½ UK
Triclabendazole	Fascioliasis: A: PO: 10 mg/kg/dose for 2 doses given 12 h apart; *max:* 20 mg/kg/d	Antiparasitic used to treat infections of worms. Contraindicated in hypersensitivity to triclabendazole and benzimidazole, irregular heartbeat, heart disease Caution: pregnancy, breastfeeding Adverse reactions: Chest pain, changes in heart rate, dizziness, palpitations, breathing problems PB: 90%, t½: 8 h

A, Adult; *d*, day; *h*, hour; *max*, maximum; *PB*, protein binding; *PO*, by mouth; *t½*, half-life; *tid*, three times a day; *UK*, unknown; *wk*, week; *y*, year; *>*, greater than; *<*, less than.

Severe Adverse Effects

High serum levels of polymyxins can cause nephrotoxicity and neurotoxicity. In nephrotoxicity, the blood urea nitrogen (BUN) and serum creatinine levels are elevated, but when the serum drug level decreases, renal toxicity is usually reversed. Signs and symptoms of neurotoxicity (toxicity of the nerves) include paresthesias—abnormal sensations such as numbness, tingling, burning, and prickling—and dizziness. Neurotoxicity is usually reversible when the drug is discontinued.

Bacitracin

Bacitracin has a polypeptide structure and acts by inhibiting bacterial cell wall synthesis and damaging the cell wall membrane, which results in death of the cell. The drug action can be bacteriostatic or bactericidal. Bacitracin is not absorbed by the GI tract; if given orally, it is excreted in the feces. Bacitracin is effective against most gram-positive bacteria and some gram-negative bacteria. Over-the-counter (OTC) bacitracin ointment is available for application to the skin. The side effects of bacitracin include skin redness and rash, nausea, and vomiting. Severe adverse reactions are renal damage and ototoxicity, and mild to severe allergic reactions that range from hives to anaphylaxis may occur.

Metronidazole

Metronidazole is a synthetic antibiotic and antiprotozoal (nitroimidazole class) that works by disrupting the bacterial DNA and inhibiting cell synthesis, which causes cell death. Metronidazole as a protozoal treats *Trichomonas vaginalis*, amebiasis, and giardiasis; as an antibiotic, it is used for anaerobic bacteria, including *Helicobacter pylori*, a pathogen in GI infections. Additionally, this drug has immunosuppressive and antiinfective properties that treat rosacea. This drug can be added to multidrug regimens to reduce antibiotic resistance, which occurs when the bacteria are not sensitive to the antibiotic. Metronidazole can be administered orally, parenterally, topically, and intravaginally. Toxic reactions include neurologic disturbances such as seizures and peripheral neuropathies. The Prototype Drug Chart: Metronidazole provides information on metronidazole.

⚡ **PATIENT SAFETY**

To avoid antibiotic resistance, use health care provider–patient/family collaboration to counsel patients in antibiotic management by:
- Checking if patient can be treated without antibiotics.
- Completing antibiotics as prescribed.
- Teaching patient correct use of the antibiotic, including not skipping doses or self-medicating with someone else's medication.
- Reinforcing self-management skills in personal hygiene.

TABLE 31.3 Antiinfectives

Generic	Route and Dosage	Uses and Considerations
Peptides		
Bacitracin	A: Topical: Apply a thin layer two or three times daily. A: Opthalmic ointment: Apply a thin film to the affected eye q 3–4 h for 7–10 d	Available topical ointment for skin infections; ophthalmic ointment for eye infections; used with caution IM for pediatric staphylococcal infections **!** **Black Box Warning:** Hypersensitivity to drug class and concurrent nephrotoxic agent use. Use caution with renal impairment and/or antibiotic-associated colitis history Monitor BUN/Cr at baseline and daily Adverse reactions: Nausea, vomiting, injection site pain, rash, proteinuria, azotemia, diarrhea PB: <20%; t½: UK
Colistimethate sodium	Dosing based on colistin base activity Severe bacterial infections (due to multidrug-resistant gram-negative bacteria, including *P. aeruginosa* and *A. baumannii*) A: IV: 300 mg x 1; then, 150–180 mg/d divided q12h Adjust dose in renal dysfunction	Gram-negative infections (*Pseudomonas aeruginosa*) Adverse reactions: Dyspepsia, tingling, slurred speech, dizziness, vertigo, paresthesia, pruritus/rash/urticaria, fever, decreased urine output, elevated BUN/Cr Use with caution if hypersensitive to drug/drug class, renal impairment, concurrent use of nephrotoxic agent, neuromuscular disease, concurrent neurotoxic agent use, and/or recent antibiotic-associated colitis Monitor BUN/Cr at baseline, then frequently Therapeutic drug level: 2 mg/L; draw just prior to next dose Use with caution in renal patients and in pregnancy PB: UK; t½: 2–3 h
Additional Antiinfective Agents		
Metronidazole	See Prototype Drug Chart: Metronidazole	
Polymyxin B	Severe bacterial infections: A: IV: 15,000–25,000 units/kg/IV divided every 12 h A: IM: 25,000–30,000 units/kg/d divided q4–6h	Polypeptide antibiotic Indicated for the treatment of infections of the urinary tract, meninges, and bloodstream, caused by susceptible strains of *Pseudomonas aeruginosa* **!** **Black Box Warning:** Hypersensitivity to drug or drug class; caution if concurrent neurotoxic or nephrotoxic agent use; caution in renal impairment; caution if recent antibiotic-associated colitis, neurotoxicity, pregnancy Administration requires specialized care setting *Adverse reactions:* Albuminuria, urinary casts, azotemia, flushing, dizziness, ataxia, drowsiness, paresthesia, fever, rash/urticaria. Serious reactions include nephrotoxicity, neurotoxicity, superinfection Polymyxin B should not be used in pregnancy unless the benefit outweighs the risk. Nursing mothers should either stop nursing or stop polymyxin B treatment depending on the risks to both the mother and child. PB: 79%–92%; t½: 6 h

A, Adult; *bid*, twice daily; *BUN*, blood urea nitrogen; *Cr*, creatinine; *d*, day; *GI*, gastrointestinal; *h*, hour; *IM*, intramuscular; *IV*, intravenous; *kg*, kilogram; *max*, maximum; *PB*, protein binding; *PO*, by mouth; *q*, every; *t½*, half-life; *UK*, unknown; *UTI*, urinary tract infection; *<*, less than; *≥*, greater than or equal to.

📄 PROTOTYPE DRUG CHART

Metronidazole

Drug Class	Dosage
Antibacterial peptide, amebicide Reduces development of drug-resistant organisms and maintains effectiveness of antimicrobial drugs Systemic, topical, and vaginal use	Trichomoniasis: A: PO: 500 mg bid x 7 d or 2 g as single dose; do not repeat treatment for 4–6 wk Amebic hepatic abscess: A: PO: 750 mg tid x 7–10 d Intestinal amebiasis (amebic dysentery): A: PO: 500–700 mg tid q 8 h for 5–10 d Serious anaerobic bacterial infections: A: IV: 15 mg/kg over 1 h loading dose; then 7.5 mg/kg/IV q 6 h, not to exceed 4 g/d; last maintenance dose should be administered 6 h after loading dose Bacterial vaginosis: A: PO: regular 500 mg bid; ext rel 750 mg/day x 7 A: Female: 1 application (5 g of 0.75% gel) intravaginally once d for 5/d

PROTOTYPE DRUG CHART—CONT'D

Contraindications	Drug-Lab-Food Interactions
Hypersensitivity to drug components, first trimester of pregnancy, breastfeeding should be withheld, hematological disease Use of disulfiram within 2 wk, use of alcohol during therapy or within 3 days of discontinuing metronidazole *Caution:* Hepatic disease, cardiac and neoplastic disease **!** **Black Box Warning:** New primary malignancy	Drug: Alcohol may cause disulfiram-type reaction. Disulfiram may increase risk of toxicity. May increase effects of oral anticoagulants Herbal: None significant Food: None known Lab: May increase serum LDH, ALT, AST; Monitor: CBC w/diff

Pharmacokinetics	Pharmacodynamics
Absorption: Well absorbed orally Distribution: Widely distributed; crosses blood-brain barrier Metabolized in liver; PB: <20%; t½: 8 h Excretion: In urine (60%–80%) and feces (6%–15%)	Administered IV, intravaginally, topically IV: Onset immediate, peak end of infusion PO: Peak 2 h

Therapeutic Effects/Uses
Produces bactericidal, antiprotozoal, amebicidal, trichomonacidal effects. Produces antiinflammatory, immunosuppressive effects when applied topically. Mechanism of Action: Diffuses into organism, interacting with DNA and causing a loss of helical DNA structure and strand breakage, inhibiting protein synthesis

Side Effects	Adverse Reactions
Anorexia, nausea, dry mouth, metallic taste, headache, dizziness, vomiting, diarrhea, abdominal cramps	Seizures, aseptic meningitis, pseudomembranous colitis, pancreatitis leukopenia, bone marrow suppression, aplasia, thrombocytopenia, Stevens-Johnson syndrome, toxic epidermal necrolysis

A, Adult; *ALT,* alanine aminotransferase; *AST,* aspartate aminotransferase; *bid,* twice daily; *CBC,* complete blood count; *d,* day; *dif,* differential; *DNA,* deoxyribonucleic acid; *ext rel,* extended release; *h,* hour; *IV,* intravenous; *LDH,* lactate dehydrogenase; *max,* maximum; *PB,* protein binding; *PO,* by mouth; *q,* every; *tid,* three times daily; *wk,* week; <, less than; >, greater than.

◎ CLINICAL JUDGMENT [NURSING PROCESS]

Antiinfectives: Peptides

Concept: Immunity
- Protective immunologic response of microbial peptides in patients with bacterial diseases

Concept: Infection
- Presence of drug-resistant bacteria causing infectious disease

Recognize Cues [Assessment]
- Obtain a health history listing all prescribed and over-the-counter (OTC) medications, medications, and medication allergies.
- Assess the patient's prior use of antibiotics, use of a multidrug regimen, and presence of untreated infections.
- Assess the patient's level of consciousness.
- Assess renal function and urinary output.
- Assess skin integrity and evaluate for skin rash and pruritus.

Analyze Cues and Prioritize Hypothesis [Patient Problems]
- Sensory-perceptual impairment: decreased hearing, decreased vision
- Disrupted fluid and electrolyte balance: nephrotoxicity
- Decreased functional ability: dizziness
- Allergic skin rash
- Need for health teaching
- Nausea and vomiting

Generate Solutions [Planning]
- The laboratory values at baseline level by assessing urine output, blood urea nitrogen (BUN), and hepatic enzymes.
- The patient's skin will be intact without pruritus, swelling, or rash.
- The patient will be able to identify dose and explain how to properly take the prescribed drug.

- The patient will describe the side effects and adverse reactions that require notification of a health care provider.

Take Action [Nursing Interventions]
- ⚡ Monitor laboratory values, including liver function tests (aspartate aminotransferase [AST], alanine aminotransferase [ALT]) and evaluation of renal function (BUN, creatinine clearance [CrCl]) and blood serum (platelet count, hemoglobin, hematocrit).
- ⚡ Check urinary function by monitoring intake and output.
- ⚡ Monitor the patient for an altered level of consciousness.

Patient Teaching
- Teach patients to read all instructions before taking medications.
- Inform patients to take all prescribed medication.
- Discuss possible side effects that can occur as a reaction to the drug.
- Instruct patients to check for signs of superinfection, such as white patches on the tongue.
- Advise patients to report all adverse reactions to a health care provider, including fever, diarrhea, trouble breathing, and decreased urination.
- Describe urinary signs that indicate impairment, such as decreased urinary flow.
- Caution patient to not replace an herbal supplement for a prescribed medication.
- Use safety measures during activities of mobility.
- Encourage self-management skills, reporting all side effects and adverse reactions.

Evaluate Outcomes [Evaluation]
- Evaluate effectiveness of treatment by absence of manifestations.
- Evaluate patient understanding of the medication regimen by encouraging patient feedback and questions.

CRITICAL THINKING CASE STUDY

A 40-year-old male has returned to the US after working in a missionary health clinic in a malaria-endemic area. He was admitted to the hospital with fever, chills, and severe unrelieved headache. A diagnosis of acute malaria was made.

Chloroquine was ordered, and the patient discharged. One week later, he returned to the emergency room with worsening symptoms and signs of confusion. The patient states he took his pills every other day then stopped because they made him sick and decided to take OTC antinausea medication. The patient was readmitted to the hospital. A care coordination meeting was scheduled with the patient, family, health care provider, and pharmacist to determine ways to improve medication adherence.

1. Which key factors should be assessed in this patient's history?
2. What is the significance of monitoring liver function tests, BUN/Cr, and CBC?
3. Describe the correct method of preventive prophylaxis when taking antimalarial drugs.

REVIEW QUESTIONS

1. An international traveler diagnosed with malaria is admitted to the emergency department and is prescribed mefloquine hydrochloride. The nurse anticipates that which laboratory test will be ordered?
   a. Liver function test (LFT)
   b. Blood glucose
   c. Sputum culture and sensitivity
   d. White blood cell count
2. A patient is admitted to the hospital with multidrug-resistant urinary tract infection. Laboratory tests show *Pseudomonas aeruginosa*. Colistimethate sodium is ordered in powder form and must be diluted for intramuscular injection. The nurse understands that which of the following is the purpose for this drug?
   a. This drug prevents toxic adverse reactions.
   b. This drug treats gram-negative bacteria.
   c. This drug is safe for patients with renal impairments.
   d. This drug prevents antibiotic resistance.
3. Which of the following is a priority to evaluate in a patient being treated for *Taenia solium* (pork tapeworm)?
   a. Increased appetite
   b. Abdominal distension
   c. Fatigue
   d. Constipation

4. A patient with a history of malaria who is being treated with chloroquine is in the clinic for a follow-up visit. What should the nurse advise the patient to do?
   a. Get frequent hearing checks.
   b. Take antimalarials before meals.
   c. Get frequent testing of stool specimens.
   d. Avoid sun exposure.
5. A 50-year-old woman is being discharged from the hospital after treatment for malaria. Which teaching topic would best inform the patient about adverse reactions?
   a. The occurrence of headaches
   b. Experiencing dizziness
   c. Developing mild pruritus
   d. Skin and eyes that appear yellowish
6. A 30-year-old woman presents with a recurrence of *Trichomonas vaginalis* infection, and metronidazole is ordered. The patient's history reveals which of the following contraindications?
   a. A recent pregnancy test is negative.
   b. She previously took metronidazole and had no side effects.
   c. She drinks a glass of wine before bedtime.
   d. She takes an oral contraceptive.

32

HIV- and AIDS-Related Drugs

http://evolve.elsevier.com/McCuistion/pharmacology

OBJECTIVES

- Identify the common risk factors for HIV transmission.
- Describe the six classifications of antiretroviral therapy and give examples of medications in each group.
- Explain specific issues of medication adherence to antiretroviral agents.
- Discuss the nurse's role in medication management and issues of adherence.

- Discuss medical management for preventing mother-to-child transmission of HIV infection during pregnancy.
- Discuss health care workers' exposure risks and relate the risk and type of exposure to recommendations.
- Apply the Clinical Judgment [Nursing Process], including teaching, to the care of patients with HIV infection.

OUTLINE

Since the acquired immunodeficiency syndrome (AIDS) epidemic began in the United States in the early 1980s, advancement of antiretroviral therapy (ART) has dramatically improved human immunodeficiency virus (HIV)-related morbidity and mortality, and has reduced perinatal and behaviorally associated HIV transmission. The Centers for Disease Control and Prevention (CDC) reports that more than 1 million people in the United States are infected with HIV; 6 in 7 persons knew they had the virus. In 2018 nearly 38,000 people were newly diagnosed with HIV. Improvement of health, prolonging lives, reducing transmission risk, and suppression of HIV necessitate the use of combination treatments with antiretroviral drugs. Current clinical guidelines recommend ART for all persons infected with HIV-1, regardless of their viral load (CD4+ cell count). Prophylactic treatment of HIV-negative partners minimizes their risk of contracting HIV. It is critical that nurses educate patients regarding ART and, in partnership with the patient, develop strategies to optimize adherence.

Although strides have been made in the treatment of HIV/AIDS, challenges remain. One important aspect is increased drug resistance to current therapies. The makeup of the HIV DNA strands allows the virus to mutate from a drug-sensitive to a drug-resistant form. To minimize resistant strains, clinical and nonclinical providers and health departments need to strive for the highest possible adherence to ART. At each health care visit, persons with HIV and their partners should receive ongoing counseling to reinforce HIV prevention measures, screening for high-risk behaviors, diagnosis and treatment of sexually transmitted infections (STIs), and reinforcement of the importance of medication adherence. Open communication between the health care provider and patient should be fostered.

The goals for initiating ART are to (1) reduce HIV-associated morbidity and mortality, (2) prolong the duration and quality of life, (3) restore and preserve immunologic function, (4) maximally and durably suppress plasma HIV viral load, and (5) prevent HIV transmission.

HIV INFECTION: PATHOPHYSIOLOGY

HIV is an RNA retrovirus. It is unable to survive and replicate unless it is inside a living human cell. HIV destroys CD4+ T cells, also called *helper T cells* or *CD4+ T lymphocytes;* these play a critical role in the human immune response through recognition of infectious and neoplastic processes. The destruction of CD4+ cells by HIV results in immune deficiency, so the CD4+ cell count is an indicator for immune function in those with HIV.

Normal CD4+ counts range from 500 to 1200 cells/mm^3. After initial infection, rapid viral replication occurs, resulting in a high level of HIV in circulation (high viral load); the virus then attacks and destroys CD4+ cells. There is a corresponding drop in CD4+ cells, which triggers an immune response that results in CD4+ cell replacement and HIV antibody production. HIV uses the CD4+ cell's apparatus to replicate itself and spread throughout the body. The CD4+ cells continue to drop as HIV viral load increases, which further weakens the person's natural immune system such that it cannot fight off infection and disease (e.g., cancer). Symptoms of HIV infection range from mild to severe and include fever, fatigue, pharyngitis, myalgia or arthralgia, lymphadenopathy, headache, and night sweats in those recently infected; these symptoms can be experienced 2 to 12 weeks after HIV exposure. This period is called *acute retroviral syndrome, acute seroconversion syndrome,* or *primary HIV infection.* At this stage, people are highly infectious, and symptoms can often be mistaken, by both patient and health care provider, for a transient flulike illness. Consequently, few people are diagnosed during this time. Additionally, the time delay from infection to a positive HIV test result—the so-called window period—averages 10 to 14 days, but some do not seroconvert for 3 to 4 weeks. Almost all patients seroconvert within 6 months. For this reason, patients who are at risk for HIV infection and test negative should be counseled to have the test repeated in 3 months (the close of the window period). If HIV is strongly suspected, an HIV RNA quantitative test can be done. A viral load of 10,000 copies/mL usually indicates the virus is adequately suppressed.

HIV TRANSMISSION

HIV is spread via intimate contact with blood, semen, vaginal fluids, and breast milk. Transmission of the virus occurs primarily by (1) sexual contact, which includes oral, vaginal, and anal sex; (2) direct blood contact including intravenous (IV) drug use with shared needles or shared drug works, shared contaminated personal care items such as razors, and blood transfusions (now extremely rare in the United States); and (3) mother-to-child contact through shared maternal-fetal blood circulation, direct blood contact during delivery, or breast milk. Included in these modes are accidental needle injury, artificial insemination with donated semen, and organ transplant. Those at highest risk include persons who engage in unprotected sex, those with multiple sexual partners (either the patient or partner[s] of the patient), IV drug users who share needles or drug works, and infants born to women with HIV. The risk of mother-to-child transmission (MTCT) is 25% without ART; the risk decreases to 1% to 2% with successful use of ART. Other factors that increase the risk of MTCT are a mother with a viral load greater than 1000 copies/mL at delivery, premature rupture of the membranes, hepatitis C virus coinfection, preterm gestation, and vaginal delivery. HIV is not spread by air or water, mosquitoes or ticks, shaking hands, hugging, sharing toilets, sharing dishes or drinking glasses, or drinking fountains.

LABORATORY TESTING

Several laboratory tests are important for initial patient evaluation upon entry to care, during follow-up evaluation for those not on ART, and before and after initiation or modification of ART to assess for immunologic and virologic efficacy of treatment.

The laboratory tests used to determine when to initiate medication therapy and to monitor efficacy of therapy and indications for changing therapy are CD4+ T-cell count, plasma HIV RNA quantitative assay (or viral load test), and HIV resistance testing.

The count reflects the number of CD4+ cells circulating in the blood. The result is listed as an absolute number and a relative percentage. The absolute count can vary in the same patient depending on the laboratory used, the time of day laboratory blood work is drawn, or acute illness. The CD4+ percentage is a more stable reflection of the immune system and is used in conjunction with the absolute count to monitor health status and response to medication therapy. The patient should be encouraged to use the same laboratory at approximately the same time of day to promote consistency of results. The nurse should monitor the laboratory used because laboratory value references vary from laboratory to laboratory. The HIV viral load is indicative of the level of virus circulating in the blood and is the best determinant of treatment efficacy. A key goal of therapy is to achieve and maintain a viral load below the limits of detection (<20 to 40 copies/mL, depending on the assay used). This goal should be achieved in 16 to 24 weeks of therapy. Resistance to ART leads to treatment failure and the risk of transmitting drug-resistant virus. Determination of the presence of a drug-resistant strain of HIV is important to prevent ineffective treatment. Individuals who experience failure of ART should have drug resistance testing, assessment of drug adherence, and a review of possible drug-drug and drug-food interactions and drug intolerability, treatment history, and HIV RNA and CD4+ cell counts.

CLASSIFICATION

HIV disease staging and classification systems are important tools for tracking and monitoring the HIV epidemic and for providing the clinician and patient with information about HIV disease stage and clinical management. The two major classification systems are the CDC staging system (revised in 2014) and the World Health Organization (WHO) system (revised in 2015).

The CDC system assesses the severity of HIV disease by CD4+ cell counts and by presence of specific HIV-related conditions; the system is based on the lowest documented CD4+ cell count (*nadir CD4+*) and on previously diagnosed HIV-related conditions. The WHO system is useful in resource-constrained settings without access to CD4+ cell measurements and classifies HIV disease based on clinical manifestations that clinicians and those with varying levels of HIV expertise and training can recognize in diverse settings.

INDICATIONS FOR ANTIRETROVIRAL THERAPY

ART has dramatically reduced HIV-associated morbidity and mortality. However, the CDC reported that, in the United States, 56% of adults and adolescents with HIV have adequate viral suppression. Many individuals with HIV infection are undiagnosed or they are not retained within the health care system for routine monitoring.

A set of guidelines was developed by the US Department of Health and Human Services Expert Panel on Antiretroviral Guidelines for Adults and Adolescents (the Panel). The Panel last updated the guidelines in 2019 and recommends ART for all HIV-infected individuals regardless of CD4+ count to reduce HIV-related morbidity and mortality and to prevent HIV transmission. The Panel also seeks to educate patients on the benefits and considerations for ART, especially the importance of adherence. The current guidelines for treatment-naïve persons with HIV include initial therapy with two nucleoside reverse transcriptase inhibitors (NRTIs) in combination with a third active antiretroviral (ARV) drug from one of three drug classes: an integrase strand transfer inhibitor (INSTI), a nonnucleoside reverse transcriptase inhibitor (NNRTI), or a protease inhibitor (PI) with a pharmacokinetic (PK) enhancer (booster) (cobicistat or ritonavir). All HIV-infected persons diagnosed with active tuberculosis (TB) should be started on antiretroviral and TB therapy. Rifamycin (rifabutin, rifampin) should be included in the TB regimen despite drug interactions. Chapter 29 further discusses antituberculars.

Suppression of HIV with ART may decrease inflammation and immune activation thought to contribute to higher rates of cardiovascular, kidney, and liver disease; neurologic complications; and malignancy in HIV-infected cohorts. If therapy is to be initiated, medications are selected based on results of genotypic resistance testing where applicable, comorbidities (e.g., liver disease, renal dysfunction, depression), potential drug-drug interactions, pregnancy status, and assessment of the patient's willingness and readiness to start therapy. Evaluation of medication readiness should include dosage regimen, pill burden, dosing frequency, food restrictions, side effects, and the patient's daily routine. Tools for promoting medication adherence (e.g., alarms, pill planners) and plans for management of potential medication side effects should be reviewed before medication initiation. The patient should be instructed in the need for a better than 95% medication adherence, the potential for development of medication resistance with less than optimal adherence, and the clinical implications of resistance.

ANTIRETROVIRAL DRUGS

NRTIs, NNRTIs, PIs, fusion (entry) inhibitors, CCR5 antagonists, and INSTIs make up the drugs used as ART. Table 32.1 lists dosages, uses, and considerations for several ARVs. More than 25 different ARVs have received US Food and Drug Administration (FDA) approval, and various combination of drugs are available in fixed-dose combinations that contain two or more HIV medications from one or more drug classes. In addition to the previously mentioned classes of antiretrovirals, PK enhancers are approved to be taken with some ARVs (e.g., PIs and certain INSTIs).

Since the 1980s, when zidovudine monotherapy showed survival benefits in advanced HIV patients, much progress has been made. Newer drugs have improved adherence (e.g., fewer pills for more convenient dosing, formulation changes that reduce dosing frequency or pill burden, combination dosage forms with two or three drugs in one pill). Other improvements include increased potency, improved side effect profile (e.g., decreased gastrointestinal [GI] effects), and PI enhancers.

ART is the standard of care in the treatment of HIV infection. Currently, there are six recommended regimens for treatment-naïve patients, five of which are INSTI based and one that is ritonavir-boosted–PI based. For treatment-naïve patients, ART generally consists of two NRTIs plus an INSTI, NNRTI, or PK-enhanced PI. Treatment-experienced patients who encounter drug resistance should begin a new regimen that includes two to three fully active drugs. Adding a single ARV is not recommended because of the increased risk of drug resistance to all ARVs. Furthermore, drug interruption is not recommended due to a risk of rapid increase of HIV RNA viral load and a decrease in CD4+ cell count.

The Panel reports that nevirapine (NVP) should not be given to ARV-naïve women whose CD4+ count is greater than 250 cells/mm^3 or to men with CD4+ greater than 400 cells/mm^3 due to a high incidence of hepatotoxicity; however, if no other ARV option is available, NVP can be administered, but patients should be closely monitored. On the other hand, the Panel reports no exceptions to stavudine plus zidovudine (antagonistic effect) and unboosted darunavir, saquinavir, or tipranavir (inadequate bioavailability).

Nucleoside/Nucleotide Reverse Transcriptase Inhibitors

Of the antiretroviral drugs, NRTIs were the first type of drug to treat HIV. NRTIs act by interfering with HIV viral RNA-dependent DNA polymerase, resulting in inhibition of viral replication. Seven NRTIs, also known as "nukes," are approved for use in the United States: zidovudine, didanosine, stavudine, lamivudine, abacavir, tenofovir, and emtricitabine. All but didanosine and stavudine are available in a fixed-dose combination with other classes of ARV drugs.

All NRTIs except didanosine can be taken without regard to food. Didanosine should be taken 30 minutes before or 2 hours after meals for optimal absorption. Fifty percent or more of NRTIs are excreted by the kidneys; therefore NRTIs require dosage adjustment in persons with renal insufficiency. With abacavir, dosage adjustment is recommended in individuals with hepatic insufficiency.

As a class, NRTIs are associated with changes in the body's metabolism secondary to mitochondrial toxicity. GI side effects such as nausea, diarrhea, and abdominal pain are transient and improve within the first 2 weeks of therapy. Rash is a common hypersensitivity reaction. Complications include peripheral neuropathy, myopathy, pancreatitis, and lipoatrophy. Lipoatrophy—or wasting of fat on the extremities, face, and buttocks—is associated with chronic NRTI administration. Rare fatalities have occurred due to lactic acidosis and hepatic steatosis associated with NRTIs. Persons coinfected with hepatitis B virus (HBV) are at risk for severe acute exacerbation of their HBV upon discontinuation of emtricitabine, lamivudine, or tenofovir disoproxil fumarate.

Drug interactions are minimal with NRTIs because these drugs are not metabolized by the cytochrome P450 (CYP450) isoenzymes. However, drug interactions can still occur: for example, ribavirin inhibiting phosphorylation of zidovudine can cause hematologic toxicities, and coadministration of ribavirin with didanosine is contraindicated because fatal hepatic failure can occur; didanosine coadministered with stavudine can worsen lactic acidosis and pancreatitis; allopurinol is contraindicated in individuals taking didanosine; and PIs can increase serum concentration of tenofovir disoproxil fumarate.

Prototype Drug Chart: Zidovudine gives pharmacologic data for zidovudine, and Prototype Drug Chart: Tenofovir Disoproxil Fumarate shows the data for tenofovir.

Nonnucleoside Reverse Transcriptase Inhibitors

Five NNRTIs are used in the United States: delavirdine, efavirenz (EFV), etravirine, NVP, and rilpivirine. NNRTIs ("non-nukes") do not require intracellular metabolism; they directly bind to the reverse transcriptase (RT) enzymes and block DNA polymerization. The primary advantage of using NNRTIs is to reserve a PI-based therapy for future use. In general, an NNRTI regimen has a lower pill burden compared with most PI-based regimens. Major disadvantages are the prevalence of NNRTI-resistant viral strains and the low genetic barrier of NNRTIs for development of resistance. (Resistance testing is recommended for treatment-naïve patients before starting therapy.)

EFV and rilpivirine are available as components of fixed-dose regimens. EFV should be taken on an empty stomach; delavirdine and NVP can be taken without regard to food; all other NNRTIs should be taken with food to enhance absorption. Except for NVP, all NNRTIs are metabolized by the liver and excreted in feces, whereas NVP is mostly excreted in urine.

TABLE 32.1 Antiretroviral Agents

Generic	Route and Dosage	Uses and Considerations
Nucleoside/Nucleotide Reverse Transcriptase Inhibitors (NRTIs)		
Abacavir (ABC) Also available as a component of fixed-dose combinations	Tablets and solution: A: PO: 300 mg bid or 600 mg once daily	Used in combination with other ARVs. Screen for HLA-B∗5701 before initiation. Hypersensitivity reactions are highest in patients who test positive for HLA-B∗5701. Avoid in persons with cardiovascular risk factors. A black-box warning exists for hepatotoxicity or lactic acidosis. May be administered without regard to meals. Metabolized by alcohol dehydrogenase and glucuronyl transferase; ethanol decreases elimination of ABC. A reduced dose is recommended in persons with hepatic impairment.
Didanosine (DDI)	Extended-release capsule and powder for oral solution: A ≥60 kg: PO: 400 mg once daily A <60 kg: PO: 250 mg once daily *Dosages are decreased if administered with TDF.*	DDI is not recommended for initial therapy due to inferior virologic efficacy. Used in combination with other ARVs. Metabolized by the liver. A black-box warning exists for hepatotoxicity or lactic acidosis and pancreatitis. Take on an empty stomach. ER capsules must be swallowed whole. Reduce the dose in persons with renal impairment.
Emtricitabine (FTC) Also available as a component of fixed-dose combinations	Capsule: A: PO: 200 mg once daily Solution: A: PO: 240 mg once daily	Used in combination with other ARVs. Metabolized by oxidation. A black-box warning exists for acute severe exacerbation of hepatitis B upon discontinuation of FTC and hepatitis or lactic acidosis. Otherwise, minimal toxicity is noted with FTC. Take without regard to meals. Reduce dose in patients with renal impairment.
Lamivudine (3TC) Also available as a component of fixed-dose combinations	Tablet and solution: A: PO: 300 mg once daily or 150 mg bid	Used in combination with other ARVs for treating HIV. Minimal toxicity with 3TC; a black-box warning exists for acute severe exacerbation of hepatitis B upon discontinuation of 3TC and hepatitis or lactic acidosis. Take without regard to meals. Adjust dosage in patients with renal insufficiency.
Stavudine (d4T)	A ≥60 kg: PO: 40 mg q12h A <60 kg: PO: 30 mg q12h	Used in combination with other ARVs for treating HIV. Crosses the blood-brain barrier. A black-box warning exists for hepatotoxicity or lactic acidosis and pancreatitis. Take without regard to meals. Adjust dosage in patients with renal insufficiency
Tenofovir (TDF)	See Prototype Drug Chart: Tenofovir Disoproxil Fumarate	
Zidovudine (ZDV) Also available as a component of fixed-dose combinations	See Prototype Drug Chart: Zidovudine	
Nonnucleoside Reverse Transcriptase Inhibitors (NNRTIs)		
Delavirdine (DLV)	A: PO: 400 mg tid	Used in combination with NRTIs. Take without regard to meals. Acidic food improves absorption, and 100-mg tablets may be dispersed in liquid before administration. DLV is metabolized extensively by the CYP450 isoenzymes.
Efavirenz (EFV) Also available as a component of fixed-dose combinations	See Prototype Drug Chart: Efavirenz	
Etravirine (ETR)	A: PO: 200 mg bid	Used in combination with NRTIs. However, patients with virologic failure on NNRTIs should not receive ETR solely with NRTIs. Administer after meals to enhance absorption. Tablets may be dispensed in water. Do not use grapefruit juice, carbonated beverages, or warm liquids. Do not add ETR to juice or milk without first adding it to water. Add more fluids to the glass to ensure the full dose is consumed. Metabolized by CYP450 enzymes; numerous drug-drug interactions exist. No dosage adjustment is needed in patients with renal insufficiency. Hypersensitivity reactions include rash, including Stevens-Johnson syndrome and hepatitis that includes hepatic necrosis.

TABLE 32.1 Antiretroviral Agents—cont'd

Generic	Route and Dosage	Uses and Considerations
Nevirapine (NVP)	Immediate release: A: PO: 200 mg/d for 14 d, then 200 mg bid. Extended release: A: PO: Initial dosing with IR as previously discussed for 14 d, then 400 mg ER once daily	NVP should not be used as an initial treatment option for treatment-naïve patients because fatal toxicities can occur. Used in combination with other ARVs (NRTIs, NNRTIs, PIs). A black-box warning exists for females whose CD4+ counts are >250/mm³ because risk of hepatotoxicity is increased. Take without regard to meals. Do not crush or chew ER tablets. Metabolized by CYP450. NVP is contraindicated in persons with hepatic impairment because of increased risk for hepatotoxicity. Numerous drug-drug interactions exist. Discontinue with hepatotoxicity or rash, including Stevens-Johnson syndrome.
Rilpivirine (RPL) Also available as a component of fixed-dose combinations	A ≥35 kg: PO: 25 mg once daily	Must be administered in combination with other ARVs. Take with a meal. Primarily metabolized by the liver. Numerous drug-drug interactions exist, and hepatotoxicity can occur. Monitor for depression, insomnia, cephalgia.
Protease Inhibitors (PIs) Atazanavir (ATV) Also available as a component of fixed-dose combinations	See Prototype Drug Chart: Atazanavir	
Darunavir (DRV) Also available as a component of fixed-dose combinations	A: PO: 600–800 mg bid	Used in combination with other ARVs. Must be administered with PK enhancer (cobicistat or low-dose ritonavir). Administer with food. DRV is metabolized by CYP450 isoenzymes. Adjust dosage in patients with hepatic insufficiency. Caution in patients with sulfa hypersensitivity. Monitor closely for rash, including Stevens-Johnson syndrome, toxic epidermal necrolysis, acute generalized exanthematous pustulosis, and erythema multiforme. Hepatotoxicity, DKA, and pancreatitis can occur. Other adverse effects include lipodystrophy, elevated transaminases, nausea, and diarrhea.
Fosamprenavir (FPV)	A: PO: 700 mg bid with ritonavir 100 mg PO bid	Used in combination with other ARVs. A PK enhancer with low-dose ritonavir and twice-daily dosing are recommended. Monitor in patients with sulfa hypersensitivity; cross-reaction can occur. Metabolized by CYP450 isoenzymes and drug transporters. Dose adjustment is required in patients with hepatic impairment. Tablets can be taken without regard to meals. Oral suspension is taken on an empty stomach in adults and with food in children. Can readminister dose if emesis occurs within 30 min of administration. Adverse effects include rash, diarrhea, nausea, vomiting, headache, hyperlipidemia, elevated transaminase levels, hyperglycemia, fat maldistribution, and possible increased bleeding in patients with hemophilia.
Indinavir (IDV)	A: PO: 800 mg q12h	Used in combination with other ARVs and PK enhancers (e.g., ritonavir). CYP450 3A4 inhibitor and substrate. Adjust dosage in patients with hepatic insufficiency. For optimal absorption, take on an empty stomach. Hydrate with at least 1.5 L of fluid during a 24-h period. Adverse effects include nephrolithiasis, GI intolerance, nausea, indirect hyperbilirubinemia, headache, asthenia, blurred vision, dizziness, rash, metallic taste, thrombocytopenia, alopecia, hemolytic anemia, hyperlipidemia, elevated transaminase levels, hyperglycemia, fat maldistribution, and risk of increased bleeding in patients with hemophilia.
Lopinavir–ritonavir (LPV/r)	A: PO: 400/100 mg bid *or* 800/200 mg once daily	Used in combination with other ARVs. CYP450 3A4 inhibitor and substrate. May take tablet with or without food; take oral solution with food. Adverse effects include GI intolerance, asthenia, PR interval prolongation, pancreatitis, hyperlipidemia, elevated transaminase levels, hyperglycemia, fat maldistribution, and risk of increased bleeding in patients with hemophilia.

Continued

TABLE 32.1   Antiretroviral Agents—cont'd

Generic	Route and Dosage	Uses and Considerations
Nelfinavir (NFV)	A: PO: 1250 mg bid or 750 mg tid	Used in combination with other ARVs. Not recommended in treatment-naïve patients as initial therapy. CYP450 3A4 inhibitor and substrate. Take with food; do not mix with acidic food or juice. Tablets can be dispersed in a small amount of water before mixing with food or juice. Nelfinavir oral powder may be added to water, milk, formula, soymilk, or dietary supplements. Do not mix nelfinavir oral powder with acidic food or juice (orange juice, apple juice, or applesauce). Do not mix nelfinavir with water in the original container. Adverse effects include diarrhea, hyperlipidemia, elevated transaminase levels, hyperglycemia, fat maldistribution, and risk of increased bleeding in patients with hemophilia. ⚡ Persons with phenylketonuria should not take nelfinavir powder as it contains phenylalanine.
Ritonavir (RTV)	Other ARVs: A: PO: 600 mg bid. Booster: A: PO: 100–400 mg in 1–2 divided doses	Used in combination with other ARVs and as a PK enhancer (booster) of other PIs. Dosage depends on use of RTV. CYP450 3A4 potent inhibitor; use extreme caution when administering other drugs, especially antihistamines, sedative hypnotics, antiarrhythmics, and ergot alkaloids. If coadministering with didanosine, separate drugs by 2 h. Take with food. Swallow tablets and capsules whole. Refrigerate capsules; RTV oral solution should not be refrigerated but left at room temperature for up to 30 days. Adverse effects include GI intolerance, paresthesias, hepatitis, asthenia, hyperlipidemia, hyperglycemia, fat maldistribution, and risk of increased bleeding in patients with hemophilia. Titrating the dosage may help reduce side effects. ⚡ RTV oral solution contains significant amounts of ethanol (43.2%) and propylene glycol (26.57%). Accidental ingestion by small children may lead to deadly ethanol or propylene glycol toxicity.
Saquinavir (SQV)	A: PO: 1000 mg bid	*Must* be dosed concurrently with low-dose ritonavir. SQV is not recommended for treatment-naïve adults due to its serious adverse effects. CYP450 3A4 inhibitor and substrate. Take with food. Adverse effects include nausea, diarrhea, headache, hyperlipidemia, elevated transaminase levels, hyperglycemia, PR and QT interval prolongation, fat maldistribution, and risk of increased bleeding in patients with hemophilia. Contraindicated in patients with PR or QT prolongation, hypokalemia, or hypomagnesemia.
Tipranavir (TPV)	A: PO: 500 mg bid	Used in combination with other ARVs; *must* be coadministered with ritonavir. TPV has a black-box warning for hepatotoxicity and intracranial bleeding. CYP450 3A4 inducer and substrate. Take with food if coadministered with RTV tablets; if administered with RTV capsules or solutions, TPV can be taken regardless of food. Adverse effects include hepatotoxicity, rash hyperlipidemia, hyperglycemia, fat maldistribution, and risk of increased bleeding in patients with hemophilia. Use with caution in patients with sulfa hypersensitivity.
Fusion (Entry) Inhibitors (FIs)		
Enfuvirtide (T20)	A: subcut: 90 mg bid	Used in treatment-experienced patients in combination with other ARVs. Administer via subcut, and rotate site. Store vial at room temperature; once reconstituted, refrigerate and use within 24 h. Adverse effects include local injection site reaction (pain, erythema, induration, nodules, cysts, pruritus, ecchymosis), increased rate of bacterial pneumonia, hypersensitivity reaction (rash, fever, nausea, vomiting, chills, rigors, hypotension, elevated transaminases), fatigue. To minimize local reactions, apply ice or heat after injection or gently massage the site to better disperse the drug.

TABLE 32.1   Antiretroviral Agents—cont'd

Generic	Route and Dosage	Uses and Considerations
Ibalizumab	A: IV: 2000 mg ×1, then 2 wk later, 800 mg every 2 wk	Used in treatment-experienced patients with multidrug-resistant virus. Before administering, must be further diluted. May store the diluted drug at room temperature for 4 hours; refrigerated for up to 24 hours. Do not administer via IVP or as bolus. Infuse first dose over 30 min. Succeeding doses can be infused over 15–30 min. Observe patient 1 hour after infusion. Common adverse reactions included diarrhea, dizziness, nausea, and rash.
CCR5 Antagonists Maraviroc (MRV)	A: PO: 150–600 mg bid	Used in combination with other ARVs. MRV is administered *only* to patients with CCR5-tropic HIV infection. Dosing depends on other drugs taken concomitantly. CYP3A substrate; drugs that inhibit or induce the enzymes will alter the pharmacokinetics of MRV. May take without regard to food. Concentration may increase in kidney dysfunction (CrCl <30); therefore caution is advised when used in renal-compromised patients; it is contraindicated in patients with CrCl <30 who are taking strong inhibitors and/or inducers of CYP3A. May need to adjust dose with concomitant CYP3A inhibitors or inducers (because of interactions) or with postural hypotension. Adverse effects include fever, upper respiratory tract infection, flatulence, orthostatic hypotension, hepatotoxicity, rash, cough, abdominal pain, and dizziness.
Integrase Strand Transfer Inhibitors (INSTIs) Dolutegravir (DTG) Also available as a component of fixed-dose combinations	A ≥40 kg: PO: 50 mg once daily	Used in treatment-naïve or -experienced patients in combination with other ARVs. Metabolized by CYP3A4 enzyme. Can be taken without regard to meals. Take polyvalent cation products (e.g., Mg++, Fe, and Ca++ salts); ASA on an empty stomach can reduce bioavailability of DTG. Adverse effects include headache, insomnia, rash, and liver injury.
Elvitegravir (EVG) Also available as a component of fixed-dose combinations	A: PO: 85–150 mg once daily depending on ritonavir and other ARVs taken concurrently	Used in treatment-naïve or -experienced patients in combination with other ARVs; unboosted EVG is not recommended. EVG is metabolized by CYP3A. Take with food. Adverse effects are rare, but nausea and vomiting can occur; suicidal ideation, albeit rare, can also occur, especially in those with a history of psychiatric illness.
Raltegravir (RTG)	A: PO: 400 mg bid	Used in treatment-naïve or -experienced patients in combination with other ARVs. Does not affect the CYP450 isoenzymes, nor is it a substrate of CYP450 enzymes. Can be taken without regard to meals. Coated tablets are not bioequivalent with chewable tablets or powder for oral suspension; swallow coated tablets whole. Adverse effects include GI symptoms, headache, pyrexia, increased total cholesterol, fatigue, rhabdomyolysis, insomnia, and rash that includes Stevens-Johnson syndrome and epidermal necrolysis.

A, Adult; *ARV,* antiretroviral; *ASA,* acetylsalicylic acid (aspirin); *bid,* twice a day; *Ca++,* calcium; *CrCl,* creatinine clearance; *CYP450,* cytochrome P450; *d,* day; *DKA,* diabetic ketoacidosis; *ER,* extended-release; *Fe,* iron; *GI,* gastrointestinal; *h,* hour; *HIV,* human immunodeficiency virus; *HLA,* human leukocyte antigen; *IR,* immediate release; *IV,* intravenous; *IVP,* intravenous push; *Mg++,* magnesium; *min,* minute; *mo,* months; *PI,* protease inhibitor; *PK,* pharmacokinetic; *PO,* by mouth; *q,* every; *subcut,* subcutaneous; *tid,* three times a day; *wk,* week; *y,* years; >, greater than; <, less than; ≥, greater than or equal to; ≤, less than or equal to.

PROTOTYPE DRUG CHART

Zidovudine (ZDV)

Drug Class	Dosage
Nucleoside/nucleotide reverse transcriptase inhibitor (NRTI) Also available as a component of fixed-dose combinations	Treatment in combination with other ARV: A: PO: 200 mg q8h or 300 mg q12h A: IV: 1 mg/kg over 1 h q4h (total daily dose: 6 mg/kg/d). Initiate oral therapy as soon as possible.

Contraindications	Drug-Lab-Food Interactions
Life-threatening allergies to ZDV or components of the preparation *Black Box Warning:* Hepatotoxicity, lactic acidosis, myopathy, bone marrow suppression *Caution:* Severe anemia (interruption of therapy or reduction in daily dose should be considered); renal impairment/failure; viral hepatitis	*Drug:* Ganciclovir, probenecid, valproic acid may increase concentration/adverse effects. Rifampin, interferon, and ritonavir may decrease concentration/effects. May potentiate hematologic toxicity with other drugs (e.g., interferon alfa, ganciclovir, primaquine, etc.), causing myelosuppression; interferon beta can increase ZDV levels, leading to drug toxicity. Can be taken without regard to food. *Lab:* May increase ALT, AST

Pharmacokinetics	Pharmacodynamics
Absorption: PO: 66%–70% Distribution: PB: <38%, crosses blood-brain barrier, crosses placenta, excreted in breast milk Metabolism: t½: 0.5–3 h; extensive first-pass effect in liver to GZDV (metabolite) Excretion: 63%–95% in urine as GZDV (metabolite)	Route: PO/IV Onset: UK Peak: 30–90 min; can be taken without regard to meals Duration: UK

Therapeutic Effects/Uses
Management of patients with HIV infection, prevention of maternal-fetal HIV transmission Mechanism of Action: Inhibits viral enzyme reverse transcriptase and thymidine kinase, enzymes necessary for viral HIV replication.

Side Effects	Adverse Reactions
Headache, malaise, nausea, anorexia, vomiting, asthenia (abnormal weakness and loss of energy), constipation, abdominal cramps/pain, arthralgia, rigors, dyspepsia, fatigue, insomnia, musculoskeletal pain, myalgia, neuropathy, elevated liver enzymes, anemia, fever, cough, hepatomegaly, rash, diarrhea, lipodystrophy, and stomatitis	Severe anemia, lactic acidosis, pancreatitis, neutropenia, pancytopenia, seizures, congestive heart failure, myelosuppression, rhabdomyolysis, anaphylaxis, hyperlipidemia, insulin resistance, Stevens-Johnson syndrome, and toxic epidermal necrolysis

A, Adult; *ALT,* alanine aminotransferase; *ARV,* antiretroviral; *AST,* aspartate aminotransferase; *bid,* twice a day; *d,* day; *GZDV,* 5'-glucuronyl zidovudine; *h,* hour; *HIV,* human immunodeficiency virus; *IV,* intravenously; *LD,* loading dose; *min,* minute; *PB,* protein binding; *PO,* by mouth; *q,* every; *t½,* half-life; *UK,* unknown; *wk,* weeks; *>,* greater than; *≥,* greater than or equal to; *<,* less than.

EFV is the first-choice drug within the NNRTI class, and it is the only NNRTI that penetrates the cerebrospinal fluid (CSF). It should be used with caution in pregnancy because neural tube defects have been reported after early human gestational exposure. Because of CSF involvement, neuropsychiatric symptoms such as dizziness, sedation, nightmares, euphoria, or loss of concentration can occur. Common complications among all the NNRTIs are rashes, which includes Stevens-Johnson syndrome. Elevated liver transaminases and hepatotoxicity, including hepatic failure, can also occur.

Drug-drug interactions are many because of the extensive metabolizing effects by cytochrome P3A4 (CYP3A4). Acid reducers (e.g., antacids, H₂-receptor antagonists, proton pump inhibitors [PPIs]) can decrease the bioavailability of rilpivirine, so coadministration of rilpivirine with PPIs is contraindicated; all other acid reducers can be taken at least 2 hours before or 4 hours after rilpivirine. Coadministration with drugs that induce or inhibit any of the CYP isoenzymes can alter the therapeutic effects of other drugs (e.g., anticonvulsants, antidepressants, anticoagulants, antiplatelets, antifungals, antimycobacterials,

statins, and calcium channel blockers [CCBs]). Other drugs used concomitantly can alter NNRTI serum levels (e.g., corticosteroids, hepatitis antivirals, and St. John's wort). NNRTIs can decrease the efficacy of hormonal contraceptives, so individuals should use alternative means of contraception or additional contraceptive methods.

Prototype Drug Chart: Efavirenz presents the pharmacologic data for EFV.

Protease Inhibitors

PI-based regimens (one or two PIs plus two NRTIs) have revolutionized the treatment of HIV infection, especially with PK enhancement (boosters such as cobicistat and ritonavir); this has led to sustained viral suppression, improved immunologic function, and prolonged patient survival. PIs that have been approved by the FDA include atazanavir (ATV), atazanavir/cobicistat (ATV/c), darunavir (DRV), darunavir/cobicistat (DRV/c), fosamprenavir (FPV), indinavir (IDV), lopinavir/ritonavir (LPV/r), nelfinavir (NFV), saquinavir (SQV), ritonavir (RTV), and tipranavir (TPV). RTV as the sole PI is not recommended;

PROTOTYPE DRUG CHART

Tenofovir Disoproxil Fumarate (TDF)

Drug Class	Dosage
Nucleoside/nucleotide reverse transcriptase inhibitor (NRTI) Also available as a component of fixed-dose combinations	HIV treatment: A ≥35 kg: PO: 300 mg once daily

Contraindications	Drug-Lab-Food Interactions
Black Box Warning: Hepatitis B exacerbation, hepatotoxicity, lactic acidosis *Caution:* Renal and hepatic dysfunction	*Drug:* Concomitant use with streptozocin is contraindicated because it can increase risk of nephrotoxicity and ototoxicity. Tenofovir can decrease levels of some drugs (e.g., dabigatran, edoxaban) and increase levels of other drugs (e.g., adefovir, bacitracin, diltiazem, metformin); acyclovir, amikacin, cisplatin, ganciclovir, and gentamicin may increase levels and adverse effects of TDF. *Lab:* May increase triglycerides, AST, ALT, ALP

Pharmacokinetics	Pharmacodynamics
Absorption: PO: 25%–40% Distribution: PB: 7.2% Metabolism: t½: 17 h; is not metabolized by CYP450 isoenzymes; converted intracellularly by hydrolysis and phosphorylated to active tenofovir diphosphate Excretion: 70%–80% primarily in urine as unchanged drug	Route: PO Onset: UK Peak: 1 h (fasting), 2 h (food) Duration: UK

Therapeutic Effects/Uses

Management of patients with HIV infection, treatment of chronic hepatitis B
Mechanism of Action: Inhibits viral enzyme reverse transcriptase, an enzyme necessary for viral HIV replication, by competing with AMP as substrate

Side Effects	Adverse Reactions
Diarrhea, nausea, vomiting, flatulence, insomnia, dizziness, depression, fever, hyperlipidemia, elevated transaminases, chest pain	Lactic acidosis, hepatomegaly, bone fractures, renal insufficiency, Fanconi syndrome

A, Adult; *ALP,* alkaline phosphatase; *ALT,* alanine aminotransferase; *AMP,* adenosine monophosphate; *AST,* aspartate aminotransferase; *CYP,* cytochrome P; *h,* hour; *HIV,* human immunodeficiency virus; *PB,* protein binding; *PO,* by mouth; *t½,* half-life; *UK,* unknown; *y,* years; ≥, greater than or equal to.

---

instead, it should be used as a boosting agent with other PIs. TPV is only approved for ARV-experienced patients. Unlike NRTIs and NNRTIs, PIs act at the end of the HIV life cycle to target viral assembly by inhibiting the activity of protease, an enzyme used to cleave nascent proteins for final assembly of new virions, resulting in formation and release of immature, defective, and noninfectious virus particles. Each PI has unique characteristics based on clinical efficacy, side effect profile, and PK properties. PIs are highly protein bound, metabolized by the liver, and primarily eliminated in feces.

The Panel's recommended PI regimen is DRV/r plus two NRTIs (tenofovir disoproxil fumarate/emtricitabine [TDF/FTC]). RTV boosting is a relatively new concept and one of the mainstays of PI therapy. The potent inhibitory effect of RTV on the cytochrome P450 3A4 isoenzyme (CYP3A4) allows the addition of 100 mg to 400 mg of RTV to other PIs as a PK booster. This helps reduce dietary restrictions, increase drug exposure, inhibit metabolism, and maximize blood levels of the coadministered PI, thus reducing dosing frequency and pill burden and overcoming viral resistance. Because "boosted" regimens may be less complex, patients may be able to follow and tolerate them better.

Selection of a PI-based regimen should consider dosing frequency, food and fluid requirements, pill burden, drug interaction potential, and side effect profile. PIs result in numerous metabolic abnormalities

that include dyslipidemia and insulin resistance; PK enhancers can alter these adverse effects. Some PIs come with a risk factor for causing myocardial infarction (MI). When initiating therapy with PIs, GI side effects (nausea, vomiting, and diarrhea) can be bothersome and may negatively affect adherence. Skin reactions such as rash, which includes Stevens-Johnson syndrome, can occur with PIs. Other adverse effects include hemolytic anemia, electrocardiogram (ECG) changes, and MI.

In patients with hepatic impairment, dosing adjustment may be necessary. All PIs inhibit the CYP450 system, which can lead to many drug-drug interactions. Drugs such as H₂-receptor antagonists (e.g., cimetidine, famotidine, or ranitidine) should be given 10 or more hours before PIs. PPIs are not recommended in PI-experienced patients, and concomitant use with anticoagulants/antiplatelets should also be avoided. Ritonavir-boosted PIs can decrease warfarin levels. Anticonvulsants (e.g., carbamazepine, phenobarbital, phenytoin) are contraindicated with certain PIs, whereas some antidepressants (e.g., bupropion, selective serotonin reuptake inhibitors [SSRIs]) may need dose adjustments. Trazodone is contraindicated with saquinavir/ritonavir, and antimycobacterials and cardiac drugs can worsen cardiac toxicities. Many PIs without the ritonavir boost can increase drug levels of hormonal contraceptives, whereas boosted PIs can decrease the levels. It is important that nurses instruct patients to use an alternative

PROTOTYPE DRUG CHART

Efavirenz (EFV)

Drug Class	Dosage
Nonnucleoside reverse transcriptase inhibitor (NNRTI) Also available as a component of fixed-dose combination.	Note: Take dose at bedtime to minimize CNS adverse effects; take on an empty stomach to reduce adverse reactions. A: PO: 600 mg at bedtime Do not crush tablets. Capsules may be opened and sprinkled into a small amount of age-appropriate soft food or formula; administer within 30 min of mixing; no additional food for 2 h after dosing.

Contraindications	Drug-Lab-Food Interactions
Life-threatening allergies to EFV or components of the preparation; concurrent use with rifapentine, St. John's wort, dasabuvir, ombitasvir, paritaprevir, simeprevir, triazolam *Caution:* Patients with history of mental illness or drug abuse; liver impairment; seizure disorder	*Drug:* EFV can increase or decrease levels of warfarin, carbamazepine, nevirapine, phenobarbital, bupropion, sertraline, phenytoin, rifampin, CCBs, hormonal contraceptives, HMG-CoA reductase inhibitors; EFV can increase the levels of triazolam. Drugs that can increase or decrease EFV include dexamethasone, boceprevir, St. John's wort. *Food:* Avoid alcohol because of liver/CNS adverse effects; high-fat meals increase absorption. *Lab:* May cause a false-positive result for cannabinoid and benzodiazepine screening assays.

Pharmacokinetics	Pharmacodynamics
Absorption: PO: Increased after high-fat meal Distribution: PB: >99%, widely distributed (found in CSF) Metabolism: $t\frac{1}{2}$: 40–76 h; metabolized in liver; CYP3A4 inducer/inhibitor Excretion: 16%–61% in feces, primarily as unchanged drug; 14%–34% in urine, primarily as metabolite	Route: PO Onset: UK Peak: 3–5 h Duration: UK

Therapeutic Effects/Uses
Treatment of HIV-1 infections Mechanism of Action: Binds directly to reverse transcriptase, blocking RNA- and DNA-dependent DNA polymerase activities, including HIV-1 replication

Side Effects	Adverse Reactions
Rash, nausea, diarrhea, CNS effects (dizziness, insomnia, abnormal dreams/thinking, impaired concentration, amnesia, agitation, hallucinations, euphoria, anxiety)	Aggressive reaction, allergic reaction, convulsion, liver failure, neuropathy, suicide, abnormal vision, hyperlipidemia

A, Adult; *CCB*, calcium channel blocker; *CNS*, central nervous system; *CSF*, cerebrospinal fluid; *CYP3A4*, cytochrome P450 3A4; *d*, day; *h*, hour; *HMG-CoA*, hydroxymethylglutaryl coenzyme A; *min*, minutes; *PB*, protein binding; *PO*, by mouth; *t½*, half-life; *UK*, unknown; ≥, greater than or equal to; >, greater than.

contraceptive method when taking boosted PIs. Rifampin and rifapentine are contraindicated with PIs, as are many other classes of drugs (e.g., antiarrhythmics, antivirals for viral hepatitis, St. John's wort, hydroxymethylglutaryl coenzyme A [HMG-CoA] reductase inhibitors, and some hypnotics) due to a decrease in PI drug levels and toxic drug levels in the other classes of drugs. Benefits of corticosteroid use should outweigh the risks with concomitant administration with corticosteroids.

Prototype Drug Chart: Atazanavir presents the pharmacologic data for ATV.

Fusion (Entry) Inhibitors

Enfuvirtide (T20) was the first approved in this class. T20 acts by a mechanism that inhibits the fusion of the virus to healthy cell membranes, thus preventing HIV entry into healthy cells. T20 is indicated only in combination with other ARVs for patients with limited treatment options who require salvage therapy. It is not indicated for HIV-2. Before initiating a fusion (entry) inhibitor, immunoassay and subsequent testing for HIV-1/HIV-2 are recommended.

Enfuvirtide T20 does not require dosage adjustment in patients with renal failure or hepatic impairment. It is not metabolized by CYP enzymes and is not associated with any CYP-mediated drug-drug interactions. Injection site reactions (e.g., subcutaneous nodules, redness) occur in up to 98% of patients. Other side effects reported include rash and diarrhea. Serious allergic reactions—including anaphylaxis, fever, and hypotension—have occurred in less than 1% of patients.

Ibalizumab is newly approved fusion inhibitors to treat HIV-1. Similar to T20, ibalizumab is indicated for patients with multiple drug-resistant infection. It is also used in combination with other ART drugs. Dose modification is not required. Reported side effects include diarrhea, dizziness, nausea, and rash.

Chemokine (CCR5) Coreceptor Antagonists

Maraviroc (MVC), the only drug in this class, blocks the CCR5 coreceptor needed for CCR5-tropic HIV entry into immune cells, thus preventing viral replication. MVC is indicated in combination with other ARVs for treatment-experienced adult patients with evidence of viral replication and HIV-1 strains resistant to multiple ART. The

PROTOTYPE DRUG CHART

Atazanavir (ATV)

Drug Class	Dosage
Protease inhibitor Also available as a component of fixed-dose combinations.	Note: HIV guidelines recommend administering concurrently with a PK enhancer (cobicistat or RTV). Capsules and powder packets are not interchangeable. Capsules: A: PO: 300 mg plus RTV 100 mg once daily Capsules must be swallowed whole. Powder may be mixed with food; use oral dosing syringe in persons unable to drink from a cup.

Contraindications	Drug-Lab-Food Interactions
Hypersensitivity to ATV or any component, concurrent use with alfuzosin, ergot derivatives, lovastatin, midazolam (oral), rifampin, simvastatin, St. John's wort *Caution:* Patients with preexisting conduction abnormalities (may prolong PR interval), hepatitis B or C, hepatic impairment, hemophilia A or B	*Drug:* Drug-drug interactions are numerous. Some known interactions include drugs that can decrease or decrease ATV; acid reducers, including H_2-receptor antagonists and PPIs; carbamazepine, phenytoin, phenobarbital, itraconazole, rifampin, boceprevir, and St. John's wort. ATV can increase or decrease levels of dabigatran, warfarin, buspirone, rifabutin, amiodarone, BBs, CCBs, digoxin, corticosteroids, hormonal contraceptives, lovastatin, and simvastatin *Lab:* May increase liver function tests, cholesterol, triglycerides, glucose *Food:* Bioavailability increases when taken with food

Pharmacokinetics	Pharmacodynamics
Absorption: PO: Rapidly, increased with food Distribution: PB: 86% Metabolism: t½: 7–8 h (9–18 h when boosted with RTV). Metabolized in the liver; inhibitor of CYP450 isoenzymes Excretion: Primarily in feces (79%) but also in urine (13%)	Route: PO Onset: UK Peak: 2–3 h Duration: UK

Therapeutic Effects/Uses
Treatment of HIV-1 infection Mechanism of Action: Inhibits HIV protease, rendering enzyme incapable of processing polyprotease precursors, thus rendering immature HIV particles noninfectious

Side Effects	Adverse Reactions
Rash, nausea, vomiting, diarrhea, cough, fever	Atrioventricular block, hyperglycemia, diabetes mellitus, jaundice, hyperlipidemia, lipodystrophy, cholelithiasis, nephrolithiasis, elevated liver transaminases

A, Adult; *BB,* beta blocker; *CCB,* calcium channel blocker; *CYP450,* cytochrome P450; *h,* hour; *H₂,* histamine 2; *HIV,* human immunodeficiency virus; *PB,* protein binding; *PK,* pharmacokinetic; *pk,* pack; *PO,* by mouth; *PPI,* proton pump inhibitor; *RTV,* ritonavir; *t½,* half-life; *UK,* unknown; *y,* year; ≥, greater than or equal to.

most common side effects are cough, pyrexia, upper respiratory tract infection, rash, abdominal pain, and dizziness. Because MVC is metabolized by the liver, drug-drug interactions exist.

MVC is metabolized by the CYP3A substrate. Coadministration with St. John's wort or rifampin or other CYP3A inducers is not recommended due to reduced effectiveness of MVC. Rifapentine and some NRTI fixed-drug combinations are contraindicated with CCR5 coreceptor antagonists. Possible drug-induced hepatotoxicity with allergy-type features has been reported. Use caution in patients with liver or heart disease or a history of orthostatic hypotension and in those on medication that lowers blood pressure. Other adverse reactions include rash, musculoskeletal symptoms, upper respiratory infections, and pyrexia.

Integrase Strand Transfer Inhibitors

INSTIs such as dolutegravir (DTG), elvitegravir (EVG), and raltegravir (RTG) exert their action by interfering with integrase, the

enzyme that HIV needs to multiply and divide, thus limiting the ability of the virus to replicate and infect new cells. INSTIs are used for the treatment of HIV-1 infections with at least two or three other ARVs in both treatment-naïve (recommended initial agent) and treatment-experienced patients. DTG and EVG are also available in fixed-dose combinations. INSTIs distribute into the CSF. DTG and RTG are metabolized by the UDP-glucuronosyltransferases (UGTs) 1A1-mediated glucuronidation pathway; EVG is metabolized by the CYP450 enzymes. Strong inducers (e.g., EFV, rifampin, rifabutin) or inhibitors (e.g., tenofovir, atazanavir) of UGT1A1 can significantly alter the concentration of RTG. DTG distributes into the CSF. Common side effects include rash, nausea, headache, insomnia, diarrhea, and pyrexia; liver injury can also occur. Caution is advised in patients at increased risk for muscle problems (e.g., myopathy, rhabdomyolysis), which includes patients who take medications that can cause these adverse effects, such as statins.

IMMUNE RECONSTITUTION INFLAMMATORY SYNDROME

Immune reconstitution inflammatory syndrome (IRIS) is related to a disease- or pathogen-specific inflammatory response in patients with ART being initiated or changed. IRIS comprises two distinct entities: *paradoxical IRIS* is an exacerbation of treated (successful or partial) opportunistic infection (OI), whereas *unmasking IRIS* is a response to undiagnosed or subclinical OI. Diagnosis is a challenge because there are no laboratory markers; it is a condition of exclusion. For example, new OI or concurrent illness must be excluded before IRIS can be diagnosed. CD4+ cells usually increase in patients with IRIS because of the acute inflammatory response. IRIS may occur in response to many diseases and pathogens, such as Kaposi sarcoma or infection with mycobacteria, viruses, bacteria, or fungi.

Risk factors for developing IRIS include a low CD4+ cell count when ART is initiated and a high baseline HIV RNA. Starting ART soon after initiation of treatment for recognized OI also increases risk for IRIS. Severity of IRIS ranges from mild to life-threatening. Treatment varies according to the specific pathogen and clinical situation but typically includes continuing ART if possible, treating the OI as indicated, and adding antiinflammatory therapy (including corticosteroids) as needed.

THE NURSE'S ROLE IN ANTIRETROVIRAL THERAPY

Thorough assessment of the patient's physiologic and psychosocial health needs and literacy levels is required initially and for the duration of care. Follow-up assessment after ART initiation should include drug side effects, adherence to the therapy regimen, and issues that affect medication adherence. Patients may confuse drug side effects with new onset of symptoms. Careful follow-up assessment can detect the need for additional medical care or drug management.

Adherence challenges are common with any drug therapy, but ART presents a greater challenge because patients are asked to achieve an adherence of 95% or greater. Nonadherence can result in HIV viral replication and can potentiate drug resistance. Multiple strategies for adherence are available and should be discussed with patients. Drug organizers, alarms on cell phones or mobile devices, medication "maps" with pictures, and drug diaries are available tools to improve adherence. Friends, family members, and personal support systems can also assist patients with adherence. Nurses can facilitate adherence by allowing sufficient time to educate patients about drugs, developing a trusting relationship, and building a partnership with the patient.

Nursing assessment for adherence should include asking the reasons for missing drug dosages. Reasons commonly include stigma, forgetting, feeling ill, side effects, not having the medicine when doses are due, pill fatigue (nonadherence due to the stress and monotony of constant pill swallowing), drug costs, loss of health insurance, and lack of transportation to the pharmacy. If barriers to adherence are identified, individualized plans should be addressed with the patient and the prescriber.

Patient education should include the purpose of each drug, the dosage schedule, food and fluid restrictions, recommended food choices, and storage of drugs. Additional suggestions include taking drugs during a daily routine, such as brushing teeth, or using a drug calendar to track drugs taken. The nurse should assess whether scheduled appointments to assist the patient with filling a drug organizer would be helpful until the patient is comfortable with completing this task.

BOX 32.1   HIV Resources

AIDS Info
The website www.aidsinfo.nih.gov provides information on HIV/AIDS clinical research, treatment, and prevention.

National HIV/AIDS Clinicians' Consultation Center
The website www.nccc.ucsf.edu provides up-to-date HIV/AIDS information to pharmacists, physicians, and nurses and is staffed by pharmacists, physicians, and nurse practitioners.

Discussion of anticipated drug side effects and management of drug side effects is necessary.

In addition to patient assessment, education, and advocacy, nurses should identify problems that require additional investigation and research. Because of individual needs, research on strategies to promote adherence is needed. Whenever drug regimens change, nurses should contribute to the ongoing evaluation of the drug regimen, any side effects, and adverse event reporting. See Box 32.1 for HIV resources.

OPPORTUNISTIC INFECTIONS

As HIV advances, patients are more vulnerable to malignancies and opportunistic infections (OIs). Since the introduction of ART, there has been a dramatic reduction in the incidence of OIs among HIV-positive patients receiving ARVs. Although hospitalizations and deaths have decreased, OIs continue to be a leading cause of morbidity and mortality among patients with HIV. Prevention and treatment of OIs remain essential. The most common HIV-related OIs include pulmonary TB, pneumococcal pneumonia, *Cryptosporidium*, fungal infections, Kaposi sarcoma, toxoplasmosis, histoplasmosis, and cytomegalovirus (CMV), among others.

Tuberculosis infection predominantly affects the lungs but can affect other organs, such as the bowel, brain, and lining of the heart, lungs, central nervous system (CNS), or integument. The CD4+ cell count is not a reliable predictor of increased risk for TB disease. Treatment for TB is discussed in Chapter 30.

Kaposi sarcoma causes dark blue lesions that can occur in a variety of locations, including the skin, mucous membranes, GI tract, lungs, or lymph nodes; they usually appear early in the course of HIV infection. Treatment depends on the symptoms and location, but chemotherapy is the preferred treatment for severe widespread disease.

Pneumocystis jiroveci pneumonia (PJP) is caused by a fungus that shares biologic characteristics with protozoa that infect the lungs. Symptoms include fever, dry cough, chest pain, and dyspnea. Even though PJP is classified as a fungal infection, it does not respond to antifungals. Trimethoprim-sulfamethoxazole (TMP-SMX), dapsone plus trimethoprim, pentamidine, or atovaquone is recommended treatment for persons with HIV and PJP.

Toxoplasmosis encephalitis caused by a protozoan can be found in uncooked meat and cat feces. Infection in the brain can cause headache, confusion, motor weakness, and fever. If left untreated, the disease progression results in seizures, stupor, and coma. Treatment includes pyrimethamine, sulfadiazine, and clindamycin. Leucovorin is added to decrease hematologic toxicities associated with pyrimethamine therapy.

Cryptosporidiosis is an infection caused by the protozoan parasite *Cryptosporidium*, usually in the bowel mucosa; in persons with low CD4+ counts, *Cryptosporidium* may involve the biliary tract or

⊚ CLINICAL JUDGMENT [NURSING PROCESS]

Antiretroviral Therapy

Concept: Drug Adherence
- The ability or lack of the ability to take drugs as prescribed

Recognize Cues [Assessment]
- Obtain an in-depth patient history and assess physiologic and psychosocial needs.
- Assess for signs and symptoms related to clinical progression of human immunodeficiency virus (HIV), and refer to medical care and psychological support as indicated.
- Perform a drug reconciliation that includes all prescription, over-the-counter (OTC), and herbal products. Assess for use of illegal and other nonprescription drugs. Report potential drug-drug or drug-herb interactions.
- Obtain a nutritional history to assess for nutritional deficits and for potential drug-food interactions. Assess for the potential need for therapeutic lifestyle change.
- Assess readiness to learn and discern the preferred method of instruction (written, verbal, pictorial).
- With each patient visit, conduct a pill count to determine treatment adherence.

Analyze Cues and Prioritize Hypothesis [Patient Problems]
- Risk for nonadherence
- Need for health teaching
- Coping
- Decreased immunity

Generate Solutions [Planning]
- The patient will adhere to the drug regimen and will report any difficulties related to adherence.
- The patient will participate in medical treatment and in the spiritual and psychological support that best fits the patient's needs and belief system; the patient will verbalize fears.
- The patient will verbalize ways of maintaining self-health management such as a daily calendar and reminders.
- The patient will verbalize ways to cope with side effects of the drug regimen.
- The patient will verbalize signs and symptoms of potential infection and can reiterate when to notify the health care provider.
- The patient will have undetectable viral load at end of therapy.
- The patient will not experience secondary or opportunistic infections (OIs).

Take Action [Nursing Interventions]
- Provide information on the necessity of adhering to the drug regimen and regular health care. Inconsistent dosing can promote drug resistance. Effectiveness and side effects of antiretroviral therapy (ART) need to be monitored and/or treated.
- Provide information on various methods of remembering to take drugs. Inconsistent dosing can increase the risk of drug resistance.

- Refer the patient for health care maintenance and appropriate health screening examinations, including Pap tests, ophthalmologic and dental examinations, and age- or risk-related colonoscopies. Side effects and adverse reactions are common in patients receiving ART.
- Refer the patient for spiritual support and for mental health or substance use counseling as needed.
- Provide opportunities for the patient and/or support persons to verbalize feelings.
- Encourage strategies to cope with the side effects of medications.
- Monitor laboratory reports for indications of decreasing CD4+ counts and/or rising viral load; inform the HIV health care provider.
- Refer the patient for nutritional counseling as needed.

Patient Teaching
General
- Educate patients about adherence to the therapeutic regimen by providing information on drugs and a timetable of dosing in patients' preferred method of learning.
- Explain common emotional responses.
- For patients of childbearing age, explain how HIV transmission to the unborn baby can occur.
- Teach about safe sex practices and other ways to prevent transmission of HIV.
- Inform patients that certain drugs—including OTC medications—and foods and herbal products may interact with antiretrovirals.
- Assist patients in developing a system for taking the correct dose of the correct drugs at the correct time.
- Counsel patients about the importance of having an adequate supply of drugs to avoid interruption in the dosing schedule. Omission of drugs may result in deterioration of the patient's condition.

Side Effects
- Explain how HIV can damage the immune system and promote infection.
- To decrease risk for exposure to infection, emphasize protective precautions as necessary, such as frequent handwashing, avoiding crowds, and receiving influenza vaccines.
- Inform the patient to report unmanageable side effects, such as nausea and diarrhea.

Evaluate Outcomes [Evaluation]
- The patient will have at least a 95% drug adherence. The patient will maintain a pill calendar or reminder to increase drug adherence.
- Viral load will decrease or become undetectable.
- The patient and/or the significant other will openly discuss any fears or concerns related to HIV and ART.
- The patient will verbalize safe sex practices and methods to reduce HIV transmission.

---

respiratory tract. GI symptoms include profuse, nonbloody, watery diarrhea, often with nausea, vomiting, and lower abdominal cramping. In addition to symptomatic therapy, treatment includes nitazoxanide or paromomycin combined with azithromycin. Treatment may be only partially effective in the setting of a low CD4+ count.

Mycobacterium avium complex (MAC) is a blood infection caused by bacteria related to *M. tuberculosis,* the pathogen in TB. MAC generally affects multiple organs with symptoms that include fever, night sweats, weight loss, fatigue, diarrhea, and abdominal pain. Localized

syndromes include pneumonitis, osteomyelitis, skin or soft tissue abscesses, or CNS infections. Treatment includes clarithromycin, azithromycin, ethambutol, amikacin, moxifloxacin, rifabutin, or rifampin.

Cytomegalovirus (CMV) infection is caused by a virus that infects the entire body, but it most commonly appears as retinitis, causing blurred vision that can lead to blindness. CMV can also affect other organs and can cause fever, diarrhea, nausea, pneumonia-like symptoms, and dementia. Treatment includes ganciclovir, valganciclovir, foscarnet, or cidofovir.

ANTIRETROVIRAL THERAPY IN PREGNANCY

Optimal drug therapy should be used for women of reproductive age and for those who are pregnant. When initiating ART for women of reproductive age, the criteria for starting therapy and the goals of treatment are identical to those for other adults and adolescents. Because of considerations related to the prevention of HIV transmission to the fetus during pregnancy, the timing of initiation of treatment and the selection of regimens for pregnant patients may differ from those for nonpregnant adults or adolescents. Women of childbearing potential should undergo a pregnancy test before initiation of EFV. If the patient expresses interest in becoming pregnant, and EFV is considered as part of the ARV regimen, a risk-benefit discussion must take place regarding the risk of neural tube defects related to EFV use in the first 5 to 6 weeks of pregnancy. EFV can be continued in pregnant patients receiving an EFV-based regimen who present for antenatal care in the first trimester, provided the regimen produces virologic suppression.

A pregnant patient infected with HIV can transmit the virus during pregnancy, labor, and delivery and through breastfeeding. To prevent mother-to-child transmission of HIV, ART is recommended in all pregnant patients who test positive for HIV infection, regardless of virologic, immunologic, or clinical parameters. Combination drug therapy is considered the standard of care for both treatment of maternal HIV infection and prophylaxis to reduce the risk for perinatal HIV transmission. The goal of ART is to achieve maximal and sustained viral suppression during pregnancy to prevent perinatal transmission of HIV. If viral load is greater than or equal to 400 copies/mL, IV zidovudine is recommended regardless of current ART. Prototype Drug Chart: Zidovudine presents the pharmacologic data for zidovudine.

OCCUPATIONAL HIV EXPOSURE AND POSTEXPOSURE PROPHYLAXIS

Treatment regimens after percutaneous exposure to HIV are called postexposure prophylaxis (PEP) regimens. Many PEP regimens are available, with varying degrees of tolerability and probability of patients completing 4 weeks of treatment. PEP management of potential HIV exposure should be initiated within 72 hours of the event and should be continued for 4 weeks. Health care workers who take PEP have reported adverse reactions, with the most common being nausea, malaise, and fatigue. More information from the Panel on the treatment of HIV/AIDS can be found at https://aidsinfo.nih.gov.

CRITICAL THINKING CASE STUDY

A 35-year-old female patient was recently diagnosed with HIV. Other than a recent "case of the flu" approximately 1 month ago, she has been healthy. She has been divorced for 2 years and has a 3-year-old child from her previous marriage. The patient tested negative for HIV in the first trimester of her pregnancy and was not retested during the third trimester. She reports that the relationship with her partner was monogamous and that they did not use "protections." She began a relationship with a new partner 1 year after her divorce, who denied having HIV, and they did not use protective barriers (the patient takes oral contraceptives for pregnancy prevention). The patient denies a history of IV drug use and other high-risk behaviors. Her baseline labs include a CD4+ count of 450 cells/mm^3 and a viral load of 75,000 copies/mL. Her genotypic resistance assay shows no baseline resistance. Her preference is for a once-a-day regimen. She may want to have another child but is not certain.

1. The patient asks the nurse when she may have become infected with HIV. What are some of the responses that the nurse should include in a discussion with the patient? What else should the nurse discuss with the patient about HIV transmission?
2. Considering the patient's preference for a daily antiretroviral regimen and in view of her history, which medication regimens could be considered? What, if any, risk-benefit discussion should occur with regard to choices?
3. The patient is told she will begin therapy with a fixed-dose combination regimen containing three different ARVs. The patient asks why she needs to be on more than one drug. How would the nurse explain the reason for the multidrug regimen?
4. At her next routine visit, the patient says that she missed two doses of her medications because she had an unplanned overnight stay during a trip. What counseling and interventions would the nurse include in discussion with the patient?

REVIEW QUESTIONS

1. During routine prenatal testing, a patient is diagnosed with human immunodeficiency virus infection. To help prevent perinatal transmission of human immunodeficiency virus to the fetus, which nursing action is best?
   a. Provide the patient with contact information for an acquired immunodeficiency syndrome support group.
   b. Educate the patient about the risks of human immunodeficiency virus disease to the fetus.
   c. Notify the Centers for Disease Control and Prevention of the patient's diagnosis.
   d. Provide written and oral education about the use of antiretroviral therapy during pregnancy.

2. A recent laboratory results indicated an "undetectable" human immunodeficiency virus viral load. Which response is best by the nurse?
   a. Inform the patient that they must be seen immediately because the undetectable viral load indicates that the medication stopped working.
   b. Have the patient reschedule the clinic visit.
   c. Congratulate the patient on the treatment success.
   d. Educate the patient about the continued need for medications and ongoing laboratory monitoring.

3. The nurse advises human immunodeficiency virus (HIV)-positive patients about blood draws to obtain a CD4+ count. Which information would be correct?
   a. Laboratory tests should be done at the same laboratory at approximately the same time of day
   b. A 10-hour fast is required for laboratory tests
   c. Laboratory tests will need to be obtained approximately 1 hour after taking antiretroviral medications
   d. It does not matter where the labs are conducted as long as it is done

4. In collaboration with a patient on antiretroviral therapy, the nurse formulates a plan of care. Which items are appropriate to include in planning? (Select all that apply.)
   a. Viral load will become and remain undetectable.
   b. The patient will not experience secondary infection.
   c. New onset of symptoms and side effects will be promptly reported.
   d. Laboratory blood work will be within normal limits.
   e. The patient will adhere to the medication regimen and will report any difficulties related to adherence.

5. A patient is to start on efavirenz. Which points are important for the nurse to include in health teaching for this patient? (Select all that apply.)
   a. The dose is given at bedtime to minimize central nervous system adverse effects.
   b. Alcohol should be avoided because of adverse effects to the liver.
   c. The dose should be taken after breakfast to minimize central nervous system adverse effects.
   d. High-fat meals can increase absorption of the medication.
   e. Hyperglycemia, jaundice, and diabetes mellitus are side effects.

33

Transplant Drugs

http://evolve.elsevier.com/McCuistion/pharmacology

OBJECTIVES

- Describe the mechanism of action of the six maintenance therapy drugs and relate the processes to the principles of immunosuppression.
- Differentiate the three drugs used in the treatment of transplant rejection.

- Calculate the absolute neutrophil count of a patient on immunosuppressive drugs and relate it to neutropenic precautions.
- Describe the issues surrounding nonadherence in transplant recipients.
- Describe the nurse's role in promoting adherence to the therapeutic drug regimen.

OUTLINE

ORGAN TRANSPLANTATION

Organ transplantation is a life-saving procedure. In cadaveric transplantation, a healthy organ donated at the time of a person's death is transplanted into the body of a patient with end-stage organ failure. In living-donor transplantation, a kidney or a portion of liver donated by a living person is transplanted into the body of a patient with end-stage kidney or liver disease. Organ transplant is an acceptable treatment option when organs fail (e.g., kidney, heart, liver, and lung). More than 122,000 people are currently waiting for an organ transplant. Every 10 minutes, another person is added to the wait list, and more than 8000 people die each year while waiting for a donor organ.

Principles of Immunosuppression

The immune system remains the biggest barrier to transplantation as a routine medical treatment because it has effective mechanisms to fight off foreign organisms. These same mechanisms are involved in the rejection of transplanted organs, which are recognized as foreign by the recipient's immune system. The underlying premise of immunosuppression is to use multiple drugs that alter different aspects of the immune system (Fig. 33.1), thereby reducing the chances of transplant rejection and enabling the use of lower doses of individual drugs, which reduces the likelihood of drug toxicity. Transplantation has revolutionized care for patients with end-stage organ failure, yet significant problems remain with treatments designed to promote transplant survival and prevent rejection. Immunosuppressant drugs are not always effective; in addition, they are expensive, must be taken daily, and are associated with toxic effects.

Immunosuppressant Drugs

Induction Therapy

Induction therapy provides intense immunosuppression with drugs designed to diminish antigen presentation and T-cell response, thus reducing the risk for acute rejection during the initial transplant period.

Basiliximab is a monoclonal antibody that inhibits activation of lymphocytes, a critical component of the cellular immune response involved in transplant rejection. By inhibiting activation of lymphocytes, it prevents the body from mounting an immune response against the transplanted organ. Basiliximab has been approved for induction therapy in kidney transplants.

Pharmacokinetics. Complete pharmacokinetic data are not available.

Pharmacodynamics. Drug half-life is known to be 7.2 days in adults and 9.5 days in children; duration of action is 36 days.

Basiliximab is administered intravenously (IV), 20 mg within 2 hours before transplant surgery, followed by a second 20-mg dose 4 days after transplantation. The second dose should be withheld if complications occur (including severe hypersensitivity reactions or loss of the transplanted organ). Children under 35 kg should receive 10 mg IV within 2 hours before transplant surgery, followed by a second 10-mg dose 4 days after transplantation; the second dose should be withheld if complications occur (including severe hypersensitivity reactions or loss of the transplanted organ); children over 35 kg should receive the adult dose.

Side effects of basiliximab include abdominal and back pain, coughing, dizziness, fever or chills, fatigue, weakness, dysuria, dyspnea, sore

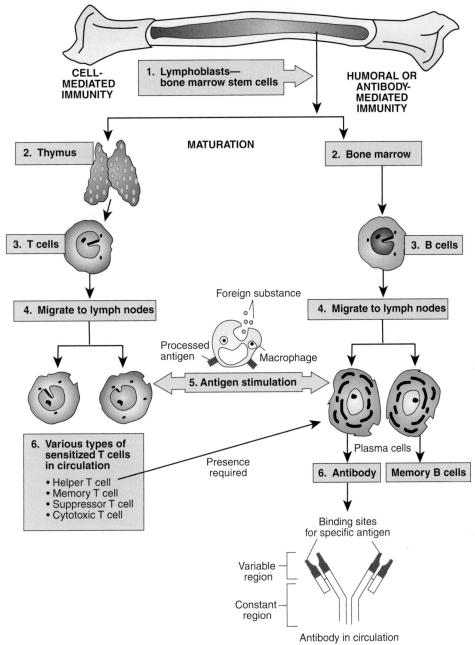

Fig. 33.1 The immune response. (From Gould, B., & Dyer, R. [2011]. *Pathophysiology for the health professions* [4th ed.]. St Louis: Saunders.)

throat, edema, tremor, nausea and vomiting, and anemia. Serious reactions include sepsis, opportunistic infections, malignancy, lymphoproliferative disorders, thrombocytopenia, leukopenia, diabetes mellitus, anaphylaxis, capillary leak syndrome, and cytokine release syndrome (Box 33.1).

Transplant recipients who receive basiliximab should not receive live vaccines because they may produce an inadequate immune response and are at risk for disseminated infection resulting from the live virus. Caution is advised when basiliximab is administered with other drugs that lower the immune response because of the increased risk of serious infection.

No adequate and well-controlled studies have been done on basiliximab's use in pregnant women, so women of childbearing potential should use effective contraceptive measures before beginning treatment, during treatment, and for 4 months after completion of therapy.

It is not known whether basiliximab is excreted in breast milk. Because of the potential for adverse drug reactions, a decision should be made whether to discontinue nursing or to discontinue the drug, taking into account the importance of the drug to the mother.

Maintenance Therapy

Calcineurin Inhibitors. The calcineurin inhibitors (CNIs) suppress the immune system by binding to cytoplasmic proteins that inhibit calcineurin phosphatase, ultimately resulting in inhibition of T-lymphocyte proliferation. There are two CNIs, cyclosporine and tacrolimus; the prototype CNI is cyclosporine (see Prototype Drug Chart: Cyclosporine [Modified]). The drug became available in 1983 and was modified to improve bioavailability in 1994. Cyclosporine carries a boxed warning for malignancies and serious infections. Additionally, the warning advises that cyclosporine oral solution

BOX 33.1   Cytokine Release Syndrome

Cytokine release syndrome is a symptom complex associated with the use of anti-T-cell antibody infusions, such as antithymocyte globulin (rabbit) and muromonab-CD3. Commonly referred to as an *infusion reaction,* cytokine release syndrome results from the release of cytokines from cells targeted by the antibody. When cytokines are released into the circulation, systemic symptoms such as fever, nausea, chills, hypotension, tachycardia, asthenia, headache, rash, scratchy throat, and dyspnea can result. In most patients, the symptoms are mild to moderate in severity and are managed easily. Premedication with corticosteroids or acetaminophen plus an antihistamine has been reported to be effective in reducing the severity of symptoms caused by cytokine release. Other management measures include reduction of the infusion rate. However, some patients may experience life-threatening reactions; therefore nurses must closely monitor patients receiving anti-T–cell antibody infusions. Patients with asthma, autoimmune disease, history of drug allergies, and previous exposure to the drug are at increased risk of developing cytokine release syndrome. During infusions, nurses must assess the patient frequently, monitoring vital signs and watching for any signs or symptoms of a reaction. Reactions are most likely to occur in the first hour, but a reaction could occur at any time. Any delay in recognition of the signs of anaphylaxis can compromise the patient's outcome.

From Vogel, W. H. (2010). Infusion reactions: Diagnosis, assessment and management. *Clinical Journal of Oncology Nursing, 14*(2), E10–E21.

USP modified and cyclosporine oral solution USP *are not* bioequivalent and *cannot* be used interchangeably.

Grapefruit and grapefruit juice affect drug metabolism, increasing blood concentration of cyclosporine; for this reason, grapefruit should be avoided. To make cyclosporine oral solution USP modified more palatable, it should be diluted with room-temperature orange or apple juice; patients should avoid switching diluents frequently. When mixed with juice, the cyclosporine solution may appear cloudy. Cyclosporine is also available as immediate-release capsules (25 mg and 100 mg) and as an IV solution (250 mg/5 mL).

Transplant recipients taking cyclosporine should not receive live vaccines because they may have inadequate immune response and are at risk for disseminated infection resulting from the live virus.

In addition to therapeutic drug monitoring (TDM; drug levels should be drawn just before the dose), patients taking cyclosporine should have frequent monitoring of blood urea nitrogen (BUN), creatinine, potassium, and magnesium levels in addition to liver function tests (LFTs) and lipid profiles.

Cyclosporine does not appear to be a major human teratogen; however, it may be associated with increased rates of prematurity. Cyclosporine is present in breast milk. Because of the potential for serious adverse drug reactions in nursing infants, a decision should be made whether to discontinue nursing or to discontinue the drug, taking into account the importance of the drug to the mother.

Tacrolimus. Approved by the US Food and Drug Administration (FDA) in 1994, tacrolimus is the second CNI approved for prophylaxis of rejection in heart, liver, and kidney transplants. It carries a boxed warning for malignancies and serious infections. Patients taking this drug are at increased risk for developing lymphoma and other malignancies. Additionally, patients taking tacrolimus are at risk for developing bacterial, viral, fungal, and protozoal infections.

Dosing for heart transplant recipients begins no sooner than 6 hours posttransplant with a continuous infusion at 0.01 mg/kg/day IV. When oral dosing begins, it should be at a dose of 0.075 mg/kg/day orally divided every 12 hours. For patients with a liver transplant, tacrolimus is administered with a continuous infusion at 0.03 to 0.05 mg/kg/day IV. When oral dosing begins, it should be dosed 0.1 to 0.15 mg/kg/day orally divided every 2 hours. Kidney transplant recipients should begin tacrolimus within 24 hours of receiving the transplanted organ. Dosing ranges from 0.1 to 0.2 mg/kg/day orally divided every 12 hours and may vary based on drugs used for induction.

For all transplant recipients, dosing is adjusted based on serum drug levels, with trough levels ranging between 5 and 20 ng/mL, depending on organ transplanted and length of time since transplant.

The drug is highly nephrotoxic and should be administered at the lowest recommended dose for those with renal impairment. For those with postoperative oliguria, use of tacrolimus may be delayed until kidney function is adequate. All patients on tacrolimus should have their kidney function monitored periodically during therapy.

Tacrolimus may prolong the QT/QTc interval and may cause torsades de pointes. Avoid tacrolimus in patients with congenital long QT syndrome. In patients with congestive heart failure, bradyarrhythmias, those taking certain antiarrhythmic medications or other medicinal products that lead to QT prolongation, and those with electrolyte disturbances such as hypokalemia, hypocalcemia, or hypomagnesemia, consider obtaining electrocardiograms and monitoring electrolytes (magnesium, potassium, calcium) periodically during treatment.

Pharmacokinetics. Tacrolimus is slowly absorbed in the gastrointestinal (GI) tract. Food, especially food high in fat, slows absorption and reduces bioavailability. Tacrolimus is highly bound (>98.8%) to plasma proteins. It is metabolized extensively in the liver and is over 90% excreted in the feces, with the remaining excreted in the urine.

Pharmacodynamics. Bioavailability averages 25%, and peak serum concentration is reached in 3 hours. Genetic variations in activity of the CYP3A5 protein can affect serum concentrations of tacrolimus. Its half-life is variable depending on organ transplanted (3.5 to 40.6 hours).

Tacrolimus has multiple common side effects, including tremor, diarrhea, headache, hypertension, nephrotoxicity, infection, insomnia, electrolyte, metabolic and lipid abnormalities, constipation, edema, fever, anemia, hyperglycemia, hepatotoxicity, anorexia, dyspepsia, dyspnea, pruritus, dizziness, cough, leukopenia, and photosensitivity. Serious reactions include malignancy, posttransplant lymphoproliferative disorder, severe infections, Stevens-Johnson syndrome, toxic epidermal necrolysis, anaphylaxis, neurotoxicity, seizures, myocardial hypertrophy, QT prolongation, torsades de pointes, pericardial effusion, diabetes, myelosuppression, DIC, thrombocytopenic purpura, and hemolytic anemia.

Persons receiving tacrolimus have absolute contraindication for live vaccines, mifepristone, pimozide, quinidine, saquinavir, streptozocin, talimogene laherparepvec (a genetically modified oncolytic viral therapy used in patients with recurrent melanoma), and ziprasidone. Multiple other drugs should be used with caution. Protease inhibitors may increase serum drug levels, as can antifungal agents, calcium channel blockers, gastric acid suppressors/antacids, and antibacterials. Anticonvulsants can decrease serum drug levels, as can St. John's wort. Patients receiving tacrolimus should avoid grapefruit juice, as it too may increase serum drug levels.

Cyclosporine (Modified)

Drug Class	Dosage (adult)
Calcineurin inhibitors	Organ transplant rejection prophylaxis (dosing protocols vary) Start: 7–9 mg/kg/day PO divided bid, give first dose 4–12 h pretransplant or postop; for heart, kidney, or liver transplant; adjust dose based on target levels, rejection status, adverse effects rheumatoid arthritis, severe (2.5–4 mg/kg/day PO divided bid) Start: 2.5 mg/kg/day PO divided bid, increase 0.5–0.75 mg/kg/day after 8 wk and after 12 wk; *max:* 4 mg/kg/day; info: use alone or with methotrexate; decrease 25%–50% prn adverse effects; D/C if no benefit by 16 wk psoriasis, severe recalcitrant plaque (2.5–4 mg/kg/day PO divided bid) Start: 2.5 mg/kg/day PO divided bid, increase 0.5 mg/kg/day q2wk after 4 wk; *max:* 4 mg/kg/day; Info: decrease 25%–50% prn adverse effects; D/C if inadequate response after 6 wk on max tolerated dose. Trough drug levels for kidney transplants: 0–3 months 200–300 ng/mL 3–6 months 150–250 ng/mL 6–12 months 100–200 ng/mL >12 months 50–100 ng/mL Recommended trough levels may vary by transplant center protocol and immunosuppressive drug regimen

Contraindications/Cautions

Hypersensitivity to drug/class/components
HTN, uncontrolled (RA or psoriasis use)
Renal impairment (RA or psoriasis use)
Malignancy (RA or psoriasis use)
PUVA/UVB treatment (psoriasis use)
Concurrent immunosuppressants (psoriasis use)
Coal tar treatment (psoriasis use)
Concomitant radiation therapy (psoriasis use)
Caution if hepatic impairment
Caution if renal impairment
Caution if concurrent nephrotoxic agent use
Caution if concurrent immunosuppressants
Caution in elderly patients

Drug-Lab-Food Interactions

Multiple drug-drug interactions, refer to package insert
Grapefruit and grapefruit juice can increase the levels of cyclosporine

Monitoring Parameters

Transplant: BUN/Cr at baseline, then cont. frequently; LFTs; K, Mg; lipid panel; serum drug levels
RA: BUN/Cr, BP × 2 at baseline, then q2wk × 3 mo, then if stable, q mo; LFTs; K, Mg; lipid panel; serum drug levels
Psoriasis: BUN/Cr × 2 at baseline, then q2wk × 3 mo, then if stable, q mo; BP × 2, CBC, K, Mg, lipid panel, uric acid at baseline, then q2wk × 3 mo, then q mo if stable, or more frequently if adjust dose; LFTs

Pharmacokinetics

Absorption: dependent on the individual patient, the patient population, and the formulation
Distribution: Distributed widely outside the blood volume; 90% bound to proteins
Metabolism: extensively metabolized by the cytochrome P-450 3A enzyme system in the liver, and to a lesser degree in the gastrointestinal tract, and the kidney
Elimination: primarily biliary with only 6% of the dose (parent drug and metabolites) excreted in urine

Pharmacodynamics

Onset: UK
Peak: oral 1.5–2 h
Duration: UK
Half-life is approximately 8.4 hours (range 5–18 hours)

Therapeutic Effects/Uses

Used to prevent organ rejection and in various autoimmune conditions

Side Effects

BUN, Cr elevated, hypertension, hirsutism, infection, tremor, gingival overgrowth, headache, hypertriglyceridemia (psoriasis use), nausea/vomiting, diarrhea, leg cramps, paresthesia, influenza-like symptoms, edema, dizziness, rash, acne, chest pain, stomatitis, hypomagnesemia, arthralgia, flushing, bronchospasm, hyperkalemia, hyperglycemia, hyperuricemia, others (see package insert)

Adverse Reactions

Hypertension, severe; immunosuppression; infection, severe; opportunistic infection; BK virus–associated nephropathy; hyperkalemia, severe; nephrotoxicity; hepatotoxicity; glomerular capillary thrombosis; diabetes mellitus; leukopenia; thrombocytopenia; hemolytic anemia; malignancy; seizures; encephalopathy; posterior reversible encephalopathy syndrome; neurotoxicity; intracranial HTN; optic disc edema; hypersensitivity reaction; myocardial infarction; depression; pancreatitis; GI bleeding

Portions excerpted from Epocrates. (2019). Cyclosporine modified (generic). Retrieved January 4, 2019, from https://online.epocrates.com/drugs/418210/cyclosporine-modified/Monograph.

bid, Twice a day; *BP,* blood pressure; *BUN,* blood urea nitrogen; *Cr,* creatinine; *d,* day; *GI,* gastrointestinal; *h,* hour; *HTN,* hypertension; *K, potassium; LFT,* liver function test; *Mg,* magnesium; *min,* minute; *mo,* month; *PO,* by mouth; *RA,* rheumatoid arthritis; *q,* every; *UK,* unknown; *wk,* weeks; *>,* greater than; *<,* less than.

PROTOTYPE DRUG CHART

Sirolimus

Drug Class	Dosage
mTOR inhibitors	Give consistently with or without food; do not cut/crush/chew tab
	Kidney Transplant Rejection Prophylaxis:
	Adult:
	Low-mod immunologic risk, <40 kg: 1 mg/m² PO qd; start: 3 mg/m² PO × 1 ASAP after transplant; *max:* 40 mg/day; refer to institution protocols for risk classification
	Low-mod immunologic risk, >40 kg: 2 mg PO qd; start: 6 mg PO × 1 ASAP after transplant; *max:* 40 mg/day; refer to institution protocols for risk classification
	High immunologic risk, <40 kg: 1 mg/m² PO qd; start: 3 mg/m² PO ×1 ASAP after transplant; *max:* 40 mg/day; refer to institution protocols for risk classification
	High immunologic risk, >40 kg: : 5 mg PO qd; start: up to 15 mg PO × 1 ASAP after transplant; *max:* 40 mg/day
	Pediatric:
	Low-mod immunologic risk, 13 y and older, <40 kg: 1 mg/m² PO qd; start: 3 mg/m² PO × 1 ASAP after transplant; *max:* 40 mg/day; refer to institution protocols for risk classification
	Low-mod immunologic risk, 13 y and older, >40 kg: 2 mg PO qd; start: 6 mg PO ×1 ASAP after transplant; *max:* 40 mg/day; Info: refer to institution protocols for risk classification
	Therapeutic Drug Levels:
	Transplant rejection prophylaxis: 16–24 ng/mL (whole blood sample) × 1 y after transplant, then 12–20 ng/mL (whole blood sample) thereafter.

Contraindications/Cautions	Drug-Lab-Food Interactions
Hypersensitivity to drug/class/component	Multiple drug-drug interactions, refer to package insert
Lung transplant use	Because grapefruit juice inhibits metabolism of sirolimus, it must not be taken with or be used to dilute sirolimus solution
Liver transplant use	Monitoring parameters lipid panel; serum drug levels; urine protein
Caution if concurrent nephrotoxic agent use	
Caution if delayed graft function	
Caution if BMI >30 kg/m²	
Caution if hepatic impairment	
Caution if renal impairment	
Caution if hyperlipidemia	

Pharmacokinetics	Pharmacodynamics
Absorption: dependent on the individual patient, the patient population, and the formulation	Onset: UK
Distribution: extensively bound (approximately 92%) to human plasma proteins	Peak: 1–3 h solution; 1–6 h tablets
Metabolism: liver extensively, GI tract; CYP450: 3A4 substrate; Info: P-gp substrate	Duration: UK
Excretion: feces 91%, urine 2.2%	Half-life: 2.5 days

Therapeutic Effects/Uses

Indicated for the prophylaxis of organ rejection in patients aged 13 years or older receiving renal transplants

Side Effects	Adverse Reactions
Peripheral edema, hyperlipidemia, hypertension, creatinine increase, constipation, pain, diarrhea, headache, fever, infection, anemia, nausea, arthralgia, thrombocytopenia, acne, dizziness, myalgia, diabetes mellitus, rash, proteinuria, tachycardia, stomatitis, leukopenia, abnormal healing, LDH increase, hypokalemia, epistaxis, pyelonephritis, ovarian cysts, menstrual disorder	Immunosuppression; malignancy; lymphoma; infection, severe; opportunistic infection; progressive multifocal leukoencephalopathy; BK virus–associated nephropathy; nephrotic syndrome; hemolytic uremic syndrome; thrombotic thrombocytopenic purpura; thrombotic microangiopathy; venous thromboembolism; myelosuppression; hypersensitivity reaction; anaphylaxis/anaphylactoid reaction; angioedema; exfoliative dermatitis; impaired wound healing; lymphocele; ascites; pericardial effusion; pleural effusion; interstitial lung diagnosis; hepatotoxicity; hypokalemia; osteonecrosis

Portions excerpted from Epocrates. (2019). Sirolimus. Retrieved January 4, 2019, from https://online.epocrates.com/drugs/247410/sirolimus/Monograph.
bid, Twice a day; *BP,* blood pressure; *BMI, body mass index; Cr,* creatinine; *d,* day; *GI,* gastrointestinal; *h,* hour; *mo,* month; *LDH,* lactate dehydrogenase; *PO,* by mouth; *q,* every; *UK,* unknown; *wk,* weeks; *>,* greater than; *<,* less than.

Costimulation Blockers. Belatacept is a first-in-class selective T-cell costimulation blocking agent indicated for use in combination with basiliximab induction, mycophenolate mofetil, and corticosteroids to prevent kidney transplant rejection. It inhibits T-cell activation and proliferation, thereby inhibiting T-lymphocyte proliferation and the production of inflammatory mediators.

The prescribed dose must be divisible by 12.5 to accurately prepare the dose from the reconstituted solution. Initial dosing is 10 mg/kg IV before surgery on the day of transplant; the dose is repeated on day 5 and at the end of weeks 2, 4, 8, and 12 after transplantation. Maintenance dosing is 5 mg/kg IV at the end of week 16 after transplantation and then every 4 weeks thereafter. Belatacept is not approved for pediatric use.

⚡ This drug carries a boxed warning for increased risk of developing posttransplant lymphoproliferative disorder (PTLD), predominantly involving the central nervous system (CNS). Additionally, recipients without immunity to Epstein-Barr virus (EBV) are at a particularly increased risk; therefore belatacept is for use in EBV-seropositive patients only.

Pharmacokinetics. Metabolism and excretion of belatacept are unknown.

Pharmacodynamics. Drug half-life is 8.2 to 9.8 days. Common side effects of belatacept include infection, anemia, diarrhea, peripheral edema, hypertension, constipation, fever, cough, nausea and vomiting, altered potassium levels, headache, leukopenia, abdominal pain, dyslipidemia, hypophosphatemia, arthralgia, hyperglycemia, proteinuria, increased creatinine, insomnia, hypocalcemia, back pain, dysuria, and anxiety. Serious reactions include PTLD, malignancy, serious infections, progressive multifocal leukoencephalopathy (PML), neutropenia, acute renal failure, nephropathy, and diabetes mellitus.

Transplant recipients receiving belatacept should not receive live vaccines because their immune response may be inadequate, and they are at risk for disseminated infection resulting from the live virus. Caution is advised when belatacept is administered with other drugs that lower the immune response because of the increased risk of serious infection.

Adverse events have been observed in animal studies with belatacept. According to the manufacturer, belatacept should not be used in pregnancy unless the potential benefit to the mother outweighs the potential risk to the fetus. ⚡ A pregnancy registry has been established to monitor outcomes of women exposed to belatacept during pregnancy (1-877-955-6877). Safety during breastfeeding is unknown; therefore a decision should be made whether to discontinue nursing or to discontinue the drug, taking into account the importance of the drug to the mother.

mTOR Inhibitors. There are two mammalian target of rapamycin (mTOR) inhibitors approved for the prevention of organ rejection in kidney transplant recipients aged 13 years and older: sirolimus and everolimus. Sirolimus is the prototype drug (see Prototype Drug Chart: Sirolimus); it inhibits T-lymphocyte activation and proliferation and inhibits antibody production.

⚡ There are two boxed warnings for sirolimus: use of sirolimus increases susceptibility to infection and the possible development of lymphoma and other malignancies, and the safety and efficacy have not been established in liver or lung transplant recipients; therefore use is not advised in liver or lung transplant recipients due to increased morbidity and mortality.

It is recommended that the maintenance dose of sirolimus tablets be reduced by approximately one-third in patients with mild or moderate hepatic impairment and by half in patients with severe hepatic impairment. Dosing should not exceed 40 mg/day.

Transplant recipients taking sirolimus should not receive live vaccines because their immune response may be inadequate, and they are at risk for disseminated infection resulting from the live virus. Caution is advised when sirolimus is administered with other drugs that lower the immune response because of the increased risk of serious infection.

No adequate and well-controlled studies of sirolimus have been done in pregnant women; therefore effective contraception must be initiated before sirolimus therapy, and it should continue during sirolimus therapy and for 12 weeks after therapy has been stopped. Sirolimus should be used during pregnancy only if the potential benefit outweighs the potential risk. Whether sirolimus is excreted in breast milk is unknown; therefore a decision should be made whether to discontinue nursing or to discontinue the drug, taking into account the importance of the drug to the mother.

Please note: Everolimus will not be discussed here, as it is used primarily in the treatment of advanced cancers.

Purine Antimetabolites. Azathioprine, a purine antimetabolite, blocks purine metabolism and DNA synthesis, thereby suppressing T- and B-lymphocyte proliferation. It is indicated for the prevention of kidney transplant rejection.

Pharmacokinetics. Azathioprine is well absorbed after oral administration. Azathioprine and its metabolite are moderately bound to serum proteins (30%) and undergo extensive metabolism in the liver; both are primarily excreted in bile.

Pharmacodynamics. Onset of action is unknown; the drug reaches peak in 1 to 2 hours; duration of action is unknown. The half-life of azathioprine is 5 hours.

⚡ Azathioprine has a boxed warning that chronic immunosuppression with azathioprine increases risk of malignancy in humans.

Dosing ranges from 1 to 3 mg/kg per day orally (an IV form is not currently available in the United States). In the setting of kidney dysfunction, the dose should be reduced by 25% for a creatinine clearance (CrCl) between 10 and 50 mL/min; if CrCl is less than 10 mL/min, the dose should be reduced by 50%.

Common side effects include leukopenia, thrombocytopenia, anemia, infection, nausea and vomiting, anorexia, diarrhea, elevated LFTs, malaise, myalgia, fever, and rash. Serious side effects include myelosuppression, PML, pancreatitis, hepatotoxicity, lymphomas, and other malignancies.

Transplant recipients taking azathioprine should not receive live vaccines because their immune response may be inadequate, and they are at risk for disseminated infection resulting from the live virus. Caution is advised when azathioprine is administered with other drugs that lower the immune response because of an increased risk of serious infection. Combining azathioprine with antihypertensive drugs increases the risk of leukopenia.

Patients who receive azathioprine should have a complete blood count (CBC), including a platelet count, taken weekly during the first month, twice monthly for the second and third months of treatment, and then monthly. Creatinine and LFTs should be monitored.

Azathioprine can cause fetal harm when given to pregnant women and should be avoided; however, maternal benefit may outweigh fetal risk in serious or life-threatening situations. Azathioprine is found in breast milk and is possibly unsafe during breastfeeding; therefore a decision should be made whether to discontinue nursing or to discontinue the drug, taking into account the importance of the drug to the mother.

Inosine Monophosphate Dehydrogenase Inhibitors. Mycophenolate mofetil blocks synthesis of purine nucleotides, thereby preventing the proliferation of T cells and lymphocytes and preventing the formation of antibodies from B cells; it also may inhibit recruitment of leukocytes to inflammatory sites.

Recommended dosing for kidney transplant recipients is 1 g orally twice daily; for heart and liver transplant recipients, the dosage is 1.5 g orally twice daily. Kidney function should be monitored; for a CrCl less than 25 mL/min, the maximum dosage is 1 g twice daily. In pediatric transplant recipients, the recommended dose of mycophenolate mofetil oral suspension is 600 mg/m^2 twice daily, up to a maximum of 1 g twice daily. The dose of mycophenolate mofetil should be reduced or interrupted for an absolute neutrophil count (ANC) of less than 1300 (Box 33.2).

Pharmacokinetics. Mycophenolate mofetil is rapidly absorbed after oral administration with 94% bioavailability, and it is protein bound (82% to 97%). It is a prodrug that is metabolized in the liver to mycophenolic acid (MPA); it is excreted in the urine (93%) and in feces (6%).

Pharmacodynamics. Oral mycophenolate mofetil reaches peak in 1.5 hours. Drug half-life for the oral formulation is 18 hours; the half-life for the IV formulation is 17 hours.

Common side effects of mycophenolate mofetil include hypertension, infection, diarrhea, edema, anemia, abdominal pain, constipation, headache, nausea and vomiting, dyspnea and cough, hypercholesterolemia, tremor, hypokalemia, acne, and insomnia. Serious reactions include thrombocytopenia, leukopenia, neutropenia, severe infection, viral reactivation, nephropathy, PML, lymphoma, lymphoproliferative disorders, malignancy, GI bleeding, acute renal failure, and interstitial lung disease.

Transplant recipients taking mycophenolate mofetil should not receive live vaccines because their immune response may be inadequate, and they are at risk for disseminated infection resulting from the live virus. Caution is advised when mycophenolate mofetil is administered with other drugs that lower the immune response because of the increased risk of serious infection. Combining mycophenolate mofetil with nonsteroidal antiinflammatory drugs (NSAIDs) increases the risk of GI bleeding.

Patients taking mycophenolate mofetil should have a baseline creatinine level drawn and should have CBCs done weekly during the first month, twice monthly for the second and third months of treatment, and then monthly throughout the first year.

Mycophenolate mofetil is associated with an increased risk of first-trimester pregnancy loss and an increased risk of congenital malformations. ⚡ Females of reproductive potential must be made aware of the increased risk of first-trimester pregnancy loss and congenital malformations and must be counseled regarding pregnancy prevention and planning. It is unknown whether mycophenolate mofetil is found in breast milk; therefore a decision should be made whether to discontinue breastfeeding or to discontinue the drug, taking into account the importance of the drug to the mother.

Corticosteroids. Prednisone, a corticosteroid, is a glucocorticoid receptor agonist. It decreases inflammation by suppression of leukocytes and reversal of increased capillary permeability. It suppresses the immune system by reducing the activity and volume of the lymphatic system; prednisone suppresses adrenal function at high doses.

In addition to their use in maintenance therapy, corticosteroids are used in high doses for the treatment of acute transplant rejection. The drug methylprednisolone sodium succinate is administered IV in doses that range from 250 mg to 500 mg daily for 3 to 5 days.

Pharmacokinetics. Prednisone is readily absorbed from the GI tract (up to 90%). Plasma protein binding is less than 50% but is concentration dependent. Prednisone is metabolized by the liver to its active metabolite, prednisolone. It is excreted in the urine as sulfate and glucuronide conjugates.

Pharmacodynamics. Prednisone reaches peak plasma concentration in 2 hours for the immediate release formulation and 6 to 6.5 hours for the delayed release formulation. Prednisone has a plasma half-life of 2 to 4 hours and should be administered after meals or with food or milk to decrease GI upset.

Common side effects of corticosteroid use include sodium retention, edema, hypokalemia, hypertension, diaphoresis, muscle atrophy, nausea and vomiting, dyspepsia, petechiae and ecchymosis, facial erythema, acne, rash, headache, dizziness and vertigo, insomnia, emotional lability, depression, anxiety, glucose intolerance, menstrual irregularities, hirsutism, appetite changes, and weight gain. Serious reactions include anaphylaxis, adrenal insufficiency, steroid psychosis, infection, diabetes mellitus, seizures, heart failure, peptic ulcer disease and GI bleeding, osteonecrosis, and tendon rupture. Long-term use may lead to impaired wound healing, skin atrophy, Cushing syndrome, glaucoma and cataracts, Kaposi sarcoma, and growth suppression in children. Cessation of corticosteroids may lead to withdrawal symptoms with high doses or long-term use.

Transplant recipients taking corticosteroids should not receive live vaccines because their immune response may be inadequate, and they are at risk for disseminated infection resulting from the live virus. Caution is advised when corticosteroids are administered with other drugs that lower the immune response because of the increased risk of serious infection. Combining corticosteroids with certain antibiotics increases the risk of QT prolongation and arrhythmias; combining corticosteroids with diuretics increases the risk of hypokalemia.

Transplant recipients taking corticosteroids should have periodic monitoring of their electrolytes, blood pressure, weight, and glucose levels. Pediatric patients should have their height monitored. Chest x-rays and ophthalmic examinations are indicated with long-term use.

Caution is advised during pregnancy, especially in the first trimester or with long-term use, because of the possible risk of low birthweight and premature birth. Corticosteroids are probably safe during breastfeeding.

Drugs for Transplant Rejection

> **TYPES OF REJECTION:** Hyperacute rejection occurs within a few minutes to hours after transplant due to preformed antibodies that attack the transplanted organ, resulting in irreversible damage.
>
> Acute rejection occurs in the first weeks to three months after transplant. It is a cell-mediated response. Symptoms include an increase in serum creatinine, hypertension, decreased urine output, flu-like symptoms, fever, and tenderness over the graft site. Acute rejection is confirmed with biopsy.
>
> Chronic rejection develops after months or years. The body's immune system slowly damages the transplanted organ and results in a slow but progressive decline in organ function. Indications of chronic rejection include hypertension and proteinuria.

Transplant rejection occurs when the immune system of the transplant recipient attacks the transplanted organ. This happens because the immune system recognizes foreign tissues and attempts to destroy

In addition to receiving treatment from your doctor, the following suggestions can help prevent infections:

- Clean your hands frequently.
- Try to avoid crowded places and contact with people who are sick.
- Do not share food, drink cups, utensils, or other personal items, such as toothbrushes.
- Shower or bathe daily and use an unscented lotion to prevent your skin from becoming dry and cracked.
- Cook meat and eggs all the way through to kill any germs.
- Carefully wash raw fruits and vegetables.
- Protect your skin from direct contact with pet bodily waste (urine or feces) by wearing vinyl or household cleaning gloves when cleaning up after your pet. Wash your hands immediately afterward.
- Use gloves for gardening.
- Clean your teeth and gums with a soft toothbrush, and if your doctor or nurse recommends one, use a mouthwash to prevent mouth sores.
- Try and keep all your household surfaces clean.
- Get the seasonal flu shot as soon as it is available.
- If you go to the emergency room, you should not sit in the waiting room for a long time; when you check in, tell them right away you are receiving immunosuppressant drugs.
- Know the signs and symptoms of an infection:
  - Fever that is 100.4°F (38°C) or higher for more than 1 hour, or a one-time temperature of 101°F or higher
  - Chills and sweats
  - Change in cough or new cough
  - Sore throat or new mouth sore
  - Shortness of breath
  - Nasal congestion
  - Stiff neck
  - Burning or pain with urination
  - Unusual vaginal discharge or irritation
  - Increased urination
  - Redness, soreness, or swelling in any area, including surgical wounds
  - Diarrhea
  - Vomiting
  - Pain in the abdomen or rectum
  - New onset of pain
  - Changes in skin, urination, or mental status

Retrieved December 23, 2016 from https://www.cdc.gov/cancer/preventinfections/pdf/neutropenia.pdf.

them, just as it attempts to destroy infecting organisms, such as bacteria and viruses. Treatment of rejection with an anti–T-cell antibody is used when corticosteroids have failed to reverse rejection or for treatment of a recurrent rejection.

Antithymocyte Globulin (Rabbit)

Antithymocyte globulin (rabbit), or *ATG rabbit,* is a polyclonal (depleting) antibody that blocks T-cell membrane proteins; this causes altered T-cell function and lysis, and prolonged T-cell depletion, which begins within 24 hours. Complete pharmacokinetic data are not available, but drug half-life is 2 to 3 days.

Dosing is 1.5 mg/kg IV each day for 7 to 14 days in adults. The first dose should be infused over 6 hours and subsequent doses over 4 hours. This drug is not approved for use in children. Dosage should be decreased by 50% if the white blood cell (WBC) count decreases to 2000 to 3000 or the platelet count is 50,000 to 75,000. Treatments

should be discontinued if the WBC count falls to less than 2000 or the platelet count falls to less than 50,000.

Common side effects of ATG rabbit include high fever, chills, nausea and vomiting, headache, diarrhea, malaise, shortness of breath, leukopenia, thrombocytopenia, peripheral edema, and increased risk for infection. Serious side effects include anaphylaxis, severe infusion reaction, cytokine release syndrome, serum sickness, sepsis, cytomegalovirus (CMV), malignancy, and lymphoproliferative disorders. Premedication with corticosteroids or acetaminophen plus an antihistamine one hour prior to each dose is recommended to reduce the severity of adverse reactions. ⚡ Close supervision of the patient is required during and after IV infusion, to include frequent vital signs and assessment of the site for signs of extravasation.

Transplant recipients receiving ATG rabbit should not receive live vaccines because their immune response may be inadequate, and they are at risk for disseminated infection resulting from the live virus. Caution is advised when ATG rabbit is administered with other drugs that lower the immune response because of the increased risk of serious infection.

Patients should have WBC and platelets monitored frequently during treatment. There are no adequate and well-controlled studies of ATG rabbit in pregnant women. Inadequate information is available to assess the risk of ATG rabbit when breastfeeding; therefore a decision should be made whether to discontinue nursing or to discontinue the drug, taking into account the importance of the drug to the mother.

Muromonab-CD3

Muromonab-CD3 is a monoclonal antibody that binds specifically to the CD3 complex on the surface of T lymphocytes; the CD3 complex is involved in antigen recognition. Immediately after administration, CD3-positive T lymphocytes are abruptly removed from circulation. Complete pharmacokinetic data are not available, but drug half-life is 18 hours.

Dosing is 5 mg IV push daily for 10 to 14 days in adults. In pediatric patients under 30 kg, dosage is 2.5 mg IV push daily for 10 to 14 days; pediatric patients over 30 kg are dosed the same as adults. ⚡ Muromonab-CD3 carries a boxed warning for the risk of anaphylactic reactions occurring with any dose, and life-threatening or lethal systemic, cardiovascular, and CNS reactions.

Common side effects of muromonab-CD3 include fever, chills, nausea and vomiting, diarrhea, headache, tachycardia, hypotension, dyspnea, tremor, rash, edema, fatigue, diaphoresis, dyspepsia, arthralgia, pruritus, leukopenia, and increased risk of infection. Serious reactions include anaphylaxis, Stevens-Johnson syndrome, cytokine release syndrome, cardiorespiratory arrest, seizures, encephalopathy, aseptic meningitis, opportunistic infection, malignancy, lymphoproliferative disorders, thrombosis, thrombocytopenia, anemia, neutropenia, and leukopenia.

Transplant recipients receiving muromonab-CD3 should not receive live vaccines because their immune response may be inadequate, and they are at risk for disseminated infection resulting from the live virus. Caution is advised when muromonab-CD3 is administered with other drugs that lower the immune response because of the increased risk of serious infection.

Transplant recipients receiving muromonab-CD3 should have BUN, creatinine, LFTs, and a CBC with differential drawn at baseline.

There are no adequate and well-controlled studies of muromonab-CD3 in pregnant women; however, potential benefits may warrant use of the drug in pregnant women despite potential risks. The drug is unsafe during breastfeeding.

Drugs for Infection

Bacterial

Pneumocystis jiroveci pneumonia (PJP) is a life-threatening illness in immunocompromised patients. Routine prophylaxis with trimethoprim-sulfamethoxazole (TMP-SMZ) has significantly reduced the morbidity and mortality of PJP after transplantation. TMP-SMZ is dosed once every morning or one tablet three times a week (Monday, Wednesday, and Friday). TMP-SMZ can make the skin more sensitive to sunlight; therefore patients should be instructed to use a lotion with a minimum sun protection factor (SPF) of 25 when in the sun. See Chapter 26 for further information regarding antibacterial drugs.

Fungal

Transplant recipients use nystatin to prevent or treat thrush in the mouth and esophagus. This is usually given when the patient is on a high-dose immunosuppression regimen and is stopped when the steroid dose is reduced below 20 mg per day. Nurses must instruct the transplant recipient in proper administration of nystatin liquid:

- Shake the preparation well before measuring the dose.
- Swish the dose around in the mouth for at least 2 minutes before swallowing.
- Allow the nystatin to coat the mouth for as long as possible.
- Do not eat or drink anything for 30 minutes after taking the medication.
  See Chapter 27 for further information regarding antifungal drugs.

Viral

One common virus that patients develop after transplantation is CMV. It may present as a viral syndrome or as invasive disease, and it plays a role in organ rejection. Transplant recipients receive antiviral prophylaxis with oral ganciclovir or valganciclovir for 3 to 6 months after surgery. If untreated, CMV can cause serious complications, particularly in the liver, intestine, kidneys, heart, lungs, and eyes. See Chapter 27 for further information regarding antiviral drugs.

PROMOTING ADHERENCE

Upon discharge from the hospital, transplant recipients begin a lifelong journey of close medical supervision that includes frequent visits to their health care provider, monitoring of blood work, and maintenance of a complex drug regimen. The 1-year survival rates are over 80% for liver transplants and over 90% for kidney transplants; most recipients experience an improved quality of life. However, long-term adherence is a problem, with reports of nonadherence ranging from a low of 2% to as high as 68%. Nonadherence to the posttransplant regimen (e.g., drug regimen, exercise and health promotion) is one of the top three reasons for transplant failure. Factors that affect adherence include episodes of rejection, comorbid illness and disease, side effects of drugs, and health care costs. Nurses play a key role in promoting adherence by incorporating education, motivational strategies, and coping skills into an individually tailored posttransplant plan of care.

◎ CLINICAL JUDGMENT [NURSING PROCESS]

Organ Transplants: Immunosuppression

Concept: Safety
- Protecting the patient from potential or actual harm; a basic human need

Concept: Immunity
- The body's protective response to infection and disease

Recognize Cues [Assessment]
- Assess for clinical signs of rejection including malaise, fever, edema, pain over the transplant site, and increased weight.
- Assess for presence of risk factors for infection, including drugs, travel, and exposure to individuals with active infections.
- Assess for signs and symptoms of infection, including redness, swelling, pain, and elevated temperature.
- Assess immunization status.
- Assess nutritional status, including weight and history of weight loss.

Analyze Cues and Prioritize Hypothesis [Patient Problems]
- Decreased immunity
- Self-concept
- Need for health teaching

Generate Solutions [Planning]
- Infection is recognized early to allow prompt treatment.
- The transplant recipient and family members will verbalize understanding of early signs and symptoms of rejection.
- The transplant recipient will remain free of infection.

Take Action [Nursing Interventions]
- Instruct the transplant recipient on the benefits of a balanced and healthy diet accompanied by exercise.
- Instruct the transplant recipient on proper adherence to the drug regimen. Teach the transplant recipient the purpose of each drug and how to administer each drug, and reinforce that each drug should be taken exactly as prescribed. Also teach the most common side effects associated with each drug and what to do if they occur.
- Patients should be instructed to avoid anyone with an active infection and to be careful not to injure themselves, which may increase the chance of acquiring a wound infection. They should stay away from anyone who has a cold, mumps, measles, chickenpox, or other communicable diseases.
- Promote health education with patients and families to recognize and minimize the risk of complications and rejection and to facilitate optimum quality of life.
- Teach the transplant recipient the signs and symptoms of rejection and infection, and instruct them on when to call their health care provider.
- Teach the transplant recipient to self-monitor vital signs, daily weights, and blood glucose (if appropriate); ensure the recipient knows when to call the health care provider.
- Transplant recipients and their families should be taught to wash hands properly, especially after toileting, before meals, and before administering drugs.

Evaluate Outcomes [Evaluation]
- Evaluate effectiveness of the plan, including adherence to the immunosuppressive drug regimen and freedom from infection and transplant rejection.

CRITICAL THINKING UNFOLDING CASE STUDY

Phase I: Induction therapy
NGN Item Type: Enhanced hot spot
Cognitive Skills: Recognize cues

A 42-year-old African American female with a six-year history of chronic kidney disease requiring hemodialysis (HD), secondary to polycystic kidney disease, is admitted for cadaveric kidney transplant. She lives alone and has been on disability for the past four years. She had become too fatigued with HD to continue her job as an elementary school teacher. She denies a history of substance use. On admission, her blood pressure (BP) is 145/90 mm Hg, temperature (T) is 98.4, respiratory rate (RR) is 18, and heart rate (HR) is 100; height 68 inches and weight 185 pounds. While receiving basiliximab 20 mg intravenously two hours prior to surgery, the patient tells the nurse that she is both excited and scared; she has a lot of questions about her induction therapy. Three days after surgery, the patient reports fatigue, headache (pain rated a 5 on a scale of 0 to 10), and dizziness. On assessment, her T is 101.6, HR 115, RR 16, and her BP is 100/62 mm Hg. Additionally, she did not eat breakfast due to nausea and abdominal discomfort. Intake and output from the previous shift are 1000 mL/250 mL.

1. **Highlight the assessment findings that require immediate follow-up.**
2. **Use an X to indicate the potential issues listed in the left column that may place this patient at risk while in the hospital.**

Potential Issues	Risk to Patient
Acute pain	
Decreased immunity	
Cognitive decline	
Social isolation	
Need for health teaching	

Answers:

A 42-year-old African American female with a six-year history of chronic kidney disease requiring hemodialysis (HD), secondary to polycystic kidney disease, is admitted for cadaveric kidney transplant. She lives alone and has been on disability for the past four years. She had become too fatigued with HD to continue her job as an elementary school teacher. She denies a history of substance use. On admission, her blood pressure (BP) is 145/90 mm Hg, temperature (T) is 98.4, respiratory rate (RR) is 18, and heart rate (HR) is 100; height 68 inches and weight 185 pounds. While receiving basiliximab 20 mg intravenously two hours prior to surgery, the patient tells the nurse that she is both excited and scared; she has a lot of questions about her induction therapy. Three days after surgery, the patient reports fatigue, headache (pain rated a 5 on a scale of 0 to 10), and dizziness. On assessment, her T is 101.6, HR 115, RR 16, and her BP is 100/62 mm Hg. Additionally, she did not eat breakfast due to nausea and abdominal discomfort. Intake and output from the previous shift are 1000 mL/250 mL.

Highlight the assessment findings that require immediate follow-up. Use an X to indicate the potential issues listed in the left column that may place this patient at risk while in the hospital.

Potential Issues	Risk to Patient
Acute pain	X
Decreased immunity	X
Cognitive decline	
Social isolation	
Need for health teaching	X

Rationale

Signs and symptoms of cytokine release syndrome resulting from basiliximab include fever, nausea, chills, hypotension, tachycardia, asthenia, headache, rash, scratchy throat, and dyspnea. Signs and symptoms of acute rejection include flu-like symptoms, fever, tenderness over kidney, decreased urine output, and hypertension.

Phase II: Discharge
NGN Type Item: Matrix
Cognitive Skills: Analyze cues

The nurse is completing final preparations for the patient's discharged home, nine days following cadaveric kidney transplant. Her discharge drugs include cyclosporine (modified), mycophenolate mofetil, and prednisone, as well as nifedipine, furosemide, sulfamethoxazole/trimethoprim, nystatin, and valganciclovir. The patient is voicing concerns about taking so many drugs and their side effects; she is worried about how she is going to pay for all of them. Her BP on discharge is 145/88 mm Hg, T 99.5, RR 16, and HR 90. This morning her creatinine is 2.0 mg/dL (was 1.7 mg/dL yesterday) and her blood urea nitrogen (BUN) is 30 mg/dL; her K 5.3 mEq/l, Na 136 mEq/l, and glucose 110 mg/dL. Her cyclosporin trough concentration is 325 ng/mL. Her adult daughter has flown in from across the country and will stay with her for a couple weeks after discharge.

1. Based on the patient's condition at discharge, which education MUST be included prior to discharge home? (Select all that apply).
   a. Information about when to call the provider about drug side effects
   b. Information on systems to promote adherence with her drug regimen
   c. Information on balanced diet accompanied by exercise
   d. Information on support groups for transplant recipients
   e. Information on drug assistance programs
   f. Information about catch up immunization schedule and pre-travel vaccines
   g. Information related to glucose monitoring

2. Place a check mark to indicate which assessment data listed in the left column may place this patient at risk during the discharge phase of treatment.

Assessment Data	Risk to Patient
Lives alone	
BP 145/88 mm Hg	
Creatinine 2.0 mg/dL	
K 5.3 mEq/l	
Glucose 110 mg/dL	
Cyclosporin trough concentration 325 ng/mL	
T 99.5	

Answers:

1. Based on the patient's condition at discharge, which education MUST be included prior to discharge home? (Select all that apply).
   a. Information about when to call the provider about drug side effects
   b. Information on systems to promote adherence with her drug regimen
   c. Information on balanced diet accompanied by exercise
   d. Information on drug assistance programs

Rationale:

The patient is voicing concerns about taking so many drugs (b) and their side effects (a); she is worried about how she is going to pay for all of them (e). Her BP and glucose are borderline; her prescribed drugs have side effects related to weight gain, hypertension, electrolyte imbalance, and elevated lipids. Diet and exercise are an important part of discharge planning (c). While the other options may be important, they are not a priority for discharge of this patient.

2. Place a check mark to indicate which assessment data listed in the left column may place this patient at risk during the discharge phase of treatment.

Continued

CRITICAL THINKING UNFOLDING CASE STUDY—CONT'D

Assessment Data	Risk to Patient
Lives alone	
BP 145/88 mm Hg	
Creatinine 2.0 mg/dL	✓
K 5.3 mEq/l	✓
Glucose 110 mg/dL	
Cyclosporin trough concentration 325 ng/mL	
T 99.5	✓

Rationale:

Living alone does not put the patient at risk during the discharge phase; although an isolated BP of 145/88 mm Hg is borderline, it can be managed as an outpatient, as can a glucose of 110 mg/dL; therefore, they do not put the patient at risk during the discharge phase. The cyclosporine trough concentration is within range for a patient immediately posttransplant. The rise in creatinine level accompanied by an elevated potassium level and low-grade fever are indicators of acute rejection and put the patient at risk during the discharge phase.

Phase III: Acute Rejection

NGN Type Item: Extended multiple response; Matrix
Cognitive Skills: Take action; Evaluate outcomes

Six months post kidney transplant surgery the patient experiences another episode of acute rejection. In addition to cyclosporine (modified), mycophenolate mofetil, and prednisone, this morning she is starting antithymocyte globulin (rabbit), having failed high-dose steroid treatment over the last three days as the initial treatment for her acute rejection. The patient tearfully admits to being scared about losing her transplant, going back on HD, and never being able to teach again. Her weight this morning is 215 pounds. She had a CBC with differential drawn; her WBC count is $3.0 \times 10^3/\mu L$, segmented neutrophils are 14.8%, and the segmented bands are 5% (absolute neutrophil count of 594 cells/μL); platelets are 100,000/μL. Her cyclosporin trough concentration is 150 ng/mL, creatinine 2.5 mg/dL, and BUN is 38 mg/dL; her K is 4.4 mEq/L, and glucose is 150 mg/dL. Her BP is 148/90, T 99.5, RR 20, and HR 106. Urine output for the last 12 hours was 336 cc.

1. Which nursing actions are appropriate for the patient at this time? (Select all that apply).
   a. Refer to counseling and psychology
   b. Refer to social work
   c. Administer acetaminophen and diphenhydramine
   d. Refer for dietary counseling
   e. Administer insulin per sliding scale
   f. Instruct on using a soft toothbrush
   g. Remove flowers from the patient's room
   h. Instruct on the side effects of antithymocyte globulin (rabbit)

2. The nurse administers the diphenhydramine/acetaminophen premedication; then, one hour later the nurse administers ATG rabbit and teaches the patient the drug side effects and when to call the health care provider. The nurse also instructs the patient regarding neutropenic precautions. **Use an X to indicate whether assessment findings in the left column indicate effectiveness, ineffectiveness or are unrelated to the nursing interventions?**

Assessment Finding	Effective	Ineffective	Unrelated
The patient requests assistance to the bathroom			
The patient reports pain 1 on scale of 0–10			

Assessment Finding	Effective	Ineffective	Unrelated
The patient reports shakes and chills			
T 98.4°F			
The patient reports bleeding gums after oral care			

Answers:

1. Which nursing actions are appropriate for the patient at this time? (Select all that apply).
   a. Administer acetaminophen and diphenhydramine
   b. Instruct on using a soft toothbrush
   c. Instruct on the side effects of antithymocyte globulin (rabbit)

Rationale:

Side effects of antithymocyte globulin (rabbit) include high fever and chills; premedication with corticosteroids or acetaminophen and antihistamines will decrease the severity. The patient is neutropenic. Neutropenic precautions include using a soft toothbrush. Safe and effective nursing care includes educating patients on the side effects of the drugs they are receiving.

2. The nurse administers the diphenhydramine/acetaminophen premedication; then, one hour later the nurse administers ATG rabbit and teaches the patient the drug side effects and when to call the healthcare provider. The nurse also instructs the patient regarding neutropenic precautions. **Use an X to indicate whether assessment findings in the left column indicate effectiveness, ineffectiveness or are unrelated to the nursing interventions?**

Assessment Finding	Effective	Ineffective	Unrelated
The patient requests assistance to the bathroom			X
The patient reports pain 1 on scale of 0–10	X		
The patient reports shakes and chills		X	
T 98.4°F	X		
The patient reports bleeding gums after oral care		X	

Rationale:

Requesting assistance to the bathroom does not reflect nursing actions taken immediately prior to drug administration. A report of pain as a 1 on scale of 0 to 10 reflects the administration of premedication. A potential side effect of antithymocyte globulin (rabbit) is headache. Experiencing shakes and chills would indicate high fever; premedication is administered to reduce the severity of adverse reactions. However, a high fever indicates administration of the premedication was not effective. A temperature of 98.4°F would indicate administration of the premedication was effective. The patient reporting bleeding gums after oral care indicates instructions regarding neutropenic precautions did not prevent bleeding, creating an access point for infection.

REVIEW QUESTIONS

1. All transplant drugs have the same advisory, to use caution when administering them with another immunosuppressant drug because of the increased risk for:
   a. Nausea and vomiting
   b. Edema
   c. Anemia
   d. Infection

2. Which virus has been associated with posttransplant lymphoproliferative disorder?
   a. Cytomegalovirus
   b. Herpes simplex virus
   c. Epstein-Barr virus
   d. Human immunodeficiency virus

3. Nurses are key to promoting adherence in transplant recipients. What factors influence whether a recipient adheres to a drug regimen? (Select all that apply.)
   a. Drug side effects
   b. Episodes of rejection
   c. Cost
   d. Infection
   e. Marital status

4. Your patient is receiving basiliximab and develops cytokine release syndrome. You would expect to see:
   a. Coughing
   b. Chills
   c. Tremors
   d. Weakness

5. Your patient taking belatacept becomes pregnant. After discussion with her partner, you, and her health care provider, she decides the best thing to do is continue taking the drug while pregnant. In addition to making this informed decision, what else should she do?
   a. Discontinue all other drugs
   b. Contact the pregnancy registry
   c. Ensure her blood level stays between 16 and 24 ng/mL
   d. Decrease her dose by 50%

34

Vaccines

OBJECTIVES

- Describe active and passive immunity as both relate to the action of vaccines used in immunizations.
- Differentiate between active natural and active acquired immunity as it relates to the human immune system.
- Identify the diseases that can be prevented with vaccines.
- Review the recommended immunization schedule for children and teens.
- Correlate the manifestations and administration routes for adult vaccines.
- Discuss contraindications to the administration of recommended immunizations.
- Apply the Clinical Judgment [Nursing Process] to include teaching for patients receiving vaccines.

OUTLINE

November 17, 2019, marked the first case of what was to become known as the COVID-19 (novel coronavirus, or 2019-nCoV, or SARS-CoV-2; Fig. 34.1) pandemic, the worst pandemic since the 1918 Spanish flu killed 50 million people worldwide. By January 9, 2020, there were 59 cases of pneumonia from this virus in Wuhan, China, where it began. It spread to the United States by January 21; by January 31 the World Health Organization (WHO) issued a Global Health Emergency. By March 11, 2020, the WHO declared COVID-19 a pandemic. Phase I vaccine trials began in March. On December 11, 2020, the Food and Drug Administration (FDA) granted emergency use authorization (EUA) for Pfizer-BioNTech's vaccine. On December 14, 2020, the first vaccine was administered in Queens, with shipments heading to all 50 states. On this date there were 16.9 million cases of COVID-19 in the United States, with 307,803 deaths.

Over the years, immunizations have prevented global epidemics, such as smallpox in 1977 and the eradication of polio in the United States in 1979. The US National Immunization Survey (NIS; https://www.cdc.gov/vaccines/imz-managers/nis/index.html) tracks vaccination coverage of children 19 to 35 months and teens 13 to 17 years. In 2017, overall vaccination rates for children between 19 and 35 months was at 70.4%. Specific vaccination rates were 83.2% for diptheria, tetanus, pertussis; 92.7% for polio; 91.5% for measles, mumps, rubella; 80.7% for haemophilus influenzae type b; 91.4% for hepatitis B; 91% for chickenpox; and 82.4% for pneumococcal conjugate vaccine. Children below the federal poverty level have lower coverage for all vaccinations compared with children at or above the poverty level, and those with insurance or Medicaid.

The NIS estimated that in 2019, among teens aged 13 to 17 years, vaccination rates continue to increase. For tetanus, diphtheria, and acellular pertussis (Tdap) coverage rates were 90.2% and 88.9% for ≥1 dose of meningococcus 4-valent conjugate (MenACWY). Vaccination coverage for human papillomavirus (HPV) continues to improve. In 2019, 71.5% of teens had received their first dose, and 54.2% had completed the series. Coverage exceeded 90% for ≥2 doses measles, mumps, and rubella vaccine (MMR), ≥3 doses of hepatitis B vaccine, and ≥1 and ≥2 doses of varicella vaccine among adolescents without a history of varicella disease. These results indicate an increase in all vaccinations for teens, with a continued need to improve HPV coverage.

IMMUNITY

Active Immunity

The body can obtain immunity in different ways. Active immunity occurs when the body's immune response is stimulated by an antigen or when a pathogen enters the body. The body recognizes this pathogen as a foreign substance and produces antibodies, also called *immunoglobulins,* which defend the body against pathogens. The immune response is slow, taking several days or weeks to develop immunity. Yet the immunity is often long-lasting. During this process, the immune system retains memory of the pathogen then produces antibodies to defend against the disease. Natural acquired active immunity occurs from exposure to a pathogen or disease. Active acquired artificial immunity occurs when a

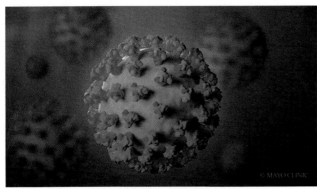

Figure 34.1 Microphotograph of the novel coronavirus.

weakened antigen or immunoglobulin (Ig) is injected into an individual as a vaccination, which then stimulates an immune response.

Passive Immunity

When an individual is unable to make antibodies and memory cells, antibodies are given from another source to provide passive immunity. These antibodies may be produced using recombinant deoxyribonucleic acid (DNA) technology or pooled antigens from several human or animal sources that have been exposed to disease-causing pathogens.

Passive immunity can be natural, in which case the body produces its own antibodies, or it can be acquired—that is, the body receives antibodies from an outside source. Either way the immunity is immediate and short-lived, lasting no more than several weeks to a few months; the recipient does not induce his or her own immune response. One example of natural immunity passively acquired is in infants, who are unable to protect against disease because of immature immune systems but instead require antibodies from an outside source, such as the mother's placenta and breast milk. Another example is receiving an Ig to provide antibodies against a specific disease. Passive acquired immunity is essential when (1) time does not permit active vaccination alone, (2) the exposed individual is at high risk for complications of the disease, or (3) the individual suffers from an immune system deficiency that renders that person unable to produce an effective immune response.

Community Immunity

Community immunity, also known as *herd immunity,* occurs when most of the community is immunized against contagious diseases, allowing protection of those not immunized. In contrast, when most of the community is *not* immunized, there is an increased risk for the spread of contagious disease within the community (Fig. 34.2). For more information, see https://www.vaccines.gov/basics/work/protection/index.html.

VACCINES

Vaccination involves the administration of a small amount of antigen that, although capable of stimulating an immune response, does not typically produce the disease. Different types of vaccines are available, but the type used in vaccinations depends on the person's immune response. The antigen in vaccines may be produced in several ways. Traditional vaccines contain the whole or components of an inactivated (killed) microorganism. Other vaccines are attenuated viruses composed of live, attenuated (weakened) microorganisms. Persons who are immunocompromised because of illness or who take medication that causes immunosuppression should avoid live vaccines. Toxoids are inactivated toxins that can no longer produce harmful diseases but do stimulate formation of antitoxins, which produces active immunity (e.g., tetanus toxoid).

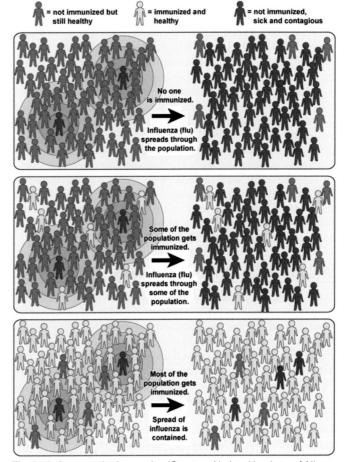

Fig. 34.2 Community immunity. (Courtesy National Institute of Allergy and Infectious Diseases.)

Newer vaccines, called conjugate vaccines, require a protein or toxoid from an unrelated organism to link to the outer coating of the disease-causing microorganism. This linkage creates a substance that can be recognized by the immature immune system of young infants. One example is *H. influenzae* type B.

Recombinant subunit vaccines involve the insertion of some of the genetic material (e.g., DNA) of a pathogen into another cell or organism, where the antigen is then produced in massive quantities. These antigens are then used as a vaccine in place of the whole pathogen. The HepB vaccine is an example of this type of vaccine.

Adenovector vaccines have been in development for the past 20 years. In these vaccines, a modified adenovirus is injected into an individual, triggering an immune response. After administration, the vaccine enters the cells and teaches the immune cells to make the desired protein. The first such adenovector vaccine approved for general use is a vaccine for ebola. Trials of adenovector vaccines are underway for HIV and Zika.

The newest vaccine in the arsenal against infectious diseases is the severe acute respiratory syndrome coronavirus 2 (SARS-CoV-2) vaccine, a messenger RNA (mRNA) vaccine. Messenger RNA vaccines have been 30 years in the making, with mRNA vaccines in development for ebola, cytomegalovirus, Zika virus, and influenza. With an mRNA vaccine, scientists synthesize an mRNA strand with an altered code, so the body does not identify it as foreign. The synthetic mRNA tells the body to create the spike protein found on the SARS-CoV-2 virus, which in turn triggers the immune system to produce cells designed to fight the spike protein, protecting the body against SARS-CoV-2

(Fig. 34.3). The CDC has launched v-safe, the after-vaccination health checker, to monitor side effects experienced by persons receiving the COVID-19 vaccine (see https://www.cdc.gov/coronavirus/2019-ncov/vaccines/safety/vsafe.html for further information).

An **adjuvant**—often an aluminum salt such as aluminum hydroxide, aluminum phosphate, or aluminum potassium sulfate—is a substance added to a vaccine to increase the body's immune response to the vaccine. One value of adding an adjuvant to a vaccine is to reduce the amount of antigen needed to produce a dose of vaccine. Vaccines with adjuvants are rigorously tested for safety before being licensed. In the United States, vaccines against measles, mumps, rubella, chickenpox, rotavirus, polio, and seasonal influenza do *not* contain adjuvants.

Regardless of the composition of the vaccine, each vaccine is designed to stimulate an immune response against a specific pathogen. Some vaccines require booster doses to maintain sufficient immunity. The immune system's memory responds rapidly to prevent disease when exposed to a booster, which provides an active albeit artificially acquired immunity.

VACCINE-PREVENTABLE DISEASES

Vaccinations maintain health by preventing disease. In the United States, more than 20 infectious diseases may be prevented by active vaccination. Many of these vaccines are routinely administered to healthy children and adults. Others are reserved for special populations such as health care providers, military personnel, immigrants, adults with special health needs, the chronically ill, and travelers to certain foreign countries. Table 34.1 provides an overview of the disease manifestations and vaccine information, including route of administration and storage temperature. Vaccine-preventable diseases for children, adolescents, and adults include—but are not limited to—anthrax, diphtheria, *H. influenzae* type B, hepatitis A and B, HPV, influenza (flu), Japanese encephalitis, measles, meningococcal disease, mumps, pertussis, pneumococcal disease, poliomyelitis, rabies, rotavirus, rubella, smallpox, tetanus, tuberculosis (TB), typhoid, varicella, yellow fever, SARS-CoV-2, and herpes zoster.

VACCINATION RECOMMENDATIONS

Immunization schedules are approved by the Advisory Committee on Immunizations (ACIP). Each schedule identifies recommended vaccinations, ages to vaccinate, dosage, and route for children, adolescents, and adults. For the most current information on childhood immunizations, consult the Centers for Disease Control and Prevention (CDC) website at www.cdc.gov/vaccines. A vaccine information statement (VIS) is also produced by the CDC for each vaccine and provides information on the (1) route of administration, (2) schedule for routine vaccine administration, (3) minimum dosing intervals, (4) contraindications, and (5) standing orders for administering vaccines.

The childhood immunization schedule from birth to 6 years recommends HepB, RV, DTaP, Hib, PCV, inactivated polio virus (IPV), MMR, varicella, and HepA. Before immunizations are administered, screen for medical conditions that put the child at risk, use of prescription and over-the-counter (OTC) drugs to include herbal preparations, and any food or drug allergies.

The adolescent immunization schedule from ages 7 to 18 years recommends Tdap, influenza, HPV, and meningococcal vaccinations. Adolescents may also need to catch up on any vaccines missed, such as MMR, HepA, HepB, IPV, and varicella (chickenpox).

A catch-up immunization schedule is available for those up to 18 years of age who fall behind or start late with immunizations. Childhood and adolescent immunization schedules are also available as a combined schedule (birth to 18 years).

Adult (19 years and older) vaccination rates remain low, which indicates a need to improve. One way is to increase awareness that routine vaccines for adults are important for well-being, to provide information on how vaccines protect from diseases, and to assess routine vaccinations for adults are important for well-being, to provide information on how vaccines protect from diseases, and to assess immunization status during clinical visits. Adult vaccines are based on factors such as age and health status and include Tdap, tetanus-diphtheria (Td) booster, influenza,

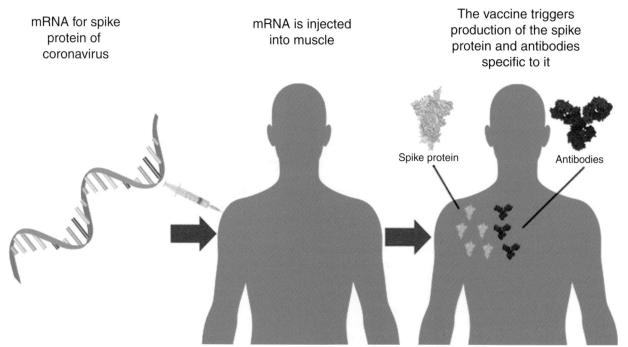

mRNA for spike
protein of
coronavirus

mRNA is injected
into muscle

The vaccine triggers
production of the spike
protein and antibodies
specific to it

Spike protein

Antibodies

Figure 34.3 COVID-19 mRNA vaccines give instructions for our cells to make **a harmless piece** of what is called the *spike protein.*

TABLE 34.1 Vaccine-Preventable Diseases

Disease, Route of Administration, Storage	Manifestations	Vaccine
Anthrax, subcut 2°C–8°C Do not freeze	*Cutaneous:* An itchy sore that may blister and form a black ulcer (eschar). The sore is usually painless but may have surrounding edema. *Gastrointestinal:* Abdominal pain, vomiting, mouth sores, bloody diarrhea, toxemia, shock, and possibly death *Inhaled:* Wool sorter's disease or associated with the use of biologic warfare: Fever, malaise, headache, cough, shortness of breath, and chest pain (due to bleeding and swelling in chest cavity) are often followed by shock within 36 hours of symptom onset due to bacteremia.	Routine vaccinations are not recommended but are administered to specific groups: laboratory workers who work with anthrax; people who handle animals or animal products, such as some veterinarians; some members of the US military. These persons should receive five shots over 18 months with annual boosters. When used as postexposure prophylaxis, the vaccine is given as a three-dose series, administered at 0, 2, and 4 weeks after exposure, along with 60 days of antibiotic therapy (ciprofloxacin and doxycycline).
Diphtheria, IM (diphtheria toxoids) 35°F–46°F (2°C–8°C) Do not freeze	Respiratory infection, blocked airway, myocardial damage, nerve damage, sore throat, weakness, swollen glands	Toxoid A single-antigen toxoid is not available. Currently combined as DTaP, Tdap, DT, and Td. DTaP is used for active immunity in those 6 wk to 6 y. Tdap (active booster) is given as a single dose for those 10 years and older.
Haemophilus influenzae type B (Hib), IM 35°F–46°F (2°C–8°C) Do not freeze	Sepsis, arthritis, skin and throat infections, meningitis, intellectual disability, epiglottitis, pneumonia, and death Increased severity is seen in those younger than 5 y and older than 65 y.	Bacterial conjugate is contained in Hib vaccine. There are different types of influenza; Hib is specific to influenza B. Not all influenza bacteria have vaccines.
Hepatitis A virus (HAV), IM 36°F–46°F (2°C–8°C) Do not freeze	Fever; can cause liver damage or failure, malaise, jaundice, anorexia, nausea, arthralgia, kidney, pancreatic, and blood disorders This acute, self-limited illness is highly contagious.	Inactivated viral antigen is available as HepA vaccine and in HepA/HepB. Routinely administered to children 12–23 mo, high-risk populations, close contacts to persons with HAV, and persons traveling to certain countries. Because it is inactivated, the vaccine can be given to immunocompromised persons.
Hepatitis B virus (HBV), IM 35°F–46°F (2°C–8°C) Do not freeze	Fever, headache, malaise, anorexia, arthralgia, arthritis, jaundice Chronic infection can occur, leading to liver cirrhosis, liver cancer, and death.	Recombinant viral antigen is available as HepB and HepA/HepB vaccines. Vaccines are recommended for at-risk infants, health care personnel, those who share injectable/IV drug needles and equipment, men who have sex with men, those whose sex partners are HBV positive, and those not in a monogamous relationship. HepB vaccine is available as a single dose and as a combined vaccine. Administer monovalent HepB to all infants at birth. Combination HepA-HepB is recommended only for those 18 y and older and for at-risk infants.
Human papillomavirus (HPV; various disease strains), IM 35°F–46°F (2°C–8°C) Protect from light, and shake well before administering Pregnancy: Administer only if needed	Sexually transmitted and seen as cervical, vaginal, anal, and oropharyngeal cancers and genital warts	The HPV vaccine is recommended for preteen boys and girls at age 11 or 12 so they are protected before ever being exposed to the virus. Women and men can receive the HPV vaccine through age 26.
Influenza, IM/ID/IN Inactivated influenza vaccine (IIV) 35°F–46°F (2°C–8°C): Administer IM/ID Live attenuated influenza vaccine (LAIV) ≤5°F (−15°C): Administer IN	Fever, chills, headaches, malaise, myalgias, nasal congestion, and cough Can cause pneumonia.	*Trivalent flu vaccine* (influenza A [H1N1 and an H3N2] and influenza B). *Quadrivalent flu vaccine* (2 influenza A and 2 influenza B). Everyone 6 months and older should have the flu vaccine annually, particularly those at high risk. Those who should NOT receive the flu shot include infants <6 months old, those with allergies to the flu vaccine or any of its components, those with allergies to eggs, and those with or who have recovered from Guillain-Barré syndrome. The IN flu vaccine should not be administered to children <2 y or adults >50 y, or children >2 or <17 y receiving aspirin-containing therapy or with asthma.
Japanese encephalitis, subcut Keep at 35°F–46°F (2°C–8°C) before and after reconstitution	Headache, vomiting, fever, myalgias, confusion, encephalitis, and possible death	Inactivated virus is given to travelers going to some Asian locations.

Continued

TABLE 34.1   Vaccine-Preventable Diseases—cont'd

Disease, Route of Administration, Storage	Manifestations	Vaccine
Measles, subcut (rubeola) 35°F–46°F (2°C–8°C) or colder; may be frozen Protect from light, and discard after 8 hours	Rash, fever, cough, nasal congestion, conjunctivitis, pneumonia Occasionally results in encephalitis	Live virus is contained in measles, MMR, and MMRV vaccines. **[!]** Contraindicated in pregnancy
Meningococcal disease, subcut/IM 35°F–46°F (2°C–8°C) Groups A, C, W, Y Meningococcal *Haemophilus influenzae* type b conjugate vaccine	Fever, sepsis, rash, meningitis	Meningococcal conjugate vaccines MenACWY: quadrivalent (protects against serogroups A, C, W, and Y). Recommended for children 2 mo to 10 y who are at increased risk and children/adolescents 11–18 y. First dose is recommended between 11 and 12 y with booster at 16 y. Also for adults after splenectomy, persons working with the pathogen, college freshmen, and military recruits. Meningococcal polysaccharide vaccine (MPSV4): quadrivalent (protects against serogroups A, C, W, and Y) meningococcal vaccine. For adults after splenectomy, persons working with the pathogen, college freshmen, and military recruits. Serogroup B meningococcal vaccine (MenB): monovalent (protects against serogroup B) meningococcal vaccine. Recommended for children/adolescents 10–18 y who are at increased risk.
Mumps, subcut 35°F–46°F (2°C–8°C), but may be frozen	Swelling of salivary glands, fever, headache, fatigue, and myalgia Can cause meningitis, encephalitis, inflammation of testicles or ovaries, deafness	Live attenuated virus is contained in MMR and MMRV. **[!]** Contraindicated in pregnancy
Pertussis ("whooping cough"), IM 35°F–46°F (2°C–8°C)	Highly contagious Severe coughing spasms; can cause pneumonia, seizures, encephalitis, and death Symptoms are more severe in infants and young children.	Antigenic components of inactivated bacteria (acellular) are contained in the two vaccines that are available, DTap and Tdap.
Pneumococcal disease, IM/subcut 35°F–46°F (2°C–8°C)	Ear infections, sinus infections, pneumonia; can cause sepsis, meningitis, and death	Pneumococcal polysaccharide vaccine (PPSV23) protects against 23 types of pneumococcal bacteria (IM/subcut). PPSV23 is recommended for all adults ≥65 y. Immunocompromised patients ≥2 but ≤64 y should also receive PPSV23. Pneumococcal conjugate vaccine (PCV13) protects against 13 types of pneumococcal bacteria (IM). PCV13 is recommended for all children <5 y as a series of 4 injections starting at 2 mo, then 4 mo, 6 mo, and between 12 and 15 mo; adults ≥65 y, and people ≥6 y with certain chronic illnesses should also receive the vaccine.
Poliomyelitis, subcut/IM 35°F–46°F (2°C–8°C)	Invades brain and spinal cord; the milder form causes fever, sore throat, nausea, and headaches; the severe form causes paralysis and death.	Children should receive a series of 4 inactive polio vaccine (IPV) injections starting at 2 mo, then at 4 mo, 6–18 mo, and a booster at 4–6 y.
Rabies, IM 35°F–46°F (2°C–8°C)	Anxiety, difficulty swallowing, seizures; almost always progresses to death	Administer killed virus to high-risk groups (e.g., veterinarians, animal handlers) and to persons traveling to areas where rabies is common. The preexposure schedule for rabies vaccination is three doses, given on the following schedule: 1st dose: before potential exposure 2nd dose: 7 days after the first dose 3rd dose: 21 days or 28 days after the second dose
Rotavirus, PO 35°F–46°F (2°C–8°C)	Acute gastroenteritis; contagious and may be particularly severe in infants and young children but mild in adults	Two vaccines are available: RV5 is given in 3 doses at ages 2 mo, 4 mo, and 6 mo RV1 is given in 2 doses at ages 2 mo and 4 mo **[!]** Due to the small increase in cases of intussusception from rotavirus vaccination, health care providers should weigh the potential risks and benefits of administering rotavirus vaccine to infants with a previous history of intussusception.

TABLE 34.1   Vaccine-Preventable Diseases—cont'd

Disease, Route of Administration, Storage	Manifestations	Vaccine
Rubella ("German measles"), subcut 35°F–46°F (2°C–8°C) May be frozen	Rash, fever, swollen lymph nodes Birth defects occur if rubella is acquired by a pregnant patient.	The rubella vaccine is a live attenuated virus. Recommended vaccination schedule: 1st dose: 12 through 15 mo 2nd dose: 4 through 6 y [!] Contraindicated in pregnancy
SARS-Cov-2 (COVID-19), IM into the deltoid muscle Pfizer-BioNTech: –70°C; can last 6 months if kept frozen at this temperature. May be thawed under refrigeration or at room temperature. Must reach room temperature before dilution. After dilution, store vials between 2°C to 25°C and is stable for 6 hours. Moderna: –20°C; can last 6 months if kept frozen at this temperature. Unpunctured vials may be stored in the refrigerator between 2°C to 8°C for up to 30 days. Do NOT refreeze thawed vaccine. Punctured vials may be stored between 2°C and 25°C for up to 12 hours. Johnson & Johnson/Janssen COVID-19 vaccine should be stored between 2°C and 8°C. Unpunctured vials are good until their expiration date; punctured vials are good for 6 hours; unused vaccine should be discarded after 6 hours.	The virus spreads by close person-to-person contact, mainly via respiratory droplets 2–14 days after exposure. Fever/chills, cough, dyspnea, fatigue, myalgia, headache, new-onset loss of taste or smell, sore throat, rhinorrhea, nausea, vomiting, or diarrhea. May progress to acute respiratory distress syndrome and death. Serious complications include arrhythmias, cardiomyopathy and acute cardiac injury, coagulation disorders, sepsis, shock, and multiorgan failure. Children may develop multisystem inflammatory syndrome. Some individuals develop COVID-19 syndrome, or "long COVID," and experience persistent symptoms including cognitive impairment, fatigue, anxiety, depression, PTSD, headaches, dizziness, persistent shortness of breath, and permanent lung damage.	Pfizer-BioNTech vaccine: Emergency Use Authorization issued 12/11/2020 by the FDA for ages 16 and older. Two IM doses (0.3 mL each) 21 days apart. On 05/10/2021, Pfizer received approval for the emergency use of the Pfizer-BioNTech COVID-19 vaccine to include adolescents 12 through 15 years of age. On 08/23/2021, Pfizer-BioNTech COVID-19 vaccine received full approval from the FDA for individuals 16 and over. The FDA is reviewing their application for a booster dose. Moderna vaccine: Application for Emergency Use Authorization has been submitted to the FDA. Two doses 28 days apart. No further information is available at this time. Moderna has submitted an application for full FDA approval, but as of 09/28/2021, the application is still pending. Their application includes approval for a booster dose. Johnson & Jonson/Janssen COVID-19 vaccine received emergency use authorization on 02/27/2021. It is a 1-shot vaccination recommended for individuals 18 years of age and over. After a brief pause in the use of the vaccine due to increased risk of thrombocytopenia syndrome (TTS) and reports of Guillain-Barré Syndrome (GBS), the FDA recommended the resumption of use on 04/23/2021, as the vaccine's known benefits outweigh the risks of not being vaccinated. Application for full approval and approval of a booster dose has not yet been submitted to the FDA.
Smallpox, percutaneous skin prick of 15 jabs using a steel bifurcated needle 35°F–46°F (2°C–8°C) Protect from light and use within 6–8 hours after reconstitution, then discard	High fever, severe headache, backache, abdominal pain, and lethargy that lasts 2–5 days; then an extensive rash develops that begins as macules and progresses to papules; then firm vesicles form; and finally, deep-seated, hard pustules form that cause significant scarring.	Smallpox vaccine (live vaccinia virus) is stockpiled in case of an outbreak and emergency. Immunization program for at-risk laboratory personnel and health care providers, emergency personnel, military personnel Vaccinate only if exposed to smallpox. [!] Contraindicated in pregnancy; can cause stillbirth. Can cause myocarditis and pericarditis.
Tetanus ("lockjaw"), IM 35°F–46°F (2°C–8°C)	Stiffness in neck and abdominal muscles, difficulty swallowing, muscle spasms, fever; can cause broken bones, breathing difficulty, and death	Toxoid conjugate contained in tetanus, DTaP, DT, Tdap, and Td vaccines. Children should receive a series of 5 doses of DTaP vaccine, beginning at 2 mo; then at 4 and 6 mo; then between 15 and 18 mo; and between 4 and 6 y. The Td booster should be given every 10 y.
Tuberculosis (TB), ID (preferred)/subcut 35°F–46°F (2°C–8°C)	Highly contagious respiratory infection Symptoms include cough lasting 3 wk or longer, pleuritic chest pain, coughing up blood or sputum, weakness or fatigue, weight loss, anorexia, fever and night sweats. May also cause meningitis and bone, joint, and skin infections	Live attenuated bacteria Called *bacille Calmette-Guérin (BCG)* Not routinely administered in the United States, it prevents severe disease but does not prevent infection with the bacterium. Should only be considered for children who have a negative tuberculin skin test and who are continually exposed, or for select health care workers.
Typhoid, subcut/PO 35°F–46°F (2°C–8°C)	Sustained high fever, headache, anorexia, abdominal pain, enlarged liver and spleen, constipation, and, later, diarrhea	Vaccine given in exposure to *Salmonella paratyphi* and *S. typhi B* is available as live attenuated bacteria (Ty21a; PO) or inactivated components of the typhoid bacterial capsule (Vi; subcut). Routine vaccinations are not required in the United States but are recommended for travelers to certain foreign countries.
Varicella (chickenpox), subcut ≤5°F (–15°C) Contraindicated in pregnancy	Fever and rash, consisting of a few to hundreds of itchy, blister-like lesions; symptoms are more severe in older children and adults. Complications may include encephalitis, bacterial skin infections, pneumonia, Reye syndrome, and death.	Varicella vaccine, live, is recommended as a two-dose series, first at 12–15 mo, then again between 4 and 6 y. [!] Contraindicated in pregnancy

Continued

TABLE 34.1 Vaccine-Preventable Diseases—cont'd

Disease, Route of Administration, Storage	Manifestations	Vaccine
Yellow fever, subcut 35°F–46°F (2°C–8°C)	Fever, jaundice, and gastrointestinal hemorrhage	Yellow fever vaccine, live A single primary dose is recommended for persons ≥9 mo traveling to, or living in, areas at risk for yellow fever virus transmission (e.g., South America and Africa). The vaccine is required by international regulations for travel to and from certain countries.
Herpes zoster (shingles), subcut ≤5°F (−15°C) Contraindicated in pregnancy	A painful, blisterlike rash in a dermatomal distribution occurs due to reactivation of varicella virus. After resolution of the rash, prolonged severe pain (postherpetic neuralgia) may occur.	Herpes zoster vaccine approved by the FDA for people ≥50 y.

DT, Diphtheria-tetanus; *DTaP,* diphtheria-tetanus–acellular pertussis; *FDA,* US Food and Drug Administration; *HepA,* hepatitis A; *HepB,* hepatitis B; *ID,* intradermal; *IM,* intramuscular; *IN,* intranasal; *IV,* intravenous; *MMR,* measles-mumps-rubella; *MMRV,* measles-mumps-rubella-varicella; *mo,* months; *PO,* by mouth; *subcut,* subcutaneous; *Td,* tetanus-diphtheria; *Tdap,* tetanus-diphtheria–acellular pertussis; *wk,* weeks; *y,* years; *>,* greater than; *≥,* greater than or equal to; *<,* less than; *≤,* less than or equal to.

pneumococcal polysaccharide vaccine (PPSV23), HPV, MMR, varicella vaccine (chickenpox), and zoster vaccine (shingles). In certain situations, adults may also be immunized with certain additional vaccines, including HepA, HepB, smallpox (2016 update: routine for laboratory personnel handling vaccine cultures), and meningococcal vaccine. Current recommendations for adult immunization can be found at www.cdc.gov/vaccines/schedules/.

⚡ PATIENT SAFETY

Do not Confuse...

- Hepatitis A, inactivated/hepatitis B (recombinant) vaccine provides active immunity against both hepatitis A virus (HAV) and hepatitis B virus (HBV) for adults >18 years of age who are at high risk for HAV and HBV.
- There are different types of **meningococcal vaccine:** MCV4 or Men-ACWY (conjugate; administered to preteens 11 to 12 years old), MenB (serogroup B; administered to teens and young adults ages 16 to 23), and MPSV4 (polysaccharide; for adults ≥56 who require a single dose [traveling or at risk due to community outbreak]).
- **HepA** and **HepB** vaccines are *dosed differently* for children, adolescents, and adults.
- Do not confuse HepB *vaccine* and HepB *immunoglobulin.*
- **Zoster vaccine,** a vaccine administered to adults to prevent shingles, and **varicella vaccine,** which prevents chickenpox and is approved for use in susceptible children and adults.
- ⚠️ **DTaP,** for active immunization in children 6 weeks to 6 years, and **Tdap,** the active booster for those aged 10 years and older; antigens in both are the same, but the amount of antigen component varies.

IMMUNIZATION BEFORE INTERNATIONAL TRAVEL

International travel warrants the updating of routine vaccines based on age and immunization history, and travelers to some areas should consider additional vaccines. For example, the CDC currently recommends US travelers 6 months and older to have an updated MMR vaccine based on the travel destination.

Travelers may need to consider vaccination against typhoid and yellow fever. Typhoid fever is caused by a bacterium, *Salmonella typhi,* which is generally spread via contaminated food and water (see Table 34.1). Risk of contracting this infection is greatest for travelers to India, Pakistan, Mexico, Bangladesh, the Philippines, and Haiti. Even stays of less than 2 weeks pose significant risk. Two forms of typhoid vaccine are available for use in the United States. Typhoid vaccine live oral contains the Ty21a strain of *S. typhi* and is a live attenuated vaccine, which can be administered to persons 6 years of age and older and consists of four capsules, one taken every 48 hours, with the series completed 1 week before potential exposure. A booster dose consisting of the same four-capsule regimen is recommended every 5 years. The other vaccine, parenteral typhoid Vi polysaccharide vaccine, is an inactivated vaccine that contains purified cell surface polysaccharide antigens extracted from *S. typhi* of the Ty2 strain and may be administered to travelers 2 years of age and older. It is administered at least 2 weeks before expected exposure as a single, intramuscular (IM) injection. A booster dose is recommended every 2 years for those who remain at risk.

Yellow fever is a mosquito-borne viral illness endemic to sub-Saharan Africa and tropical South America. The vaccine is administered as a single injection for persons older than 9 months. Boosters are no longer recommended (ACIP and World Health Organization [WHO], 2016) except for persons at risk. In the United States the vaccine is administered only at authorized vaccine centers throughout the country. Other vaccines needed for travel may include those for meningococcus, rabies, hepatitis A and B, and Japanese encephalitis. Current vaccine recommendations and related travel information, such as with the Zika virus and cholera, are available from the CDC at 1-800-CDC-INFO or www.cdc.gov/travel.

VACCINE SAFETY: REPORTING DISEASES AND ADVERSE REACTIONS

Vaccines are generally safe, although mild reactions include swelling at the injection site and low-grade fever. Awareness of the contraindications for use of vaccines decreases the incidence of serious adverse reactions. Contraindications include moderate or severe illness or anaphylaxis, a serious, life-threatening allergic reaction to a specific vaccine or vaccine component. Therefore it is important to review vaccine-specific contraindications before administering any vaccine. In general, vaccines may be given in cases of mild acute illness or the convalescent phase of illness, antimicrobial therapy, exposure to infectious disease, or premature birth.

Health care providers are responsible for reporting cases of vaccine-preventable diseases and adverse reactions after immunizations. These data identify whether an outbreak is occurring and assess the effect of immunization policies and procedures. Providers must report adverse reactions to the Vaccine Adverse Events Reporting System (VAERS). Information and forms are available at http://vaers.hhs.gov/index. VAERS is a surveillance system that receives and acts on reports of adverse events. The National Childhood Vaccine Injury Act of 1986 initiated the National Vaccine Injury Compensation Program (NVICP), which provides compensation for injury or death caused by a vaccination. More information is available

PROTOTYPE DRUG CHART

Varicella Vaccine

Drug Class	Dosage
Vaccine	0.5 mL subcut × 2 doses First dose: 12–15 mo; second dose: 4–6 y Catch-up initiated any time after 12–15 mo <13 y, space doses at least 3 mo apart ≥13 y, space doses 4–8 wk apart *For varicella prophylaxis; for outbreak control of local epidemics of wild-type varicella virus in susceptible persons after varicella exposure,* consult the current recommendations of the CDC (www.cdc.gov/chickenpox/outbreaks.html)
Contraindications	**Drug-Lab-Food Interactions**
Previous anaphylaxis to this vaccine or to any of its components; pregnancy or possibility of pregnancy within 1 mo; immunocompromised vaccine recipient; presence of moderate to severe acute illness; active untreated tuberculosis	Drug: Separate from other live virus vaccines (e.g., MMR, intranasal flu) by 4 wk if not given on the same day; delay VV for up to 11 mo after blood transfusion or Ig; delay Ig for 2 mo after VV, high-dose immunosuppressant medications; avoid salicylates for 6 wk after VV
Pharmacokinetics	**Pharmacodynamics**
Not applicable	Seroconversion rates: 12 mo–12 y: >98% at 4–6 wk after vaccination ≥13 y: ~75% 4 wk after first dose and 99% 4 wk after second dose
Therapeutic Effects/Uses	
For prevention of chickenpox; when administered to susceptible individuals, vaccine results in complete protection from chickenpox for the majority of persons. For the minority in whom breakthrough chickenpox develops after vaccination, the disease is typically very mild. The vaccine may also provide prophylaxis protection if administered within 3–5 d of exposure to chickenpox. Mechanism of Action: Stimulates active immunity against natural disease	
Side Effects	**Adverse Reactions**
Pain and redness at injection site, fever, chickenpox-like rash (generalized or confined to area surrounding injection site)	Anaphylaxis, thrombocytopenia, encephalitis, Stevens-Johnson syndrome

CDC, Centers for Disease Control and Prevention; *d*, day; *Ig*, immunoglobulin; *MMR*, measles-mumps-rubella; *mo*, month; *subcut*, subcutaneous; *VV*, varicella vaccine; *wk*, week; *y*, year; <, less than; >, greater than; ≥, greater than or equal to; ~, approximately.

at www.hrsa.gov/vaccinecompensation. To provide safety through communication, the NVICP requires providers to distribute a VIS before vaccines are administered. Federal law requires health care providers to provide information to those receiving vaccines. These information statements include indications, age recommendations, schedule of doses, side effects, special circumstances, and resources to notify if an adverse reaction occurs. For more information, visit www.cdc.gov/vaccines/hcp/vis.

VARICELLA VACCINE

Before the development of the varicella vaccine in 1995, about 4 million people came down with varicella zoster virus (VZV), resulting in 10,600 hospitalizations and close to 150 deaths per year. Since implementation of the varicella vaccine, cases of VZV have declined more than 75%, hospitalizations have declined more than 90%, and deaths from VZV have been reduced by 85% or more.

Prototype Drug Chart: Varicella Vaccine provides the pharmacologic data for varicella vaccine.

Pharmacokinetics. Biologic products such as vaccines do not undergo the pharmacokinetic processes associated with other drug therapy.

Pharmacodynamics. Seroconversion is the acquisition of detectable levels of antibodies in the bloodstream. In the case of

varicella vaccine, seroconversion occurs in more than 98% of 12-month-old to 12-year-old recipients approximately 6 weeks after receiving a single dose of vaccine. Susceptible persons 13 years of age and older who receive two doses of varicella vaccine 4 to 8 weeks apart show a seroconversion rate of approximately 75% 4 weeks after the first dose and 99% 4 weeks after the second dose. Despite the high rate of initial seroconversion among children 12 months to 12 years of age, clinical trials have shown that, over a 10-year period, the vaccine's effectiveness in preventing disease was 94% for children who received one dose of vaccine and 98% for those who received two doses. Therefore beginning in 2007, a second dose of varicella vaccine was recommended for all susceptible individuals, including children.

Contraindications

Varicella vaccine should be avoided in patients with a history of previous anaphylaxis to this vaccine or to any of its components, including gelatin and neomycin. It is also contraindicated in the presence of moderate to severe acute illness or active untreated TB.

Although varicella infection can cause fetal harm, the possible effects of the vaccine on fetal development are currently unknown. Therefore varicella vaccine is contraindicated during pregnancy. Pregnancy should also be avoided for at least 1 month after each dose of the vaccine. It is important to note that this recommendation differs from the product package insert, which suggests a 3-month delay in pregnancy.

Patients who are immunocompromised because of malignancies, high-dose systemic steroids, or other immunosuppressive therapy should avoid varicella vaccine. Likewise, the vaccine is generally contraindicated in the presence of primary or acquired immunodeficiencies. However, vaccination may be considered in children with certain classes of human immunodeficiency virus (HIV) infection.

Drug Interactions

Frequently, a patient is eligible for several immunizations at a visit. A patient receiving varicella vaccine may receive all other vaccines concurrently as long as each is administered at a separate site. If the MMR or other live virus vaccine is not given the same day as the varicella vaccine, administration of the two vaccines should be separated by at least 4 weeks.

If a patient has received a transfusion of blood or blood products, including Ig, administration of the varicella vaccine will need to be deferred for as long as 11 months. Likewise, such blood products should be avoided for at least 2 months after vaccination if possible. Blood products and Ig interfere with the body's production of antibodies specific to chickenpox, thereby decreasing the likelihood that active immunity will develop.

Reye syndrome has occasionally occurred in children after natural chickenpox infection. The majority of these children were also receiving salicylate medications (e.g., aspirin). Therefore it is generally recommended that patients avoid salicylates for 6 weeks after vaccination.

FUTURE DEVELOPMENTS IN VACCINES

A small outbreak of anthrax cases in the United States in 2001 increased the level of awareness of the anthrax vaccine. Anthrax is caused by the bacteria *Bacillus anthracis*. A serious disease, cutaneous anthrax is the most common form (95% of cases). Anthrax can also occur in the gastrointestinal (GI) tract and lungs. As a biologic weapon, anthrax is highly lethal. It is easily produced, stored, and spread over large areas. Proper vaccination is an essential part of protection against this disease. Approved by the US Food and Drug Administration (FDA) in 1970, anthrax vaccine adsorbed (AVA) has been routinely and safely administered to laboratory and military personnel, livestock farmers, and veterinarians. The vaccine requires five injections over 18 months with annual boosters. No serious side effects have been reported, but the vaccination is contraindicated during pregnancy. In the event of a bioterrorism attack, persons exposed to anthrax should receive three doses of vaccine over 4 weeks and be given ciprofloxacin and doxycycline for 60 days to prevent anthrax. Additional information is available at www.cdc.gov/anthrax/medical-care/prevention.html.

Smallpox, caused by the variola virus, is transmitted through human body fluids or contaminated materials. Smallpox was eradicated in the United States by 1972 and worldwide by 1977; therefore the United States discontinued routine childhood immunization against smallpox in 1972. The vaccine is no longer in use except in persons who have a high risk of exposure. When the vaccine is administered, most people usually have a mild reaction, such as a sore arm, fever, and body aches. However, persons with a weakened immune system may experience more serious side effects, including death. Since the events of September 2001, concern has arisen that smallpox could be used as a bioterrorist weapon. A smallpox immunization response plan is available for outbreaks or emergencies (https://www.cdc.gov/smallpox/bioterrorism/public/index.html).

It has long been known that immunity to pertussis, or "whooping cough," weakens over time and that adolescents and adults are often responsible for transmitting this infection to vulnerable, incompletely immunized infants and young children. In 2018, there were over 15,500 cases of pertussis in the United States. Pertussis in infants is associated with significant morbidity and mortality; a quarter of infants with pertussis

develop pneumonia, and 1 in 100 infants die. Tdap contains tetanus and diphtheria toxoids along with acellular pertussis; these are licensed for use in older children and adults. Tdap may be used as an active booster for people 11 to 64 years of age, and DTaP is approved for use in children 6 weeks to 6 years. Each vaccine contains the same antigens, but the quantities of diphtheria and acellular pertussis vary. It is recommended that, for booster immunization, adolescents and adults receive a one-time dose of Tdap in lieu of the Td vaccine. Research is underway to update the current vaccine, as the causative bacterium, *Bordetella pertussis,* has undergone genetic changes.

Herpes zoster, commonly known as *shingles* or *zoster,* occurs as the result of reactivation of the varicella virus. After a primary varicella infection (chickenpox), the virus persists but becomes dormant in the body, usually settling in a dorsal root ganglion. Zoster often occurs decades after the primary varicella infection. It appears that development of zoster may be related to a decline in immunity to the VZV. Zoster is characterized by a painful rash that presents in a dermatomal distribution. Especially in older adults, resolution of the rash may be followed by a chronic, severe, sometimes debilitating pain, referred to as *postherpetic neuralgia*. A live attenuated vaccine (zoster vaccine, live) is licensed for use as a one-time injection in adults 50 years of age and older. The vaccine has been shown to boost VZV immunity among vaccine recipients. In clinical trials, zoster vaccine prevented zoster in about 50% of people who received the vaccine. Effectiveness appears to decrease with increasing age of the vaccine recipient. In those who received the vaccine yet went on to develop zoster, the duration of pain was reduced.

Rotavirus is a leading cause of severe acute gastroenteritis in infants and young children. Rotavirus vaccine, live oral, containing five strains of rotavirus, is effective in protecting against severe gastroenteritis and significantly reduces the need for hospitalization among infected children. The vaccine is administered as a three-dose series at 2, 4, and 6 months of age. It is recommended that the third dose be administered before 8 months.

HPV is a sexually transmitted virus that causes cancer of the cervix, vagina, vulva, and penis and can cause genital warts. It also causes anal and oropharyngeal cancers in both men and women. There are more than 100 different types of this disease. Two vaccines are approved as routine prophylaxis to prevent HPV disease: HPV quadrivalent vaccine (recombinant) and HPV 9-valent vaccine (recombinant).

Both HPV vaccines are administered as a three-dose series to 9- to 26-year-old males and females. The HPV vaccine is contraindicated in pregnancy. The FDA denied Merck's request for expanded use in women 27 to 45 years of age. Because HPV is sexually transmitted, the vaccine is most effective if administered before initiation of sexual intercourse.

The pneumococcal vaccine provides protection against multiple strains of *Streptococcus pneumoniae* (pneumococcus). Pneumococcal disease includes serious infections of the blood, brain, and lungs. Each year in the United States, around 22,000 persons (both children and adults) die of this vaccine-preventable disease. Two forms of the vaccine are available: pneumococcal 23-valent polysaccharide vaccine (PPV) targeting 23 of the most common serotypes, and pneumococcal 13-valent conjugate vaccine (PCV13) targeting 13 serotypes. PPV is indicated in high-risk persons between the ages of 2 and 65 years (e.g., those undergoing splenectomy, cochlear implant, or immunosuppression) and in all persons older than 65 years. PPV should be repeated after 5 years. PCV13 is recommended for all high-risk persons and for all persons older than 65 years. Since initiation of pneumococcal vaccination, the incidence of antibiotic-resistant disease has dropped significantly.

Bacterial meningitis is a potentially life-threatening infection. Annually, more than 1000 cases occur in the United States; 10% to 15% of patients die and one out of five who live have permanent disability, including brain damage, hearing loss, amputations, or loss of kidney function. ACIP recommends routine vaccination to prevent meningococcal infection for those aged 2 to 55 years. The quadrivalent meningococcal conjugate vaccine (MCV4) and meningococcal polysaccharide vaccine (MPSV4) are approved in the United States. MCV4 is preferred for those between the ages of 2 and 55 years; MPSV4 should be used for those over 55 years of age. For those receiving MCV4, the first dose should be given at 11 or 12 years, with a booster at 16 years. For those who receive the first dose between 13 and 15 years, a one-time booster should be given between 16 and 18 years. If the first dose of MCV4 is given after 16 years, a booster is not needed unless the individual remains at high risk (e.g., microbiologists exposed to *Neisseria meningitidis*, military recruits, those traveling outside the United States, or those with asplenia).

◎ CLINICAL JUDGMENT [NURSING PROCESS]

Vaccines

Concept: Safety
- Protection of the patient from potential or actual harm; is a basic human need

Concept: Health, Wellness, and Illness
- Health, wellness, and illness are dynamic responses to a continuum of biopsychosocial states experienced through all stages of life.

Recognize Cues [Assessment]
- Identify benefits and barriers to timely and complete immunization (e.g., beliefs that vaccine-preventable diseases no longer exist, misunderstanding of true contraindications to immunization, concerns regarding vaccine safety and efficacy, fear of multiple injections, cost).
- Obtain a medical history, including history of malignancy or other immune deficiency.
- Determine history of pregnancy or possible pregnancy within the next month. Many vaccines are contraindicated during pregnancy.
- Obtain a drug history that includes high-dose immunosuppressants, blood transfusions, and Ig.
- Obtain a list of complementary and alternative therapies used, and in the case of a breast-fed infant, include herbal products used by the mother.
- Determine a complete allergy history that includes drugs, vaccines, food, and environmental allergies.
- Assess for adverse reactions (other than allergic) to previous doses of vaccine or any vaccine component.
- Assess for symptoms of moderate to severe acute illness with or without fever.
- Screen for unvaccinated or immunocompromised household contacts at every visit.
- Obtain an immunization history and a history of vaccine-preventable diseases to determine current vaccine needs. For example, a person with a reliable history of chickenpox or herpes zoster (shingles) does not need the varicella vaccine; natural immunity is assumed.

Analyze Cues and Prioritize Hypothesis [Patient Problems]
- Need for health teaching
- Potential for decreased adherence

Generate Solutions [Planning]
- The patient or the patient's parent or guardian will possess knowledge of vaccine-preventable diseases and risks and benefits of vaccination.
- The patient or the patient's parent or guardian will adhere to the recommended immunization schedule for vaccine-preventable diseases unless contraindications exist.
- The patient will be free of adverse reactions.

Take Action [Nursing Interventions]
- Strictly adhere to individual vaccine storage requirements to ensure potency of the product.

- Upon preparation, including reconstitution of a given vaccine, administer within the time limits stated in the package insert to ensure potency.
- ⚡ Administer at separate sites all vaccines for which a patient is eligible at the time of the visit. Do *not* mix vaccines in the same syringe.
- ⚡ Document in a patient's record the vaccination date, route, and site of administration; the vaccine type, manufacturer, lot number, and expiration date; and the name, business address, and title of the person administering the vaccine.
- ⚡ Observe the patient for signs and symptoms of adverse reactions to vaccines.
- Keep epinephrine readily available for immediate use in case of an anaphylactic reaction.
- Provide the patient with a record of immunizations administered.
- Modify communications to meet the cultural needs of the patient and the patient's family.
- Use a professional interpreter when necessary.
- Provide the patient and the patient's family with a VIS in the patient's preferred language (available at www.immunize.org).
- Discuss vaccine-preventable diseases with the patient and/or the patient's family, including manifestations and risk of contracting the disease.
- Answer all questions regarding vaccine safety, effectiveness, and risk factors in clear, understandable language.
- Advise female patients of childbearing age to avoid pregnancy for 1 month, depending on the vaccines administered.
- Advise patients to avoid contact with immunocompromised persons, depending on the vaccines to be administered.
- Provide the patient or the patient's family with a current vaccine information statement (VIS), available from the Centers for Disease Control and Prevention (CDC), for each vaccine before its administration as required by federal law.
- Remind the patient or the patient's family to maintain a vaccine immunization record and to bring it to all visits.
- Provide the patient or the patient's family with a return date for the next vaccination(s) based on assessment of the immunization history.
- Discuss common side effects of vaccines, such as injection site soreness, fever, and side effects specific to individual vaccines.
- Offer suggestions for management of common side effects (e.g., cold compresses for injection site soreness, acetaminophen for soreness or fever).
- Advise the patient or the patient's family to contact the health care provider if signs of a serious reaction are noted.

Evaluate Outcomes [Evaluation]
- Evaluate patient and family understanding of rationale for immunizations.
- Evaluate patient adherence to the recommended immunization schedule.
- Evaluate whether the patient is free from adverse reactions.

⚡ PATIENT SAFETY

  Don't Wait! Vaccinate!

Use the SHARE method (see https://www.cdc.gov/vaccines/hcp/adults/downloads/standards-immz-practice-recommendation.pdf):
Share reasons why the vaccine is right for the patient.

Highlight positive experiences.
Address the patient's questions about the vaccine.
Remind the patient that vaccines protect against diseases.
Explain the costs and consequences of getting the disease.

CRITICAL THINKING CASE STUDY

A 22-year-old college student is in the wellness clinic with her 3-month-old daughter and her 13-year-old sister. They live with her grandmother, who is 68 years old. She requests immunizations for her daughter and asks if there are any immunizations she and her sister need.

1. The patient says her daughter needs her "regular shots." The infant received her first hepatitis B vaccine while in the newborn nursery but has not had any shots since coming home. What is the hepatitis B vaccine catch-up schedule for the infant? What is the routine schedule for hepatitis B vaccine in infants?

2. The patient is worried that she will need to start her immunizations over because "she's so far behind." How should the nurse respond to her concern? When would her infant be due for another series of immunizations?

3. Which vaccines is the daughter due for today?

4. The nurse asks the patient about her vaccine history. She says she had her "baby shots" a long time ago but did not keep her personal vaccine record; however, she remembers receiving a flu shot 2 years ago. What immunizations will she need at this point? How can she best keep track of her immunizations?

5. After administering the patient's meningitis vaccine, her 13-year-old sister mentions that she heard that high school students should get a vaccination for human papillomavirus (HPV). She wants to know if she should get one or if it is too late. Who is eligible to receive the HPV vaccine, and what assessment questions would the nurse ask? What type and dosage of vaccine would the nurse administer?

6. After the visit, how does the nurse ensure that the vaccines were safely administered?

REVIEW QUESTIONS

1. The father of a 4-month-old infant calls in to the clinic reporting that his child is having a reaction to immunizations. What is the most important piece of information the nurse should elicit?
   a. The time the immunization was received
   b. Whether the father has given the infant any acetaminophen
   c. The signs and symptoms the infant is experiencing
   d. The sites used to administer the immunizations

2. The nurse is preparing to administer varicella vaccine to a young woman. Which of the following findings has the greatest implication for this young woman's care?
   a. The patient tells the nurse she is "deathly afraid of needles."
   b. The medical record indicates that the patient is allergic to eggs.
   c. The medical history indicates that the patient had leukemia as a young child.
   d. The patient appears to be pregnant.

3. A 38-year-old migrant farm worker is seen in the clinic with a cut to his arm from an old metal drum. The patient has sutures placed, and a tetanus, diphtheria, and acellular pertussis vaccine is given. What is the nurse's most important action after the vaccine has been administered?
   a. The nurse provides the patient with a vaccine information statement about the tetanus, diphtheria, and acellular pertussis vaccine in the patient's primary language.
   b. The nurse determines the exact date of the patient's last tetanus booster.
   c. The nurse documents that the patient did not experience any side effects immediately after immunization.
   d. The nurse provides the patient with a record of the immunization administered at the visit.

4. The nurse is preparing to administer routine, recommended immunizations to an immunocompromised 1-year-old child. What is the most important information to know before administering a vaccination?
   a. The type of vaccine to be administered to the child
   b. The child presents with a temperature of 99.8°F.
   c. The child's vaccine report shows immunizations were received on time.
   d. The child did not experience adverse reactions to prior immunizations.

5. A 14-year-old girl requests a vaccination for human papillomavirus. After the nurse administers the first dose, which of the following is important to include in the patient's teaching?
   a. Human papillomavirus prevents all sexually transmitted diseases.
   b. Pap smears are no longer needed after the human papillomavirus vaccination.
   c. The patient needs to notify the health care provider about pain at the injection site.
   d. The date the patient needs to return to the clinic for the next human papillomavirus dose.

6. Which of the following patients would be eligible to receive the influenza vaccine?
   a. The patient who is taking care of her son with human immunodeficiency virus
   b. The patient who is pregnant
   c. The patient with an egg allergy
   d. The child who is 18 months old

7. With the help of an interpreter, the nurse has just immunized a 35-year-old woman with the tetanus, diphtheria, and acellular pertussis vaccine and the vaccine against measles, mumps, and rubella. It is essential that the nurse proceed with which action(s)? (Select all that apply.)
   a. Provide a vaccine information statement in the patient's preferred language for each vaccine received.
   b. Document in the patient's record the date; site and route of administration; vaccine type, manufacturer, lot number, and expiration date; and the name, business address, and title of the person administering the vaccine.
   c. Administer a dose of ibuprofen to prevent postimmunization fever.
   d. Instruct the patient to call about any injection site soreness.
   e. Administer a dose of acetaminophen to prevent postimmunization fever.

8. It would be of greatest priority to notify the health care provider if a live vaccine was prescribed for a person in which situation?
   a. Child whose parent is receiving chemotherapy
   b. A child with an active viral infection
   c. A patient undergoing chemotherapy
   d. An HIV-positive patient with no active infections

35

Anticancer Drugs

http://evolve.elsevier.com/McCuistion/pharmacology

OBJECTIVES

- Define chemotherapy as an anticancer drug.
- Discuss ways the nurse can avoid exposure to anticancer drugs.
- Differentiate between cell cycle–specific and cell cycle–nonspecific anticancer drugs.
- Compare the uses and considerations for alkylating compounds, antimetabolites, antitumor antibiotics, hormones, and biotherapy agents.

- Prioritize appropriate nursing interventions to use while patients receive anticancer drugs.
- Develop a focused teaching plan on the uses and side effects of anticancer drugs.

OUTLINE

Cancer-related deaths rank second only to deaths by heart disease in the United States. Even though cancer-related mortality has decreased since the early 1990s, 39.5% of the population are projected to develop cancer over their lifetime. Excluding basal and squamous cell skin cancers, the highest incidences of cancer in men are prostate, lung, and colorectal cancer. In women, the highest frequency includes breast, lung, and colorectal cancers. Cancer mortality continues to be higher among men than women. Lung cancer remains the leading cause of cancer-related death regardless of gender.

The incidences and mortality rates of cancer differ by ethnicity. Non-Hispanic blacks (henceforth "African Americans") have higher incidences (except breast cancer) and higher death rates from cancer (except breast and lung) than any racial or ethnic group. African American women have lower incidences of breast cancer but higher mortality rates than Caucasian women do. Hispanics have the lowest incidences and mortality rates of lung cancer. Incidences and mortality rates for liver and stomach cancers due to hepatitis B virus (HBV) and *Helicobacter pylori (H. pylori)* are the highest among Asians and Pacific Islanders. Incidences of cancer increase among all immigrants as they adopt a more westernized lifestyle.

BOX 35.1 Environmental, Infective, and Dietary Influences on Cancer Development

Environmental

Tobacco
Gastric cancers and cancer of the bladder, cervix, colon, esophagus, head and neck, kidney and ureter, liver, lung, pancreas, trachea and bronchus, and acute myeloid leukemia

Asbestos
Lung cancer

Benzene
Acute myelogenous leukemia

Formaldehyde
Cancer of the nose, throat, and trachea

Vinyl Chloride
Sarcoma, leukemia

Arsenic
Cancer of the lung and skin, sarcoma

Ionizing Radiation
Leukemia; cancer of the thyroid, breast

Ultraviolet Rays
Skin cancer

Aflatoxin
Liver cancer

Infective

Herpes Simplex 2 Virus (Genital Herpes)
Cervical and penile cancer

Hepatitis B and C Viruses
Cancer of the liver

Epstein-Barr Virus
Non-Hodgkin lymphoma, Hodgkin disease, nasopharyngeal cancers

Human Papillomavirus (HPV)
Cancer of the cervix, vulva, vagina, anus, penis, head and neck

Human Immunodeficiency Virus (HIV)
Kaposi sarcoma, non-Hodgkin lymphoma, cervical cancer

Human T-Cell Lymphotropic Virus
T-cell leukemia

Helicobacter pylori
Cancer of the stomach, gastric mucosa-associated lymphoid tissue (MALT) lymphoma

Dietary
Animal Fat
Cancer of the colon, rectum, breast, uterus, prostate, ovary

Heterocyclic Amines (found in some smoked meats)
Cancer of the stomach, colon, rectum, pancreas, breast

Alcohol
Cancer of the mouth, throat, esophagus, liver, breast

Cancer is a group of diseases in which abnormal cells grow out of control and can spread to other areas of the body. DNA is the genetic substance in the body cells that transfers information necessary for the production of enzymes and protein synthesis. In most cases cancer is caused by damage to the DNA within the cell. Although some cancers are inherited, most develop when genes in a normal cell become damaged or lost. More than one mutation is required before a malignancy can develop; therefore the development of cancer is a multistep process that may take years to complete.

Pharmaceuticals are often used to destroy cancer cells and are called by different names, including *anticancer drugs, cancer chemotherapeutic agents*, antineoplastic drugs, or cytotoxic therapy. In the 1970s combination chemotherapy—the use of two or more chemotherapy agents to treat cancer—was adopted and led to improved response rates and increased survival times. Chemotherapy may be used as the only treatment of cancer, or it may be used in conjunction with other modalities such as radiation, surgery, and biologic response modifiers (BRMs). Chemotherapy is the use of chemicals to kill cancer cells. Combination chemotherapy increases the chance for months to years of cancer remission. If cancer can no longer be controlled, palliative treatment with chemotherapy may be used to relieve disease-related symptoms and improve quality of life.

GENETIC, INFLAMMATORY, INFECTIVE, ENVIRONMENTAL, AND DIETARY INFLUENCES

Cancer can be influenced by genetic mutations, inflammation, infectious organisms, environment, and an unhealthy diet. Box 35.1 gives examples of environmental substances, viruses, and foods that have a carcinogenic effect in humans. Genes provide the instructions for the production and function of cellular proteins essential for normal cellular activities. Genetic defects may occur in a variety of ways, including deletion, translocation, duplication, inversion, or insertion of genetic material. When defects cannot be effectively repaired, cells exhibit abnormal characteristics and unregulated growth. More than 2000 genes have been causally implicated in the formation of cancer. Cancers with a proven genetic influence include breast, ovarian, prostate, endometrial, colon, pancreatic, and lung cancers; retinoblastoma; and malignant melanoma, to name a few. Many more genetic influences are expected to be found as cancer research continues.

Genes can cause cells to become cancerous in several ways. Proto-oncogenes are normal genes involved in cell differentiation and division, and they regulate cell death, also known as apoptosis. These processes are necessary for healthy tissues and organs. An oncogene is a mutation in a proto-oncogene that affects cellular growth-control proteins and triggers unregulated cell division. Some genes, called antioncogenes, protect others. One such gene is the tumor-suppressor (TS) genes that signal a cell to cease multiplying and stop the action of oncogenes. Uncontrollable cell growth can occur if TS genes become lost or dysfunctional. Other genes repair damage to DNA. If these DNA-repair genes are damaged, mutations are not corrected and are subsequently passed on to the next generation of daughter cells. These and other gene mutations can take place over a long time before cancer develops. As a result, cancers more commonly occur in older individuals.

Inflammation is a normal physiologic process to heal injured tissues. Chronic inflammation, such as chronic inflammatory bowel disease (IBD), is an ongoing inflammatory process. The continued inflammation can lead to DNA damage and can result in cancer.

A number of viruses are associated with the development of cancer. The human papillomavirus (HPV) has been found in most women with invasive cervical cancer. Individuals with human immunodeficiency virus (HIV) may develop lymphomas and rectal or genital cancers. The Epstein-Barr virus (EBV) is found in almost all people with Burkitt lymphoma in central Africa and has been implicated in the development of nasopharyngeal cancer. Hepatocellular carcinoma (liver cancer) is linked to hepatitis B and C viruses. Other viruses linked to cancer include human T-cell lymphotropic virus (HTLV) and Kaposi sarcoma–associated herpesvirus.

Bacteria can play a role in the development of cancer. The presence of *H. pylori* in the stomach is associated with an increased risk of gastric cancer. Some reports have indicated a link between certain bacteria and cancer of the gallbladder, colon, and lung. However, no clear evidence supports a link between bacterial infection and other cancers.

Environmental factors associated with the development of cancer include tobacco use, poor diet, decreased physical activity, chemicals, and excessive sun and radiation exposures. According to the Centers for Disease Control and Prevention (CDC), 80% to 90% of lung cancers occur due to smoking. In 2019, a sharp increase in the use of electronic cigarettes (e-cigs) increased smoking-associated lung injury and death from these injuries. The CDC continues to research the long-term health effects from e-cigs. Other cancer-causing environmental agents include alcohol consumption on a regular basis, which raises the risk of mouth, larynx, and throat cancers; being overweight or obese, which increases the risk of uterine, breast, prostate, and colorectal cancers; and excessive exposure to sun and other forms of ultraviolet (UV) rays, which promotes skin cancers. Many of these cancers can be prevented. According to the American Cancer Society (ACS), about 606,520 people were expected to succumb to cancer during the year 2020.

CELL CYCLE–NONSPECIFIC AND CELL CYCLE–SPECIFIC ANTICANCER DRUGS

The cell cycle progress through five distinct phases or cycles, four of which are directed toward cell replication and a fifth phase in which the cell stops dividing. The five phases include *gap I* (G_1), *synthesis* (S), *gap 2* (G_2), *mitosis* (M), and *gap 0* (G_0). G_0 is a dormant phase, and most cells in the human body are in the G_0 phase. Fig. 35.1 illustrates the cell cycle.

Anticancer drugs stop or slow the growth of cancer cells by interfering with cell replication and are classified according to their action. Cell cycle–nonspecific (CCNS) drugs act during any phase of the cell cycle, including the G_0 phase. CCNS drugs include most alkylating drugs, antitumor antibiotics, and hormones. Cell cycle–specific (CCS) drugs exert their influence during a specific phase of the cell cycle and are most effective against rapidly growing cancer cells. The CCS drugs include antimetabolites, some alkylating agents, and vinca alkaloids. Fig. 35.2 shows selected categories of anticancer drugs and the phase of the cell cycle in which they are most effective.

Growth fraction and doubling time are two factors that play a major role in how the cancer cells respond to anticancer drugs. Growth fraction, the percent of actively dividing cells, decreases as the tumor enlarges, and doubling time increases. Doubling time is defined as the time it takes for a tumor to double in size. Anticancer drugs are more effective against neoplastic cells that have a high growth fraction. Leukemia and some lymphomas have high growth fractions and thus respond well to anticancer drug therapy.

Solid tumors have a large percentage of their cell mass in the G_0 phase; thus they generally have a low growth fraction and are less sensitive to anticancer drugs. As the tumor grows, the blood supply decreases, thereby slowing the growth rate. High-dose chemotherapy results in better tumor-killing (tumoricidal) effects. Depending on the type of cancer, malignant cell growth is usually faster in the earlier

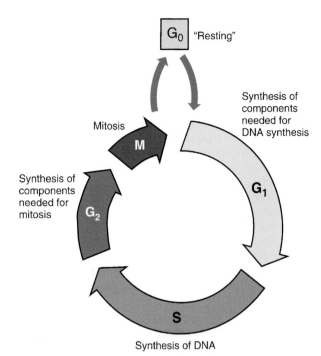

Fig. 35.1 Cell cycle G_1 phase (postmitotic gap): Production of RNA, protein, and enzymes for DNA synthesis; the G_1 phase lasts 15 to 18 hours. S phase (synthesis): All the components of DNA are synthesized, and the cells have doubled; the S phase lasts 10 to 20 hours. G_2 phase (premitotic gap): The cell continues to grow and ensures it is not defective; the G_2 phase lasts approximately 3 hours. M phase (mitosis): Cell growth has stopped, and the cell divides into two identical (daughter) cells; the M phase lasts approximately 1 hour. G_0 phase (resting): Cells remain in this phase and leave the cell cycle or return to the cell cycle for cell replication. Cells in this phase are not as sensitive to many antineoplastic drugs. The cells must pass through a series of checkpoints to continue through the cycle. Defective cells undergo apoptosis (self-destruction). (From Burcham, J., & Rosenthal, L. [2016]. *Lehne's pharmacology for nursing care* [9th ed.]. St Louis: Elsevier.)

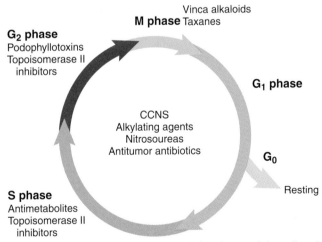

Fig. 35.2 Selected anticancer drugs and the phases of the cell cycle in which they are most effective. *CCNS,* cell cycle nonspecific.

stages of tumor development. Adequate vascularization is needed for the anticancer drugs to be effective. Anticancer drugs are more effective against small, fast-growing tumors with sufficient blood supply. The vascularization in solid tumors can be inconsistent. Some areas of tumor may have an adequate blood supply, whereas other areas are poorly perfused. This characteristic may make some large tumors resistant to anticancer drugs and therefore difficult to treat.

CANCER CHEMOTHERAPY

Anticancer drugs do not affect just cancer cells; instead, the drugs affect both cancer and healthy cells. The side effects of chemotherapy are largely related to the toxic effects on these healthy cells. Healthy cells are able to repair themselves and continue to grow; thus the side effects of chemotherapeutic agents are often temporary. Chemotherapy is usually administered systemically for cancer that has spread to other parts of the body, for cancers in multiple sites, or for cancers too large to be removed by other means (e.g., surgery). The most common route of chemotherapy administration is through intravenous (IV) infusion, although other routes may be used and include oral, intramuscular, subcutaneous, intraperitoneal, intraventricular (intrathecal), intrapleural, intravesicular, intraarterial, and topical routes.

Some types of cancer can be cured with chemotherapy (e.g., Hodgkin disease, Burkitt lymphoma, and testicular cancer). Other types of cancer (e.g., breast and colon cancer) may be treated with surgery first, followed by chemotherapy to eliminate any residual cancer cells (microscopic metastases) that may remain in the body. This is referred to as adjuvant therapy. Sometimes neoadjuvant chemotherapy may be given first to help shrink a large tumor, so that it can be surgically removed. Palliative chemotherapy, used to relieve symptoms associated with advanced disease (e.g., pain and shortness of breath), can improve quality of life.

Chemotherapy administration is guided by specific protocols based on the results of controlled research studies. The length of treatment is determined by the type and extent of the malignancy, the type of chemotherapy given, expected side effects of the drugs, and the amount of time that normal cells need to recover. Chemotherapy is usually given in cycles to improve the likelihood that cancer cells will be destroyed and that normal cells can recover. The duration, frequency, and number of chemotherapy cycles are based on the cancer type and size, the spread of the disease to other areas of the body (metastasis), and the condition of the patient. Chemotherapy treatment may consist of one drug or a combination of drugs. Combination chemotherapy may be

---

BOX 35.2 Anticancer Drugs by Classification[a]

High-Alert Medications

All chemotherapeutic agents are categorized as high-alert medications for all routes of drug delivery.

Alkylating Agents
Nitrogen Mustard Gas Derivatives
Bendamustine
Chlorambucil
Cyclophosphamide
Estramustine
Ifosfamide
Mechlorethamine hydrochloride
Melphalan

Nitrosoureas
Carmustine (bis-chloroethylnitrosourea [BCNU])
Lomustine (1-[2-chloroethyl]-3-cyclohexyl-1-nitrosourea [CCNU])
Streptozocin

Alkyl Sulfonates
Busulfan

Alkylating-Like Agents
Altretamine
Carboplatin
Cisplatin
Dacarbazine
Oxaliplatin

Antimetabolites
Folic Acid Antagonists
Methotrexate
Pemetrexed disodium

Pyrimidine Analogues
Azacitidine
Capecitabine
Cytarabine
Floxuridine

Fluorouracil injection (5-Fluorouracil [5-FU])
Gemcitabine hydrochloride

Purine Analogues
Cladribine
Clofarabine
Fludarabine
Mercaptopurine (6-MP)
Nelarabine
Pentostatin
Thioguanine (6-TG)

Ribonucleotide Reductase Inhibitors (Enzyme Inhibitors)
Hydroxyurea

Antitumorals
Anthracyclines
Daunorubicin hydrochloride
Daunorubicin liposomal
Doxorubicin
Epirubicin
Idarubicin
Mitoxantrone
Valrubicin

Other Antitumor Antibiotics
Bleomycin sulfate
Dactinomycin
Doxorubicin liposomal
Mitomycin

Plant Alkaloids
Antimicrotubules and Taxanes
Docetaxel
Paclitaxel

Camptothecin Analogues
Irinotecan
Topotecan

BOX 35.2 Anticancer Drugs by Classification[a]—cont'd

Epipodophyllotoxins
Etoposide
Teniposide

Immunomodulators
Alemtuzumab
Interleukin 2 (IL-2)
Rituximab
Thalidomide

Retinoids
Bexarotene

Vinca Alkaloids
Vinblastine sulfate
Vincristine sulfate
Vincristine, liposomal
Vinorelbine

Sex Hormones, Hormonal Agonists and Antagonists, Selective Estrogen Receptor Modulators, Luteinizing Hormone–Releasing Hormone Agonists, Aromatase Inhibitors, Enzymes, and Vaccines
Androgens
Fluoxymesterone

Hormonal Agonists and Antagonists
Abiraterone
Anastrozole
Bicalutamide
Enzalutamide
Exemestane
Flutamide
Fulvestrant
Goserelin acetate
Histrelin acetate implant
Letrozole
Leuprolide acetate
Medroxyprogesterone
Megestrol acetate
Mitotane
Nilutamide
Raloxifene
Tamoxifen citrate
Toremifene citrate

Enzymes
Asparaginase *Erwinia chrysanthemi*
Pegaspargase

Vaccines
Hepatitis B
Quadrivalent human papillomavirus subtypes 6, 11, 16, and 18
Human papillomavirus bivalent vaccine

[a] See Chapter 33 for monoclonal antibodies and targeted therapies and Chapter 34 for biologic therapies.

administered in 1 day or may be spread out over several days. The duration of treatment is based on the protocol being followed; it can vary from minutes to days and may be repeated weekly, biweekly, or monthly. Selected anticancer drugs are listed in Box 35.2 according to classification.

Combination Chemotherapy

Single-agent drug therapy is not usually used to treat cancer because combination therapy with two or more anticancer drugs has demonstrated more effective tumoricidal activity. Combination therapy increases the likelihood of affecting cancer cells in all phases of the cell cycle.

To maximize cell death, CCNS and CCS drugs are often combined to increase synergistic effects. Each individual drug used in combination therapy should have a proven tumoricidal activity, a different mechanism of action, and different dose-limiting toxicities. A combination of antineoplastic drugs has the advantage of decreasing drug resistance while increasing cancer cell destruction. Table 35.1 presents some of the combined anticancer drugs.

General Side Effects and Adverse Reactions

Anticancer drugs exert adverse effects on rapidly growing normal cells, such as skin and hair. These drugs can also affect cells in the gastrointestinal (GI) tract, mucous membranes, bone marrow, and reproductive system. Myelosuppression can occur when there is a significant decrease in the bone marrow activity that results in decreased white blood cells, platelets, and red blood cells. After chemotherapy administration, the nadir—the time at which the blood count is at the lowest—typically occurs 7 to 10 days after treatment.

Table 35.2 lists the general adverse effects anticancer drugs exert on the fast-growing cells of the body. Selected nursing measures and considerations are included. Because of the toxic effects of chemotherapy, care in handling of such drugs must be considered, and protective gear that includes gloves specific for handling chemotherapy drugs must be used.

Anticancer Therapy in Outpatient Settings

The administration of anticancer drugs in outpatient settings, such as in homes and oncology clinics, is both cost-effective and convenient. Although chemotherapy regimens have become increasingly aggressive, most patients are not hospitalized unless they require close monitoring or become very ill. Patients receiving highly potent drugs will need to be closely monitored for severe adverse effects. When a chemotherapy drug is given, a health care provider qualified to administer anticancer drugs follows the policies provided by the oncologist and the health care agency. By following strict protocols, the nurse reduces exposure to hazardous chemotherapy drugs during administration.

ALKYLATING DRUGS

One of the largest groups of anticancer drugs is the alkylating compounds. Alkylating drugs damage the cell's DNA by cross-linkage of DNA strands, abnormal base pairing, or DNA strand breaks, thus preventing the reproduction of cancer cells. Drugs in this group belong to the CCNS category and kill cells in all phases of the cell cycle. They are used to treat many different types of cancer, including leukemia, lymphoma, multiple myeloma, sarcoma, and solid tumors such as those

TABLE 35.1 Selected Combinations of Anticancer Drugs

Generic	Acronym[a]	Selected Uses
Cytarabine, daunorubicin, etoposide	ADE	Acute myelogenous leukemia
Fluorouracil, doxorubicin, cyclophosphamide	FAC	Breast cancer
Leucovorin, fluorouracil, irinotecan	FOLFIRI	Colorectal cancer
Leucovorin, fluorouracil, oxaliplatin	FOLFOX	
Capecitabine, irinotecan	XELIRI	Esophageal cancer, gastric cancer
Bortezomib (PS-341), doxorubicin, dexamethasone	PAD	Multiple myeloma
Carboplatin, paclitaxel	CARBOPLATIN-TAXOL	Non–small cell lung cancer
Cyclophosphamide, doxorubicin, vincristine, prednisone	CHOP	Non-Hodgkin lymphoma
Rituximab, cyclophosphamide, doxorubicin, vincristine, prednisone	R-CHOP	
Gemcitabine, cisplatin	(None)	Pancreatic cancer
Gemcitabine, fluorouracil, leucovorin	OFF	
Bleomycin, etoposide, cisplatin	BEP	Testicular cancer
Vinblastine, ifosfamide, cisplatin	VIP	

[a]Acronyms are based on the generic or trade name of the chemotherapy drugs used in a specific protocol (e.g., ABVD [Adriamycin, bleomycin, vinblastine, dacarbazine], FAC [fluorouracil, Adriamycin, cyclophosphamide]). Not all acronyms for combination chemotherapy treatments are listed.

TABLE 35.2 General Adverse Reactions to Anticancer Drugs[a]

Adverse Reactions	Nursing Measures and Considerations
Bone Marrow Suppression, Myelosuppression	
Low RBC count (anemia)	Assess for fatigue, shortness of breath, low blood pressure, increased heart rate, increased respiratory rate, and oliguria. Assess for cyanosis. Plan rest periods. Administer oxygen as prescribed. Elevate the head of the bed to facilitate breathing. Provide pain mediation if pain is increasing oxygen consumption. Provide assistance with activities. Monitor for mental status changes. Anemia may be treated with ferrous sulfate or infusions of RBCs. EPO may be administered to stimulate RBC production. Monitor RBCs, hemoglobin, and hematocrit.
Low WBC count (leukopenia)	Susceptibility to infection increases as WBCs decrease. Patients should avoid people with infections and report fever, chills, URIs, or sore throat to their HCP. Hand hygiene before and after contact with the patient is important. Monitor for changes in body temperature; elevated temperature is considered a sign of infection. Avoid medications that may mask fever. Immediately report temperatures of 101°F (38.3°C) or above to the HCP. Appropriate cultures (e.g., blood, urine, sputum) are collected before antibiotics are started if applicable, and an antibiotic regimen is initiated. Assess for localized infections. Auscultate breath sounds. Colony-stimulating factors (e.g., filgrastim) may be administered to stimulate WBC production. Monitor WBCs, especially ANCs.
Low platelet count (thrombocytopenia)	Petechiae, bruising, bleeding of gums, and nosebleeds are signs of a low platelet count; report these signs to a HCP. Assess for bleeding, petechiae, and ecchymosis. Assess for occult bleeding in urine, feces, and emesis. Apply pressure to injection sites until bleeding has stopped. Platelet transfusions may be needed. Avoid medications that may promote bleeding (aspirin, heparin). Avoid invasive procedures (injections, indwelling urinary catheters, rectal temperature, and suppositories). Monitor platelet counts and bleeding time.
Gastrointestinal Disturbances	
Anorexia	Loss of appetite may be related to anemia, pain, fatigue, or altered taste caused by chemotherapy drugs. Provide small, frequent meals that are high in calories and protein. Plan rest periods. Address issues of pain control. Hard candy or ice chips may help relieve bitter taste.
Nausea and vomiting	Antineoplastic drugs often stimulate the CTZ, leading to nausea and vomiting, which can be caused by irritation of the GI tract; effects of radiation to chest, abdomen, or brain; anxiety; constipation; pain; electrolyte imbalances; or other medications. Grading scales are useful to assess severity. Provide antiemetics before, during, and after chemotherapy. Assess for GI upset, and medicate appropriately. Minimize noise, stimulation, and odors. Frequent mouth care is recommended. Monitor fluid balance and serum electrolytes.
Diarrhea	Diarrhea may be one of three types: *osmotic* (absorption defects), *secretory* (bacterial infection or neoplasm), or *exudative* (secondary to chemotherapy). Chemotherapeutic drugs most commonly associated with diarrhea are alkylating agents, antitumor antibiotics, and antimetabolites. Treatment (e.g., medications, diet changes) will depend on cause and severity. Diarrhea may be caused by other medications, such as antibiotics, comorbid conditions (e.g., Crohn disease), or enteral (tube) feedings. Assess normal bowel habits, and monitor for electrolyte imbalances and dehydration. Administer appropriate antidiarrheal medications (antibiotics, anticholinergics, antispasmodics, psyllium, kaolin and pectin, or octreotide acetate). Teach patients to eat small, frequent meals; follow a low-residue diet; limit spicy, fatty foods; limit intake of salty foods, whole grains, fresh fruits and vegetables, and caffeinated and carbonated drinks; and avoid very hot or very cold foods (may stimulate peristalsis). Monitor intake and output.

TABLE 35.2   General Adverse Reactions to Anticancer Drugs[a]—cont'd

Adverse Reactions	Nursing Measures and Considerations
Mucositis (stomatitis)	Many antineoplastic drugs cause changes in oral mucosa that generally occur 2–14 days after initiation of therapy. Assess for taste changes, tissue swelling, redness, pain, dry mouth, white patches, or a white coating on the oral mucosa. Mucositis ranges from mild to severe. Symptomatic treatment may include frequent mouth rinses, topical anesthetics, antibiotics, antifungal medication, saliva substitutes, and pain medication. Patients should avoid commercial mouthwashes that contain alcohol. A soft toothbrush is recommended. Offer ice chips or ice pops to help relieve pain. Assess intake and output. Evaluate caloric needs. A grading scale may be useful to assess severity.
Other Alopecia	Not all chemotherapeutic drugs cause hair loss. Hair thinning, patchy baldness, or complete alopecia may occur, depending on the drug. Hair on all areas of the body is affected. Hair loss may be gradual, progressing with each cycle of chemotherapy, or rapid. Hair regrowth usually occurs once chemotherapy is completed, although the texture may be changed. Before therapy, discuss potential hair loss and ways to address the discomforts (e.g., baldness and scalp hypothermia) due to hair loss (wigs, scarves, hats, or turbans). Assess for body image changes and concerns.
Fatigue	Fatigue may be caused by chemotherapy, sleep disturbances, emotional distress, depression, bone marrow suppression, infection, pain, or electrolyte imbalances. Assess fatigue using a visual analogue grading scale (0 = no fatigue; 10 = worst fatigue). Address conditions that might be contributing to fatigue (lack of sleep, pain, depression). Plan ways to help patients conserve energy. Plan a well-balanced diet, and encourage participation in regular (but not strenuous) exercise and stress reduction measures, such as relaxation and guided imagery.
Infertility	If infertility occurs, it may be permanent. Pretreatment counseling is advised.

ANC, Absolute neutrophil count; *CTZ,* chemoreceptor trigger zone; *EPO,* erythropoietin; *GI,* gastrointestinal; *HCP,* health care provider; *RBC,* red blood cell; *URI,* upper respiratory infection; *WBC,* white blood cell.
[a]The list in the table is not all-inclusive. Some more serious reactions are discussed in the Prototype Drug Charts.

of the breast, ovary, uterus, lung, bladder, and stomach. Even though alkylating drugs are effective in all phases of the cell cycle, they are most effective in the G_0 phase. Alkylating drugs are divided into five different classes: (1) nitrogen mustards, (2) nitrosoureas, (3) alkyl sulfonates, (4) triazines, and (5) ethylenimines. Table 35.3 lists some of the alkylating drugs, their uses, and considerations. Of the alkylating drugs, nitrosoureas cross the blood-brain barrier, making them useful in the treatment of brain cancer. General adverse effects to anticancer drugs are discussed in Table 35.2. Additionally, alkylating drugs given in high doses can cause long-term damage to the bone marrow, resulting in acute leukemia. The platinum (alkylating-like) drugs—cisplatin, carboplatin, and oxaliplatin—kill cells in a similar fashion but are less likely to cause leukemia later.

Cyclophosphamide

Cyclophosphamide, an alkylating drug, is an analogue of nitrogen mustard and has activity against many neoplastic diseases including Hodgkin and non-Hodgkin lymphoma (NHL), acute and chronic lymphocytic leukemia (CLL), multiple myeloma, breast and ovarian carcinoma, lung cancer, and retinoblastoma. The drug is also used for immunologic disorders such as lupus nephritis and has been shown to prevent progressive renal scarring, preserve renal function, induce renal remission, and decrease end-stage renal failure. This drug is a severe vesicant that causes tissue necrosis if it infiltrates into the tissues. Cyclophosphamide can be administered orally or intravenously. The patient should be well hydrated while taking cyclophosphamide to prevent hemorrhagic cystitis (bleeding due to severe bladder inflammation). Sodium 2-mercaptoethanesulfonate is a chemoprotectant drug often given with high-dose cyclophosphamide to inactivate urotoxic metabolites to reduce the incidence of hemorrhagic cystitis.

> **⚡ PATIENT SAFETY**
>
> Patients should be well hydrated before and during therapy.
> **Do not confuse...**
> - **Myleran** with **Alkeran**
> - **Cisplatin** with **carboplatin**
> - **Paraplatin** with **Platinol**
> - **Cyclophosphamide** with **cyclosporine**

Pharmacokinetics. Oral cyclophosphamide is well absorbed in the GI system. Cyclophosphamide is a prodrug that is activated and extensively metabolized by the liver. About 5% to 25% of the drug is eliminated by the kidney as unchanged, and its elimination half-life is 3 to 12 hours. Approximately 20% is bound to plasma protein, and this is not dose dependent. Some cyclophosphamide metabolites are greater than 60% protein bound. Less than 10%, mostly in the form of metabolites, is excreted in feces.

Pharmacodynamics. Cyclophosphamide is an early antineoplastic drug used alone or with other drugs to treat a variety of cancers. Average time to peak plasma concentration (T_{max}) is 1 hour. Several drug interactions can occur with cyclophosphamide. Patients should report all medications they are taking, including over-the-counter (OTC) medicines and herbal supplements. Anthracycline (e.g., doxorubicin) has been reported to induce cardiotoxicity when taken with cyclophosphamide, and it exacerbates hemorrhagic cystitis. Other serious drug interactions can occur when taking cyclophosphamide concomitantly with aspirin, allopurinol, phenobarbital, warfarin, thiazide diuretics, and some psychiatric medications. The Complementary and Alternative Therapies box lists herbal supplements that may also interact with cyclophosphamide.

TABLE 35.3   Antineoplastics: Alkylating Drugs

- Visually inspect parenteral products for particulate matter and discoloration before use.
- Observe and exercise precautions when handling, preparing, and administering cytotoxic drugs.
- The correct dose of chemotherapeutic drugs will vary from protocol to protocol. Consult appropriate references to verify doses.

Drug	Route and Dosage	Uses and Considerations
Nitrogen Mustards		
Bendamustine	CLL: A: IV: 100 mg/m^2 on days 1 and 2, repeated q28d for up to 6 cycles NHL: A: IV: 120 mg/m^2 on days 1 and 2, repeated q21d for up to 8 cycles	For CLL and NHL. Monitor for bone marrow depression. Assess for tumor lysis syndrome and skin reactions PB: 94%–96%; t½: 40 min
Chlorambucil	Palliative CLL, Hodgkin disease, and NHL: A: PO: 0.1–0.2 mg/kg/d (4–10 mg/d) for 3–6 wk	For CLL, Hodgkin disease, and NHL. Monitor for bone marrow suppression or pancytopenia PB: 99%; t½: 1.5 h
Estramustine	A: PO: 14 mg/kg/d or 600 mg/m^2/d in 3–4 divided doses	For palliative treatment of prostate cancer. Gynecomastia and impotence may occur PB: UK; t½: 20–24 h
Ifosfamide	A: IV: 1.2–2 g/m^2/d for 5 d in combination with mesna; repeat every 3 wk after recovery from hematologic toxicity. Mesna is usually given concomitantly to prevent hemorrhagic cystitis	For testicular cancer. Monitor for hemorrhagic cystitis PB: negligible; t½: 7–15 h
Mechlorethamine hydrochloride	Hodgkin disease: A: IV: 0.2 mg/kg or 6 mg/m^2 as single dose CLL: A: IV: 6 mg/m^2 q4wk CML: A: IV: 0.4 mg/kg or 6 mg/m^2 monthly Other dosing regimen and routes are available	For Hodgkin disease, leukemias, solid tumors, and effusions caused by cancer. This drug is contraindicated in patients with active infections PB: UK; t½: Minutes
Melphalan	Multiple myeloma: A: PO: 6 mg daily for 2–3 wk; *maint:* 2 mg/d; adjust 1–3 mg/d based on hematologic response A: IV: 16 mg/m^2 q2wk for 4 doses; *maint:* 16 mg/m^2 q4wk Ovarian cancer: A: PO: 200 mcg/kg/d for 5 d; repeat q4–5wk based on hematologic response	For multiple myeloma and ovarian cancer. *Do not confuse Alkeran with Leukeran or Myleran* PB: 20%–30%; t½: 1.25–1.5 h
Nitrosoureas		
Carmustine (BCNU)	A: IV: 150–200 mg/m^2 single dose q6wk or 75–100 mg/m^2/d for 2 days q6wk	For Hodgkin disease, NHL, multiple myeloma, and brain tumors. Monitor for bone marrow suppression and pulmonary symptoms PB: UK; t½: 5–30 min
Lomustine (CCNU)	Hodgkin disease and malignant glioma: A: PO: 100–130 mg/m^2 q6wk	For Hodgkin disease and malignant gliomas. Monitor for bone marrow suppression and liver function PB: UK; t½: 16 h-2 d
Streptozocin	A: IV: 500 mg/m^2/d for 5 d q4–6wk; doses above 500 mg/m^2 are not recommended	*Do not confuse with streptomycin.* For pancreatic cancer PB: UK; t½: 30–45 min
Alkyl Sulfonates		
Busulfan	A: PO: 4–8 mg/d	For myelocytic leukemia. Monitor for seizures and cerebral hemorrhage PB: 32%; t½: 2.5 h
Alkylating-Like Drugs		
Altretamine	A: PO: 260 mg/m^2/d in 4 divided doses after meals and at bedtime for 14 or 21 d in a 28-d cycle; drug holiday for ≥14 d then restart at 200 mg/m^2/d	For ovarian cancer PB: Weakly; t½: 4.7–10.2 h
Carboplatin	New cancer: A: IV: 300 mg/m^2 in combination with cyclophosphamide q4wk for 6 cycles Recurrent cancer: A: IV: 360 mg/m^2 q4wk	For advanced ovarian cancer. Usually given as combination therapy PB: UK; t½: 1.5–2.5 h

TABLE 35.3 Antineoplastics: Alkylating Drugs—cont'd

Drug	Route and Dosage	Uses and Considerations
Cisplatin	Bladder cancer: A: IV: 50–70 mg/m^2 q3–4wk Ovarian cancer: A: IV: 50–75 mg/m^2 q21d Testicular cancer: A: IV: 20 mg/m^2 for 5 d; repeat q3wk for 2 more cycles	For bladder, ovarian, testicular, and NSCLC. Monitor for CNS function; reversible posterior leukoencephalopathy may occur PB: 90%; t½: 30–100 h, dose related
Dacarbazine	Melanoma: A: IV: 250 mg/m^2/d for 5 d repeated q3wk Hodgkin disease: A: IV: 375 mg/m^2 days 1 and 15 q28d	For Hodgkin disease and malignant melanoma. Monitor hepatic function PB: Minimal; t½: 5 h
Oxaliplatin	A: IV: 85 mg/m^2 on day 1 q2wk for 12 cycles	For metastatic colorectal cancer. Used with 5-FU and leucovorin (FOLFOX4). Assess for pulmonary complications PB: >90%; t½: 391 h

Note: Chemotherapeutic doses and schedules will vary depending on protocol, body surface area (m^2), age, functional status, and comorbid conditions. For a full discussion of body surface area in dosage calculation, see Chapter 11.

5-FU, 5-Fluorouracil; *A,* adult; *CLL,* chronic lymphocytic leukemia; *CML,* chronic myelogenous leukemia; *CNS,* central nervous system; *d,* day; *h,* hour; *IV,* intravenous; *maint,* maintenance; *min,* minute; *NHL,* non-Hodgkin lymphoma; *NSCLC,* non–small cell lung cancer; *PB,* protein binding; *PO,* by mouth; *q,* every; *t½,* half-life; *UK,* unknown; *wk,* week; *>,* greater than; *≥,* greater than or equal to.

🌿 COMPLEMENTARY AND ALTERNATIVE THERAPIES

Cyclophosphamide

- Use cautiously with garlic (antiplatelet activity), ginkgo (increased antiplatelet effect), echinacea (decreased effects of immunosuppressive drugs), ginseng (altered bleeding time), St. John's wort (may interfere with chemotherapy), and kava kava (increased risk for bleeding). Toxicity and actions of both cyclophosphamide and vitamin A are altered if given together. *Do not use with mistletoe because it may promote cancer growth.*
- Astragalus (Huang-qi; milk vetch root) stimulates the immune system and may help speed recovery from immunosuppressive chemotherapy. Astragalus has blood clot–fighting properties and may increase risk of bleeding when given with cyclophosphamide.

Side Effects and Adverse Reactions

The side effects of cyclophosphamide reflect those seen in the general class of antineoplastic drugs. (For the general side effects, see Table 35.2.) Hemorrhagic cystitis is a serious problem that can arise when high doses of cyclophosphamide are given. Patients who receive a high dose should be assessed for cardiomyopathy and syndrome of inappropriate antidiuretic hormone (SIADH) during treatment with this drug. In addition, cyclophosphamide may increase pigmentation of the skin or nail beds. Prototype Drug Chart: Cyclophosphamide details the pharmacologic behavior of cyclophosphamide.

ANTIMETABOLITES

Molecularly, antimetabolites resemble natural substances, building blocks that not only synthesize but also recycle and break down organic compounds used by the body. However, antimetabolites interfere with various substances needed for normal cell function. Most antimetabolites are classified as CCS, and they exert their effects during the S phase (DNA synthesis and metabolism) of the cell cycle. Few antimetabolites (e.g., 5-fluorouracil [5-FU], floxuridine) have cytotoxic effects in multiple phases of the cell cycle. Antimetabolites are classified according to the substances with which they interfere. Substances can include folate, pyrimidine, purine analogues, and ribonucleotide reductase inhibitors. Table 35.4 lists the antimetabolite drugs, uses, and considerations.

Methotrexate, a folate antimetabolite, is used to treat malignant and nonmalignant conditions (e.g., rheumatoid arthritis, psoriasis). Methotrexate affects cells that have high metabolic rates, such as neoplasms, hair follicles, endothelium, cells of the GI tract, fetal cells, and bone marrow; it is used to treat leukemias and cancers of the GI tract, head and neck, breast, and ovaries. Because methotrexate causes apoptosis to fetal cells, it can be used for ectopic pregnancies. Methotrexate inhibits the biosynthesis of a purine nucleotide, 5-aminoimidazole-4-carboxamide ribonucleotide (AICAR) transformylase, which provides antiinflammatory properties that result in metabolites; AICARs are immunotoxic. Leucovorin can be given 12 to 24 hours after methotrexate administration (not simultaneously) to reduce AICAR concentrations, thereby diminishing the adverse effects of methotrexate. Leucovorin should not be referred to as *folinic acid* because it can be confused with *folic acid,* which can lead to severe methotrexate toxicity. Other interactions are seen with methotrexate. Nonsteroidal antiinflammatory drugs (NSAIDs) given just before, concomitantly with, or after intermediate or high doses of methotrexate have resulted in severe hematologic and GI toxicity. Furthermore, NSAIDs may mask fever, swelling, and other signs and symptoms of infection. Several corticosteroids can reduce the cytotoxicity of methotrexate. Protein-bound drugs such as salicylates (aspirin), sulfonylureas (glyburide), hydantoin (phenytoin) anticonvulsants, and sulfonamides can induce methotrexate toxicity. Penicillins, proton pump inhibitors, and probenecid, among other drugs, can cause methotrexate toxicity. Acidic food and drink can also cause elevated methotrexate concentrations.

Fluorouracil

Fluorouracil (5-FU), an antimetabolite agent similar to uracil with an addition of fluoride, is a component of chemotherapy for many cancers, including breast, colorectal, GI, and head and neck. 5-FU is administered intravenously to treat solid tumors and is applied topically for superficial basal cell carcinoma and actinic keratosis. A microsponge delivery system for a cream-based 5-FU was approved in 2000 to provide a sustained-release formulation administered once daily. It is not administered orally because of the inconsistent bioavailability.

🖹 PROTOTYPE DRUG CHART

Cyclophosphamide

Drug Class	Dosage
Alkylating drug: Nitrogen mustard Generic Name: Cyclophosphamide	Acute lymphocytic leukemia (ALL): A: IV: 40–50 mg/kg/d A: PO: 1–5 mg/kg/d Breast cancer: A: IV: 500–1000 mg/m² q15d Various protocols exist, including combination therapy. Dosage varies based on indicated use and response. Adjust dose if bone marrow suppression (myelosuppression) occurs.
Contraindications	**Drug-Lab-Food Interactions**
Absolute contraindications: Hypersensitivity, severe urinary outflow obstruction, bladder obstruction *Caution:* Myelosuppression, tumor lysis syndrome, liver or kidney disease, hemorrhagic cystitis, or heart failure. Many other precautions are necessary when administering cyclophosphamide.	Drug: Doxorubicin may potentiate cardiac toxicity, and busulfan may potentiate lung toxicity. Other antineoplastic and immunosuppressive drugs may have an additive effect on immunosuppressive activity. Drugs metabolized via cytochrome P450 can increase toxic effects of cyclophosphamide. Doxorubicin decreases digoxin level and increases drug action of barbiturates, chloramphenicol half-life, and effects of anticoagulant drugs. Duration of leukopenia may be prolonged if given with thiazide diuretics. Actions and toxicities of allopurinol, probenecid, colchicine, phenothiazines, potassium iodide, imipramine, warfarin, and succinylcholine are altered if given with cyclophosphamide. Toxicity is increased if given with corticosteroids, phenytoin, or sulfonamides. Many other possible drug-drug interactions are not listed here. Lab: Suppresses positive reaction to uric acid, purified protein derivative, mumps, *Candida*. Cyclophosphamide may cause Papanicolaou test (Pap smear) to be falsely positive.
Pharmacokinetics	**Pharmacodynamics**
Absorption: PO: Well absorbed Distribution: PB: 20%, not dose dependent Metabolism: t½: 3–12 h Excretion: 5%–25% in urine unchanged; 4% in feces mostly as metabolites	PO/IV: Onset: 7 d PO/IV: Peak: 7–15 d PO/IV: Duration: 21 d
Therapeutic Effects/Uses	
Leukemias, breast and ovarian cancer, lymphomas, multiple myeloma, lung cancer, and retinoblastoma Mechanism of Action: Cell cycle–nonspecific alkylating drugs inhibit the protein synthesis by interfering with DNA replication by alkylation of DNA.	
Side Effects	**Adverse Reactions**
Nausea, vomiting, diarrhea, anorexia, leukopenia, febrile neutropenia, fever, weight loss, alopecia, amenorrhea, gonadal suppression, impaired wound healing, stomatitis, pain	Anaphylaxis, hematologic toxicity, pulmonary toxicity (pneumonitis, pulmonary fibrosis, pulmonary thrombosis), hemorrhagic cystitis, urotoxicity, nephrotoxicity, secondary neoplasm, cardiotoxicity, hepatotoxicity, tumor lysis syndrome

Note: Chemotherapy drug doses are based on body weight and are prescribed either as milligrams per kilogram (mg/kg) or milligrams per meter squared (mg/m²). Doses will also vary based on drug protocol, type and stage of cancer, age, functional status, and comorbid conditions (e.g., heart disease).

A, Adult; *d,* day; *DNA,* deoxyribonucleic acid; *h,* hour; *IV,* intravenous; *q,* every; *PB,* protein binding; *PO,* by mouth; *t½,* half-life.

⚡ PATIENT SAFETY

Obtain a complete medication list that includes OTC, herbal preparations, and other alternative therapies.

Do not confuse...

- **Hydroxyurea** with **hydroxychloroquine**
- **Xeloda** with **Xenical**

Pharmacokinetics. 5-FU crosses the blood-brain barrier and is distributed widely throughout the body tissues. The concentration of 5-FU can be sustained for several hours in the cerebrospinal fluid (CSF). It is also effective for ascites and pleural effusions. The bioavailability and elimination half-life of IV 5-FU is nonlinear with high dosages, most likely due to saturation of metabolic processes. Approximately 15% is protein bound, and the rest (85%) is distributed throughout

CLINICAL JUDGMENT [NURSING PROCESS]

Alkylating Drug: Cyclophosphamide

Concept: Immunity
- The protective response of the body toward inflammation and infection

Recognize Cues [Assessment]
- To avoid drug-drug interactions, obtain a detailed medication history that includes prescriptions, over-the-counter (OTC) medicines, antacids, dietary supplements, vitamins, and herbal supplements.
- Obtain a list of the patient's drug and food allergies.
- Obtain baseline information about the patient's physical status. Include height, weight, vital signs, cardiopulmonary assessment, intake and output, skin assessment, nutritional status, and information on any underlying disease.
- Assess baseline laboratory values (complete blood count [CBC], uric acid, chemistry panel) for future comparisons.
- Assess baseline results of pulmonary function tests, chest radiographs, electrocardiography (ECG), and renal and liver function studies.
- Assess the patient's current level of comprehension.

Analyze Cues and Prioritize Hypothesis [Patient Problems]
- Decreased immunity
- Need for patient teaching

Generate Solutions [Planning]
- The patient will verbalize understanding of the signs and symptoms of infection.
- The patient will maintain adequate white blood cell (WBC), red blood cell (RBC), and platelet counts.
- The patient will remain free from infection and hemorrhagic cystitis.
- The patient will demonstrate understanding of protection from sun exposure.
- The patient/family/caregiver will demonstrate understanding of chemotherapeutic protocol (e.g., dose administration).

Take Action [Nursing Interventions]
- Monitor labs (CBC, blood urea nitrogen [BUN], creatinine, liver panel, and electrolytes) before drug administration and during treatment.
- Monitor the IV site frequently for irritation and phlebitis.
- Maintain strict medical asepsis during dressing changes and invasive procedures.
- Encourage small, frequent meals high in calories and protein.
- Monitor fluid intake and output and nutritional intake during therapy.
- Encourage patients to drink at least 2 L of fluid per day to promote excretion of cellular breakdown products and to reduce the risk of hemorrhagic cystitis.
- Assess the need for IV hydration.
- Maintain hydration before and during chemotherapy.
- Assess for signs and symptoms of hematuria, urinary frequency, or dysuria.

- Administer premedications as ordered 30 to 60 minutes before giving drugs.
- Provide drug information verbally and in print to the patient/family/caregiver.
- Encourage patients to use sunblock with a sun protection factor (SPF) of 50 or greater and to use other means to protect skin from sun exposure.

Patient Teaching
General
- Teach patients to take cyclophosphamide early in the day to prevent accumulation of drug in the bladder during the night.
- Remind patients to consult with a health care provider before administration of any vaccines.
- Advise patients to promptly report signs of infection (e.g., elevated temperature, fever, chills, sore throat, frequent urination or burning on urination, and redness/swelling/pain near a wound), bleeding (e.g., bleeding gums, petechiae, bruises, hematuria, blood in the stool), and anemia (e.g., increased fatigue, dyspnea, and orthostatic hypotension).
- Advise patients not to visit anyone who has a respiratory infection. A decreased WBC count puts patient at high risk for acquiring an infection.
- Emphasize protective precautions as necessary (e.g., hand washing and personal hygiene).
- Teach patients to empty their bladder every 2 to 3 hours.
- Teach methods of sun protection (e.g., sunblock with SPF 50 or greater, brimmed hats, and lightweight, long-sleeved shirts).

Side Effects
- Advise patients about good oral hygiene with a soft toothbrush for stomatitis; have patients use a soft toothbrush when the platelet count is less than $50,000/mm^3$.
- Assess for use of alternative and complementary therapies that may interact with chemotherapy drugs.
- Advise patients to report any signs of bleeding.

Diet
- Advise patients to follow a diet low in purines—such as organ meats, beans, and peas—to alkalize urine.
- Advise patients to avoid citric acid.
- Offer patients food and fluids that may decrease nausea (e.g., cola, crackers, and ginger ale).
- Plan small, frequent meals.

Evaluate Outcomes [Evaluation]
- The patient is free from infection.
- The patient does not develop hemorrhagic cystitis.
- The patient/family/caregiver education needs are met.

---

the body, including in the liver, GI mucosa, and peripheral WBCs. The major catabolizer is the liver; however, with continuous IV infusion, significant extrahepatic metabolism occurs. After IV administration, the mean elimination half-life is 16 minutes, with a range of 8 to 20 minutes, and it is dose dependent. A small amount of unchanged 5-FU is eliminated by the biliary and renal systems. After topical administration, approximately 6% is absorbed systemically. Also, 5-FU can be administered to patients with hepatic impairment with serum bilirubin less than 5 mg/dL without reducing the dose. No dose adjustments are needed for patients with renal impairment.

Pharmacodynamics. 5-FU converts into multiple active metabolites, inhibiting normal cell growth by interfering with the cell's RNA and DNA. Cytotoxicity involving the DNA is noted during the S phase of the cell cycle during the first 24 hours after drug exposure. The cell's RNA is affected after 24 hours during the G_1 phase. 5-FU is used alone or with other anticancer drugs and has a low therapeutic index. Dosing of 5-FU can vary from protocol to protocol. High IV boluses of 5-FU can result in severe hemorrhagic colitis or bone marrow suppression. Administering high doses as continuous therapy has reduced the incidences of hematologic toxicity. The Complementary and Alternative Therapies box lists herbal supplements that may interact with 5-FU.

TABLE 35.4 Antineoplastics: Antimetabolites

- Visually inspect parenteral products for particulate matter and discoloration before use.
- Observe and exercise precautions when handling, preparing, and administering cytotoxic drugs.
- Chemotherapeutic drug dosages will vary from protocol to protocol. Consult appropriate references to verify doses.

Drug	Route and Dosage	Uses and Considerations
Folic Acid Antagonists		
Methotrexate	ALL: A: PO/IM/IV: 3.3 mg/m^2/d for 4–6 wk followed by maintenance dosing NHL: A: IV: 200 mg/m^2 days 8 and 15 q21d in a combination regimen Head/Neck: A: IV: 40 mg/m^2 days 1 and 15 q21d A: PO: 25–50 mg/m^2 q7d Osteogenic sarcoma: A: IV: 12 g/m^2 q2wk	For ALL, NHL, sarcomas, solid tumors, head and neck cancers, choriocarcinomas, lymphomas, and some autoimmune disorders. Older adults may be more sensitive to toxicity and adverse events. PB: 50%–60%; t½: 10–12 h Leucovorin is used with high doses of methotrexate as rescue therapy to prevent fatal toxicity
Pemetrexed	A: IV: 500 mg/m^2 day 1 of a 21-d cycle	For mesothelioma and non–small cell lung cancer. Folic acid and vitamin B$_{12}$ IM injections are recommended to prevent hematologic and GI adverse reactions PB: 81%; t½: 3.5 h
Pyrimidine Analogues		
Azacitidine	A: IV/Subcut: 75 mg/m^2/d for 7 d q4wk	For myelomonocytic syndrome (MDS). Absolutely contraindicated in those with mannitol hypersensitivity PB: UK; t½: 4 h
Capecitabine	Breast cancer and colorectal cancer: A: PO: 1250 mg/m^2/d twice daily for 2 wk, repeated q3wk for a total of 8 cycles	For breast and colorectal cancer. Usually reserved for patients resistant to anthracyclines. Converted in tissue to 5-FU. Monitor for GI symptoms PB: <60%; t½: 0.75 h
Cytarabine	AML: A: IV: 100–200 mg/m^2/d continuous infusion for 7 d A: Subcut (maint): 100 mg/m^2/d for 5 d q28d ALL: A: IV: 1–3 g/m^2 every 12 h for 8–12 doses CML: A: IV: 200 mg/m^2/d continuous infusion for 9 d, but other doses have been used Carcinomatous meningitis: A/C: Intrathecal: 5–70 mg/m^2	For ALL, AML, CML, carcinomatous meningitis. Use preservative-free diluent PB: 15%; t½: 3–6 h in plasma; 2–11 h in CSF
Floxuridine	A: Intraarterial: 0.1–0.6 mg/kg/d continuous infusion	For colorectal cancer with liver metastasis. Given as an intraarterial infusion into the hepatic artery; catabolized to 5-FU PB: UK; t½: UK, but CSF concentrations can be sustained for several hours
5-Fluorouracil (fluorouracil, 5-FU)	See Prototype Drug Chart: 5-Fluorouracil (5-FU)	
Gemcitabine hydrochloride	NSCLC and breast cancer: A: IV: 1250 mg/m^2 on days 1 and 8 of a 21-d cycle (usually given with another chemotherapeutic drug) Pancreatic cancer: A: IV: 1000 mg/m^2 weekly for up to 7 wk followed by 1 wk of rest Ovarian cancer: A: IV: 1000 mg/m^2 days 1 and 8 of a 21-d cycle	For breast, ovarian, pancreatic, and NSCLC. Pulmonary and cardiac toxicity may occur PB: 10%; t½: 32–94 min (sex and dose dependent)
Purine Analogues		
Cladribine	A: IV: 0.09 mg/kg/d continuous infusion for 7 d	For hairy cell leukemia. Chemical conversion to the active form takes place intracellularly PB: 20%; t½: 7 h
Fludarabine	A: IV: 25 mg/m^2/d for 5 d q28d	For CLL. Absolutely contraindicated in those with hemolytic anemia and renal disease PB: UK; t½: 7–12 h

TABLE 35.4   Antineoplastics: Antimetabolites—cont'd

Drug	Route and Dosage	Uses and Considerations
Mercaptopurine (6-MP)	A: PO: 1.5–2.5 mg/kg/d followed by maintenance dosage	For ALL. Significant first-pass metabolism occurs after oral administration; significant metabolic variability PB: UK; t½: 1–2 h
Nelarabine	A: IV: 1500 mg/m² on days 1, 3, and 5 repeated q21d	For T-cell leukemia/lymphoma. Assess for neurologic symptoms PB: <25%; t½: 0.5–1 h
Pentostatin	A: IV: 4 mg/m² every other wk	*Do not confuse with pentosan.* For hairy cell leukemia. Monitor pulmonary, hepatic, and renal function; assess for seizures. Concomitant use with fludarabine is not recommended PB: 4%; t½: 2.6–15 h
Thioguanine (6-TG)	A: PO: 100 mg/m² q12h for 5–10 d	For AML. Not recommended for maintenance therapy or long-term continuous treatments due to liver toxicity PB: UK; t½: Variable
Ribonucleotide Reductase Inhibitors (Enzyme Inhibitors)		
Hydroxyurea	CML: A: PO: 20–30 mg/kg/d Head and neck: A: PO: 80 mg/kg q3d	For CML and head and neck cancer. Monitor for infection and bone marrow suppression PB: UK; t½: 3.5–4.5 h

Note: Chemotherapeutic doses and schedules will vary depending on protocol, body surface area (m²), age, functional status, and comorbid conditions. For a full discussion of body surface area in dosage calculation, see Chapter 11.

5-FU, 5-Fluorouracil; *A,* adult; *ALL,* acute lymphocytic leukemia; *AML,* acute myelogenous leukemia; *CLL,* chronic lymphocytic leukemia; *CSF,* cerebrospinal fluid; *CML,* chronic myelogenous leukemia; *d,* day; *GI,* gastrointestinal; *h,* hour; *IM,* intramuscular; *IV,* intravenous; *maint,* maintenance dose; *min,* minute; *NHL,* non-Hodgkin lymphoma; *NSCLC,* non–small cell lung cancer; *PB,* protein binding; *PO,* by mouth; *q,* every; *subcut,* subcutaneous; *t½,* half-life; *UK,* unknown; *WBC,* white blood cell; *wk,* weeks; *>,* greater than; *<,* less than ; *≤,* less than or equal to.

🌸 COMPLEMENTARY AND ALTERNATIVE THERAPIES

Fluorouracil

- Use cautiously with ginseng and St. John's wort (may interfere with chemotherapy). *Do not use with mistletoe because it may promote cancer growth.*
- Astragalus stimulates the immune system and may help speed recovery from immunosuppressive chemotherapy. Astragalus has blood clot–fighting properties and may increase risk of bleeding when given with 5-fluorouracil (5-FU).

Side Effects and Adverse Reactions

See Table 35.2 for general side effects. GI bleeding and bone marrow suppression can occur with high bolus doses of 5-FU, and patients who previously received myelosuppressive therapy and/or radiation treatment have increased risk for bone marrow suppression. 5-FU can potentiate the effects of radiation therapy and should be discontinued at the first visible sign of WBCs less than 3500/mm³, a rapidly falling WBC count, or a platelet count below 100,000/mm³. Prototype Drug Chart: Fluorouracil, 5-Fluorouracil (5-FU) details the pharmacologic behavior of 5-FU.

ANTITUMOR ANTIBIOTICS

Antitumor antibiotics are similar to natural antibiotics; however, they do *not* treat infections; instead, they interfere with DNA replication and RNA transcription of cancer cells. All antitumor antibiotics except for bleomycin have their major effects in all phases of the cell cycle (cell cycle nonspecific). Bleomycins affect cells during the G₂ phase. Types of antitumor antibiotics are anthracyclines (daunorubicin, doxorubicin,

epirubicin, and idarubicin) and other antitumor antibiotics (actinomycin D, bleomycin, mitomycin C, and mitoxantrone). Antitumor antibiotics are used to treat leukemias and many solid tumors. Table 35.5 lists the antitumor antibiotics, and their uses and considerations.

Adverse reactions to the antitumor antibiotics are similar to those of other antineoplastics and include alopecia, nausea, vomiting, stomatitis, and myelosuppression. Antitumor antibiotics are capable of causing vesication (blistering of tissue); exceptions to this are bleomycin and plicamycin. General adverse reactions to chemotherapeutic drugs are listed in Table 35.2.

Anthracyclines: Doxorubicin

Doxorubicin is an anthracycline antitumor antibiotic antineoplastic agent used to treat many solid and hematogenous tumors except for acute myelogenous leukemias (AMLs), due to the increased incidences of stomatitis and cardiotoxicity compared with other anthracyclines. Doxorubicin is a component of many combination chemotherapy treatments because of its broad antitumor activity and flexible dosing schedule. However, patients receiving IV doxorubicin must be monitored for cardiotoxicity. Doxorubicin has a maximum dose of 550 mg/m² due to cardiotoxicity. Patients taking other cardiotoxic drugs, who are older, who have preexisting cardiac problems, or who have had radiation therapy to the chest are at increased risk for cardiotoxicity. Dexrazoxane, a chemoprotectant, is administered before anthracyclines to prevent cardiotoxicity. Cardiac function should be assessed before administering doxorubicin or other anthracyclines. Liposomal doxorubicin was developed to be carried by a liposomal carrier, which decreases the incidence of severe toxicity; however, the dosages vary greatly from conventional doxorubicin, and the indications for use are different.

📄 PROTOTYPE DRUG CHART

Fluorouracil, 5-Fluorouracil (5-FU)

Drug Class	Dosage
Antimetabolite	A: IV: 300–1000 mg/m^2/d for 4–5 d continuous infusion q4wk Topical: 1%–5% cream once or twice daily for 3–12 wk Various protocols exist, including topical; IV drugs are often used with other chemotherapeutic drugs.

Contraindications	Drug-Lab-Food Interactions
Bone marrow suppression, dihydropyrimidine dehydrogenase deficiency, infection, malnutrition, pregnancy *Caution:* GI bleeding, liver and renal impairment, biliary tract disease, coronary artery disease Many other precautions are present when administering fluorouracil.	Drug: Bone marrow depressants increase chances of toxicity. Avoid live virus vaccines, which may potentiate infection. Leucovorin may potentiate adverse effects of 5-FU. Drugs that can increase the systemic cytotoxicity of 5-FU include cimetidine, dipyridamole, interferon-alfa, and levamisole. Metronidazole may cause blood dyscrasias. Synergistic reaction can occur with cisplatin and 5-FU. Lab: May decrease albumin; may increase excretion of 5-HIAA in urine

Pharmacokinetics	Pharmacodynamics
Absorption: IV and topical: 5%–10% Distribution: PB: 15%; readily crosses the blood-brain barrier Metabolism (IV): t½: 8–20 min, dose dependent Excretion: 7%–20% via urine unchanged within 6 h; inactive metabolites via respiratory system as CO_2 and the urinary system as urea	IV onset: 1–9 d Topical onset: 2–3 d IV peak: 9–21 d Topical peak: 2–6 wk IV duration: 30 d Topical duration: 1–2 mo This information provides two examples of pharmacodynamics. Clinical pharmacology is complex and is dependent on route of administration and patient condition.

Therapeutic Effects/Uses
Basal cell carcinoma; breast, colorectal, pancreas, and gastric cancers; given in combination with levamisole after surgical resection in patients with Duke stage C colon cancer Mechanism of Action: Some cell cycle–specific effects during the S and G$_1$ phases; prevention of thymidine synthase production interferes with RNA synthesis and function and has some effects to DNA

Side Effects	Adverse Reactions
Nausea, vomiting, anorexia, leukopenia, febrile neutropenia, fever, weight loss, alopecia, amenorrhea, gonadal suppression, impaired wound healing, stomatitis, pain, dry/cracked skin	Bone marrow suppression, bleeding, stomatitis, esophagopharyngitis, intractable vomiting, diarrhea, palmar-plantar erythrodysesthesia (hand and foot syndrome), cardiac toxicity, thrombocytopenia, myelosuppression, renal failure

5-FU, Fluorouracil; *5-HIAA*, 5-hydroxyindoleacetic acid; *A*, adult; *CO₂*, carbon dioxide; *d*, day; *GI*, gastrointestinal; *h*, hour; *IV*, intravenous; *min*, minute; *mo*, months; *PB*, protein binding; *q*, every; *RNA*, ribonucleic acid; *t½*, half-life; *UK*, unknown; *wk*, week.

Pharmacokinetics. Doxorubicin is administered intravenously and is distributed throughout the body tissues but does not cross the blood-brain barrier. It is extensively bound to DNA, 75% bound to plasma proteins, and not dose dependent up to 1.1 mcg/mL. Doxorubicin does not cross the placenta but appears to pass into breast milk. It is extensively metabolized by the liver into active (doxorubicinol) and inactive (hydroxylated conjugates or glucuronide) metabolites. Clearance of doxorubicinol from the blood decreases as the dose of conventional doxorubicin increases. The metabolites are excreted in the bile (50%), feces, and urine (<10%).

Pharmacodynamics. Doxorubicin is part of standard regimens for breast, lung, gastric, and ovarian cancers; Hodgkin and non-Hodgkin lymphomas; sarcoma and myeloma; and acute lymphocytic leukemia (ALL). The terminal half-life for doxorubicin is 30 to 50 hours. The clearance of doxorubicin was found to be reduced in patients with elevated serum bilirubin levels; therefore dose reduction is recommended in patients with a bilirubin level greater than 1.2 mg/dL. Clearance was also reduced in patients whose weight was greater than 130% of ideal body weight. Administration of doxorubicin is not recommended to patients who received the maximum allowable dose of other anthracyclines. Cardiotoxicity is a major concern with doxorubicin. Mitochondrial damage to cardiac cells can be extensive and can cause cardiomyopathy, dysrhythmias, congestive heart failure (CHF), and cardiogenic shock. Mitochondrial damage occurs because superoxide radicals cannot be converted back to oxygen; the heart is nearly devoid of glutathione peroxidase, an enzyme necessary for the conversion. Dexrazoxane is a parenteral chemoprotectant agent used to decrease anthracycline-associated cardiomyopathies; it is administered 30 minutes before the doxorubicin infusion. It is also used to treat anthracycline extravasation and is administered intravenously close to the affected area. The Complementary and Alternative Therapies box lists herbal supplements that may also interact with doxorubicin.

◎ CLINICAL JUDGMENT [NURSING PROCESS]

Antimetabolite: Fluorouracil

Concept: Immunity
- The protective response of the body toward inflammation and infection

Recognize Cues [Assessment]
- To avoid drug-drug and drug-supplement interactions, conduct a detailed current medication history that includes prescriptions, over-the-counter (OTC) medicines, antacids, dietary supplements, vitamins, and herbal supplements.
- Obtain a list of drug and food allergies.
- Obtain baseline information about the patient's physical status. Include height, weight, vital signs, cardiopulmonary assessment, intake and output, skin assessment, daily activities status, nutritional status, and any underlying disease.
- Obtain baseline laboratory values (complete blood count [CBC], uric acid, and chemistry panel) to compare with future laboratory results.
- Assess baseline results of pulmonary function tests, chest radiographs, electrocardiograms (ECGs), and renal and hepatic studies.
- Assess the ability for comprehension.

Analyze Cues and Prioritize Hypothesis [Patient Problems]
- Decreased immunity
- Need for patient teaching

Generate Solutions [Planning]
- The patient will be free of infection.
- The patient will remain free from signs and symptoms of bleeding.
- The patient/family/caregiver will demonstrate understanding of chemotherapeutic protocol (dose, administration, side effects, and adverse reactions).

Take Action [Nursing Intervention]
- Monitor the intravenous (IV) site frequently. Extravasation produces severe pain and can promote infection.
- Maintain strict medical asepsis during dressing changes and invasive procedures.
- Monitor blood counts and laboratory values.
- Administer an antiemetic 30 to 60 minutes before the drug to prevent nausea and emesis.
- Monitor fluid intake and output and nutritional intake.
- Offer the patient food and fluids that may decrease nausea (e.g., crackers, cola, and ginger ale).
- Assist with the planning of small, frequent meals.
- Record the number and consistency of stools; monitor perineal skin condition.

Patient Teaching
General
- Advise patients to promptly report signs of infection (fever, sore throat, chills, urinary frequency or burning on urination; redness, swelling, or pain near a wound), bleeding (bleeding gums, petechiae, bruises, hematuria, or blood in the stool), or signs of anemia (increased fatigue, dyspnea, or orthostatic hypotension).
- Teach patients to examine their mouth daily and report signs of stomatitis (soreness, ulcerations, or white patches in the mouth).
- Advise patient not to visit anyone who has a respiratory infection.
- Emphasize protective precautions such as hand washing and personal hygiene.
- Emphasize the importance of maintaining sound nutrition, and assist in the development of small, frequent meals high in calories and protein.

Side Effects
- Advise patients about good oral hygiene with a soft toothbrush for mucositis/stomatitis; have patients use a soft toothbrush when the platelet count is 50,000/mm³ or less. Instruct patients to rinse their mouth every 2 hours with saline solution of 1/4 teaspoon of salt in 1 cup of water and to avoid use of commercial mouthwashes that contain alcohol.
- Assess for use of alternative or complementary therapies that may interact with chemotherapy.

Diet
- Encourage small, frequent meals to decrease incidences of nausea and emesis.
- Encourage use of cool, bland foods when the patient is nauseated.
- Offer ice chips or ice pops to help relieve mouth pain.
- Encourage foods high in calories and protein.

Evaluate Outcomes [Evaluation]
- The patient is free from infection.
- Oral mucosa is free from erythema and swelling.
- Skin integrity remains intact.
- Patient/family/caregiver education needs are met.
- The patient's weight is maintained at the desired level.

❀ COMPLEMENTARY AND ALTERNATIVE THERAPIES

Doxorubicin

- St. John's wort is a potent cytochrome P450 inducer and moderate P-glycoprotein inducer that may decrease the concentration of doxorubicin.
- Grapefruit is a potent cytochrome P3A4 inhibitor that may increase the concentration and effect of doxorubicin.
- Black cohosh and Dong-quai should be avoided in estrogen-dependent tumors.
- Many complementary therapies—such as acupuncture, art therapy, and music therapy—have been used to improve patients' sense of well-being.

⚡ PATIENT SAFETY

Monitor for cardiac toxicity and infection.
Do not confuse...
- **Doxorubicin** with **daunorubicin, doxorubicin liposomal,** or **idarubicin**

Side Effects and Adverse Reactions

Doxorubicin has adverse drug effects similar to those of other chemotherapeutic agents. Table 35.2 lists the common side effects and adverse reactions. One common side effect of doxorubicin includes a change of the urine color to pink or light red. Life-threatening effects include cardiotoxicity, CHF, severe myelosuppression, and ECG abnormalities. The amount of myelosuppression tends to be dose dependent, dose limiting, and reversible. Prototype Drug Chart: Doxorubicin presents the pharmacologic data for doxorubicin.

PLANT ALKALOIDS

Plant alkaloids are derived from plants and are cell cycle specific; they block cell division at the M phase of the cell cycle. The **vinca alkaloids** (vinblastine, vincristine, and vinorelbine) and the **taxanes** (docetaxel and paclitaxel) are considered antimicrotubule compounds that cause disruption and interference with vital cell functions when cells are dividing (mitosis), which leads to cell apoptosis. Microtubules also involve many nonmitotic functions and thereby affect malignant and nonmalignant cells.

TABLE 35.5 Antineoplastics: Antitumorals

- Visually inspect parenteral products for particulate matter and discoloration before use.
- Observe and exercise precautions when handling, preparing, and administering cytotoxic drugs.
- Dosages of chemotherapeutic drugs vary from protocol to protocol. Consult appropriate references to verify dosages.

Drug	Route and Dosage	Uses and Considerations
Anthracyclines		
Daunorubicin	AML: A ≤60 y: IV: 45 mg/m²/d for 3 d for first course, then 2 d for subsequent courses A ≥60 y: IV: 30 mg/m²/d for 3 d for first course, then 2 d for subsequent courses ALL: A: IV: 45 mg/m²/d on days 1–3.	*Do not confuse with doxorubicin.* For ALL and AML. Given with other antineoplastic drugs. Monitor for cardiotoxicity PB: 80%; t½: 45–55 h
Doxorubicin	See Prototype Drug Chart: Doxorubicin	*Do not confuse with daunorubicin*
Epirubicin	A: IV: 75 mg/m² q21d for 4 cycles	Adjuvant treatment for breast cancer. Assess for signs of infection PB: 77%; t½: 30 h
Idarubicin	AML and APL: A: IV: 12 mg/m²/d for 3 d	For AML and APL. May cause red or orange urine discoloration PB: 97%; t½: 22 h
Mitoxantrone	AML: A: IV: 12 mg/m²/d; duration of treatment is different for induction and consolidation therapy Prostate cancer: A: IV: 12–14 mg/m² q21d	*Do not confuse with mitomycin.* For AML and prostate cancer PB: 78%; t½: 23–215 h
Valrubicin	Intravesicular: A: 800 mg q1wk for 6 wk; *max:* 800 mg intravesically	For bladder cancer. Systemic exposure is dependent on the integrity of the bladder wall PB: UK; t½: UK
Other Antitumor Antibiotics		
Bleomycin	Hodgkin disease and cervical, head and neck, and vulvar cancers: A: IV/IM/subcut: 5–20 units/m² 1 or 2 times/wk; other dosing is available NHL and testicular cancer: A: IV/IM/subcut: 10–20 units/m² once a wk 1 or 2 times/wk	For head and neck cancer; Hodgkin disease; NHL; cervical, penile, testicular, and vulvar cancer; and malignant effusion. Monitor for pulmonary complications PB: 10%; t½: 2–4 h
Dactinomycin, actinomycin D	Testicular cancer: A: IV: 1000 mcg/m² q3wk for 12 wk Malignant melanoma: A: IA: 50 mcg/kg for legs; 35 mcg/kg for arms Other dosing regimen available	For testicular cancer, Ewing sarcoma, Wilms tumor, malignant melanoma, and rhabdomyosarcoma. Nausea and vomiting may occur during first 24 h. Absolutely contraindicated with herpes infection or varicella PB: UK; t½: 36 h
Mitomycin	A: IV: 20 mg/m² q6–8wk	For gastric and pancreatic cancer. Monitor for pulmonary complications PB: UK; t½: 0.25–1.5 h

Note: Chemotherapeutic doses and schedules vary depending on protocol, body surface area (m²), age, functional status, and comorbid conditions. For a full discussion of body surface area in dosage calculation, see Chapter 11.
A, Adult; *ALL,* acute lymphocytic leukemia; *AML,* acute myelocytic leukemia; *APL,* acute promyelocytic leukemia; *d,* day; *h,* hour; *IA:* intraarterial; *IM,* intramuscular; *IV,* intravenous; *max,* maximum dosage; *NHL,* non-Hodgkin lymphoma; *PB,* protein binding; *q,* every; *subcut,* subcutaneous; *t½,* half-life; *UK,* unknown; *wk,* week; ≥, greater than or equal to; ≤, less than or equal to.

The vinca alkaloids are derived from the periwinkle plant, and taxanes are derived from the yew tree. When the natural resources became scarce, a semisynthetic form of taxanes was developed. Epipodophyllotoxins (etoposide, teniposide) come from apple trees and interfere with topoisomerases, enzymes that separate strands of DNA during the S phase of the cell cycle. Another group of plant alkaloids, camptothecin analogues (irinotecan, topotecan) isolated from a Chinese tree, are water soluble and have a broad range of antitumor properties. Retinoids (bexarotene), a natural derivative of vitamin A, are an important regulator for cell reproduction, proliferation, and differentiation. However, retinoids do not convert into the rhodopsin needed for night vision. Retinoids are given orally or topically. Table 35.6 lists the plant alkaloids and their uses and considerations.

Adverse reactions to plant alkaloids include leukopenia, hypersensitivity reactions, partial to complete alopecia, constipation, nausea,

PROTOTYPE DRUG CHART

Doxorubicin

Drug Class	Dosage
Antitumor antibiotic: Anthracycline	A: IV: 60–75 mg/m² once q21d as a single agent, 20–75 mg/m² q21–28d if used in combination with other drugs Various protocols exist, including combination therapy. Dose varies based on indicated use and response. Adjust dose with hepatic impairment.

Contraindications	Drug-Lab-Food Interactions
Anthracycline hypersensitivity, hepatic disease, myocardial infarction or severe myocardial insufficiency, neutropenia, those who received the maximum dose of doxorubicin or daunorubicin. *Caution:* Bone marrow suppression, extravasation, heart failure, impaired hepatic or renal function	Drug: Other cytotoxic drugs combined with doxorubicin may increase hematologic and GI toxicities. Cardiotoxicity may results with concomitant use with paclitaxel and verapamil. Hematologic toxicity can occur when used with cyclosporine and cyclophosphamide. Secondary malignancies have been noted with use of progesterone. Cytarabine has been known to cause necrotizing colitis. Lab: Abnormal hepatic function tests; may induce tumor-lysis syndrome and hyperuricemia, ECG changes; increases uric acid and may reduce neutrophil and RBC counts

Pharmacokinetics	Pharmacodynamics
Absorption: IV Distribution: PB: 70% Metabolism: t½: 20–48 h Excretion: 40% in bile and 5%–12% in urine	IV: Onset: 10 d Peak: 14 d Duration: 21–24 d

Therapeutic Effects/Uses	
Breast, gastric, lung, and ovarian cancers; hematogenous tumors; soft tissue and bone sarcomas; leukemias; lymphomas Mechanism of Action: Inhibits DNA and RNA synthesis; has immunosuppressant activity; it is cell cycle specific for the S phase.	

Side Effects	Adverse Reactions
Complete alopecia, stomatitis, anorexia, nausea, vomiting, diarrhea, rash, reddish-colored urine, hyperpigmentation of nail beds, dermal creases, fever, chills Dexrazoxane, a cytoprotectant drug, is used to treat extravasation and reduce the incidence and/or severity of cardiotoxicity due to anthracycline toxicity.	Cardiotoxicity (cardiomyopathy, dysrhythmias, CHF, and cardiogenic shock); myelosuppression (hematologic toxicity [leukopenia, anemia, and thrombocytopenia])

A, Adult *CHF*, congestive heart failure; *d*, day; *DNA*, deoxyribonucleic acid; *ECG*, electrocardiogram; *GI*, gastrointestinal; *h*, hour; *IV*, intravenous; *PB*, protein binding; *q*, every; *RBC*, red blood cell; *RNA*, ribonucleic acid; *t½*, half-life.

vomiting, diarrhea, and phlebitis. The plant alkaloids damage peripheral nerve fibers and may cause reversible or irreversible neurotoxicity. Signs and symptoms of neurotoxicity include a decrease in muscular strength numbness and tingling of fingers and toes (**stocking-glove syndrome**), constipation, and motor instability. Other adverse effects of these drugs include loss of deep tendon reflexes, muscle weakness, joint pain, and bone marrow suppression. Docetaxel may cause fluid retention. General adverse effects to chemotherapeutic drugs are listed in Table 35.2.

Vincristine

Vincristine was developed from the periwinkle plant and has an increased cellular retention compared with vinblastine. Neurotoxicity is a dose-limiting adverse effect of vincristine, whereas other vinca alkaloids have a dose-limiting myelosuppression. Vincristine is used for leukemias, breast carcinoma, NHL, multiple myeloma, soft tissue and osteogenic sarcomas, and brain tumors.

Pharmacokinetics. Vincristine is given parenterally. It is distributed widely throughout many tissues and binds to RBCs and platelets. Approximately 50% is metabolized by the liver and is excreted as metabolites or as the parent drug in the bile and feces. Approximately three-fourths of the drug is eliminated through the biliary tree within 72 hours. The final elimination half-life is between 23 and 85 hours. Patients with significant biliary obstruction may need dose adjustment.

Pharmacodynamics. Vincristine exerts cytotoxic effects by interfering with microtubules in the M phase in addition to having other effects, such as inhibition of RNA, DNA, and protein synthesis; inhibition of glycolysis; and disruption of cell membrane integrity. It has a high-volume distribution and rapid distribution half-life of less than 5 minutes due to extensive tissue binding. Vincristine does not cross the blood-brain barrier. The Complementary and Alternative Therapies box lists herbal supplements that may also interact with vincristine.

CLINICAL JUDGMENT [NURSING PROCESS]

Antitumor Antibiotic: Doxorubicin

Concept: Perfusion
- The ability for the cardiopulmonary and vascular systems to deliver oxygen and nutrients to body tissues

Recognize Cues [Assessment]
- Conduct a detailed medication history that lists all concurrent medications and includes prescriptions, over-the-counter (OTC) medicines, antacids, dietary supplements, vitamins, and herbal supplements to avoid drug-drug and drug supplement interactions.
- Obtain baseline information about the patient's physical status. This should include height, weight, vital signs, cardiopulmonary assessment, intake and output, skin assessment, daily activities status (e.g., sleep-wake cycle, ability to perform activities of daily living [ADLs]), nutritional status, presence or absence of any underlying disease, and past or current use of medications and treatment.
- Assess laboratory values (complete blood count [CBC] with differentials, uric acid, electrolytes, serum bilirubin, and hepatic and renal studies) and electrocardiogram (ECG) for comparison with future labs.
- Assess patient and family knowledge related to the therapeutic regimen.

Analyze Cues and Prioritize Hypothesis [Patient Problems]
- Decreased tissue perfusion, general
- Risk for dysrhythmias
- Need for patient teaching

Generate Solutions [Planning]
- The patient will remain free from infection.
- The patient will be free from cardiac abnormalities.
- The patient will have intact skin.
- The patient/family/caregiver will demonstrate understanding of the chemotherapy regimen, including side effects.
- The patient/family/caregiver will exhibit behavior appropriate for the chemotherapeutic protocol.

Take Action [Nursing Interventions]
- Maintain strict medical asepsis during dressing changes and invasive procedures.

- Assess cardiac status and check for any ECG abnormalities before and during treatment. Prepare to administer dexrazoxane.
- Monitor the intravenous (IV) site frequently, and stop the infusion immediately if signs of extravasation are apparent.
- Give drug through a large-bore, quickly running IV infusion. Monitor blood counts and laboratory values.
- Handle the drug with care during preparation, and avoid direct skin contact with the drug.

Patient Teaching
General
- Teach patients/family/caregivers when to call the health care provider.
- Explain to patients that the anticancer drug can decrease immune response and blood count.
- Emphasize protective precautions such as hand washing, personal hygiene, and avoiding people with respiratory infection.

Side Effects
- Teach patients about changes in urine color (pink or red) caused by this drug.
- Advise patients when to call a health care provider about cardiac abnormalities (chest pain, shortness of breath, or palpitations).
- Advise patients to promptly report signs of infection (fever, sore throat), bleeding (bleeding gums, petechiae, bruises, hematuria, or blood in stool), and anemia (increased fatigue, dyspnea, or orthostatic hypotension).
- Stress to patients the importance of notifying their health care provider immediately if burning or pain is experienced at the IV site.

Diet
- Encourage small, frequent, bland meals high in calories and protein.

Evaluate Outcomes [Evaluation]
- The patient is free from infection.
- Cardiac function is maintained.
- The patient and family educational needs are met.
- Side effects of therapy are controlled.

 COMPLEMENTARY AND ALTERNATIVE THERAPIES

Vincristine

St. John's wort and echinacea are cytochrome P450 inducers, which cause decreased levels of vincristine. Many complementary therapies—such as acupuncture, art therapy, and music therapy—have been used to improve patients' sense of well-being.

Side Effects and Adverse Reactions

Vincristine is associated with neurotoxicity with an intracellular concentration above a certain critical threshold. Continuous infusion is associated with longer tissue exposure above the critical cytotoxic level. Neurotoxicity is a dose-limiting adverse effect, and neuropathy may occur with single weekly vincristine doses but usually resolves within a week. If the total calculated dose is administered in divided doses, more severe neuritic pain occurs. Sensory loss, paresthesias, difficulty

walking, hyporeflexia, and muscle wasting may occur and may become progressively worse as therapy continues. Neurologic symptoms usually resolve within 6 months; however, residual effects have been prolonged in some patients. Other adverse effects from vincristine include bronchospasm, hepatic venoocclusive disease, transient cortical blindness and optic atrophy with blindness, and bladder atony. Glutamic acid given with vincristine has been known to decrease the adverse effects. Nonneurologic symptoms are similar to those of other anticancer drugs.

Vincristine is a substrate for the cytochrome P450 system. Several drug interactions may occur with vincristine, so the patient should report all medications being taken, including OTC medicines and herbal supplements. Other CYP3A4 inhibitors—including L-asparaginase, calcium channel blockers, amiodarone, statin drugs, proton pump inhibitors, and grapefruit juice—can decrease metabolism of vincristine, thereby increasing tissue exposure. CYP3A4 inducers such as phenytoin, barbiturates, and nafcillin decrease vincristine efficacy. Prototype Drug Chart: Vincristine details the pharmacologic behavior of vincristine.

TABLE 35.6 Antineoplastics: Plant Alkaloids

- Visually inspect parenteral products for particulate matter and discoloration before use.
- Observe and exercise precautions when handling, preparing, and administering cytotoxic drugs.
- Antineoplastic drug dosages vary from protocol to protocol. Consult appropriate references to verify doses.

Drug	Route and Dosage	Uses and Considerations
Antimicrotubules/Taxanes		
Docetaxel	Breast cancer: A: IV: 60–100 mg/m² day 1, repeat q3wk All other cancers: A: IV: 75 mg/m² q3wk	For breast, gastric, prostate, and head and neck cancers and NSCLC. Monitor for pulmonary and cardiac complications PB: 94%; t½: 11 h
Paclitaxel	Breast cancer: A: IV: 175 mg/m² q3wk Ovarian, NSCLC, and Kaposi sarcoma: A: IV: 135 mg/m² q3wk	*Do not confuse Taxol with Taxotere.* For breast and ovarian cancers, NSCLC, and Kaposi sarcoma PB: 95%–98%; t½: 19 h
Camptothecin Analogues		
Irinotecan	A: IV: 125 mg/m² once a week for 4 wk Other dosing regimen is available	For colorectal cancer. Consider lower doses in older adults PB: 30%–68%; t½: 6–12 h
Topotecan	Ovarian cancer and SCLC: A: IV: 1.5 mg/m²/d for 5 d q21d Cervical cancer: A: IV: 0.75 mg/m² for 3 d q3wk	For cervical and ovarian cancers and SCLC. Do not give for severe renal impairment (creatinine >1.5 mg/dL) PB: >35%; t½: 2–6 h (route dependent)
Epipodophyllotoxins		
Etoposide	SCLC: A: IV: 35–50 mg/m²/d for 4–5d q21d for 4 cycles Testicular cancer: A: IV: 100 mg/m²/d for 5 d, repeat q3–4wk Other dosing regimen is available	For testicular cancer and SCLC. Contraindicated in known benzyl alcohol intolerance PB: 95%; t½: 5–10 h
Teniposide	A: IV: 165 mg/m² on days 1, 4, 8, and 11.	For ALL. Contraindicated with polyoxyethylated castor oil hypersensitivity PB: 99%; t½: 5 h
Immunomodulators		
Thalidomide	ENL: A: PO: 100–300 mg/d at bedtime Multiple myeloma: A: PO: 200 mg/d at bedtime	For multiple myeloma and ENL. Do not administer to pregnant patients; severe birth defects have occurred PB: 55%–66%; t½: 5.5–7.3 h
Retinoids		
Bexarotene	A: PO: 300 mg/m²/d (round to nearest 75 mg)	For cutaneous T-cell lymphoma. Do *not* administer to pregnant patients PB: >99%; t½: 7 h
Vinca Alkaloids		
Vinblastine	Breast cancer: A: IV: 4.5 mg/m²/d every 21 d NHL: A: IV: 4 mg/m² days 1 and 2, repeated q28d for 3 cycles Hodgkin disease: A: IV: 6 mg/m² days 1 and 15, repeated q28d Other dosing regimen is available	For solid organ cancers, choriocarcinoma, cutaneous T-cell lymphoma, Hodgkin disease, and NHL. Usually given with combination therapy. Monitor for any pulmonary complications PB: 50%; t½: 23–85 h
Vincristine	See Prototype Drug Chart: Vincristine	
Vinorelbine	A: IV: 30 mg/m²/wk	For NSCLC. Dose must be adjusted with hepatic impairment PB: 79.6%–91.2%; t½: 27.7–43.6 h

Note: Chemotherapeutic doses and schedules vary depending on protocol, body surface area (m²), age, functional status, and comorbid conditions. For a full discussion of body surface area in dosage calculation, see Chapter 11.

A, Adult; *ALL,* acute lymphocytic leukemia; *d,* day; *ENL,* erythema nodosum leprosum; *h,* hour; *IV,* intravenous; *NHL,* non-Hodgkin lymphoma; *NSCLC,* non–small cell lung cancer; *PB,* protein binding; *PO,* by mouth; *q,* every; *SCLC,* small cell lung cancer; *t½,* half-life; *UK,* unknown; *wk,* week; >, greater than; ≥, greater than or equal to.

IMMUNOMODULATORS

Chapter 25 provides information on other immunomodulators used as antiinflammatories. Thalidomide has antiangiogenic, immunomodulatory, and antitumor properties. The exact mechanism of action is unknown; however, thalidomide selectively reduces levels of tumor necrosis factor alpha (TNF-α), inhibits interleukin 12 (IL-12), increases IL-2, and increases interferon (IFN) gamma. Thalidomide is used to treat moderate to severe erythema nodosum leprosum (ENL; leprosy), and it is used with dexamethasone to treat patients with multiple myeloma. Thalidomide is well known for its teratogenicity; hence availability is limited. Other immunomodulators include monoclonal antibody therapy (rituximab, alemtuzumab, and nonspecific immunotherapies and adjuvants such as IL-2 and interferon-alfa) designed to strengthen the immune system to attack cancer cells. Table 35.2 provides information for general adverse effects from chemotherapeutic drugs.

PATIENT SAFETY

Serious drug interactions can occur. Obtain a complete medication list that includes over-the-counter (OTC) preparations and herbal supplements.

Do not confuse...
- **Taxol** with **Taxotere** or **Paxil**
- **Vincristine** with **vinblastine**

PATIENT SAFETY

Thalidomide is a known human teratogen.

Do not confuse...
- **Thalomide** and **thalidomide** with **thiamine**

PROTOTYPE DRUG CHART

Vincristine

Drug Class	Dosage
Plant alkaloid/vinca alkaloid	A: IV: 1.4 mg/m² q7d for 4 wk Various protocols exist, including combination therapy. Dosage varies based on indicated use and response. Adjust dose if hepatic impairment.

Contraindications	Drug-Lab-Food Interactions
Demyelinating form of Charcot-Marie-Tooth syndrome, hypersensitivity to vincristine, pregnancy *Caution:* Liver impairment, history of viral infections, neurotoxicity, electrolyte imbalances, patients receiving radiation through ports (including liver), elderly *Hyaluronidase* may be given for extravasation.	Drug: Many drug-drug interactions exist. Vincristine can increase serum concentrations of methotrexate and bleomycin. Neurotoxicity can result if asparaginase or pegaspargase is coadministered with vincristine. Many drugs increase the concentration of vincristine; some include amiodarone, statin drugs, proton pump inhibitors, and testosterone. All these drugs inhibit the P-glycoprotein system. Lab: May increase serum uric acid, may cause leukopenia, may cause hyponatremia

Pharmacokinetics	Pharmacodynamics
Absorption: IV Distribution: PB: 44% Metabolism: Liver; t½: triphasic 19–155 h Excretion: 80% in feces; 10%–20% in urine	Onset: UK Peak: 4 d Duration: 7 d

Therapeutic Effects/Uses

Hodgkin disease, non-Hodgkin lymphoma, neuroblastoma, rhabdomyosarcoma, Wilms tumor, acute lymphocytic leukemia
Mechanism of Action: Affects cells in the M and S phase of the cell cycle by inhibiting microtubule formation; inhibits cell division and RNA, DNA, and protein synthesis

Side Effects	Adverse Reactions
Peripheral neuropathy, loss of deep tendon reflexes, phlebitis, constipation, cramps, nausea, vomiting, muscle weakness, reversible alopecia *Glutamic acid* may decrease adverse effects. *Leucovorin* may be given as a cytoprotectant from the toxic effects of vincristine.	Hepatic venoocclusive disease, neurotoxicity (dose dependent), sensory loss, hypotension, visual disturbances, ptosis, ileus, SIADH, hyponatremia, hyperuricemia, severe local reaction with extravasation, fever *Life-threatening:* Intestinal necrosis, seizures, coma, acute bronchospasm, bone marrow suppression

A, Adult; *d,* day; *DNA,* deoxyribonucleic acid; *h,* hour; *IV,* intravenous; *PB,* protein binding; *q,* every; *RNA,* ribonucleic acid; *SIADH,* syndrome of inappropriate antidiuretic hormone; *t½,* half-life; *UK,* unknown; *wk,* weeks; <, less than; ≥, greater than or equal to.

CLINICAL JUDGMENT [NURSING PROCESS]

Plant Alkaloid: Vincristine

Concept: Sensory Perception
- Receiving and interpreting various stimuli for functional nervous system pathways to the brain

Recognize Cues [Assessment]
- Conduct a detailed medication history that lists all concurrent medications and includes prescriptions, over-the-counter (OTC) medicines, antacids, dietary supplements, vitamins, and herbal supplements to avoid drug interactions.
- Obtain baseline information about the patient's physical status. This should include height, weight, vital signs, cardiopulmonary assessment, intake and output, skin assessment, daily activities status (i.e., ability to perform activities of daily living [ADLs]), sleep-wake cycle, nutritional status, presence or absence of underlying symptoms of disease, and the use of current or past medications and treatments. Be especially aware of evidence of neurotoxicity such as peripheral neuropathy (numbness or tingling in fingers or toes), loss of deep tendon reflexes, foot drop, slapping gait, and difficulty walking.
- Assess baseline laboratory values (complete blood count [CBC], liver and renal function tests, serum sodium, and serum bilirubin) for comparison with future values.
- Monitor for acute bronchospasm.
- Monitor bowel and urinary function. Autonomic neuropathy may lead to constipation, paralytic ileus, and bladder atony.
- Obtain baseline data regarding psychosocial status that include the patient's educational level, ability and desire to learn, support systems, past coping strategies, presence or absence of emotional difficulties, and self-care abilities.

Analyze Cues and Prioritize Hypothesis [Patient Problems]
- Risk for reduced sensory perception
- Risk for constipation
- Risk for urinary elimination
- Need for teaching

Generate Solutions [Planning]
- The patient will be free from neuropathic dysfunction.
- The patient will be free from respiratory complications (bronchospasm).
- The patient will maintain adequate bowel function.
- The patient will maintain adequate urinary function.
- The patient/family/caregiver will demonstrate understanding of the chemotherapy regimen, including side effects.

Take Action [Nursing Interventions]
- Assess for signs of respiratory distress during and after drug administration.

- Monitor for signs of peripheral neuropathy (numbness or tingling in hands or feet, sensory loss, loss of deep tendon reflexes, paresthesia, foot drop or wrist drop, ataxia).
- Assess the intravenous (IV) site carefully. Give drug through a large-bore, quickly running IV infusion.
- Monitor the IV site for extravasation, and if it occurs, stop the infusion immediately and follow the drug protocol for extravasation.
- Monitor blood counts and laboratory values.
- Maintain strict medical asepsis during dressing changes and invasive procedures.
- Administer stool softener or laxative as prescribed.
- Monitor fluid intake and output and nutritional intake.

Patient Teaching

General
- Teach patients the signs and symptoms of neurotoxicity: numbness or tingling in hands or feet, sensory loss, loss of deep tendon reflexes, paresthesia, foot or wrist drop, and ataxia.
- Emphasize the importance of notifying the health care provider of any breathing difficulties such as wheezing, shortness of breath, and anxiety.
- Advise patients to promptly report signs of infection (fever, sore throat), bleeding (bleeding gums, petechiae, bruises, hematuria, blood in the stool), and anemia (increased fatigue, dyspnea, orthostatic hypotension).
- Emphasize protective precautions such as hand washing and personal hygiene.

Side Effects
- Teach patients the signs of peripheral neuropathy.
- Teach patients the signs of respiratory compromise.
- Teach patients to report constipation, abdominal pain, and difficulty with urination.
- Teach patients the signs of drug extravasation into tissue, which can occur 3 to 4 weeks after administration of the drug.

Diet
- Encourage bulky high-fiber foods and moderate exercise to reduce the risk of constipation.
- Encourage adequate hydration to prevent electrolyte imbalances and renal toxicity.

Evaluate Outcomes [Evaluation]
- Bowel function is maintained.
- Electrolytes and renal function are maintained.
- Peripheral neuropathy did not occur.
- Patient/family/caregiver educational needs are met.

TARGETED THERAPIES

Targeted therapy is a relatively new approach to treating cancers. Targeted therapy attacks specific cells with less harm to healthy cells. Chapter 36 provides in-depth information on this treatment modality.

LIPOSOMAL CHEMOTHERAPY

A more recent change in the delivery of chemotherapy involves the use of anticancer drugs packaged inside synthetic fat globules called **liposomes**. The fatty coating helps the chemotherapy drug remain in the system longer and increases the duration of therapeutic effects; it also decreases side effects such as hair loss, nausea, and cardiotoxicity. Encapsulated forms of liposomal doxorubicin, daunorubicin, vincristine, and cytarabine are examples of liposomal chemotherapy.

HORMONES AND HORMONAL AGONISTS AND ANTAGONISTS

Although hormones are not considered true chemotherapeutic agents, several classes of hormonal agents are used in the treatment of cancer. These hormones do not work in the same ways as standard chemotherapy drugs. Instead, the hormones mask the cancer cells and prevent them from using or producing hormones. These include corticosteroids, estrogens, antiestrogens, aromatase inhibitors, gonadotropin-releasing hormone, progestins, and antiandrogens.

Corticosteroids

Corticosteroids are natural hormones and hormone-like drugs used to treat many types of cancer and noncancerous illnesses. They are divided into glucocorticoids and mineralocorticoids. These steroids should not be confused with anabolic steroids. *Glucocorticoids* assist with protein metabolism; examples of such steroids are prednisone, methylprednisolone, hydrocortisone, and dexamethasone. Steroids suppress the inflammatory process associated with tumor growth. Additionally, they are also considered immunosuppressives, which depress the patient's immune system. Steroids are used to treat leukemias, multiple myeloma, IBD, and transplant rejection, among other diseases. Because steroids suppress both the immune and the inflammatory systems, they can mask infection. Other common adverse effects include delirium, elevated serum glucose, insomnia, irritability, and other psychological problems. Because of its deleterious effects, it is recommended to avoid the use of prednisone among older adults who are at high risk for delirium. Prednisone is the most common steroid prescribed and is four times as potent as a glucocorticoid. Prednisone has little mineralocorticoid activity. Other adverse effects include fluid retention, muscle weakness, irregular menstrual bleeding, atherosclerosis, and thrombosis, among others. It is metabolized in the liver to the active metabolite prednisolone, and the drug is excreted in the urine.

Sex Hormones

The sex hormones (estrogen, androgen) and hormone-like drugs are used to slow the growth of hormone-dependent tumors (e.g., prostate cancer and breast cancer). Exogenous estrogens maintain all the properties of endogenous estrogens, and estrogen therapy is a palliative treatment used to slow the progression of prostatic cancer by decreasing testosterone production. Estrogen has also been used for the improvement of bone metastasis. An example of this group of drugs is conjugated estrogens. Synthetic progestin (e.g., hydroxyprogesterone caproate, megestrol, and medroxyprogesterone acetate) is used for renal and endometrial cancers. Both estrogen and progesterone are mainly metabolized by the liver, excreted through the biliary system, and eliminated by the kidneys. Adverse effects of estrogens and progestins include fluid retention, thrombosis, menstrual irregularities, and osteoporosis, among others. Testosterone is the primary androgen synthesized by the cells in the testes, ovaries, and adrenal cortex. Exogenous androgen opposes the activity of estrogen and is most effective for palliative treatment of breast cancer among postmenopausal women.

Table 35.7 lists sex hormones, hormonal agonists and antagonists, selective estrogen receptor modulators, luteinizing hormone–releasing hormone agonists, aromatase inhibitors, miscellaneous enzymes, and vaccines, and their uses and considerations.

Antiandrogens

Antiandrogens, such as bicalutamide and flutamide, and antiestrogens such as fulvestrant block the effects of testosterone and estrogen, respectively, thereby slowing or shrinking cancers.

Selective Estrogen Receptor Modulators

Selective estrogen receptor modulators (SERMs) such as tamoxifen and raloxifene have both estrogenic and antiestrogenic effects on various tissues. Tamoxifen is primarily used for breast cancer in both men and women. Raloxifene produces estrogenic effects in bone and lipids and has an antiestrogenic property in mammary tissues. It is used as a prophylactic against breast cancer in high-risk postmenopausal women with osteoporosis.

Luteinizing Hormone–Releasing Hormone Agonists

Luteinizing hormone–releasing hormone (LHRH), also known as *gonadotropin-releasing hormone* (GnRH) analogues or agonists (leuprolide, goserelin), suppresses the secretion of follicle-stimulating hormone and luteinizing hormone from the pituitary gland. In men, the continued suppression of the male hormone decreases the size of the prostate gland and produces an improvement in symptoms. In women, continued suppression of LHRH decreases serum estradiol and reduces the size and function of the ovaries, uterus, and mammary glands.

Aromatase Inhibitors

Aromatases are enzymes that convert other hormones into estrogen, and aromatase inhibitors are drugs that stop the enzyme from converting other hormones into estrogen. For example, in postmenopausal women, the ovaries no longer produce estrogen, but aromatase converts androgen to estrogen in this group of women. The aromatase inhibitors block the peripheral conversion of androgens to estrogens, thus suppressing the postmenopausal synthesis of estrogen and slowing tumor growth. Aromatase inhibitors are used in the treatment of hormonally sensitive breast cancer in postmenopausal women and premenopausal women who have had their ovaries removed. Anastrozole, letrozole, and exemestane are examples of aromatase inhibitors currently in use. Increasingly these agents are being used before tamoxifen in postmenopausal women with hormonally responsive metastatic breast cancer. Table 35.7 lists hormonal agents and their uses and considerations.

BIOLOGIC RESPONSE MODIFIERS

Biologic response modifiers (BRMs) enhance the body's immune system. Drugs that are BRMs are discussed further in Chapter 37.

MISCELLANEOUS CHEMOTHERAPY AGENTS

This category includes a number of antineoplastic agents in which the mechanism of action is unclear. Table 35.7 describes two, asparaginase and pegaspargase.

VACCINES

Vaccines used to prevent cancer can be considered specific immunotherapy. Recombinant vaccines include hepatitis B to prevent infection with HBV, which can cause liver cancer, and HPV quadrivalent, HPV-9 valent, and HPV bivalent, given to males and females aged 9 to 26 years to prevent HPV infections that can cause cervical cancer in females and genital warts in males. Sipuleucel-T is composed of autologous blood mononuclear cells and antigen-presenting cells (APCs) fused in protein, and it is given to stimulate T-cell immunity against the prostate cancer antigen prostatic acid phosphatase. Sipuleucel-T is the first immunotherapy to treat prostate cancer.

TABLE 35.7 Antineoplastics: Sex Hormones, Hormonal Agonists and Antagonists, Selective Estrogen Receptor Modulators, Luteinizing Hormone–Releasing Hormone Agonists, Aromatase Inhibitors, Enzymes, and Vaccines

- Visually inspect parenteral products for particulate matter and discoloration before use.
- Observe and exercise precautions when handling, preparing, and administering cytotoxic drugs.
- Antineoplastic drug dosages will vary from protocol to protocol. Consult appropriate references to verify doses.

Drug	Route and Dosage	Uses and Considerations
Sex Hormones		
Androgens		
Fluoxymesterone	Women: PO: 10–40 mg/d in divided doses	For breast cancer. Do *not* give to pregnant patients. PB: UK; t½: 9.2 h
Hormonal Agonists and Antagonists		
Abiraterone	Men: PO: 1 g/d	For prostate cancer. Assess liver function. PB: 99%; t½: 7–17 h
Anastrozole	A: PO: 1 mg/d	For advanced breast cancer. Monitor for cardiac toxicity and angioedema. PB: 40%; t½: 50 h
Bicalutamide	Men: PO: 50 mg/d	For prostate cancer. Monitor for hepatotoxicity. PB: 99%; t½: 6–10 d
Enzalutamide	A: PO: 160 mg/d	For prostate cancer. Given after docetaxel failure. PB: 97%; t½: 2.8–10.2 d
Exemestane	Postmenopausal women: PO: 25 mg/d	For breast cancer. Adjuvant treatment for those who have estrogen receptor–positive early disease that and received tamoxifen. PB: 90%; t½: 24 h
Flutamide	A: PO: 250 mg q8h; max daily dose: 750 mg	For prostate cancer. Assess for any suicidal thoughts or tendencies. Do not use with MAOIs. PB: 95%; t½: UK
Fulvestrant	A: IM: 500 mg on days 1, 15, and 29 and once monthly thereafter	For breast cancer. Avoid IV administration. PB: 99%; t½: UK
Goserelin acetate	Subcut: 3.6 mg q28d Implants available for prostate cancer	For breast and prostate cancers. Slow absorption for first 8 days of therapy. PB: <30%; t½: 4.2 h
Histrelin acetate implant	A men: Subcut implant: 50 mg q12mo	For prostate cancer. Contraindicated in children, females, and pregnancy. Proper surgical technique is critical to minimize adverse events. PB: UK; t½: 3.92 h
Letrozole	Postmenopausal women: PO: 2.5 mg/d	For breast cancer. Dose adjustment is needed for severe hepatic impairment. PB: UK; t½: 2 d
Leuprolide	Leuprolide acetate lyophilisate: A: Subcut: 1 mg/d Leuprolide acetate suspension: IM: Depot 7.5 mg q1mo	For prostate cancer. Cardiac, pulmonary, and hepatic toxicity can occur. PB: 43%–49%; t½: 3 h
Medroxyprogesterone	A: IM: Depot 400–1000 mg/wk; attempt to decrease to 400 mg/mo	For endometrial and renal cell cancers. Monitor hepatic and renal function. PB: >90%; t½: 30–50 d (dose dependent)
Megestrol acetate	Breast: A: PO: 40 mg qid Endometrial: A: PO: 40–320 mg/d divided doses	For breast and endometrial cancers. Risk for thromboembolism increases. PB: >90%; t½: 15–105 h
Mitotane	A: PO: 2–6 g/d in 3–4 divided doses, then 9–10 g/d	For adrenocortical cancer. Monitoring parameters include neurologic function and serum cortisol and potassium. PB: UK; t½: 18–159 d
Nilutamide	A: PO: 300 mg/d for 30 d, then 150 mg/d maintenance dose	For prostate cancer. Absolutely contraindicated in hepatic and respiratory disease. Use with caution in Asians. PB: UK; t½: 38–59 h
Raloxifene	Postmenopausal women: PO: 60 mg/d	For breast cancer prophylaxis. Increases risk of embolism and thromboembolism with estrogen products. PB: UK; t½: 25.8–86.6 h
Tamoxifen citrate	A: PO: 20–40 mg bid	For breast cancer. May cause abnormal Papanicolaou and vaginal smears; regular gynecologic examinations should be performed; uterine malignancy can occur. PB: UK; t½: 5–7 d
Toremifene citrate	Women: PO: 60 mg/d	For breast cancer. Absolutely contraindicated in those with hypokalemia, hypomagnesemia, and prolonged QT intervals. PB: >99%; t½: 5 d
Miscellaneous Enzymes		
Asparaginase *Erwinia chrysanthemi*	To substitute pegaspargase: A: IV: 25,000 u/m² 3/wk for 6 doses To substitute L-asparaginase *Escherichia coli*: A: IV: 25,000 u/m² for each scheduled dose of L-asparaginase	For ALL. Used as part of combination treatment. Assess for any pancreatic complications. PB: UK; t½: 8–30 h

Continued

TABLE 35.7   Antineoplastics: Sex Hormones, Hormonal Agonists and Antagonists, Selective Estrogen Receptor Modulators, Luteinizing Hormone–Releasing Hormone Agonists, Aromatase Inhibitors, Enzymes, and Vaccines—cont'd

Drug	Route and Dosage	Uses and Considerations
Pegaspargase	A: IV/IM: 2500 units/m² q14d	For ALL. Assess for any pancreatic complications or seizures. PB: UK; t½: 3.24–5.07 d
Vaccines		
Hepatitis B virus (HBV)	A: IM: Given in a series of 3 doses at 0, 1, and 3 mo	As prophylaxis against HBV. Contraindicated with known yeast hypersensitivity. PB: UK; t½: UK
Quadrivalent human papillomavirus (HPV; types 6, 11, 16, and 18) recombinant vaccine	A: IM: 0.5 mL given in a series of 3 doses (0, 2, and 6 mo)	As prophylaxis against HPV types 6, 11, 16, and 18 for prevention of cervical cancer. Contraindicated with known yeast hypersensitivity. PB: UK; t½: UK
HPV bivalent vaccine	IM: 0.5 mL given in a series of 3 shots (0, 1, and 6 mo) in deltoid region of upper arm	As prophylaxis against HPV for prevention of cervical cancer and precancerous lesions associated with the most common cancer-causing HPV types. PB: UK; t½: UK

Note: Chemotherapeutic doses and schedules vary depending on protocol, body surface area (m²), age, functional status, and comorbid conditions. For a full discussion of body surface area in dosage calculation, see Chapter 11.

A, Adult; *ALL,* acute lymphocytic leukemia; *bid,* twice daily; *d,* day; *h,* hour; *IM,* intramuscular; *IV,* intravenous; *MAOI,* monoamine oxidase inhibitor; *max,* maximum; *mo,* month; *PB,* protein binding; *PO,* by mouth; *q,* every; *qid,* four times daily; *subcut,* subcutaneous; *t½,* half-life; *UK,* unknown; *wk,* week; *>,* greater than; *<,* less than.

CRITICAL THINKING SINGLE EPISODE CASE STUDY

SLO: Apply knowledge of drug pharmacodynamics to determine which medication effects require a follow-up by the nurse.
NGN Item Type: Extended multiple response
Cognitive Skills: Recognize cues

A 43-year-old female with metastatic colorectal cancer has been receiving Bolus-IFL, which consists of irinotecan, fluorouracil (5-FU), and leucovorin 5 mg/kg IV every 2 weeks. The patient weighs 140 pounds. The patient presents to the oncology unit for the third round of treatment. Before starting treatment, the nurse documents the assessment findings.

Assessment
Temperature of 99.3°F
Blood pressure of 118/60 mm Hg
Heart rate at 94 beats per minute with occasional irregularities
Respiratory rate of 19 breaths per minute
Complains of right upper quadrant abdominal pain
Reports being able to walk down the driveway to retrieve mail
States nausea but is able to tolerate oral intake
Weight gain of 2 pounds in one week
Electrocardiogram with premature ventricular contractions
States hands and feet have felt hot since last treatment

Place a check mark next to the assessment data that requires a follow-up by the nurse.

Answers:

	Assessment
X	Temperature of 99.3°F for 5 days
	Blood pressure of 118/60 mm Hg
X	Heart rate at 94 beats per minute with occasional irregularities
	Respiratory rate of 19 breaths per minute
X	Complains of right upper quadrant abdominal pain
	Reports being able to walk down the driveway to retrieve mail
	States nausea but is able to tolerate oral intake
	Weight gain of 2 pounds in one week
X	Electrocardiogram with premature ventricular contractions
X	States hands and feet have felt hot since last treatment

Rationale:

Fluorouracil (5-FU) is an antimetabolite used to treat colorectal cancer. The mechanism of action of 5-FU affects cells during the S and G_1 phases of the cell cycle and interferes with healthy and cancer cell RNA synthesis. Anticancer drugs such as 5-FU can result in many side effects and adverse drug reactions because of their effect on healthy cells. Some of 5-FU negative effects include leukopenia, including neutropenia, increasing patient's risk for infection. Fever is usually the first hallmark sign of an infection. Therefore, the nurse would follow up for any elevated temperature. A temperature of 99.3°F is slightly elevated. Anticancer drugs can also cause serious adverse drug reactions, such as hematologic toxicity, cardiotoxicity, and hepatotoxicity. Cardiac rhythm irregularities, such as skipped beats on palpation and

premature ventricular contractions on electrocardiogram, would need further investigation. If these cardiac abnormalities are new, the dose of 5-FU may need to be adjusted. 5-FU is metabolized by the liver and a report of right upper quadrant abdominal pain can indicate hepatic involvement. Reports of hands and feet feeling hot can indicate palmar-plantar erythrodysesthesia, an adverse hand-foot syndrome that includes erythema, swelling, and intense pain to the palms of the hands and soles of the feet. If the hand-foot syndrome is severe, the dose of 5-FU may need to be adjusted.

Reference:
Chidharia A, Kanderi T, Kasi A. Nov 24, 2020. Chemotherapy acral erythema. *StatPearls [Internet].* Retrieved from https://www.ncbi.nlm.nih.gov/books/NBK459375/.

REVIEW QUESTIONS

1. A patient is to receive a chemotherapy protocol that includes an alkylating agent, an antimetabolite, and an antitumor antibiotic. Which response by the nurse would be best when the patient asks the nurse why so much chemotherapy is needed?
   a. Combination of chemotherapeutic drugs works in the S phase to kill cells.
   b. Combination chemotherapy increases the extent of tumor cell killing.
   c. Combination chemotherapy uses drugs that work the same way.
   d. Combination chemotherapy has no dose-limiting toxicities.

2. A patient is scheduled to receive chemotherapy drugs that will cause myelosuppression. Which action by the nurse would be most important?
   a. Monitor for a change in temperature.
   b. Evaluate gastrointestinal function.
   c. Assess for evidence of cardiac compromise.
   d. Question the patient about changes in sense of taste.

3. The nurse is caring for a patient with colorectal cancer who is to receive fluorouracil. Which symptom would be most important for the nurse to report to the health care provider?
   a. Nausea
   b. Decreased appetite
   c. Bleeding gums
   d. Constipation

4. A patient in the outpatient oncology clinic complains of fatigue after receiving chemotherapy. Which initial nursing action would be most appropriate?
   a. Assess for other factors contributing to her fatigue, such as trouble sleeping.
   b. Encourage a high-protein, high-calorie diet, and design it with the patient.
   c. Refer the patient to a physical therapist to develop a strenuous exercise program.
   d. Encourage the patient to sleep as much as possible during the day to ease fatigue.

5. A patient in the outpatient oncology clinic has developed mucositis after receiving fluorouracil. Which statement made by the patient indicates the need for additional teaching about mucositis?
   a. I will frequently rinse out my mouth with normal saline.
   b. To relieve my mouth pain, I will use ice pops or ice chips.
   c. I will use mouthwash with alcohol to clean my mouth.
   d. Using a soft toothbrush will clean my teeth and freshen my breath.

6. A patient is scheduled to receive high-dose cyclophosphamide via an intravenous infusion as treatment for cancer. Which patient teaching would be most important for the nurse to include on cyclophosphamide?
   a. An indwelling urinary catheter will be placed.
   b. Drink at least 2 liters of fluid per day.
   c. Empty the bladder every 4 to 6 hours.
   d. Limit fluid intake during chemotherapy.

7. A nurse is administering doxorubicin to a patient in the outpatient oncology clinic. Which information would be most important for the nurse to include in patient teaching?
   a. Blood counts will most likely remain normal.
   b. Complete alopecia rarely occurs with this drug.
   c. Report any shortness of breath, palpitations, or edema to the health care provider.
   d. Tissue necrosis usually occurs 2 to 3 days after administration.

8. A patient diagnosed with cancer is scheduled to receive vincristine. Which assessment would have the highest priority when providing care for this patient?
   a. Degree of alopecia
   b. Increased digoxin levels
   c. Decreased phenytoin effects
   d. Peripheral neuropathy

9. A patient is experiencing mucositis (stomatitis) after receiving chemotherapy. Which symptomatic treatment will be appropriate? (Select all that apply.)
   a. Frequent mouth rinses
   b. Antiemetics
   c. Topical anesthetics
   d. Stress reduction
   e. Antibiotics

10. A nurse is teaching a patient who will receive chemotherapy that can cause thrombocytopenia. Which instructions would the nurse include in the patient's teaching plan? (Select all that apply.)
    a. Use an electric razor when shaving.
    b. Use a soft-bristled toothbrush.
    c. Use aspirin for pain or headache.
    d. Monitor oral temperature daily.
    e. Report any bleeding (gums, petechiae, bruises, hematuria, melena) to the health care provider.

36

Targeted Therapies to Treat Cancer

http://evolve.elsevier.com/McCuistion/pharmacology

OBJECTIVES

- Identify the different forms of targeted therapy for cancers.
- Compare the mechanisms of action of targeted therapies for cancer with those of standard chemotherapy drugs.
- Explain the pharmacokinetics and pharmacodynamics for the different types of targeted therapy.

- Incorporate the Clinical Judgment [Nursing Process] related to the needs of patients receiving targeted therapies for cancer.
- Evaluate a focused teaching plan for patients, family, and caregivers for the different types of targeted therapies for cancer.

OUTLINE

Genes, inflammatory processes, infection, environment, and diet can influence cancer cells. Cancer cells grow out of control and can spread to distant parts of the body, invading normal tissues to the extent that tissues and vital organs can no longer function normally.

As discussed in Chapter 35, traditional chemotherapy is systemic, and its chemical makeup is cytotoxic such that it directly damages or kills normal, healthy cells and cancer cells. Chemotherapeutic drugs inhibit mitosis, which can damage the RNA and DNA and thus prevent cell division, eventually causing apoptosis, or programmed cell death. Even though traditional chemotherapy treatments improve cancer control and increase long-term survival, adverse effects of traditional chemotherapy can be life-threatening. Furthermore, traditional chemotherapy's cancer cell–killing effect is limited by the dosages and scheduling regimens needed to reduce toxic side effects on normal cells. Drugs that molecularly target cells associated with cancer are currently the focus of much research.

In 1998 targeted therapy was first recognized as a potential cancer therapy against certain cell receptors. Targeted therapy for cancer treatment differs from traditional cancer chemotherapy in that targeted therapies are specific, deliberate, and cytostatic, whereas most standard chemotherapies are not specific but rather are cytotoxic to normal and abnormal cells. Targeted therapy is the cornerstone of precision medicine because it directs the treatment according to the person's genes and proteins. The National Cancer Institute (NCI) defines *targeted therapy* as drugs or other substances that block the growth and spread of cancer by interfering with specific molecules involved in tumor growth, progression, and spread.

The ability to treat cancers with targeted therapy continues to expand. Currently, there are three approaches to targeted therapy. One approach compares individual proteins in cancer cells with those of normal cells. An example of a differentially expressed target is the human epidermal growth factor receptor 2 protein (*ERBB2*), which is expressed at high levels in breast and gastric cancers. Targeted therapy directed at *ERBB2*

includes trastuzumab, which has been approved by the US Food and Drug Administration (FDA) to treat certain breast and gastric cancers. A second approach identifies mutant proteins that can cause cancer progression. An example of a mutant cell is the *BRAF* gene in its altered form, *BRAF V600E,* in melanomas. Vemurafenib targets this altered form of *BRAF* and has been approved to treat metastatic or inoperable melanomas. A third approach looks for abnormal chromosomes present in cancer cells but not in normal cells. Chromosomal abnormalities can result in gene fusion, wherein parts of two different genes are incorporated as one gene. These fusion proteins can increase cancer development. Imatinib mesylate is one example of a therapy that targets the *BCR-ABL1* fusion protein responsible for the growth of some leukemic cells.

According to the American Cancer Society, targeted therapies have five ways to attack cancer cells. One way is for the drug to block or turn off chemical signals; this prevents cancer cells from growing and dividing. Second, targeted drugs can change proteins within the cancer cells causing cell lysis. Third, targeted drugs can prevent cancer cells from angiogenesis, formation of new vessels. Fourth, targeted therapies can trigger the immune system to kill cancer cells. Lastly, targeted therapy is toxic to cancer cells but not to noncancerous cells.

Targeted therapies do have limitations. One limitation is that cancers that do not have sufficient quantities of the specific molecular targets will not respond to targeted therapy. Another limitation involves cancer cells mutating and becoming drug resistant. Finally, yet another limitation of targeted therapy is the difficulty of developing drugs for some identified targets.

TARGETED THERAPY DRUGS

Once a cell receives signals, the signal is relayed to other cells by a series of biochemical reactions. In cancer cells, the cells are stimulated to divide continuously without being prompted by external growth factors. Signal transduction inhibitors (STIs) block signals to cancerous cells by blocking signals passed from one molecule to another. They work at sites that are on the cell surface, at the intracellular level, or in the extracellular domain. Blocking various signals can affect cell division and can ultimately cause cell death. Targeted cancer therapies are STIs that block signal transduction among specific molecules, which blocks the growth and spread of cancerous cells. Drugs that target specific cells inhibit cancer cell division by blocking cancer membrane receptors and tyrosine kinase (TK) activities, interfering with signal transduction, stimulating immune system attacks on cancer cells, or inducing cells to undergo apoptosis. Targeted drugs may be used as monotherapy (a single agent), in combination with traditional chemotherapy, and with radiotherapy.

Targeted therapies are more selective for specific molecular targets than cytotoxic anticancer drugs; thus they are able to kill cancer cells with less damage to normal cells compared with chemotherapy. They are the cornerstone of precision medicine that uses a person's genes and proteins to prevent, diagnose, and treat cancer. Targeted therapies are sometimes known as *molecular targeted drugs* and *precision medicines*. Most targeted therapies consist of either small molecules or large molecules. Small molecular drugs enter cancer cells while large molecules affect the surfaces of cancer cells. Drug classes used for targeted therapies include angiogenesis inhibitors, epidermal growth factor receptor (EGFR)-TK inhibitors, BCR-ABL1 TK inhibitors, monoclonal antibodies (mAbs) and proteasome inhibitors. Small-molecule drugs are *not* antibodies. Most generic small-molecule drugs have -*nib* or -*mib* suffixes, such as imatinib and bortezomib. mAbs generally have -*mab* suffixes, such as rituximab. Table 36.1 identifies other suffixes common to small-molecule drugs and mAbs. Small-molecule drugs are usually administered orally, whereas mAbs are given intravenously. All targeted therapies are categorized as high-alert medications.

Targeted therapies differ from standard chemotherapy in several ways. Targeted therapies (1) act on specific molecular targets associated with cancer, (2) are deliberately designed to interact with a specific target, and (3) often are cytostatic by blocking tumor cell proliferation.

However, targeted therapy does have drawbacks. Cancer cells can become resistant, and drugs for some targets are difficult to develop. Side effects and risks associated with targeted therapy include diarrhea, hepatitis, thrombus formation, poor wound healing, hypertension, fatigue, stomatitis, and skin changes, among others.

The rapid identification of specific cancer cell targets in recent years has led to an increased development of targeted therapies. Management of patient issues related to targeted therapies is an evolving area of study. With many targeted therapies being new to the market, costs can be prohibitive.

Small-Molecule Compounds

Small-molecule compounds are one of the two main types of targeted therapy. Like most other types of drugs, they are chemicals that are small enough to have an intracellular effect, targeting the internal structures of cells. Small-molecule drugs are classified according

TABLE 36.1 Suffixes of Targeted Cancer Therapies

Suffix	Meaning
-mab	A monoclonal antibody
-momab	A monoclonal antibody composed of only murine (mouse) proteins
-imab	A monoclonal antibody composed of more human proteins (>60%) than murine proteins (~30%)
-zumab	A monoclonal antibody composed of mostly human proteins (95% or more) and only a few murine proteins (<5%)
-umab	A monoclonal antibody composed of only human proteins and no murine proteins
-nib	A tyrosine kinase inhibitor
-mib	A proteasome inhibitor

to their actions; these include inhibiting enzymes, inducing apoptosis, and inhibiting formation of new vasculatures (angiogenesis). Table 36.2 lists the small-molecule inhibitors (SMIs) and their dosages, routes, uses, and considerations.

Angiogenesis Inhibitors/Vascular Endothelial Growth Factor Receptor Inhibitors

Angiogenesis inhibitors prevent new blood vessels from forming, which is required for tumors to grow. Some angiogenesis inhibitors interfere with the action of vascular endothelial growth factor (*VEGF*), a substance that stimulates new blood vessel formation. Others prevent the formation of platelet-derived growth factor (*PDGF*) that is intricate in the formation of new blood vessels and in the growth of preexisting blood vessels. Some angiogenesis inhibitors are also considered mAbs, such as bevacizumab. Prototype Drug Chart: Bevacizumab lists specific drug information for bevacizumab.

Ziv-Aflibercept. Ziv-aflibercept is a fully humanized recombinant fusion protein that inhibits angiogenesis. It is indicated in combination with 5-fluorouracil (5-FU), leucovorin, and irinotecan (FOLFIRI) for the treatment of metastatic colorectal cancer that is resistant to or has progressed after receiving an oxaliplatin-containing regimen.

Pharmacokinetics. Ziv-aflibercept is administered by intravenous (IV) infusion. Its elimination half-life is approximately 6 days, which appears to be dose dependent. The steady state is also dose dependent, with the average steady state reached by the second dose in a 2-week regimen. The metabolic and elimination pathways are unknown. However, free ziv-aflibercept does not seem to be affected by mild to moderate hepatic or renal impairment.

Pharmacodynamics. Ziv-aflibercept is an angiogenesis inhibitor that acts as a soluble receptor to bind VEGFs A and B and placental growth factors 1 and 2, which prevents other native receptors from binding. This action can result in decreased neovascularization and decreased vascular permeability.

Side Effects and Adverse Reactions. Ziv-aflibercept can cause severe bleeding, including gastrointestinal (GI) bleeding, intractable bleeding, and pulmonary hemorrhage. GI perforations, some fatal, have also been reported. Other adverse events include compromised wound healing and/or wound dehiscence, reversible posterior leukoencephalopathy syndrome (RPLS), hypertensive crisis, nephrotic syndrome, or thrombotic microangiopathy. Common side effects include diarrhea, dizziness, asthenia, weight loss, and dehydration.

Drug Interactions. No interactions have been reported.

TABLE 36.2 Small-Molecule Inhibitors

Drug Name and Type	Route and Dosage	Uses and Considerations
Angiogenesis Inhibitors/Vascular Endothelial Growth Factor Receptor Inhibitors		
Bevacizumab (*VEGFR*/mAb; prototype)	See Prototype Drug Chart: Bevacizumab	
Ziv-aflibercept (VEGFR)	A: IV: 4 mg/kg over 1 h, followed by FOLFIRI Steady state is reached by the second dose.	For metastatic colorectal cancer. Fully humanized angiogenesis inhibitor. Monitor ANC and UA. Discontinue for severe bleeding, GI perforation, fistula formation, wound dehiscence, hypertensive crisis/hypertensive encephalopathy, arterial thromboembolic events, and reversible posterior leukoencephalopathy syndrome. PB: UK; t½: 6 d
Epidermal Growth Factor Receptor Inhibitors		
Erlotinib (prototype)	See Prototype Drug Chart: Erlotinib	
Gefitinib	A: PO: 250 mg once daily Steady state is achieved in 10 d.	For NSCLC. Monitor LFTs, and increase the dose if used concomitantly with strong CYP3A4 inducers. Drug may be held for up to 14 d if patient develops poorly managed diarrhea, worsening ocular or pulmonary disorders, or worsening rash. Discontinue if GI perforation or interstitial lung disease is present. PB: 90%; t½: 48 h
Osimertinib	A: PO: 80 mg/d	For NSCLC. Dose adjustment is required for treatment-related toxicities. Contraindicated in patients with interstitial lung disease/pneumonitis and symptomatic heart failure. Monitor ECG, ejection fraction, and serum electrolytes. PB: likely high based on physiochemical properties; t½: 48 h
Tyrosine Kinase Inhibitors/Multikinase Inhibitors		
Alectinib (TKI)	A: PO: 600 mg bid with food until disease progression or unacceptable toxicity occurs	For *ALK*-positive metastatic NSCLC in a patient who has progressed or is intolerant to crizotinib. Monitor LFTs, worsening respiratory symptoms, heart rate and blood pressure, and CPK levels. PB: >99%; t½: 31–33 h
Dasatinib (MKI)	A: PO: Advanced CML, resistance or intolerance to prior therapy: 100–140 mg/d; can be increased to 180 mg/d if response is inadequate with the initial dose. Newly diagnosed CML: 100 mg/d; may be increased to 140 mg/d if response is inadequate.	For Ph+ CML and ALL. Adjust dose with concomitant use of a strong CYP3A4 inhibitor/inducer. Avoid grapefruit juice and concomitant use with H₂-receptor antagonists or proton pump inhibitors. Monitor CBC, serum electrolytes, and uric acid. PB: 96%; t½: 3–5 h
Imatinib mesylate, STI-571 (TKI) prototype	See Prototype Drug Chart: Imatinib Mesylate, STI-571	
Nilotinib (TKI)	A: PO: Resistance or intolerance to imatinib: 400 mg bid on an empty stomach Newly diagnosed Ph+ CML: 300 mg bid on an empty stomach	For Ph+ CML. No food should be given 1 hour after or 2 hours before dose is taken. Capsule may be opened and dispersed in 1 teaspoon of applesauce. Monitor ECG, CBC, electrolytes, LFTs, pancreatic functions, uric acid, and weight. *Absolute contraindications:* Hypokalemia, hypomagnesemia, long QT syndrome, and QT prolongation. PB: 98%; t½: 17 h
Sorafenib (MKI)	A: PO: 400 mg bid; administer without food, at least 1 h before or 2 h after meal.	For hepatocellular, renal cell, and thyroid cancers. Adjust the dose if use is concomitant with a strong CYP3A4 inhibitor/inducer. Monitor CBC and LFTs. PB: 99.5%; t½: 25–48 h
Sunitinib (MKI)	GIST and RCC: A: PO: 50 mg/d on a schedule of 4 wk on treatment followed by 2 wk off treatment PNET: A: PO: 37.5 mg/d; administer with or without food.	For GIST, PNET, and advanced RCC. Avoid concomitant use with a strong CYP3A4 inhibitor/inducer. Monitor UA and cardiac function. PB: sunitinib 95%; metabolite 90%; t½: sunitinib 40–60 h, major metabolite 80–110 h

TABLE 36.2   Small-Molecule Inhibitors—cont'd

Drug Name and Type	Route and Dosage	Uses and Considerations
mTOR Kinase Inhibitors (mTOR)/Proteasome Inhibitors (PIs)		
Bortezomib (prototype)	See Prototype Drug Chart: Bortezomib	
Carfilzomib (PI)	A: IV: Progressive disease on or within 60 d after completing therapy: Cycle 1: 20 mg/m^2 on days 1 and 2; if tolerated, increase to 27 mg/m^2 on days 8, 9, 15, and 16. Treatment cycles are repeated q28d. Cycles 2–12: 27 mg/m^2 on days 1, 2, 8, 9, 15, and 16. Cycles 13 and beyond: 27 mg/m^2 on days 1, 2, 15, and 16 Relapsed multiple myeloma: Give carfilzomib as discussed earlier with lenalidomide daily for 21 d of each cycle and dexamethasone on days 1, 8, 15, and 22 of each cycle. Treatment cycles are repeated q28d.	For relapsed multiple myeloma refractory to previous one to three lines of therapy, in combination with lenalidomide and dexamethasone. Premedicate with dexamethasone 30 min to 4 h before carfilzomib. Prehydrate and maintain hydration with oral and IV fluids. Monitor CBC, liver and renal function, and uric acid. PB: 97%; t½: ≤1 h
Ixazomib (PI)	A: PO: 4 mg on days 1, 8, and 15 in combination with lenalidomide on days 1 through 21 and dexamethasone on days 1, 8, 15, and 22. Repeat treatment cycles q28d.	For relapsed multiple myeloma refractory to one previous therapy. Give with lenalidomide and dexamethasone, and adjust dose for hepatic or renal impairment. Adjust or hold dose for hematologic toxicity, moderate-grade rash, peripheral neuropathy, and other nonhematologic toxicity. PB: 99%; t½: 9.5 d
Temsirolimus (mTOR)	A: IV: 25 mg given over 30–60 min once per wk	For advanced RCC. Premedicate with antihistamine intravenously approximately 30 min before the start of infusion. Two dilutions are required before IV infusion; use only the supplied diluent for initial dilution. Avoid strong CYP3A4 inducers/inhibitors. Dose reduction is required in patients with mild hepatic impairment. *Contraindication:* Moderate to severe hepatic impairment. PB: UK; t½: 17 h

A, Adult; *ALL*, acute lymphoblastic leukemia; *ANC*, absolute neutrophil count; *bid*, twice daily; *CBC*, complete blood count; *CML*, chronic myelogenous leukemia; *CPK*, creatine phosphokinase; *CYP3A4*, cytochrome P3A4; *d*, day; *ECG*, electrocardiograph; *FOLFIRI*, folinic acid, fluorouracil, and irinotecan; *GI*, gastrointestinal; *GIST*, gastrointestinal stromal tumor; *h*, hour; *IV*, intravenous; *LFT*, liver function test; *mAb*, monoclonal antibody; *min*, minutes; *MKI*, multikinase inhibitor; *mTOR*, mechanistic target of rapamycin; *NSCLC*, non–small cell lung cancer; *PB*, protein bound; *Ph+*, Philadelphia chromosome positive; *PI*, proteasome inhibitor; *PNET*, pancreatic neuroendocrine tumor; *PO*, oral; *q*, every; *RCC*, renal cell carcinoma; *t½*, half-life; *TKI*, tyrosine kinase inhibitor; *UA*, urinalysis; *UK*, unknown; *VEGFR*, vascular endothelial growth factor receptor; *wk*, week; *>*, greater than; *≤*, less than or equal to.

Epidermal Growth Factor Receptor Inhibitors

The largest class of targeted therapy that attacks one particular molecular target is EGFR inhibitors. These receptors are overexpressed, dysregulated, or mutated in many epithelial cancers. *EGFR* expression has been associated with poor prognosis, metastasis, chemotherapy resistance, hormonal therapy, and radiation therapy. The activation of *EGFRs* is important in cancer cell growth and proliferation. Most EGFR inhibitors also inhibit TK indirectly. However, two other classes of EGFR inhibitors target *EGFR* extracellularly (mAbs) and also target the receptor catalytic domain of *EGFR* (TK inhibitors). These two classes are further discussed under the headings *Monoclonal Antibodies* and *Tyrosine Kinase Inhibitors and Multikinase Inhibitors*. The EGFR inhibitors that inhibit TK indirectly include erlotinib, gefitinib, and osimertinib. The growth factor receptors on the cell membrane can activate TKs, which then turn on signal transduction pathways that promote cell division. The EGFR inhibitors bind to different areas of the *EGFR*, blocking its activity so that it cannot activate TK. As a result, the downstream signal transduction pathway for promotion of cell division is inhibited, and cell proliferation is severely limited.

Table 36.2 lists the EGFR inhibitors and their dosages, routes, uses, and considerations. Prototype Drug Chart: Erlotinib lists the specific drug information for erlotinib.

Gefitinib. Gefitinib is a synthetic anilinoquinazoline that selectively inhibits the epidermal growth factor receptor tyrosine kinase (EGFR-TK). It is most commonly used in the management of locally or advanced metastatic non–small cell lung cancer (NSCLC).

Pharmacokinetics. Gefitinib is taken orally and is absorbed slowly in the GI tract, with 60% reaching systemic circulation. Peak plasma level occurs 3 to 7 hours after dosing. No significant alteration in its bioavailability was noted when gefitinib was taken with food. It is metabolized mainly by the hepatic system primarily through the CYP3A4 enzyme. Gefitinib is primarily excreted in the feces, mostly in the form of its metabolites. The elimination half-life is approximately 48 hours.

Pharmacodynamics. Gefitinib reversibly binds to the adenosine triphosphate (ATP) binding site and completely inhibits autophosphorylation by EGFR-TK; EGFR-TK functions as a mediator of cell growth, differentiation, and death. This action results in blockage

---

📄 **PROTOTYPE DRUG CHART**

Bevacizumab

Drug Class	Dosage
Monoclonal antibody/angiogenesis inhibitor (VEGF inhibitor)	A: IV: *Colorectal cancer:* 5 or 10 mg/kg q2wk in combination with 5-FU; or 5 or 7.5 mg/kg q2–3wk with fluoropyrimidine and irinotecan or fluoropyrimidine and oxaliplatin. *NSCLC:* 15 mg/kg q3wk with carboplatin and paclitaxel. *Metastatic RCC:* 10 mg/kg q2wk in combination with interferon-alfa. *Progressive glioblastoma:* 10 mg/kg q2wk on a 28-d cycle. *Ovarian cancer:* 10 mg/kg q2wk in combination with paclitaxel, topotecan, or pegylated liposomal doxorubicin. *Cervical cancer:* 15 mg/kg with cisplatin on day 2 in combination with paclitaxel q3wk. Other treatment protocols exist (see full prescriber's information).

Contraindications	Drug-Lab-Food Interactions
No absolute contraindications. Warnings and precautions during treatment include serious bleeding (e.g., GI, intracranial), GI obstruction/perforation, wound dehiscence, and nephrotic syndrome. *Caution:* Known murine protein hypersensitivity, hamster protein hypersensitivity, or sensitivity to any other component of the drug; preexisting hypertension, cardiovascular disease, renal disease, history of glaucoma (see full prescriber's information for a complete list).	Drug: When used as combination therapy with irinotecan, incidence of grade 3–4 diarrhea and neutropenia increased and serum concentration of irinotecan active metabolites increased. Concomitant use with sunitinib increased incidences of microangiopathic hemolytic anemia. Concomitant use with daunorubicin, doxorubicin, and epirubicin, among others, has an increased risk of cardiotoxicity. Lab: None known Food: None known

Pharmacokinetics	Pharmacodynamics
Absorption: IV, bioavailability UK Distribution: PB: UK; steady-state levels achieved at approximately 100 d Metabolism: UK; t½: 11–50 d, dose dependent Excretion: Clearance of drug varies by weight, sex, and tumor burden	Onset: UK Peak: UK Duration: UK

Therapeutic Effects/Uses

For cervical, colorectal, and ovarian cancers; metastatic RCC; NSCLC; and relapsed glioblastoma multiforme

Mechanism of Action: Recombinant humanized monoclonal antibody binds to VEGF and prevents the binding of VEGF with its receptors, which are found on the surface of endothelial cells. The role of VEGF is critical in angiogenesis, the formation of new blood vessels. In human cancers, increased VEGF expression is associated with increased microvascular density, tumor growth, metastasis, and poor prognosis. The result of bevacizumab therapy is the reduction of microvascular growth and inhibition of metastatic disease progression.

Side Effects	Adverse Reactions
Hypertension, proteinuria, cephalgia, rhinitis, taste alteration, dry skin, rectal hemorrhage, lacrimation disorder, back pain, and exfoliative dermatitis	Perforation or fistula, thromboembolic events, hypertensive crisis/encephalopathy, nephrotic syndrome, infusion reactions, embryonic/fetal toxicity, ovarian failure, PRES, exogenous endophthalmitis, gallbladder perforation, and congestive heart failure have been associated with bevacizumab (see full prescriber's information for a complete list)

5-FU, 5-Fluorouracil; *A,* adult; *d,* day; *GI,* gastrointestinal; *IV,* intravenous; *NSCLC,* non–small cell lung cancer; *PB,* protein bound; *PRES,* posterior reversible encephalopathy syndrome; *q,* every; *RCC,* renal cell cancer; *t½,* half-life; *UK,* unknown; *VEGF,* vascular endothelial growth factor; *wk,* week.

---

of downstream EGFR-TK–mediated signal transduction pathways, cell cycle arrest, and inhibition of angiogenesis.

Side Effects and Adverse Reactions. Common side effects include skin reactions, diarrhea, anorexia, vomiting, and elevated transaminases. Gefitinib can cause conjunctivitis and abnormal eyelash growth, and rash occurs in about 47% of patients. Patients can also experience acne, pruritus, and nail disorders. Interstitial lung disease and GI perforation were also reported.

Drug Interactions. Gefitinib is extensively metabolized by CYP3A4. Other drugs metabolized by the hepatic system can affect the concentrations of gefitinib and other drugs. Drugs that inhibit CYP3A4, increasing the gefitinib level, include thioridazine, amiodarone, bupropion, diphenhydramine, promethazine, and metoclopramide. Other CYP3A4 inhibitors, such as venlafaxine, may decrease the levels

of gefitinib. Gefitinib can increase the concentration of other drugs that have a narrow therapeutic index, such as amitriptyline, warfarin, and eliglustat. Patients taking warfarin concomitantly with gefitinib had an elevated international normalized ratio (INR) and/or hemorrhage. CYP3A4 inducers—such as acetaminophen, butalbital, caffeine, and aspirin—can increase gefitinib metabolism, thereby decreasing concentrations of the drug. When given concomitantly with gefitinib, drugs that decrease gastric pH (e.g., omeprazole and lansoprazole) can lower plasma concentrations of gefitinib.

Osimertinib. Osimertinib is one of the newest FDA-approved EGFR-TK inhibitors for *T790M* mutation–positive NSCLC. It is currently being studied in the treatment of other types of cancer.

Pharmacokinetics. Osimertinib is taken orally, and absorption is dose dependent. High-fat, high-calorie meals increase the absorption

PROTOTYPE DRUG CHART

Erlotinib

Drug Class	Dosage
Epidermal growth factor receptor inhibitor	*NSCLC:* 150 mg PO once daily *Pancreatic cancer:* 100 mg PO once daily as combination therapy. Take without food, 1 h before or 2 h after meal.

Contraindications	Drug-Lab-Food Interactions
No absolute contraindications. Precautions are warranted in patients who may become pregnant, are pregnant, or are breastfeeding; who have preexisting respiratory problems (pulmonary fibrosis may occur); or who are dehydrated or have liver impairment. Use cautiously in patients with history of peptic ulcer disease or diverticulitis (increases risk for GI perforation). Advise smokers to stop smoking while taking erlotinib; tobacco decreases the effectiveness of the drug.	Drug: Concomitant use with drugs that alter the pH of the upper GI tract is contraindicated (e.g., esomeprazole, lansoprazole, omeprazole, or pantoprazole). CYP3A4 inhibitors such as ketoconazole, atazanavir, clarithromycin, indinavir, itraconazole, nefazodone, nelfinavir, ritonavir, saquinavir, telithromycin, and voriconazole increase blood levels of erlotinib and may lead to increased adverse reactions or toxicities. Concomitant use with competitive inhibitors of CYP3A4, such as midazolam and statin drugs, can increase the competitor's concentration. CYP3A4 inducers such as rifampicin, dexamethasone, phenytoin, carbamazepine, phenobarbital, St. John's wort, H_2-receptor blockers, and proton pump inhibitors reduce the effectiveness of erlotinib. Lab: Erlotinib may increase INR and can lead to increased risk for bleeding. Food: Drug must be given on an empty stomach; administering with food increases the risk of side effects.

Pharmacokinetics	Pharmacodynamics
Absorption: Bioavailability is 60%. Distribution: 93% PB. Steady-state levels are achieved in 7–8 d. Metabolism: Liver (CYP3A4 and CYP1A2 enzymes); $t\frac{1}{2}$: 36 h. Excretion: Mainly in feces, some renal elimination; 24% higher among smokers	Give drug on an empty stomach, either 1 h before or 2 h after meals (administering with food increases risk for side effects). Administer at the same time each day between meals. Increase dose if used concomitantly with strong CYP3A4 inducers. Onset: Slowly absorbed with oral dosage with 60% bioavailability. Peak: 4 h; duration: UK

Therapeutic Effects/Uses
Approved for treatment of NSCLC and pancreatic cancer. Mechanism of Action: Erlotinib selectively inhibits activation of *EGFR* tyrosine kinase, possibly blocking angiogenesis and cellular proliferation.

Side Effects	Adverse Reactions
Diarrhea, skin changes (acne vulgaris, acneiform rash), alopecia, anorexia, anxiety, bone pain, cough, constipation, anorexia, diarrhea, fatigue, vomiting, pruritus	Ocular changes (inflammation, corneal perforation), GI perforation, skin desquamation, renal failure, hepatic failure, interstitial pulmonary disease

CYP, Cytochrome P; *d*, day; *GI*, gastrointestinal; *h*, hour; *H₂*, histamine 2; *INR*, international normalized ratio; *NSCLC*, non–small cell lung cancer; *PB*, protein bound; *PO*, by mouth; *t½*, half-life; *UK*, unknown.

rate by 14%. It is metabolized primarily by the hepatic system through the CYP3A isoenzyme and by oxidation and dealkylation. Osimertinib is primarily excreted in the feces and to a lesser extent in the urine. The elimination half-life is approximately 48 hours.

Pharmacodynamics. Osimertinib is a CYP3A4 and CYP1A2 inducer that irreversibly binds to certain mutant forms of *EGFR* (*T790M, L858R,* and *exon 19* deletion). In vitro, it exhibits inhibition of *ERBB2, ERBB3, ERBB4, ACK1,* and *BLK* receptors.

Side Effects and Adverse Reactions. Common side effects include pancytopenia, rash, dry skin, anorexia, constipation, hyponatremia, nausea, pruritus, fatigue, cough, back pain, and stomatitis. Other side effects include eye disorders and cephalgia. Adverse reactions include venous thromboembolism, interstitial lung disease, pneumonitis, increased QTc, and cardiomyopathy.

Drug Interactions. Osimertinib is a CYP3A inducer. Drugs metabolized by the liver can affect their concentrations and the osimertinib plasma level. Osimertinib can cause a prolonged QT interval. Other drugs that can prolong QT intervals, causing torsade

de pointes, should be avoided or monitored closely when used concomitantly with osimertinib (e.g., thioridazine, beta agonists, chlorpromazine, ofloxacin, desipramine, moxifloxacin, metronidazole, promethazine, and trimethoprim or sulfamethoxazole-trimethoprim). CYP3A inhibitors such as aldesleukin, alfentanil, and ethanol can alter osimertinib concentration. Osimertinib can alter plasma concentration of other drugs, which can worsen adverse reactions and can alter the efficacy of drugs such as acetaminophen, amlodipine, amitriptyline, and alprazolam.

Tyrosine Kinase Inhibitors and Multikinase Inhibitors

Several types of targeted therapies inhibit TKs. Specific drugs that cause this action as their main mechanism are referred to as TK inhibitors (TKIs). TKIs primarily exert their effects on an enzyme known as *BCR-ABL TK.* The *BCR-ABL* gene is an important pathogenesis for chronic myelogenous leukemia (CML). CML cells make abnormal active *BCR-ABL TK* enzyme. *BCR-ABL TK* enzymes are present in cancer cells that have a specific gene mutation known as the *Philadelphia chromosome.*

CLINICAL JUDGMENT [NURSING PROCESS]

Angiogenesis Inhibitors, Vascular Endothelial Growth Factor Receptor Inhibitors, and Epidermal Growth Factor Receptor Inhibitors

Concept: Cellular Regulation

- The ability for cells to maintain homeostasis, including its responses to extracellular signals.

Recognize Cues [Assessment]

- Obtain a detailed medication history that includes current prescriptions, over-the-counter (OTC) medicines, antacids, dietary supplements, vitamins, and herbal supplements and compare them to the targeted therapy for possible drug reactions.
- Obtain a list of all drug and food allergies.
- Obtain baseline information about the patient's physical status that includes height, weight, vital signs, cardiopulmonary assessment, intake and output, skin assessment, nutritional status, and any underlying diseases.
- Obtain baseline laboratory values (complete blood count [CBC], uric acid, chemistry panel) before and during treatment.
- Assess baseline results of pulmonary function tests, chest radiographs, electrocardiographs (ECGs), and renal and liver function studies.
- Assess patient's and caregiver's current level of comprehension related to the therapeutic regimen.

Analyze Cues and Prioritize Hypothesis [Patient Problems]

- Altered potential for inflammation
- Potential for altered clotting
- Potential for decreased immunity
- Need for teaching

Generate Solutions [Planning]

- The patient will remain free of skin breakdown.
- The patient will remain free from infection.
- The patient and family will verbalize understanding of targeted therapy as part of an anticancer treatment regimen.
- The patient and family will verbalize strategies to minimize risks related to targeted therapy–related side effects.
- The patient and family will demonstrate understanding of the importance of reporting targeted therapy–related side effects and adverse reactions.
- The patient will have tolerable side effects.

Take Action [Nursing Interventions]

- Examine the patient's skin closely at each visit for the presence of erythema, rash, peeling, or blister formation; rate the severity of dermatologic reactions.
- Monitor for any evidence of infection, such as fever, chills, leukocytosis or leukopenia, and neutropenia.
- Assess for evidence of thromboembolic events.

- Monitor for any signs of perforation, such as abdominal pain/distension, absent bowel sounds, and changes in blood pressure and heart rate.
- Monitor laboratory values, such as renal function, hepatic function, CBC, chemistry, and urinalysis.
- Administer prescribed premedications according to established protocols for specific targeted therapies.
- Assess for any cardiac events, such as new chest pain and ECG changes.
- Assess for any pulmonary complications, such as dyspnea or cough.

Patient Teaching
General

- Advise patients to notify the health care provider if foaming of urine occurs (an indication of protein in the urine).
- Teach patients to avoid taking nonsteroidal antiinflammatory drugs (NSAIDs) such as aspirin, celecoxib, ibuprofen, and naproxen to decrease the risk of bleeding.
- Teach patients ways to promote venous return and avoid deep venous thrombosis (DVT), such as avoiding dehydration, constrictive clothing, and smoking cigarettes.

Side Effects

- Advise patients to immediately report worsening of skin rash; severe or persistent diarrhea, nausea, anorexia, or vomiting; onset or worsening of unexplained shortness of breath or cough; or eye irritation.
- Teach patients to avoid direct sunlight and tanning beds to prevent worsening of skin side effects.
- Advise patients to seek medical help immediately if chest pain, severe abdominal pain, or swelling associated with redness or pain in one leg occurs.
- Report symptoms of adverse effects or severe side effects promptly, especially fever, chills, persistent sore throat, swelling, weight gain, or increasing shortness of breath.
- Report symptoms of bleeding immediately, including black stools, coffee ground emesis, and easy bleeding or bruising.

Evaluate Outcomes [Evaluation]

- Patient, family, and caregiver education needs are met.
- The patient, family, and caregivers understand therapy-related side effects and adverse reactions.
- The patient, family, and caregivers understand strategies to minimize side effects and adverse reactions.
- Side effects are managed effectively.
- The patient is free from infection.
- The patient is free from injury, perforation, or internal fistula.

When activated and expressed, *BCR-ABL TK* turns on a strong pro-cell-division signal transduction pathway that leads to the proliferation of cancer cells. TKIs prevent activation of TKs, which then inhibits further activation of the signal transduction pathway and stops the proliferation of cancer cells. This action can control the disease but cannot eradicate it alone. Receptors on the cell membrane can activate TKs, which then turn on signal transduction pathways that promote cell division. Table 36.2 lists some of the TKI drugs and their uses and considerations. Of the TKIs, alectinib and nilotinib are further discussed under those headings in text. Prototype Drug Chart: Imatinib Mesylate, STI-571 lists specific drug information about the TKI imatinib.

The multikinase inhibitors (MKIs) are chemicals that directly inhibit the activity of multiple kinase enzymes in cancer cells. (Recall that kinases are enzymes that activate other proteins, including those that activate signal transduction pathways that promote cancer cell division.) Table 36.2 lists some of the MKIs and their dosages, routes, uses, and considerations. Of the MKIs, dasatinib, sorafenib, and sunitinib are discussed.

Alectinib. Alectinib is a TKI that targets anaplastic lymphoma kinase (*ALK*) and the RET proto-oncogene (*RET*). It is indicated for the treatment of patients with *ALK*-positive metastatic NSCLC whose disease has progressed on or who are intolerant to crizotinib.

PROTOTYPE DRUG CHART

Imatinib Mesylate, STI-571

Drug Class	Dosage
Signal transduction inhibitor/tyrosine kinase inhibitor	A: PO: For Ph+ leukemias, myelodysplastic syndrome, myeloproliferative disease, GI stromal tumors (GISTs), hypereosinophilic syndrome (HES) or chronic eosinophilic leukemia (CEL), aggressive systemic mastocytosis, metastatic dermatofibrosarcoma protuberans. Dose depends on disease; starting dose is 400 mg/d; may increase if no serious adverse reactions occur. Other protocols exist, including twice-daily dosing.

Contraindications	Drug-Lab-Food Interactions
Contraindicated among patients who may be or could become pregnant or who are breastfeeding. *Caution:* Patients with renal impairment, cardiac disease, hepatic impairment, bone marrow suppression, or infection, and in children. Avoid concomitant strong CYP3A4 inducers. *See full prescriber's information for a complete list of contraindications.*	Drug: Any drug that *inhibits* CYP450 or CYP3A4 (e.g., nefazodone, itraconazole, fluvoxamine, fluconazole, erythromycin) can decrease the metabolism of imatinib and increases the concentration, leading to an increased incidence of adverse reactions. Any drug that *induces* CYP450 (e.g., St. John's wort, phenytoin, fosphenytoin, rifampin, barbiturates, dexamethasone, phenobarbital) can increase the metabolism of imatinib and decrease imatinib concentrations and clinical effects. Imatinib is a CYP450 inhibitor and serum concentrations of any drug that is metabolized by CYP450 (e.g., ergot alkaloids, carbamazepine, cyclosporine, quinidine, clonazepam, fentanyl, calcium channel blockers, sertraline, acetaminophen) can increase. Taking imatinib with thrombolytic agents, NSAIDs, platelet inhibitors, aspirin, and other anticoagulants/antiplatelets may increase risk of bleeding. Concomitant use of flibanserin and moderate CYP3A4 inhibitors, such as imatinib, is contraindicated due to severe hypotension and syncope. Lab: May affect serum levels of liver enzymes, CBC, electrolytes, renal function, and uric acid Food: Grapefruit juice increases imatinib plasma concentrations.

Pharmacokinetics	Pharmacodynamics
Absorption: Bioavailability is 98%. Distribution: 95% PB with extensive distribution. Metabolism: Mainly by CYP3A4; inhibits CYP2D6 and CYP3A4; t½: imatinib is 18 h, major metabolite is 40 h. Clearance is 8–14 L/h. Excretion: Mainly in the feces as metabolites	Well absorbed after oral administration with Cmax achieved within 2–4 h. Imatinib should be taken with food and a large glass of water to decrease the risk of GI irritation. Drug may be dispersed in water or apple juice for patients who cannot swallow tablets. Suspension should be administered immediately after complete disintegration of the tablets. Onset: UK Peak: 2–4 h Duration: UK

Therapeutic Effects/Uses

Approved for ALL, CEL, CML, dermatofibrosarcoma protuberans, GIST, HES, myelodysplastic syndrome, and systemic mastocytosis.

Mechanism of Action: Imatinib competitively inhibits the ATP binding site on *BCR-ABL* tyrosine kinase (TK) that results in inhibition of proliferation and induces apoptosis in *BCR-ABL*–positive cell lines and in fresh leukemic cells of Philadelphia chromosome–positive CML. Receptors for TKs include various growth factors (e.g., *EGF, PDGF, SGF, VEGF, NGF*). Imatinib also acts as a mediator for many nonreceptor TKs (e.g., G-protein–coupled receptors, B- and T-cell receptors, and interferon gamma receptors). Imatinib also interacts with lipids, proteins, and DNA. Imatinib inhibits proliferation in vitro and induces apoptosis in GIST cells, which express an activating *KIT* mutation. Imatinib inhibits CYP2C9, CYP2D6, and CYP3A4.

Side Effects	Adverse Reactions
Edema, fluid retention, GI irritation, nausea, vomiting, hematologic dyscrasias, hepatotoxicity, electrolyte abnormalities	The most common adverse reactions include cerebral edema, cardiac tamponade, increased ICP and papilledema, pleural effusions, heart failure, renal failure, GI perforation and bleeding, avascular necrosis, cardiac events, and tumor lysis syndrome.

A, Adult; *ALL,* acute lymphoblastic leukemia; *ATP,* adenosine triphosphate; *CBC,* complete blood count; *CEL,* chronic eosinophilic leukemia; *Cmax,* maximum serum concentration; *CML,* chronic myelogenous leukemia; *CYP3A4,* cytochrome P3A4; *CYP450,* cytochrome P450; *d,* day; *EGF,* epidermal growth factor; *h,* hour; *GI,* gastrointestinal; *GIST,* gastrointestinal stromal tumor; *HES,* hypereosinophilic syndrome; *ICP,* intracranial pressure; *NGF,* nerve growth factor; *NSAID,* nonsteroidal antiinflammatory drug; *PDGF,* platelet-derived growth factor; *PB,* protein bound; *Ph+,* Philadelphia chromosome positive; *PO,* oral; *SGF,* sarcoma growth factor; *t½,* half-life; *UK,* unknown; *VEGF,* vascular endothelial growth factor; *y,* year; *>,* greater than; *≤,* less than or equal to.

Pharmacokinetics. Alectinib is administered orally. Alectinib and its major metabolite, M4, are more than 99% bound to plasma proteins. Steady state is reached by day 7 of administration. Alectinib is metabolized by CYP3A4 to its major active metabolite, M4. The elimination half-lives for alectinib and M4 are 33 and 31 hours, respectively. Alectinib and its metabolite are excreted in the feces (84% and 6%, respectively). No significant effect was noted in patients with mild to moderate hepatic and renal impairment.

Pharmacodynamics. Alectinib is a TKI that targets *ALK* and *RET.* Alectinib is a central nervous system (CNS)-active and highly selective

ALK inhibitor that inhibits *ALK* phosphorylation and *ALK*-mediated activation of the downstream signaling proteins.

Side Effects and Adverse Reactions. Common side effects include anemia, elevated transaminases, fatigue, constipation, bradycardia, edema, hypocalcemia, hypokalemia, and myalgia. Serious adverse events include hepatotoxicity, pneumonitis, bradycardia, and elevated creatine phosphokinase (CPK).

Drug Interactions. No interactions with alectinib that require dose adjustment have been identified.

Nilotinib. Nilotinib is a TKI that has a high affinity for the ATP binding site of *BCR-ABL* kinase, inhibiting cell proliferation in cell lines and in primary Philadelphia chromosome–positive (Ph+) CML cells. It is indicated for the treatment of Ph+ CML that is resistant or intolerant to imatinib in the chronic or accelerated phase.

Pharmacokinetics. Nilotinib is administered orally, and approximately 98% is protein bound in plasma. The elimination half-life is approximately 17 hours. Peak serum concentration occurs 3 hours after oral administration, and steady state is achieved on day 8. The bioavailability of the drug is significantly increased with food. Nilotinib is metabolized in the liver by CYP3A4; no active metabolites have been identified. The primary metabolic pathways are oxidation and hydroxylation. The majority of the drug is eliminated mainly in the feces within 7 days. Caution is advised in administering nilotinib to patients with hepatic impairment.

Pharmacodynamics. Nilotinib is an oral TK that selectively inhibits *BCR-ABL* kinase. It is a competitor inhibitor at the ATP-binding site of *BCR-ABL* and prevents tyrosine phosphorylation of downstream intracellular signal transduction proteins. Blocking the TK prevents proliferation of cancer cells and induces cell death.

Side Effects and Adverse Reactions. The most common adverse effects are pancytopenia, rash, pruritus, nausea, fatigue, cephalgia, and constipation. Severe adverse events include dysrhythmias due to prolonged QT interval, which can cause sudden cardiac death. Pulmonary toxicity has been reported in patients with CML.

Drug Interactions. Concomitant administration of strong CYP3A4 inhibitors or inducers may significantly alter nilotinib concentrations. If CYP3A4 inhibitor drugs (e.g., ketoconazole, clarithromycin, ritonavir, fluoroquinolones, ibutilide, lithium) are unavoidable, dose reduction should be considered, and the QT interval should be monitored on a frequent basis. Electrolyte imbalances should be corrected before administering nilotinib.

Dasatinib. Dasatinib is an MKI approved for newly diagnosed Ph+ CML and acute lymphocytic leukemia (ALL); Ph+ CML in chronic, accelerated, or myeloid or lymphoid blast phases resistant or intolerant to prior therapy, including imatinib; and Ph+ ALL with resistance or intolerance to prior therapy.

Pharmacokinetics. Dasatinib is an oral drug that is readily absorbed from the GI tract, and it can be taken with or without food. Dasatinib and its active metabolite are highly protein bound (96% and 93%, respectively). The drug is extensively metabolized in the liver by the CYP3A4 isoenzyme. Dasatinib is also a weak time-dependent inhibitor of CYP3A4. Unlike other tyrosine inhibitors, dasatinib does not have the multidrug-resistant protein P-glycoprotein. Dasatinib is eliminated primarily through feces, with only minimal amounts recovered in the urine. Antacids slow the absorption.

Pharmacodynamics. Dasatinib specifically targets *BCR-ABL TK*, *SRC* family kinases, and imatinib-resistant mutations mostly found in CML and ALL, possibly blocking angiogenesis and cell proliferation. Inhibiting the activity of these enzymes further inhibits activation of the signal transduction pathway, thereby stopping the proliferation of cancer cells. The drug has the greatest effects on Ph+-expressing cancer cells.

Side Effects and Adverse Reactions. Dasatinib often causes electrolyte imbalances, especially hypokalemia, hypocalcemia, and hypophosphatemia. Other common side effects include diarrhea, cephalgia, fatigue, skin rash, nausea, vomiting, anorexia, arthralgia, pyrexia, and dyspnea, among others. Hemorrhage, vascular disorders, and severe dermatologic reactions have been associated with dasatinib. Another adverse reaction includes ECG abnormalities, especially prolonged QT intervals, and development of arrhythmias. Hematologic side effects of myelosuppression with anemia, thrombocytopenia, and neutropenia are relatively common and are usually reversible. Bleeding, including GI and intracranial bleeding, was reported that required treatment interruptions and transfusions.

Drug Interactions. CYP3A4 enzyme inhibitors decrease dasatinib metabolism, resulting in an increased serum concentration and increased risk for toxicity. Other drugs that strongly increase the serum concentration of dasatinib include atazanavir, clarithromycin, indinavir, itraconazole, ketoconazole, nefazodone, nelfinavir, telithromycin, triazolobenzodiazepines, and voriconazole.

Drugs that enhance the activity of the CYP3A4 enzyme decrease dasatinib serum levels and reduce its effectiveness. Such drugs include aminoglutethimide, barbiturates, carbamazepine, dexamethasone, griseofulvin, nafcillin, phenytoin, primidone, and rifampin. Other drugs that appear to reduce the effectiveness of dasatinib include antacids, histamine 2 (H_2) receptor blockers, and proton pump inhibitors. Dasatinib may interfere with the metabolism of other drugs that use the CYP3A4 enzyme system, such as alfentanil, terfenadine, cisapride, cyclosporine, fentanyl, quinidine, tacrolimus, and ergot alkaloids.

Sorafenib. Sorafenib is an MKI that specifically targets serine/threonine and receptor TKs, which are activated because of gene mutations. Gene mutations are most commonly found in pancreatic cancer, colon cancer, and NSCLC. In addition, the drug may be used in hepatocellular carcinomas and renal cell carcinomas (RCCs) that overexpress the target.

Pharmacokinetics. Sorafenib is an oral drug whose absorption and bioavailability are inhibited when taken with a high-fat meal. The drug is metabolized in the liver, mainly by the CYP3A4 enzyme system. It is 99.5% protein bound and reaches steady state within 7 days. The peak plasma level is about 3 hours; the mean half-life is 25 to 48 hours. Eight metabolites have been identified, with pyridine *N*-oxide being the major circulating active metabolite. The drug is eliminated in the feces unchanged and in the urine as glucuronidated metabolites (77% and 19%, respectively).

Pharmacodynamics. Sorafenib inhibits multiple kinase receptors to inhibit cell proliferation and angiogenesis. Some of the targeted kinases include *RAF* kinase, *VEGF* receptors, platelet-derived growth factor receptor (*PDGFR*), and *RET*. When cytokines or growth factors activate these TK receptors, a protein kinase–mediated cascade starts that leads to uncontrolled cellular proliferation. The inhibition of these signaling pathways decreases cancer cellular proliferation. In addition, sorafenib specifically inhibits two *VEGF* receptors, thereby inhibiting angiogenesis.

Side Effects and Adverse Reactions. Sorafenib has many common adverse effects, such as hypertension, cephalgia, alopecia, pruritus, xerosis, exfoliative dermatitis, acne, flush, anorexia, nausea/vomiting, diarrhea, constipation, abdominal pain, dyspepsia, dysphagia, hand and foot syndrome, and mild neutropenia. More severe adverse events include QT prolongation, especially in patients with heart failure or electrolyte abnormalities and in those taking other drugs that prolong QT interval. Other severe adverse events were hemorrhage, especially in patients taking anticoagulants or antiplatelets; cardiac ischemia/infarction; GI perforation; and pulmonary toxicity.

Drug Interactions. Sorafenib levels are not increased by the presence of other drugs, even those that inhibit the enzyme that metabolizes sorafenib. However, drugs that induce metabolizing enzyme activity can reduce the blood levels and the effectiveness of sorafenib. These include primidone, phenobarbital, rifampicin, phenytoin, carbamazepine, and dexamethasone. If drugs that prolong QT intervals—such as methadone, daunorubicin, epirubicin, and doxorubicin—are coadministered with sorafenib, close ECG monitoring is warranted. Sorafenib can increase the blood levels of repaglinide, amiodarone, ibuprofen, loperamide, irinotecan, propofol, and warfarin.

Sunitinib. Sunitinib is an MKI with antiangiogenic and antitumor activities. It selectively inhibits several receptor TKs (RTKs). This inhibition results in regression of tumor growth, especially in advanced RCC; gastrointestinal stromal tumors (GISTs); and progressive, well-differentiated pancreatic neuroendocrine tumors in patients with unresectable or metastatic disease.

Pharmacokinetics. Sunitinib is an oral MKI that is well absorbed with or without food. Sunitinib and its active metabolites are highly protein bound (95% and 90%, respectively). Sunitinib reaches peak plasma level in 6 to 12 hours. The drug and its metabolite are metabolized in the liver, mainly by the CYP3A4 enzyme system; elimination half-life is 40 to 60 hours, and the drug is eliminated primarily in the feces. No dose adjustment is warranted in patients with renal impairment or in patients with mild to moderate hepatic impairment.

Pharmacodynamics. Sunitinib inhibits more than 80 RTKs, including PDGFR, vascular endothelial growth factor receptor (*VEGFR*), stem cell factor receptor, and glial cell line–derived neurotrophic factor receptor. Additionally, it inhibits the phosphorylation of RTKs, and it has demonstrated inhibition of tumor growth, tumor regression, and tumor angiogenesis. Several adverse effects of sunitinib, including hair and skin discoloration, are associated with the inhibition of the multiple signaling pathways.

Side Effects and Adverse Reactions. Side effects and adverse reactions are more widespread as a result of the number of different types of kinases sunitinib inhibits. Cardiovascular effects include hypertension, peripheral edema, left ventricular dysfunction, prolonged QT interval, and venous thromboembolism. GI effects include nausea, vomiting, diarrhea, stomatitis, and dyspepsia. Neuromuscular effects include fatigue, asthenia, headache, dizziness, peripheral neuropathy, mild arthralgia, limb pain, myalgia, and back pain. Liver impairment may occur with elevated liver enzymes and jaundice of the skin and sclera. Common integumentary changes include depigmentation of the skin, skin discoloration, rash, dry skin, and palmar-plantar erythrodysesthesia. Endocrine changes may include hypothyroidism and adrenal insufficiency, hematologic changes may include myelosuppression, and respiratory effects may include mild dyspnea and cough.

Drug Interactions. Plasma concentration and the activity of sunitinib are increased by drugs that inhibit CYP3A4 enzyme levels, including atazanavir, clarithromycin, ketoconazole, itraconazole, nefazodone, nelfinavir, telithromycin, diltiazem, and verapamil. When these drugs are used during sunitinib therapy, side effects of sunitinib are more common and more severe. Drugs that increase sunitinib elimination and reduce its effectiveness include rifampin, phenytoin, phenobarbital, carbamazepine, dexamethasone, rifabutin, and rifapentine.

mTOR Kinase Inhibitors and Proteasome Inhibitors

Mechanistic target of rapamycin (mTOR) is an atypical serine/threonine protein kinase that helps regulate cell growth, proliferation, and survival. Inhibitors of mTOR lead to G_1 arrest and apoptosis. They are not without adverse effects, which are common and include weakness, rash, mucositis, nausea, edema, anorexia, and fever. Effects on laboratory values include pancytopenia, hyperglycemia, hypercholesterolemia, hypertriglyceridemia, and hypophosphatemia. Severe adverse events include hepatic necrosis, pericardial effusion, cardiac tamponade, nephrotic syndrome, hemolytic uremic syndrome, and exfoliative dermatitis. Like other targeted drugs, adverse effects of mTOR and other CYP3A4 inhibitor drugs are increased when mTOR is administered concomitantly. CYP3A4 inducers can cause drug levels to decrease.

Proteasomes are multienzyme complexes that degrade proteins intracellularly. The degraded proteins can accumulate and can disrupt a cell's physiologic properties, such as regulating transcription, cell adhesion, apoptosis, and progression of mitosis. In cancer cells, proteasome inhibitors promote the accumulation of proteins that promote programmed cell death. It has limited action on normal, healthy cells. Table 36.2 lists the mTOR kinase inhibitors and the proteasome inhibitors. Prototype Drug Chart: Bortezomib lists specific drug information on bortezomib.

Temsirolimus. Temsirolimus is an inhibitor of mTOR. When temsirolimus or sirolimus binds to the intracellular protein *FKBP-12*, a protein-drug complex forms that directly inhibits the activity of mTOR. Inhibition of mTOR greatly reduces the concentration of VEGF. In addition, by its inhibition of mTOR, a variety of downstream pro-cell-division signal transduction pathways are disrupted, especially in RCC cells. This drug is most commonly used to treat advanced RCC.

Pharmacokinetics. Temsirolimus is administered by IV infusion. It is extensively metabolized in the liver by CYP3A4 into five active metabolites, including sirolimus. The half-life of temsirolimus is 17 hours, and the half-life of sirolimus is 54 hours. Temsirolimus and its metabolites are primarily excreted in the feces. Approximately 82% of total radioactivity is eliminated within 14 days. Serum concentration of the metabolite, sirolimus, peaks at 0.5 to 2 hours. Caution is advised in patients with mild hepatic impairment. In patients with moderate to severe hepatic impairment, the drug is contraindicated.

Pharmacodynamics. Temsirolimus and its metabolites bind to an intracellular protein to form a drug-protein complex that inhibits the activity of mTOR, and mTOR regulates messenger RNA (mRNA) translation through phosphorylation. Inhibition of mTOR activity results in G_1 growth arrest in treated RCC cells.

Side Effects and Adverse Reactions. Hypersensitivity reactions to temsirolimus are common, and premedication with an IV antihistamine (e.g., diphenhydramine) is recommended. Adverse effects are common and include weakness, rash, mucositis, nausea, edema, anorexia, dyspnea, pain, elevated transaminases, pancytopenia, hyperlipidemia, diarrhea, hypophosphatemia, hypercholesterolemia, and hypertriglyceridemia. Hyperglycemia is also common in patients receiving temsirolimus; patients may require treatment with oral antidiabetic agents or with insulin. Respiratory adverse effects of interstitial pneumonitis or other interstitial lung disease are possible. Liver impairment and renal impairment have been reported. Cardiovascular effects of edema formation, chest pain, hypertension, venous thromboembolism, and thrombophlebitis are possible.

Drug Interactions. Drugs that inhibit the CYP3A4 enzyme can lead to increased serum levels of temsirolimus, which increases the risk for severe side effects. These drugs include ketoconazole, clarithromycin, indinavir, itraconazole, nefazodone, telithromycin, voriconazole, diltiazem, fluconazole, verapamil, and cimetidine.

Drugs that induce CYP3A4 enzyme activity may lower temsirolimus blood serum levels and can reduce its effectiveness. These drugs include rifampin, carbamazepine, and phenytoin.

⊙ CLINICAL JUDGMENT [NURSING PROCESS]

Tyrosine Kinase Inhibitors and Multikinase Inhibitors for Cancer Treatment

Concept: Cellular Regulation
- The ability for cells to maintain homeostasis, including responses to extracellular signals.

Recognize Cues [Assessment]
- Obtain a detailed current medication history that includes prescriptions, over-the-counter (OTC) medicines, antacids, dietary supplements, vitamins, and herbal supplements and compare with the targeted therapy drug for possible drug-drug interactions.
- Obtain a list of drug and food allergies.
- Obtain baseline information about the patient's physical status that includes height, weight, vital signs, cardiopulmonary assessment, intake and output, skin assessment, nutritional status, and any underlying diseases.
- Assess baseline laboratory values (complete blood count [CBC], uric acid, chemistry panel) to compare with future ones.
- Assess baseline results of pulmonary function tests, chest radiographs, electrocardiograms (ECGs), and renal and liver function studies.
- Assess the patient's and caregiver's current level of comprehension ability related to the therapeutic regimen.

Analyze Cues and Prioritize Hypothesis [Patient Problems]
- Potential for altered clotting
- Potential for decreased immunity
- Need for teaching

Generate Solutions [Planning]
- The patient/family member/caretaker will verbalize understanding of the signs and symptoms of infection.
- The patient will maintain white blood cell, red blood cell, and platelet counts in the desired range.
- The patient will remain free from infection and from pulmonary, cardiac, and gastrointestinal (GI) complications.
- The patient will verbalize ways to decrease GI disturbances to improve nutrition intake.
- The patient/family/caregiver will demonstrate understanding of the chemotherapeutic protocol (e.g., dose administration).

Take Action [Nursing Interventions]
- Monitor labs (CBC, blood urea nitrogen [BUN], creatinine, liver panel, and electrolytes) before administration and during treatment.
- Monitor for any signs of bleeding.
- Monitor for any dysrhythmias, decreased cardiac output, heart rate, and blood pressure.
- Monitor intravenous (IV) site frequently for irritation and phlebitis.
- Maintain strict medical asepsis during dressing changes and invasive procedures.

- Encourage small, frequent meals that are high in calories and protein.
- Monitor fluid intake and output, weight, and nutritional intake during therapy.
- Assess the need for IV hydration.
- Administer premedications as ordered 30 to 60 minutes before giving the drug.
- Provide drug information—such as therapeutic effects, side effects, and drug-drug/drug-food interactions—verbally and in print to the patient/family/caregiver.
- Monitor for any vision changes.

Patient Teaching
General
- Teach patients when to take medications as it relates to food intake.
- Teach patient to weigh daily and report a weight gain of more than 2 pounds in 1 day or 4 pounds in 1 week to the health care provider.
- Remind women with childbearing potential to avoid pregnancy throughout treatment and for up to 12 months after treatment is complete.
- Advise breastfeeding patients to stop breastfeeding during and for 60 days after therapy.
- Teach patients to avoid using St. John's wort while on treatment.

Side Effects
- Avoid alcohol and nonessential drugs that are metabolized by the liver or that have hepatotoxic effects (e.g., acetaminophen).
- Report symptoms of adverse effects or severe side effects promptly, especially fever, chills, persistent sore throat, swelling, weight gain, or increasing shortness of breath.
- Report symptoms of bleeding immediately, including black stools, coffee ground emesis, or easy bleeding or bruising.
- Report symptoms of stomach or abdominal pain, yellowing of eyes or skin, dark urine, or unusual fatigue.
- Teach patients to avoid grapefruit juice, which can increase blood levels of drug to a dangerous level, leading to worsening side effects or adverse events.

Evaluate Outcomes [Evaluation]
- Patient, family, and caregiver education needs are met.
- The patient, family, and caregivers understand therapy-related side effects and adverse reactions.
- The patient, family, and caregivers understand strategies to minimize side effects and adverse reactions.
- Side effects are managed effectively.
- The patient is free from infection.
- The patient's fluid balance and electrolytes are maintained at expected normal ranges.

Patients taking antihypertensive drugs such as angiotensin-converting enzyme (ACE) inhibitors or angiotensin II–receptor antagonists during temsirolimus therapy are at increased risk for angioedema of the face and upper airways. The combination of temsirolimus and sunitinib may result in dose-limiting integumentary toxicities of erythematous maculopapular rash and gout/cellulitis that require hospitalization. The use of live vaccines such as intranasal influenza; measles, mumps, rubella; oral polio; bacille Calmette-Guérin (BCG); yellow fever; varicella; and typhoid vaccines should be avoided during treatment with temsirolimus.

Carfilzomib. Carfilzomib is a proteasome inhibitor that prevents the proliferation of cancerous cells and promotes apoptotic activity in solid and hematologic tumor cells. Carfilzomib is indicated in the treatment of multiple myeloma.

Pharmacokinetics. Carfilzomib is administered intravenously, and in vitro, 97% of the drug is protein bound. Its metabolites have no known biologic activity. The elimination half-life is 1 hour or less. Carfilzomib is extensively metabolized in the plasma rather than in the liver. The drug clearance exceeds hepatic blood flow, suggesting a large extrahepatic clearance. About 25% of the drug's metabolite is excreted in the feces.

PROTOTYPE DRUG CHART

Bortezomib

Drug Class	Dosage
Proteasome inhibitor	A: IV or Subcut: *Mantle cell lymphoma:* 1.3 mg/m² on days 1, 4, 8, and 11 followed by a 10-d rest period (days 12–21) for six 3-wk cycles in combination with rituximab, cyclophosphamide, doxorubicin, and prednisone. *Multiple myeloma* (FDA-designated orphan drug for multiple myeloma): Treatment is administered for nine 6-wk cycles. Cycles 1–4: Admin 1.3 mg/m²/dose on days 1, 4, 8, and 11 followed by a 10-d rest period (days 12–21); then 1.3 mg/m²/dose on days 22, 25, 29, and 32 followed by another 10-d rest period (days 33–42) in combination with melphalan and prednisone. Cycles 5–9: Admin 1.3 mg/m²/dose on days 1, 8, 22, and 29 in combination with melphalan and prednisone. Other protocols exist. See full prescribing information. At least 72 h should elapse between consecutive doses of bortezomib. IV doses should be given as a bolus over 3–5 s. Subcut injections should be administered in the thigh or abdomen; rotate sites and *do not* admin to areas that are tender, bruised, erythematous, or indurated. Dose adjustment is needed for moderate to severe hepatic impairment; no adjustments are needed with renal impairment. Admin bortezomib after dialysis procedure; dialysis may reduce bortezomib blood levels.

Contraindications	Drug-Lab-Food Interactions
Absolute contraindications: Intrathecal administration, patients with mannitol, bortezomib, or boron hypersensitivity Avoid during pregnancy; breastfeeding should be discontinued. *Caution:* Cardiac, pulmonary, and liver disorders; bleeding dyscrasias; pancytopenia; dehydration; diabetes mellitus; herpes infection; bleeding; history of tumor lysis syndrome; and in neonates and children.	Drug: Dialysis may reduce bortezomib drug level; bortezomib may increase serum levels of eliglustat, amobarbital, axitinib, and tamsulosin by inducing CYP2D6 metabolism. CYP3A4 inhibitor drugs (e.g., idelalisib, mefloquine, cimetidine, clarithromycin, cyclosporine, erythromycin, fluconazole, nifedipine) can increase the serum level of bortezomib if given concomitantly. CYP2C19 inhibitor drugs can decrease the effects of clopidogrel and diazepam. Drugs metabolized by CYP3A4 (e.g., dexamethasone, diazepam, St. John's wort, phenobarbital) can decrease the level or effect of bortezomib. Bortezomib may increase the level or effect of omeprazole and pantoprazole through CYP2C19 metabolism. *See full prescriber's information for a complete list of drug interactions.* Lab: Bortezomib may alter other drug levels if given concomitantly (e.g., phenytoin and phenobarbital). Food: Green tea decreases bortezomib's effects; grapefruit juice may increase the level of bortezomib.

Pharmacokinetics	Pharmacodynamics
Absorption: Bioavailability is unknown. Distribution: Range, 498–1884 L/m² distributed widely into peripheral tissues; >83% PB. Metabolism: CYP3A4, CYP2C19, and CYP1A2; t½: 40–193 h; dose dependent. Excretion: UK	Onset: UK Peak: 509 ng/mL Duration: UK

Therapeutic Effects/Uses

Mantle cell lymphoma (MCL) and multiple myeloma.

Mechanism of Action: Bortezomib is a signal transduction inhibitor and a reversible inhibitor of the 26S proteasome in mechanistic cells. Proteasome is a large multiprotein particle present in the cytosol and cell nucleus that regulates protein expression and degradation of damaged or obsolete proteins within the cell; it regulates the expression of proteins that mediate cell cycle progression, oncogenes, and apoptosis. Proteasome inhibition affects malignant cells more so than normal cells.

Side Effects	Adverse Reactions
See full prescriber's information for a complete list. Nausea, vomiting, diarrhea, constipation, anorexia, abdominal pain, dyspepsia, dysgeusia, hypotension, neuropathy, pancytopenia, rash, urticaria, vasculitis, pruritus, injection site reaction (e.g., pain, erythema, hematoma, skin irritation, and phlebitis), arthralgia, myalgia, back pain, bone pain, bone fractures, hyperglycemia, hypoglycemia, fatigue, fever, insomnia	*See full prescriber's information for a complete list.* Severe sensory and peripheral neuropathy, cardiotoxicity, heart failure, QT prolongation, arrhythmias, pulmonary hypertension, acute respiratory distress syndrome, pneumonitis, interstitial pneumonia, GI perforation, GI toxicity, hepatotoxicity, toxic epidermal necrolysis, acute febrile neutrophilic dermatosis (Sweet syndrome)

A, Adult; *admin*, administer; *CYP*, cytochrome P; *d*, day; *FDA*, US Food and Drug Administration; *GI*, gastrointestinal; *h*, hour; *IV*, intravenous; *PB*, protein bound; *s*, second; *Subcut*, subcutaneous; *t½*, half-life; *UK*, unknown; *wk*, week; >, greater than.

Pharmacodynamics. Carfilzomib irreversibly binds to the *N*-terminal threonine-containing active sites of the 20S proteasome, unlike bortezomib. Carfilzomib may be more selective for the chymotrypsin protease, leading to more sustained and selective proteasome activity. It has minimal cross-reactivity with other protease classes.

Side Effects and Adverse Reactions. Adverse effects include fatigue, pancytopenia, dyspnea, diarrhea, pyrexia, cephalgia, cough, peripheral edema, nausea, vomiting, arthralgia, hypertension, asthenia, insomnia, and back pain. Cardiac toxicity (e.g., congestive heart failure, cardiac arrest, myocardial ischemia/infarction) has been reported. Pulmonary arterial hypertension and pulmonary edema were noted in some patients. Renal and hepatic toxicity was also noted; therefore close monitoring of renal and hepatic functions is warranted.

Drug Interactions. Specific drug interactions have not been reported with this drug. Because carfilzomib is not metabolized by the liver, it is unlikely to be affected by concomitant administration of cytochrome P450 (CYP450) inhibitors and inducers.

Ixazomib. Ixazomib is a reversible proteasome inhibitor that binds and inhibits 20S proteasome. It is indicated for the treatment of multiple myeloma in patients who have received at least one prior therapy.

Pharmacokinetics. Ixazomib is administered orally and is highly bound to plasma proteins (99%) with distribution into erythrocytes. Terminal half-life is 9.5 days. The drug is metabolized by CYP450 isoenzymes and non-CYP proteins. Approximately 62% of the dose radioactivity is recovered in the urine and 22% in the feces. The concentration of the drug is decreased with food; therefore the drug should be given at least 1 hour before or at least 2 hours after food consumption.

Pharmacodynamics. Ixazomib is a reversible proteasome inhibitor that preferentially binds to the beta-5 subunit of the 20S proteasome, and it inhibits its chymotrypsin-like activity. It induces apoptosis of multiple myeloma cells and has a cytotoxic effect on myeloma cells in patients who relapse after receiving prior therapies with other drugs.

Side Effects and Adverse Reactions. Ixazomib causes multiple adverse effects that include pancytopenia, diarrhea, peripheral neuropathies, peripheral edema, back pain, upper respiratory tract infection, nausea, vomiting, dry eye, and grade 3 rash. Severe adverse effects include drug-induced hepatotoxicity, Stevens-Johnson syndrome, and grade 3 or 4 GI toxicity.

Drug Interactions. Ixazomib is metabolized by CYP3A4; levels of ixazomib can be altered by drugs that induce or inhibit CYP3A4. Such drugs include carbamazepine, fosphenytoin, primidone, rifabutin, rifampin, and St. John's wort.

Large-Molecule Compounds

Monoclonal antibodies (mAbs) are larger molecules that exert their effects mostly on specific cell membrane surface proteins. Some mAbs act more like immunotherapy drugs because of their effects in improving the person's immune system to find and attack cancer cells. Chapter 37 provides more information on immunotherapies. All FDA-approved mAbs currently used in cancer treatment are given intravenously because the GI tract could alter the drug's structure and render it inactive. Ideal target antigens for cancer treatment should (1) be specific to tumor cells, (2) be located on the surface of the tumor cell and not shed into the bloodstream, (3) occur in high numbers, and (4) play a role in tumor cell survival.

mAb therapy is aimed specifically at tumor cells that express the target antigen. The side effects of mAbs are related to activation of the immune system, location of the target antigen, and the type of mAb.

Binding of a mAb to its specific target antigen on the cancer cell inactivates or destroys the cell by one or more of the following mechanisms:

- Causing neutralization of tumor cell growth by direct interference with normal biologic activities of the antigen, such as signal transduction of cell growth messages. This cytostatic process can slow growth of the tumor cells.
- Promoting antibody-dependent cell-mediated cytotoxicity (ADCC) that recruits effector cells such as phagocytes, T cells, and natural killer cells of the immune system to release cytokines that destroy the target cell.
- Initiating complement-dependent cytotoxicity (CDC) that activates the complement system, a cascade of naturally circulating blood proteins, thus enhancing immune system destruction of antibody-bound cells.
- Directly inducing apoptosis, or programmed cell death.

Fully human antibodies are engineered to contain only human antibody protein sequences. Murine mAbs are derived from mice. Mouse antibodies have a very short half-life in the human body, are not as effective as human antibodies in eliciting a response from the CDC and ADCC systems, and can cause development of human anti-mouse antibodies (HAMAs) that neutralize the mouse antibodies and render them ineffective against the tumor. Chimeric mAbs contain both human and mouse protein sequences (typically 70% human and 30% mouse). Humanized mAbs also contain human and gene mouse sequences; however, they are not considered chimeric because they contain more human sequences than do chimeric mAbs, usually 90% to 95% human and 5% to 10% mouse.

mAbs can also be transporters for other anticancer agents (e.g., chemotherapy agents, toxins, or radioisotopes). Although agents attached to conjugated antibodies specifically target tumor cells, nearby healthy cells can still be negatively affected, especially if radioisotopes are used. If the specific target antigen is found on normal cells, these antibodies also cause damage to these cells.

Table 36.3 lists some of the mAbs currently in use. Bevacizumab has angiogenesis-inhibiting properties. Prototype Drug Chart: Bevacizumab lists specific information on bevacizumab. Prototype Drug Chart: Rituximab lists specific drug information on rituximab.

Alemtuzumab

Alemtuzumab is an unconjugated, humanized mAb against the cell surface antigen CD52 that promotes antigen-dependent cell lysis of leukemic cells. CD52 is found on most B and T lymphocytes; on the majority of monocytes, macrophages, and natural killer (NK) cells; and on some granulocytes, stem cells, and mature spermatozoa. Although normal cells may express this antigen, malignant cells are much more sensitive to the destructive activity of this antibody. This drug is most commonly used for management of chronic lymphocytic leukemia (CLL) and multiple sclerosis (MS). However, alemtuzumab should be reserved for patients who have had an inadequate response to two or more drugs for the treatment of MS.

Pharmacokinetics. Alemtuzumab is administered as an IV infusion. Its average half-life is 12 days, and steady-state levels are reached by about 6 weeks. Alemtuzumab is largely confined to blood and interstitial spaces. mAbs bind to target cell surfaces and are destroyed along with the target cell; they are then cleared as debris from the blood and are eliminated in the feces.

Pharmacodynamics. Alemtuzumab binds to leukemic cells that express the CD52 cell surface antigen and induces antibody-dependent lysis. Alemtuzumab seems to have preferential effects in the blood and bone marrow, as opposed to the spleen or lymph nodes, which indicates that alemtuzumab is most effective in hematologic disease. As an unconjugated mAb, this drug relies on inducing apoptotic signals

TABLE 36.3 Monoclonal Antibodies

Drug Name and Type	Route and Dosage	Uses and Considerations
Alemtuzumab	Chronic lymphocytic leukemia: A: IV: Initially, 3 mg over 2 h once daily. When tolerated, escalate dose to 10 mg/d until infusion reactions are grade 2 or less, then start maintenance dose: 30 mg 3 × weekly on alternate days (e.g., Monday, Wednesday, Friday). Total therapy duration including dose escalation is 12 wk. MS with inadequate response to two or more previous treatments: A: IV: First treatment: 12 mg daily for 5 d Second treatment: 12 months later, 12 mg daily for 3 d (Not FDA approved for subcut use).	For CLL and MS. Premedicate 30 min before infusion with diphenhydramine and acetaminophen and an antiinfective prophylaxis to reduce risk of opportunistic infection. Monitor for infusion-related reaction. *Absolute contraindication:* HIV PB: UK; t½: 12 d
Bevacizumab (*VEGFR*/mAb; prototype)	See Prototype Drug Chart: Bevacizumab	
Cetuximab	A: IV: Initial infusion dose is 400 mg/m² over 2 h, then continue weekly infusions of 250 mg/m² over 60 min.	For colorectal and head and neck cancers. Monitor for infusion-related reactions and worsening symptoms of cardiac or respiratory problems. PB: UK; t½: 41–213 h
Ibritumomab tiuxetan	A: IV: Given in two steps: Step 1: Day 1, admin rituximab 250 mg/m² with initial rate at 50 mg/h; increase as tolerated to a max of 400 mg/h. Step 2: Day 7, 8, or 9 repeat rituximab; within 4 h of second rituximab infusion, give ibritumomab 0.4 mCi/kg over 10 min; *max:* 32 mCi. Adjust dose for thrombocytopenia.	For untreated or relapsed/refractory follicular B-cell NHL. Premedicate with diphenhydramine and acetaminophen 30 min before each rituximab dose. Use actual body weight to calculate dose, not to exceed 32 mCi. *Do not* exceed 10% of the prescribed dose. *Do not* give Y-90 ibritumomab tiuxetan if platelets are <100,000 cells/mm³. Monitor CBC and platelet count. PB: UK; t½: 30 h
Panitumumab	A: IV: 6 mg/kg admin over 60 min given once q2wk.	Fully human Ab against EGFR colorectal cancer. Not indicated for *RAS* mutation–positive or *RAS* mutation–unknown cancers. Monitor for acute or worsening dermatologic changes; monitor serum electrolytes. PB: nonlinear, dose dependent; t½: 7.5 d
Trastuzumab	A: IV: Breast cancer: Week 1: 4 mg/kg over 90 min Week 2: If patient tolerates initial infusion, admin 2 mg/kg over 30 min once weekly. Other treatment protocols exist (see full prescriber's information). Gastric/GEJ adenocarcinoma given in combination with other chemotherapeutic drugs: Day 1: 8 mg/kg over 90 min. Day 22: 6 mg/kg over 30–90 min every 21 d.	*ERBB2*-positive metastatic breast cancer and not previously treated *ERBB2*-metastatic gastric or GEJ adenocarcinoma. *Do not* substitute trastuzumab for or with ado-trastuzumab emtansine. Monitor CBC and cardiac function; hold or adjust dose for LVEF ≥16% absolute decrease from baseline; may need to permanently discontinue. Monitor for infusion-related reactions such as fever, chills, and dyspnea. PB: UK; t½: dose dependent, 6–16 d

A, Adult; *Ab,* antibody; *admin,* administer; *CBC,* complete blood count; *CLL,* chronic lymphocytic leukemia; *d,* day; *EGFR,* epidermal growth factor receptor; *FDA,* US Food and Drug Administration; *GEJ,* gastroesophageal junction; *h,* hour; *HIV,* human immunodeficiency virus; *IV,* intravenous; *LVEF,* left ventricular ejection fraction; *mAb,* monoclonal antibody; *max,* maximum dosage; *mCi,* millicurie; *min,* minutes; *MS,* multiple sclerosis; *NHL,* non-Hodgkin lymphoma; *PB,* protein bound; *q,* every; *subcut,* subcutaneous, *t½,* half-life; *UK,* unknown; *VEGFR,* vascular endothelial growth factor receptor; *wk,* week; *Y-90,* yttrium-90; <, less than; ≥, greater than or equal to.

and activation of mechanisms such as complement or T cells to attack and kill the target cells. Alemtuzumab is also associated with the release of tumor necrosis factor, interleukin 6, and interferon gamma.

Side Effects and Adverse Reactions. The most common side effect of alemtuzumab that is not related to infusion reactions or pancytopenia is fatigue. Another common side effect is flulike symptoms. Subcutaneous injections, compared with IV infusion, have been shown to decrease the incidence of flulike symptoms. Additional reactions include nausea, blood pressure changes, hyperglycemia, and hypoxia; these are common and often require premedication with antihistamines and acetaminophen. Alemtuzumab can cause severe lymphopenia and a rapid, sustained lymphocyte count decrease in addition to fatal autoimmune pancytopenia and prolonged myelosuppression. Because of severe lymphopenia, patients are at increased risk for infections. Other adverse events include nonlethal arrhythmias, heart failure, cardiomyopathy, and decreased ejection fraction along with infusion reactions and rash. Some patients have reduced reactions with subsequent infusions.

Drug Interactions. Specific drug interactions have not been reported with this drug; however, concomitant administration of drugs with similar pharmacologic effects may cause additive side effects, including toxicity.

Cetuximab

Cetuximab is a recombinant human/mouse chimeric mAb that binds specifically to the extracellular domain of the human *EGFR*. However, cetuximab differs in mechanism of action from small-molecule TK inhibitors (e.g., imatinib) that inhibit the TK activity of *EGFR* by interfering with ATP binding; cetuximab blocks the *EGFR* receptor. It is most commonly used for the management of colorectal and head and neck cancers.

Pharmacokinetics. Cetuximab is administered as an IV infusion, and it exhibits nonlinear pharmacokinetics. The mean half-life ranges from 41 to 213 hours. Steady-state half-life ranges from 75 to 188 hours. The pharmacokinetics do not seem to have any effect on patients with renal or hepatic impairments.

Pharmacodynamics. Cetuximab still contains about 30% mouse protein. It binds specifically to *EGFR* on both normal and tumor cells and prevents formation of a ligand that usually attaches epidermal growth factor (*EGF*) to the receptor. This action prevents the receptor from binding to agonists that activate it. As a result, *EGFR*-TKs are not activated, and the signals are not conducted downstream. Other effects of this drug include inhibition of cell growth, induction of apoptosis, decreased proinflammatory cytokine and vascular growth factor production, and internalization of the *EGFR*. Cetuximab may make cancer cells more vulnerable to other cancer chemotherapy agents and radiation therapy. The drug is most effective in causing regression in tumors that have the wild-type *KRAS* oncogene and overexpress *EGFR*.

Side Effects and Adverse Reactions. Cetuximab carries a black-box warning for infusion reactions, usually with the initial dosing, although severe reactions also have been reported during later infusions. Manifestations include rapid onset of airway obstruction, including bronchospasm, stridor, hoarseness, urticaria, and hypotension. Cetuximab is associated with dermatologic changes that typically involve the face, upper chest, and back. An acneiform rash occurred in 90% of patients, usually within the first 2 weeks of therapy. Most patients continued to have the rash for at least 28 days after therapy was discontinued.

Drug Interactions. Minimal information is available on drug interactions, although cisplatin and radiation therapy increased the incidence of adverse events.

Ibritumomab Tiuxetan

Ibritumomab tiuxetan is a conjugated murine mAb. Yttrium-90 (Y-90), a pure beta-radionuclide ibritumomab, binds specifically to the human B lymphocytes that express the CD20 cell surface antigen. This drug is most commonly used for management of B-cell types of non-Hodgkin lymphoma (NHL).

Pharmacokinetics. Ibritumomab tiuxetan is administered as an IV infusion. Its physical half-life is 64 hours, and its biologic half-life (determined by radioactivity detection) is 30 hours. The drug is excreted to a slight degree by the kidneys (7.2%) but is mostly eliminated in the feces. Y-90 decays by emission of beta particles with a half-life of 64.1 hours.

Pharmacodynamics. Ibritumomab tiuxetan binds to the CD20 antigen on B lymphocytes and lymphoma cells. After binding with the CD20 antigen, beta-wave radioactive emissions from the attached radionuclide, Y-90, induce cellular damage by the formation of free radicals in the target and neighboring cells. This cellular damage prevents cells from dividing.

Side Effects and Adverse Reactions. Ibritumomab tiuxetan carries a black-box warning for infusion reactions, bone marrow suppression, and exfoliative dermatitis. Severe infusion reactions warrant discontinuing the drug. Less severe infusion reactions may be managed using premedication with antihistamines and acetaminophen.

Some patients experienced reduced reactions with the second and subsequent infusions. Common adverse effects include pancytopenia, asthenia, fever, chills, nausea, vomiting, cephalgia, abdominal pain, and infections.

Drug Interactions. Ibritumomab tiuxetan increases the risk for bleeding or hemorrhage when used along with anticoagulant or antiplatelet drugs, including NSAIDs, aspirin, salicylate derivatives, thrombolytic therapy, and anticoagulants. Immunization with live viruses is not recommended for 12 months after therapy because of the patient's immunosuppressed state. No other formal studies have been conducted with other drugs to determine specific drug interactions.

Panitumumab

Panitumumab is a fully human mAb with a high affinity for the *EGFR* extracellularly. It is most commonly used in the management of advanced metastatic colorectal carcinomas that express or overexpress *EGFR*.

Pharmacokinetics. Panitumumab is administered as an IV infusion. It is a small immunoglobulin that appears to be eliminated in the feces. The half-life ranges from 3.6 to 10.9 days, and the steady state is reached by the third infusion. Mild to moderate hepatic and renal impairment do not affect the drug's action.

Pharmacodynamics. Panitumumab binds strongly to the *EGFR* when it is overexpressed on malignant cells. It binds specifically to the *EGFR* on both normal and tumor cells. As a result, *EGFR*-TKs are not activated, and the signals are not conducted downstream. Other effects of this drug include inhibition of cell growth, induction of apoptosis, and decreased proinflammatory cytokine and vascular growth factor production. Tumors must express *EGFR* for patients to be candidates for panitumumab.

Side Effects and Adverse Reactions. Panitumumab carries a black-box warning for dermatologic toxicity. Manifestations usually occur within the first 2 weeks of therapy and include dry skin, skin fissures, erythema, acneiform rash, pruritus, exfoliation, and paronychia and other nail disorders. Electrolyte imbalances, specifically hypomagnesemia and hypocalcemia, may occur and require replacement. Severe diarrhea can occur when panitumumab is given along with irinotecan. Severe infusion reactions, including angioedema and anaphylaxis, have occurred with hypotension and bronchospasm. Although this reaction is rare, patients should be monitored closely throughout the infusion. Full resuscitative equipment should be available during infusion, including epinephrine, corticosteroids, IV antihistamines, bronchodilators, and oxygen.

Drug Interactions. Panitumumab is not recommended for use in combination with other antineoplastic drug regimens because of the increased toxic reactions. No other information on drug interactions is available.

Tositumomab

Tositumomab is a murine mAb conjugated with the radioactive isotope Iodine I-131. Like rituximab and ibritumomab tiuxetan, the antibody portion of this drug binds specifically to the human B lymphocytes that express the CD20 cell surface antigen. This drug is most commonly used to manage B-cell NHL that does not respond to rituximab.

Pharmacokinetics. Tositumomab is administered as four IV infusions in two distinct steps. It has a median blood clearance of 68.2 mg/h (with a 485-mg dosage). The mean total-body effective half-life is 67 hours. The Iodine I-131 decays with beta and gamma emissions with a half-life of 8.04 days. The elimination of Iodine I-131 occurs by decay and is excreted in the urine. Whole-body clearance was 67% of the injected dose, with elimination occurring mostly in the urine. Patients with high tumor burden, splenomegaly, or bone marrow

PROTOTYPE DRUG CHART

Rituximab

Drug Class	Dosage
Humanized monoclonal antibody	*Relapsed/refractory low-grade or follicular CD20-positive B-cell NHL:* A: IV: 375 mg/m^2 once weekly for 4 doses; may be retreated for an additional 4 doses Combination chemotherapy treatment: A: IV: Day 1 of each cycle, 375 mg/m^2 for up to 8 infusions Maintenance therapy with Y-90 ibritumomab: Day 1, admin 250 mg/m^2; day 7, 8, or 9, admin second rituximab dose within 4 h after Y-90 ibritumomab. *CD20-positive CLL in combination with fludarabine and cyclophosphamide:* Cycle 1: 375 mg/m^2 1 d before fludarabine and cyclophosphamide Cycles 2–6: 500 mg/m^2 plus fludarabine 25 mg/m^2/d on days 1–3 and cyclophosphamide 250 mg/m^2/d on days 1–3, repeated every 28 d for 6 cycles *RA, in combination with methotrexate:* 1000 mg on days 1 and 15. Admin subsequent courses every 16–24 wk based on clinical evaluation. Admin methylprednisolone 30 min before each infusion for RA. Premedicate 30 min before rituximab with diphenhydramine and acetaminophen.

Contraindications	Drug-Lab-Food Interactions
Patients who are or may become pregnant and those who are breastfeeding; those who have previously had hepatitis B; have active bacterial or viral infection; those who have moderate to severe renal, liver, and/or cardiac disease; and those with preexisting pulmonary fibrosis.	Drug: Hypotension is potentiated when drug is coadministered with antihypertensive drugs. Bone marrow suppression is potentiated when drug is coadministered with drugs that also cause bone marrow suppression, increasing risk for infection and bleeding. Rituximab reduces effectiveness of vaccinations. Lab: None known Food: None known

Pharmacokinetics	Pharmacodynamics
Absorption: Bioavailability is 100% after IV infusion. Distribution: Throughout extracellular fluid, bone marrow, and secondary lymphoid tissues (primarily the spleen); t½: first infusion, 76.3 h; fourth infusion, 205.8 h. Metabolism: Degraded by circulating and liver-based phagocytic cells. Excretion: As cellular debris in feces.	Antibody binding specifically to the CD20 cell surface antigen on B lymphocytes

Therapeutic Effects/Uses

Relapsed or refractory, low-grade, or follicular CD20-positive B-cell NHL, CLL, RA, Wegener granulomatosis.
Mechanism of Action: Binds to CD20-positive B lymphocytes and lymphoma cells, leading to complement-dependent cytotoxicity, antibody-dependent cellular cytotoxicity, and apoptosis.

Side Effects	Adverse Reactions
Bone marrow suppression with pancytopenia, tumor lysis syndrome, hypotension, night sweats, joint and muscle aches, headaches, soreness at injection site	Infusion reactions, pulmonary fibrosis, cardiac dysrhythmias, heart failure, reactivation of dormant viruses

A, Adult; *admin*, administer; *CLL*, chronic lymphocytic leukemia; *d*, day; *h*, hour; *IV*, intravenous; *min*, minute; *NHL*, non-Hodgkin lymphoma; *RA*, rheumatoid arthritis; *t½*, half-life; *wk*, week; *Y-90*, yttrium-90.

involvement had faster clearance, shorter terminal half-life, and larger volume distribution.

Pharmacodynamics. A tositumomab therapeutic regimen is administered as a two-step process. Each step consists of unlabeled tositumomab administered intravenously followed by Iodine I-131 tositumomab. The unlabeled tositumomab is given to decrease splenic targeting and to increase the terminal half-life of the Iodine I-131 tositumomab. The regimen induces cytotoxicity by combining the immunologic effects of antibody binding to nonmalignant B lymphocytes in the circulation, liver, and spleen. Actions of the antibody include the induction of complement-mediated cytolysis, antibody-dependent cellular cytotoxicity, and apoptosis. Radiation

activity is cytotoxic not only to the cells bound by the radiolabeled antibody but also to adjacent normal cells, a process called the *cross-fire effect*. Together, these actions result in sustained depletion of circulating CD20-positive lymphocytes and lymphoma cells.

Side Effects and Adverse Reactions. Tositumomab carries a black-box warning for fetal damage when used during pregnancy, for severe hypersensitivity reactions (anaphylaxis), severe bone marrow suppression, and radiation exposure. Specific tositumomab side effects and adverse effects include asthenia, headache, hypotension, nausea, vomiting, abdominal pain, diarrhea, hypothyroidism, cough, dyspnea, pleural effusion, and pneumonia. Toxicities associated with radioimmunotherapy can be acute, delayed, or long term. The

◎ CLINICAL JUDGMENT [NURSING PROCESS]

mTOR Inhibitors, Proteasome Inhibitors, and Monoclonal Antibodies

Concept: Cellular Regulation
- The ability for cells to maintain homeostasis, including responses to extracellular signals

Recognize Cues [Assessment]
- Obtain a detailed current medication history that includes prescription drugs, over-the-counter (OTC) medicines, antacids, dietary supplements, vitamins, and herbal supplements and check for possible drug–drug interactions with targeted therapy drugs.
- Obtain a list of the patient's drug and food allergies.
- Obtain baseline information about the patient's physical status. Include height, weight, vital signs, cardiopulmonary assessment, intake and output, skin assessment, nutritional status, and any underlying diseases.
- Assess baseline laboratory values (complete blood count [CBC], uric acid, chemistry panel) to compare with future ones.
- Assess baseline results of pulmonary function tests, chest radiographs, electrocardiograms (ECGs), and renal and liver function studies.
- Assess patient, family, and caregiver knowledge related to the therapeutic regimen.

Analyze Cues and Prioritize Hypothesis [Patient Problems]
- Disrupted fluid and electrolyte balance
- Potential for altered clotting
- Potential for decreased immunity
- Need for teaching

Generate Solutions [Planning]
- The patient will remain free from infection.
- The patient and family will verbalize understanding of targeted therapy as part of an anticancer treatment regimen.
- The patient and family will verbalize strategies to minimize risks related to targeted therapy–related side effects.
- The patient and family will demonstrate understanding of the importance of reporting targeted therapy–related side effects and adverse reactions.
- The patient's side effects will be managed to a tolerable level and are not life-threatening.

Take Action [Nursing Interventions]
- Assess for any cardiac events, such as new chest pain and ECG changes.
- Monitor appropriate labs according to established protocol for specific targeted therapy (e.g., CBC with differential, electrolytes, renal and hepatic function, glucose, phosphate).
- Assess for any bleeding, especially if the patient is taking anticoagulants, antiplatelets, or NSAIDs.
- Monitor liver function tests and renal function tests at baseline and at least once monthly during therapy.

- Examine the patient's skin closely at each visit for the presence of erythema, rash, peeling, or blister formation; rate the severity of dermatologic reactions, and determine whether infection is present in any nonintact skin.
- Administer prescribed premedications according to established protocols for specific targeted therapies (e.g., allopurinol, antiinfectives, antivirals, antihistamines).
- Have resuscitative equipment on standby as per protocol.
- Ensure appropriate supervising personnel are present according to protocols for specific targeted therapy.

Patient Teaching
General
- Ensure patient understands to avoid alcohol and nonessential drugs that are cleared by the liver or that have hepatotoxic effects (e.g., acetaminophen).
- Remind women with childbearing potential to avoid pregnancy throughout treatment and for up to 12 months after treatment is completed.
- Advise breastfeeding patients to stop breastfeeding during and for 60 days after therapy.
- Teach diabetic patients to monitor their glucose more frequently, and advise them when to seek medical help.
- Teach proper waste disposal to patients receiving monoclonal antibodies conjugated to radioisotopes (ibritumomab tiuxetan and tositumomab) to prevent unnecessary radiation exposure.

Side Effects
- Report symptoms of bleeding immediately, including black stools, vomit that looks like coffee grounds, and easy bleeding or bruising.
- Report symptoms of adverse effects or severe side effects promptly, especially fever, chills, persistent sore throat, swelling, weight gain, or increasing shortness of breath.
- Report symptoms of liver impairment immediately, including stomach/abdominal pain, yellowing eyes or skin, dark urine, or unusual fatigue.
- Advise the patient or a family member to immediately report convulsions, persistent headache, reduced eyesight, increased blood pressure, or blurred vision.

Evaluate Outcomes [Evaluation]
- Patient, family, and caregiver education needs are met.
- The patient, family, and caregiver understand therapy-related side effects and adverse reactions.
- The patient, family, and caregiver understand strategies to minimize side effects and adverse reactions.
- Side effects are managed effectively.
- The patient is free from infection.
- The patient's fluid balance and electrolytes are maintained at expected normal ranges.

---

most common acute toxicities are fever, rigors, fatigue, headache, and nausea, whereas hypotension and allergic reactions are less common. Delayed toxicities include shortness of breath, fever, signs of infection, inflammation, pain with urination, rash, sore joints, and bone marrow suppression. Long-term toxicities are myelodysplasia or acute leukemia, secondary malignancies, and hypothyroidism. Just as with other mAbs, this drug causes profound bone marrow suppression that may require dose interruptions or reductions, based on severity, and is more profound in patients who are also receiving standard cytotoxic chemotherapy. In addition, infusion reactions with fever, nausea, chills, blood pressure changes, hyperglycemia, and hypoxia

are common and often require premedication with antihistamines and acetaminophen. Some patients have reduced reactions with subsequent infusions.

Drug Interactions. Tositumomab increases the risk for bleeding or hemorrhage when used along with anticoagulant or antiplatelet therapy. When patients are immunosuppressed, immune response to vaccines and toxoids is decreased, and higher doses or more frequent boosters may be required. Other specific drug interactions have not been reported with this drug; however, concomitant administration of drugs with similar pharmacologic effects may cause additive side effects, including toxicity.

Trastuzumab

Trastuzumab is an mAb that binds to the *ERBB2* protein on the surface of cancer cells. The *ERBB2* receptor is structurally related to *VEGFR*. The *ERBB2* receptor is overexpressed in some breast, ovarian, and colon cancers. Proliferation and angiogenesis of cancer cells are increased with the overexpression of *ERBB2* receptors. When the VEGF pathway is inhibited, tumor growth is suppressed. Trastuzumab is most commonly used in combination with chemotherapy agents to manage breast and gastric cancers that have demonstrated overexpression of the *ERBB2* receptor. Trastuzumab and ado-trastuzumab emtansine are not interchangeable.

Pharmacokinetics. Trastuzumab is administered as a weekly IV infusion. Its half-life is 6 days. The steady state is reached within 9 weeks in patients with gastric cancer and 12 weeks in breast cancer patients. Elimination is unknown.

Pharmacodynamics. Trastuzumab is a mostly humanized mAb that binds to the *ERBB2* protein on the surface of breast, ovarian,

---

⚡ PATIENT SAFETY

Do not confuse...
• **Trastuzumab** with **ado-trastuzumab emtansine**

---

and colon cancer cells that overexpress this receptor. This drug specifically inhibits the proliferation of cancer cells that overexpress *ERBB2* receptors. In addition, binding of trastuzumab to the cancer cell receptor increases killing of these cells through attack by immune system cells, especially NK cells and monocytes.

Side Effects and Adverse Reactions. Trastuzumab carries a black-box warning for cardiomyopathy manifesting as congestive heart failure when the drug is used as a monotherapy. This risk is increased when the drug is given in combination with other drugs that cause cardiotoxicity, such as the anthracyclines and cyclophosphamide. Another black-box warning includes infusion-related reactions (anaphylaxis) and pulmonary toxicity. Hypersensitivity reactions, including anaphylaxis, may occur but are not common. Trastuzumab is associated with headache, dizziness, hypotension, fever, chills, and nausea during the initial infusion. After the initial infusion, these symptoms typically do not recur. Other common side effects include headache, muscle aches, and loss of appetite.

Drug Interactions. Trastuzumab can increase the incidence and severity of cardiac dysfunction in patients who receive trastuzumab in combination with anthracyclines and cyclophosphamide. Elevated INR can occur in patients taking warfarin concomitantly with trastuzumab. This drug may increase the myelosuppressive effects of other antineoplastic agents.

▌ CRITICAL THINKING CASE STUDY

A 64-year-old is diagnosed with stage III B-cell non-Hodgkin lymphoma (NHL). The patient is scheduled to receive rituximab and a traditional chemotherapy regimen of cyclophosphamide, doxorubicin, vincristine, and prednisolone, a combination known as "CHOP." The dosage and schedule of rituximab for the patient is 375 mg/m^2 IV on day 1 before the first CHOP chemotherapy cycle, which will be administered on day 8. The next two doses will be administered 2 days before the third and fifth cycles, and the remaining two cycles of rituximab will be administered after the sixth cycle of CHOP on days 134 and 141. The patient has a friend who is taking imatinib daily as an oral drug for CML and asks why rituximab must be taken intravenously through the implanted port. The patient also asks if

a family member, who is a licensed practical nurse, could administer it at home rather than having to travel to the clinic for the chemotherapy.

1. What is nurse's best response about why rituximab must be administered intravenously?
2. How are rituximab and imatinib different?
3. Why can the patient's family member *not* administer rituximab at home?
4. What side effects are specific for rituximab?
5. What are the most common adverse effects of rituximab?
6. What would the nurse teach the patient specifically in relation to rituximab therapy?

▌ REVIEW QUESTIONS

1. A patient undergoing chemotherapy for breast cancer asks why she is not receiving trastuzumab like her sister. Which response by the nurse is correct?
   a. Your breast cancer cells are estrogen receptor positive, and targeted therapy is not needed.
   b. You are much older than your sister and would not tolerate the treatment well.
   c. The drug is expensive, and your insurance does not cover it.
   d. Your cancer cells do not have the target for trastuzumab.
2. Which instruction is important for the nurse to include when teaching a patient about imatinib therapy?
   a. Do not drink grapefruit juice while taking this drug.
   b. Go immediately to the emergency department if you develop a headache.
   c. This drug will only work for about 2 months.
   d. Be sure to take this drug on an empty stomach.
3. Which patient problem is a priority for patients receiving epidermal growth factor receptor inhibitors?
   a. Potential for decreased clotting related to bone marrow suppression and neutropenia

   b. Potential for tissue injury related to skin side effects
   c. Potential for injury related to reduced platelet activity
   d. Disturbed self-concept related to alopecia
4. Which class of targeted therapy would cause the nurse the most concern in regard to a possible infusion reaction?
   a. Tyrosine kinase inhibitors
   b. Multikinase inhibitors
   c. Monoclonal antibodies
   d. Proteasome inhibitors
5. A patient taking sunitinib reports that the skin on the hands and feet is red and painful, and has some blisters. Which action is appropriate for the nurse to take?
   a. The only action needed is to document the finding because this is a mild side effect.
   b. Advise the patient to wear gloves and mittens when going outdoors in cold weather.
   c. Advise the patient to avoid getting hands wet and touching food.
   d. Notify the oncologist to determine whether a dosage reduction is needed.

6. Which action is most important for the nurse to teach a patient who is taking tositumomab?
   a. Avoid drinking alcohol for 1 week after receiving this drug.
   b. Avoid smoking cigarettes for the entire treatment period.
   c. Use a separate bathroom and sit while urinating for 1 week after receiving this drug.
   d. Be sure to take this drug on an empty stomach, either 1 hour before or 2 hours after eating.

7. Which activity has a higher priority for the nurse to advise the patient to avoid while taking ixazomib?
   a. Drinking alcoholic beverages
   b. Taking aspirin or aspirin-containing drugs
   c. Socializing in crowds or with persons who are ill
   d. Taking the drug 1 hour before or 2 hours after food

8. A patient receiving a targeted therapy asks the nurse why St. John's wort must be avoided. Which response by the nurse is most appropriate?
   a. This herbal drug increases blood levels of most targeted therapies and increases the risk for severe side effects or adverse reactions.
   b. This herbal drug decreases blood levels of most targeted therapies and reduces their effectiveness.
   c. Targeted therapies increase blood levels of St. John's wort, increasing the risk of an overdose of this herbal agent.
   d. Targeted therapies bind with St. John's wort in the intestinal tract, preventing absorption of both the drug and the herbal agent.

9. A patient taking imatinib voices concern about gaining 5 pounds in the past week. Which statement is correct about imatinib and weight gain?
   a. Weight gain is an expected side effect of this drug because it increases the appetite.
   b. Weight gain is an indication of slow metabolism and possible hypothyroidism.
   c. Weight gain is an indication of water retention and possible renal impairment.
   d. Weight gain is an indication of a drug interaction between imatinib and loop diuretics.

Biologic Response Modifiers

OBJECTIVES

- Compare the mechanisms of action of drugs classified as *biologic response modifiers* with those of standard chemotherapy drugs.
- Distinguish among the different types of biologic response modifiers with regard to indications, common side effects and adverse effects, route of administration, and nursing responsibilities.

- Discuss three common side effects of interferons, colony-stimulating factors, and interleukin 2.
- Incorporate the Clinical Judgment [Nursing Process] related to the needs of patients receiving biologic response modifiers.

OUTLINE

The immune system recognizes and protects the body from foreign invaders, such as bacteria or viruses; it also destroys damaged, diseased, or abnormal cells, including cancer cells. When the body detects an invader, an immune response is triggered, and substances such as white blood cells (WBCs), cytokines, and natural killer cells (NKCs) provide a certain level of protection. Biologic response modifiers (BRMs), also called *immunotherapies,* are a class of pharmacologic drugs used to enhance, direct, or restore the body's immune system. BRMs consist of substances naturally made in the body and those developed in the laboratory. They can kill cancer cells directly or indirectly. BRMs that target cancer cells directly are also called *targeted therapy,* and these are discussed in Chapter 36. Indirect therapies stimulate the body's immune system and do not directly target cancer cells. Biologic therapies are used to treat the cancer or the side effects caused by other cancer treatments. Recombinant DNA, the genetic engineering process that combines two human DNA strands artificially, and hybridoma technology, the process that genetically makes monoclonal antibodies, are two advances that have led to commercial mass production of BRMs (Fig. 37.1). Interferons (IFNs; alfa, beta, and gamma), tumor necrosis factor (TNF), erythropoietin (EPO), vaccine therapy, colony-stimulating factors (CSFs), interleukins, and monoclonal antibodies (mAbs) are some currently known BRMs. With the exception of monoclonal antibodies, BRMs are a complex set of proteins produced by the immune system (Fig. 37.2). Monoclonal antibodies are considered for targeted therapies and are further discussed in Chapter 36. Like chemotherapy, BRMs suppress the immune system; people in an immunocompromised state are at risk for complications such as infection. BRMs assist the immune system in several ways:

- They enhance the immune system's ability to kill abnormal cells (immunomodulation).
- They change cancer cells to make them behave more like healthy cells.
- They inhibit normal cells from changing into cancer cells.
- They enhance the body's ability to repair or replace damaged cells caused by other cancer treatments.
- They prevent cancer cells from metastasizing (spreading to other parts of the body).

New BRMs are always under development and investigation for clinical effectiveness. One newly emerged method of immunotherapy is chimeric antigen receptor T cell (CAR T cell), A person's T cells are removed and genetically modified to grow more of the T cells in a laboratory. These T cells are then infused to recognize and attack specific cancer cells and kill them. According to the American Society of Clinical Oncology (ASCO), the US Food and Drug Administration (FDA) has approved two CAR T-cell therapies to treat children and young adults with acute lymphoblastic leukemia and diffuse large B-cell lymphoma in adults. The drugs were approved in late 2017 and include tisagenlecleucel and axicabtagene ciloleucel. Other categories of BRMs have been approved by the FDA. Of the BRMs, IFNs, CSFs, and interleukin 2 (IL-2) are further discussed later in this chapter.

INTERFERONS

Interferons (IFNs) are a family of cytokines that occur naturally in the body. They are also produced in the laboratory. Various subtypes of IFNs have different mechanisms of action, with some overlapping actions. IFNs work directly on cancer cells to slow their growth or cause cancer cells to behave more like normal cells. Some IFNs also stimulate certain types of WBCs to fight cancer, which includes NKCs, T cells, and macrophages. The two main types of IFNs are type I and type II. *Type I interferons* include IFN-α (leukocyte IFN) and IFN-β

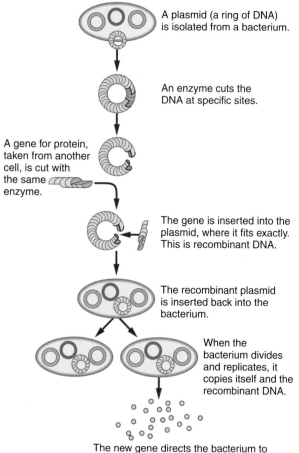

A plasmid (a ring of DNA) is isolated from a bacterium.

An enzyme cuts the DNA at specific sites.

A gene for protein, taken from another cell, is cut with the same enzyme.

The gene is inserted into the plasmid, where it fits exactly. This is recombinant DNA.

The recombinant plasmid is inserted back into the bacterium.

When the bacterium divides and replicates, it copies itself and the recombinant DNA.

The new gene directs the bacterium to make a new protein product, such as interferon.

Fig. 37.1 Recombinant DNA.

(fibroblast and epithelial cell IFN). *Type II interferon* includes IFN-γ produced by CD4+, CD8+, NKCs, and lymphokine-activated killer (LAK) cells. Table 37.1 provides information on IFNs with their dosages, uses, and considerations.

Interferon Alfa

B-lymphocyte cells; non–B- and non–T-lymphocyte cells; and macrophages (mature monocytes) produce interferon alfa-2b (IFN-α-2b) endogenously in response to viral infection and other various exogenous inducers. Exogenous α-2b IFNs used as BRMs are considered second-generation IFNs. IFN-α-2a, a first-generation IFN, is currently not being marketed; however, both subtypes have similar actions. IFNs bind to cell receptors for biologic activities followed by activation of the tyrosine kinases (TKs). IFNs have been shown to have antiviral, antiproliferative, and immunomodulatory effects, and they affect cellular differentiation, regulation of cell surface major histocompatibility complex (MHC) antigen expression, and cytokine induction.

IFN-α-2b is approved for hairy cell leukemia, AIDS-related Kaposi sarcoma, malignant melanoma, and non-Hodgkin lymphoma (NHL); hepatitis B and C viruses; and human papillomavirus (HPV) infection. Additionally, it has been used in combination with antiviral or anticancer drugs in patients with Philadelphia chromosome– positive (Ph+) chronic myelogenous leukemia (CML), renal cell cancer (RCC), and T-cell leukemia/lymphoma.

Pharmacokinetics. IFN-α-2b is administered parenterally via intravenous (IV), intramuscular (IM), or subcutaneous routes. Mean serum concentrations after IM and subcutaneous administration were similar. IFN is catabolized by the renal system. Maximum concentration occurs in 3 to 12 hours, and elimination half-life is 2 to 3 hours. After the IV route, the half-life is reached in about 2 hours and is undetectable in the serum in about 4 hours. IFN-α-2b is not cleared by hemodialysis.

Pharmacodynamics. IFN-α-2b has similar actions to native IFN-α. Endogenous IFNs are secreted by leukocytes in response to viral infection or various synthetic and biologic inducers. Once the IFN binds to cell surface receptors, TKs are activated, which produce several IFN-stimulated enzymes that cause antiviral, antiproliferative, and immunomodulatory effects; cellular differentiation; regulation of cell surface MHC antigen expression; and cytokine induction. Antiviral effects include inhibiting viral replication by inhibiting translation of

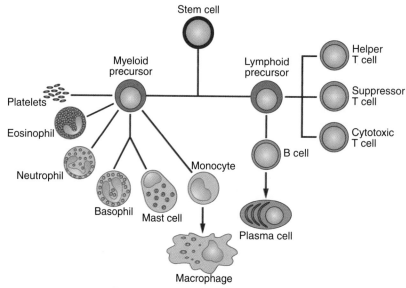

Fig. 37.2 Cells of the immune system.

TABLE 37.1 Biologic Response Modifiers: Interferons

Generic Drug Name	Route and Dosage	Uses and Considerations
Interferon alfa-2b	Hairy cell leukemia: A: IM/Subcut: 2 million units/m^2 3 times/wk for up to 6 mo Kaposi sarcoma: A: IM/Subcut: Initially: 30 million units/m^2 3 times/wk until severe intolerance or maximal response after 16 wk Malignant melanoma as adjuvant treatment: A: IV: Induction: 20 million units/m^2 for 5 consecutive d/wk for 4 wk Subcut: *Maint:* 10 million units/m^2 3 times/wk for 48 wk Non-Hodgkin's lymphoma (NHL): A: Subcut: 5 million units 3 times/wk for up to 18 mo	For hairy cell leukemia, adjuvant to surgical resection of malignant melanoma, follicular NHL, condyloma acuminata, AIDS-related Kaposi sarcoma, and chronic hepatitis B and non-A hepatitis. Monitor CBC, AST, ALT, ALP, LDH. PB: UK; t½: 2–3 h
Interferon gamma	Body surface area: >0.5 m^2: A: Subcut: 50 mcg/m^2 3 times/wk Body surface area: <0.5 m^2: A: Subcut: 1.5 mcg/kg/dose 3 times/wk	For chronic granulomatous disease and malignant osteopetrosis. PB: UK; t½: 0.5–6 h
Interferon beta-1b	Relapsing-remitting forms of MS: A: Subcut 250 mcg every other day. Incremental titration q2wk is recommended at 62.5 mcg every other day during wk 1 and 2, 125 mcg every other day during wk 3 and 4, and 187.5 mcg every other day during wk 5 and 6.	For MS. PB: UK; t½: 8 min–4.3 h

A, Adult; *AIDS,* acquired immunodeficiency syndrome; *ALP,* alkaline phosphatase; *ALT,* alanine aminotransferase; *AST,* aspartate aminotransferase; *CBC,* complete blood count; *d,* day; *h,* hour; *IM,* intramuscular; *IV,* intravenous; *LDH,* lactate dehydrogenase; *maint,* maintenance; *min,* minute; *mo,* month; *MS,* multiple sclerosis; *NHL,* non-Hodgkin lymphoma; *PB,* protein binding; *q,* every; *subcut,* subcutaneous; *t½,* half-life; *UK,* unknown; *wk,* week; *y,* year; >, greater than; <, less than.

TABLE 37.2 Adverse Effects and Dosage Modifications for Biologic Response Modifiers

Drug Class	Side Effects/Adverse Effects	Dose Adjustment or Discontinuation
Colony-stimulating factors: Erythropoietin (EPO)	Hypertension, flulike symptoms, rash, anaphylactoid reactions, antibody formation, arthralgia, myalgia, cephalgia, edema, red cell aplasia, thromboembolism, injection site reaction, urticaria, bronchospasm, cough, encephalopathy.	Stop treatment: Anaphylactoid reactions, red cell aplasia secondary to antibody formation Adjust dosage: Hgb rise >1 g/dL in 2 wk, CKD
Colony-stimulating factors: Granulocyte colony-stimulating factor (G-CSF), granulocyte-macrophage colony-stimulating factor (GM-CSF)	Peripheral edema, flulike symptoms, chest pain, splenomegaly, anaphylactoid reactions, elevated hepatic enzymes, rash, cardiac arrhythmia, cephalgia, arthralgia, leukocytosis, asthenia, antibody formation, pulmonary disorders, capillary leak syndrome.	Stop treatment: Anaphylactoid reaction, capillary leak syndrome, ANC >10,000/mm^3; ARDS, splenic involvement, sickle cell crisis, alveolar hemorrhage Adjust dosage: Vasculitis, renal disorders
Erythropoietin-stimulating drugs (ESAs; interferons)	Flulike symptoms (fever, chills, tachycardia, malaise, myalgia, cephalgia), chest pain, fatigue, depression, drowsiness, dizziness, irritability, paresthesia, insomnia, alopecia, skin rash, amenorrhea, nausea, diarrhea, vomiting, xerostomia, abdominal pain, pancytopenia, dyspnea, cough, pharyngitis, infection.	Stop treatment: Severe depression, hypersensitivity reactions, hematologic toxicity (ANC <500/mm^3 or platelets <25,000/mm^3); severe hepatic decompensation Adjust dosages for other hematologic toxicity.
Interleukin (IL-2)	Hypotension, peripheral edema, tachycardia, SVT, flulike symptoms, rash, pruritus, electrolyte imbalances, diarrhea, vomiting, nausea, weight gain, anorexia, abdominal pain, pancytopenia, elevated liver function tests, weakness, renal impairment, respiratory disorders, antibody formation, infection.	See Table 37.5.

ANC, Absolute neutrophil count; *ARDS,* acute respiratory distress syndrome; *CKD,* chronic kidney disease; *Hgb,* hemoglobin; *SVT,* supraventricular tachycardia; *wk,* week; >, greater than; <, less than.

viral proteins; inhibition of viral penetration and uncoating and/or viral assembly and release; and enhancement of the lytic (killing) effects of cytotoxic T lymphocytes. Viruses affected include hepatitis B, C, and D; herpes simplex virus types 1 and 2; human immunodeficiency virus (HIV); HPV; and rhinovirus, among others.

Antineoplastic effects may result from IFN's ability to induce a host response to the tumor (e.g., immunomodulatory effects), cause a cyto-static effect on tumor cells, and slow the rate of cell proliferation by enhancing or inhibiting the synthesis of specific proteins, modifying cell surface antigen expression, and/or modulating the immune system. IFNs prolong all phases of the cell cycle and promote cells to enter the G_0 (resting) phase, which is thought to be important in treating hairy cell leukemia.

Side Effects and Adverse Reactions

Side effects are not usually severe but, when present, persons may report flulike symptoms, fatigue, and loss of appetite. Table 37.2 lists the common adverse effects for BRMs, including IFNs, and any

TABLE 37.3   US Food and Drug Administration Black-Box Warnings for Interferon, Interleukin 2, and Erythropoietin

Interferon	Aldesleukin (IL-2)	Erythropoietin
Autoimmune disorders	Cardiac disease	Hgb concentration >11 g/dL
Infectious disorders	Coma	Myocardial infarction
Ischemic disorders	Capillary leak syndrome	Neoplastic disease
Neuropsychiatric disorders	Infection	Surgery
	Pulmonary disease	Thromboembolic disease
	Treatment requires a specialized setting and experienced clinician.	

Hgb, Hemoglobin; *IL*, interleukin; >, greater than.

dosage adjustments or discontinuation of the drug for toxicity. The black-box warning includes the risk of fatal or life-threatening neuropsychiatric, autoimmune, ischemic, and infectious disorders. Patients must be closely monitored with periodic clinical and laboratory evaluations. Table 37.3 compares the black-box warnings for IFN, IL-2, and EPO. While taking IFN-α, close monitoring of complete blood count (CBC), chest radiography (CXR), electrocardiography (ECG), liver function tests (LFTs), triglycerides, and thyroid function tests (TFTs) should be conducted.

Drug Interactions

It is unknown whether IFN-α-2b is metabolized by the liver; therefore caution is advised when IFN-α-2b is taken with other drugs metabolized through the hepatic cytochrome P450 enzyme system. The effect of IFN on the CYP450 system might increase enzyme degradation or inhibit CYP450 system. IFN-α-2b with concomitant use of theophylline may result in a 100% increase in theophylline concentrations. Caution is also warranted when taking drugs (e.g., antiretroviral nonnucleoside reverse transcriptase inhibitors [NNRTIs] and antiretroviral protease inhibitors) that can cause liver toxicity because IFNs also can cause liver damage. Hearing loss has been associated with IV eflornithine in combination with IFN-α-2b. Other drugs that may interact with IFN include barbiturates, colchicine, chemotherapy, and hydroxyurea. No information is available on drug-food or drug-herbal interactions.

Interferon Beta

Interferon beta (IFN-β) is a type I IFN produced by fibroblasts, macrophages, and epithelial cells. It has both antiviral and immune regulatory activities, especially against herpesvirus, HPV, hepatitis B and C, and HIV. IFN-β-1a is indicated for the treatment of multiple sclerosis (MS); IFN-β-1a inhibits the proinflammatory cytokines responsible for triggering the autoimmune reaction that leads to MS. IFN-β-1a also reduces T-cell migration across the blood-brain barrier and increases the production of nerve growth factor, which promotes axonal recovery; this may result in remyelination.

Interferon Gamma

Interferon gamma (IFN-γ) is a type II IFN produced endogenously by targeting macrophages, T lymphocytes, and NKCs, and it is genetically produced from *Escherichia coli*. IFN-γ regulates the immune system and interacts with other interleukins, and it has direct and indirect antiviral activities by affecting attachment, penetration, uncoating, transcription, assembly, and maturation of viruses. It is also the primary factor for macrophage activation to kill parasites and cancer cells. IFN-γ enhances antigen processing and presentation by increasing the expression of MHC. It also increases humoral immunity and the expression of tumor suppressor genes, and it enhances recruitment of leukocytes to the sites of inflammation. IFN-γ is used for the treatment of chronic granulomatous disease and osteopetrosis.

COLONY-STIMULATING FACTORS

Hematopoietic colony-stimulating factors (CSFs) are proteins that stimulate or regulate the growth, maturation, and differentiation of bone marrow stem cells. Like IFNs, CSFs are a subgroup of cytokines. Although CSFs are not directly tumoricidal, they are useful in cancer treatment. Chemotherapy depletes normal stem cells and the blood cells that they produce; CSFs promote the growth of these blood cells, which increases the opportunity to continue with chemotherapy. More specifically, CSFs have other functions:

- CSFs decrease the length of posttreatment neutropenia—the length of time neutrophils, a type of WBC, are decreased secondary to chemotherapy—thereby reducing the risk, incidence, and duration of infection.
- CSFs permit the delivery of higher doses of chemotherapy drugs. Myelosuppression, suppression of bone marrow activity, is often a dose-limiting toxicity of chemotherapy. Higher, possibly tumoricidal doses of these drugs cannot be administered because of potentially life-threatening side effects. CSFs can minimize the myelosuppressive toxicity, thus allowing the delivery of the higher doses.
- CSFs reduce bone marrow recovery time after bone marrow transplantation.
- CSFs enhance macrophage or granulocyte tumor-, virus-, and fungus-destroying abilities.
- CSFs prevent severe thrombocytopenia after myelosuppressive chemotherapy.

CSFs have been used to treat patients with neutropenia secondary to disease or treatment and can be administered both intravenously and subcutaneously. The CSFs that are FDA approved for clinical use are erythropoietin-stimulating agents (ESAs), granulocyte colony-stimulating factors (G-CSFs), and granulocyte-macrophage colony-stimulating factors (GM-CSFs).

Erythropoietin-Stimulating Agents

Erythropoietin (EPO) is a glycoprotein produced by the kidney; it stimulates red blood cell (RBC) production in the bone marrow. Specifically, EPO stimulates the division and differentiation of committed RBC progenitors (parent cells destined to become circulating RBCs) in the bone marrow. RBCs contain hemoglobin, which is necessary to transport oxygen in the body.

Erythropoietin-stimulating agents (ESAs) include epoetin alfa and darbepoetin alfa. These recombinant ESAs are used when blood transfusions are not an option. ESAs are administered as an injection to stimulate RBC production in the bone marrow. They must be used cautiously and only as indicated because of the potential for serious complications (e.g., myocardial infarction, stroke, venous thromboembolism, thrombosis of vascular access, and tumor progression or recurrence) and even death. Table 37.2 lists the common adverse effects for BRMs, including ESAs, dosage adjustments, and whether discontinuation of the drug is warranted. Prototype Drug Chart: Epoetin Alfa (Erythropoietin) provides specific drug information for epoetin alfa.

Pharmacokinetics. EPO can be administered either subcutaneously or intravenously. The IV route for either drug results in a more rapid peak, whereas the subcutaneous route, with its delayed systemic absorption, gives a more sustained response. Serum half-life for darbepoetin alfa after IV administration is 22.1 hours in patients without chronic renal failure (CRF). With subcutaneous injections, peak plasma concentrations occur at 71 to 123 hours (in CRF, peak is 24–72 hours), and the half-life of darbepoetin alfa in patients with CRF ranges from 27 to 89 hours. The pharmacokinetics in children suggests darbepoetin is absorbed more rapidly after subcutaneous injection compared with adults.

Pharmacodynamics. EPO stimulates erythropoiesis as endogenous EPO. Exogenous EPO stimulates the bone marrow in the production of RBCs to transport oxygen.

Side Effects and Adverse Reactions

Absolute contraindications for EPO include hypertension or hypersensitivity to albumin, hamster protein, or polysorbate 80. Black-box warnings include patients with a hemoglobin (Hgb) concentration greater than 11 g/dL, those who have had myocardial infarction (MI) or stroke, and patients with neoplastic or thromboembolic disease, because of the increased risk of death. Other side effects and adverse reactions are similar to those of epoetin alfa. Table 37.3 compares the black-box warnings for IFNs, IL-2, and EPO.

Drug Interactions

Darbepoetin alfa and epoetin alfa should not be used concomitantly because of the danger of adverse reactions. Concurrent administration of androgens can increase the patient's

---

PROTOTYPE DRUG CHART

Epoetin Alfa (Erythropoietin)

Drug Class	Dosage
Biologic response modifier	*Black Box Warning:* ESAs increase the risk for death when given to target Hgb >11 g/dL in cancer patients. A: Modify dose to keep target Hgb <11 g/dL. CKD: A/Adol ≥17 y: IV/Subcut: 50–100 units/kg 3 times/wk Dialysis patients: Initiate IV treatment when Hgb <10 g/dL Anemia as a result of myelosuppression: A: Subcut: 150 units/kg 3 times/wk or 40,000 units once/wk

Contraindications	Drug-Lab-Food Interactions
Absolute contraindications: Benzyl alcohol hypersensitivity *Black Box Warning:* Hgb concentration >11 g/dL; myocardial infarction; stroke; neoplastic disease; surgery; thromboembolic disease *Precautions:* Hypertension, anticoagulant therapy, cardiac disease, coagulopathy, dialysis, folate deficiency, heart failure, electrolyte imbalance, hyperparathyroidism, iron-deficiency hematologic disease, renal disease, seizure disorders, vitamin B$_{12}$ deficiency	Drug: Use with darbepoetin alfa has additive effects that increase adverse reactions. Androgens have an additive effect to epoetin alfa. Probenecid and amphotericin B may inhibit the response of epoetin. Lab: Inadequate iron stores interfere with the therapeutic response to epoetin alfa. Monitor transferrin saturation and serum ferritin before and during treatment. Administer iron therapy when serum ferritin is <100 mcg/L or when transferrin saturation is <20%. Food: None known

Pharmacokinetics	Pharmacodynamics
Absorption: Subcut, IV Distribution: PB: UK Metabolism: t½: Affected by renal function; 4–13 h in patients with CKD (IV); 20% less in those with normal renal function Excretion: Majority in feces, 10% in urine; dialysis does not remove EPO	Onset: Several days Peak: 5–24 h (subcut); IV with more rapid peak Duration: UK

Therapeutic Effects/Uses

Approved for use in the treatment of anemia to increase the Hgb concentration to the lowest level sufficient to avoid the need for RBC transfusions.
Mechanism of Action: Regulates the production of RBCs by stimulating the committed erythroid progenitor cells to divide and differentiate in the bone marrow to maintain optimal red cell mass for oxygen transport.

Side Effects	Adverse Reactions
Injection site reaction, myalgia, arthralgia, cephalgia, nausea, emesis, pruritus, cough, urticaria, dizziness, insomnia, anemia, fever, hypokalemia	Anaphylactoid reactions, angioedema, bronchospasm, MI, seizures, stroke, thromboembolism, red cell aplasia, hypertension, antibody formation, heart failure, encephalopathy

A, Adult; *Adol*, adolescent; *CKD*, chronic kidney disease; *EPO*, erythropoietin; *ESA*, erythropoietin-stimulating agent; *h*, hour; *Hgb*, hemoglobin; *IV*, intravenous; *MI*, myocardial infarction; *PB*, protein binding; *RBC*, red blood cell; *subcut*, subcutaneous; *t½*, half-life; *UK*, unknown; *wk*, week; *y*, year; <, less than; >, greater than; ≥, greater than or equal to.

📄 PROTOTYPE DRUG CHART

Filgrastim

Drug Class	Dosage
Granulocyte colony-stimulating factor	Chronic neutropenia, chemotherapy-induced neutropenia prophylaxis, after induction or consolidation therapy for AML; prophylaxis in nonmyeloid cancer A: IV/subcut: 5 mcg/kg/d HIV or drug therapy-induced neutropenia: A: Subcut: 5–10 mcg/kg/d 1–3 times weekly to maintain ANC of 2000–10,000/mm^3 Refer to specific protocols.
Contraindications	**Drug-Lab-Food Interactions**
Absolute: Hypersensitivity to *Escherichia coli*–derived proteins or 24 h before or after cytotoxic chemotherapy *Precautions:* Pregnancy, lactation, latex hypersensitivity, leukemia, leukocytosis, obstetric delivery, pulmonary bleeding, radiation therapy, respiratory distress syndrome, sickle cell disease, vasculitis, thrombocytopenia	Drug: No clinically important drug interactions have been noted, but drugs that can increase the release of neutrophils (e.g., lithium) should be used with caution. Lab: Leukocytosis, thrombocytopenia, proteinuria, elevated LDH, and increased ALP Food: None known
Pharmacokinetics	**Pharmacodynamics**
Absolute bioavailability with subcut route is 60%–70%. Absorption: Subcut: Well absorbed Distribution: PB: UK Metabolism: t½: 1.8–3.5 h Excretion: Mainly by the kidneys; clearance is nonlinear and dependent on drug concentration and neutrophil count	Onset: UK Peak: 2–8 h Duration: ANC decreases to baseline in approximately 4 d.
Therapeutic Effects/Uses	
To decrease incidence of infection in patients with MDS; in those receiving myelosuppressive chemotherapeutic drugs, including patients with AML undergoing induction or consolidation therapy; in aplastic anemia; and for mobilization of progenitor stem cells used in autologous transplant; also for treatment of patients with severe chronic neutropenia Mechanism of Action: Increases production, maturation, and activation of neutrophils and enhances their migration and cytotoxicity	
Side Effects	**Adverse Reactions**
Most common side effects include nausea, vomiting, arthralgia, alopecia, diarrhea, fever, fatigue, skin rash, anorexia, cephalgia, cough, chest pain, sore throat, constipation, dizziness, and dyspnea.	Splenomegaly, thrombocytopenia, MI, ARDS, splenic rupture, capillary leak syndrome, anaphylactoid reactions, glomerulonephritis, pulmonary bleeding/alveolar hemorrhage, and cutaneous vasculitis

A, Adult; *ALP,* alkaline phosphatase; *AML,* acute myelogenous leukemia; *ANC,* absolute neutrophil count; *ARDS,* acute respiratory distress syndrome; *d,* day; *h,* hour; *IV,* intravenous; *LDH,* lactate dehydrogenase; *MDS,* myelodysplastic syndrome; *MI,* myocardial infarction; *PB,* protein binding; *subcut,* subcutaneous; *t½,* half-life; *UK,* unknown.

response to EPO. In addition, the patient's iron stores should be repleted because inadequate iron interferes with EPO's therapeutic response.

Granulocyte Colony-Stimulating Factor

Endogenous granulocyte colony-stimulating factor (G-CSF) is produced by macrophages, endothelium, and other immune cells, and stimulates the synthesis of neutrophils. Neutrophils are the most abundant WBCs that take part in the inflammatory response system, and their main function is to detect and destroy harmful bacteria. Recombinant DNA technology can produce CSFs for human granulocytes to be used for myelodysplastic syndrome (MDS) and for patients receiving myelosuppressive cancer chemotherapy, induction or consolidation chemotherapy for acute myeloid leukemia (AML), and bone marrow transplantation for cancer; for severe, chronic neutropenia; and to increase the hematopoietic stem cells in stem cell donors before leukapheresis. Two commercially available forms are filgrastim and pegfilgrastim.

Unlike filgrastim, pegfilgrastim is administered once per chemotherapy cycle. Prototype Drug Chart: Filgrastim provides specific drug information for filgrastim.

Granulocyte-Macrophage Colony-Stimulating Factor

Granulocyte-macrophage colony-stimulating factor (GM-CSF), or *sargramostim,* belongs to a group of growth factors that support survival, proliferation, and differentiation (maturation) of hematopoietic progenitor cells. It induces partially committed progenitor (parent) cells to divide and differentiate in the granulocyte-macrophage pathway. GM-CSF, unlike G-CSF, is a multilineage factor that promotes proliferation of myelomonocytic, megakaryocytic, and erythroid progenitors. It is primarily produced by the bone marrow, B and T lymphocytes, and monocytes (immature macrophages). Commercially prepared GM-CSF came about through recombinant DNA technology and is FDA approved for use to reduce neutropenia and promote myeloid recovery in patients receiving myelosuppressive chemotherapy or bone marrow transplant (BMT), for mobilization of autologous

PROTOTYPE DRUG CHART

Sargramostim

Drug Class	Dosage
Granulocyte-macrophage colony-stimulating factor	After reinfusion of BMT: A: 250 mcg/m²/d subcut or IV over 2 h After failed or delayed engraftment from BMT: A: 250 mcg/m²/d subcut or IV over 2 h for 14 d; may repeat after having 7 d off therapy. If a third dose is warranted, give 500 mcg/m²/d for 14 d after 7 d off therapy. Other dosing protocols are available.

Contraindications	Drug-Lab-Food Interactions
Absolute: Concomitant use with chemotherapy and/or radiation therapy or within 24 h of chemotherapy administration or within 12 h after last dose of radiation therapy; yeast hypersensitivity; excessive leukemic blasts (≥10%) in the bone marrow or peripheral blood *Caution:* Pregnancy, lactation, cardiac arrhythmias, heart failure, leukemia, mannitol hypersensitivity, neonates, pulmonary disorders, leukocytosis	Drug: Drugs having synergistic effects may increase leukocytosis (e.g., lithium and corticosteroids); however, formal drug interaction data are currently not available. Sargramostim may increase the activity of zidovudine. Lab: Leukocytosis including neutrophilia, hyperbilirubinemia, elevated transaminases and serum creatinine Food: None known

Pharmacokinetics	Pharmacodynamics
Absorption: IV: Essentially complete Distribution: PB: UK Metabolism: t½: 1 h (IV); 2.7 h (subcut) Excretion: Mostly in urine as inactive protein fragments	Onset: 7–14 d Peak: 1–3 h (subcut) Duration: Baseline WBCs within 1 wk of stopping therapy

Therapeutic Effects/Uses	
To accelerate growth and development of myeloid cell lines to shorten neutropenic state, to mobilize peripheral blood progenitor cells for collection, and for bone marrow graft failure or engraftment delay Mechanism of Action: Stimulates the proliferation and differentiation of myeloid cell lines to enhance immune defense mechanism; enhances the function of mature granulocytes and monocytes; enhances bacteriocidal activity of neutrophils	

Side Effects	Adverse Reactions
Generally well tolerated, but SEs may occur. Common SEs include arthralgia, myalgia, diarrhea, fatigue, chills, weakness, asthenia, cephalgia, malaise, unspecified chest pain, local irritation at injection site, peripheral edema, rash, and fever.	Pleural/pericardial effusion, capillary leak syndrome, anaphylactoid reactions, rigors, GI hemorrhage, dyspnea, hypotension

A, Adult; *BMT,* bone marrow transplant; *d,* day; *GI,* gastrointestinal; *h,* hour; *IV,* intravenous; *PB,* protein binding; *SEs,* side effects; *subcut,* subcutaneous; *t½,* half-life; *UK,* unknown; *WBC,* white blood cell; *wk,* week; ≥, greater than or equal to.

TABLE 37.4   Interleukin 2ᵃ

Generic	Route and Dosage	Uses and Considerations
Aldesleukin	Two 5-d treatment periods are separated by a rest period. A: IV: 600,000 units/kg (0.037 mg/kg) over 15 min q8h; *max:* 14 doses. After 9 d of rest, repeat the schedule for another 14 doses; *max:* 28 doses per course	For metastatic renal cancer and metastatic melanoma *Do not* give dexamethasone during treatment unless absolutely necessary; it may negate the effects of IL-2.

A, Adult; *d,* day; *h,* hour; *IL,* interleukin; *IV,* intravenous; *max,* maximum; *min,* minute; *q,* every.

ᵃPatients receiving IL-2 by any route, in any dose, and in any setting—inpatient or outpatient—should be monitored closely for signs of toxicity.

peripheral blood progenitor cells, and in BMT failure or delayed engraftment. Prototype Drug Chart: Sargramostim provides specific drug information for sargramostim.

INTERLEUKIN 2

Interleukins are a group of signaling molecule proteins produced by leukocytes, more specifically by T lymphocytes. Because interleukins are hormone-like glycoproteins manufactured by T lymphocytes, they are sometimes called lymphokines. Interleukins also increase the growth and activity of other T cells and B cells, which affects the immune response system. One of the most widely studied interleukins is IL-2. Table 37.4 provides information on IL-2 and includes dosages, uses, and considerations.

IL-2 is produced commercially through recombinant DNA technology as aldesleukin. It is FDA approved for treatment of metastatic renal cell carcinoma and metastatic melanoma by inducing proliferation and differentiation of B and T cells along with other cells involved in the immune system. Table 37.2 lists common adverse effects with IL-2 therapy.

Pharmacokinetics. Aldesleukin is administered intravenously or subcutaneously and is rapidly distributed to the extravascular and extracellular spaces and to the liver, spleen, kidneys, and lungs. After IV administration, the serum distribution and elimination half-life is 13 and 85 minutes, respectively. After subcutaneous injection, the serum levels were slightly prolonged. Aldesleukin is cleared from the systemic circulation by the kidneys and is then metabolized into amino acids by the renal cells; the drug is also affected by the cytochrome P450 isoenzymes.

Pharmacodynamics. Aldesleukin has essentially identical effects to those of endogenous IL-2. The interaction of the drug with the IL-2 receptors stimulates the cytokine cascade and involves various IFNs, interleukins, and TNFs. Along with these other cytokines, aldesleukin induces proliferation and differentiation of B and T lymphocytes, monocytes, macrophages, and NKCs, among others.

Side Effects and Adverse Reactions

The black-box warning includes patients with cardiac disease, coma, capillary leak syndrome, infection, and pulmonary disease, and warns that the drug must be administered in a specialized care setting by an experienced clinician. Table 37.3 compares the black-box warnings for IFNs, IL-2, and EPO. Box 37.1 lists absolute contraindications for aldesleukin.

> ### ⚡ BOX 37.1 Absolute Contraindications for Aldesleukin
>
> | | |
> |---|---|
> | Angina | Organ transplant |
> | Cardiac arrhythmias | Psychosis |
> | Cardiac disease | Pulmonary disease |
> | Cardiac tamponade | Renal failure |
> | Coma | Respiratory insufficiency |
> | Gastrointestinal bleeding | Seizures |
> | Gastrointestinal perforation | Ventricular tachycardia |
> | Myocardial infarction | |

⚠ Conventional high-dose IV bolus aldesleukin is associated with significant adverse reactions that affect almost every organ system. Many of the adverse effects may be due to capillary leak syndrome, which results from extravasation of plasma proteins and fluid into the extravascular space, which leads to vascular atony. Vascular tone is lost within 2 to 12 hours of starting aldesleukin and causes decreased arterial pressure and decreased organ perfusion, resulting in multiorgan dysfunction that leads to death. Once the drug is discontinued, the capillary leak syndrome resolves within a few hours. Other side effects and adverse reactions include hyperglycemia, diabetes, metabolic and respiratory acidosis, and electrolyte imbalance (e.g., hypomagnesemia and hypocalcemia). Because of the many potential adverse effects, patients must be selected with care, and those with significant cardiac, pulmonary, renal, hepatic, or central nervous system impairments must be excluded. Table 37.5 provides information on aldesleukin for dose interruption or discontinuation for drug toxicity.

Drug Interactions

Because of the number of serious adverse effects associated with aldesleukin therapy, almost any other drug represents a potential interaction. Aldesleukin is associated with kidney and liver toxicity, and other drugs known to cause such toxicity can exacerbate the impairment caused by aldesleukin (e.g., vancomycin, cyclosporine, nonsteroidal antiinflammatory drugs [NSAIDs], methotrexate, isoniazid [INH], and ethanol). Antihypertensives (e.g., beta blockers and calcium channel blockers) can worsen hypotension. The immune response from vaccines may be decreased if given to those who are immunocompromised and receiving aldesleukin.

> ### ⚡ PATIENT SAFETY
>
> **Do not Confuse...**
> - **Interferon alfa-2a** with **interferon alfa-2b**
> - **Interferon alfa** with **interferon beta** or **interferon gamma**
> - **Interleukin 2** with **interferon 2**
> - **Darbepoetin alfa** with **epoetin alfa**

TABLE 37.5 Aldesleukin[a] Dose Interruption or Discontinuation

Body System	Interruption[b]	Discontinue Permanently
Mental health	Any changes to mental status, including confusion or agitation	Coma or toxic psychosis lasting more than 48 h, poorly managed seizures
Skin, hair, and nails	New bullous dermatitis or worsening of preexisting skin condition; may treat with antihistamines; *do not* treat with topical steroids.	
⚠ Cardiovascular	Atrial fibrillation, SVT, or bradycardia that is persistent, recurrent, or needs treatment SBP <90 mm Hg if it requires vasopressors ECG changes consistent with MI, ischemia, or myocarditis	Sustained ventricular tachycardia ≥5 beats Uncontrolled cardiac rhythm disturbances ECG changes that show MI or cardiac tamponade
Pulmonary	O₂ saturation <90%	Requiring intubation >72 h
Endocrine	Hypoglycemia	
Hematology	Sepsis	
GI/GU	Stool guaiac repeatedly >3–4+; serum creatinine >4.5 mg/dL or ≥4 mg/dL with severe volume overload, acidosis, or hyperkalemia; persistent oliguria, UO <10 mL/h for 16–24 h with increasing serum creatinine	Renal failure that requires dialysis >72 h; bowel ischemia or perforation or GI bleeding that requires surgery
Hepatobiliary	Hepatic failure, including encephalopathy, ascites, liver pain, hypoglycemia	

ECG, Electrocardiograph; *GI/GU*, gastrointestinal/genitourinary; *h*, hours; *MI*, myocardial infarction; *O₂*, oxygen; *SBP*, systolic blood pressure; *SVT*, supraventricular tachycardia; *UO*, urine output; *<*, less than; *>*, greater than; *≥*, greater than or equal to.

⚠ [a]Aldesleukin must be withheld or interrupt a dose due to drug toxicity; *do not reduce dose.*

[b]May be resumed with dose adjustment once toxicity has resolved.

◎ CLINICAL JUDGMENT [NURSING PROCESS]

Biologic Response Modifiers

Concept: Immunity
- The protective response of the body toward inflammation and infection

Recognize Cues [Assessment]
- Conduct a detailed current medication history that includes prescriptions, over-the-counter (OTC) medicines, antacids, dietary supplements, vitamins, and herbal supplements.
- Obtain a list of the patient's drug and food allergies.
- Obtain baseline information about physical status that includes height, weight, vital signs, cardiopulmonary assessment, intake and output, skin assessment, nutritional status, and any underlying diseases.
- Obtain baseline laboratory values (complete blood count [CBC] with differentials and platelet count, uric acid, chemistry panel, lipid panel, and thyroid panel) before and during treatment.
- ⚡ With erythropoietin-stimulating agents, assess serum ferritin and serum iron–transferrin saturation. Most patients will need supplemental iron.
- Assess baseline results of pulmonary function tests, chest radiographs, electrocardiogram (ECG), and kidney and liver function studies.
- Assess patient's and caregiver's level of comprehension and physical ability related to the therapeutic regimen.

Analyze Cues and Prioritize Hypothesis [Patient Problems]
- Decreased immunity
- Need for teaching

Generate Solutions [Planning]
- The patient and caregivers will verbalize signs and symptoms of significant reactions (e.g., wheezing; chest pain; swelling of face, neck, lips, throat, or tongue; emotional instability; altered speaking or thinking; and excessive weight gain or loss).
- The patient and caregivers will verbalize when to notify the health care provider or seek emergency treatment.
- The patient will remain free from infection.
- The patient and caregivers will verbalize understanding of immunotherapy as part of an anticancer treatment regimen.

Take Action [Nursing Interventions]
- Assess for any cardiac events, such as new chest pain and ECG changes.
- ⚡ Monitor appropriate labs according to established protocol for the specific immunotherapy (e.g., CBC with differential, electrolytes, renal and hepatic function, and glucose).
- Assess for bleeding, especially in patients taking anticoagulants, antiplatelets, or nonsteroidal antiinflammatory drugs (NSAIDs).

- Monitor renal and hepatic function at baseline and per treatment protocol.
- Examine the patient's skin closely at each visit for the presence of erythema, rash, peeling, or blister formation, and rate the severity of any dermatologic reactions.
- ⚡ During treatment, monitor patients for any indications of adverse effects such as fever, chills, hypoxia, wheezing, bradycardia or tachycardia, hypotension or hypertension, arrhythmia, or seizures.
- Premedicate patients with acetaminophen to reduce chills and fever, and with diphenhydramine to reduce histamine effects.
- Have resuscitative equipment on standby as per protocol.
- Actively listen to patient and caregiver concerns, and explain in laymen's terms the immunotherapy being used as part of the patient's cancer treatment regimen.

Patient Teaching
General
- Report flulike symptoms, such as chills, fever, myalgia, and weakness.
- Report unmanageable nausea and vomiting.
- Instruct patient to not receive vaccines with live viruses.
- Inform patient of the need for frequent laboratory tests.
- Teach patient to avoid crowds and people with infection.

Side Effects
- Report symptoms of bleeding immediately; these include black stools, vomit that looks like coffee grounds, easy bleeding/bruising, or hematuria.
- Report symptoms of adverse effects or severe side effects promptly, especially chest pain; swelling of the face, neck, tongue, or lips; weight gain or loss; increasing shortness of breath; fever or chills; convulsions; or difficulty speaking.
- Advise patients and caregivers to immediately report convulsions, persistent headache, reduced eyesight, increased blood pressure, decreased urine output, or blurred vision.

Evaluate Outcomes [Evaluation]
- The patient is free of further injury related to immunotherapy.
- Side effects are managed effectively.
- The patient is free from infection.
- Patient, family, and caregiver education needs are met.
- The patient, family, and caregivers understand therapy-related side effects and adverse reactions.
- The patient, family, and caregivers understand strategies to minimize side effects and adverse reactions.

▮ CRITICAL THINKING CASE STUDY

A 75-year-old patient has metastatic non–small cell cancer of the lung. The patient's past treatment regimen included external-beam chest irradiation and combination chemotherapy. Two weeks before hospitalization, the patient received a course of carboplatin and paclitaxel as an outpatient, with subsequent admission to the hospital with neutropenia, thrombocytopenia, and anemia. Upon assessment, the patient was cachectic and weak but was able to perform activities of daily living with only minimal assistance. Admitting laboratory data were hemoglobin (Hgb) 6.9 g/dL, hematocrit (Hct) 20.6%, platelets $16 \times 10^3/\mu L$, a WBC count of $6 \times 10^3/\mu L$ with an absolute neutrophil count (ANC) of $0.096 \times 10^3/\mu L$. The patient was prescribed units subcutaneously once a week and filgrastim, G-CSF 5 mcg/kg/day given subcutaneously. Parenteral antibiotic therapy was also initiated.

1. Why were filgrastim and erythropoietin (EPO) indicated?
2. What must be monitored closely in patients receiving EPO and why?
3. List three patient problems for this patient.
4. Identify three nursing actions for each of the patient problems identified in Question 3.

REVIEW QUESTIONS

1. Which action is primary for interferon alfa?
   a. Enhancing immune function and producing antigen/antibody reaction
   b. Causing allergic reactions, producing red blood cells, and producing interferon
   c. Immunomodulation, causing cytotoxic/cytostatic effects, and differentiating stem cells
   d. Producing cytokines, producing interleukin, and fighting infection

2. A patient diagnosed with malignant melanoma, a skin cancer, is treated with interferon alfa-2a. The nurse teaches this patient about which side effect?
   a. Increase in white blood cells
   b. Increase in red blood cells
   c. Flulike syndrome
   d. Gastrointestinal symptoms

3. The nurse reviews the list of medications and is aware that red blood cell production can be stimulated with which drug for anemia?
   a. Epoetin alfa
   b. Filgrastim
   c. Interleukin 2
   d. Sargramostim

4. Which drug must be administered intravenously?
   a. Epoetin alfa
   b. Interleukin 2
   c. Granulocyte colony-stimulating factor
   d. Granulocyte-macrophage colony-stimulating factor

5. In developing a plan of care for the patient, the nurse understands that the order for pegfilgrastim was prescribed for which reason?
   a. Pegfilgrastim is eliminated via the kidneys.
   b. Pegfilgrastim is a pegylated filgrastim.
   c. Pegfilgrastim is not easily eliminated from the body.
   d. Pegfilgrastim requires injection once per chemotherapy cycle.

6. A patient receiving erythropoietin-stimulating drug has the following laboratory values: hemoglobin, 12.8 mg/dL; platelet count, 148,000/mm^2; white blood cell count, 4800/mm^2. Which action is most appropriate for the nurse to implement?
   a. Discuss with the health care provider the potential need for a colony-stimulating factor such as granulocyte colony-stimulating factor based on the laboratory results.
   b. Contact the health care provider to discuss the laboratory results and a possible discontinuation of the ordered erythropoietin-stimulating agent.
   c. Discuss the laboratory values with the health care provider to determine whether a colony-stimulating factor such as interleukin 2 should be given.
   d. Discuss with the health care provider the potential need for more laboratory tests before administration of the erythropoietin-stimulating agent.

Upper Respiratory Disorders

http://evolve.elsevier.com/McCuistion/pharmacology

OBJECTIVES

- Compare antihistamine, decongestant, antitussive, and expectorant drug groups.
- Differentiate between rhinitis, sinusitis, and pharyngitis.

- Describe the side effects of nasal decongestants and how they can be avoided.
- Apply the Clinical Judgment [Nursing Process] for drugs used to treat the common cold.

OUTLINE

INTRODUCTION

The respiratory tract is divided into two major parts: the *upper respiratory tract,* which consists of the nares, nasal cavity, pharynx, and larynx, and the *lower respiratory tract,* which consists of the trachea, bronchi, bronchioles, alveoli, and alveolar-capillary membrane. Air enters through the upper respiratory tract and travels to the lower respiratory tract, where gas exchanges occur. Fig. 38.1 illustrates these components.

Ventilation and *respiration* are distinct terms and should not be used interchangeably. Ventilation is the movement of air from the atmosphere through the upper and lower airways to the alveoli. *Respiration* is the process whereby gas exchange occurs at the alveolar-capillary membrane. Respiration has three phases:

- *Ventilation* is the phase in which oxygen passes through the airways. With every inspiration, air is moved into the lungs, and with every expiration, air is transported out of the lungs.
- *Perfusion* involves blood flow at the alveolar-capillary bed. Perfusion is influenced by alveolar pressure. For gas exchange to occur, the perfusion of each alveolus must be matched by adequate ventilation. Factors such as mucosal edema, secretions, and bronchospasm increase resistance to air flow and decrease ventilation and diffusion of gases.
- *Diffusion,* the movement of molecules from higher to lower concentrations, takes place when oxygen passes into the capillary bed to be

circulated and carbon dioxide leaves the capillary bed and diffuses into the alveoli for ventilatory excretion.

Upper respiratory infections (URIs) include the common cold, acute rhinitis, sinusitis, and acute pharyngitis. The common cold is the most prevalent type of URI. Adults have an average of 2 to 4 colds per year, and children have an average of 4 to 12 colds per year. Incidence is seasonally variable: approximately 50% of the population experiences a winter cold and 25% experience a summer cold. A cold is not considered a life-threatening illness, but it does cause physical and mental discomfort and lost time at work and school. The common cold is an expensive illness in the United States—more than $60 billion is spent each year on over-the-counter (OTC) cold and cough preparations in addition to missed time at work and school.

COMMON COLD, ACUTE RHINITIS, AND ALLERGIC RHINITIS

The common cold is caused by the rhinovirus and affects primarily the nasopharyngeal tract. Acute rhinitis, acute inflammation of the mucous membranes of the nose, usually accompanies the common cold. Acute rhinitis is not the same as allergic rhinitis, often called *hay fever,* which is caused by pollen or a foreign substance such as animal dander. Nasal secretions increase in both acute and allergic rhinitis.

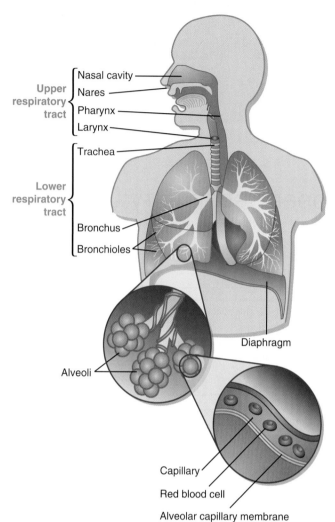

Upper respiratory tract
- Nasal cavity
- Nares
- Pharynx
- Larynx

Lower respiratory tract
- Trachea
- Bronchus
- Bronchioles

Diaphragm

Alveoli

Capillary
Red blood cell
Alveolar capillary membrane

Fig. 38.1 Basic structures of the respiratory tract.

A cold is most contagious 1 to 4 days before the onset of symptoms (the incubation period) and during the first 3 days of the cold. Transmission occurs more frequently from touching contaminated surfaces and then touching the nose or mouth than it does from contact with viral droplets released by sneezing.

The groups of drugs used to manage cold symptoms include antihistamines (H_1 blockers), decongestants (sympathomimetic amines), antitussives, and expectorants. These drugs can be used singly or in combination preparations.

Symptoms of the common cold include rhinorrhea (watery nasal discharge), nasal congestion, cough, and increased mucosal secretions. If a bacterial infection secondary to the cold occurs, infectious rhinitis may result, and nasal discharge becomes tenacious, mucoid, and yellow or yellow green. The nasal secretions are discolored by white blood cells and cellular debris that are by-products of the fight against the bacterial infection. Antibiotics used to treat bacterial respiratory infections are discussed in Chapter 26.

Antihistamines

Antihistamines, H_1 blockers or H_1 antagonists, compete with histamine for receptor sites and prevent a histamine response. The two types of histamine receptors, H_1 and H_2, cause different responses. When the H_1 receptor is stimulated, the extravascular smooth muscles—including

those lining the nasal cavity—are constricted. With stimulation of the H_2 receptor, an increase in gastric secretions occurs, which is a cause of peptic ulcer (see Chapter 46). These two types of histamine receptors should not be confused. Antihistamines decrease nasopharyngeal secretions by blocking the H_1 receptor.

Although antihistamines are commonly used as cold remedies, these agents can also treat seasonal allergies that cause allergic rhinitis. However, antihistamines are not useful in an emergency situation such as anaphylaxis. Most antihistamines are rapidly absorbed in 15 minutes, but they are not potent enough to combat anaphylaxis.

First-Generation Antihistamines

The antihistamine group can be divided into first and second generations. Most *first-generation antihistamines* cause drowsiness, dry mouth, and other anticholinergic symptoms, whereas *second-generation antihistamines* have fewer anticholinergic effects and a lower incidence of drowsiness. Many OTC cold remedies contain a first-generation antihistamine, which can cause drowsiness; therefore patients should be alerted not to drive or operate dangerous machinery when taking such medications. The anticholinergic properties of most antihistamines cause dryness of the mouth and decreased secretions, making them useful in treating rhinitis caused by the common cold. Antihistamines also decrease the nasal itching and tickling that cause sneezing.

The first-generation antihistamine diphenhydramine has been available for years and is frequently combined with other ingredients in cold remedy preparations. Its primary use is to treat rhinitis. Prototype Drug Chart: Diphenhydramine lists the pharmacologic behavior of diphenhydramine.

Pharmacokinetics. Diphenhydramine can be administered orally, intramuscularly (IM), or intravenously (IV). It is well absorbed from the gastrointestinal (GI) tract, but systemic absorption from topical use is minimal. It is highly protein bound (98%) and has an average half-life of 2 to 8 hours. Diphenhydramine is metabolized by the liver and is excreted as metabolites in the urine.

Pharmacodynamics. Diphenhydramine blocks the effects of histamine by competing for and occupying H_1 receptor sites. It has anticholinergic effects and should be used with caution by patients with closed-angle glaucoma. Drowsiness is a major side effect of the drug; in fact, it is sometimes used in sleep aid products. Diphenhydramine is also used as an antitussive to alleviate cough. Its onset of action can occur in as few as 15 minutes when taken orally and IM. Intravenous administration results in an immediate onset of action. The duration of action is 4 to 7 hours.

Diphenhydramine can cause central nervous system (CNS) depression if taken with alcohol, narcotics, hypnotics, or barbiturates.

⚡ **PATIENT SAFETY**

Do not confuse…
- **Benadryl,** an antihistamine, with **benazepril,** an angiotensin-converting enzyme (ACE) inhibitor

---

Side Effects of Most First-Generation Antihistamines. The most common side effects of first-generation antihistamines are drowsiness, dizziness, fatigue, and disturbed coordination. Skin rashes and anticholinergic symptoms such as dry mouth, urine retention, blurred vision, and wheezing may also occur.

PROTOTYPE DRUG CHART

Diphenhydramine

Drug Class	Dosage
Antihistamine	Allergic reaction: A: PO: 25–50 mg q4–6h; *max:* 300 mg/d A: IM/IV: 10–50 mg as single dose IV or IM q4–6h; *max:* 400 mg/d

Contraindications	Drug-Lab-Food Interactions
Breastfeeding *Caution:* Asthma, hepatic disease, COPD, neonate, prostatic hypertrophy, pregnancy, urinary retention, GI obstruction, increased intraocular pressure, older adults	Drug: Increased CNS depression with alcohol, opioids, hypnotics, and barbiturates; avoid use with MAOIs

Pharmacokinetics	Pharmacodynamics
Absorption: PO: Well absorbed Distribution: PB: 98% Metabolism: t½: 2–8 h Excretion: In urine as metabolites	PO: Onset: 15–30 min Peak: 2–4 h Duration: 4–6 h IM: Onset: 15–30 min Peak: 1–4 h Duration: 4–7 h IV: Onset: Immediate Peak: 0.5–1 h Duration: 4–7 h

Therapeutic Effects/Uses

To treat insomnia and allergic reactions including allergic rhinitis, the common cold, cough, sneezing, pruritus, and urticaria and to prevent motion sickness
Mechanism of Action: Competes with histamine for binding at H_1-receptor sites and antagonizes histamine effects

Side Effects	Adverse Reactions
Drowsiness, dizziness, headache, weakness, insomnia, fatigue, urinary retention, blurred vision, dry mouth, dermatitis, rash, paresthesia, abdominal pain, restlessness, confusion, diarrhea, constipation	Seizures *Life-threatening:* thrombocytopenia

A, Adult; *CNS,* central nervous system; *COPD,* chronic obstructive pulmonary disease; *d,* day; *h,* hour; *IM,* intramuscular; *IV,* intravenous; *MAOI,* monoamine oxidase inhibitor; *max,* maximum; *min,* minute; *PB,* protein binding; *PO,* by mouth; *q4–6h,* every 4 to 6 hours; *t½,* half-life; *y,* years; *>,* greater than.

Second-Generation Antihistamines

The second-generation antihistamines are frequently called *nonsedating antihistamines* because they have little to no sedative effect. In addition, these antihistamines cause fewer anticholinergic symptoms. Although a moderate amount of alcohol and other CNS depressants may be taken with second-generation antihistamines, many clinicians advise against such use.

The second-generation antihistamines cetirizine, fexofenadine, azelastine, desloratadine, and loratadine have half-lives between 3 and 30 hours and are administered by nasal spray. Table 38.1 lists the first- and second-generation antihistamines used to treat allergic rhinitis.

Nasal and Systemic Decongestants

Nasal congestion results from dilation of nasal blood vessels caused by infection, inflammation, or allergy. With this dilation, a transudation of fluid into the tissue spaces occurs that results in swelling of the nasal cavity. Nasal decongestants (sympathomimetic amines) stimulate the alpha-adrenergic receptors, producing vascular constriction (vasoconstriction) of the capillaries within the nasal mucosa. The result is shrinking of the nasal mucous membranes and a reduction in fluid secretion (runny nose).

Nasal decongestants are administered by nasal spray or drops or in tablet, capsule, or liquid form. Frequent use of decongestants, especially nasal spray or drops, can result in tolerance and rebound nasal congestion, rebound vasodilation instead of vasoconstriction. Rebound nasal congestion is caused by irritation of the nasal mucosa.

Systemic decongestants (alpha-adrenergic agonists) are available in tablet, capsule, and liquid form, and are used primarily for allergic rhinitis, including hay fever and acute coryza (profuse nasal discharge). Examples of systemic decongestants are tetrahydrozoline, phenylephrine, oxymetazoline, and pseudoephedrine. In the past, phenylpropanolamine was used in many cold remedies; however, the US Food and Drug Administration (FDA) ordered its removal from OTC cold remedies and weight loss aids because reports suggest that the drug might cause stroke, hypertension, renal failure, and cardiac dysrhythmias. Pseudoephedrine is frequently combined with an antihistamine, analgesic, or antitussive in oral cold remedies. The advantage of systemic decongestants is that they relieve nasal congestion for a longer period than nasal decongestants; however, long-acting nasal decongestants are now available. Nasal decongestants usually act promptly and cause fewer side effects than systemic decongestants.

National regulatory measures control pseudoephedrine drug sales with individual limits of 3.6 g/day and 9 g within 30 days. Identifications are scanned with each purchase. The database is linked nationally and keeps a 2-year tally. Table 38.2 lists systemic and nasal decongestants and their dosages, uses, and considerations.

TABLE 38.1 Antihistamines for Treatment of Allergic Rhinitis

Drug	Route and Dosage	Uses and Considerations
First-Generation Antihistamines		
Alkylamine Derivatives		
Brompheniramine tannate	Extended release: A: PO: 6–12 mg q12h; *max:* 24 mg/d	For allergic rhinitis, rhinorrhea, and conjunctivitis. May cause drowsiness, dizziness, restlessness, euphoria, irritability, blurred vision, dry mouth, constipation, urinary retention, palpitations, and tachycardia. PB: 39%–49%; t½: 11.8–34.7 h
Chlorpheniramine	Immediate release: A: PO: 4 mg q4–6h; *max:* 24 mg/d Extended release: A: 8–12 mg bid; *max:* 24 mg/d	For allergic rhinitis and conjunctivitis. May cause drowsiness, dizziness, headache, dry mouth, blurred vision, confusion, ataxia, weakness, constipation, restlessness, tachycardia, palpitations, and urinary retention. PB: 70% t½: 21–24 h
Ethanolamine Derivatives		
Clemastine fumarate	A: PO: 1 tab (1.34 mg) q12h; *max:* 2 tabs/d	For common cold, allergic rhinitis, pruritus, and urticaria. May cause drowsiness, dizziness, restlessness, euphoria, headache, confusion, dry mouth, constipation, palpitations, tachycardia, blurred vision, and urinary retention. PB: UK; t½: 4–6 h
Diphenhydramine	See Prototype Drug Chart: Diphenhydramine	
Piperidine Derivatives		
Cyproheptadine	A: Initially 4 mg tid; *maint:* 4–20 mg/d in divided doses; *max:* 32 mg/d	For allergies rhinitis, conjunctivitis, pruritus, and urticaria. May cause drowsiness, dry mouth, constipation, dizziness, excitability, euphoria, blurred vision, restlessness, wheezing, hypotension, tachycardia, and urinary retention. PB: UK; t½: 1–4 h
Piperazine Derivatives		
Levocetirizine	A: PO: 2.5–5 mg/d in the evening; *max:* 5 mg/d	For allergic rhinitis and chronic urticaria. May cause drowsiness, dizziness, blurred vision, fever, hypotension, tachycardia, palpitations, fatigue, nasal congestion, urinary retention, dry mouth, diarrhea, and constipation. PB: 91%–92%; t½: 8–9 h
Chlorcyclizine	A: PO: 25 mg q6–8h PRN; *max:* 75 mg/d	For allergic rhinitis and hay fever. May cause blurred vision, dry mouth, weakness, dizziness, drowsiness, confusion, constipation, euphoria, headache, restlessness, tachycardia, and urinary retention. PB: 85%–90%; t½: 12 h
Combination Antihistamines		
Azelastine and fluticasone	A: Nasal spray: 1 spray per nostril bid; *max:* 2 sprays/nostril/d	For allergic rhinitis. May cause drowsiness, dizziness, blurred vision, headache, tachycardia, palpitations, dysphonia, dysgeusia, rhinitis, nasal irritation, and epistaxis. PB: 88% azelastine, 91% fluticasone; t½: 25 h azelastine, 7.8 h fluticasone
Second-Generation Antihistamines		
Azelastine	Nasal spray: A: 1–2 sprays in each nostril q12h; *max:* 4 sprays/nostril/d	For allergic rhinitis and pruritus. May cause drowsiness, headache, confusion, fatigue, blurred vision, pharyngitis, ocular irritation, dry mouth, palpitations, tachycardia, and urinary retention. PB: 88%; t½: 25 h
Cetirizine	A: PO: 5–10 mg/d; *max:* 10 mg/d Older A>77 y: PO: 5 mg/d; *max:* 5 mg/d	For allergic rhinitis and urticaria. May cause drowsiness, dizziness, headache, insomnia, fatigue, euphoria, ataxia, dry mouth, pharyngitis, cough, epistaxis, hearing loss, blurred vision, urinary retention, diarrhea, and abdominal pain. PB: 93%; t½: 6.5–10 h
Fexofenadine	A: PO: 60 mg q12h; *max:* 120 mg/d	For allergic rhinitis and chronic urticaria. May cause dizziness, fever, fatigue, headache, restlessness, cough, dyspepsia, vomiting, and diarrhea. PB: 60%–70%; t½: 14.4 h
Loratadine	A: PO: 10 mg/d; *max:* 10 mg/d	For allergic rhinitis, pruritus, and urticaria. May cause drowsiness, confusion, headache, blurred vision, dry mouth, vomiting, constipation, urinary retention, palpitations, wheezing, and tachycardia. PB: 97%; t½: 3–20 h
Desloratadine	A: PO: 5 mg/d; *max:* 5 mg/d	For allergic rhinitis, chronic urticaria, and pruritus. May cause drowsiness, dizziness, headache, fever, infection, irritability, cough, restlessness, insomnia, dry mouth, tachycardia, palpitations, nausea, vomiting, and diarrhea. PB: 82%–87%; t½: 20–30 h

A, Adult; *bid*, twice a day; *d*, day; *GI*, gastrointestinal; *h*, hour; *max*, maximum; *PB*, protein binding; *PO*, by mouth; *q*, every; *qd*, every day; *t½*, half-life; *tid*, three times a day; *UK*, unknown; *y*, years; *>*, greater than; *≥*, greater than or equal to; *<*, less than.

Side Effects and Adverse Reactions

The incidence of side effects is low with topical preparations such as nose drops. However, decongestants can make a patient nervous or restless. These side effects decrease or disappear as the body adjusts to the drug.

Use of nasal decongestants for as little as 3 days could result in rebound nasal congestion. Instead of the nasal membranes constricting, vasodilation occurs, causing increased stuffy nose and nasal congestion. The nurse should emphasize the importance of limiting the use of nasal sprays and drops.

As with any alpha-adrenergic drug such as decongestants, blood pressure and blood glucose levels can increase. These drugs are contraindicated or used with extreme caution in patients with hypertension, cardiac disease, hyperthyroidism, and diabetes mellitus.

⊙ CLINICAL JUDGMENT [NURSING PROCESS]

Antihistamine: Diphenhydramine

Concept: Gas Exchange
- The lungs deliver oxygen to the pulmonary capillaries, carried by hemoglobin to body cells, and carbon dioxide is carried away from body cells to the lungs and exhaled from the body.

Recognize Cues [Assessment]
- Determine baseline vital signs.
- Obtain a drug history, and report if a drug-drug interaction is probable.
- Assess for signs and symptoms of urinary dysfunction, including retention, dysuria, and altered frequency.
- Note complete blood count (CBC) during drug therapy.
- Assess cardiac and respiratory status.
- Obtain a history of environmental exposures that includes drugs, recent foods eaten, and stress.

Analyze Cues and Prioritize Hypothesis [Patient Problems]
- Airway obstruction
- Decreased gas exchange
- Hypoxemia
- Discomfort

Generate Solutions [Planning]
- Patient will have decreased nasal congestion, mucosal secretions, and cough.
- Patient will sleep 6 to 8 hours per night.

Take Action [Nursing Interventions]
- Give the oral form of the drug with food to decrease gastric distress.
- Administer the intramuscular form in a large muscle. *Avoid subcutaneous injection.*

Patient Teaching
General
- ⚡ Warn patients to avoid driving a motor vehicle and performing other dangerous activities if drowsiness occurs or until stabilized on the drug.
- ⚡ Advise patients to avoid alcohol and other central nervous system (CNS) depressants.
- Encourage patients to take drugs as prescribed. Notify a health care provider if confusion or hypotension occurs.
- Teach patients on prophylaxis for motion sickness to take the drug at least 30 minutes before the offending event, and also before meals and at bedtime during the event.
- Inform breastfeeding mothers that small amounts of drug pass into breast milk. Because children are more susceptible to the side effects of antihistamines (e.g., unusual excitement or irritability), breastfeeding is not recommended while using these drugs.

Side Effects
- Advise family members or parents that children are more sensitive to the effects of antihistamines. Nightmares, nervousness, and irritability are more likely to occur in children.
- Inform older adults that they are more sensitive to the effects of antihistamines and are more likely to experience confusion, difficult or painful urination, dizziness, drowsiness, feeling faint, and dryness of the mouth, nose, or throat.
- Suggest using sugarless candy or gum, ice chips, or a saliva substitute for temporary relief of mouth dryness.

Evaluate Outcomes [Evaluation]
- Evaluate effectiveness of the drug in relieving allergic symptoms or as a sleep aid.

TABLE 38.2 Systemic and Nasal Decongestants (Sympathomimetic Amines)

Drug	Route and Dosage	Uses and Considerations
Oxymetazoline hydrochloride	A: gtt or spray; 2–3 sprays in each nostril q10–12h PRN; *max:* 2 doses/d for no more than 3 d	For nasal congestion, pruritus, and facial erythema due to acne. May cause nasal irritation, blurred vision, dry eyes, ocular pain/irritation, keratitis, conjunctival hyperemia, and headache. Limit use to less than 3 days to avoid rebound congestion. PB: 57%; t½: 5.6–13.9 h
Phenylephrine hydrochloride	A: Sol (0.25%) 2–3 sprays/gtt in each nostril q4h PRN <3 d A: PO: 10–20 mg q4–6h; *max:* 60 mg/d	For nasal congestion. May cause nasal irritation, excitability, blurred vision, nausea, dyspnea, hypertension, and headache. PB: UK; t½: 2.1–3.4 h
Pseudoephedrine	Regular release: A: PO: 60 mg q4–6h; *max:* 240 mg/d Extended release: A: PO: 120 mg q12h; *max:* 240 mg/d	For rhinitis, nasal congestion, and the common cold. May cause dizziness, headache, photophobia, restlessness, insomnia, palpitations, dysrhythmia, hypertension, tachycardia, and nausea. PB: UK; t½: 9–16 h
Tetrahydrozoline	A: Nasal: 2–4 drops (0.1% sol) each nostril q3h PRN	For nasal congestion and eye redness. May cause drowsiness, headache, blurred vision, insomnia, nasal irritation, and palpitations. PB: UK; t½: UK

A, Adult; *bid*, twice a day; *d*, day; *GI*, gastrointestinal; *gtt*, drops; *h*, hour; *max*, maximum; *PB*, protein binding; *PO*, by mouth; *PRN*, as necessary; *q4h*, every 4 hours; *sol*, solution; *t½*, half-life; *UK*, unknown; *y*, year; *>*, greater than; *<*, less than.

Drug Interactions

When using decongestants with other drugs, drug interactions can occur. Pseudoephedrine may decrease the effect of beta blockers. Taken together with monoamine oxidase inhibitors (MAOIs), decongestants may increase the possibility of hypertension or cardiac dysrhythmias. The patient should also avoid large amounts of caffeine (coffee, tea) because it can increase restlessness and palpitations caused by decongestants.

Intranasal Glucocorticoids

Intranasal glucocorticoids and steroids are effective for treating allergic rhinitis because they have an antiinflammatory action, thus decreasing the allergic rhinitis symptoms of rhinorrhea, sneezing, and congestion. The following are examples of intranasal steroids:

- Beclomethasone
- Budesonide
- Flunisolide

TABLE 38.3   Intranasal Glucocorticoids

Drug	Route and Dosage	Uses and Considerations
Beclomethasone	Rhinitis: A: 1–2 sprays (42 mcg/spray) each nostril bid	For allergic rhinitis, nasal polyps, and asthma. May cause headache, nasopharyngitis, candidiasis, dysphonia, hoarseness, epistaxis, and ocular hypertension. PB: 87%; t½: 15 h
Budesonide	Rhinitis: A: 1–2 sprays/d each nostril	For rhinitis and asthma. May cause dizziness, headache, weakness, fatigue, dyspepsia, nausea, diarrhea, cough, and epistaxis. PB: 90%; t½: 2–3.6 h
Flunisolide	A: 2 sprays each nostril bid; *max:* 8 sprays/d each nostril	For allergic rhinitis. May cause nasal irritation, dysgeusia, headache, pharyngitis, epistaxis, ocular hypertension, and candidiasis. PB: UK; t½: 1.8–2 h
Fluticasone	A: 2 sprays/d each nostril week 1, then 1–2 sprays each nostril qd PRN	For allergic rhinitis and asthma. May cause headache, blurred vision, fatigue, insomnia, arthralgia, epistaxis, pharyngitis, nasal candidiasis/irritation, dysphonia, malaise, nasal congestion, nausea, and vomiting. PB: 91%; t½: 7.8 h
Mometasone furoate	Allergic rhinitis prophylaxis: A: 2 sprays/d each nostril	For allergic rhinitis, asthma, nasal congestion, and nasal polyps. May cause headache, candidiasis, pharyngitis, cough, fatigue, sinusitis, wheezing, arthralgia, and epistaxis. PB: 98%–99%; t½: 5–6 h
Triamcinolone	A: 2 sprays/d each nostril	For allergic rhinitis, ocular inflammation, and asthma. Common side effects are ocular hypertension, rash, pruritus, arthralgia, erythema, and nasal irritation. PB: UK; t½: 88 min

A, Adult; *bid,* twice a day; *d,* day; *GI,* gastrointestinal; *h,* hour; *IOP,* intraocular pressure; *max,* maximum; *PB,* protein binding; *t½,* half-life; *UK,* unknown; *y,* year; *>,* greater than.

PROTOTYPE DRUG CHART

Dextromethorphan Hydrobromide

Drug Class	Dosage
Antitussive	Immediate release: A: PO: 10–20 mg q4h PRN or 30 mg q6–8h PRN; *max:* 120 mg/d Extended release: A: PO: 60 mg q12h; *max:* 120 mg/d

Contraindications	Drug-Lab-Food Interactions
Hypersensitivity, MAOI therapy *Caution:* Asthma, emphysema, hepatic disease, older adults, pregnancy, breastfeeding, tobacco smoking	No significant drug interactions occur with this drug.

Pharmacokinetics	Pharmacodynamics
Absorption: PO: Rapidly absorbed Distribution: PB: 60%–70% Metabolism: t½: 2–24 h Excretion: In urine	PO: Onset: 15–30 min Peak: 2–3 h Duration: 3–6 h

Therapeutic Effects/Uses

For temporary cough relief, especially a nonproductive cough due to sore throat, irritation, or the common cold
Mechanism of Action: Decreases excitability of cough center in the medulla

Side Effects	Adverse Reactions
Dizziness, drowsiness, confusion, fatigue, ataxia, nausea, vomiting, restlessness	Psychosis, tachycardia, seizures *Life-threatening:* Respiratory depression, serotonin syndrome

A, Adult; *d,* day; *GI,* gastrointestinal; *h,* hour; *max,* maximum; *min,* minute; *PB,* protein binding; *PO,* by mouth; *PRN,* as necessary; *q4h,* every 4 hours; *t½,* half-life; *UK,* unknown; *y,* year; *>,* greater than.

- Fluticasone
- Mometasone
- Triamcinolone

These drugs may be used alone or in combination with an H₁ antihistamine. The spray should be directed away from the nasal septum, and the patient should sniff gently. With continuous use, dryness of the nasal mucosa may occur. Common side effects include headache, nasal irritation, pharyngitis, fatigue, insomnia, and candidiasis.

Intranasal glucocorticoids undergo rapid deactivation after absorption. Most allergic rhinitis is seasonal; therefore the drugs are for short-term use unless otherwise indicated by the health care provider.

Table 38.3 lists the intranasal glucocorticoids and their dosages, uses, and considerations.

Antitussives

Antitussives act on the cough control center in the medulla to suppress the cough reflex. The cough is a naturally protective way to clear the airway of secretions or any collected material. A sore throat may cause coughing that increases throat irritation. If the cough is nonproductive and irritating, an antitussive may be taken. Hard candy may decrease the constant, irritating cough. Dextromethorphan, a nonnarcotic antitussive, is widely used in OTC cold remedies. Prototype Drug

TABLE 38.4 Antitussives and Expectorants

Drug	Route and Dosage	Uses and Considerations
Opioid Antitussives		
Codeine CSS II	Cough: A: PO: 10–20 mg q4–6h; *max:* 120 mg/d	For cough and pain. May cause drowsiness, dizziness, euphoria, orthostatic hypotension, weakness, nausea, diarrhea, constipation, dependence, tolerance, withdrawal, and respiratory depression. PB: 7%–25%; t½: 3 h
Dextromethorphan	See Prototype Drug Chart: Dextromethorphan Hydrobromide	
Guaifenesin 200 mg and codeine 9 mg CSS V	A: PO: 2 capsules q4h PRN; *max:* Codeine 120 mg/d and guaifenesin 2400 mg/d	For cough and the common cold. May cause drowsiness, dizziness, headache, euphoria, hypotension, dependence, nausea, vomiting, constipation, abdominal pain, urinary retention, and respiratory depression. PB: Guaifenesin UK, codeine 7%–25%; t½: guaifenesin 1 h, codeine 3 h
Homatropine 1.5 mg and hydrocodone 5 mg CSS III	A: PO: Hydrocodone 5 mg and homatropine 1.5 mg q4–6h PRN; *max:* hydrocodone 30 mg and homatropine 9 mg/d	For cough. May cause drowsiness, dizziness, euphoria, headache, blurred vision, dry mouth, nausea, vomiting, urinary retention, constipation, and dependence. PB: UK; t½: 4 h; hydrocodone, UK homatropine
Nonopioid Antitussives		
Benzonatate	A: PO: 100–200 mg tid; *max:* 600 mg/d	For cough. May cause drowsiness, dizziness, headache, confusion, nausea, constipation, and ocular irritation. PB: UK; t½: UK
Expectorants		
Guaifenesin	Immediate release: A: PO: 200–400 q4h PRN; *max:* 2400 mg/d Extended release: A: PO: 600–1200 mg q12h PRN; *max:* 2.4 g/d	For cough associated with URI and the common cold. May cause drowsiness, dizziness, headache, nausea, vomiting, and diarrhea. PB: UK; t½: 1 h
Combinations of Antitussives and Expectorants		
Guaifenesin and dextromethorphan	Immediate release: A: PO: Guaifenesin 200–400 mg and dextromethorphan 20 mg q4h PRN; *max:* guaifenesin 2400 mg and dextromethorphan 120 mg/d Extended release: A: PO: 30–60 mg dextromethorphan, 200 mg guaifenesin q12h; *max:* 2 doses/d	For common cold. May cause drowsiness, dizziness, headache, confusion, irritability, nausea, and respiratory depression. PB: Guaifenesin UK, dextromethorphan 60%–70%; t½: Guaifenesin 1 h, dextromethorphan 2–24 h

A, Adult; *CSS,* Controlled Substances Schedule; *d,* day; *GI,* gastrointestinal; *h,* hour; *max,* maximum; *PB,* protein binding; *PO,* by mouth; *PRN,* as necessary; *q6h,* every 6 hours; *t½,* half-life; *tid,* three times a day; *UK,* unknown; *y,* year; *>,* greater than.

Chart: Dextromethorphan Hydrobromide lists the drug data related to dextromethorphan.

The three types of antitussives are nonopioid, opioid, or combination preparations. Antitussives are usually used in combination with other agents (Table 38.4).

Pharmacokinetics. Dextromethorphan is available in numerous cold and cough remedy preparations in syrup or liquid form, chewable capsules, and lozenges. The drug is rapidly absorbed and exerts its effects 15 to 30 minutes after oral administration. Its protein-binding percentage is 60% to 70%, and the half-life is 13 hours. Dextromethorphan is metabolized by the liver and is excreted in the urine.

Pharmacodynamics. Dextromethorphan, an antitussive, provides temporary cough relief, especially for nonproductive cough due to sore throat, irritation, or the common cold. This drug acts by decreasing the excitability of the cough center in the medulla.

Dextromethorphan has a duration of 3 to 6 hours. Usually preparations that contain dextromethorphan can be used several times a day.

Expectorants

Expectorants loosen bronchial secretions so they can be eliminated by coughing. They can be used with or without other pharmacologic agents. Expectorants are found in many OTC cold remedies along with analgesics, antihistamines, decongestants, and antitussives. The most common expectorant in such preparations is guaifenesin. Hydration is the best natural expectorant. When taking an expectorant, patients should increase fluid intake to at least 8 glasses per day to help loosen mucus. Table 38.4 lists the dosages, uses, and considerations for antitussives and expectorants.

SINUSITIS

Sinusitis is an inflammation of the mucous membranes of one or more of the maxillary, frontal, ethmoid, or sphenoid sinuses. A systemic or nasal decongestant may be indicated. Acetaminophen, fluids, and rest may also be helpful. For acute or severe sinusitis, an antibiotic may be prescribed.

ACUTE PHARYNGITIS

Acute pharyngitis, inflammation of the throat or "sore throat," can be caused by a virus, beta-hemolytic streptococci ("strep throat"), or other bacteria. It can occur alone or with the common cold and rhinitis or acute sinusitis. Symptoms include elevated temperature and cough. A throat culture should be obtained to rule out beta-hemolytic

◎ CLINICAL JUDGMENT [NURSING PROCESS]

Nasal Decongestant: Oxymetazoline

Concept: Gas Exchange

- The lungs deliver oxygen to the pulmonary capillaries, carried by hemoglobin to the body cells, and carbon dioxide is carried away from body cells to the lungs and exhaled from the body.

Recognize Cues [Assessment]

- Determine whether the patient has a history of hypertension, especially if a decongestant is an ingredient in the cold remedy being taken.
- Note baseline vital signs. An elevated temperature of 99°F to 101°F (37.2°C to 38.3°C) may indicate a viral infection caused by a cold.
- Obtain a drug history, and report if a drug-drug interaction is probable. Dextromethorphan hydrochloride (HCl) given with monoamine oxidase inhibitors (MAOIs), narcotics, sedative-hypnotics, barbiturates, antidepressants, and alcohol may increase toxicity.
- Assess cardiac and respiratory status.

Analyze Cues and Prioritize Hypothesis [Patient Problems]

- Airway obstruction
- Decreased gas exchange
- Hypoxemia
- Discomfort
- Fatigue

Generate Solutions [Planning]

- Patient's cough will be eliminated or diminished.
- Patient will be free from a secondary bacterial infection.

Take Action [Nursing Interventions]

- Monitor vital signs. Blood pressure can become elevated when a decongestant is taken, and dysrhythmias can also occur.
- Observe the color of bronchial secretions. Yellow or green mucus is indicative of a bronchial infection. Antibiotics may be needed.
- Warn patients that codeine preparations for cough suppression can lead to tolerance and physical dependence.

Patient Teaching
General

- Tell patients that hypotension and hyperpyrexia may occur when dextromethorphan is taken with MAOIs.
- Teach patients about proper use of nasal sprays and proper use of "puff" or squeeze products.

- Caution patients not to use more than 3 days, because rebound congestion can occur with overuse.
- ⚡ Advise patients to read labels on over-the-counter (OTC) drugs and to check with a health care provider before taking cold remedies. This is especially important when taking other drugs or when a patient has a major health problem such as hypertension or hyperthyroidism. Also, acetaminophen may be in many products, promoting an overdose.
- Inform patients that antibiotics are *not* helpful in treating common cold viruses. However, they may be prescribed if a secondary infection occurs.
- Encourage older patients with heart disease, asthma, emphysema, diabetes mellitus, or hypertension to contact a health care provider concerning the selection of drug, including OTC drugs.
- Direct patients not to drive during initial use of a cold remedy containing an antihistamine because drowsiness is common.
- Tell patients to maintain adequate fluid intake. Fluids liquefy bronchial secretions to ease elimination with coughing.
- Teach patients not to take a cold remedy before or at bedtime. Insomnia may occur if it contains a decongestant.
- Encourage patients to get adequate rest.
- Inform patients that common cold and flu viruses are transmitted frequently by hand-to-hand contact or by touching a contaminated surface. Cold viruses can live on the skin for several hours and on hard surfaces for several days.
- Advise patients to avoid environmental pollutants, fumes, smoking, and dust to lessen irritating cough.
- Teach patients to perform three effective coughs before bedtime to promote uninterrupted sleep.
- Direct patients and parents to store drugs out of reach of children; request childproof caps.
- Advise patients to contact a health care provider if cough persists for more than 1 week or is accompanied by chest pain, fever, or headache.

Self-Administration

- Teach patients to self-administer medications such as nose drops and inhalants.
- Encourage patients to cough effectively, to take deep breaths before coughing, and to be in an upright position.

Evaluate Outcomes [Evaluation]

- Evaluate effectiveness of drug therapy. Determine that the patient is free from nonproductive cough, has adequate fluid intake and rest, and is afebrile.

---

streptococcal infection. If the culture is positive for beta-hemolytic streptococci, a 10-day course of antibiotics is often prescribed. Saline gargles, lozenges, and increased fluid intake are usually indicated.

Acetaminophen may be taken to decrease elevated temperature. Antibiotics are *not* effective for viral pharyngitis.

■ CRITICAL THINKING CASE STUDY

A 35-year-old patient has allergic rhinitis. Her prescriptions include loratadine 5 mg/day and fluticasone, two nasal inhalations per day. Previously, she had taken OTC drugs and asked if she should continue to take the OTC drug with her prescriptions. She has never used a nasal inhaler before.

1. What additional information is needed from the patient concerning her health problem?
2. What is your response to the patient concerning the use of OTC drugs with her prescription drugs?

3. How would you instruct the patient to use a nasal inhaler? Explain your answer.
4. What are the similarities and differences between loratadine and diphenhydramine? Could one of these antihistamines be more effective than the other? Explain your answer.
5. What could you suggest to decrease allergens such as dust mites in the home?

REVIEW QUESTIONS

1. A patient tells the nurse that he has started to take an over-the-counter antihistamine, diphenhydramine. In teaching about side effects, what is most important for the nurse to tell the patient?
   a. To avoid insomnia, do not to take this drug at bedtime.
   b. Avoid driving a motor vehicle until stabilized on the drug.
   c. Nightmares and nervousness are more likely in an adult.
   d. Medication may cause excessive secretions.

2. A patient complains of a sore throat and has been told it is due to beta-hemolytic streptococcal infection. The nurse anticipates that the patient has which acute condition?
   a. Rhinitis
   b. Sinusitis
   c. Pharyngitis
   d. Rhinorrhea

3. A patient is prescribed a decongestant nasal spray that contains oxymetazoline. What will the nurse teach the patient?
   a. Take this drug at bedtime because it may cause drowsiness.
   b. Directly spray the medication away from the nasal septum and gently sniff.
   c. This drug may be used in maintenance treatment for asthma.
   d. Limit use of the drug to 3 days to prevent rebound nasal congestion.

4. A patient has been prescribed guaifenesin. The nurse understands that the purpose of the drug is to accomplish what?
   a. Treat allergic rhinitis and prevent motion sickness
   b. Loosen bronchial secretions so coughing can eliminate them
   c. Compete with histamine for receptor sites, thus preventing a histamine response
   d. Stimulate alpha-adrenergic receptors, thus producing vascular constriction of capillaries in nasal mucosa

5. Beclomethasone has been prescribed for a patient with allergic rhinitis. What should the nurse teach the patient regarding this medication?
   a. This may be used for an acute attack.
   b. An oral form is available if the patient prefers to use it.
   c. Avoid large amounts of caffeine intake because an increased heart rate may occur.
   d. With continuous use, dryness of the nasal mucosa/lining may occur.

6. The nurse is teaching a patient about diphenhydramine. Which instructions should the nurse include in the patient's teaching plan? (Select all that apply.)
   a. Take medication on an empty stomach to facilitate absorption.
   b. Avoid alcohol and other central nervous system depressants.
   c. Notify a health care provider if confusion or hypotension occurs.
   d. Use sugarless candy, gum, or ice chips for temporary relief of dry mouth.
   e. Avoid handling dangerous equipment or performing dangerous activities until stabilized on the medication.

39

Lower Respiratory Disorders

http://evolve.elsevier.com/McCuistion/pharmacology

OBJECTIVES

- Compare chronic obstructive pulmonary disease (COPD) and restrictive lung disease.
- Differentiate the drug groups used to treat COPD and asthma and the desired effects of each.
- Compare the side effects of beta$_2$-adrenergic agonists and methylxanthines.
- Describe the therapeutic serum or plasma theophylline level and the toxic level.

- Contrast the therapeutic effects of leukotriene antagonists, glucocorticoids, cromolyn, and antihistamines for COPD and asthma.
- Apply the Clinical Judgment [Nursing Process] for the patient taking drugs commonly used for COPD, including asthma, and for restrictive lung disease.

OUTLINE

INTRODUCTION

The chest cavity is a closed compartment bounded by 12 ribs, the diaphragm, thoracic vertebrae, sternum, neck muscles, and intercostal muscles between the ribs. The pleurae are membranes that encase the lungs. The lungs are divided into lobes; the right lung has three lobes, and the left lung has two lobes. The heart, which is not attached to the lungs, lies on the mid-left side in the chest cavity.

LUNG COMPLIANCE

Lung compliance is the lung volume based on the pressure in the alveoli. This volume determines the lung's ability to stretch. Factors that influence lung compliance include (1) connective tissue (collagen and elastin) and (2) surface tension in the alveoli, which is controlled by surfactant. Surfactant lowers the surface tension in the alveoli and prevents interstitial fluid from entering. Increased lung compliance is present with chronic obstructive pulmonary disease (COPD), and decreased lung compliance occurs with restrictive pulmonary disease. With low compliance, there is decreased lung volume resulting from increased connective tissue or increased surface tension. The lungs become "stiff," and it takes greater-than-normal pressure to expand lung tissue.

CONTROL OF RESPIRATION

Oxygen (O_2), carbon dioxide (CO_2), and hydrogen (H^+) ion concentrations in the blood influence respiration. *Chemoreceptors* are sensors that are stimulated by changes in these gases and ions. The central chemoreceptors, located in the medulla near the respiratory center and cerebrospinal fluid, respond to an increase in CO_2 and a decrease in pH by increasing ventilation. However, if the CO_2 level remains elevated, the stimulus to increase ventilation is lost.

Peripheral chemoreceptors, located in the carotid and aortic bodies, respond to changes in oxygen (P_{O_2}) levels. A low blood oxygen level (P_{O_2} <60 mm Hg) stimulates the peripheral chemoreceptors, which in turn stimulate the respiratory center in the medulla, and ventilation is increased. If oxygen therapy increases the oxygen level in the blood, the P_{O_2} may be too high to stimulate the peripheral chemoreceptors, and ventilation will be depressed.

BRONCHIAL SMOOTH MUSCLE

The tracheobronchial tube is composed of smooth muscle whose fibers spiral around the tracheobronchial tube, becoming more closely spaced as they near the terminal bronchioles (Fig. 39.1). Contraction of these muscles constricts the airway. The sympathetic and parasympathetic nervous systems affect the bronchial smooth muscle in opposite ways. The vagus nerve (parasympathetic nervous system) releases acetylcholine, which causes bronchoconstriction. The sympathetic nervous system releases epinephrine, which stimulates the $beta_2$ receptor in the bronchial smooth muscle, resulting in bronchodilation. These two nervous systems counterbalance each other to maintain homeostasis.

Cyclic adenosine monophosphate (cAMP) in the cytoplasm of bronchial cells increases bronchodilation by relaxing the bronchial smooth muscles. The pulmonary enzyme phosphodiesterase can inactivate cAMP. Drugs of the methylxanthine group (theophylline) inactivate phosphodiesterase, thus permitting cAMP to function.

This chapter discusses drugs used to alleviate and control airway obstruction. These include the sympathomimetics (adrenergics), particularly the $beta_2$ adrenergics; methylxanthines such as theophylline; leukotriene receptor antagonists; glucocorticoids; cromolyn sodium; and mucolytics.

Chronic obstructive pulmonary disease (COPD) and restrictive pulmonary disease are the two major categories of lower respiratory tract disorders. COPD is caused by airway obstruction with increased airway resistance of airflow to lung tissues. Four major pulmonary disorders cause COPD: (1) chronic bronchitis, (2) bronchiectasis, (3) emphysema, and (4) asthma. Chronic bronchitis, bronchiectasis, and emphysema frequently result in irreversible lung tissue damage. The lung tissue changes that result from an acute asthmatic attack are normally reversible; however, if the attacks are frequent and asthma becomes chronic, irreversible changes in the lung tissue may result. Patients with COPD usually have a decrease in forced expiratory volume in 1 second (FEV_1) as measured by pulmonary function tests.

Restrictive lung disease is a decrease in total lung capacity as a result of fluid accumulation or loss of elasticity of the lung. Pulmonary edema, pulmonary fibrosis, pneumonitis, lung tumors, thoracic deformities (scoliosis), and disorders that affect the thoracic muscular wall, such as myasthenia gravis, are among the types and causes of restrictive pulmonary disease.

Drugs discussed in this chapter are primarily used to treat COPD, particularly asthma. These drugs include bronchodilators (sympathomimetics [primarily $beta_2$-adrenergic agonists], methylxanthines [xanthines]), leukotriene antagonists, glucocorticoids, cromolyn, and anticholinergics. Some of these drugs may also be used to treat restrictive pulmonary diseases.

CHRONIC OBSTRUCTIVE PULMONARY DISEASE

Asthma is an inflammatory disorder of the airway walls associated with a varying amount of airway obstruction. This disorder is triggered by stimuli such as stress, allergens, and pollutants. When activated by stimuli, the bronchial airways become inflamed and edematous, leading to constriction of air passages. Inflammation aggravates airway hyperresponsiveness to stimuli, causing bronchial cells to produce more mucus, which obstructs air passages. This obstruction contributes to wheezing, coughing, dyspnea (breathlessness), chest tightness, and bronchospasm, particularly at night or in the early morning.

Bronchial asthma, one of the COPD lung diseases, is characterized by bronchospasm (constricted bronchioles), wheezing, mucous secretions, and dyspnea. There is resistance to airflow caused by obstruction

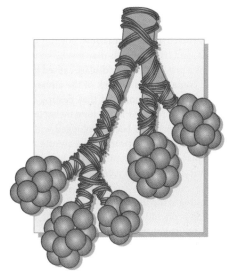

Fig. 39.1 Bronchial smooth muscle fibers become more closely spaced as they near the alveoli.

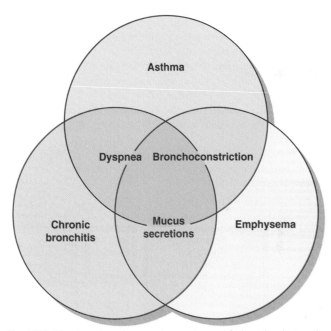

Fig. 39.2 Overlapping signs and symptoms of chronic obstructive pulmonary disease (COPD) conditions.

of the airway. In acute and chronic asthma, minimal to no changes are seen in the structure and function of lung tissues when the disease process is in remission. In chronic bronchitis, emphysema, and bronchiectasis, irreversible damage is done to the physical structure of lung tissue. Symptoms are similar to those of asthma in these three pulmonary disorders, except wheezing does not occur. Fig. 39.2 shows the overlapping symptoms of COPD conditions. Frequently, a steady deterioration occurs over a period of years.

Chronic bronchitis is a progressive lung disease caused by smoking or chronic lung infections. Bronchial inflammation and excessive mucous secretion result in airway obstruction. Productive coughing is a response to excess mucus production and chronic bronchial irritation. Inspiratory and expiratory rhonchi may be heard on auscultation. Hypercapnia (increased carbon dioxide retention) and hypoxemia (decreased blood oxygen) lead to respiratory acidosis.

In **bronchiectasis**, dilation of the bronchi and bronchioles is abnormal secondary to frequent infection and inflammation. The bronchioles become obstructed by the breakdown of the epithelium of the bronchial mucosa, and tissue fibrosis may result.

Emphysema is a progressive lung disease caused by cigarette smoking, atmospheric contaminants, or lack of the alpha$_1$-antitrypsin protein that inhibits proteolytic enzymes that destroy alveoli (air sacs). Proteolytic enzymes are released in the lung by bacteria or phagocytic cells. The terminal bronchioles become plugged with mucus, causing a loss in the fiber and elastin network in the alveoli. Alveoli enlarge as many of the alveolar walls are destroyed. Air becomes trapped in the overexpanded alveoli, leading to inadequate gas exchange (oxygen and carbon dioxide).

Cigarette smoking is the most common risk factor for COPD, especially with chronic bronchitis and emphysema. There is no currently known cure for COPD; however, it remains preventable in most cases. Because cigarette smoking is the most directly related cause, not smoking significantly prevents COPD from developing. Quitting smoking will slow the disease process.

Medications frequently prescribed for COPD include the following:

- Bronchodilators such as sympathomimetics (adrenergics), parasympatholytics (anticholinergic drugs, ipratropium bromide), and methylxanthines (caffeine, theophylline) are used to assist in opening narrowed airways.
- Glucocorticoids (steroids) are used to decrease inflammation.
- Leukotriene modifiers reduce inflammation in the lung tissue, and cromolyn acts as an antiinflammatory agent by suppressing the release of histamine and other mediators from the mast cells.
- Expectorants are used to assist in loosening mucus from the airways.
- Antibiotics may be prescribed to prevent serious complications from bacterial infections.

Bronchial Asthma

Bronchial asthma is a COPD characterized by periods of bronchospasm resulting in wheezing and difficulty breathing. **Bronchospasm**, or bronchoconstriction, results when the lung tissue is exposed to extrinsic or intrinsic factors that stimulate a bronchoconstrictive response. Factors that can trigger an asthmatic attack (bronchospasm) include humidity, air pressure changes, temperature changes, smoke, fumes (exhaust, perfume), stress, emotional upset, exercise, and allergies to animal dander, dust mites, food, and drugs (e.g., aspirin, ibuprofen, beta-adrenergic blockers). Reactive airway disease (RAD) is a cause of asthma that results from sensitivity stimulation from allergens, dust, temperature changes, and cigarette smoking.

Pathophysiology

Mast cells found in connective tissue throughout the body are directly involved in the asthmatic response, particularly to extrinsic factors. Allergens attach themselves to mast cells and basophils, resulting in an antigen-antibody reaction on the mast cells in the lung; thus the mast cells stimulate the release of chemical mediators such as histamines, cytokines, serotonin, eosinophil chemotactic factor of anaphylaxis (ECF-A), and leukotrienes. Eosinophil counts are usually elevated during an allergic reaction, which indicates that an inflammatory process is occurring. These chemical mediators stimulate bronchial constriction, mucus secretions, inflammation, and pulmonary congestion. Histamine and ECF-A are strong bronchoconstrictors. Bronchial smooth muscles are wrapped spirally around the bronchioles and contract as they are stimulated by these mediators. Exposure to an allergen results in bronchial hyperresponsiveness, epithelial shedding of the bronchial wall, mucous gland hyperplasia and hypersecretion, leakage of plasma that leads to swelling, and bronchoconstriction.

Fig. 39.3 shows factors that contribute to bronchoconstriction. Cyclic AMP, or cAMP, a cellular signaling molecule, is involved in many cellular activities and is responsible for maintaining bronchodilation.

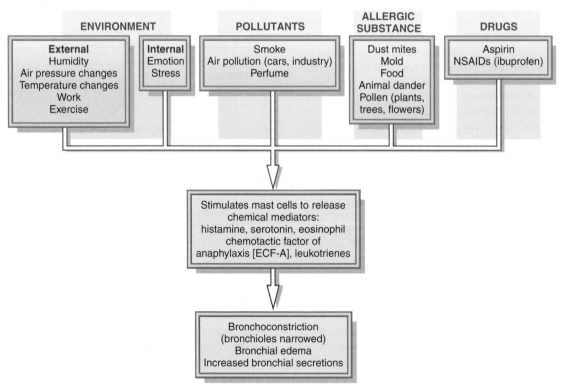

Fig. 39.3 Factors that contribute to bronchoconstriction. *NSAIDs,* Nonsteroidal antiinflammatory drugs.

When histamine, ECF-A, and leukotrienes inhibit the action of cAMP, bronchoconstriction results. The sympathomimetic (adrenergic) bronchodilators and methylxanthines increase the amount of cAMP in bronchial tissue cells.

In an acute asthmatic attack, the short-acting sympathomimetics (beta$_2$-adrenergic agonists) are the first line of defense. They promote cAMP production and enhance bronchodilation. Long-acting sympathomimetics are used for maintenance. Sympathomimetics (adrenergics) are also discussed in Chapter 15.

SYMPATHOMIMETICS: ALPHA- AND BETA$_2$-ADRENERGIC AGONISTS

Sympathomimetics increase cAMP, causing dilation of the bronchioles. In an acute bronchospasm caused by anaphylaxis from an allergic reaction, the nonselective sympathomimetic epinephrine—an alpha$_1$, beta$_1$, and beta$_2$ agonist—is given subcutaneously to promote bronchodilation and elevate blood pressure. Epinephrine is administered in emergency situations to restore circulation and increase airway patency (see Chapter 55).

For bronchospasm associated with chronic asthma or COPD, selective beta$_2$-adrenergic agonists are given by aerosol or as a tablet. These drugs act primarily on the beta$_2$ receptors; therefore side effects are less severe than those of epinephrine, which acts on alpha$_1$, beta$_1$, and beta$_2$ receptors.

Albuterol

The newer beta-adrenergic drugs for asthma are more selective for beta$_2$ receptors. High doses or overuse of the beta$_2$-adrenergic agents for asthma may cause some degree of beta$_1$ response, such as nervousness, tremor, and increased pulse rate. The ideal beta$_2$ agonist is one that has a rapid onset of action, longer duration of action, and few side effects. Albuterol is a selective beta$_2$ drug that is effective for treatment and control of asthma by causing bronchodilation with a long duration of action. (See Prototype Drug Chart: Albuterol for drug data related to albuterol.)

PROTOTYPE DRUG CHART

Albuterol

Drug Class	Dosage
Beta$_2$-adrenergic agonist	Acute bronchospasm: A: MDI: 2 puffs (90–180 mcg/inhal) q4–6h; *max:* 12 puffs/d Bronchospasm prophylaxis: Immediate release: A: PO: 2–4 mg q6–8h; *max:* 32 mg/d Extended release: A: PO: 4–8 mg q12h; *max:* 32 mg/d

Contraindications	Drug-Lab-Food Interactions
Hypersensitivity, milk protein hypersensitivity *Caution:* Cardiac dysrhythmia, heart failure, cardiac disease, hypo/hyperthyroidism, diabetes mellitus, rheumatoid arthritis, hypokalemia, hypocalcemia, older adults, seizures, MAOI therapy, pregnancy	Drug: Increased effect with other sympathomimetics; may increase effect with MAOIs and TCAs Antagonize effect with beta blockers Lab: May increase glucose level slightly; may decrease serum potassium level

Pharmacokinetics	Pharmacodynamics
Absorption: Well absorbed from the GI tract after oral administration; well absorbed from respiratory tract after inhalation Distribution: PB: 10% Metabolism: t½: Oral inhal: 3.8–5 h, PO: 2.7–6 h 100% excreted in the urine	Immediate release: PO: Onset: 30 min Peak: 2–3 h Duration: 4–6 h Extended release: PO: Onset: UK Peak: UK Duration: 8–12 h Inhal: Onset: 5–15 min Peak: 0.5–2 h Duration: 2–6 h

Therapeutic Effects/Uses

To treat asthma and for prophylaxis and treatment of bronchospasm
Mechanism of Action: Stimulates beta$_2$-adrenergic receptors in the lungs, which relaxes the bronchial smooth muscle, thus causing bronchodilation

Side Effects	Adverse Reactions
Tremor, dizziness, drowsiness, restlessness, agitation, anxiety, excitability, ataxia, headache, nasopharyngitis, insomnia, weakness, dry mouth, nausea, vomiting, diarrhea, edema, urinary retention, muscle cramps, rhinitis, throat irritation, tooth discoloration, hyperhidrosis	Palpitations, tachycardia, hypo/hypertension, infection, hyperglycemia, hypokalemia, chest pain, dyspnea *Life-threatening:* Dysrhythmia, angioedema, bronchospasm, Stevens-Johnson syndrome

A, Adult; *d,* day; *GI,* gastrointestinal; *h,* hour; *inhal,* inhalation; *MAOI,* monoamine oxidase inhibitor; *MDI,* metered-dose inhaler; *min,* minute; *PB,* protein binding; *PO,* by mouth; *q4–6h,* every 4 to 6 hours; *qid,* four times a day; *t½,* half-life; *TCA,* tricyclic antidepressant; *tid,* three times a day; *UK,* unknown; *y,* year.

Metaproterenol

The beta-adrenergic agent metaproterenol has some beta₁ effect but is primarily used as a beta₂ agent. It can be administered orally or by inhalation with a metered-dose inhaler (MDI) or a nebulizer.

For long-term asthma treatment, beta₂-adrenergic agonists are frequently administered by inhalation. This route of administration usually delivers more of the drug directly to the constricted bronchial site. The effective inhalation drug dose is less than it would be by the oral route, and there are also fewer side effects using this route. The onset of action is 1 minute by oral inhalation, 5 to 30 minutes by nebulization, and 15 to 30 minutes when taken orally. The peak for inhalation and oral administration is 1 hour with a duration of 4 hours.

Use of an Aerosol Inhaler

If the beta₂ agonist is given by MDI or dry-powder inhaler (DPI), correct use of the inhaler and dosage intervals need to be explained to the patient. If the patient does not receive effective relief from the inhaler, either the technique is faulty or the canister is empty. A spacer device may be attached to the inhaler to improve drug delivery to the lung with less deposition in the mouth. If the patient does not use the inhaler properly to deliver the drug dose, the medication may be trapped in the upper airways. Because of drug inhalation, mouth dryness and throat irritation could result.

Excessive use of the aerosol drug can lead to tolerance and loss of drug effectiveness. Occasionally, severe paradoxic airway resistance (bronchoconstriction) develops with repeated excessive use of sympathomimetic oral inhalation. Frequent dosing can cause tremors, nervousness, and increased heart rate. Table 39.1 lists the sympathomimetics used as bronchodilators.

Side Effects and Adverse Reactions

The side effects and adverse reactions of epinephrine include tremors, dizziness, hypertension, tachycardia, palpitations, dysrhythmias, and angina. The patient needs to be closely monitored when epinephrine is administered.

The side effects associated with beta₂-adrenergic drugs, such as albuterol, include tremors, headaches, restlessness, increased pulse rate, and palpitations (high doses). The beta₂ agonists may increase blood glucose levels, so patients with diabetes should be taught to closely monitor their serum glucose levels. Side effects of beta₂ agonists may diminish after 1 week or longer. The bronchodilating effects may decrease with continued use. It is believed that tolerance to these drugs can develop; if this occurs, the dose may need to be increased. Failure to respond to a previously effective dose may indicate worsening asthma that requires reevaluation before increasing the dose.

ANTICHOLINERGICS

Tiotropium is an anticholinergic drug used for maintenance treatment of bronchospasms associated with COPD. This drug is administered by inhalation only with the HandiHaler device (DPI). Patients should discard any capsules that are opened and not used immediately. HandiHalers should be washed with warm water and dried. The most common adverse effects of tiotropium

---

📄 **PROTOTYPE DRUG CHART**

Tiotropium

Drug Class	Dosage
Anticholinergic	COPD: A: Oral inhalation: 2 inhal/d (2.5 mcg/actuation) at the same time qd; *max:* 2 inhal/d

Contraindications	Drug-Lab-Food Interactions
Hypersensitivity *Caution:* Lactose hypersensitivity, narrow-angle glaucoma, bladder obstruction, renal impairment, cardiac dysrhythmias, breastfeeding, older adults	Drug: Increased anticholinergic effects with phenothiazines; decreased action of prokinetics (cisapride, metoclopramide, parasympathomimetics)

Pharmacokinetics	Pharmacodynamics
Absorption: Minimally absorbed PO Distribution: 72% PB Metabolism: t½: 5–6 d Excretion: In urine as metabolites	Inhalation: PO: Onset: 30 min Peak: 1–4 h Duration: UK

Therapeutic Effects/Uses

For maintenance treatment of asthma and COPD
Mechanism of Action: Blocks muscarinic cholinergic receptors and antagonizes acetylcholine action by inhibiting M3 receptor response to acetylcholine, thereby relaxing smooth muscle of bronchi; dilates bronchi

Side Effects	Adverse Reactions
Insomnia, dizziness, depression, headache, sinusitis, nasopharyngitis, cough, dry mouth, vomiting, abdominal pain, constipation, urinary retention, arthralgia, myalgia, peripheral edema, blurred vision, oral ulceration, candidiasis, infection	Tachycardia, ileus, dehydration, hyperglycemia, chest pain, GI obstruction, cataracts *Life-threatening:* Dysrhythmias, anaphylaxis, angioedema

A, Adult; *COPD,* chronic obstructive pulmonary disease; *d,* day; *h,* hour; *inhal,* inhalations; *min,* minutes; *PB,* protein binding; *PO,* by mouth; *qd,* every day; *t½,* half-life; *URI,* upper respiratory infection; *UTI,* urinary tract infection.

TABLE 39.1   Adrenergic Bronchodilators and Anticholinergics

Drug	Route and Dosage	Uses and Considerations
Alpha- and Beta-Adrenergics		
Epinephrine Alpha$_1$, beta$_1$, beta$_2$	Mild bronchospasm: A: Inhalation: 1 inhal (0.125 mg), may repeat after 1 min if needed, then wait 4 h between doses; *max:* 0.25/dose, 1 mg/d	For acute bronchospasm, anaphylaxis, angioedema, nasal congestion, asthma, and cardiac arrest. May cause restlessness, tremors, dizziness, diaphoresis, weakness, paresthesia, infection, hypo/hyperglycemia, angina, palpitations, tachycardia, hypertension, and dysrhythmias. PB: UK; t½: <5 min
Revefenacin	A: Inhal: 175 mcg/d by nebulizer; *max:* 1 dose/d	For treatment of bronchospasm associated with COPD including bronchitis, and emphysema. May cause headache, cough, infection, pharyngitis, dizziness, hypertension, and back pain. PB: 71%; t½: 22 h
Beta-Adrenergics		
Albuterol Beta$_2$	See Prototype Drug Chart: Albuterol	
Formoterol Beta$_2$	A: Inhalation: Inhale 20 mcg (one 2 mL unit) via nebulizer q12h; max: 40 mcg/d	For chronic bronchitis, COPD, and emphysema. May cause dizziness, insomnia, tachycardia, chest pain, palpitations, hypokalemia, pharyngitis, sinusitis, infection, nausea, diarrhea, and hyperglycemia. PB: 61%–64%; t½: 10 h
Levalbuterol Beta$_2$	Nebulizer inhalation: A: Inhalation: 0.63–1.25 mg q6–8h PRN; *max:* 3 doses/d (3.75 mg/d)	For bronchospasm, prophylaxis, and acute bronchospasm due to asthma and COPD. May cause dizziness, weakness, nasopharyngitis, nausea, vomiting, diarrhea, headache, chest pain, hyperglycemia, hypokalemia, tachycardia, fever, candidiasis, and tremors. PB: UK; t½: 3.3–4 h
Metaproterenol sulfate Beta$_1$ (some) and beta$_2$	A: PO: 20 mg tid/qid; *max:* 80 mg/d A: Nebulizer: 1 vial (0.4%) tid/qid PRN	For bronchospasm due to asthma and COPD. May cause headache, dizziness, insomnia, nausea, diarrhea, fatigue, blurred vision, chest pain, hypokalemia, tremor, tachycardia, and palpitations. PB: UK; t½: UK
Salmeterol Beta$_2$	A: Inhal: 1 puff (50 mcg) q12h Prevention of exercise-induced bronchospasm: A: Inhal MDI: 1 puff at least 30 min before exercise	For asthma, COPD, and exercise-induced bronchospasm prophylaxis. May cause headache, pharyngitis, nasal congestion, palpitations, tachycardia, hypokalemia, hyperglycemia, dizziness, hypertension, influenza, and musculoskeletal pain. PB: 94%–98%; t½: 5.5 h
Terbutaline sulfate Beta$_2$	A: PO: 2.5–5 mg tid; *max:* 15 mg/d A: Subcut: 0.25–0.5 mg, may repeat in 15–30 min; *max:* 0.5 mg/4 h	For asthma, COPD, bronchospasm prophylaxis, and acute bronchospasm. May cause dizziness, drowsiness, weakness, headache, chest pain, dyspnea, tremors, nausea, vomiting, palpitations, tachycardia, and hypokalemia. PB: 25%; t½: 2.9–14 h
Arformoterol tartrate Beta$_2$	A: Inhal nebulizer: 15 mcg q12h; *max:* 30 mcg/d	For COPD. May cause headache, sinusitis, muscle cramps, dyspnea, peripheral edema, back pain, rash, tremor, hyperglycemia, chest pain, tachycardia, and diarrhea. PB: 52%–65%; t½: 26 h
Indacaterol Beta$_2$	A: Oral inhal: 1 inhal/d (75 mcg in 1 capsule) at same time every day; *max:* 75 mcg/d	For COPD. May cause cough, headache, nasopharyngitis, hyperglycemia, nausea, hypertension, and tachycardia. PB: 94%–96%; t½: 45.5–126 h
Olodaterol Beta$_2$	A: Inhal: 2 inhal/d (2.5 mcg each) at the same time every day; *max:* 5 mcg/d	For COPD. May cause cough, nasopharyngitis, hypokalemia, hyperglycemia, dizziness, back pain, diarrhea, constipation, and infection. PB: 60%; t½: 45 h
Anticholinergics		
Ipratropium bromide	COPD: A: Inhal MDI: 2 puffs tid/qid, *max:* 12 inhal/d	For allergic rhinitis, common cold, and bronchospasm due to COPD prophylaxis. May cause headache, blurred vision, tachycardia, palpitations, epistaxis, nasopharyngitis, dyspnea, urinary retention, dry mouth, and back pain. PB: UK; t½: 2 h
Aclidinium	A: Oral MDI inhal: 1 inhal (400 mcg aclidinium) bid; *max:* 2 inhal/d	For COPD. May cause headache, blurred vision, ocular hypertension, cough, diarrhea, and nasopharyngitis. PB: UK; t½: 5–8 h
Tiotropium	See Prototype Drug Chart: Tiotropium	
Umeclidinium	A: Inhal: 1 inhal (62.5 mcg)/d at the same time every day	For COPD. May cause nasopharyngitis, blurred vision, cough, depression, tachycardia, urinary retention, arthralgia, and infection. PB: 89%; t½: 11 h
Monoclonal Antibody		
Omalizumab	A: Subcut: 150–300 mg q4wk; dose and frequency based upon body weight and total IgE serum levels	For asthma and chronic urticaria. May cause dizziness, headache, pharyngitis, sinusitis, arthralgia, bone fractures, peripheral edema, nausea, fatigue, injection site reaction, and infection. Do not give more than 150 mg/injection site. PB: UK; t½: 24–26 d
Reslizumab	A: IV: 3 mg/kg infusion q4wk	For asthma. May cause pharyngitis, musculoskeletal pain, dyspnea, antibody formation, hypotension, and malignancy. PB: UK; t½: 24 d

Continued

TABLE 39.1   Adrenergic Bronchodilators and Anticholinergics—cont'd

Drug	Route and Dosage	Uses and Considerations
Dupilumab	A: Subcut: Initially 400 mg, followed by 200 mg q2wk, followed by 300 mg q2wk	For moderate to severe asthma. May cause injection site reaction, ocular pruritus, conjunctivitis, blepharitis, keratitis, xerophthalmia, and antibody formation. PB: UK; t½: UK
Combination Beta-Adrenergics and Anticholinergics		
Ipratropium and albuterol	A: Inhaled spray: 1 inhal (120 mcg albuterol, 20 mcg ipratropium) q6h; *max:* 6 inhal/d	For COPD. May cause headache, blurred vision, pharyngitis, angina, cough, sinusitis, hyperglycemia, infection, hypokalemia, and dyspnea. PB: 9% ipratropium, 10% albuterol; t½: 2 h ipratropium, 3.8–5 h albuterol
Indacaterol and glycopyrrolate	A: Inhal: 1 capsule (27.5 mcg indacaterol and 15.6 mcg glycopyrrolate) bid; *max:* 2 capsules/d	For COPD. May cause hypertension, chest pain, tachycardia, palpitations, blurred vision, headache, hyperglycemia, hypokalemia, edema, and pharyngitis. PB: 38%–41% glycopyrrolate, 94%–96% indacaterol; t½: 33–53 h glycopyrrolate, 45.5–126 h indacaterol
Olodaterol and tiotropium	A: Inhal: 2 inhal/d (2.5 mcg olodaterol and 2.5 mcg tiotropium) at same time every day; *max:* 2 inhal/d	For COPD. May cause blurred vision, ocular hypertension, peripheral edema, nasopharyngitis, headache, insomnia, palpitations, chest pain, tachycardia, hyperglycemia, hypokalemia, abdominal pain, myalgia, and constipation. PB: 60% olodaterol, 72% tiotropium; t½: olodaterol 45 h, tiotropium 5–6 d
Umeclidinium and vilanterol	A: Inhal: 1 inhal/d (62.5 mcg umeclidinium and 25 mcg vilanterol) at same time every day; *max:* 1 inhal/d	For COPD. May cause pharyngitis, hypokalemia, hyperglycemia, blurred vision, palpitations, chest pain, urinary retention, constipation, and diarrhea. PB: 89% umeclidinium, 94% vilanterol; t½: 11 h umeclidinium, 21.3 h vilanterol
Glycopyrrolate and formoterol	A: Inhal: 2 inhal (9 mcg glycopyrrolate and 4.8 mcg formoterol) morning and evening; *max:* 2 inhal/d	For COPD. May cause dizziness, blurred vision, cough, chest pain, palpitations, infection, hyperglycemia, hypokalemia, ocular hypertension, and urinary retention. PB: 38%–41% glycopyrrolate, 46%–58% formoterol; t½: 33–53 h glycopyrrolate, 10 h formoterol
Aclidinium bromide and formoterol fumarate	A: Inhalation: 1 oral inhal (400 mcg aclidinium and 12 mcg formoterol) morning and evening	For COPD. May cause dizziness, headache, blurred vision, insomnia, muscle cramps, pharyngitis, hoarseness, hyperglycemia, hypokalemia, and infection. PB: UK aclidinium, 46%–58% formoterol; t½: 12 h aclidinium, 10 h formoterol

A, Adult; *bid,* two times a day; *COPD,* chronic obstructive pulmonary disease; *d,* day; *GI,* gastrointestinal; *h,* hour; *IgE,* immunoglobulin E; *IM,* intramuscular; *inhal,* inhalation; *IV,* intravenous; *max,* maximum; *MDI,* metered-dose inhaler; *min,* minute; *PB,* protein binding; *PO,* by mouth; *PRN,* as needed; *q,* every; *qd,* every day; *qid,* four times a day; *sol,* solution; *subcut,* subcutaneous; *t½,* half-life; *tid,* three times a day; *UK,* unknown; *URI,* upper respiratory infection; *wk,* week; *y,* year; *>,* greater than; *<,* less than.

include dry mouth, constipation, vomiting, dyspepsia, abdominal pain, depression, insomnia, headache, joint pain, and peripheral edema. Chest pain has been reported after tiotropium administration. Prototype Drug Chart: Tiotropium lists the drug data related to tiotropium.

The anticholinergic drug ipratropium bromide is used to treat asthmatic conditions by dilating the bronchioles. Unlike other anticholinergics, ipratropium bromide has few systemic effects. It is administered by MDI.

The combination of ipratropium bromide with albuterol sulfate is used to treat COPD. The combination is more effective and has a longer duration of action than either agent used alone. These two agents combined increase the FEV_1, the index used to evaluate asthma and obstructive lung disease and the patient's response to bronchodilator therapy. Table 39.2 lists the inhalants for asthma control.

METHYLXANTHINE (XANTHINE) DERIVATIVES

The second major group of bronchodilators used to treat asthma is the methylxanthine (xanthine) derivatives, which include aminophylline, theophylline, and caffeine. Xanthines also stimulate the central nervous system (CNS) and respiration, dilate coronary and pulmonary vessels, and cause diuresis. Because of their effect on respiration and pulmonary vessels, xanthines are used in the treatment of asthma.

TABLE 39.2   Inhalants for Asthma Control

Categories	Inhalant Agents
Adrenergics	
Beta₂ and some beta₁	Metaproterenol sulfate
Beta₂	Albuterol
	Salmeterol
	Terbutaline sulfate
	Formoterol
	Indacaterol
	Olodaterol
	Arformoterol tartrate
Anticholinergics	Ipratropium bromide
	Aclidinium
	Tiotropium
	Umeclidinium
Antiinflammatory Drugs	
Cromolyn	Cromolyn
Glucocorticoids (corticosteroids)	Beclomethasone
	Budesonide
	Flunisolide
	Fluticasone

Aminophylline-Theophylline

Aminophylline-theophylline relaxes the smooth muscles of the bronchi, bronchioles, and pulmonary blood vessels by inhibiting the enzyme phosphodiesterase, resulting in an increase in cAMP, which promotes bronchodilation.

Theophylline has a low therapeutic index and a narrow desired therapeutic range (5 to 15 mcg/mL). The serum or plasma theophylline concentration level should be monitored frequently to avoid severe adverse effects. Toxicity is likely to occur when the serum level is greater than 20 mcg/mL. Certain theophylline preparations can be given with sympathomimetic (adrenergic) agents, but the dose may need to be adjusted.

Theophylline was once used as the first-line drug for treating patients with chronic asthma and other COPDs. However, theophylline use has declined sharply because of a potential danger of serious adverse effects—including dysrhythmias, seizures, and cardiac arrest—and efficacy has not been found to be greater than that of beta agonists or glucocorticoids. Because of its numerous adverse reactions, drug-drug interactions, and narrow therapeutic drug range, theophylline is prescribed mostly for maintenance therapy in patients with chronic stable asthma and other COPDs when other drugs have failed to show improvement. Theophylline drugs are *not* prescribed for patients with seizure disorders or cardiac, renal, or liver disease. Patients who receive theophylline preparations need to be closely monitored for serious side effects and drug interactions.

Table 39.3 lists aminophylline-theophylline and its dosages, uses, and considerations.

Pharmacokinetics. Aminophylline is usually well absorbed after oral administration, but absorption may vary according to the specific dosage form. Aminophylline is also well absorbed from oral liquids and uncoated plain tablets. Sustained-release dosage forms are slowly absorbed. Food and antacids may decrease the rate but not the extent of absorption; large volumes of fluid and high-protein meals may increase the rate of absorption. The protein binding capacity of aminophylline is 40%. The dose size can also affect the rate of absorption: larger doses are absorbed more slowly. Aminophylline can also be administered in intravenous (IV) fluids.

Aminophylline drugs are metabolized by liver enzymes, and 90% of the drug is excreted by the kidneys. Tobacco smoking increases metabolism of theophylline drugs, thereby decreasing the half-life. The half-life is also shorter in children. With a short half-life, theophylline is readily excreted by the kidneys, so the dose may need to be increased to maintain a therapeutic serum/plasma range. In nonsmokers and older adults, the average half-life of theophylline is 6.5 to 10.5 hours, and the dose requirements may be decreased. However, in smokers and children, the half-life is 4 to 5 hours, and the dose requirement may be increased. In premature infants, the half-life is 9.4 to 43 hours. In patients with heart failure (HF), cor pulmonale, COPD, or liver disease, the half-life is 24 hours. Kidney function may be decreased in older adults, so caution should be used regarding the theophylline dosage to avoid drug toxicity.

Pharmacodynamics. Theophylline increases the level of cAMP, resulting in bronchodilation. The average onset of action is 30 minutes for oral preparations and 1 to 2 hours for sustained-release (SR) capsules. The peak action is 30 minutes for IV administration and 1 to 2 hours when taken orally.

Side Effects and Adverse Reactions

Side effects and adverse reactions to theophylline include anorexia, nausea, vomiting, diarrhea, gastric pain caused by increased gastric acid secretion, hematemesis, dysrhythmias, tachycardia, palpitations, and marked hypotension. Adverse CNS reactions—headaches, irritability, restlessness, insomnia, dizziness, and seizures—are often more severe in children than in adults. To decrease the potential for side effects, patients should not take other xanthines while taking theophylline.

Theophylline toxicity is most likely to occur when serum concentrations exceed 20 mcg/mL. Theophylline can cause hyperglycemia, decreased clotting time, and, rarely, increased white blood cell count (leukocytosis). Because of the diuretic effect of xanthines, including theophylline, patients should avoid caffeinated products such as coffee, tea, cola, and chocolate, and they should increase fluid intake.

Rapid IV administration of aminophylline, a theophylline product, can cause dizziness, flushing, hypotension, severe bradycardia, and palpitations. To avoid severe adverse effects, IV theophylline preparations *must be administered slowly* via an infusion pump.

Drug Interactions

Beta blockers, cimetidine, propranolol, and erythromycin decrease the liver metabolism rate and increase the half-life and effects of theophylline; barbiturates and carbamazepine decrease its effects. In both situations, the theophylline dosage would need adjustment. Theophylline increases the risk of digitalis toxicity and decreases the effects of lithium. Phenytoin decreases theophylline levels. If theophylline and a beta-adrenergic agonist are given together, a synergistic effect can occur that can result in cardiac dysrhythmias.

LEUKOTRIENE RECEPTOR ANTAGONISTS AND SYNTHESIS INHIBITORS

Leukotriene (LT) is a chemical mediator that can cause inflammatory changes in the lung. The *cysteinyl leukotrienes* promote an increase in eosinophil migration, mucous production, and airway wall edema that results in bronchoconstriction. LT receptor antagonists and LT synthesis inhibitors, called *leukotriene modifiers,* are effective in reducing the inflammatory symptoms of asthma triggered by allergic and environmental stimuli. These drug groups are *not* recommended for treatment of acute asthmatic attacks; rather, they are used for exercise-induced asthma. Three leukotriene modifiers—zafirlukast, zileuton, and montelukast—are available in the United States. These drugs are listed in Table 39.4.

Zafirlukast was the first drug in the class of leukotriene modifiers. It acts as a leukotriene receptor antagonist, reducing the inflammatory

TABLE 39.3	**Theophylline Preparations**	
Drug	**Route and Dosage**	**Uses and Considerations**
Aminophylline-theophylline	A: 18–59 y: IV: 0.4 mg/kg/h infusion; *max:* 900 mg/d Older adults >60 y: IV: 0.2–0.3 mg/kg/h infusion Individual titration is based on serum theophylline levels. Therapeutic range: 5–15 mcg/L.	For bronchospasm due to asthma or COPD. May cause restlessness, headache, insomnia, GERD, dizziness, nausea, vomiting, diarrhea, hypokalemia, hypercalcemia, palpitations, and tachycardia. PB: 40%; t½: 6.5–10.5 h

A, Adult; *COPD,* chronic obstructive pulmonary disease; *h,* hour; *IV,* intravenous; *PB,* protein binding; *t½,* half-life; *y,* year; *>,* greater than.

PROTOTYPE DRUG CHART

Montelukast

Drug Class	Dosage
Bronchodilator: Leukotriene receptor antagonist	A: PO: 10 mg/d in the evening or at least 2 h before exercise; *max:* 10 mg/d

Contraindications	Drug-Lab-Food Interactions
Hypersensitivity *Caution:* Hepatic disease, depression, suicidal ideation, breastfeeding, pregnancy, corticosteroid withdrawal, status asthmaticus, acute bronchospasm, alcohol abuse, older adults	Aspirin and NSAIDs block drug action; telithromycin, gemfibrozil, clopidogrel increase drug levels Lab: Abnormal liver function tests (ALT, AST)

Pharmacokinetics	Pharmacodynamics
Absorption: Well absorbed Distribution: 99% PB Metabolism: t½: 2.7–5.5 h Elimination: In feces and urine	PO: Onset: UK Peak: 3–4 h Duration: 24 h

Therapeutic Effects/Uses

For treatment of allergic rhinitis and asthma, for exercise-induced bronchospasm prophylaxis
Mechanism of Action: Binds with leukotriene receptors to inhibit smooth muscle contraction and bronchoconstriction

Side Effects	Adverse Reactions
Headache, dizziness, drowsiness, cough, nasal congestion, fatigue, infection, agitation, restlessness, insomnia, confusion, depression, influenza, edema, palpitations, muscle cramps	Bleeding, seizures *Life-threatening:* Anaphylaxis, suicidal ideation, thrombocytopenia, Stevens-Johnson syndrome, angioedema

A, Adult; *ALT,* alanine aminotransferase; *AST,* aspartate aminotransferase; *d,* day; *h,* hour; *NSAID,* nonsteroidal antiinflammatory drug; *PB,* protein bound; *PO,* by mouth; *t½,* half-life; *UK,* unknown; *y,* year; *>,* greater than.

TABLE 39.4   Antiinflammatory Drugs for Chronic Obstructive Pulmonary Disease and Asthma

Drug	Route and Dosage	Uses and Considerations
Leukotriene Modifiers (Do Not Administer for Acute Asthmatic Attack)		
Leukotriene Receptor Antagonists Zafirlukast	A: PO: 20 mg bid 1 h before or 2 h after meals; *max:* 40 mg/d	For asthma. May cause headache, dizziness, myalgia, infection, restlessness, hyperbilirubinemia, peripheral neuropathy, nausea, vomiting, and diarrhea. PB: 99%; t½: 10 h
Montelukast	See Prototype Drug Chart: Montelukast	
Leukotriene Synthesis Inhibitors Zileuton	Immediate release: A: PO: 600 mg qid with meals and at bedtime Extended release: A: PO: 1200 mg bid within 1 h after morning and evening meal; *max:* 2400 mg/d	For asthma. May cause headache, chills, asthenia, fatigue, myalgia, abdominal pain, dyspepsia, nausea, constipation, sinusitis, insomnia, and elevated hepatic enzymes. PB: 93%; t½: 1–2.3 h
Phosphodiesterase-4 Inhibitor Roflumilast	A: PO: Initially 250 mcg/d for 4 wk; *maint:* 500 mcg/d; *max:* 500 mcg/d	For COPD. May cause depression, headache, anorexia, nausea, diarrhea, weight loss, and back pain. PB: 99%; t½: 17 h
Glucocorticoids (Corticosteroids)		
Intranasal Spray (See Chapter 35.) Beclomethasone Budesonide Flunisolide Fluticasone Mometasone furoate Triamcinolone		

TABLE 39.4 Antiinflammatory Drugs for Chronic Obstructive Pulmonary Disease and Asthma—cont'd

Drug	Route and Dosage	Uses and Considerations
Aerosol Inhalation (See Chapter 46.) Beclomethasone Flunisolide Budesonide Fluticasone		
Oral and Intravenous Administration (See Chapter 46.) Cortisone acetate Dexamethasone Fludrocortisone acetate Hydrocortisone Methylprednisolone Prednisolone Prednisone		
Combination Drugs: Glucocorticoid and Beta$_2$ Agonist		
Fluticasone and salmeterol	COPD: A: Inhal DPI diskus: 1 inhal (250 mcg fluticasone and 50 mcg salmeterol) q12h; *max:* 2 inhal/d	For asthma and COPD. May cause headache, fever, throat irritation, cough, pharyngitis, diarrhea, infection, oral candidiasis, nausea, vomiting, and musculoskeletal pain. PB: 99% fluticasone, 94%–98% salmeterol; t½: 7.8 h fluticasone, 12.6 h salmeterol
Fluticasone furoate and vilanterol	COPD: A: Inhal: 1 inhalation/d (100 mcg fluticasone and 25 mcg vilanterol) at same time every day	For asthma and COPD. May cause headache, nasopharyngitis, candidiasis, fatigue, infection, fever, cough, and arthralgia. PB: 99% fluticasone, 93.9% vilanterol; t½: 7.8 h fluticasone, 21.3 h vilanterol
Mast Cell Stabilizer		
Cromolyn sodium	Asthma maintenance: A: Inhal: 20 mg nebulizer q6h	For allergic rhinitis and conjunctivitis and exercise-induced bronchospasm prophylaxis. May cause headache, cough, hoarseness, nausea, diarrhea, rash, pruritus, and myalgia. Do not use for acute asthma attack. PB: UK; t½: 80–90 min

A, Adult; *bid,* twice a day; *COPD,* chronic obstructive pulmonary disorder; *d,* day; *DPI,* dry-powder inhaler; *GI,* gastrointestinal; *h,* hour; *inhal,* inhalation; *max,* maximum; *MDI,* metered-dose inhaler; *min,* minute; *PB,* protein binding; *PO,* by mouth; *q,* every; *qd,* every day; *t½,* half-life; *UK,* unknown; *y,* years; *>,* greater than.

process and decreasing bronchoconstriction. It is administered orally, is absorbed rapidly, and has a moderate to moderately long half-life; it is given twice a day. Zileuton is a leukotriene synthesis inhibitor. It decreases the inflammatory process and decreases bronchoconstriction. Zileuton has a short half-life of 1 to 2.3 hours. Montelukast has a short half-life of 2.7 to 5.5 hours and is considered safe for use in children 2 years of age and older (Prototype Drug Chart: Montelukast).

Leukotriene receptor antagonists and synthesis inhibitors should not be used during an acute asthmatic attack. They are only for prophylactic and maintenance drug therapy for chronic asthma.

🌿 COMPLEMENTARY AND ALTERNATIVE THERAPIES

Lower Respiratory Disorders
- Ephedra may increase the effect of the theophylline group and may cause theophylline toxicity.
- St. John's wort may decrease montelukast concentration

GLUCOCORTICOIDS (STEROIDS)

Glucocorticoids, members of the corticosteroid family, are used to treat respiratory disorders, particularly asthma. These drugs have an antiinflammatory action and are indicated if asthma is unresponsive to bronchodilator therapy or if the patient has an asthmatic attack while on maximum doses of theophylline or an adrenergic drug. It is thought that glucocorticoids have a synergistic effect when given with a beta$_2$ agonist.

Glucocorticoids can be given using the following methods:
- *MDI inhaler:* Beclomethasone
- *Tablet:* Dexamethasone, prednisone
- *Intravenous:* Dexamethasone

Inhaled glucocorticoids are not helpful in treating a severe asthmatic attack because it may take 1 to 4 weeks for an inhaled steroid to reach its full effect. When maintained on inhaled glucocorticoids, asthmatic patients demonstrate an improvement in symptoms and a decrease in asthmatic attacks. Inhaled glucocorticoids are more effective for controlling symptoms of asthma than are beta$_2$ agonists, particularly in the reduction of bronchial hyperresponsiveness. The use of an oral inhaler minimizes the risk for adrenal suppression associated with oral systemic glucocorticoid therapy. Inhaled glucocorticoids are preferred over oral preparations unless they fail to control the asthma.

The National Asthma Education and Prevention Program guidelines recommend systemic glucocorticoids—prednisone, prednisolone, dexamethasone, or methylprednisolone—for management of moderate to severe asthma exacerbations. Oral or IV administration of methylprednisolone 40 to 80 mg per day in 1 to 2 divided doses may be given for 3 to 10 days. With a single dose or short-term use, glucocorticoids may be discontinued abruptly after symptoms are controlled. Suppression of adrenal function does not usually occur within 1 to 2 weeks.

When severe asthma requires prolonged glucocorticoid therapy, weaning or tapering of the dose may be necessary to prevent an exacerbation of asthma symptoms and suppression of adrenal function. Previously, alternate-day therapy (ADT) with oral prednisone was used in some asthmatic patients. Currently, inhaled glucocorticoids are thought to be preferable in the treatment of most patients with asthma. Glucocorticoid preparations are discussed in detail in Chapter 46.

Glucocorticoids can irritate the gastric mucosa and should be taken with food to avoid ulceration. A combination inhalation drug containing the glucocorticoid fluticasone propionate and salmeterol is effective in controlling asthma symptoms by alleviating airway constriction and inflammation. This combination is used every day but requires only one inhalation in the morning and one at night. This drug does not replace fast-acting inhalers for sudden symptoms.

◎ CLINICAL JUDGMENT [NURSING PROCESS]

Bronchodilators

Concept: Oxygenation
- The addition of oxygen to the body

Recognize Cues [Assessment]
- Obtain a medical and drug history; report probable drug-drug interactions.
- Note baseline vital signs and pulse oximetry for abnormalities and future comparisons.
- Assess for wheezing, decreased breath sounds, cough, and sputum production.
- Assess sensorium for confusion and restlessness caused by hypoxia and hypercapnia.
- Determine hydration; diuresis may result in dehydration in children and older adults.
- Assess serum theophylline levels. Toxicity occurs at a higher frequency with levels greater than 20 mcg/mL.

Analyze Cues and Prioritize Hypothesis [Patient Problems]
- Airway obstruction
- Decreased gas exchange
- Dyspnea
- Fatigue

Generate Solutions [Planning]
- The patient will be free from wheezing, and lung fields will be clear within 2 to 5 days.
- The patient will self-administer oral drugs and will use an inhaler as prescribed.

Take Action [Nursing Interventions]
- Monitor vital signs. Blood pressure and heart rate can increase greatly. Check for cardiac dysrhythmias.
- Provide adequate hydration. Fluids help loosen secretions.
- Monitor drug therapy.
- Observe for side effects.
- Administer medication after meals to decrease gastrointestinal (GI) distress.
- Administer medication at regular intervals around the clock to have a sustained therapeutic level.
- Do *not* crush enteric-coated (EC) or sustained-released (SR) tablets or capsules.
- ⚡ Check serum theophylline levels (normal level is 5 to 15 mcg/mL).

Patient Teaching
General
- Teach patients to monitor their pulse rate.
- Encourage patients to monitor the amount of medication remaining in the canister.

- Advise patients not to take over-the-counter (OTC) preparations without first checking with a health care provider. Some OTC products may have an additive effect.
- Encourage patients contemplating pregnancy to seek medical advice before taking a theophylline preparation.
- Advise patients to avoid smoking. Avoid marked sudden changes in smoking amounts, which could affect theophylline blood levels. Smoking increases drug elimination, which may require an increased drug dose.
- Discuss ways to alleviate anxiety, such as relaxation techniques and music.
- ⚡ Advise patients having asthmatic attacks to wear an identification bracelet or MedicAlert tag.
- Inform patients that certain complementary and alternative therapies may interact with theophylline.
- ⚡ Advise patients to notify a health care provider of aggressive or altered behavior and suicidal thoughts.

Self-Administration
- Teach patients to correctly use the inhaler or nebulizer. Caution against overuse because side effects and tolerance may result.
- Teach patients to monitor pulse rate and report to a health care provider any irregularities in comparison with baseline values.

Diet
- Advise patients that a high-protein, low-carbohydrate diet increases theophylline elimination. Conversely, a low-protein, high-carbohydrate diet prolongs half-life; dosage may need adjustment.

Correct Use of a Metered-Dose Inhaler to Deliver Beta$_2$ Agonist
- Insert the medication canister into the plastic mouthpiece.
- Shake the inhaler well before use.
- Remove the cap from the mouthpiece.
- Hold the mouthpiece 1 to 2 inches from the mouth or place the inhaler mouthpiece in the mouth. A spacer may be used; discuss technique with a health care provider.
- Breathe out through the mouth, then take a *slow deep* breath in through the mouth; at the same time, push the top of the medication canister once.
- Hold the breath for a few seconds; exhale slowly through pursed lips.
- Wait 2 minutes if a second dose is required, and then repeat the procedure by first shaking the inhaler with the mouthpiece cap in place.
- Do a test spray into the air before administering the metered dose of a new inhaler or when the inhaler has not been used recently.

Evaluate Outcomes [Evaluation]
- Evaluate the effectiveness of the bronchodilator. The patient should be breathing without wheezing and should be unharmed from the side effects of the drug.
- Determine serum theophylline levels to ensure a therapeutic range.

Side Effects and Adverse Reactions

Side effects associated with orally inhaled glucocorticoids are generally local (e.g., throat irritation, hoarseness, dry mouth, coughing) rather than systemic. Oral, laryngeal, and pharyngeal fungal infections have occurred but can be reversed with discontinuation and antifungal treatment. *Candida albicans* oropharyngeal infections may be prevented by using a spacer with the inhaler to reduce drug deposits in the oral cavity, rinsing the mouth and throat with water after each dose, and washing the apparatus (cap and plastic nose or mouthpiece) daily with warm water.

Oral and injectable glucocorticoids have many side effects when used long term, but short-term use usually causes no significant side effects. Most adverse reactions are seen within 2 weeks of glucocorticoid therapy and are usually reversible. Side effects that may occur include headache, euphoria, confusion, diaphoresis, insomnia, nausea, vomiting, weakness, and menstrual irregularities. Adverse effects include depression, peptic ulcer, loss of bone density and development of osteoporosis, and psychosis.

When oral and IV steroids are used for prolonged periods, electrolyte imbalance, fluid retention (puffy eyelids, edema in the lower extremities, moon face, weight gain), hypertension, thinning of the skin, purpura, abnormal subcutaneous fat distribution, hyperglycemia, and impaired immune response are likely to occur.

◎ CLINICAL JUDGMENT [NURSING PROCESS]
Leukotriene Receptor Antagonists

Concept: Oxygenation
- The addition of oxygen to the body.

Recognize Cues [Assessment]
- Obtain a medical, drug, and herbal history; report probable drug-drug or drug-herb interactions.
- Note baseline vital signs for identifying abnormalities and for future comparisons.
- Assess for wheezing, decreased breath sounds, cough, and sputum production.
- Assess sensorium for confusion and restlessness caused by hypoxia and hypercapnia.
- Assess for a history of phenylketonuria when montelukast is prescribed because children's chewable tablets contain phenylalanine.
- Determine hydration; diuresis may result in dehydration in children and older adults.

Analyze Cues and Prioritize Hypothesis [Patient Problems]
- Airway obstruction
- Decreased gas exchange
- Dyspnea
- Fatigue

Generate Solutions [Planning]
- The patient will be free from wheezing, or wheezing will have significantly improved.
- The patient's lung fields will be clear within 2 to 5 days.
- The patient will take medications as prescribed.

Take Action [Nursing Interventions]
- Monitor respirations for rate, depth, rhythm, and type.
- Monitor lung sounds for rhonchi, wheezing, or rales.
- Observe lips and fingernails for cyanosis.
- Monitor drug therapy for effectiveness.
- Observe for side effects.
- Provide adequate hydration; fluids help loosen secretions.
- Monitor liver function tests; aspartate transaminase (AST) and alanine transaminase (ALT) may be elevated with zafirlukast and montelukast.
- Provide pulmonary therapy by chest clapping and postural drainage as appropriate.

Patient Teaching
General
- Advise patients that if an allergic reaction occurs (i.e., rash, urticaria), the drug should be discontinued, and a health care provider should be notified.
- Monitor hepatic function tests periodically.
- Direct patients not to take St. John's wort without first checking with a health care provider because this product may decrease montelukast concentration.
- Warn patients that black or green tea and guarana taken with montelukast and zafirlukast may cause increased stimulation.
- Encourage patients to stop smoking.
- Discuss ways to alleviate anxiety (relaxation techniques, music).
- ⚡ Advise patients who have frequent or severe asthmatic attacks to wear an identification bracelet or a MedicAlert tag.
- Encourage patients contemplating pregnancy to seek medical advice before taking montelukast.
- Caution patients and their significant others not to open oral granule packets until they are ready to use them. After opening a packet, the dose must be administered within 15 minutes. If mixed with baby formula or an approved food (applesauce, carrots, rice, or ice cream), do *not* store for future use.
- Advise patients with known aspirin sensitivity to avoid a bronchoconstrictor response by avoiding aspirin and nonsteroidal antiinflammatory drugs (NSAIDs) while taking montelukast.

Self-Administration
- Teach patients not to use montelukast for reversal of an acute asthmatic attack because it is only recommended for prevention of acute attacks and for treatment of chronic asthma.
- Advise patients to continue to use the usual regimen of inhaled prophylaxis and short-acting rescue medication for exercise-induced bronchospasm.
- ⚡ Encourage patients to inform a health care provider if short-acting inhaled bronchodilators are needed more often than usual with montelukast.
- Tell patients to comply with the medication regimen even during symptom-free periods.
- Advise patients, especially children, that chewable tablets are to be chewed thoroughly because swallowing whole may alter absorption.

Diet
- Tell patients to take leukotriene receptor antagonists in the evening for maximum effectiveness.

Evaluate Outcomes [Evaluation]
- Evaluate the effectiveness of the bronchodilators. The patient should be breathing without wheezing and without side effects of the drug.
- Evaluate tolerance to activity.

CROMOLYN

Cromolyn sodium is used for prophylactic treatment of bronchial asthma, and it must be taken daily. It is not used for acute asthmatic attacks. Cromolyn does not have bronchodilator properties but instead acts by inhibiting release of histamine and other inflammatory mediators from mast cells to prevent an asthma attack. Its most common side effects include postnasal drip, irritation of the nose and throat, and a cough. These effects can be decreased by drinking water before and after using the drug.

Cromolyn is administered by oral inhalation via MDI or nebulizer and nasal inhalation via metered spray. It can be used with beta adrenergics and xanthine derivatives. Rebound bronchospasm is a serious side effect of cromolyn. The drug should not be discontinued abruptly because a rebound asthmatic attack can result.

Cromolyn has a low incidence of side effects but the drug is only moderately effective, and many newer drugs have replaced cromolyn use. Table 39.4 lists antiinflammatory drugs for COPD, including LT receptor antagonists, LT synthesis inhibitors, phosphodiesterase-4 inhibitors, glucocorticoids, combination drugs (glucocorticoid and beta₂ agonist), and cromolyn.

DRUG THERAPY FOR ASTHMA ACCORDING TO SEVERITY

Chronic asthma may be controlled through a long-term medical treatment program and by a quick-relief program during an acute phase. The long-term program may vary according to the symptoms of the asthma and its severity, whereas the quick-relief therapy is the same for all classes of asthma.

DRUG THERAPY FOR ASTHMA ACCORDING TO AGE

Young Children

Cromolyn is used to treat the inflammatory effects of asthma in children. Oral glucocorticoids may be prescribed for the young child to control a moderate to severe asthmatic state. An inhalation dose of a glucocorticoid should be about 1 to 2 inhalations 4 times a day. If the condition is severe, selected young children may be ordered an oral beta₂-adrenergic agonist.

Older Adults

Drug selection and dosage need to be considered for the older adult with an asthmatic condition. Beta₂-adrenergic agonists and methylxanthines such as theophylline can cause tachycardia, nervousness, and tremors in older adults, especially those with cardiac conditions. Frequent use of glucocorticoids can increase the risk of the patient developing cataracts, osteoporosis, and diabetes mellitus. If a theophylline drug is ordered, dosages of glucocorticoids are normally decreased.

ANTIMICROBIALS

Antibiotics are used only if a bacterial infection results from retained mucous secretions. Trimethoprim-sulfamethoxazole is effective for the treatment of mild to moderate acute exacerbations of chronic bronchitis (AECBs) from infectious causes.

CRITICAL THINKING SINGLE EPISODE CASE STUDY

Cognitive Skill: Prioritize hypothesis.

A 45-year-old female patient with a diagnosis of asthma was feeling short of breath. Earlier in the morning she performed outside gardening work. She used the rescue inhaler prescribed by her doctor. After not receiving any relief the symptoms worsened, so she went to the emergency department. Her oxygen saturation was 91% on room air. They immediately placed her on oxygen and called for the respiratory therapist who started her on albuterol breathing treatment. After about 1 hour she started to improve. Upon discharge she received an order for the anticholinergic drug tiotropium bromide, two inhalations once a day, with instructions to continue her prescribed medications and to follow-up with her respiratory doctor.

During the discharge teaching, the nurse reviewed the new drug tiotropium inhaler its therapeutic effectiveness and side effects.

Tiotropium is used to treat _____(1). The therapeutic response of tiotropium is to _____(1) and _____(1). The side-effects include _____(2), _____(2), _____(2), and _____(2).

Options for 1	Options for 2
Increases wheezing	Insomnia
Relaxes smooth muscle	Muscle cramping
Asthma	Tremor
Increases shortness of breath	Sinusitis
Dilate the bronchi	Coughing

Options for 1	Options for 2
Promotes drowsiness	Headache
Sore throat	Increased appetite
Hypokalemia	Blurred vision

Answers:

Tiotropium is used to treat asthma (1). The therapeutic response of tiotropium is to relax smooth muscle (1) and dilate the bronchi (1). The side-effects include insomnia (2), sinusitis (2), headache (2), and blurred vision (2).

Rationale:

Asthma is an inflammatory disorder of the airway walls associated with varying amount of airway obstruction. The patient's asthma was triggered by stimuli such as stress, allergens, and pollutants. When activated by stimuli, the bronchial airways become inflamed and edematous, leading to constriction of air passages. Inflammation aggravates airway hyperresponsiveness to stimuli, causing bronchial cells to produce more mucus, which obstructs air passages. Tiotropium blocks muscarinic cholinergic receptors and antagonizes acetylcholine action by inhibiting M3 receptor response to acetylcholine, thereby relaxing smooth muscle of bronchi and dilating the bronchi.

Reference:

Pharmacology, McCuistion, et al. Pharmacology, Chapter 39 (Tiotropium Prototype Drug Chart); J. R. Burchum, et al, Lehne's Pharmacology for Nursing Care, (9th ed) Chapter 76, p. 930.

REVIEW QUESTIONS

1. Fluticasone propionate and salmeterol combination inhalation is ordered for a patient with chronic obstructive pulmonary disease. What does the nurse know about this medication? (Select all that apply.)
   a. It can be used to treat an acute attack.
   b. It is delivered as a dry-powder inhaler.
   c. It contains a beta1 agonist and cromolyn.
   d. It is taken as one puff two times a day.
   e. It promotes bronchodilation.

2. A patient with chronic obstructive pulmonary disease has an acute bronchospasm. The nurse anticipates that the health care provider will prescribe which medication?
   a. Zafirlukast
   b. Epinephrine
   c. Dexamethasone
   d. Beclomethasone

3. A patient is prescribed aminophylline-theophylline. For what adverse effect should the nurse monitor the patient?
   a. Drowsiness
   b. Hypoglycemia
   c. Increased heart rate
   d. Decreased white blood cell count

4. A patient is receiving intravenous aminophylline. The nurse checks the patient's laboratory values and sees the serum theophylline level is 32 mcg/mL. What action should the nurse take?
   a. Assess the patient's breath sounds for improvement.
   b. Increase the dosage per sliding scale directions.
   c. Notify the health care provider of the level.
   d. Have the laboratory collect another sample to verify the results.

5. A patient with chronic obstructive pulmonary disease is taking the leukotriene antagonist montelukast. The nurse is aware that this medication is given for which purpose?
   a. Maintenance treatment of asthma
   b. Treatment of acute asthmatic attack
   c. Reversing bronchospasm associated with chronic obstructive pulmonary disease
   d. Treatment of inflammation in chronic bronchitis

40

Cardiac Glycosides, Antianginals, and Antidysrhythmics

http://evolve.elsevier.com/McCuistion/pharmacology

OBJECTIVES

- Differentiate the actions of cardiac glycosides, antianginal drugs, and antidysrhythmic drugs.
- Describe the signs and symptoms of digitalis toxicity.
- Compare the side effects and adverse reactions of nitrates, beta blockers, calcium channel blockers, quinidine, and procainamide.

- Apply the Clinical Judgment [Nursing Process], including patient teaching, related to cardiac glycosides, antianginal drugs, and antidysrhythmic drugs.

OUTLINE

INTRODUCTION

The cardiovascular system includes the heart, blood vessels (arteries and veins), and blood flow. Blood that is abundant in oxygen (O_2), nutrients, and hormones moves through vessels called *arteries,* which narrow to arterioles and then to capillaries. Capillaries transport nourished blood to body cells and absorb waste products, such as carbon dioxide (CO_2), urea, creatinine, and ammonia. The deoxygenated blood returns to the circulation by small venules and larger veins to be eliminated by the lungs and kidneys with other waste products (Fig. 40.1).

The heart's pumping action serves as the energy source that circulates blood to the cells of the body. Blockage of vessels can inhibit blood flow.

HEART

The heart is composed of four chambers, including the right and left atria and the right and left ventricles (Fig. 40.2). The right atrium

receives deoxygenated blood from the circulation, and the right ventricle pumps blood through the pulmonary artery to the lungs for gas exchange (carbon dioxide for oxygen). The left atrium receives oxygenated blood, and the left ventricle pumps the blood into the aorta for systemic circulation.

The heart muscle, called the *myocardium,* surrounds the ventricles and atria. The ventricles have thick walls, especially the left ventricle, to produce the muscular force needed to pump blood to the pulmonary and systemic circulations. The atria have thin walls, have less pumping action, and receive blood from the circulation and lungs.

The heart has a fibrous covering called the *pericardium,* which protects it from injury and infection. The *endocardium* is a three-layered membrane that lines the inner part of the heart chambers. Four valves—two atrioventricular (tricuspid and mitral) and two semilunar (pulmonic and aortic)—control blood flow between the atria and ventricles, and between the ventricles and the pulmonary artery and the aorta. There are two main coronary arteries: the right coronary artery

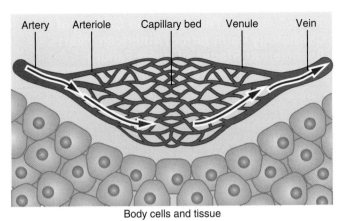

Fig. 40.1 Basic structures of the vascular system.

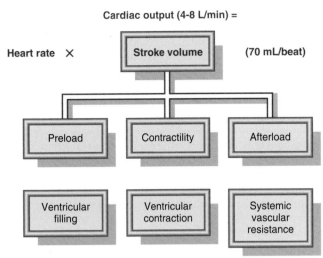

Fig. 40.3 Cardiac Output and Stroke Volume. Three groups of drugs—cardiac glycosides, antianginals, and antidysrhythmics—are discussed in this chapter. Drugs in these groups regulate heart contraction, heart rate and rhythm, and blood flow to the myocardium (heart muscle).

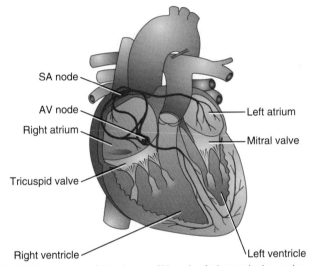

Fig. 40.2 Anatomy of the heart. *AV node,* Atrioventricular node; *SA node,* sinoatrial node.

divides into branches that supply blood to the right atrium and both ventricles of the heart, and the left coronary artery divides near its origin to form the left circumflex artery and the anterior descending artery, which supply blood to the left atrium and both ventricles of the heart. Blockage to one of these arteries can result in a myocardial infarction (MI), or heart attack.

CONDUCTION OF ELECTRICAL IMPULSES

The myocardium can generate and conduct its own electrical impulses. The cardiac impulse normally originates in the *sinoatrial (SA) node* located in the posterior wall of the right atrium. The SA node is frequently called the *pacemaker* because it regulates the heartbeat (firing of cardiac impulses), which is approximately 60 to 80 beats/min in the normal adult. The *atrioventricular (AV) node,* located in the posterior right side of the interatrial septum, has a continuous tract of fibers called the *bundle of His,* or the AV bundle. The AV node has an adult rate of 40 to 60 beats/min. If the SA node fails, the AV node takes over as the pacemaker, thus causing a slower heart rate; the AV node sends impulses to the ventricles. These two conducting systems, the SA and AV nodes, can act independently of each other. The ventricle can contract independently 30 to 40 times per minute.

Drugs that affect cardiac contraction include calcium, digitalis preparations, and quinidine and its related preparations. The autonomic nervous system (ANS) and drugs that stimulate or inhibit it

influence heart contractions. The sympathetic nervous system and drugs that stimulate it *increase* heart rate; the parasympathetic nervous system and drugs that stimulate it *decrease* heart rate.

REGULATION OF HEART RATE AND BLOOD FLOW

The heart beats approximately 60 to 80 times per minute in an adult, pumping blood into the systemic circulation. As blood travels, resistance to blood flow develops, and arterial pressure increases. The average systemic arterial pressure, known as *blood pressure,* is 120/80 mm Hg. Arterial blood pressure is determined by peripheral resistance and *cardiac output,* which is the volume of blood expelled from the heart in 1 minute, calculated by multiplying the heart rate by the stroke volume. The average cardiac output is 4 to 8 L/min. *Stroke volume,* the amount of blood ejected from the left ventricle with each heartbeat, is approximately 70 mL/beat.

Three factors—preload, contractility, and afterload—determine the stroke volume (Fig. 40.3). *Preload* refers to the blood flow force that stretches the ventricle at the end of diastole. However, an increase in preload can increase stroke volume, and a decrease in preload can decrease stroke volume. *Contractility* is the force of ventricular contraction, and afterload is the resistance to ventricular ejection of blood, which is caused by opposing pressures in the aorta and systemic circulation. If afterload *increases,* stroke volume will *decrease,* and if afterload *decreases,* stroke volume will *increase.*

Specific drugs can increase or decrease preload and afterload, affecting both stroke volume and cardiac output. Most vasodilators decrease preload and afterload, thus decreasing arterial pressure and cardiac output.

CIRCULATION

There are two types of circulation, pulmonary and systemic. With *pulmonary circulation,* the heart pumps deoxygenated blood from the right ventricle through the pulmonary artery to the lungs. The pulmonary artery carries blood that has a high concentration of carbon dioxide. Oxygenated blood returns to the left atrium by the pulmonary vein.

With *systemic circulation,* also called *peripheral circulation,* the heart pumps blood from the left ventricle to the aorta and into the general circulation. Arteries and arterioles carry the blood to capillary beds. Nutrients in the capillary blood are transferred to cells in exchange for waste products. Blood returns to the heart through venules and veins.

BLOOD

Blood is composed of plasma, red blood cells (RBCs; erythrocytes), white blood cells (WBCs; leukocytes), and platelets. Plasma, made up of 90% water and 10% solutes, constitutes 55% of the total blood volume. The solutes in plasma include glucose, protein, lipids, amino acids, electrolytes, minerals, lactic and pyruvic acids, hormones, enzymes, oxygen, and carbon dioxide.

The major function of blood is to provide nutrients, including oxygen, to body cells. Most of the oxygen is carried on the hemoglobin of RBCs. WBCs are the major defense mechanism of the body and act by engulfing microorganisms. They also produce antibodies. The platelets are large cells that cause blood to coagulate. RBCs have a life span of approximately 120 days, whereas the life span of a WBC is only 2 to 24 hours.

Three groups of drugs (cardiac glycosides, antianginals, and antidysrhythmics) are discussed in this chapter. Drugs in these groups regulate heart contraction, heart rate, heart rhythm, and blood flow to the myocardium.

LABORATORY TESTS TO DIAGNOSE HEART FAILURE

Atrial Natriuretic Hormone or Peptide

Reference values: 20 to 77 pg/mL; 20 to 77 ng/L (SI units). An elevated atrial natriuretic hormone (ANH) or atrial natriuretic peptide (ANP) may confirm heart failure (HF). ANH is secreted from the atria of the heart and acts as an antagonist to renin and aldosterone. Released during expansion of the atrium, it produces vasodilation and increases glomerular filtration rate (GFR). Results of ANH secretion include a large volume of urine that decreases blood volume and blood pressure.

Brain Natriuretic Peptide

Reference values: Desired value is less than 100 pg/mL; positive value is greater than 100 pg/mL. The brain natriuretic peptide (BNP) is primarily secreted from atrial cardiac cells and, when tested, aids in the diagnosis of HF. Diagnosing HF is difficult in persons with lung disease who are experiencing dyspnea and in those who are obese or older. An elevated BNP helps differentiate that dyspnea is due to HF rather than to lung dysfunction. Frequently the BNP is higher than 100 pg/mL in women who are 65 years of age or older. An 80-year-old woman may have a BNP of 160 pg/mL; however, the BNP is markedly higher (i.e., 400 pg/mL) in HF. BNP is considered a more sensitive test than ANP for diagnosing HF. Today, a bedside/emergency department machine can be used to measure BNP.

NONPHARMACOLOGIC MEASURES TO TREAT HEART FAILURE

Nondrug therapy is an integral part of the regimen for controlling HF. The nondrug component of the regimen should be tailored to meet the needs of each patient, but the following are some general recommendations. The patient should limit salt intake to 2 g/day, approximately 1 teaspoon. Alcohol intake should be either decreased to 1 drink per day or completely avoided because excessive alcohol use can lead to cardiomyopathy. Fluid intake may be restricted. Smoking should be avoided because it deprives the heart of oxygen (O_2). Obesity may increase cardiovascular problems if it is associated with unhealthy behaviors; thus obese patients should modify their behaviors as needed. Saturated fat intake should be decreased. Mild exercise, such as walking or bicycling, is recommended.

TABLE 40.1 The American College of Cardiology Foundation/American Heart Association Stages of Heart Failure

Stage	Characteristics According to Stage
A	At high risk for heart failure but without structural heart disease or symptoms of heart failure
B	Structural heart disease but without signs or symptoms of heart failure
C	Structural heart disease with prior or current symptoms of heart failure
D	Refractory heart failure requiring specialized interventions

Data from Maddox, T. M., Januzzi, J. L., Allen, L. A., et al.; (2021). Update to the 2017 ACC Expert Consensus Decision Pathway for Optimization of Heart Failure Treatment: Answers to 10 Pivotal Issues About Heart Failure With Reduced Ejection Fraction: A Report of the American College of Cardiology Solution Set Oversight Committee. Journal of the American College of Cardiology, 77(6), 772-810.

AGENTS USED TO TREAT HEART FAILURE

Cardiac Glycosides

Digitalis use began as early as CE 1200, making it one of the oldest drugs. It is still used in a purified form. Digitalis is obtained from the purple and white foxglove plant, and it can be poisonous. Digitalis preparations have come to be known for their effectiveness in treating HF, also known as *cardiac failure* (CF), and previously referred to as congestive heart failure (CHF). When the heart muscle (*myocardium*) weakens and enlarges, it loses its ability to pump blood through the heart and into the systemic circulation. This is called heart failure, *pump failure,* or *chronic heart failure.* When compensatory mechanisms fail and the peripheral and lung tissues are congested, the condition is called *acute heart failure.* The causes of HF include chronic hypertension, MI, coronary artery disease (CAD), valvular heart disease, congenital heart disease, and arteriosclerosis.

HF can be left-sided or right-sided. The patient has *left-sided HF* when the left ventricle does not contract sufficiently to pump the blood returned from the lungs and left atrium out through the aorta into the peripheral circulation; this causes excessive amounts of blood to back up into the lung tissue. Usually the patient has shortness of breath (SOB) and dyspnea. *Right-sided HF* occurs when the heart does not sufficiently pump the blood returned into the right atrium from the systemic circulation. As a result, the blood and its constituents are backed up into peripheral tissues, causing peripheral edema. Left-sided HF may lead to right-sided HF and vice versa. Myocardial hypertrophy resulting in *cardiomegaly,* increased heart size, can be a major problem associated with chronic HF.

In the cardiac physiology of HF, an increase in *preload* and *afterload* occurs. The increased preload results from an excess of blood volume in the ventricle at the end of diastole. This occurs because of a pathologic increase in the stretching and thickening of the ventricular walls, which allows a greater filling pressure associated with a weakened heart. Increased afterload is an additional pressure or force in the ventricular wall caused by excess resistance in the aorta. This resistance must be overcome to open the aortic valve so blood can be ejected into the circulation. The American College of Cardiology Foundation (ACCF) and the American Heart Association (AHA) have classified HF in stages according to its severity. Table 40.1 lists the stages of HF according to the ACCF/AHA. In the early stage of HF, there are no symptoms, and no structural heart damage occurs. Detailed information related to the staging process of HF can be found at http://www.heart.org/HEARTORG/Conditions/HeartFailure/Heart-Failure_UCM_002019_SubHomePage.jsp.

Naturally occurring cardiac glycosides are found in several plants, including *Digitalis.* Also called *digitalis glycosides,* this group of drugs inhibits the sodium-potassium pump, which results in an increase in intracellular sodium. This increase leads to an influx of calcium, which causes the cardiac muscle fibers to contract more efficiently. Digitalis preparations have three effects on heart muscle: (1) a positive inotropic action *increases* myocardial contraction stroke volume, (2) a negative chronotropic action *decreases* heart rate, and (3) a negative dromotropic action *decreases* conduction of heart cells. The increase in myocardial contractility strengthens cardiac, peripheral, and kidney function by enhancing cardiac output, decreasing preload, improving blood flow to the periphery and kidneys, decreasing edema, and promoting fluid excretion. As a result, fluid retention in the lungs and extremities is decreased. Digoxin does not prolong life; rather, it acts by increasing the force and velocity of myocardial systolic contraction.

Digoxin is a secondary drug for HF. First-line drugs used to treat acute HF include intravenous (IV) inotropic agents (dopamine and dobutamine) and phosphodiesterase (PDE) inhibitors, such as milrinone. Other drugs prescribed for HF include oral diuretics, beta blockers, angiotensin-converting enzyme (ACE) inhibitors, angiotensin-receptor blockers (ARBs), calcium channel blockers (CCBs), and vasodilators, all of which are more convenient to self-administer. Oral administration allows the patient to go home on these medications.

Cardiac glycosides are also used to correct atrial fibrillation, cardiac dysrhythmia with rapid uncoordinated contractions of atrial myocardium, and atrial flutter, cardiac dysrhythmia with rapid contractions of 200 to 300 beats/min. This is accomplished by the negative chronotropic effects (decreased heart rate) and negative dromotropic effects (decreased conduction through the atrioventricular [AV] node).

When digoxin cannot convert atrial fibrillation to normal heart rhythm, the goal is to slow the heart rate by decreasing electrical impulses through the AV node. For management of atrial fibrillation, a CCB such as verapamil may be prescribed. To prevent thromboemboli resulting from atrial fibrillation, warfarin is prescribed concurrently with other drug therapy. Warfarin is discussed in Chapter 40.

Digoxin

Prototype Drug Chart: Digoxin gives the pharmacologic data for digoxin, a cardiac glycoside.

Pharmacokinetics. The absorption rate of digoxin in oral tablet form is 70% to 80%. The rate is 75% to 85% in liquid form. The protein-binding power for digoxin is 20% to 30%. The half-life is 30 to 40 hours. Because of its long half-life, drug accumulation can occur. Side effects should be closely monitored to detect digitalis toxicity. Patients should be made aware of side effects that need to be reported to the health care provider. Serum digoxin levels are most commonly drawn when actual digitoxicity is suspected. This allows the health care provider to ascertain the extent of such toxicity and to confirm elimination of the drug after it is stopped or decreased in dosage (see the Digitalis [Digoxin] Toxicity section later in this chapter).

Thirty percent of digoxin is metabolized by the liver, and 70% is excreted by the kidneys mostly unchanged. Kidney dysfunction can

PROTOTYPE DRUG CHART

Digoxin

Drug Class	Dosage
Cardiac glycoside	Atrial fibrillation: A: PO: LD 10–15 mcg/kg in 3 divided doses (give 50% LD for dose 1, 25% for doses 2 and 3); *maint:* 3.4–5.1 mcg/kg/d A: IV/IM: LD 8–12 mcg/kg/d in 3 divided doses; *maint:* 2.4–3.6 mcg/kg/d TDM: 0.8–2 ng/mL

Contraindications	Drug-Lab-Food Interactions
Ventricular fibrillation, hypersensitivity *Caution:* AMI, AV block, ventricular tachycardia, hypertension, thyroid disorder, renal/hepatic dysfunction, bradycardia, electrolyte imbalance, cardiomyopathy, breastfeeding, older adults	Drug: Increased digoxin serum level with quinidine, flecainide, verapamil, indomethacin; decreased digoxin absorption with antacids, kaolin, pectin, psyllium, acarbose, colestipol; increased risk for digoxin toxicity with thiazide diuretics, loop diuretics, proton pump inhibitors Lab: Hypokalemia, hypomagnesemia, hypercalcemia can increase digitalis (digoxin) toxicity

Pharmacokinetics	Pharmacodynamics
Absorption: PO tablet: 70%–80%; PO liquid: 75%–85% Distribution: PB: 20%–30% Metabolism: t½: 36–48 h Excretion: 70% in urine; 30% by liver metabolism	PO: Onset: 30 min-2 h Peak: 2–6 h Duration: 3–4 d IV: Onset: 5–30 min Peak: 1–6 h Duration: UK

Therapeutic Effects/Uses

To treat heart failure, atrial fibrillation
Mechanism of Action: Inhibits sodium-potassium ATPase, promoting increased force of cardiac contraction, cardiac output, and tissue perfusion; decreases ventricular rate

Side Effects	Adverse Reactions
Anorexia, nausea, vomiting, diarrhea, abdominal pain, headache, blurred or yellow vision, dizziness, weakness, confusion, visual impairment, anxiety	Bradycardia, hallucinations, bowel necrosis, palpitations *Life-threatening:* Dysrhythmias, thrombocytopenia

A, Adult; *AMI,* acute myocardial infarction; *ATPase,* adenosine triphosphatase; *AV,* atrioventricular; *d,* day; *h,* hour; *IM,* intramuscular; *IV,* intravenous; *LD,* loading dose; *maint,* maintenance; *min,* minute; *PB,* protein binding; *PO,* by mouth; *t½,* half-life; *TDM,* therapeutic drug monitoring; *UK,* unknown; *y,* year; *>,* greater than.

! TABLE 40.2   Cardiac Glycosides and Inotropic Agents

Drug	Route and Dosage	Uses and Considerations
Rapid-Acting Digitalis		
Digoxin	See Prototype Drug Chart: Digoxin	
Phosphodiesterase Inhibitors (Positive Inotropic Bipyridines)		
Milrinone lactate	A: IV: LD: 50 mcg/kg infusion over 10 min; *maint:* 0.125–0.75 mcg/kg/min infusion; *max:* 0.75 mcg/kg/min infusion	For acute decompensated heart failure. May cause headache, hypotension, tachycardia, dysrhythmias, injection site reaction, tremor, nausea, vomiting, hypokalemia, thrombocytopenia, and angina. PB: 70%; t½: 2.4 h
Atrial Natriuretic Peptide Hormones		
Nesiritide	A: IV bolus: 2 mcg/kg; *maint:* 0.01 mcg/kg/min infusion; *max:* 0.03 mcg/kg/min continuous infusion	For acute decompensated heart failure. May cause orthostatic hypotension, headache, drowsiness, anxiety, nausea, tachycardia, back pain, bradycardia, angina, insomnia, hypoglycemia, and dysrhythmias. PB: UK; t½: 18 min
Antidote for Digitalis Toxicity		
Digoxin-immune Fab	A: IV: 800 mg IV as a single dose or 400 mg, then 400 mg more if needed	For digitalis overdose and toxicity and cardiac glycoside–induced dysrhythmias. May cause anaphylaxis, orthostatic hypotension, atrial fibrillation, heart failure exacerbation, angioedema, wheezing, infusion site reactions, phlebitis, and hypokalemia. PB: UK; t½: 15 h
Guanylate Cyclase Stimulant		
Vericiguat	A: PO: 2.5 mg/d with food; *maint:* 10 mg/d; *max:* 10 mg/d	For heart failure and ejection fraction less than 45%. May cause hypotension, anemia, syncope, and birth defects. PB: 98%; t½: 30 h

A, Adult; *h,* hours; *IV,* intravenous; *maint,* maintenance; *max,* maximum; *min,* minute; *PB,* protein binding; *t½,* half-life; *UK,* unknown.

affect the excretion of digoxin. Thyroid dysfunction can alter the metabolism of cardiac glycosides. For patients with hypothyroidism, the dose of digoxin should be decreased; in hyperthyroidism, the dose may need to be increased.

Pharmacodynamics. In patients with a failing heart, cardiac glycosides increase myocardial contraction, which increases cardiac output and improves circulation and tissue perfusion. Because these drugs decrease conduction through the AV node, the heart rate decreases. The onset and peak actions of oral and IV digoxin vary. The digoxin **therapeutic serum level** for dysrhythmias is 0.8 to 2.0 ng/mL. The target therapeutic serum level for HF is 0.5 to 1.0 ng/mL.

Digoxin can be administered orally or by the IV route. Table 40.2 lists the digitalis preparations and their dosages, uses, and considerations.

Digitalis (Digoxin) Toxicity

Overdose or accumulation of digoxin causes digitalis toxicity. Signs and symptoms include anorexia, diarrhea, nausea and vomiting, **bradycardia** (pulse rate below 60 beats/min), premature ventricular contractions, cardiac dysrhythmias, headaches, malaise, blurred vision, visual illusions (white, green, or yellow halos around objects), confusion, and delirium. Older adults are more prone to toxicity.

Cardiotoxicity is a serious adverse reaction to digoxin, and ventricular dysrhythmias result. Three cardiac-altered functions can contribute to digoxin-induced ventricular dysrhythmias: (1) suppression of AV conduction, (2) increased automaticity, and (3) a decreased refractory period in ventricular muscle. The antidysrhythmics phenytoin and lidocaine are effective in treating digoxin-induced ventricular dysrhythmias. Lidocaine should be limited to short-term treatment.

Antidote for Cardiac/Digitalis Glycosides

Digoxin-immune Fab may be given to treat severe digitalis toxicity. This agent binds with digoxin to form complex molecules that can be excreted in the urine; thus digoxin is unable to bind at the cellular site of action. Serum digoxin levels should be closely monitored, and signs and symptoms of digoxin toxicity should be reported promptly

to the health care provider. Digitalis toxicity may result in first-degree, second-degree, or complete heart block.

🌿 COMPLEMENTARY AND ALTERNATIVE THERAPIES

Cardiac Glycosides, Antihypertensives, and Antidysrhythmics

- Ginseng may falsely elevate digoxin levels.
- St. John's wort decreases absorption of digoxin and thus decreases serum digoxin level.
- Psyllium may decrease digoxin absorption.
- Hawthorn may increase the effect of digoxin and hypotensive drugs.
- Licorice can potentiate the effect of digoxin; it promotes potassium loss (hypokalemia), which increases the effect of digoxin, and it may cause digitalis toxicity. Licorice also decreases the effectiveness of antihypertensives.
- Aloe may increase the risk of digitalis toxicity. It increases potassium loss, which increases the effect of digoxin.
- Ma-huang, or ephedra, increases the risk of digitalis toxicity.
- Goldenseal may decrease the effects of cardiac glycosides and may increase the effects of antidysrhythmics.
- Coleus may potentiate effects of antihypertensives.
- Ginger may cause a synergistic antiplatelet effect with nifedipine.
- Ginkgo may increase drug levels or side effects of nifedipine.
- Korean ginseng may decrease effectiveness of antihypertensives.
- Laxative (anthraquinone-containing) herbs may potentiate cardiac glycosides and antidysrhythmics.
- Milk thistle may delay absorption rate of nifedipine.

Drug Interactions

Drug interaction with digitalis preparations can cause digitalis toxicity. Many of the potent diuretics, such as furosemide and hydrochlorothiazide, promote the loss of potassium from the body. The resultant **hypokalemia**, low serum potassium level, increases the effect of digoxin at its myocardial cell site of action, resulting in digitalis toxicity. Cortisone

CLINICAL JUDGMENT [NURSING PROCESS]

! *Cardiac Glycosides: Digoxin*

Concept: Perfusion
- The passage of blood flow through the arteries and capillaries that deliver oxygen and nutrients to body cells

Recognize Cues [Assessment]
- Obtain a drug and herbal history. Report if a drug-drug or drug-herb interaction is probable. If a patient is taking digoxin and a potassium-wasting diuretic or cortisone drug, hypokalemia can result, causing digitalis toxicity. A low serum potassium level enhances the action of digoxin. Patients taking a thiazide and/or cortisone with digoxin should take a potassium supplement.
- Obtain a baseline pulse rate for future comparisons. Apical pulse should be taken for a full minute and should be greater than 60 beats/min.
- Assess for signs and symptoms of digitalis toxicity. Common symptoms include anorexia, nausea, vomiting, bradycardia, cardiac dysrhythmias, and visual disturbances. Report symptoms immediately to the health care provider.

Analyze Cues and Prioritize Hypothesis [Patient Problems]
- Decreased gas exchange
- Decreased tissue perfusion
- Hypoxemia
- Ischemia

Generate Solutions [Planning]
- The patient will demonstrate checking their pulse rate before taking digoxin.
- The patient will state that it is important to report the pulse rate when it is less than 60 beats/min or when a marked decline in pulse rate occurs.
- The patient will list six foods high in potassium to maintain a desired serum potassium level (see Patient Teaching and Diet sections).

Take Action [Nursing Interventions]
- ⚡ Ascertain apical pulse rate before administering digoxin. Do *not* administer if pulse rate is below 60 beats/min.
- Determine signs of peripheral and pulmonary edema, which indicate HF is present.

- ⚡ Monitor serum digoxin level (normal therapeutic drug range is 0.8 to 2 ng/mL). A serum digoxin level greater than 2 ng/mL is indicative of digitalis toxicity.
- ⚡ Monitor serum potassium level (normal range is 3.5 to 5.0 mEq/L), and report if hypokalemia (<3.5 mEq/L) is present.

Patient Teaching
General
- Explain to patients the importance of adherence to drug therapy. A visiting nurse may ensure that medications are taken properly.
- Advise patients to avoid adverse drug interactions by not taking over-the-counter (OTC) drugs without first consulting a health care provider.
- Keep drugs out of reach of small children and request childproof bottles.
- Teach patients and caregivers to check the pulse rate before administering drugs.
- Inform patients of possible herb-drug interactions.

Self-Administration
- Teach patients how to check the pulse rate before taking digoxin and to notify a health care provider if the pulse rate is irregular or less than 60 beats/min.

Side Effects
- ⚡ Instruct patients to report side effects: pulse rate less than 60 beats/min, nausea and vomiting, headache, diarrhea, and visual disturbances, including diplopia.

Diet
- Advise patients to eat foods high in potassium, such as fresh and dried fruits, fruit juices, and vegetables, including potatoes.

Evaluate Outcomes [Evaluation]
- Evaluate the effectiveness of digoxin by noting the patient's response to a drug (decreased heart rate, decreased rales) and absence of side effects. Continue monitoring the pulse rate.

---

preparations taken systemically promote sodium retention and potassium excretion or loss and can also cause hypokalemia. Patients who take digoxin along with a potassium-wasting diuretic or a cortisone drug should consume foods rich in potassium or take potassium supplements to avoid hypokalemia and digitalis toxicity. Antacids can decrease digitalis absorption if taken at the same time. To prevent this problem, doses should be staggered.

! Phosphodiesterase Inhibitors

PDE inhibitors are another positive inotropic group of drugs given to treat acute HF. This drug group inhibits the enzyme PDE, which promotes a positive inotropic response and vasodilation. A drug in this group is milrinone lactate. This drug increases stroke volume and cardiac output and promotes vasodilation. It is administered intravenously for no longer than 48 to 72 hours. Severe cardiac dysrhythmias might result from the use of PDE inhibitors, so the patient's electrocardiogram (ECG) and cardiac status should be closely monitored. Milrinone is a high-alert medication that may cause significant harm to a patient when given inappropriately.

Other Agents Used to Treat Heart Failure

Vasodilators, ACE inhibitors, angiotensin II–receptor antagonists (blockers), diuretics (thiazides, furosemide), spironolactone, nesiritide, and some beta blockers are other drug groups prescribed to treat HF.

Vasodilators can be used to treat HF. The vasodilators decrease venous blood return to the heart and result in a decrease in cardiac filling, ventricular stretching (preload), and oxygen demand on the heart. Arteriolar dilators act in three ways: they (1) reduce cardiac afterload, which increases cardiac output; (2) dilate the arterioles of the kidneys, which improves renal perfusion and increases fluid loss; and (3) improve circulation to the skeletal muscles.

ACE inhibitors are usually prescribed for HF. ACE inhibitors dilate venules and arterioles, which improves renal blood flow and decreases blood fluid volume. ACE inhibitors also moderately decrease the release of aldosterone, which in turn reduces sodium and fluid retention.

ACE inhibitors can increase potassium levels, so serum potassium levels should be monitored, especially if potassium-sparing diuretics such as spironolactone are being taken concurrently. Angiotensin II–receptor blockers (ARBs) such as valsartan and candesartan have been approved for HF in patients who cannot tolerate ACE inhibitors. Refer to Chapter 39 for a complete discussion of ACE inhibitors and ARBs.

Diuretics are the first-line drug treatment for reducing fluid volume. They are frequently prescribed with digoxin or other agents.

Spironolactone, a potassium-sparing diuretic, is used in treating moderate to severe HF. Aldosterone secretions are increased in HF. This promotes body loss of potassium and magnesium needed by the heart and increases sodium and water retention. Spironolactone blocks the production of aldosterone. This drug improves heart rate

TABLE 40.3   Effects of Antianginal Drug Groups on Angina

Drug Groups	Variant (Vasospastic) Anginas	Classic (Stable) Anginas
Nitrates	Relaxation of coronary arteries, which decreases vasospasms and increases oxygen supply	Dilation of veins, which decreases preload and decreases oxygen demand
Beta blockers	Not effective	Decrease heart rate and contractility, which decreases oxygen demand
Calcium channel blockers	Relaxation of coronary arteries, which decreases vasospasms and increases oxygen supply	Dilation of arterioles decreases afterload and decreases oxygen demand. Verapamil and diltiazem decrease heart rate and contractility.

variability and decreases myocardial fibrosis by its cardioprotective effect of blocking aldosterone in the heart and blood vessels to promote cardiac remodeling. The recommended dose for HF is 12.5 to 25 mg/day. Occurrence of hyperkalemia (excess serum potassium) is rare unless the patient is receiving 50 mg/day and has renal insufficiency. However, the serum potassium level should be closely monitored.

In the past, all beta blockers were contraindicated for patients with HF because this drug class reduces cardiac contractility. With dosage control, beta blockers (carvedilol, metoprolol, and bisoprolol) have been shown to improve cardiac performance. Doses should be low initially and gradually increased. It may take 1 to 3 months for a beneficial effect to develop. Refer to Chapters 15 and 39 for more information on beta blockers.

Nesiritide is an atrial natriuretic peptide hormone that inhibits antidiuretic hormone (ADH) by increasing urine sodium loss. Its effect in correcting HF is achieved by promoting vasodilation, natriuresis, and diuresis. It is useful for treating patients who have acute decompensated HF with dyspnea at rest or who have dyspnea with little physical exertion.

A combination of hydralazine (for blood pressure) and isosorbide dinitrate (a dilator to relieve heart pain) has received US Food and Drug Administration (FDA) approval for treating HF, especially in African Americans, who have more than twice the rate of HF as Caucasians; a research study has shown this drug to be effective in treating HF in the African American population.

The newest drug to treat HF is vericiguat, a guanylate cyclase stimulant. Vericiguat acts to help regulate vascular tone, cardiac contractility, and cardiac remodeling. It is used for the reduction of cardiovascular mortality and reduction of HF hospitalizations associated with HF and ejection fraction less than 45%. This drug is contraindicated in pregnancy due to serious birth defects. A female of child-bearing age must have a negative pregnancy test before treatment and use effective contraception. Vericiguat is not recommended with coadministration of phosphodiesterase type 5 inhibitors due to potentiated hypotension. Some side effects of vericiguat include hypotension, anemia, syncope, and serious birth defects.

ANTIANGINAL DRUGS

Antianginal drugs are used to treat angina pectoris, a condition of acute cardiac pain caused by inadequate blood flow to the myocardium due to either plaque occlusions within or spasms of the coronary arteries. With decreased blood flow, there is a decrease in oxygen to the myocardium, which results in pain. Anginal pain is frequently described by the patient as tightness, pressure in the center of the chest, and pain radiating down the left arm. Referred pain felt in the neck and left arm commonly occurs with severe angina pectoris. Anginal attacks may lead to MI (heart attack). Anginal pain usually lasts for only a few minutes. Stress tests, echocardiogram, cardiac profile laboratory tests, and cardiac catheterization may be needed to determine the degree of blockage in the coronary arteries and then also to treat the condition.

Types of Angina Pectoris

The frequency of anginal pain depends on many factors, including the type of angina. There are three types of angina:

- *Classic (stable) angina* occurs with predictable stress or exertion.
- *Unstable (preinfarction) angina* occurs frequently with progressive severity unrelated to activity and is unpredictable regarding stress/exertion and intensity.
- *Variant (Prinzmetal, vasospastic) angina* occurs during rest.

The first two types are caused by a narrowing or partial occlusion of the coronary arteries; variant angina is caused by vessel spasm (vasospasm). It is common for a patient to have both classic and variant angina. Unstable angina often indicates an impending MI; it is an emergency that needs immediate medical intervention.

Nonpharmacologic Measures to Control Angina

A combination of pharmacologic and nonpharmacologic measures is usually necessary to control and prevent anginal attacks. Nonpharmacologic methods of decreasing anginal attacks are to avoid heavy meals, smoking, extreme weather changes, strenuous exercise, and emotional upset. Proper nutrition, moderate exercise (only after consulting with a health care provider), adequate rest, and relaxation techniques are used as preventive measures.

Types of Antianginal Drugs

Antianginal drugs increase blood flow either by increasing oxygen supply or by decreasing oxygen demand by the myocardium. Three types of antianginals are (1) nitrates, (2) beta blockers, and (3) CCBs. The major systemic effect of nitrates is a reduction of venous tone, which decreases the workload of the heart and promotes vasodilation. Beta blockers and CCBs decrease the workload of the heart and decrease oxygen demands.

Nitrates and CCBs are effective in treating variant (vasospastic) angina pectoris; beta blockers are not effective for this type of angina and may aggravate it. With stable angina, beta blockers can effectively be used to prevent angina attacks. Table 40.3 lists the effects of antianginal drug groups on angina.

With unstable angina, immediate medical care is necessary. Nitrates are usually given sublingually and intravenously as needed. If the cardiac pain continues, a beta blocker is given intravenously, and if the patient is unable to tolerate beta blockers, a CCB may be substituted.

Nitrates

Nitrates were the first agents used to relieve angina. They affect coronary arteries and blood vessels in the venous circulation. Nitrates cause generalized vascular and coronary vasodilation, which increases blood flow through the coronary arteries to the myocardial cells. This group of drugs reduces myocardial ischemia but can cause hypotension.

⚡ PATIENT SAFETY

Do not confuse…
- **Nitrostat**, a nitroglycerin drug that promotes coronary vasodilation and thus increases blood flow to the coronary arteries, with **Nystatin**, an antifungal antibiotic that has fungistatic and fungicidal activity against yeasts and fungi

The sublingual (SL) nitroglycerin tablet, which is absorbed under the tongue, comes in various dosages, but the average prescribed dose is 0.4 mg after cardiac pain. If pain has not subsided, then 911 should be called. The effects of SL nitroglycerin last for 30 to 60 minutes. The SL tablets decompose when exposed to heat and light, so they must be kept in their original, airtight glass containers. The tablets themselves are normally dispensed in these original glass containers, which have screw-cap tops that are *not* childproof to facilitate emergency use by older adults who may have reduced manual dexterity and are experiencing an anginal attack. After a dose of nitroglycerin, the patient may experience dizziness, faintness, or headache as a result of the peripheral vasodilation. If pain persists, the patient should immediately call for medical assistance.

SL nitroglycerin is the most commonly used nitrate. It is not swallowed, because it undergoes first-pass metabolism by the liver, which decreases its effectiveness. Instead, it is readily absorbed into the circulation through the SL vessels. Nitroglycerin is also available in other forms: topical (ointment, transdermal patch), translingual, oral extended-release capsule and tablet, aerosol spray (inhalation), and IV. Prototype Drug Chart: Nitroglycerin summarizes the action of nitroglycerin (nitrates).

Among the various types of organic nitrates is *isosorbide dinitrate*, which can be administered in an SL tablet form and is also available as a chewable tablet, immediate-release tablet, and sustained-release tablet or capsule. *Isosorbide mononitrate* can be given orally in immediate- and sustained-release tablets.

📄 PROTOTYPE DRUG CHART

Nitroglycerin

Drug Class	Dosage
Antianginal	Angina: A: SL: 1 tab of 0.3, 0.4, or 0.6 mg; repeat q5min × 3 as needed or 5–10 min before strenuous activities Extended release: A: PO: 2.5–6.5 mg, 3–4 times/d Topical ointment: 15–30 mg (2.5–5 cm or 1–2 inches) q6–8h while awake, remove at bedtime to provide 12-h nitrate-free interval Transdermal patch: 1 Patch qd, allow 10- to 12-h nitrate-free interval Translingual spray: 1–2 sprays on or under tongue at onset of attack, may repeat q5min Hypertensive emergency: IV: Initially: 5 mcg/min infusion, titrate up by 5 mcg/min q3–5 min up to 20 mcg/min until control is achieved

Contraindications	Drug-Lab-Food Interactions
Increased intracranial pressure, AMI, cardiomyopathy, cardiac tamponade, shock, constrictive pericarditis *Caution:* Hepatic disease, hypotension, hypovolemia, anemia, diabetes mellitus, head trauma, pregnancy, breastfeeding, older adults	Drug: Increased effect with alcohol, beta blockers, calcium channel blockers, antihypertensives, aspirin, benzodiazepines, vasodilators; decreased effects of heparin Herbs: Hawthorn increases nitroglycerin levels.

Pharmacokinetics	Pharmacodynamics
Absorption: SL: Greater than 75% absorbed; ointment and patch: slow absorption Distribution: PB: 60% Metabolism: t½: 1–3 min Excretion: Liver and urine	SL: Onset: 1–3 min Peak: 5 min Duration: 30–60 min ER cap: Onset: 20–45 min Duration: 8–12 h Topical ointment: Onset: 20–60 min Peak: 1 h Duration: 4–8 h Transdermal patch: Onset: 40–60 min Peak: 2 h Duration: 18–24 h IV: Onset: Immediate Duration: 3 min

Therapeutic Effects/Uses

To control angina, AMI, hypertensive emergency, pulmonary edema, and heart failure
Mechanism of Action: Decreases myocardial demand for oxygen; decreases preload by dilating veins, indirectly decreasing afterload

Side Effects	Adverse Reactions
Headache, blurred vision, dizziness, syncope, weakness, diaphoresis, flushing, nausea, vomiting, dry mouth, paresthesia, peripheral edema, rash, pharyngitis, tolerance	Orthostatic hypotension, chest pain, dyspnea, tachycardia, bradycardia, palpitations, methemoglobinemia *Life-threatening:* MI, pulmonary edema

A, Adult; *AMI,* acute myocardial infarction; *cap,* capsule; *d,* day; *ER,* extended release; *h,* hour; *IV,* intravenous; *max,* maximum; *min,* minute; *PB,* protein binding; *PO,* by mouth; *q,* every; *qd,* every day; *qid,* four times daily; *SL,* sublingual; *t½,* half-life; *tab,* tablet.

Pharmacokinetics. When taken sublingually, nitroglycerin is absorbed rapidly and directly into the internal jugular vein and the right atrium. Nitrates absorbed through the gastrointestinal (GI) tract are inactivated by first-pass metabolism in the liver. The nitroglycerin in the ointment and in the patch is absorbed slowly through the skin and is excreted primarily in the urine. The protein binding is 60%, and the half-life is 1 to 3 minutes.

Pharmacodynamics. Nitroglycerin acts directly on the smooth muscle of blood vessels, causing relaxation and dilation. It decreases cardiac preload (amount of blood in the ventricle at the end of diastole) and afterload (peripheral vascular resistance) and reduces myocardial O_2 demand. With dilation of the veins, there is less blood return to the heart, and with dilation of the arteries, there is less vasoconstriction and resistance.

The onset of action of nitroglycerin depends on the method of administration. With SL use, the onset of action is rapid (1 to 3 minutes); it is slower with the transdermal method (40 to 60 minutes). The duration of action of the transdermal nitroglycerin patch is approximately 18 to 24 hours. Because nitroglycerin ointment is effective for only 4 to 8 hours, it must be reapplied three to four times a day. The use of nitroglycerin ointment has declined since the advent of the transdermal nitroglycerin patch, which is applied only once a day. It is important to note that the patch should be removed nightly to allow for an 8- to 12-hour nitrate-free interval. This is also true for most other forms of nitroglycerin. This is necessary to avoid tolerance associated with uninterrupted use or continued dosage increases of nitrate preparations. Table 40.4 lists the nitrates and their dosages, uses, and considerations.

Side Effects and Adverse Reactions. Headaches are one of the most common side effects of nitroglycerin, but they may become less frequent with continued use. Otherwise, acetaminophen may provide some relief. Other side effects include hypotension, dizziness, flushing, weakness, and faintness. When nitroglycerin ointment or transdermal patches are discontinued, the dose should be tapered over several weeks to prevent the rebound effect of severe pain caused by myocardial ischemia, lack of blood supply to the heart muscle. In addition, *reflex tachycardia* may occur if the nitrate is given too rapidly. The heart rate increases greatly because of overcompensation of the cardiovascular system.

Drug Interactions. Beta blockers, CCBs, vasodilators, and alcohol can enhance the hypotensive effect of nitrates. IV nitroglycerin may antagonize the effects of heparin.

⚠ Beta Blockers

Beta-adrenergic blockers block the beta$_1$- and beta$_2$-receptor sites. Beta blockers decrease the effects of the sympathetic nervous system by blocking the action of the catecholamines, epinephrine and norepinephrine, thereby decreasing the heart rate and blood pressure. Beta blockers are used as antianginal, antidysrhythmic, and antihypertensive drugs. Beta blockers are effective as antianginals because by decreasing the heart rate and myocardial contractility they reduce the need for oxygen consumption and consequently reduce anginal pain. These drugs are most useful for classic (stable) angina.

Beta blockers should *not* be abruptly discontinued. The dose should be tapered over a specified number of days to avoid reflex tachycardia and recurrence of anginal pain. Patients who have decreased heart rate and blood pressure usually cannot take beta blockers. Patients who have second- or third-degree AV block should not take beta blockers.

Beta blockers, discussed in detail in Chapters 15 and 39, are subdivided into *nonselective* beta blockers that block beta$_1$ and beta$_2$ and *selective* (cardiac) beta blockers that only block beta$_1$. Examples of nonselective beta blockers are propranolol, nadolol, and pindolol. These drugs decrease the heart rate and can cause bronchoconstriction. The cardioselective beta blockers act more strongly on the beta$_1$ receptor, which decreases heart

rate but avoids bronchoconstriction because of their lack of activity at the beta$_2$ receptor. Examples of selective beta blockers are atenolol and metoprolol. Selective beta blockers are the group of choice for controlling angina pectoris. Table 40.4 lists the beta blockers most frequently used for angina and their dosages, uses, and considerations.

Pharmacokinetics. Beta blockers are well absorbed orally. Absorption of sustained-release capsules is slow. The half-life of propranolol is 2 to 6 hours. Of the selective beta blockers, atenolol has a half-life of 6 to 7 hours, and metoprolol has a half-life of 3 to 7 hours. Propranolol and metoprolol are metabolized and excreted by the liver. Half an *oral* dose of atenolol is absorbed from the GI tract, with the remainder excreted unchanged in feces.

Pharmacodynamics. Because beta blockers decrease the force of myocardial contraction, oxygen demand by the myocardium is reduced. Therefore the patient can tolerate increased exercise with less oxygen requirement. Beta blockers are effective for classic (stable) angina.

The onset of action of the nonselective beta blocker propranolol is 30 minutes, its peak action is reached in 2 to 4 hours, and its duration is 12 to 24 hours. For the cardioselective beta blockers, the onset of action of atenolol is 60 minutes, its peak action occurs in 2 to 4 hours, and its duration of action is 24 hours. The onset of action of selective metoprolol is reached in 30 to 60 minutes, and the duration of action is approximately 3 to 6 hours.

Side Effects and Adverse Reactions. Both nonselective and selective beta blockers cause a decrease in heart rate and blood pressure. For the nonselective beta blockers, bronchospasm, agitation, dizziness, drowsiness, confusion, cool extremities, and erectile dysfunction (with use of propranolol) are potential adverse reactions.

Vital signs need to be closely monitored in the early stages of beta blocker therapy. When discontinuing use, the dosage should be tapered for 1 or 2 weeks to prevent a rebound effect such as reflex tachycardia or life-threatening cardiac dysrhythmias.

Calcium Channel Blockers

Calcium channel blockers (CCBs), or *calcium blockers*, were introduced in 1982 for the treatment of stable and variant angina pectoris, certain dysrhythmias, and hypertension. Calcium activates myocardial contraction, increasing the workload of the heart and the need for more oxygen. CCBs relax coronary artery spasm (variant angina) and relax peripheral arterioles (stable angina), decreasing cardiac oxygen demand. They also decrease cardiac contractility (negative inotropic effect that relaxes smooth muscle), afterload, and peripheral resistance, and they reduce the workload of the heart, which decreases the need for oxygen. CCBs achieve their effect in controlling variant (vasospastic) angina by relaxing coronary arteries and in controlling classic (stable) angina by decreasing oxygen demand. Fig. 40.4 shows the suggested steps for treating classic and variant angina pectoris. Table 40.4 presents the drug data for the CCBs used to treat angina and their dosages, uses, and considerations.

Pharmacokinetics. Three CCBs—verapamil, nifedipine, and diltiazem—have been effectively used for the long-term treatment of angina. Eighty to ninety percent of CCBs are absorbed through the GI mucosa. However, first-pass metabolism by the liver decreases the availability of free circulating drug, and only 20% of verapamil, 45% to 65% of diltiazem, and 35% to 40% of nifedipine are bioavailable. All three drugs are highly protein bound (70% to 98%), and their half-lives are usually 2 to 12 hours.

Several other CCBs are available, such as nicardipine hydrochloride (HCl), amlodipine, felodipine, and nisoldipine. All are highly protein bound (greater than 93%). Nicardipine has the shortest half-life at 8.6 hours.

Pharmacodynamics. Bradycardia is a common problem with the use of verapamil, the first calcium blocker. Nifedipine, the most potent

⚠ TABLE 40.4   Antianginals

Drug	Route and Dosages	Uses and Considerations
Nitrates		
Short Acting Nitroglycerin	See Prototype Drug Chart: Nitroglycerin	
Long Acting Isosorbide dinitrate	Immediate release: A: PO: Initially 5–20 mg bid/tid; *maint:* 10–60 mg bid/tid; *max:* 480 mg/d Sustained release: A: PO: Initially 40 mg/d; *maint:* 40–160 mg/d; *max:* 160 mg/d A: Sublingual: 2.5–5 mg 15 min before angina-causing activity	To prevent and treat angina. May cause headaches, dizziness, dry mouth, orthostatic hypotension, tachycardia, bradycardia, nausea, vomiting, methemoglobinemia, syncope, and flushing. PB: 28%; t½: 1 h
Isosorbide mononitrate	Immediate release: A: PO: 5–20 mg bid; *max:* 40 mg/d Extended release: A: PO: 30–60 mg in a.m.; *maint:* 30–120 mg/d *max:* 240 mg/d	To prevent angina. May cause headache, dizziness, flushing, fatigue, cough, anxiety, hypotension, dry mouth, abdominal pain, nausea, vomiting, rash, pruritus, chest pain. PB: <4%; t½: 5 h
Beta-Adrenergic Blockers		
Atenolol (beta₁)	Angina: Regular release: A: PO: Initially 50 mg/d; *max:* 200 mg/d	To treat angina, hypertension, and AMI. May cause hypotension, bradycardia, fatigue, dizziness, nausea, diarrhea, depression, peripheral vasoconstriction, tachycardia, edema, and heart failure. PB: 10%; t½: 6–7 h
Metoprolol tartrate (beta₁)	Angina: Regular release: A: PO: 25–50 mg bid; *maint:* 100–400 mg/d in divided doses; *max:* 450 mg/d Extended release: A: PO: 100 mg/d; *max:* 400 mg/d	To treat angina, AMI, hypertension, and heart failure. May cause dizziness, fatigue, drowsiness, blurred vision, depression, rash, pruritus, diarrhea, peripheral edema, erectile dysfunction, bradycardia, hypotension, heart failure, and palpitations. PB: 10%–12%; t½: 3–7 h
Nadolol (beta₁ and beta₂)	Angina: A: PO: Initially 40 mg/d; *maint:* 40–80 mg/d; *max:* 240 mg/d	For angina and hypertension. May cause dizziness, drowsiness, headache, bradycardia, hypotension, palpitations, peripheral vasoconstriction, erectile dysfunction, and fatigue. PB: 30%; t½: 10–24 h
Propranolol hydrochloride (beta₁ and beta₂)	Angina: Immediate release: A: PO: Initially 10–20 mg bid/qid; *maint:* 160–320 mg/d in 2–4 divided doses; *max:* 320 mg/d Extended release: A: PO: Initially 80 mg/d; *maint:* 160–320 mg/d; *max:* 320 mg/d	For angina, hypertension, AMI, HF, dysrhythmias, and migraine prophylaxis. May cause dizziness, headache, visual impairment, bradycardia, depression, weakness, hyperkalemia, agitation, fatigue, erectile dysfunction, and bronchospasm. PB: 90%; t½: 2–6 h
Calcium Channel Blockers		
Amlodipine	Angina: A: PO: Initially 5–10 mg/d; *maint:* 10 mg/d; *max:* 10 mg/d	For angina, CAD, and hypertension. May cause peripheral edema, dizziness, palpitations, flushing, bradycardia, orthostatic hypotension, constipation, nausea, hyperglycemia, peripheral neuropathy, visual impairment, edema, weakness, drowsiness, erectile dysfunction, and fatigue. PB: 93%; t½: 30–50 h
Diltiazem hydrochloride	Angina: Immediate release: A: PO: Initially 30 mg qid; *maint:* 180–360 mg/d in 3–4 divided doses; *max:* 480 mg/d Extended release: A: PO: 120–180 mg/d; *max:* 540 mg/d	For angina, PSVT, atrial flutter or fibrillation, and hypertension. May cause headache, peripheral edema, dizziness, weakness, bradycardia, hypotension, dyspnea, fatigue, rhinitis, pharyngitis, infection, constipation, and dyspepsia PB: 70%–80%; t½: 3.5–9 h
Felodipine	Angina: A: PO: Initially 5–10 mg/d; *max:* 10 mg/d Older A: Initially 2.5 mg/d; *max:* 10 mg/d	To treat hypertension and angina. May cause peripheral edema, palpitations, dizziness, weakness, infection, hypotension, erectile dysfunction, cough, rash, and headache. PB: >99%; t½: 11–16 h
Isradipine	Angina: Regular release: A: PO: Initially 2.5 mg tid; *max:* 20 mg/bid	To treat hypertension and angina. May cause headache, palpitations, peripheral edema, fatigue, flushing, hypotension, tachycardia, angina, abdominal pain, erectile dysfunction, and dizziness. PB: 95%; t½: 8 h

Continued

⚠ TABLE 40.4 Antianginals—cont'd

Drug	Route and Dosages	Uses and Considerations
Nicardipine hydrochloride	Angina: A: PO: Initially 20 mg tid; *maint:* 20–40 mg tid; *max:* 120 mg/d	For angina and hypertension. May cause peripheral edema, headache, dizziness, hypotension, palpitations, weakness, tachycardia, flushing, angina, nausea, and vomiting. PB: 95%; t½: 8.6 h
Nifedipine	Angina: Immediate release: A: PO: Initially 10 mg tid; *max:* 180 mg/d Extended release: A: PO: 30–60 mg/d; *max:* 90 mg/d	For angina and hypertension. May cause dizziness, flushing, headache, peripheral edema, nausea, constipation, hypotension, pyrosis, tremor, muscle cramps, cough, fatigue, dyspnea, heart failure, erectile dysfunction, nasal congestion, and weakness. PB: 92%–98%; t½: 2–5 h
Nisoldipine	Angina: Extended release: A: PO: Initially 17–34 mg/d; *maint:* 8.5–34 mg/d; *max:* 34 mg/d Older A: PO: Initially 8.5 mg/d; *max:* 34 mg/d	For hypertension and angina. May cause headache, dizziness, flushing, sinusitis, pharyngitis, orthostatic hypotension, palpitations, tachycardia, hypokalemia, visual impairment, and peripheral edema. PB: 99%; t½: 7–12 h
Verapamil hydrochloride	Angina: Immediate release: A: PO: 80–120 mg q8h; *max:* 480 mg/d in 3–4 divided doses Older A: PO: Initially 40 mg q8h; *max:* 480 mg/d Extended release: A: PO: Initially 180 mg/d at bedtime; *max:* 540 mg/d	For angina, cardiac dysrhythmias, and hypertension. May cause dizziness, weakness, peripheral edema, nausea, constipation, tachycardia, headache, confusion, bradycardia, fatigue, blurred vision, erectile dysfunction, and orthostatic hypotension. PB: 90%; t½: 2–10 h

A, Adult; *a.m.*, in the morning; *AMI*, acute myocardial infarction; *bid*, twice a day; *CAD*, coronary artery disease; *d*, day; *GI*, gastrointestinal; *h*, hour; *maint*, maintenance; *max*, maximum; *min*, minute; *PB*, protein binding; *PO*, by mouth; *PSVT*, paroxysmal supraventricular tachycardia; *q8h*, every 8 hours; *qid*, four times a day; *SL*, sublingual; *SR*, sustained release; *tid*, three times a day; *t½*, half-life; *>*, greater than.

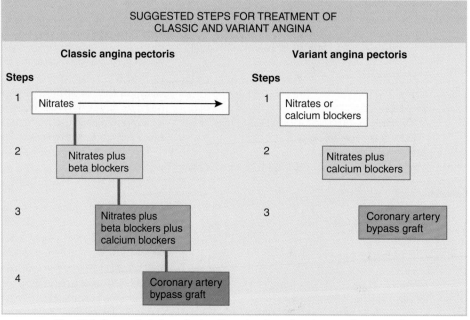

Fig. 40.4 Suggested steps for treating classic and variant angina pectoris.

of the calcium blockers, promotes vasodilation of the coronary and peripheral vessels, and hypotension can result. The onset of action is 10 minutes for verapamil and 30 minutes for nifedipine and diltiazem. Verapamil's duration of action is 6 to 8 hours when given orally and 10 to 20 minutes when given intravenously. The duration of action for nifedipine and diltiazem is 6 to 8 hours.

Side Effects and Adverse Reactions. The side effects of calcium blockers include headache, hypotension (more common with nifedipine and less common with diltiazem), dizziness, and flushing of the skin.

Reflex tachycardia can occur as a result of hypotension. Peripheral edema may occur with several CCBs, including nicardipine, nifedipine, and verapamil. CCBs can cause changes in liver and kidney function, and serum liver enzymes should be checked periodically. CCBs are frequently given with other antianginal drugs such as nitrates to prevent angina.

In its immediate-release form (10- and 20-mg capsules), nifedipine has been associated with an increased incidence of sudden cardiac death, especially when prescribed in high doses for outpatients. This is not true of the sustained-release preparations. For this reason,

CLINICAL JUDGMENT [NURSING PROCESS]

Antianginals

Concept: Perfusion
- The passage of blood flow through the arteries and capillaries that deliver oxygen and nutrients to body cells.

Recognize Cues [Assessment]
- Obtain baseline vital signs for future comparisons.
- Obtain health and drug histories. Nitroglycerin is contraindicated for marked hypotension or acute myocardial infarction (AMI).

Analyze Cues and Prioritize Hypothesis [Patient Problems]
- Dyspnea
- Myocardial tissue injury
- Pain
- Decreased tissue perfusion
- Hypoxemia
- Anxiety
- Reduced functional ability

Generate Solutions [Planning]
- The patient will report that angina pain is controlled by nitroglycerin or other antianginals.

Take Action [Nursing Interventions]
- Monitor vital signs. Hypotension is associated with most antianginal drugs.
- Position the patient sitting or lying down when administering a nitrate for the first time. After administration, check vital signs while the patient is lying down and then sitting up. Have the patient rise slowly to a standing position.
- Offer sips of water before giving sublingual (SL) nitrates; dryness may inhibit drug absorption.
- ⚡ Monitor effects of intravenous (IV) nitroglycerin. Report angina that persists.
- Apply nitroglycerin ointment to a designated mark on paper. Do *not* use fingers because drug can be absorbed; use tongue blade or gloves. When using a nitroglycerin patch, do not touch the medication portion.
- Do *not* apply nitroglycerin ointment or a nitroglycerin patch in any area on the chest in the vicinity of defibrillator-cardioverter paddle placement. Explosion and skin burns may result.

Patient Teaching
General
- ⚡ Administer SL nitroglycerin tablet if chest pain occurs. If pain has not subsided or has worsened in 5 minutes, call 911.
- Advise patients not to ingest alcohol while taking nitroglycerin to avoid hypotension, weakness, and faintness.
- Advise patients to notify a health care provider if chest pain is not completely alleviated. Tolerance to nitroglycerin can occur.
- ⚡ Inform patients not to discontinue beta blockers and calcium blockers without a health care provider's approval. Withdrawal symptoms (reflex tachycardia and pain) may be severe.

Self-Administration
- Demonstrate how SL nitroglycerin tablets are taken. The tablet is placed under the tongue for quick absorption. A stinging or biting sensation indicates that the tablet is fresh; however, with newer SL nitroglycerin tablets, the biting sensation may not be present.
- Teach patients to store medication bottles away from light in a dry place and to keep the drug in its original screw-cap, amber glass bottle. The amber color provides light protection, and the screw-cap closure protects from moisture in the air, which can easily reduce tablet potency.
- Teach patients about nitroglycerin patches, applied once a day, usually in the morning. Rotate skin sites. The patch is usually applied to the chest wall, but the thighs and arms may also be used. Avoid hairy areas.
- Advise patients to seek medical attention if nitroglycerin does not relieve pain.

Side Effects
- Suggest acetaminophen to patients for relief of headache, which commonly occurs when first taking nitroglycerin products and lasts about 30 minutes.
- ⚡ Place patients in a supine position with legs elevated if hypotension results from SL nitroglycerin.
- Instruct patients how to check their pulse rate.
- Advise patients taking beta blockers and calcium blockers to notify a health care provider if dizziness or faintness occurs because it may indicate hypotension.

Evaluate Outcomes [Evaluation]
- Evaluate the patient's response to nitrate products for relieving anginal pain. Note headache, dizziness, or faintness.

---

immediate-release nifedipine is usually prescribed only as needed in the hospital setting for acute increases in blood pressure.

⚠ ANTIDYSRHYTHMIC DRUGS

Cardiac Dysrhythmias

A cardiac dysrhythmia (arrhythmia) is defined as any deviation from the normal rate or pattern of the heartbeat. This includes heart rates that are too slow (bradycardia), too fast (tachycardia), or irregular. The terms *dysrhythmia* (disturbed heart rhythm) and *arrhythmia* (absence of heart rhythm) are used interchangeably despite the slight difference in meaning.

The ECG identifies the type of dysrhythmia. The *P wave* of the ECG reflects atrial activation, the *QRS complex* indicates ventricular depolarization, and the *T wave* reflects ventricular repolarization (return of cell membrane potential to resting after depolarization). The *PR interval* indicates AV conduction time, and the *QT interval* reflects ventricular action potential duration. Atrial dysrhythmias prevent proper filling of the ventricles and decrease cardiac output by 33%. Ventricular

dysrhythmias are life-threatening because ineffective filling of the ventricle and ineffective pumping result in decreased or absent cardiac output. With ventricular tachycardia, ventricular fibrillation is likely to occur, followed by death. Cardiopulmonary resuscitation (CPR) is necessary to treat these patients.

Cardiac dysrhythmias frequently follow an MI (heart attack) or can result from hypoxia (lack of oxygen to body tissues), hypercapnia (increased carbon dioxide in the blood), thyroid disease, CAD, cardiac surgery, excess catecholamines, or electrolyte imbalance.

Cardiac Action Potentials

Electrolyte transfer occurs through the cardiac muscle cell membrane. When sodium and calcium enter the cardiac cell, depolarization (myocardial contraction) occurs. Sodium enters rapidly to start the depolarization, and calcium enters later to maintain it. Calcium influx leads to an increased release of intracellular calcium from the sarcoplasmic reticulum, resulting in cardiac contraction. In the presence of myocardial ischemia, the contraction can be irregular.

Cardiac action potentials are transient depolarizations followed by repolarizations of myocardial cells. Fig. 40.5 illustrates the action potential of a ventricular cardiac cell (myocyte) during a heartbeat. There are five phases: phase 0 is the rapid depolarization caused by an influx of sodium ions; phase 1 is initial repolarization, which coincides with termination of sodium ion influx; phase 2 is the plateau and is characterized by the influx of calcium ions, which prolong the action potential and promote atrial and ventricular muscle contraction; phase 3 is rapid repolarization caused by influx of potassium ions; and phase 4 is the resting membrane potential between heartbeats and is normally flat in ventricular muscle, but it begins to rise in the cells of the SA node as they slowly depolarize toward the threshold potential just before depolarization occurs, initiating the next heartbeat.

Types of Antidysrhythmic Drugs

The desired action of antidysrhythmic (antiarrhythmic) drugs is to restore the cardiac rhythm to normal. Box 40.1 describes the various mechanisms by which this is accomplished. Antidysrhythmics are high-alert drugs that may cause significant harm to the patient when given inappropriately.

The antidysrhythmics are grouped into four classes: (1) sodium (fast) channel blockers IA, IB, and IC; (2) beta blockers; (3) drugs that prolong repolarization; and (4) calcium (slow) channel blockers. Table 40.5 lists the classes, actions, and indications for cardiac antidysrhythmic drugs. Table 40.6 lists the commonly administered antidysrhythmics and their dosages, uses, and considerations.

Class I: Sodium Channel Blockers

A sodium channel blocker decreases sodium influx into cardiac cells. Responses to the drug are decreased conduction velocity in cardiac tissues; suppression of automaticity, which decreases the likelihood of ectopic foci; and increased recovery time (repolarization or refractory period). There are three subgroups of sodium channel blockers: those in *class IA* slow conduction and prolong repolarization (quinidine, procainamide, disopyramide); those in *class IB* slow conduction and shorten repolarization (lidocaine, mexiletine HCl); and *class IC*

drugs prolong conduction with little to no effect on repolarization (flecainide).

Lidocaine, a class IB sodium channel blocker, was used in the 1940s as a local anesthetic and is still used for this purpose. It was later discovered to have antidysrhythmic properties as well. Lidocaine is still used by some cardiologists to treat acute ventricular dysrhythmias. It slows conduction velocity and decreases action potential amplitude. Onset of action (IV) is rapid. About one-third of lidocaine reaches the general circulation, and a bolus of lidocaine is short-lived. Another class IB sodium channel blocker is mexiletine.

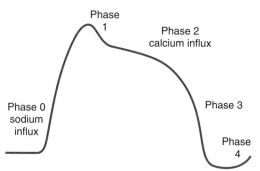

Fig. 40.5 Action potential of a ventricular myocyte during the course of a heartbeat.

BOX 40.1   Pharmacodynamics of Antidysrhythmics

Mechanisms of Action
- Blocks adrenergic stimulation of the heart
- Depresses myocardial excitability and contractility
- Decreases conduction velocity in cardiac tissue
- Increases recovery time (repolarization) of the myocardium
- Suppresses automaticity (spontaneous depolarization to initiate beats)

TABLE 40.5   Classes, Actions, and Indications of Antidysrhythmic Drugs

Classes	Actions	Indications
Class I		
Sodium Channel Blockers		
IA	Slow conduction and prolong repolarization	Atrial and ventricular dysrhythmias, paroxysmal atrial tachycardia (PAT), supraventricular dysrhythmias
IB	Slow conduction and shorten repolarization	Acute ventricular dysrhythmias
IC	Prolong conduction with little to no effect on repolarization	Life-threatening ventricular dysrhythmias
Class II		
Beta blockers	Reduce calcium entry Decrease conduction velocity, automaticity, and recovery time (refractory period)	Atrial flutter and fibrillation, tachydysrhythmias, ventricular and supraventricular dysrhythmias
Class III		
Drugs that prolong repolarization	Prolong repolarization during ventricular dysrhythmias Prolong action potential duration	Life-threatening atrial and ventricular dysrhythmias resistant to other drugs
Class IV		
Calcium channel blockers	Block calcium influx Slow conduction velocity Decrease myocardial contractility (negative inotropic) Increase refraction in atrioventricular node	Supraventricular tachydysrhythmias; prevention of paroxysmal supraventricular tachycardia (PSVT)

⚠ TABLE 40.6 Antidysrhythmics

Drug	Route and Dosage	Uses and Considerations
Class I		
Sodium Channel Blockers IA		
Disopyramide phosphate	Immediate release: A >18 y >50 kg: PO: 150–300 mg q6h; *max:* 800 mg/d A >18 y <50 kg: PO: 100 mg q6h; *max:* 800 mg/d Extended release: A >50 kg: PO: 300 mg q12h; *max:* 800 mg/d A <50 kg: PO: 200 mg q12h; *max:* 800 mg/d TDM: 2–5 mcg/mL	For life-threatening dysrhythmias, such as ventricular tachycardia. May cause dizziness, headache, fatigue, blurred vision, dry mouth, urinary urgency/frequency/retention, nausea, flatulence, abdominal pain, and constipation. PB: 90%; t½: 4–10 h
Procainamide hydrochloride	Ventricular tachycardia: Loading dose: A: IV: 20–50 mg/min, then wait 10 min; *maint:* 1–4 mg/min infusion if needed	For ventricular tachycardia and cardiopulmonary resuscitation. May cause anorexia, nausea, dyspepsia, vomiting, abdominal pain, and diarrhea. PB: 15%; t½: 2.5–5.2 h
Quinidine sulfate	Immediate release: A: PO: Initially 200–300 mg q6–8h Extended release: A: PO: 300–600 mg q8–12h TDM: 2–6 mcg/mL	For atrial, ventricular, and supraventricular dysrhythmias. May cause headache, dizziness, fatigue, weakness, palpitations, fever, nausea, vomiting, esophagitis, pyrosis, diarrhea, and rash. PB: 80%–90%; t½: 6–8 h
Sodium Channel Blockers IB		
Lidocaine	Dysrhythmias: A: IV: LD: 1–1.5 mg/kg/LD, follow with 1–4 mg/min infusion	For ventricular dysrhythmias. May cause erythema, pruritus, edema, injection site reaction, petechiae, dizziness, nausea, and vomiting. PB: 60%–80%; t½: 1.5–2 h
Mexiletine hydrochloride	A: PO: Initially 200 mg q8h; *maint:* 200–300 mg q8h; *max:* 1200 mg/d	For ventricular dysrhythmias. May cause weakness, nausea, pyrosis, vomiting, diarrhea, tremor, dizziness, headache, blurred vision, palpitations, chest pain, and ataxia. PB: 50%–60%; t½: 10–12 h
Sodium Channel Blockers IC		
Flecainide	PSVT: A: PO: Initially 50 mg q12h as needed; *max:* 300 mg/d TDM: 200–1000 ng/mL	For atrial, ventricular, and supraventricular dysrhythmias. May cause dizziness, palpitations, headache, fatigue, visual impairment, tremor, dyspnea, dysrhythmia exacerbation, weakness, chest pain, HF, nausea, and constipation. PB: 40%–50%; t½: 12–30 h
Propafenone hydrochloride	Ventricular tachycardia: Immediate release: A: PO: Initially 150 mg q8h; *max:* 900 mg/d	For atrial, ventricular, and supraventricular dysrhythmias. May cause dizziness, fatigue, headache, weakness, chest pain, anxiety, dyspnea, dysgeusia, nausea, vomiting, constipation, edema, infection, influenza, and blurred vision. PB: 85%–97%; t½: 2–10 h
Class II		
Beta-Adrenergic Blockers		
Acebutolol hydrochloride (beta₁ blocker)	See Prototype Drug Chart: Acebutolol Hydrochloride	
Esmolol (beta₁ blocker)	PSVT: A: IV: LD: 50 mcg/kg/min continuous infusion; *maint:* 25–200 mcg/kg/min; *max:* 300 mcg/kg/min	To treat atrial flutter and fibrillation, PSVT, and HTN. May cause bradycardia, hypotension, dizziness, drowsiness, wheezing, infusion-site reaction, headache, confusion, agitation, and nausea. PB: 55%; t½: 9 min
Propranolol hydrochloride (beta₁ and beta₂ blocker)	PSVT: Immediate release: A: PO: Initially 10–30 mg tid/qid; *max:* 320 mg/d A: IV: 1–3 mg at 1mg/min, may repeat after 2 min, then may repeat q4h PRN	For atrial and supraventricular dysrhythmias; PSVT, AMI; angina; and HTN. May cause dizziness, agitation, headache, weakness, depression, fatigue, visual impairment, bradycardia, hyperkalemia, bronchospasm, and erectile dysfunction. PB: 90%; t½: 2–6 h
Sotalol hydrochloride (beta₁ and beta₂ blocker; also class III)	Atrial flutter/fibrillation: A: PO: Initially 80 mg bid; *max:* 320 mg/d A: IV: Initially 75 mg bid; *max:* 600 mg/d	For atrial flutter and fibrillation and ventricular tachycardia. May cause bradycardia, chest pain, hyperhidrosis, diarrhea, musculoskeletal pain, fatigue, dizziness, headache, palpitations, weakness, abdominal pain, nausea, vomiting, and dyspnea. PB: 0%; t½: 12 h

Continued

! TABLE 40.6   Antidysrhythmics—cont'd

Drug	Route and Dosage	Uses and Considerations
Class III		
Drugs That Prolong Repolarization		
Adenosine	PSVT: A: IV: Initially 6 mg rapid bolus (1–2 s); follow with 12 mg rapid bolus twice if needed, follow each dose with 20 mL saline flush; *max:* 12 mg/dose, 30 mg total	For PSVT and Wolff-Parkinson-White syndrome. May cause headache, dizziness, flushing, dyspnea, hypotension, nausea, and paresthesia. PB: UK; t½: <10 s
Amiodarone hydrochloride	A: PO: Initially 800–1600 mg/d for 1–3 wk, then 600–800 mg/d for 1 month; then reduce to lowest effective dose (usually 400 mg/d) A: IV: 150 mg over 10 min, then 1 mg/min infusion for 6 h; then 0.5 mg/min for 18 h; *maint:* 0.5 mg/min	For life-threatening ventricular tachycardia and fibrillation. May cause corneal deposits, anorexia, nausea, vomiting, constipation, hypo/hyperthyroidism, injection site reaction, bradycardia, hypotension, and photosensitivity. PB: >99%; t½: 26–107 d
Dofetilide	A: PO: Dose usually individualized based on ECG and renal function tests, *max:* 1000 mcg/d	For atrial flutter and fibrillation. May cause headache, dizziness, insomnia, chest pain, infection, dyspnea, influenza, tachycardia, and nausea. Monitor renal function. PB: 60%–70%; t½: 10 h
Ibutilide	A >60 kg: IV: 1 mg over 10 min; may repeat with 1 mg in 10 min; *max:* 2 mg over 20 min A <60 kg: IV: 0.01 mg/kg given over 10 min; may repeat after 10 min if no response; *max:* 2 mg in 20 min	For atrial flutter and fibrillation. May cause headache, palpitations, nausea, tachycardia, bradycardia, orthostatic hypotension, and dysrhythmia exacerbation. PB: 40%; t½: 2–12 h
Sotalol	Ventricular tachycardia: A: PO: Initially 80 mg bid; *maint:* 160–320 mg/d; *max:* 640 mg/d A: IV: Initially 75 mg q12h; *maint:* 150–300 mg/d; *max:* 600 mg/d	For atrial flutter and fibrillation and ventricular tachycardia. May cause bradycardia, hyperhidrosis, musculoskeletal pain, diarrhea, chest pain, abdominal pain, fatigue, dizziness, headache, palpitations, weakness, nausea, vomiting, and dyspnea. PB: 0%; t½: 12 h
Class IV		
Calcium Channel Blockers		
Verapamil hydrochloride	PSVT prophylaxis: Regular release: A: PO: 240–480 mg/d in 3–4 divided doses	For angina, cardiac dysrhythmias, PSVT, and hypertension. May cause peripheral edema, constipation, dizziness, fatigue, weakness, nausea, confusion, headache, blurred vision, erectile dysfunction, bradycardia, and orthostatic hypotension. PB: 90%; t½: 2–10 h
Diltiazem	PSVT: A: IV: 0.25 mg/kg IV bolus over 2 min, then after 15 min give 0.35 mg/kg bolus over 2 min if needed, then 10 mg/h inf if needed; *max:* 24 h continuous inf at 15 mg/h	For angina, PSVT, atrial flutter or fibrillation, and hypertension. May cause headache, peripheral edema, dizziness, weakness, bradycardia, hypotension, fatigue, infection, dyspnea, pharyngitis, rhinitis, constipation, and dyspepsia. PB: 70%–80%; t½: 3.5–9 h
Others		
Digoxin	See Prototype Drug Chart: Digoxin	
Dronedarone	A: PO: 400 mg bid with morning and evening meals; *max:* 800 mg/d	For atrial fibrillation. Discontinue class I or III drugs before dronedarone. May cause rash, pruritus, nausea, diarrhea, vomiting, abdominal pain, weakness, bradycardia, HF, and prolonged QT interval. Avoid grapefruit and grapefruit juice. PB: 98%; t½: 13–19 h

A, Adult; *AMI,* acute myocardial infarction; *bid,* two times a day; *d,* day; *ECG,* electrocardiogram; *GI,* gastrointestinal; *h,* hour; *HF,* heart failure; *HTN,* hypertension; *inf,* infusion; *IV,* intravenous; *LD,* loading dose; *maint,* maintenance; *max,* maximum; *min,* minute; *PB,* protein binding; *PO,* by mouth; *PSVT,* paroxysmal supraventricular tachycardia; *q,* every; *qd,* every day; *qid,* four times a day; *s,* second; *SVT,* supraventricular tachycardia; *t½,* half-life; *TDM,* therapeutic drug monitoring; *tid,* three times a day; *UK,* unknown; *wk,* week; *y,* year; *>,* greater than; *<,* less than.

Class II: Beta Blockers

The drugs in the second class, beta blockers, decrease conduction velocity, automaticity, and recovery time (refractory period). Examples are propranolol, acebutolol, esmolol, and sotalol. Beta blockers are more frequently prescribed for dysrhythmias than are sodium channel blockers. This drug class should be gradually reduced in dose upon discontinuation. Prototype Drug Chart: Acebutolol Hydrochloride lists the drug data related to the beta blocker acebutolol hydrochloride, which can be prescribed to treat recurrent stable ventricular dysrhythmias.

PROTOTYPE DRUG CHART

! *Acebutolol Hydrochloride*

Drug Class	Dosage
Beta₁ blocker: Cardioselective beta-adrenergic antagonist	Premature ventricular contractions: A: PO: Initially 200 mg q12h; *maint:* 600–1200 mg/d in 2 divided doses; *max:* 1200 mg/d Older A: PO: 200–400 mg/d; *max:* 800 mg/d

Contraindications	Drug-Lab-Food Interactions
Hypersensitivity, AV block, bradycardia, heart failure, cardiogenic shock *Caution:* Surgery, renal/hepatic impairment, diabetes mellitus, thyroid disorder, asthma, bronchitis, COPD, pulmonary edema, PVD, myasthenia gravis, acute bronchospasm, cerebrovascular disorder, depression, older adults, pregnancy, breastfeeding	Drug: Increased effects with diuretics, adenosine, amiodarone, class IC antidysrhythmics, cardiac glycosides, disopyramide; prolongs hypoglycemic effects of insulin and oral antidiabetics; antagonist effect with albuterol, metaproterenol, terbutaline Lab: May increase ALT, AST, ALP, ANA titer, BUN, lipoproteins, and potassium.

Pharmacokinetics	Pharmacodynamics
Absorption: Well absorbed Distribution: PB: 26% Metabolism: t½: 3–4 h Excretion: 80%–100% in bile, feces, and urine	Ventricular dysrhythmias: PO: Onset: 1–2 h Peak: 2.5–3.5 h Duration: 12–24 h

Therapeutic Effects/Uses	
To aid in treatment of premature ventricular contractions and hypertension Mechanism of Action: Blocks beta₁-adrenergic receptors in cardiac tissues	

Side Effects	Adverse Reactions
Dizziness, headache, fatigue, insomnia, nightmares, anxiety, visual impairment, depression, arthralgia, myalgia, weakness, abdominal pain, flatulence, anorexia, nausea, vomiting, dyspepsia, constipation, diarrhea, edema, diaphoresis, erectile dysfunction	Palpitations, bradycardia, hypo/hypertension, tachycardia, chest pain, hyper/hypoglycemia, diabetes mellitus, lupus-like symptoms, hyperbilirubinemia, dyspnea *Life-threatening:* Agranulocytosis, thrombocytopenia, HF

A, Adult; *ALP,* alkaline phosphatase; *ALT,* alanine aminotransferase; *ANA,* antinuclear antibody; *AST,* aspartate aminotransferase; *AV,* atrioventricular; *BUN,* blood urea nitrogen; *COPD,* chronic obstructive pulmonary disease; *d,* day; *h,* hour; *maint,* maintenance; *max,* maximum; *PB,* protein binding; *PO,* by mouth; *PVD,* peripheral vascular disease; *q12h,* every 12 hours; *t½,* half-life.

Pharmacokinetics. The cardioselective beta drug acebutolol is well absorbed in the GI tract. It is metabolized in the liver to active metabolites; 80% to 100% of the drug is eliminated in the bile via feces and in the urine. The half-life for the drug is 3 to 4 hours.

Pharmacodynamics. Acebutolol is prescribed for ventricular dysrhythmias as well as for angina pectoris and hypertension. As an antidysrhythmic drug, the onset of action is 1 to 2 hours; peak time is 2.5 to 3.5 hours, and duration of action is 12 to 24 hours.

Class III: Drugs That Prolong Repolarization

Drugs in the third class prolong repolarization and are used in emergency treatment of ventricular dysrhythmias when other antidysrhythmics are ineffective. Amiodarone increases the refractory period (recovery time) and prolongs the action potential duration (cardiac cell activity).

Class IV: Calcium Channel Blockers

The fourth class consists of the calcium channel blockers verapamil and diltiazem. Verapamil is a slow (calcium) channel blocker that blocks calcium influx, thereby decreasing the excitability and (negative inotropic) contractility of the myocardium. It increases the refractory period of the AV node, which decreases ventricular response. Verapamil is contraindicated for patients with AV block or HF.

Side Effects and Adverse Reactions With Antidysrhythmic Drugs

Quinidine, the first drug used to treat cardiac dysrhythmias, has many side effects, which include nausea, vomiting, diarrhea, confusion, and hypotension. It can also cause heart block and neurologic and psychiatric symptoms. Procainamide causes less cardiac depression than quinidine.

High doses of lidocaine can cause cardiovascular depression, bradycardia, hypotension, seizures, blurred vision, and double vision. Less serious side effects may include dizziness and confusion. The use of lidocaine is contraindicated in patients with advanced AV block, and it should be used with caution in patients with hepatic disorders or HF. Mexiletine has side effects similar to lidocaine, and both drugs are contraindicated for use in patients with cardiogenic shock or in those with second- or third-degree heart block.

The side effects of beta blockers are bradycardia and hypotension. Bretylium tosylate and amiodarone can cause nausea, vomiting, hypotension, and neurologic problems. The side effects of calcium blockers include nausea, vomiting, hypotension, and bradycardia.

It should be noted that *all* antidysrhythmic drugs are potentially prodysrhythmic. This is because of both the pharmacologic activity of the drug on the heart and the inherently unpredictable activity of a diseased heart, with or without the use of drugs. In some cases, life-threatening ventricular dysrhythmias can result from appropriate and skillful attempts at drug therapy to treat patients with heart disease. For these reasons, antidysrhythmic drug therapy is often initiated during continuous cardiac monitoring of the patient's heart rhythm in a hospital setting.

CLINICAL JUDGMENT [NURSING PROCESS]
! *Antidysrhythmics*

Concept: Perfusion
- The passage of blood flow through the arteries and capillaries that deliver oxygen and nutrients to body cells

Recognize Cues [Assessment]
- Obtain health and drug histories. The history may include shortness of breath, heart palpitations, coughing, chest pain (type, duration, and severity), previous angina or cardiac dysrhythmias, and drugs the patient currently takes.
- Obtain baseline vital signs and electrocardiogram (ECG) for future comparisons.
- Monitor early cardiac enzyme results (aspartate aminotransferase [AST], lactate dehydrogenase [LDH], creatine phosphokinase) and cardiac-specific troponins for future comparisons.

Analyze Cues and Prioritize Hypothesis [Patient Problems]
- Decreased gas exchange
- Dysrhythmia
- Decreased tissue perfusion
- Hypoxemia
- Anxiety

Generate Solutions [Planning]
- The patient will be in normal sinus rhythm.
- The patient will comply with the antidysrhythmic drug regimen.

Take Action [Nursing Interventions]
- ⚡ Monitor vital signs because hypotension can occur.

- ⚡ Administer drug by IV push or bolus over a period of 2 to 3 minutes or as prescribed.
- Monitor ECG for abnormal patterns, and report findings such as premature ventricular contractions (PVCs), increased PR and QT intervals, and/or widening of the QRS complex. Increased QT interval is a risk factor for *torsades de pointes*.

Patient Teaching
General
- Teach patients to take prescribed drugs as ordered because drug compliance is essential.
- Provide specific instructions for each drug (e.g., photosensitivity for amiodarone).

Side Effects
- Tell patients to report side effects and adverse reactions to a health care provider, including dizziness, faintness, nausea, and vomiting.
- ⚡ Advise patients to avoid alcohol, caffeine, and tobacco. Alcohol can intensify a hypotensive reaction, caffeine increases catecholamine levels, and tobacco promotes vasoconstriction.

Evaluate Outcomes [Evaluation]
- Evaluate effectiveness of prescribed antidysrhythmics by comparing heart rates with baseline rates and assessing the patient's response to the drug.
- Report side effects and adverse reactions. Drug regimens may need to be adjusted, and drug-induced dysrhythmias may occur that can require discontinuation of a drug.

CRITICAL THINKING UNFOLDING CASE STUDY

Question 1:

Cognitive Skill: Recognize cues (enhanced hot spot)

A 64-year-old-female patient with a diagnosis of heart failure has been admitted to the emergency department. Her medication profile includes furosemide 20 mg/d, digoxin 0.25 mg/d, and potassium chloride (KCl) 20 mEq/d. The patient has experienced three days of flulike symptoms, including anorexia, nausea, vomiting, and diarrhea. Her fluid and food intake are diminished, and she refused to take the KCl, stating, "This drug makes me sick." The nurse's assessment includes:
- Normal skin turgor
- Complaints of stress
- Muscle weakness
- Pulse rate 90 beats per minute (bpm), irregular
- Hypoactive bowel sounds
- Complaints of feeling lightheaded
- Pedal pulses strong and palpable
- Patient alert and oriented

Highlight or place a check mark next to the patient's assessment data that needs an immediate response by the nurse.

Answers:
- Normal skin turgor
- Complaints of stress

- Muscle weakness
- Pulse rate 90 beats per minute (bpm), irregular
- Hypoactive bowel sounds
- Complaints of feeling lightheaded
- Pedal pulses strong and palpable
- Patient alert and oriented

Rationale:

The patient has refused to take her ordered dose of potassium chloride. Signs and symptoms of hypokalemia are flulike symptoms: anorexia, nausea, vomiting, and diarrhea.

References:

Lewis S, et al (10th ed). *Medical Surgical Nursing*, Ch 16. McCuistion L, et al (10th ed). *Pharmacology*, Ch 37.

Question 2:

Cognitive Skill: Analyze cues (extended multiple response)

A 64-year-old patient with a diagnosis of heart failure has been admitted to the emergency department. Her medication profile includes furosemide 20 mg/d, digoxin 0.25 mg/d, and potassium chloride (KCl) 20 mEq/d. The patient has experience three days of flulike symptoms, including anorexia, nausea, vomiting, and diarrhea. Her fluid and food intake are diminished, and she refused to take the KCl, stating, "This drug makes me sick." The nurse's assessment includes:

CRITICAL THINKING UNFOLDING CASE STUDY—CONT'D

- Normal skin turgor
- Complaints of stress
- Muscle weakness
- Pulse rate 90 beats per minute (bpm), irregular
- Hypoactive bowel sounds
- Complaints of feeling lightheaded
- Pedal pulses strong and palpable
- Patient alert and oriented

The nurse draws blood for STAT samples. Indicate which labs require priority intervention by placing an "X" next to the correct answers.

_____a. Potassium (K) 3.0 mEq/L
_____b. Sodium (Na) 135 mEq/L
_____c. Creatinine 1.0 mg/dL
_____d. Chloride (Cl) 90 mEq/L
_____e. Blood urea nitrogen (BUN) 10 mg/dL
_____f. Digoxin 3 ng/mL
_____g. Hematocrit 38%
_____h. B-type natriuretic peptide (BNP) 1000 pg/mL

Answers:

__X__ a. Potassium (K) 3.0 mEq/L
_____ b. Sodium (Na) 135 mEq/L
_____ c. Creatinine 1.0 mg/dL
__X__ d. Chloride (Cl) 90 mEq/L
_____ e. Blood urea nitrogen (BUN) 10 mg/dL
__X__ f. Digoxin 3 ng/mL
_____ g. Hematocrit 38%
__X__ h. B-type natriuretic peptide (BNP) 1000 pg/mL

Rationale:
The abnormal labs are potassium 3.0mE/L (normal 3.5–5.0mEq/L; a low potassium level will exacerbate digoxin toxicity), chloride 90 mEq/L (normal 96–106 mEq/L; a low chloride level can cause vomiting), digoxin 3 ng/mL (normal 0.8–2.0ng/mL; a high digoxin level indicates digoxin toxicity); BNP 1000 pg/mL (normal <100 pg/mL; a BNP >900 indicates heart failure).

References:
Lewis S, et al (10th ed). *Medical Surgical Nursing*, Appendix C, Laboratory Reference Intervals; McCuistio, L, et al (10th ed). *Pharmacology*, Ch 37.

Question 3:

Cognitive Skill: Prioritize hypotheses (Cloze)
The 64 year-old-female patient is admitted to the Telemetry Unit of the hospital for further care. She will receive cardiac monitoring, nausea medication, and sodium chloride 0.9% IV.

Based on the options below, which problems should the nurse consider priority?
The patient has a diagnosis of heart failure and is experiencing _____(1)_____. The patient's history indicates a problem with _____(2)_____. The nurse recognizes the patient's lab indicates _____(3)_____.

Option 1	Option 2	Option 3
hyperkalemia	bowel incontinence	hyponatremia
hypokalemia	osteoarthritis	digoxin toxicity
hypotension	peptic ulcer disease	increased calcium levels
myocardial infarction	medication compliance	hypernatremia
tachycardia	high-protein diet	high blood sugar levels

Answers:
The patient has a diagnosis of heart failure and is experiencing hypokalemia (1). The patient's history indicates a problem with medication compliance (2). The nurse recognizes the patient's digoxin lab indicates digoxin toxicity (3).

Rationale:
In the state of hypokalemia, or low potassium, digitalis toxicity is worsened because digoxin normally binds to the ATPase pump on the same site as potassium. When potassium levels are low, digoxin can more easily bind to the ATPase pump, exerting the inhibitory effects.

Reference:
Cummings E, and Swoboda H. (2021). *Digoxin toxicity*. StatPearlsPublishing, Treasure Island (Fl). https:// www.ncbi.nlm.nih.gov/books/NBK470568; McCuistion L, et al (10th ed). *Pharmacology*, Ch 37.

Question 4:

Cognitive Skill: Generate solutions (matrix)
The provider orders much needed medications to be administered STAT. Use an X for the medication indicated for this patient that is most effective; if the medication is not recommended for this patient and could be harmful, place an X in the ineffective box. If the medication does not apply to this patient, place an X in the unrelated box.

Nursing Intervention	Effective	Ineffective
20 mEq (IV) potassium chloride over 4 h STAT		
400 mg single dose digoxin immune fab IV STAT		
1 g ceftriaxone IV over 3 h STAT		
5 mcg/kg/min dopamine IV STAT		

Answers:

Nursing Intervention	Effective	Ineffective
20 mEq (IV) potassium chloride over 4 h STAT	X	
400 mg single dose digoxin immune fab IV STAT	X	
1 g ceftriaxone IV over 3 h STAT		X
5 mcg/kg/min dopamine IV STAT		X

Rationale:
The antidote for digitalis toxicity is digoxin-immune fab. This agent binds with digoxin to form complex molecules that can be excreted in the urine, and so digoxin is unable to bind at the cellular site of action. The patient has a low potassium level which can add to the toxicity, so more potassium is being ordered. Ceftriaxone and dopamine are not indicated for this patient and are considered ineffective.

References:
McCuistion L. *Pharmacology* (10th ed) Chs 37, 40.

Question 5:

Cognitive Skill: Generate solutions (extended multiple response)
The patient is taking digoxin for heart failure and is experiencing digoxin toxicity and hypokalemia.

The nurse is instructing the patient about hypokalemia. Which of the following information is most important to prevent hypokalemia? Select all that apply.
_____a. Never skip your daily dose of potassium
_____b. You do not need to report dizziness to your doctor
_____c. Bananas and strawberries are high in potassium
_____d. Weigh yourself daily

Continued

CRITICAL THINKING UNFOLDING CASE STUDY—CONT'D

_____ e. Leg cramping is a sign of low potassium

_____ f. Drink 4 L of water each day

_____ g. Muscle weakness is a sign of low potassium

_____ h. It's OK to skip your potassium, just double the next dose

_____ i. Antacids can lower the amount of potassium in your blood if taken at same time

Answers:

__X__ a. Never skip your daily dose of potassium

_____ b. You do not need to report dizziness to your doctor

__X__ c. Bananas & strawberries are high in potassium

__X__ d. Weigh yourself daily

__X__ e. Leg cramping is a sign of low potassium

_____ f. Drink 4 L of water each day

__X__ g. Muscle weakness is a sign of low potassium

_____ h. It's okay to skip your potassium, just double the next dose

__X__ i. Antacids can lower the dose of potassium in your blood if taken at same time

Rationale:

Hypokalemia can alter the resting membrane potential, which will cause a negative pressure within the cells and impaired muscle contraction. This change can affect the cardiac muscle. Hypokalemia also increases the risk for digoxin toxicity. It is important for the nurse to instruct the patient in how to avoid the risk of hypokalemia.

Reference:

Lewis S, et al. (10th ed). _Medical Surgical Nursing_, Ch 16, Table 16-6. McCuistion L. _Pharmacology_ (10th ed), Ch 37.

Question 6:

Cognitive Skills: Evaluate outcomes (extended drag and drop)

In anticipation of discharge, the nurse is preparing to instruct the patient concerning furosemide, digoxin, and signs and symptoms of digoxin toxicity.

Indicate which nursing response listed in the far-left column is appropriate for the patient's questions by placing the number of the question under the appropriate nurse's response.

Nurse's Responses	Patient Questions	Appropriate Nurse's Response for Each Patient Question
1. Your digoxin dose will remain as 0.25 mg/d	Why is the doctor putting me back on digoxin after experiencing toxicity?	
2. Can you explain how digoxin works on your heart to improve the heart failure?	I do not know but would like to learn.	
3. Name a side effect of digoxin toxicity.	The only side effects I know are nausea, vomiting, and diarrhea.	
4. You must follow your provider's orders for blood-work.	Why must I have my blood drawn?	
5. You will have to take your pulse rate before taking digoxin. I will be happy to show you how it is done.	Why must I count my pulse rate before taking digoxin?	
6. It may affect your vision and can cause blurred or yellow vision.		
7. Digoxin increases the force of your heart's contraction and decreases the heart rate. It increases your cardiac output.		
8. The provider will request periodic lab draws to ensure your digoxin level and potassium level are within normal limits to prevent digoxin toxicity and hypokalemia.		
9. You received digoxin immune fab IV, which lowers the toxic level of digoxin in the blood. Your digoxin level this morning is in the normal range (1.8 ng/mL).		
10. If your pulse rate is less than 60 beats per minute, you must hold digoxin and notify your health provider.		

CRITICAL THINKING UNFOLDING CASE STUDY—CONT'D

Answers:

Nurse's Responses	Patient Questions	Appropriate Nurse's Response for each patient question
1. Your digoxin dose will remain as 0.25 mg/d	Why is the doctor putting me back on digoxin after experiencing toxicity?	9. You received digoxin immune fab IV, which lowers the toxic level of digoxin in the blood. Your digoxin level this morning is in the normal range (1.8 ng/mL).
2. Can you explain how digoxin works on your heart to improve heart failure?	I do not know but would like to learn.	7. Digoxin increases the force of your heart's contraction and decreases the heart rate. It increases your cardiac output.
3. Name a side effect of digoxin toxicity.	The only side effects I know are nausea, vomiting, and diarrhea.	6. It may affect your vision and can cause blurred or yellow vision.
4. You must follow your provider's orders for bloodwork.	Why must I have my blood drawn?	8. The provider will request periodic lab draws to ensure your digoxin level and potassium levels are within normal limits to prevent digoxin toxicity and hypokalemia.
5. You will have to take your pulse rate before taking digoxin. I will be happy to show you how it is done.	Why must I count my pulse rate before taking digoxin?	10. If your pulse is less than 60 beats per minute, you must hold digoxin and notify your health provider.

Rationale:
The nurse is instructing the client in medication compliance. Digoxin affects the heart by increasing the force of the contraction and decreasing the heart rate. The nurse explains the severity of digoxin toxicity. This is why she received digoxin immune fab IV. It is most important for the patient to be compliant with all of her health care provider-prescribed medications. Also, the patient must know the signs and symptoms of digoxin toxicity to report to the provider. It is important for the patient to be taught how to count the pulse and, if it's under 60 bpm, not to take the digoxin and to notify the provider.

Reference:
McCuistion L. *Pharmacology* (10th ed), Ch 37. Lewis S, et al (10th ed). *Medical Surgical Nursing*, Ch 34.

REVIEW QUESTIONS

1. The patient is receiving digoxin for treatment of heart failure. Which finding would suggest to the nurse that the heart failure is improving?
   a. Pale and cool extremities
   b. Absence of peripheral edema
   c. Urine output of 60 mL every 4 hours
   d. Complaints of increasing dyspnea

2. The patient's serum digoxin level is 3.0 ng/mL. What does the nurse know about this serum digoxin level?
   a. It is in the high (elevated) range.
   b. It is in the low (decreased) range.
   c. It is within the normal range.
   d. It is in the low-average range.

3. The nurse is assessing a patient for possible evidence of digitalis toxicity. Which of these is included in the signs and symptoms for digitalis toxicity?
   a. Apical pulse rate of 100 beats/min
   b. Apical pulse of 72 beats/min with an irregular rate
   c. Apical pulse of 90 beats/min with an irregular rate
   d. Apical pulse of 48 beats/min with an irregular rate

4. A patient is taking a potassium-depleting diuretic and digoxin. The nurse expects that a low potassium level (hypokalemia) could have what effect on digoxin?
   a. Increases serum digoxin sensitivity level
   b. Decreases serum digoxin sensitivity level
   c. No effect on serum digoxin sensitivity level
   d. Causes a low-average serum digoxin sensitivity level

5. A patient takes an initial dose of a nitrate. Which symptom(s) will the nurse expect to occur?
   a. Nausea and vomiting
   b. Headaches
   c. Stomach cramps
   d. Irregular pulse rate

6. A patient is prescribed a beta blocker. Beta blockers are as effective as antianginals because they do what?
   a. Increase oxygen to the systemic circulation
   b. Maintain heart rate and blood pressure
   c. Decrease heart rate and decrease myocardial contractility
   d. Decrease heart rate and increase myocardial contractility

7. The health care provider is planning to discontinue a patient's beta blocker. Which instruction will the nurse give the patient regarding the beta blocker?
   a. The beta blocker should be abruptly stopped when another cardiac drug is prescribed.
   b. The beta blocker should not be abruptly stopped; the dose should be tapered down.
   c. The beta blocker dose should be maintained while taking another antianginal drug.
   d. Half the beta blocker dose should be taken for the next several weeks.

8. The beta blocker acebutolol is prescribed for dysrhythmias. What is the primary purpose of the drug?
   a. Increase beta$_1$ and beta$_2$ receptors in cardiac tissues
   b. Increase the flow of oxygen to cardiac tissues
   c. Block beta$_1$-adrenergic receptors in cardiac tissues
   d. Block beta$_2$-adrenergic receptors in cardiac tissues

9. A patient who has angina is prescribed nitroglycerin. Which are appropriate nursing interventions for nitroglycerin? (Select all that apply.)
   a. Have the patient sit or lie down when taking a nitroglycerin sublingual tablet.
   b. Teach the patient who has taken nitroglycerin to call 911 if chest pain persists.
   c. Apply the nitroglycerin patch to a hairy area to protect skin from burning.
   d. Call the health care provider after taking five tablets if chest pain persists.
   e. Warn the patient against ingesting alcohol while taking nitroglycerin.
   f. Advise the patient not to drink water before taking nitroglycerin.

41

Diuretics

http://evolve.elsevier.com/McCuistion/pharmacology

OBJECTIVES

- Compare the action and uses of thiazide, loop, and potassium-sparing diuretics.
- Differentiate side effects and adverse reactions related to thiazide, loop, and potassium-sparing diuretics.

- Explain the nursing interventions—including patient teaching—related to thiazide, loop, and potassium-sparing diuretics.
- Apply the Clinical Judgment [Nursing Process] for the patient taking thiazide, loop, and potassium-sparing diuretics.

OUTLINE

Diuretics are used for two main purposes: to decrease hypertension (lower blood pressure) and to decrease edema, typically peripheral and pulmonary, in heart failure (HF) and renal or liver disorders. **Hypertension** is an elevated blood pressure greater than 120/80 mm Hg. Diuretics discussed in this chapter are used either alone or in combination to decrease blood pressure and edema.

Diuretics produce increased urine flow, or **diuresis**, by inhibiting sodium and water reabsorption from the kidney tubules. Most sodium and water reabsorption occur throughout the renal tubular segments (proximal, loop of Henle [descending loop and ascending loop], and collecting tubule). Diuretics can affect one or more segments of the renal tubules. Fig. 41.1 illustrates the renal tubule along with the normal process of water and electrolyte reabsorption and diuretic effects on the tubules.

Every 1.5 hours, the total volume of the body's extracellular fluid (ECF) goes through the kidneys (glomeruli) for cleansing; this is the first process for urine formation. Small particles such as electrolytes, drugs, glucose, and waste products from protein metabolism are filtered in the glomeruli. Larger products such as protein and blood cells are not filtered with normal renal function, and they remain in the circulation. Sodium and water are the largest filtrate substances.

Normally, 99% of the filtered sodium that passes through the glomeruli is reabsorbed; 50% to 55% of sodium reabsorption occurs in the proximal tubules, 35% to 40% occurs in the loop of Henle, 5% to 10% occurs in the distal tubules, and less than 3% occurs in the collecting tubules. Diuretics that act on the tubules closest to the glomeruli have the greatest effect in causing **natriuresis**, sodium loss in the urine. A classic example is the osmotic diuretic mannitol. The diuretic effect depends on the drug reaching the kidneys and its concentration in the renal tubules.

Diuretics have an **antihypertensive** effect because they promote sodium and water loss by blocking sodium and chloride reabsorption. This causes a decrease in fluid volume, which lowers blood pressure.

With fluid loss, edema—fluid retention in body tissues—should decrease, but if sodium is retained, water is also retained, and blood pressure increases.

Many diuretics cause the loss of other electrolytes, including potassium, magnesium, chloride, and bicarbonate. The diuretics that promote potassium excretion are classified as **potassium-wasting diuretics**, and those that promote potassium retention are called **potassium-sparing diuretics**.

The following five categories of diuretics are effective in removing water and sodium:

- Thiazide and thiazide-like diuretics
- Loop diuretics
- Osmotic diuretics
- Carbonic anhydrase inhibitors
- Potassium-sparing diuretics

Thiazide, loop, and potassium-sparing diuretics are most frequently prescribed for hypertension and for edema associated with HF. Except for those in the potassium-sparing group, all diuretics are potassium wasting.

Combination diuretics that contain both potassium-wasting and potassium-sparing drugs have been marketed primarily for the treatment of hypertension. Combinations have an additive effect in reducing blood pressure and are discussed in more detail in the Potassium-Sparing Diuretics section later in this chapter. Chapter 39 takes a closer look at the combinations of antihypertensive agents with hydrochlorothiazide.

THIAZIDES AND THIAZIDE-LIKE DIURETICS

Chlorothiazide was the first thiazide marketed and hydrochlorothiazide was the second. There are numerous thiazide and thiazide-like preparations. Thiazides act on the distal convoluted renal tubule, beyond the loop of Henle, to promote sodium, chloride, and water excretion. Thiazides are

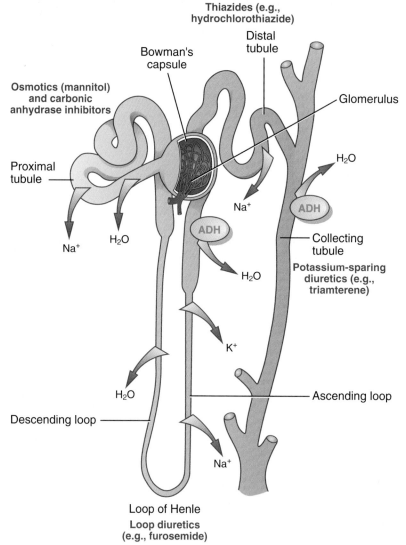

Fig. 41.1 Diuretics act on different segments of the renal tubule. Osmotic, mercurial, and carbonic anhydrase inhibitor diuretics affect the proximal tubule; loop diuretics affect the loop of Henle; thiazides affect the distal tubule; and potassium-sparing diuretics act primarily on the collecting tubules. *ADH*, Antidiuretic hormone; *H₂O*, water; *K⁺*, potassium; *Na⁺*, sodium.

used to treat hypertension and peripheral edema. They are not effective for immediate diuresis and should not be used to promote fluid loss in patients with severe renal dysfunction. Table 41.1 lists thiazide and thiazide-like diuretics and their dosages, uses, and considerations. Drug dosages for hypertension and edema are similar.

Thiazide diuretics are used primarily for patients with normal renal function. If the patient has a renal disorder and creatinine clearance is less than 30 mL/min, the effectiveness of the thiazide diuretic is greatly decreased. Thiazides cause a loss of sodium, potassium, and magnesium, but they promote calcium reabsorption. Hypercalcemia (calcium excess) may result, and the condition can be hazardous to the patient who is digitalized or has cancer that causes hypercalcemia. Thiazides affect glucose tolerance, so hyperglycemia can also occur. Thiazides should be used cautiously in patients with diabetes mellitus. Laboratory test results, such as electrolytes and glucose, need to be monitored.

Hydrochlorothiazide has been combined with selected angiotensin-converting enzyme (ACE) inhibitors, beta blockers, alpha blockers, angiotensin II blockers, and centrally acting sympatholytics to control hypertension. Prototype Drug Chart: Hydrochlorothiazide outlines the pharmacologic data for hydrochlorothiazide.

Pharmacokinetics. Thiazides are well absorbed from the gastrointestinal (GI) tract. Hydrochlorothiazide has moderate protein-binding power. The half-life of the thiazide drugs is longer than that of the loop diuretics. For this reason, thiazides should be administered in the morning to avoid nocturia (nighttime urination) and sleep interruption.

Pharmacodynamics. Thiazides act directly on arterioles to cause vasodilation, which can lower blood pressure. Other action includes the promotion of sodium chloride and water excretion, resulting in a decrease in vascular fluid volume and a concomitant decrease in cardiac output and blood pressure. The onset of action of hydrochlorothiazide occurs within 2 hours. Peak concentration times are long (4 hours). Thiazides are divided into three groups according to their duration of action: (1) short acting (duration <12 hours), (2) intermediate acting (duration 12 to 24 hours), and (3) long acting (duration >24 hours).

Side Effects and Adverse Reactions

Side effects and adverse reactions of thiazides include electrolyte imbalances (hypokalemia, hypercalcemia and hypomagnesemia), hyperglycemia (elevated blood glucose), hyperuricemia (elevated serum uric acid level), and hyperlipidemia (elevated blood lipid level).

TABLE 41.1 Diuretics

Drug	Route and Dosage	Uses and Considerations
Thiazides		
Short Acting		
Chlorothiazide	Edema: A: PO: 500–1000 mg/d in 1–2 divided doses; *max:* 1 g/d A: IV: 500–1000 mg qd/bid in 1–2 divided doses given slowly or as an infusion; *max:* 2 g/d	For hypertension, edema, HF, ascites, and nephrotic syndrome. May cause headache, dizziness, blurred vision, orthostatic hypotension, constipation, hypokalemia, hypomagnesemia, hyponatremia, hypochloremia, hypercholesterolemia, hypercalcemia, hyperglycemia, and hyperuricemia. PB: UK; t½: 45–120 min
Hydrochlorothiazide	See Prototype Drug Chart: Hydrochlorothiazide	
Intermediate Acting		
Bendroflumethiazide with nadolol	A: PO: Initially 1 tablet/d (40 mg nadolol and 5 mg bendroflumethiazide); *max:* 80 mg nadolol/5 mg bendroflumethiazide	For hypertension. May cause dizziness, fatigue, hypokalemia, hyponatremia, hypomagnesemia, hypochloremia, hypercalcemia, hypercholesterolemia, hyperuricemia, photosensitivity, and bradycardia. PB: nadolol: 30%; bendroflumethiazide: 95%; t½: nadolol: 10–24 h; bendroflumethiazide: 3 h
Long Acting		
Methyclothiazide	A: PO: 2.5–5 mg/d or qod; *max:* 5 mg/d for hypertension; 10 mg/d for edema	For hypertension and edema. May cause orthostatic hypotension, headache, dizziness, blurred vision, diarrhea, constipation, hypokalemia, hypomagnesemia, hyponatremia, hypochloremia, hypercalcemia, hypercholesterolemia, hyperuricemia, and hyperglycemia. PB: UK; t½: UK
Thiazide-Like Diuretics		
Chlorthalidone	Edema: A: PO: Initially 50–100 mg/d; *maint:* 50–200 mg/d; *max:* 200 mg/d	For hypertension and edema. May cause dizziness, headache, diarrhea, constipation, orthostatic hypotension, hypomagnesemia, hyponatremia, hypokalemia, hypochloremia, hypercalcemia, hyperglycemia, hyperuricemia, and hypercholesterolemia. PB: 75%; t½: 40–60 h
Indapamide	Edema: A: PO: 2.5 mg/d or qod; *max:* 5 mg/d	For hypertension and edema. May cause dizziness, headache, dry mouth, orthostatic hypotension, diarrhea, constipation, hypokalemia, hyperglycemia, hyperuricemia, hypochloremia, hyponatremia, hypercalcemia, and hypercholesterolemia. PB: 71%–79%; t½: 14–18 h
Metolazone	Edema: A: PO: 5–20 mg/d; *max:* 20 mg/d	For hypertension and edema. May cause blurred vision, constipation, orthostatic hypotension, hypokalemia, hypochloremia, hypomagnesemia, hyponatremia, hyperglycemia, hyperuricemia, hypercalcemia, hypophosphatemia, and hypercholesterolemia. PB: 33%; t½: 14 h

A, Adult; *bid,* twice a day; *d,* day; *GI,* gastrointestinal; *h,* hour; *HF,* heart failure; *IV,* intravenous; *maint,* maintenance; *max,* maximum; *min,* minute; *PB,* protein binding; *PO,* by mouth; *qd,* every day; *qod,* every other day; *t½,* half-life; *UK,* unknown; *y,* year; *<,* less than.

📄 PROTOTYPE DRUG CHART

Hydrochlorothiazide

Drug Class	Dosage
Thiazide diuretic	Hypertension: A: PO: 12.5–50 mg/d; *max:* 50 mg/d Edema: A: PO: 25–100 mg/d in single or divided doses; *max:* 100 mg/d

Contraindications	Drug-Lab-Food Interactions
Anuria, hypersensitivity *Caution:* Hepatic/renal dysfunction, diabetes mellitus, gout, asthma, hypotension, electrolyte imbalance, older adults, breastfeeding, hypovolemia, hypokalemia, hyponatremia, hypomagnesemia, hypochloremia	Drug: Increased digitalis toxicity with digitalis if hypokalemia is present; increased renal toxicity with aspirin; increased potassium loss with steroids; decreased effect of antidiabetics; decreased thiazide absorption and effects with NSAIDs, cholestyramine, and colestipol Lab: Increased serum calcium, glucose, uric acid; decreased serum potassium, sodium, magnesium

Pharmacokinetics	Pharmacodynamics
Absorption: Readily absorbed from GI tract Distribution: PB: 40%–68% Metabolism: t½: 5.6–14.8 h Excretion: In urine	PO: Onset: 2 h Peak: 4 h Duration: 6–12 h

Continued

PROTOTYPE DRUG CHART—cont'd

Therapeutic Effects/Uses

To increase urine output and to treat hypertension and edema due to HF, nephrotic syndrome, and ascites

Mechanism of Action: Action is on the renal distal tubules, promoting sodium, potassium, and water excretion and decreasing preload and cardiac output; also decreases edema; acts on arterioles and causes vasodilation, thus decreasing blood pressure

Side Effects	Adverse Reactions
Dizziness, headache, blurred vision, anorexia, nausea, vomiting, diarrhea, abdominal cramps, constipation, rash, photosensitivity, paresthesias, weakness, erectile dysfunction	Orthostatic hypotension, hyponatremia, hypomagnesemia, hypochloremia, hyperglycemia, hypercalcemia, hyperuricemia, hypercholesterolemia, hypertriglyceridemia, metabolic alkalosis, pulmonary edema, ocular hypertension, gout *Life-threatening:* Hypokalemia, aplastic anemia, leukopenia, hemolytic anemia, thrombocytopenia, agranulocytosis, renal failure, Stevens-Johnson syndrome

A, Adult; *d,* day; *GI,* gastrointestinal; *h,* hour; *HF,* heart failure; *max,* maximum; *mo,* month; *NSAID,* nonsteroidal antiinflammatory drug; *PB,* protein binding; *PO,* by mouth; *t½,* half-life; *>,* greater than; *<,* less than.

TABLE 41.2   Serum Chemistry Abnormalities Associated With Thiazides

Serum Chemistry Parameter	Abnormal Results
Electrolytes, Normal Levels	
Potassium, 3.5–5.0 mEq/L	Hypokalemia (low serum potassium); potassium is excreted from the distal renal tubule.
Magnesium, 1.5–2.5 mEq/L	Hypomagnesemia (low serum magnesium); potassium and sodium loss prompt magnesium loss.
Calcium, 8.6–10.2 mg/dL	Hypercalcemia (elevated serum calcium); thiazides may block calcium excretion.
Chloride, 96–106 mEq/L	Hypochloremia (low serum chloride); sodium and potassium losses produce chloride loss.
Bicarbonate, 24–28 mEq/L	Minimal bicarbonate loss occurs from the proximal tubule.
Uric acid, 2.8–8.0 mg/dL	Hyperuricemia (elevated uric acid); thiazides can block uric acid excretion.
Blood glucose, 70–99 mg/dL	Hyperglycemia (increased blood glucose); thiazides increase fasting blood glucose levels and those of the prediabetic state.
Blood Lipids	
Cholesterol: <200 mg/dL LDL: <100 mg/dL Triglyceride: <150 mg/dL	Elevated cholesterol, LDL, and triglycerides

LDL, Low-density lipoprotein.

Signs and symptoms of hypokalemia should be assessed, and serum potassium levels must be closely monitored. Potassium supplements are frequently needed. Serum calcium and uric acid levels should be checked because thiazides block calcium and uric acid excretion. Thiazides affect the metabolism of carbohydrates, and hyperglycemia can result, especially in patients with high to high-normal blood glucose levels. Thiazides can increase serum cholesterol, low-density lipoprotein, and triglyceride levels. A drug may be ordered to lower blood lipids. Other side effects include dizziness, headache, nausea, vomiting, constipation, and blood dyscrasias (rare). Table 41.2 summarizes the serum chemistry abnormalities that can occur with thiazide use.

Contraindications

Thiazides are contraindicated for use in renal failure. Symptoms of severe kidney impairment or shutdown include oliguria, a marked decrease in urine output; elevated blood urea nitrogen (BUN); and elevated serum creatinine.

Drug Interactions

Of the numerous thiazide drug interactions, the most serious occurs with digoxin. Thiazides can cause hypokalemia, which enhances the action of digoxin, and digitalis toxicity can occur. Potassium supplements are frequently prescribed, and serum potassium levels are

monitored. Thiazides also induce hypercalcemia, which enhances the action of digoxin, resulting in possible digitalis toxicity. Signs and symptoms of digitalis toxicity—bradycardia, nausea, vomiting, and visual changes—should be reported. Thiazides enhance the action of lithium, and lithium toxicity can occur. Thiazides potentiate the action of other antihypertensive drugs, which may be used to advantage in combination drug therapy for hypertension.

COMPLEMENTARY AND ALTERNATIVE THERAPIES
Diuretics

- When taken with a potassium-wasting diuretic such as a thiazide, aloe can decrease the serum potassium level, thereby causing hypokalemia.
- Ginkgo may increase blood pressure when taken with a thiazide diuretic.
- Licorice can increase potassium loss, leading to hypokalemia.
- Hawthorn may potentiate hypotension.

LOOP DIURETICS

The loop diuretics act on the thick ascending loop of Henle to inhibit chloride transport of sodium into the circulation and inhibit passive reabsorption of sodium. Sodium and water are lost, together with

⊙ CLINICAL JUDGMENT [NURSING PROCESS]

Diuretics: Thiazides

Concept: Elimination
- Excretion of body waste products through the urinary system.

Recognize Cues [Assessment]
- Assess vital signs, weight, urine output, and serum chemistry values (electrolytes, glucose, uric acid) for baseline levels.
- Check peripheral extremities for the presence of edema. Note pitting edema.
- Obtain a history of drugs and herbal supplements taken daily. Review for drugs and herbs that may cause a drug interaction (digoxin, corticosteroids, antidiabetics, ginkgo, licorice).

Analyze Cues and Prioritize Hypothesis [Patient Problems]
- Disrupted fluid and electrolyte imbalance
- Fluid overload
- Hypokalemia
- Hypernatremia
- Elimination

Generate Solutions [Planning]
- The patient's blood pressure will be decreased or will return to a normal value.
- The patient's edema will be decreased.
- The patient's serum chemistry levels will remain within normal ranges.

Take Action [Nursing Interventions]
- ⚡ Monitor vital signs and serum electrolytes, especially potassium, glucose, uric acid, and cholesterol levels. Report changes. If a patient is taking digoxin and hypokalemia occurs, digitalis toxicity frequently results.
- Observe for signs and symptoms of hypokalemia such as muscle weakness, leg cramps, and cardiac dysrhythmias.
- Monitor the patient's weight at the same time every day with the same type of clothing. A weight gain of 2.2 lb is equivalent to 1 L of body fluids.
- Note urine output to determine fluid loss or retention.
- Observe for signs and symptoms of hyperglycemia.

Patient Teaching

General
- Emphasize the need for adherence to the therapy plan. The patient may not feel better for some time or may not feel worse if treatment is missed or discontinued.
- Suggest that the patient take the drug early in the morning to avoid sleep disturbance resulting from nocturia.
- Instruct patients to keep drugs out of reach of small children. Request a child-proof bottle.
- Inform patients that certain herbal products may interact with thiazide diuretics.

Self-Administration
- Instruct patients or family members on how to take blood pressure and record daily results.

Side Effects
- ⚡ Instruct patients to slowly change positions from lying to standing because dizziness may occur as a result of orthostatic (postural) hypotension.
- Advise patients who may be prediabetic to have blood glucose checked periodically because large doses of hydrochlorothiazide increase blood glucose levels.
- Suggest that patients use sunblock when in direct sunlight to prevent photosensitivity.

Diet
- Teach patients to eat foods rich in potassium (fruits, fruit juices, and vegetables). Potassium supplements may be ordered.
- Instruct patients to take drugs with food to avoid gastrointestinal (GI) upset (anorexia, nausea, vomiting, diarrhea).

Evaluate Outcomes [Evaluation]
- Evaluate the effectiveness of drug therapy. The patient's blood pressure and edema will be reduced, and blood chemistry will remain within normal range.
- Determine an absence of side effects and adverse reactions to therapy.

---

potassium, calcium, and magnesium. Loop diuretics can affect blood glucose and can increase uric acid levels. Drugs in this group are extremely potent and cause marked depletion of water and electrolytes. The effects of loop diuretics are dose related; that is, increasing the dose increases the effect and response of the drug. More potent than thiazides for promoting diuresis, inhibiting reabsorption of sodium two to three times more effectively, loop diuretics are less effective as antihypertensive agents.

Loop diuretics should not be prescribed if a thiazide could alleviate body fluid excess. If furosemide alone is not effective in removing body fluid, a thiazide may be added. Furosemide is usually administered as an oral dose in the morning or intravenously when the patient's condition warrants immediate removal of body fluid; for example, in cases of acute HF or pulmonary edema.

Loop diuretics can increase renal blood flow up to 40%. Furosemide is a frequently prescribed diuretic for patients whose creatinine clearance is less than 30 mL/min and for those with end-stage renal disease. This group of diuretics causes excretion of calcium, unlike thiazides, which inhibit calcium loss.

The first loop diuretic marketed was ethacrynic acid, followed by furosemide and then bumetanide, which is more potent than furosemide on a milligram-for-milligram basis. Furosemide and bumetanide are derivatives of sulfonamides. Ethacrynic acid, a phenoxyacetic acid derivative, is a seldom-chosen loop diuretic. It is usually reserved for patients who are allergic to sulfa drugs. Prototype Drug Chart: Furosemide lists the drug data for the loop diuretic furosemide.

Pharmacokinetics. Loop diuretics are rapidly absorbed by the GI tract. These drugs are highly protein bound with half-lives that vary from 0.5 to 5 hours. Loop diuretics compete for protein-binding sites with other highly protein-bound drugs.

Pharmacodynamics. Loop diuretics have a great saluretic (sodium chloride–losing) or natriuretic (sodium-losing) effect and can cause rapid diuresis, decreasing vascular fluid volume and causing a decrease in cardiac output and blood pressure. Because furosemide is more potent than thiazide diuretics, it causes a vasodilatory effect; thus renal blood flow increases before diuresis. Furosemide is used when other conservative measures, such as sodium restriction and use of less potent diuretics, fail. The oral dose of furosemide is usually twice that of an intravenous (IV) dose.

The onset of action of loop diuretics occurs within 30 to 60 minutes. The onset of action for IV furosemide is 5 minutes. The duration of action is shorter than that of the thiazides.

PROTOTYPE DRUG CHART

Furosemide

Drug Class	Dosage
Loop diuretic	Peripheral edema: A: PO: Initially 20–80 mg single dose/d; may repeat in 6–8 h; *maint*: 40–120 mg/d; *max*: 600 mg/d A: IM/IV: 20–40 mg; increase by 20 mg q2h PRN; *max*: 6 g/d IV

Contraindications	Drug-Lab-Food Interactions
Hypersensitivity, anuria *Caution:* HF, electrolyte imbalance, diabetes mellitus, orthostatic hypotension, systemic lupus erythematosus, gout, hearing impairment, older adults, breastfeeding, hyperuricemia, renal/hepatic disease, thyroid disease	Drug: Increased orthostatic hypotension with alcohol; increased ototoxicity with aminoglycosides; increased bleeding with anticoagulants; increased potassium loss with steroids, amphotericin B, amiodarone; increased digitalis toxicity and cardiac dysrhythmias with digoxin and hypokalemia; increased lithium toxicity; increased amphotericin B ototoxicity and nephrotoxicity Food: Licorice may increase potassium loss. Lab: Increased BUN, blood/urine glucose, serum uric acid, ammonia; decreased potassium, sodium, calcium, magnesium, chloride serum levels Complementary and Alternative Therapies: Hawthorn may potentiate hypotension, and ginseng may decrease the action of loop diuretics.

Pharmacokinetics	Pharmacodynamics
Absorption: PO: Absorbed erratically from oral dose Distribution: PB: 95% Metabolism: t½: 0.5–1 h Excretion: In urine, some in feces; crosses the placenta	PO: Onset: 30–60 min Peak: 1–2 h Duration: 6–8 h IV: Onset: 5 min Peak: 20–30 min Duration: 2 h

Therapeutic Effects/Uses

To treat HF, renal dysfunction, hypertension, nephrotic syndrome, and acute pulmonary and peripheral edema
Mechanism of Action: Inhibition of sodium and water reabsorption from loop of Henle and distal renal tubules; increases excretion of potassium, chloride, magnesium, ammonium, phosphate, and calcium

Side Effects	Adverse Reactions
Nausea, anorexia, diarrhea, dizziness, tinnitus, abdominal cramps, constipation, rash, headache, weakness, blurred vision, muscle cramps, photosensitivity, paresthesias, injection site reaction	Hypokalemia, hyponatremia, hypocalcemia, hypomagnesemia, hypochloremia, metabolic alkalosis, hypovolemia, thromboembolism, orthostatic hypotension, diabetes mellitus, hyperglycemia, hyperuricemia, hypertriglyceridemia, hearing loss, hypercholesterolemia, gout *Life-threatening:* Aplastic anemia, hemolytic anemia, eosinophilia, leukopenia, thrombocytopenia, agranulocytosis, Stevens-Johnson syndrome

A, Adult; *BUN*, blood urea nitrogen; *d*, day; *GI*, gastrointestinal; *h*, hour; *HF*, heart failure; *IM*, intramuscular; *IV*, intravenous; *maint*, maintenance dose; *max*, maximum; *min*, minute; *PB*, protein binding; *PO*, by mouth; *q6–12h*, every 6 to 12 hours; *t½*, half-life.

Side Effects and Adverse Reactions

The most common side effects of loop diuretics are fluid and electrolyte imbalances such as hypokalemia, hyponatremia, hypocalcemia, hypomagnesemia, and hypochloremia. Hypochloremic metabolic alkalosis may result, which can worsen hypokalemia, and orthostatic hypotension can occur. Thrombocytopenia, skin disturbances, and transient hearing loss are rarely seen. Table 41.3 lists the physiologic and laboratory changes associated with loop diuretics.

Drug Interactions

The major drug interaction is with digitalis preparations. If the patient takes digoxin with a loop diuretic, digitalis toxicity can result. Hypokalemia enhances the action of digoxin and increases the risk for digitalis toxicity. The patient needs potassium replacement with food or supplements. Serum potassium levels should be closely monitored, especially when the patient is taking high dosages of loop diuretics. Table 41.4 lists the data for the four loop diuretics.

OSMOTIC DIURETICS

Osmotic diuretics increase the osmolality (concentration) and sodium reabsorption in the proximal tubule and loop of Henle. Sodium, chloride, potassium (to a lesser degree), and water are excreted. This group of drugs is used to decrease intracranial pressure (ICP, such as in cerebral edema) and decrease intraocular pressure (IOP, such as in glaucoma), and to promote excretion of toxic substances. Mannitol is a potent osmotic potassium-wasting diuretic frequently used in emergency situations such as ICP and IOP. In addition, mannitol can be used with cisplatin and carboplatin in cancer chemotherapy to induce a frank diuresis and decrease side effects of treatment.

Mannitol is the most frequently prescribed osmotic diuretic, followed by urea. Diuresis occurs within 1 to 3 hours after IV administration. Table 41.4 describes mannitol.

Side Effects and Adverse Reactions

The side effects and adverse reactions of mannitol include fluid and electrolyte imbalance, pulmonary edema from rapid shift of fluids, nausea

TABLE 41.3   Physiologic and Laboratory Changes Associated With Loop Diuretics

Physiologic/Laboratory Changes	Possible Effects of Loop (High-Ceiling) Diuretics
Physiologic Changes	
Hypotension	Postural (orthostatic) hypotension can result because of ECFV deficit.
Ototoxicity	Hearing impairment, although rare, may occur. It is more common with use of ethacrynic acid. Diuretics in other categories are not considered ototoxic. *Caution:* Avoid taking a loop diuretic with a drug that can be ototoxic, such as an aminoglycoside.
Skin disturbances	Pruritus, urticaria, exfoliative dermatitis, and purpura may occur in some persons allergic to the drug or when taking a loop diuretic in high doses over a long period.
Photosensitivity	When exposed to sun or a sunlamp for a prolonged time, severe sunburn could result. Patient should use sunblock and avoid long sun exposures.
Hypovolemia	Excess extracellular fluid is lost through increased urine excretion.
Laboratory Changes	
Hypokalemia, hypomagnesemia, hyponatremia, hypocalcemia, hypochloremia	Potassium, magnesium, sodium, calcium, and chloride are lost from the body from increased urine excretion. Chloride, an anion, is attached to the cations potassium and sodium; thus chloride is lost along with potassium and sodium.
Hyperglycemia	Increased glycogenolysis may contribute to elevated blood glucose level. Patients with diabetes should closely monitor blood glucose levels when taking a loop diuretic.
Hyperuricemia	Elevated uric acid levels are common in patients susceptible to gout.
Elevated BUN and creatinine	These elevations may result from ECFV loss. Hemoconcentration can cause elevated BUN and creatinine levels, which are reversible when fluid volume returns to normal levels.
Thrombocytopenia, leukopenia	Decreases in platelet and white blood cell counts are rare, but they should be closely monitored.
Elevated lipids	Loop diuretics can decrease HDL and increase LDL. Patients with elevated cholesterol levels should have their HDL and LDL levels checked. Regardless of the lipid effects, loop diuretics are useful for patients with serious fluid retention caused by a cardiac condition such as HF.

BUN, Blood urea nitrogen; *ECFV,* extracellular fluid volume; *HDL,* high-density lipoprotein; *HF,* heart failure; *LDL,* low-density lipoprotein.

TABLE 41.4   Diuretics: Loop, Osmotics, and Carbonic Anhydrase Inhibitors

Drug	Route and Dosage	Uses and Considerations
Loop		
Bumetanide	Edema: A: PO: Initially 0.5–1 mg/d; *max:* 10 mg/d A: IM/IV: Initially 0.5–1 mg/dose slowly over 2 min when IV; may give a 2nd and 3rd dose at 2- to 3-h intervals if needed; *max:* 10 mg/d	For edema and HF. May cause orthostatic hypotension, hypokalemia, hyponatremia, hypochloremia, hypocalcemia, hypovolemia, hyperglycemia, hyperuricemia, polyuria, and azotemia. PB: 96%; t½: 1–1.5 h
Ethacrynic acid	Pulmonary edema: A: IV: 0.5–1 mg/kg/dose, may repeat after 1 h; *max:* 100 mg/dose	For pulmonary and peripheral edema. May cause blurred vision, injection site reaction, orthostatic hypotension, hyperglycemia, hyperuricemia, hypochloremia, hypokalemia, hypomagnesemia, hyponatremia, hypocalcemia, and hearing loss. PB: 95%; t½: 2–4 h
Furosemide	See Prototype Drug Chart: Furosemide	
Torsemide	Hypertension: A: PO: Initially: 5 mg/d; *maint:* 5–10 mg/d; *max:* 10 mg/d HF/edema: A: PO/IV: 10–20 mg/d; *max:* 200 mg/d	For hypertension, edema, and ascites. May cause constipation, headache, orthostatic hypotension, tachycardia, hypokalemia, hypovolemia, hyperglycemia, hypercholesterolemia, hyperuricemia, and hearing loss. PB: 99%; t½: 3.5 h
Osmotics		
Mannitol	Cerebral edema: A: IV: 0.25–2 g/kg/dose over 30–60 min; may repeat q6–8h PRN	For edema, cerebral edema, IOP, increased ICP, acute renal failure, and excretion of toxic substances. May cause blurred vision, polyuria, hypo/hypernatremia, hypo/hypertension, headache, cough, hemoptysis, nausea, hypovolemia, dizziness, injection site reaction, tachycardia, and hypo/hyperkalemia. PB: UK; t½: 30–150 minutes
Carbonic Anhydrase Inhibitors		
Acetazolamide	Edema: A: PO/IV: 250–375 mg or 5 mg/kg in morning for 2 d; allow 1–2 d drug free, then give qod; *max:* 1000 mg/d	For edema, seizures, altitude sickness, and glaucoma. May cause dizziness, headache, hyper/hypoglycemia, hypokalemia, hyponatremia, hyperchloremia, injection site reaction, crystalluria, and metabolic acidosis. PB: 90%; t½: 10–15 h

A, Adult; *bid,* twice a day; *d,* day; *GI,* gastrointestinal; *h,* hour; *HF,* heart failure; *ICP,* intracranial pressure; *IM,* intramuscular; *IOP,* intraocular pressure; *IV,* intravenous; *maint,* maintenance dose; *max,* maximum; *min,* minute; *PB,* protein binding; *PO,* by mouth; *q4h,* every 4 hours; *qod,* every other day; *t½,* half-life; *tid,* three times a day; *UK,* unknown.

CLINICAL JUDGMENT [NURSING PROCESS]

Diuretics: Loop

Concept: Elimination
- Excretion of body waste products through the urinary system

Recognize Cues [Assessment]
- Obtain a history of drugs taken daily. Note if the patient is taking a drug that may interact with a loop diuretic, such as alcohol, aminoglycosides, anticoagulants, corticosteroids, lithium, amphotericin B, or digitalis. Recognize that furosemide is highly protein bound and can displace other protein-bound drugs such as warfarin.
- Assess vital signs, serum electrolytes, weight, and urine output for baseline levels.
- Compare the patient's drug dose with the recommended dose and report any discrepancy.
- Note whether the patient is hypersensitive to sulfonamides.

Analyze Cues and Prioritize Hypothesis [Patient Problems]
- Disrupted fluid and electrolyte imbalance
- Fluid overload
- Hypokalemia
- Hypernatremia

Generate Solutions [Planning]
- The patient's edema will be reduced.
- The patient's blood pressure will be decreased.
- The patient's serum chemistry levels will remain within normal ranges.

Take Action [Nursing Interventions]
- Monitor urinary output to determine body fluid gain or loss. Urinary output should be at least 30 mL/h or 600 mL/24 h.
- Notify a health care provider if urine output does not increase; a severe renal disorder may be present.

- Weigh the patient at the same time every day with the same type of clothing to determine fluid loss or gain. A loss of 2.2 lb is equivalent to a fluid loss of 1 L.
- Monitor vital signs and be alert for marked decreases in blood pressure.
- Administer IV furosemide slowly; hearing loss may occur if it is rapidly injected.
- ⚡ Observe for signs and symptoms of hypokalemia (<3.5 mEq/L), such as muscle weakness, abdominal distension, leg cramps, and/or cardiac dysrhythmias.
- Monitor serum potassium levels, especially when a patient is taking digoxin. Hypokalemia enhances the action of digitalis, causing digitalis toxicity.

Patient Teaching
General
- Advise patients to take furosemide in the morning and *not* in the evening to prevent sleep disturbance and nocturia. Advise patient to request childproof medication bottle if children are around.

Side Effects
- Teach patients to rise slowly from lying or sitting to standing to prevent dizziness resulting from fluid loss.

Diet
- Suggest taking furosemide with food to avoid nausea.

Evaluate Outcomes [Evaluation]
- Evaluate effectiveness of the drug action, such as decreased fluid retention or fluid overload, decreased respiratory distress, and increased cardiac output.
- Check for side effects and increased urine output.

---

and vomiting, tachycardia from rapid fluid loss, and acidosis. Crystallization of mannitol in the vial may occur when the drug is exposed to a low temperature; the vial should be warmed to dissolve the crystals. The mannitol solution should not be used for IV infusion if crystals are present and have not been dissolved.

Contraindications

Mannitol must be given with extreme caution to patients who have heart disease and HF. It should be immediately discontinued if the patient develops HF or renal failure.

CARBONIC ANHYDRASE INHIBITORS

The carbonic anhydrase inhibitor acetazolamide blocks the action of the enzyme *carbonic anhydrase,* which is needed to maintain the body's acid-base balance (hydrogen and bicarbonate ion balance). Inhibition of this enzyme causes increased sodium, potassium, and bicarbonate excretion. With prolonged use, metabolic acidosis can occur.

This group of drugs is used primarily to decrease IOP in patients with open-angle (chronic) glaucoma. Other uses include diuresis, management of epilepsy, and treatment of high-altitude or acute mountain sickness. Table 41.4 presents the drug data for carbonic anhydrase inhibitor diuretics. Such drugs may also be used for patients in metabolic alkalosis who need a diuretic. Carbonic anhydrase inhibitors may be alternated with a loop diuretic.

Side Effects and Adverse Reactions

Acetazolamide can cause fluid and electrolyte imbalance, metabolic acidosis, nausea, vomiting, anorexia, confusion, orthostatic hypotension, and crystalluria. Hemolytic anemia and renal calculi can also occur. These drugs are contraindicated during the first trimester of pregnancy.

POTASSIUM-SPARING DIURETICS

Potassium-sparing diuretics, which are weaker than thiazides and loop diuretics, are used as mild diuretics or in combination with another diuretic such as hydrochlorothiazide or an antihypertensive drug. Continuous use of potassium-wasting diuretics requires a daily oral potassium supplement because the kidneys excrete potassium, sodium, and body water. However, potassium supplements are *not* used when the patient takes a potassium-sparing diuretic; in fact, serum potassium excess, called hyperkalemia, results when a potassium supplement is taken with a potassium-sparing diuretic. The serum potassium should be periodically monitored when the patient continuously takes a potassium-sparing diuretic. If the serum potassium level is greater than 5.0 mEq/L, the patient should discontinue the potassium-sparing diuretic and restrict foods high in potassium.

Potassium-sparing diuretics act primarily in the collecting duct renal tubules and late distal tubule to promote sodium and water excretion and potassium retention. The drugs interfere with the sodium-potassium pump controlled by the mineralocorticoid hormone aldosterone (sodium retained and potassium excreted).

Spironolactone, an aldosterone antagonist, was the first potassium-sparing diuretic. Aldosterone is a mineralocorticoid hormone that promotes sodium retention and potassium excretion. Spironolactone blocks the action of aldosterone and inhibits the sodium-potassium pump (i.e., potassium is retained, and sodium is excreted). Spironolactone has been prescribed by cardiologists for patients with cardiac disorders because of its potassium-retaining effect. As a result of the action of spironolactone, the heart rate is more regular, and the possibility of myocardial fibrosis is decreased. The effects of spironolactone may take 48 hours.

Amiloride, triamterene, and eplerenone are additional commonly prescribed potassium-sparing diuretics. Amiloride and eplerenone are effective as antihypertensive agents. Triamterene is useful in the treatment of edema caused by HF or cirrhosis of the liver. Low doses of spironolactone and eplerenone are effective for chronic HF. Spironolactone, amiloride, triamterene, and eplerenone should not be taken with ACE inhibitors and angiotensin II receptor blockers (ARBs) because they can also increase serum potassium levels. Prototype Drug Chart: Spironolactone provides the pharmacologic data for spironolactone.

When potassium-sparing diuretics are used alone, they are less effective than when used in combination to reduce body fluid and sodium. These drugs are usually combined with a potassium-wasting diuretic, primarily hydrochlorothiazide or a loop diuretic. The combination of potassium-sparing and potassium-wasting diuretics intensifies the diuretic effect and prevents potassium loss. The common combination diuretics contain spironolactone and hydrochlorothiazide, amiloride and hydrochlorothiazide, and triamterene and hydrochlorothiazide. Table 41.5 lists the potassium-sparing diuretics and the combination potassium-wasting and potassium-sparing diuretics.

Side Effects and Adverse Reactions

The main side effect of potassium-sparing diuretics is hyperkalemia. Caution must be used when giving potassium-sparing diuretics to patients with poor renal function because the kidneys excrete 80% to 90% of potassium. Urine output should be at least 600 mL/day. Patients should *not* use potassium supplements while taking potassium-sparing diuretics, unless the serum potassium level is low. If a potassium-sparing diuretic is given with antihypertensive ACE inhibitors, hyperkalemia could become severe or life threatening because both drugs retain potassium. Monitoring serum potassium levels is essential to safe drug therapy. Headache, dizziness, asthenia (weakness), GI disturbances (anorexia, nausea, vomiting, diarrhea) hyperuricemia, muscle cramps, paresthesia (numbness and tingling of the hands and feet) can occur.

📄 PROTOTYPE DRUG CHART

Spironolactone

Drug Class	**Dosage**
Potassium-sparing diuretic	Edema: A: PO: Initially 100 mg/d in single or divided doses, *maint:* 25–200 mg/d in divided doses; *max:* 400 mg/d Hypertension: A: PO: 25–100 mg/d in single or divided doses; *max:* 400 mg/d
Contraindications	**Drug-Lab-Food Interactions**
Renal failure, hyperkalemia, adrenal insufficiency *Caution:* Renal/hepatic dysfunction, diabetes mellitus, HF, acid-base imbalance, acidosis/alkalosis, breastfeeding, pregnancy, older adults	Drug: Increased serum potassium level with potassium supplements; increased effects of antihypertensives and lithium *Life-threatening:* Hyperkalemia if given with an ACE inhibitor Lab: Increased serum potassium level; may increase BUN, AST, alkaline phosphatase levels; decreased serum sodium, chloride
Pharmacokinetics	**Pharmacodynamics**
Absorption: PO: Rapidly absorbed from GI tract Distribution: PB: 90% Metabolism: t½: 1–2 h Excretion: In urine, mostly as metabolites and bile	PO: Onset: UK Peak: 0.5–1.5 h Duration: 2–3 d or longer

Therapeutic Effects/Uses

For edema, hypertension, HF, hypokalemia, and hyperaldosteronism
Mechanism of Action: Inhibits aldosterone effects on distal renal tubules to promote sodium and water excretion and potassium retention

Side Effects	**Adverse Reactions**
Nausea, vomiting, diarrhea, abdominal cramps, dizziness, drowsiness, headache, confusion, weakness, muscle cramps, gout, paresthesia, dehydration, ataxia, erectile dysfunction	Hyperkalemia, hypomagnesemia, hyponatremia, hypocalcemia, hypovolemia, hyperglycemia, hyperuricemia, orthostatic hypotension, bradycardia, metabolic acidosis/alkalosis *Life-threatening:* Agranulocytosis, leukopenia, thrombocytopenia, renal/hepatic failure, Stevens-Johnson syndrome

A, Adult; *ACE,* angiotensin-converting enzyme; *AST,* aspartate aminotransferase; *BUN,* blood urea nitrogen; *d,* day; *GI,* gastrointestinal; *h,* hour; *HF,* heart failure; *max,* maximum; *PB,* protein binding; *PO,* by mouth; *t½,* half-life; *UK,* unknown.

TABLE 41.5   Diuretics: Potassium-Sparing

Drug	Route and Dosage	Uses and Considerations
Single Agents		
Amiloride hydrochloride	A: PO: 5–10 mg/d; *max:* 20 mg/d	For hypokalemia, hypertension, HF, and edema. May cause dizziness, headache, cough, orthostatic hypotension, constipation, hyperkalemia, hypochloremia, hyponatremia, anorexia, nausea, vomiting, and diarrhea. PB: 40%; t½: 6–9 h
Eplerenone	A: PO: 25–50 mg/d; *max:* 100 mg/d for hypertension; 50 mg/d for HF	For hypertension and HF. May cause hyperkalemia, hyponatremia, dizziness, hyperuricemia, hypertriglyceridemia, and hypercholesterolemia. PB: 50%; t½: 4–6 h
Spironolactone	See Prototype Drug Chart: Spironolactone	
Triamterene	A: PO: Initially 100 mg bid; *max:* 300 mg/d	For peripheral edema. May cause headache, dizziness, weakness, bradycardia, hypo/hyperkalemia, hyponatremia, hyperuricemia, and metabolic acidosis. PB: 67%; t½: 1–2 h
Combinations		
Amiloride hydrochloride and hydrochlorothiazide	A: PO: 1–2 tab/d (amiloride 5 mg/HCTZ 50 mg); *max:* 10 mg amiloride, 100 mg HCTZ	For hypertension and edema. May cause dizziness, headache, orthostatic hypotension, hypomagnesemia, hyponatremia, hypochloremia, hypovolemia, hypo/hyperkalemia, hypercalcemia, hyperglycemia, metabolic acidosis, hyperuricemia, anorexia, nausea, and rash. PB: 40% amiloride, 40%–60% HCTZ; t½: 6–9 h amiloride, 5.6–14.8 h HCTZ
Spironolactone and hydrochlorothiazide	Hypertension: A: PO: Initially 1 tab/d (25 mg spironolactone/25 mg HCTZ); *maint:* 50–100 mg/d of each; *max:* 200 mg/d of each	For edema and hypertension. May cause dizziness, headache, hyperkalemia, hypercalcemia, hyperuricemia, hyperglycemia, hypercholesterolemia, hypomagnesemia, hyponatremia, hypovolemia, anorexia, and muscle cramps. PB: 90% spironolactone, 40%–60% HCTZ; t½: 1–2 h spironolactone, 5.6–14.8 h HCTZ
Triamterene and hydrochlorothiazide	A: PO: Initially 1 cap/d pc (37.5 mg triamterene, 25 mg hydrochlorothiazide; *maint:* 1–2 cap/d pc; *max:* 75 mg triamterene, 50 mg HCTZ	For edema and HTN. May cause dizziness, headache, orthostatic hypotension, hyperglycemia, hypo/hyperkalemia, hypercalcemia, hypochloremia, hypomagnesemia, hyponatremia, hypovolemia, hyperuricemia, and hypercholesterolemia. PB: 67% triamterene, 40%–60% HCTZ; t½: 1–2 h triamterene, 5.6–14.8 h hydrochloride

A, Adult; *bid*, twice a day; *cap*, capsule; *d*, day; *GI*, gastrointestinal; *h*, hour; *HCTZ*, hydrochlorothiazide; *HF*, heart failure; *HTN*, hypertension; *maint*, maintenance dose; *max*, maximum; *MI*, myocardial infarction; *PB*, protein binding; *pc*, after meals; *PO*, by mouth; *t½*, half-life; *tab*, tablet.

◎ CLINICAL JUDGMENT [NURSING PROCESS]

Diuretics: Potassium-Sparing

Concepts: Elimination
- Excretion of body waste products through the urinary system

Recognize Cues [Assessment]
- Obtain a history of drugs taken daily. Note whether the patient is taking a potassium supplement or using a salt substitute.
- Assess vital signs, serum electrolytes, weight, and urinary output for baseline levels.
- Compare the patient's drug dose with the recommended dose, and report any discrepancy.

Analyze Cues and Prioritize Hypothesis [Patient Problems]
- Fluid overload
- Hyperkalemia
- Diarrhea
- Nausea

Generate Solutions [Planning]
- The patient blood pressure will be decreased.
- The patient's serum electrolytes will remain within normal ranges.

Take Action [Nursing Interventions]
- Note the half-life of spironolactone. With a long half-life, the drug is usually administered once a day, sometimes twice a day.
- Monitor urinary output; it should increase. Report if urine output is less than 30 mL/h or less than 600 mL/day.
- Weigh the patient at the same time every day with the same type of clothing to determine fluid loss or gain. A loss of 2.2 lb is equivalent to a fluid loss of 1 L.

- Record vital signs and report any abnormal changes.
- ⚡ Observe for signs and symptoms of hyperkalemia (serum potassium >5.0 mEq/L). Nausea, diarrhea, abdominal cramps, numbness and tingling of the hands and feet, leg cramps, tachycardia and later bradycardia, peaked narrow T wave on electrocardiogram, or oliguria may signal hyperkalemia.
- Administer spironolactone in the morning and not in the evening to avoid nocturia.

Patient Teaching
General
- Teach patients to take spironolactone with or after meals to avoid nausea.
- Encourage patients not to discontinue the drug without consulting a health care provider.

Side Effects
- Caution patients to avoid exposure to direct sunlight because spironolactone can cause photosensitivity.
- Advise patients to report possible side effects such as rash, dizziness, weakness, and gastrointestinal (GI) upset.

Diet
- Advise patients with high serum potassium levels to avoid foods rich in potassium when taking potassium-sparing diuretics.

Evaluate Outcomes [Evaluation]
- Evaluate the effectiveness of potassium-sparing diuretics (e.g., triamterene). Fluid retention (edema) should be decreased or absent.
- Determine whether urine output has increased and whether serum potassium level is within the normal range.

CRITICAL THINKING CASE STUDY

A 58-year-old patient has been recently diagnosed with hypertension. His resting blood pressure is 158/92. He is prescribed hydrochlorothiazide 50 mg/day and is told to eat foods rich in potassium.

1. How does hydrochlorothiazide differ from furosemide? What are their similarities and differences?
2. Why is it necessary for the patient to eat foods rich in potassium when taking hydrochlorothiazide? Explain your answer.
3. What nursing interventions should be considered while the patient takes hydrochlorothiazide?

After 1 month on hydrochlorothiazide therapy, the patient becomes weak and complains of nausea and vomiting. His muscles are "soft," and his serum potassium level is 3.3 mEq/L. The patient's diuretic is changed to triamterene and hydrochlorothiazide. Again, he is advised to eat foods rich in potassium.

4. Explain the rationale for changing the patient's diuretic.
5. Should the patient receive a potassium supplement? Explain your answer.
6. What nursing interventions should the nurse follow for the patient?
7. What care plan should the nurse develop for the patient in relation to patient teaching?
8. What medical follow-up care is needed for the patient?

REVIEW QUESTIONS

1. A patient is taking hydrochlorothiazide 50 mg/day and digoxin 0.25 mg/day. The nurse plans to monitor the patient for which potential electrolyte imbalance?
   a. Hypocalcemia
   b. Hypokalemia
   c. Hyperkalemia
   d. Hypermagnesemia
2. The nurse knows that which statement is correct regarding nursing care of a patient receiving hydrochlorothiazide? (Select all that apply.)
   a. Monitor patients for signs of hypoglycemia.
   b. Administer ordered potassium supplements.
   c. Monitor serum potassium and uric acid levels.
   d. Assess blood pressure before administration.
   e. Notify the health care provider if a patient has had oliguria for 24 hours.
   f. Assess for decreased cholesterol and triglyceride levels.
3. A patient has heart failure, and a high dose of furosemide is ordered. What suggests a favorable response to furosemide?
   a. A decrease in level of consciousness occurs, and the patient sleeps more.
   b. Respiratory rate decreases from 28/min to 20/min, and the depth increases.
   c. Breath sounds reveal increased congestion and the patient complains of shortness of breath.
   d. Urine output is 50 mL/4 hours, and intake is 200 milliliters.

4. What does the nurse know to be correct concerning the use of mannitol in patients?
   a. It decreases intracranial pressure.
   b. It increases intraocular pressure.
   c. It causes sodium and potassium retention.
   d. It causes diuresis in several days.
5. What should the nurse do when a patient is taking furosemide?
   a. Instruct the patient to change positions quickly when getting out of bed.
   b. Assess blood pressure before administration.
   c. Administer the drug at bedtime for maximum effectiveness.
   d. Teach the patient to avoid fruits to prevent hyperkalemia.
6. For the patient taking a diuretic, a combination such as triamterene and hydrochlorothiazide may be prescribed. The nurse realizes that this combination is ordered for which purpose?
   a. To decrease serum potassium level
   b. To maintain serum potassium level
   c. To decrease glucose level
   d. To increase glucose level
7. The patient has been receiving spironolactone 50 mg/day for heart failure. The nurse should closely monitor the patient for which condition?
   a. Hypokalemia
   b. Hyperkalemia
   c. Hypoglycemia
   d. Hypermagnesemia

42

Antihypertensives

http://evolve.elsevier.com/McCuistion/pharmacology

OBJECTIVES

- Differentiate the pharmacologic action of the various categories of antihypertensive drugs.
- Compare the side effects and adverse reactions to sympatholytics, direct-acting vasodilators, and angiotensin antagonists.
- Apply the Clinical Judgment [Nursing Process] related to antihypertensives, including nursing interventions and teaching.
- Describe the blood pressure guidelines for determining hypertension.

OUTLINE

HYPERTENSION

Hypertension is the most common condition leading to myocardial infarction (MI), stroke, renal failure, and death. Essential hypertension is the most common type of hypertension and affects 95% of persons with high blood pressure (BP). The exact origin of essential hypertension is unknown; however, contributing factors may include hyperlipidemia, African American race, diabetes, aging, stress, excessive alcohol ingestion, smoking, obesity, and a family history of hypertension. Thirty percent of hypertension cases are attributable to obesity. Five percent of hypertension cases are related to renal and endocrine disorders and are classified as secondary hypertension.

Guidelines for Hypertension

BP data collected should be based upon an average of more than two readings on more than two occasions. BP guidelines for determining hypertension have been revised and are contained in the Eighth Report of the Joint National Committee on Prevention, Detection, Evaluation, and Treatment of High Blood Pressure, or JNC 8, from 2017. The purpose of these guidelines is to decrease the risk of cardiovascular disease (CVD) in the American population. The guideline for normal BP is less than 120/80 mm Hg. *Elevated blood pressure* is defined as systolic blood pressure (SBP) of 120 to 129 and diastolic blood pressure (DBP) of less than 80. *Stage 1 hypertension* falls between 130/80 and 139/89, and *stage 2 hypertension* is 140/90 or greater.

Two out of three patients with hypertension have uncontrolled BP or are not optimally treated. SBP is more important than DBP as a CVD risk. According to the JNC 8, a BP of 140/90 is the goal for the population younger than 60 years, with a target of 150/90 for those above 60.

Selected Regulators of Blood Pressure

The kidneys and blood vessels strive to regulate and maintain a "normal" BP. The kidneys regulate BP by control of fluid volume and via the renin-angiotensin-aldosterone system (RAAS; Fig. 42.1). Kidneys control sodium and water elimination and retention, which affects cardiac output and systemic arterial BP. Renin from the renal cells stimulates production of angiotensin II, a potent vasoconstrictor that causes the release of aldosterone, an adrenal hormone that promotes sodium retention and thereby water retention. Retention of sodium and water causes fluid volume to increase, elevating BP.

The baroreceptors in the aorta and carotid sinus and the vasomotor center in the medulla also assist in the regulation of BP. Catecholamines such as norepinephrine, released from the sympathetic nerve terminals, and epinephrine, released from the adrenal medulla, increase BP through vasoconstrictive activity.

Other hormones that contribute to BP regulation are antidiuretic hormone (ADH), atrial natriuretic peptide (ANP) hormone, and brain

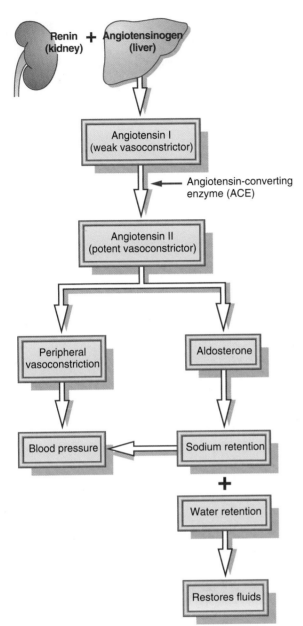

Fig. 42.1 The Renin-Angiotensin-Aldosterone System (RAAS). Renin, an enzyme located in the juxtaglomerular cells of the kidney, is released when blood pressure decreases. This diagram shows how the RAAS restores fluid balance and stabilizes blood pressure.

natriuretic peptide (BNP) hormone. ADH is produced by the hypothalamus and is stored and released by the posterior pituitary gland (neurohypophysis). This hormone stimulates the kidneys to conserve and retain water when there is a fluid volume deficit. When there is fluid overload, ADH secretion is inhibited, and the kidneys then excrete more water.

Physiologic Risk Factors

Certain physiologic risk factors contribute to hypertension. A diet high in saturated fat and simple carbohydrates can increase BP. Carbohydrate intake can affect sympathetic nervous activity. Alcohol increases renin secretions, causing the production of angiotensin II. Obesity affects the sympathetic and cardiovascular systems by increasing cardiac output, stroke volume, and left ventricular filling. Two-thirds of hypertensive persons are obese. Normally weight loss can decrease hypertension, as can mild to moderate sodium restriction.

Cultural Responses to Antihypertensive Agents

African Americans are more likely to develop hypertension at an earlier age than Caucasians. African Americans also have a higher mortality rate from hypertension than the Caucasian population. The use of beta-adrenergic blockers (beta blockers) and angiotensin-converting enzyme (ACE) inhibitors is less effective for the control of hypertension in African Americans unless the drug is combined or given with a diuretic. This group is susceptible to low-renin hypertension; therefore they do not respond well to beta blockers and ACE inhibitors. The antihypertensive drugs that are effective for African Americans are alpha$_1$ blockers and calcium channel blockers (calcium blockers). African American patients do respond to diuretics as the initial monotherapy for controlling hypertension. Caucasian patients usually have high-renin hypertension and respond well to all antihypertensive agents.

Asian Americans are twice as sensitive as Caucasians to beta blockers and other antihypertensives. A reduction in antihypertensive dosing is frequently needed. Native Americans have a reduced or lower response to beta blockers compared with Caucasians. Monitoring BP and drug dosing should be an ongoing assessment for patients in these cultural groups.

Hypertension in Older Adults

Approximately 70 million American adults have hypertension, which is 46% of the adult population. Of individuals over 60 years of age, 65% have developed hypertension, or two in three people. Only approximately 48% of hypertensive individuals have this condition under control. Typically, in the age range of 18 to 49, males have more prevalence of hypertension than females. Both systolic and diastolic hypertension are associated with increased cardiovascular morbidity and mortality. With antihypertensive therapy, the greatest decrease in cardiovascular disorders is 34% for stroke and 19% for coronary heart disease.

One of the troublesome side effects of the use of antihypertensive agents in older adults, especially frail or institutionalized persons, is orthostatic (postural) hypotension. This episode of sudden low BP presents as dizziness due to blood pooling in the lower extremities when an individual repositions to an upright position. In older adults, the sympathetic nervous system does not respond as quickly to correct the situation, especially when potentiated by antihypertensive drug administration. If orthostatic hypotension occurs, the antihypertensive drug dose may need to be decreased or another antihypertensive drug may need to be used. Older adults with hypertension should be instructed to modify their lifestyle and activities. This includes restricting dietary sodium to 2400 mg daily, avoiding tobacco, modifying diet, exercising, and decreasing stress.

NONPHARMACOLOGIC CONTROL OF HYPERTENSION

A sufficient decrease in BP can be accomplished by nonpharmacologic methods. There are many nonpharmacologic ways to decrease BP, but if the systolic pressure is greater than 140 mm Hg, antihypertensive drugs are generally ordered. Nondrug methods to decrease BP include stress-reduction techniques, exercise, salt restriction, decreased alcohol ingestion, and smoking cessation.

When hypertension cannot be controlled by nonpharmacologic means, antihypertensive drugs are prescribed. However, nonpharmacologic methods should be combined with antihypertensive drugs to control hypertension.

PHARMACOLOGIC CONTROL OF HYPERTENSION

An individualized approach to the treatment of hypertension is used by many health care providers. All drugs are considered *initial agents* when first prescribed for hypertension. Reduction of other cardiovascular risk factors and the use of fewer drugs (i.e., substituting instead of adding drugs) at the lowest effective doses are emphasized. Often more than one antihypertensive is used to control BP, which also may lead to fewer adverse effects.

Antihypertensive drugs, used either singly or in combination with other drugs, are classified into six categories: (1) diuretics, (2) sympatholytics (sympathetic depressants), (3) direct-acting arteriolar vasodilators, (4) ACE inhibitors, (5) angiotensin II–receptor blockers (ARBs), (6) direct renin inhibitors, and (7) calcium channel blockers.

Diuretics

Diuretics promote sodium depletion, which decreases extracellular fluid volume (ECFV). Diuretics are effective as first-line drugs for treating mild hypertension. Hydrochlorothiazide is the most frequently prescribed diuretic for controlling mild hypertension by decreasing excess fluid volume. It can be used alone for recently diagnosed or mild hypertension, or it can be used with other antihypertensive drugs. Many antihypertensive drugs can cause fluid retention; therefore diuretics are often administered together with antihypertensive agents. The various types of diuretics are discussed in Chapter 38.

Thiazide diuretics are not recommended for patients with renal insufficiency (creatinine clearance <30 mL/min). The loop (high-ceiling) diuretics such as furosemide are usually recommended because they do not depress renal blood flow. Loop diuretics are not used if hypertension is the result of RAAS involvement because they tend to immediately elevate serum renin level. Instead of a single thiazide drug, a combination of potassium-wasting and potassium-sparing diuretics may be useful; less potassium excretion would occur. In addition, thiazides can be combined with other antihypertensive drugs to increase their effectiveness. Box 42.1 lists the combinations of thiazides with other drugs. Many drug products on the market include combinations of thiazide diuretics and potassium-sparing diuretics, beta blockers, ACE inhibitors, or ARBs. ACE inhibitors tend to increase serum potassium (K) levels, so when they are combined with a thiazide diuretic, serum potassium loss is minimized.

Sympatholytics (Sympathetic Depressants)

The sympatholytics comprise five groups of drugs: (1) beta-adrenergic blockers, (2) centrally acting alpha$_2$ agonists, (3) alpha-adrenergic blockers, (4) adrenergic neuron blockers (peripherally acting sympatholytics), and (5) alpha$_1$- and beta$_1$-adrenergic blockers. Beta-adrenergic blockers block the beta receptors, and alpha-adrenergic blockers block the alpha receptors.

⚠ Beta-Adrenergic Blockers

Beta-adrenergic blockers, frequently called *beta blockers*, are used as antihypertensive drugs or in combination with a diuretic. Beta blockers are also used as antianginals and antidysrhythmics and are discussed in this context in Chapter 37.

Beta (β+ and β−)-adrenergic blockers reduce cardiac output by diminishing the sympathetic nervous system response to decrease basal sympathetic tone. With continued use of beta blockers, vascular resistance is diminished, and BP is lowered. Beta blockers reduce heart rate, contractility, and renin release. The hypotensive response is greater in patients with higher renin levels.

African American hypertensive patients do not respond well to beta blockers alone for the control of hypertension. Instead, hypertension in the African American population can be controlled by combining beta blockers with diuretics.

There are many types of beta blockers. Nonselective beta blockers, such as propranolol and carvedilol, inhibit beta$_1$ (heart) and beta$_2$ (bronchial) receptors. Heart rate slows, BP decreases secondary to the decrease in heart rate, and bronchoconstriction occurs because of unopposed parasympathetic tone. Cardioselective beta blockers are preferred because they act mainly on the beta$_1$—rather than the

---

BOX 42.1 Combination of Thiazides With Antihypertensive Drugs and Other Combinations

Thiazide With Potassium-Sparing Diuretics
- Hydrochlorothiazide with spironolactone
- Hydrochlorothiazide with amiloride
- Hydrochlorothiazide with triamterene

Thiazide With Beta Blockers
- Hydrochlorothiazide with bisoprolol fumarate
- Hydrochlorothiazide with metoprolol
- Bendroflumethiazide with nadolol

Tenoretic
- Chlorthalidone (thiazide-like diuretic) with atenolol

Thiazide With Angiotensin-Converting Enzyme Inhibitors
- Hydrochlorothiazide with benazepril
- Hydrochlorothiazide with captopril
- Hydrochlorothiazide with enalapril maleate
- Hydrochlorothiazide with fosinopril
- Hydrochlorothiazide with lisinopril
- Hydrochlorothiazide with moexipril
- Hydrochlorothiazide with quinapril

Thiazide With Angiotensin II Antagonists
- Hydrochlorothiazide with candesartan
- Hydrochlorothiazide with eprosartan
- Hydrochlorothiazide with irbesartan
- Hydrochlorothiazide with losartan
- Hydrochlorothiazide with olmesartan
- Hydrochlorothiazide with telmisartan
- Hydrochlorothiazide with valsartan

Thiazide With Centrally Acting Alpha$_2$ Agonist
- Chlorthalidone with clonidine
- Hydrochlorothiazide with methyldopa

Combination of Angiotensin-Converting Enzyme Inhibitors With Calcium Channel Blocker
- See Table 42.3

Combination of Calcium Channel Blocker With Statin Drug
- Amlodipine with atorvastatin

---

beta$_2$—receptors, and bronchoconstriction is less likely to occur. Acebutolol, atenolol, betaxolol, bisoprolol, and metoprolol are cardioselective beta blockers that block beta$_1$ receptors.

Cardioselectivity does not confer absolute protection from bronchoconstriction. In tests measuring forced expiratory volume in 1 second (FEV$_1$) as a measure of β− reactivity, only atenolol demonstrated true protection. Other cardioselective beta blockers were only partially effective. Studies also show that, at the upper end of the dosage range, cardioselectivity is less effective. In patients with preexisting bronchospasm or other pulmonary disease, beta blockers—even those considered to be cardioselective—should be used with caution. Some experts regard this as a relative contraindication. The real value of beta selectivity is in maintaining renal blood flow and minimizing the hypoglycemic effects of beta blockade.

The combination of beta blockers with hydrochlorothiazides is packaged together in tablet form (see Box 42.1). Usually the hydrochlorothiazide dose is 12.5 to 25 mg.

PROTOTYPE DRUG CHART

! *Metoprolol*

Drug Class	Dosage
Antihypertensive: beta₁ blocker	Hypertension: Regular release: A: PO: Initially 100 mg/d in divided doses; *maint:* 100–450 mg in divided doses; *max:* 450 mg/d in divided doses Extended release: A: PO: 25–100 mg/d; *max:* 400 mg/d

Contraindications	Drug-Lab-Food Interactions
Hypersensitivity, heart block, cardiogenic shock, hypotension, acute HF, bradycardia *Caution:* Hepatic or thyroid dysfunction, asthma, peripheral vascular disease, diabetes mellitus, COPD, cerebrovascular disease, depression	Drug: Increases bradycardia and heart block with digitalis, clonidine, SSRIs, MAOIs, cimetidine; increased hypotensive effect with other antihypertensives, alcohol, anesthetics; NSAIDs decrease effect of beta blockers. Lab: Increased hepatic enzymes

Pharmacokinetics	Pharmacodynamics
Absorption: PO: 95% Distribution: PB: 10%–12% Metabolism: t½: 3–7 h Excretion: In urine	Immediate release: PO: Onset: 30–60 min Peak: 1–2 h Duration: 6.4 h Extended release: PO: Onset UK Peak: 7 h Duration: 24 h

Therapeutic Effects/Uses

To control hypertension, acute myocardial infarction, angina, and HF
Mechanism of Action: Promotes blood pressure reduction via a beta₁-blocking effect.

Side Effects	Adverse Reactions
Fatigue, dizziness, dysgeusia, dry mouth, nausea, vomiting, diarrhea, insomnia, nightmares, drowsiness, headache, blurred vision, rash, pruritus, peripheral edema, tinnitus, erectile dysfunction, depression	Bradycardia, hypotension, palpitations, stroke, thrombocytopenia, diabetes mellitus *Life-threatening:* Dysrhythmias, bronchospasm, agranulocytosis, HF

A, Adult; *AV,* atrioventricular; *COPD,* chronic obstructive pulmonary disease; *d,* day; *h,* hour; *HF,* heart failure; *maint,* maintenance; *MAOI,* monoamine oxidase inhibitor; *max,* maximum; *min,* minute; *NSAID,* nonsteroidal antiinflammatory drug; *PB,* protein binding; *PO,* by mouth; *SSRI,* selective serotonin reuptake inhibitor; *t½,* half-life; *UK,* unknown; *y,* year.

Beta blockers tend to be more effective in lowering BP in patients who have an elevated serum renin level. The cardioselective prototype drug metoprolol is presented in Prototype Drug Chart: Metoprolol. Beta blockers should not be used by patients with second- or third-degree atrioventricular (AV) block or sinus bradycardia. A noncardioselective beta blocker such as propranolol should not be given to a patient with chronic obstructive pulmonary disease (COPD).

Pharmacokinetics. Metoprolol is well absorbed from the gastrointestinal (GI) tract. Its half-life is short, and its protein-binding power is low.

Pharmacodynamics. Cardioselective beta-adrenergic blockers block beta₁ receptors, thereby decreasing heart rate and BP. The nonselective beta blockers block beta₁ and beta₂ receptors, which can result in bronchial constriction. Beta blockers cross the placental barrier and are excreted in breast milk.

The onset of action of immediate-release metoprolol is usually 60 minutes or less. The peak is 1 to 2 hours for immediate release and usually 7 hours for extended release. The duration is typically 6.4 hours for immediate release and 24 hours for extended release.

Side Effects and Adverse Reactions. Side effects and adverse reactions include decreased pulse rate, markedly decreased BP, and, with noncardioselective beta₁ and beta₂ blockers, bronchospasm.

Beta blockers should not be abruptly discontinued because rebound hypertension, angina, dysrhythmias, and MI can result. Beta blockers can cause dizziness, insomnia, depression, fatigue, nightmares, and

❀ COMPLEMENTARY AND ALTERNATIVE THERAPIES

Antihypertensives

- Ma-huang (ephedra) decreases or counteracts the effect of antihypertensive drugs. When taken with beta blockers, hypertension may continue or increase.
- Ephedra increases hypertension when taken with beta blockers.
- Black cohosh increases the hypotensive effect of antihypertensive drugs.
- Hawthorn may increase the effects of beta blockers and angiotensin-converting enzyme (ACE) inhibitors.
- Licorice, Korean ginseng, and milk thistle decrease the effects of antihypertensive drugs.
- Goldenseal may increase the effects of antihypertensive drugs.
- Parsley may potentiate hypotension when taken with an antihypertensive drug.
- Cayenne may cause drug-induced cough with ACE inhibitors.
- Chinese skullcap may increase losartan levels.
- Coleus may potentiate effects of antihypertensives.
- St. John's wort decreases effects of calcium channel blockers, especially nifedipine and verapamil.

CLINICAL JUDGMENT [NURSING PROCESS]

! Antihypertensives: Beta Blockers

Concept: Perfusion
- The passage of blood flow through the arteries and capillaries that deliver oxygen and nutrients to body cells

Recognize Cues [Assessment]
- Obtain a medication and herbal history from the patient. Report if a drug-drug or drug-herbal interaction is probable.
- Obtain vital signs. Report abnormal blood pressure (BP) and bradycardia and compare vital signs with baseline findings.
- Check laboratory values related to renal and liver function periodically. Elevated blood urea nitrogen (BUN) and serum creatinine may be caused by beta blockers or a cardiac disorder. Elevated cardiac enzymes, such as aspartate transaminase (AST) and lactate dehydrogenase (LDH), may be caused by beta blockers or cardiac disorder.

Analyze Cues and Prioritize Hypothesis [Patient Problems]
- Hypertension
- Fatigue

Generate Solutions [Planning]
- The patient's BP will be 120/80 or below.
- The patient will take medication as prescribed.

Take Action [Nursing Interventions]
- Monitor vital signs, especially BP and pulse.
- Monitor laboratory results, especially BUN, serum creatinine, AST, and LDH.

Patient Teaching
General
- ⚡ Encourage patients to comply with the drug regimen. Advise that abrupt discontinuation of antihypertensive drugs may cause rebound hypertension.
- Inform patients that herbs can interfere with beta blockers.
- ⚡ Advise patients to avoid over-the-counter (OTC) drugs without first checking with a health care provider. Many OTC drugs carry warnings against use in presence of hypertension or concurrent use with antihypertensives.

- Suggest that patients wear a MedicAlert bracelet or carry a card indicating their health problem and prescribed drugs.
- Teach patients in trauma situations to inform a health care provider of drugs taken daily, such as a beta blocker. Beta blockers block compensatory effects of the body to the shock state. Glucagon may be needed to reverse the effects so the patient can be resuscitated.

Self-Administration
- Teach patients or family members how to take a radial pulse and BP and to report abnormal findings to a health care provider.

Side Effects
- Advise patients that antihypertensives may cause dizziness (orthostatic hypotension). Warn patients to rise slowly from lying or sitting to a standing position.
- Advise patients to report dizziness, slow pulse rate, changes in BP, heart palpitation, confusion, or gastrointestinal (GI) upset to a health care provider.
- Alert patients with diabetes mellitus to possible hypoglycemic symptoms.
- Inform patients that antihypertensives may cause sexual dysfunction (e.g., impotence).

Diet
- Teach patients and family members nonpharmacologic methods to decrease BP, such as a low-salt diet, relaxation techniques, exercise, smoking cessation, and decreased alcohol ingestion (limit to one drink for females and two drinks for males daily).
- Advise patients to report constipation. Foods high in fiber, a stool softener, and increased water intake (except in patients with heart failure) are usually indicated.

Evaluate Outcomes [Evaluation]
- Evaluate the effectiveness of the drug therapy (decreased BP, absence of side effects).
- Determine that the patient is adhering to the drug regimen.

---

erectile dysfunction. Table 42.1 lists the beta blockers used to treat hypertension and their dosages, uses, and considerations.

Noncardioselective beta blockers inhibit the liver's ability to convert glycogen to glucose in response to hypoglycemia. Because of this side effect, beta blockers should be used with caution in patients with diabetes mellitus. In addition, bradycardia is a very common adverse effect of beta blockers.

Centrally Acting Alpha₂ Agonists

Centrally acting alpha₂ agonists decrease the sympathetic response from the brainstem to the peripheral vessels. They stimulate the alpha₂ receptors, which in turn decreases sympathetic activity, increases vagus activity, decreases cardiac output, and decreases serum epinephrine, norepinephrine, and renin release. All of these actions result in reduced peripheral vascular resistance and increased vasodilation. This group of drugs has minimal effects on cardiac output and blood flow to the kidneys. Beta blockers are not given with centrally acting sympatholytics because accentuation of bradycardia during therapy can occur, as can rebound hypertension upon discontinuing therapy.

Drugs in this group include methyldopa, clonidine, and guanfacine. Methyldopa was one of the first drugs widely used to control hypertension. In high doses, methyldopa and clonidine can cause sodium and water retention. Frequently, methyldopa and clonidine are administered with diuretics. Clonidine is available in a transdermal preparation that provides a 7-day duration of action. Transdermal patches are replaced every 7 days and may be left on while bathing; skin irritations may occur. Guanfacine has effects similar to clonidine. Guanfacine has a long half-life and usually is taken once a day. Table 42.1 lists centrally acting alpha₂ agonists along with beta blockers.

Side Effects and Adverse Reactions. Side effects and adverse reactions of alpha₂ agonists include drowsiness, dry mouth, dizziness, and slow heart rate (bradycardia). Methyldopa should not be used in patients with impaired liver function, and serum liver enzymes should be monitored periodically in all patients. This group of drugs must not be abruptly discontinued because a rebound hypertensive crisis can result. If the drug needs to be stopped immediately, another antihypertensive drug is usually prescribed to avoid rebound hypertensive symptoms such as restlessness, tachycardia, tremors, headache, and increased BP. Rebound hypertension is less likely to occur with guanfacine. The nurse should emphasize the need to take the medication as prescribed. This group of drugs can cause sodium and water retention, resulting in peripheral edema. A diuretic may be ordered with methyldopa or clonidine to decrease water and sodium retention (edema). Patients who are pregnant or contemplating

⚠ TABLE 42.1 Antihypertensives: Beta Blockers and Central Alpha₂ Agonists

Drug	Route and Dosage	Uses and Considerations
Beta-Adrenergic Blockers		
Acebutolol hydrochloride Cardioselective beta₁	Hypertension: A: PO: Initially 400 mg/d in 1–2 divided doses; *maint:* 400–800 mg/d; *max:* 1200 mg/d Older A: Initially 200 mg/d; *max:* 800 mg/d	For hypertension and dysrhythmias. May cause dizziness, headache, fatigue, hypotension, bradycardia, palpitations, nausea, and constipation/diarrhea, dyspnea, and visual impairment. Closely monitor vital signs. PB: 26%; t½: 3–4 h
Atenolol Cardioselective beta₁	Hypertension: A: PO: Initially 25–50 mg/d; *max:* 100 mg/d	For hypertension, angina, and prophylaxis and treatment of AMI. May cause hypotension, heart failure, bradycardia, depression, fatigue, dizziness, nausea, diarrhea, and peripheral vasoconstriction. PB: 10%; t½: 6–7 h
Betaxolol hydrochloride Cardioselective beta₁	Hypertension: A: PO: Initially 10 mg/d; *maint:* 10–20 mg/d; *max:* 20 mg/d Older A: PO: Initially 5 mg/d; *max:* 20 mg/d	For hypertension and glaucoma. May cause headache, dizziness, bradycardia, palpitations, ocular irritation, erectile dysfunction, fatigue, insomnia, arthralgia, nausea, and chest pain. Discontinue over a 2-week period. PB: 50%; t½: 15 h
Bisoprolol fumarate Beta₁ blocker	A: PO: Initially 2.5–5 mg/d; *max:* 20 mg/d	For hypertension. May cause dizziness, headache, fatigue, bradycardia, peripheral edema, orthostatic hypotension, diarrhea, weakness, elevated hepatic enzymes, and arthralgia. PB: 30%; t½: 9–12 h
Carvedilol Alpha blocker, nonselective beta₁ and beta₂	Hypertension: Regular release: A: PO: Initially 6.25 mg bid for 7–14 d; *max:* 50 mg/d Extended release: A: PO: Initially 20 mg/d in the morning for 7–14 d; *max:* 80 mg/d	For treating hypertension, AMI, and heart failure. May cause dizziness, drowsiness, weakness, orthostatic hypotension, headache, weight gain, diarrhea, bradycardia, fatigue, dyspnea, peripheral edema, and hypo/hyperglycemia. PB: 98%; t½: 7–11 h
Metoprolol Cardioselective beta₁	See Prototype Drug Chart: Metoprolol	
Nadolol Nonselective beta₁ and beta₂	Hypertension: A: PO: Initially 40 mg/d; *maint:* 40–80 mg/d; *max:* 320 mg/d	For hypertension and angina. May cause dizziness, drowsiness, fatigue, bradycardia, hypotension, palpitations, peripheral vasoconstriction, and erectile dysfunction. PB: 30%; t½: 10–24 h
Pindolol Nonselective beta₁ and beta₂	A: PO: Initially 5 mg bid; *maint:* 10–30 mg/d in 2–3 divided doses; *max:* 60 mg/d	For hypertension. May cause dizziness, fatigue, visual impairment, myalgia, edema, bradycardia, dyspnea, hypotension, arthralgia, elevated hepatic enzymes, and weakness. PB: 40%–60%; t½: 3–4 h
Propranolol Nonselective beta₁ and beta₂	Hypertension: Immediate release: A: PO: Initially 40 mg bid; *maint:* 160–480 mg/d in 2–3 divided doses; *max:* 640 mg/d Extended release: A: PO: 80 mg/d; *maint:* 120–160 mg/d; *max:* 640 mg/d	For hypertension, AMI, angina, HF, dysrhythmias, and migraine prophylaxis. May cause dizziness, visual impairment, fatigue, bradycardia, headache, weakness, depression, erectile dysfunction, hyperkalemia, seizures, and agitation. Bronchospasm may occur due to the beta₂-blocker effect. PB: 90%; t½: 2–6 h
Central Alpha₂ Agonists		
Clonidine hydrochloride	A: PO: Initially 0.1 mg bid; *maint:* 0.2–0.6 mg/d; *max:* 2.4 mg/d A: Transdermal patch: Initially 1 patch (0.1 mg/24 h) q7d	For hypertension. May cause fatigue, drowsiness, dizziness, confusion, headache, irritability, nightmares, erythema, infection, anorexia, edema, anxiety, dry mouth, nausea, vomiting, constipation, abdominal pain, bradycardia, orthostatic hypotension, and pruritus. PB: 20%–40%; t½: 12–16 h PO, 20 h transdermal
Guanfacine hydrochloride	Immediate release: A: PO: Initially 1 mg/d at bedtime; *maint:* 2–3 mg/d; *max:* 4 mg/d	For hypertension. May cause drowsiness, dry mouth, headache, dizziness, fatigue, weakness, insomnia, irritability, nausea, abdominal pain, constipation, diarrhea, erectile dysfunction, orthostatic hypotension, and bradycardia. PB: 70%; t½: 10–30 h
Methyldopa	A: PO: Initially 250 mg bid-tid; maint: 500–2000 mg/d in 2–4 divided doses; *max:* 3 g/d Hypertensive urgency/emergency: IV: 250–500 mg q6h over 30–60 min; *max:* 4 g/d	For hypertension, hypertensive urgency, and emergency. May cause orthostatic hypotension, drowsiness, bradycardia, depression, dizziness, angina, peripheral edema, erectile dysfunction, and constipation. Take with food if GI upset occurs. Use has declined due to its adverse effects. PB: 10%–15%; t½: 2 h

A, Adult; *AMI,* acute myocardial infarction; *bid,* twice a day; *d,* day; *GI,* gastrointestinal; *h,* hour; *HTN,* hypertension; *IV,* intravenous; *maint,* maintenance; *max,* maximum; *min,* minutes; *PB,* protein binding; *PO,* by mouth; *PVCs,* premature ventricular contractions; *q,* every; *t½,* half-life; *tid,* three times a day.

pregnancy should avoid clonidine. Methyldopa is frequently used to treat chronic or pregnancy-induced hypertension; however, it crosses the placental barrier, and small amounts may enter the breast milk of a lactating patient.

Alpha-Adrenergic Blockers

This group of drugs blocks the alpha-adrenergic receptors (alpha blockers), resulting in vasodilation and decreased BP. They help maintain the renal blood flow rate. Alpha blockers are useful in treating hypertension in patients with lipid abnormalities. They decrease the very-low-density lipoprotein (VLDL) and the low-density lipoprotein (LDL) responsible for the buildup of fatty plaques in the arteries (atherosclerosis). In addition, they increase high-density lipoprotein (HDL) levels. Alpha blockers are safe for patients with diabetes because they do not affect glucose metabolism. They also do not affect respiratory function. Nonselective alpha adrenergic blockers—phenoxybenzamine and phentolamine—should not be given to patients with coronary artery disease because of their stimulating effects and resultant increase in myocardial oxygen demand.

The selective alpha$_1$-adrenergic blockers—prazosin, terazosin, and doxazosin—are used mainly to reduce BP and can be used to treat benign prostatic hypertrophy (BPH). Prazosin is a commonly prescribed drug. Terazosin and doxazosin have longer half-lives than prazosin, and they are normally given once at bedtime. When prazosin is taken with alcohol or other antihypertensives, the hypotensive state can be intensified. These drugs, like the centrally acting alpha$_2$ agonists, cause sodium and water retention with edema; therefore diuretics are frequently given concomitantly to decrease fluid accumulation in the extremities.

Pharmacokinetics. Prazosin is absorbed through the GI tract, but a large portion of prazosin is lost during hepatic first-pass metabolism. The half-life is short, so the drug should be administered twice a day. Prazosin is highly protein bound, and when it is given with other highly protein-bound drugs, the patient should be assessed for adverse reactions.

Pharmacodynamics. Selective alpha-adrenergic blockers dilate the arterioles and venules, decreasing peripheral resistance and lowering BP. With prazosin, the heart rate is only slightly increased, whereas with nonselective alpha blockers such as phenoxybenzamine, the BP is greatly reduced, and reflex tachycardia can occur. Nonselective alpha blockers are more effective for acute hypertension; selective alpha blockers are more useful for long-term essential hypertension.

The onset of action of prazosin occurs between 30 minutes and 2 hours. The duration of action of prazosin is less than 24 hours. Table 42.2 presents drug data for selective and nonselective alpha blockers.

Side Effects and Adverse Reactions. Side effects of prazosin, doxazosin, and terazosin include orthostatic hypotension (dizziness, faintness, lightheadedness, and increased heart rate, which may occur with first dose), nausea, headache, drowsiness, nasal congestion caused by vasodilation, edema, and weight gain.

Side effects of phentolamine include hypotension, reflex tachycardia caused by the severe decrease in BP, nasal congestion caused by vasodilation, and GI disturbances.

Drug Interactions. Drug interactions occur when alpha-adrenergic blockers are taken with antiinflammatory drugs and nitrates, such as nitroglycerin taken for angina. Peripheral edema is intensified when prazosin and an antiinflammatory drug are taken daily. Nitroglycerin taken for angina lowers BP. If prazosin is taken with nitroglycerin, syncope (faintness) caused by a decrease in BP can occur. The selective alpha-adrenergic blocker prazosin is shown in Prototype Drug Chart: Prazosin Hydrochloride.

Adrenergic Neuron Blockers (Peripherally Acting Sympatholytics)

Adrenergic neuron blockers are potent antihypertensive drugs that block norepinephrine release from the sympathetic nerve endings, causing a decrease in norepinephrine release that results in a lowering of BP. A decrease occurs in both cardiac output and peripheral vascular resistance. Reserpine, the most potent drug, is used to control severe hypertension. Orthostatic hypotension is a common side effect, so the patient should be advised to rise slowly from a reclining or sitting position. The adrenergic neuron blockers are considered the last choices for treatment of chronic hypertension because these drugs can cause orthostatic hypotension. Use of reserpine may cause pseudoparkinsonism, nightmares, and suicidal ideation. The drugs in this group can cause sodium and water retention, and they can be taken alone or with a diuretic to decrease peripheral edema.

⚠️ Alpha$_1$- and Beta$_1$-Adrenergic Blockers

This group of drugs blocks both the alpha$_1$ and beta$_1$ receptors. Labetalol is an example of an alpha/beta blocker. Blocking the alpha$_1$ receptor causes vasodilation, which decreases resistance to blood flow. The effect on the alpha receptor is stronger than the effect on

---

◎ CLINICAL JUDGMENT [NURSING PROCESS]

Antihypertensives: Alpha-Adrenergic Blockers

Concept: Perfusion
- The passage of blood flow through the arteries and capillaries that deliver oxygen and nutrients to body cells

Recognize Cues [Assessment]
- Obtain a medication history from the patient that includes current drugs. Report if drug-drug or drug-herbal interaction is probable. Prazosin is highly protein bound and can displace other highly protein-bound drugs.
- Obtain baseline vital signs and weight for future comparisons.
- Check urinary output. Report if it is decreased (less than 600 mL/day) because the drug is contraindicated if renal disease is present.

Analyze Cues and Prioritize Hypothesis [Patient Problems]
- Hypertension
- Fatigue

Generate Solutions [Planning]
- The patient's blood pressure (BP) will decrease to 120/80 or below.
- The patient will follow the proper drug regimen.

Take Action [Nursing Interventions]
- Monitor vital signs. The desired therapeutic effect of prazosin may not fully occur for 4 weeks. A sudden marked decrease in BP and tachycardia should be reported.
- Check daily for fluid retention in extremities and weight gain. Prazosin may cause sodium and water retention.

Patient Teaching
General
- ⚡ Advise patients to adhere to the drug regimen. Explain that abrupt discontinuation of antihypertensive drugs may cause rebound hypertension.

Antihypertensives: Alpha-Adrenergic Blockers

- Inform patients that orthostatic hypotension may occur. Explain that before rising, patients should sit and dangle their feet. Drugs may be taken at bedtime to avoid orthostatic hypotension.
- Teach patients to self-monitor daily weights. Prazosin may lead to edema.

Self-Administration
- Teach patients or family members how to take and record BP. A BP chart should be established, and BP changes should be reported.

Side Effects
- Caution patients that dizziness, lightheadedness, and drowsiness may occur, especially when a drug is first initiated. If these symptoms occur, a health care provider should be notified.
- Inform male patients that impotence may occur if high doses of drug are prescribed. This problem should be reported to the health care provider.

- Tell patients to report if edema is present in the morning. Water retention is a problem with alpha blockers.
- ⚡ Inform patients not to take over-the-counter (OTC) cold, cough, or allergy medications without first contacting the health care provider.

Diet
- Encourage patients to decrease salt intake unless otherwise indicated by the health care provider.

Evaluate Outcomes [Evaluation]
- Evaluate the effectiveness of the drug in controlling BP; side effects should be absent.
- Evaluate the patient's adherence to the medication schedule.
- Evaluate the patient's knowledge of the medication.

! TABLE 42.2 Antihypertensives: Sympatholytics—Alpha-Adrenergic and Peripherally Acting Blockers and Direct-Acting Vasodilators

Drug	Route and Dosage	Uses and Considerations
Selective Alpha-Adrenergic Blockers		
Doxazosin mesylate	Hypertension: A: PO: Initially: 1 mg/d at bedtime; *max:* 16 mg/d	For hypertension and BPH. May cause orthostatic hypotension, headache, dizziness, drowsiness, fatigue, edema, weakness, palpitations, visual impairment, and erectile dysfunction. PB: 98%; t½: 22 h
Prazosin hydrochloride	See Prototype Drug Chart: Prazosin Hydrochloride	
Terazosin hydrochloride	Hypertension: A: PO: Initially: 1 mg at bedtime; *maint:* 1–5 mg/d; *max:* 20 mg/d in divided doses q12h	For hypertension and BPH. May cause dizziness, drowsiness, nasal congestion, headache, weakness, nausea, orthostatic hypotension, palpitations, peripheral edema, and erectile dysfunction. PB: 90%–94%; t½: 12 h
Nonselective Alpha-Adrenergic Blockers		
Phenoxybenzamine hydrochloride	A: PO: Initially: 10 mg bid; *maint:* 20–40 mg bid/tid	For hypertension associated with pheochromocytoma. May cause drowsiness, dizziness, fatigue, orthostatic hypotension, tachycardia, weakness, gastritis, ejaculatory dysfunction, and nasal congestion. PB: UK; t½: 24 h
Phentolamine	Hypertension: A: IM/IV: 5 mg before surgery; may repeat during surgery	For hypertension before and during pheochromocytomectomy, pheochromocytoma diagnosis, and prevention and treatment of IV drug extravasation. May cause dental pain, bradycardia, tachycardia, headache, vomiting, diarrhea, abdominal pain, and paresthesias. PB: UK; t½: 19 min
Adrenergic Neuron Blockers (Peripherally Acting Sympatholytics)		
Reserpine	A: PO: Initially: 0.05–0.1 mg/d for 1–2 wk; *maint:* 0.1–0.25 mg/d; *max:* 0.5 mg/d for adults, 0.25 mg/d for older adults	For hypertension. May cause dizziness, drowsiness, depression, dyspnea, hearing loss, hypotension, bradycardia, peripheral edema, erectile/ejaculatory dysfunction, and pseudoparkinsonism. Use has declined due to its adverse effects. PB: 96%; t½: 50–100 h
Alpha₁- and Beta₁-Adrenergic Blockers		
Labetalol hydrochloride	Hypertension: A: PO: Initially: 100 mg bid; *maint:* 200–400 mg bid; *max:* 2.4 g/d in 2–3 divided doses	For hypertension. May cause orthostatic hypotension, dizziness, hyperhidrosis, erectile/ejaculation dysfunction, fatigue, nasal congestion, paresthesia, nausea, and depression. PB: 50%; t½: 6–8 h
Direct-Acting Vasodilators		
Hydralazine hydrochloride	A: PO: Initially: 10 mg qid; *maint:* 50 mg qid; *max:* 300 mg/d A: IM: 10–50 mg q4–6h Hypertensive urgency/emergency: A: IV: 10–20 mg bolus, may repeat q4–6h	For hypertension, hypertensive urgency and emergency, preeclampsia, and eclampsia. May cause headaches, anorexia, nausea, vomiting, diarrhea, reflex tachycardia, edema, paresthesia, nasal congestion, lupus-like symptoms, hypotension, angina, and palpitations. Closely monitor vital signs. PB: 87%; t½: 3–7 h
Minoxidil	Hypertension: A: PO: Initially: 5 mg/d; *maint:* 10–40 mg/d; *max:* 100 mg/d	For hypertension and alopecia. May cause headache, hypotension, reflex tachycardia, angina, peripheral edema, erythema, pericardial effusion, and excess hair growth. PB: 0%; t½: 4 h
Nitroprusside	Hypertensive emergency: A: IV: Initially: 0.3–0.5 mcg/kg/min in D₅W infusion till stable; *max:* 10 mcg/kg/min for 10 min	For hypertensive urgency and emergency and for HF. May cause hypotension, bradycardia, tachycardia, restlessness, flushing, dizziness, headache, and palpitations. PB: UK; t½: 2 min

A, Adult; *bid,* twice a day; *BPH,* benign prostatic hyperplasia; *d,* day; *D₅W,* dextrose 5% in water; *GI,* gastrointestinal; *h,* hour; *HF,* heart failure; *IV,* intravenous; *maint,* maintenance; *max,* maximum; *min,* minute; *PB,* protein binding; *PO,* by mouth; *PRN,* as needed; *q,* every; *qid,* four times a day; *t½,* half-life; *tid,* three times a day; *UK,* unknown; *wk,* week; *y,* year; *<,* less than.

PROTOTYPE DRUG CHART

Prazosin Hydrochloride

Drug Class	Dosage
Antihypertensive: Alpha-adrenergic blocker	A: PO: Initially 1 mg bid/tid; *maint:* 6–15 mg/d; *max:* 20 mg/d in divided doses Older A: PO: Initially 1 mg qd/bid; *max:* 20 mg/d

Contraindications	Drug-Lab-Food Interactions
Hypersensitivity *Caution:* Angina, orthostatic hypotension, syncope, ocular surgery, priapism, older adults, pregnancy, breastfeeding	Drug: Increased hypotensive effect with other antihypertensives, nitrates, diuretics, alcohol; decreased effects with NSAIDs Lab: Increased hepatic enzymes

Pharmacokinetics	Pharmacodynamics
Absorption: GI: 60% (5% to circulation) Distribution: PB: 97% Metabolism: t½: 2–4 h Excretion: In bile and feces, 10% in urine	PO: Onset: 0.5–2 h Peak: 2–4 h Duration: <24 h

Therapeutic Effects/Uses
To control hypertension Mechanism of Action: Dilates peripheral blood vessels by blocking alpha-adrenergic receptors.

Side Effects	Adverse Reactions
Dizziness, drowsiness, blurred vision, anxiety, fatigue, weakness, headache, nasal congestion, depression, syncope, dry mouth, nausea, vomiting, diarrhea, abdominal pain, rash, constipation, peripheral edema, erectile dysfunction, urinary frequency/incontinence, edema, weakness	Orthostatic hypotension, palpitations, tachycardia, pancreatitis, elevated liver enzymes, dyspnea

A, Adult; *bid*, twice a day; *d*, day; *h*, hour; *GI*, gastrointestinal; *maint*, maintenance; *max*, maximum; *NSAID*, nonsteroidal antiinflammatory drug; *PB*, protein binding; *PO*, by mouth; *qd*, every day; *t½*, half-life; *tid*, three times a day; <, less than.

the beta receptor; therefore BP is lowered, and pulse rate is moderately decreased. By blocking the cardiac beta$_1$ receptor, both heart rate and AV contractility are decreased. Large doses of alpha/beta blockers could block beta$_2$-adrenergic receptors, thus increasing airway resistance. Patients who have severe asthma should *not* take large doses of labetalol. Table 42.2 lists alpha/beta blockers.

Common side effects of these drugs include orthostatic hypotension, dizziness, paresthesia, nasal congestion, nausea, and fatigue. Large doses of labetalol may cause atrioventricular (AV) heart block.

Direct-Acting Arteriolar Vasodilators

Vasodilators are potent antihypertensive drugs. Direct-acting vasodilators act by relaxing the smooth muscles of the blood vessels, mainly the arteries, causing vasodilation. Vasodilators promote an increase in blood flow to the brain and kidneys. With vasodilation, the BP decreases and sodium and water are retained, resulting in peripheral edema. Diuretics can be given with a direct-acting vasodilator to decrease the edema.

Two direct-acting vasodilators, hydralazine and minoxidil, are used for moderate to severe (dose-related) hypertension. These two drugs cause little orthostatic hypotension because of minimum dilation of the arterioles. However, reflex tachycardia and release of renin can occur secondary to vasodilation and decreased BP. Beta blockers are frequently prescribed with arteriolar vasodilators to decrease the heart rate; this counteracts the effect of reflex tachycardia.

⚠ Nitroprusside is prescribed for acute hypertensive emergency. This is a very potent vasodilator that rapidly decreases BP. Nitroprusside acts on both arterial and venous vessels. Table 42.2 lists direct-acting vasodilators.

Side Effects and Adverse Reactions. The effects of hydralazine are numerous and include reflex tachycardia, palpitations, edema, nasal congestion, headache, dizziness, lupus-like symptoms, and neurologic symptoms (tingling, numbness). Minoxidil has similar side effects, as well as tachycardia, edema, and excess hair growth. In addition, it can precipitate an anginal attack.

Nitroprusside can cause reflex tachycardia, palpitations, restlessness, agitation, nausea, and confusion. Nitroprusside is discussed in greater detail in Chapter 55.

Angiotensin-Converting Enzyme Inhibitors

When ACE is inhibited, it in turn inhibits the formation of angiotensin II (vasoconstrictor) and blocks the release of aldosterone. Aldosterone promotes sodium retention and potassium excretion. When aldosterone is blocked, sodium is excreted along with water, and potassium is retained. ACE inhibitors cause little change in cardiac output or heart rate, and they lower peripheral resistance. (Fig. 42.1 illustrates the RAAS.) These drugs can be used in patients who have elevated serum renin levels.

The ACE inhibitors are used primarily to treat hypertension; some of these agents are also effective in treating heart failure. The ACE inhibitors are benazepril, captopril, enalapril maleate, fosinopril, lisinopril, moexipril, perindopril, quinapril, ramipril, and trandolapril, which are all presented in Table 42.3. These drugs can be used for first-line antihypertensive therapy, but thiazide diuretics are recommended by JNC 8.

African Americans and older adults do not respond to ACE inhibitors with the desired reduction in BP, but when taken with a diuretic, BP will usually be lowered. ACE inhibitors should not be given during pregnancy because they reduce placental blood flow. For patients with renal insufficiency, reduction of the drug dose (except for fosinopril) is necessary.

With the exception of moexipril, which should be taken on an empty stomach for maximum effectiveness, ACE inhibitors can be administered with food.

CLINICAL JUDGMENT [NURSING PROCESS]

Antihypertensives: Angiotensin-Converting Enzyme Inhibitors

Concept: Perfusion
- The passage of blood flow through the arteries and capillaries that deliver oxygen and nutrients to body cells.

Recognize Cues [Assessment]
- Obtain a drug and herbal history from the patient of current drugs taken. Report if a drug-drug or drug-herb interaction is probable.
- Obtain baseline vital signs for future comparisons.
- Check laboratory values for serum protein, albumin, blood urea nitrogen (BUN), creatinine, potassium, and white blood cell count to compare with future serum levels.

Analyze Cues and Prioritize Hypothesis [Patient Problems]
- Hypertension
- Anxiety
- Fatigue

Generate Outcomes [Planning]
- Patient's blood pressure (BP) will decrease to 120/80 or below.
- Patient will rise to an upright position slowly to avoid orthostatic hypotension.

Take Action [Nursing Interventions]
- Monitor BP. A sudden drop in BP should be reported.
- Monitor laboratory tests related to renal function (BUN, creatinine, protein) and blood glucose levels. *Caution:* Watch for hypoglycemic reactions in patients with diabetes mellitus. Urine protein may be checked in the morning using a dipstick.
- Report to a health care provider any bruising, petechiae, or bleeding. These may indicate a severe adverse reaction to an angiotensin antagonist such as captopril.

Patient Teaching
General
- ⚡ Warn patients not to abruptly discontinue use of captopril without notifying a health care provider. Rebound hypertension could result.

- Inform patients not to take over-the-counter (OTC) drugs such as cold medications without first contacting a health care provider.
- Advise patients not to use salt substitutes that contain potassium.
- ⚡ Warn pregnant patients and those contemplating becoming pregnant not to take angiotensin-converting enzyme (ACE) inhibitors or angiotensin II–receptor blockers (ARBs); they can cause harm to the fetus.
- Teach patients to rise slowly to avoid orthostatic hypotension.

Self-Administration
- Teach patients or family members how to take and record BP. A BP chart should be established, and BP changes should be reported.

Side Effects
- ⚡ Explain to patients that dizziness and/or lightheadedness may occur during the first week of captopril therapy. If dizziness persists, a health care provider should be notified.
- Monitor the patient for the following side effects: angioedema, cough dysgeusia, weakness, hyperkalemia, orthostatic hypotension, and renal impairment.
- Advise patients to report any occurrence of bleeding.

Diet
- Teach patients to take captopril 20 minutes to 1 hour before a meal. Food decreases 35% of captopril absorption.
- Warn patients that the taste of food may be diminished during the first month of drug therapy.
- Advise patients to avoid foods high in potassium because hyperkalemia is an adverse effect of ACE inhibitors.

Evaluate Outcomes [Evaluation]
- Evaluate the effectiveness of the drug therapy (absence of severe side effects, BP returns to desired range).
- Evaluate the patient's renal function.

Side Effects and Adverse Reactions. The primary side effect of ACE inhibitors is a constant, irritated cough. Other side effects include nausea, vomiting, diarrhea, headache, dizziness, fatigue, insomnia, serum potassium excess (hyperkalemia), and tachycardia. The persistent, nonproductive "ACE cough" may be relieved upon discontinuance of the drug. Often an ARB may be substituted without cough as a side effect. The major adverse effects are first-dose hypotension and hyperkalemia. Hypotension results because of the vasodilating effect. First-dose hypotension is more common in patients also taking diuretics. Angioedema—swelling of the face, tongue, lips, mucous membranes, and larynx and extremity edema—is rare but may occur due to hypersensitivity and has a higher incidence in African Americans. This may occur within hours or 1 week after the first dose. Angioedema may be reversed with drug discontinuance. When laryngeal edema occurs, the patient may require rescue epinephrine.

Contraindications. ACE inhibitors should not be given during pregnancy because harm to the fetus due to reduction in placental blood flow could occur. This group of drugs should not be taken with potassium-sparing diuretics such as spironolactone or with salt substitutes that contain potassium because of the risk of hyperkalemia (serum potassium excess).

Angiotensin II–Receptor Blockers

ARBs are similar to ACE inhibitors in that they prevent the release of aldosterone, a sodium-retaining hormone. They act on the RAAS. The difference between ARBs and ACE inhibitors is that ARBs block angiotensin II from the angiotensin I (AT₁) receptors found in many tissues, whereas ACE inhibitors inhibit the angiotensin-converting enzyme in the formation of angiotensin II. ARBs cause vasodilation and decrease peripheral resistance. They do not cause the constant, irritated cough ACE inhibitors can. Like ACE inhibitors, ARBs should not be taken during pregnancy.

Losartan, valsartan, irbesartan, candesartan, eprosartan, olmesartan, azilsartan, and telmisartan are examples of ARBs. These agents block the vasoconstrictor effects of angiotensin II at the receptor site. The combination of losartan potassium and hydrochlorothiazide

⚡ **PATIENT SAFETY**

Do not confuse...
- **Diovan** (valsartan), an angiotensin II–receptor blocker, and **Dioval** (estradiol), an estrogen hormone. If both drugs are in the home, caution must be taken to select the correct drug, especially by the male patient taking Diovan and the female patient taking Dioval.

TABLE 42.3 Antihypertensives: Angiotensin-Converting Enzyme Inhibitors and Angiotensin II–Receptor Blockers

Drug	Route and Dosage	Uses and Considerations
Angiotensin Antagonists (ACE Inhibitors)		
Benazepril hydrochloride	A: PO: Initially 10 mg/d; *maint:* 20–40 mg/d in 1–2 divided doses; *max:* 80 mg/d	To treat hypertension. May cause headache, dizziness, hypotension, fatigue, palpitations, peripheral edema, erectile dysfunction, hyperkalemia, nausea, constipation, flushing, and angina. PB: 95%; t½: 10–11 h
Captopril	Hypertension: A: PO: Initially 12.5–25 mg bid/tid; *maint:* 25–150 mg bid/tid; *max:* 450 mg/d	For hypertension, post MI, diabetic nephropathy, and HF. May cause cough, dizziness, hypotension, tachycardia, anorexia, constipation, dyspnea, dysgeusia, pallor, pruritus, and fatigue. PB: 25%; t½: 2 h
Enalapril maleate	A: PO: Initially 2.5–5 mg/d; *maint:* 10–40 mg/d in 1–2 divided doses; *max:* 40 mg/d	For hypertension and HF. May cause orthostatic hypotension, dizziness, headache, fatigue, weakness, syncope, cough, anorexia, hyperkalemia, hyponatremia, rash, tachycardia, and palpitations. PB: 50%; t½: 11 h
Fosinopril	Hypertension: A: PO: Initially 10 mg/d; *maint:* 20–40 mg/d in 1–2 divided doses; *max:* 80 mg/d	For hypertension and HF. May cause dizziness, cough, weakness, peripheral edema, rash, hyperkalemia, palpitations, flushing, and orthostatic hypotension. PB: 99.4%; t½: 11.5 h
Lisinopril	Hypertension: A: PO: Initially 10 mg/d; *maint:* 20–40 mg/d; *max:* 80 mg/d	For hypertension, AMI, and HF. May cause orthostatic hypotension, blurred vision, weakness, headache, dizziness, syncope, cough, and hyperkalemia. PB: UK; t½: 12 h
Moexipril	A: PO: Initially 7.5 mg/d; *maint:* 7.5–30 mg/d; *max:* 30 mg/d in divided doses	For hypertension. May increase serum lithium levels, causing toxicity. May cause dizziness, diarrhea, fatigue, chest pain, palpitations, constipation, cough, hyperkalemia, hyponatremia, flushing, rash, myalgia, and orthostatic hypotension. PB: 50%; t½: 1.3 h
Perindopril erbumine	Hypertension: A: PO: Initially 4 mg/d; *maint:* 4–8 mg/d in 1–2 divided doses; *max:* 16 mg/d Older A: Initially 4 mg/d; *max:* 8 mg/d	For hypertension and to prevent MI. May cause cough, headache, dizziness, weakness, back pain, elevated hepatic enzymes, orthostatic hypotension, and hyperkalemia. PB: 60%; t½: 0.8–1 h
Quinapril hydrochloride	Hypertension: A: PO: Initially 10–20 mg/d; *maint:* 20–80 mg/d in 1–2 divided doses; *max:* 80 mg/d Older A: PO: Initially 5–10 mg/d; *max:* 80 mg/d	For hypertension and HF. May cause dizziness, fatigue, headache, cough, orthostatic hypotension, tachycardia, hyperkalemia, nausea, vomiting, chest pain, dyspnea, and edema. PB: 97%; t½: 1–3 h
Ramipril	Hypertension: A: PO: Initially 2.5 mg/d; *max:* 20 mg/d	For hypertension, AMI, HF, and prevention of stroke. May cause dizziness, headache, cough, orthostatic hypotension, palpitations, angina, syncope, weakness, nausea, vomiting, and hyperkalemia. PB: 73%; t½: 3–17 h
Trandolapril	Hypertension: A: PO: Initially 1 mg/d for Caucasians, 2 mg/d for African Americans: *maint:* 2–4 mg/d; *max:* 8 mg/d	For hypertension, AMI, and HF. May cause dizziness, syncope, cough, dyspepsia, bradycardia, hypotension, hyperkalemia, hypocalcemia, myalgia, weakness, palpitations, and hyperuricemia. PB: 80%; t½: 6 h
Combinations of ACE Inhibitors With Calcium Blockers		
Benazepril with amlodipine	A: PO: Initially amlodipine 2.5–10 mg/d and benazepril 10–40 mg/d; *max:* amlodipine 10 mg/d and benazepril 40 mg/d	For hypertension. May cause headache, hypotension, dizziness, peripheral edema, hyperkalemia, and cough. PB: amlodipine 93%, benazepril 95%; t½: amlodipine 30–50 h, benazepril 10–11 h
Trandolapril and verapamil	A: PO: Trandolapril 2–8 mg/d and verapamil 180–240 mg/d; *max:* 8 mg/d trandolapril and 240 mg/d verapamil	For hypertension. May cause dizziness, headache, cough, hypotension, bradycardia, chest pain, hyperkalemia, fatigue, constipation, ileus, arthralgia, and edema. PB: trandolapril 80%, verapamil 90%; t½: trandolapril 6 h, verapamil 2–12 h
Perindopril arginine and amlodipine besylate	A: PO: Initially perindopril 3.5 mg/d and amlodipine 2.5 mg/d for 1–2 wk; *max:* perindopril 14 mg/d and amlodipine 10 mg/d	For hypertension. May cause dizziness, headache, cough, peripheral edema, tachycardia, bradycardia, hypotension, chest pain, depression, dyspnea, visual impairment, constipation, and hyperkalemia. PB: perindopril 60%%, amlodipine 93%; t½: perindopril 0.8–1 h, amlodipine 30–50 h
Angiotensin II–Receptor Blockers (ARBs)		
Candesartan	Hypertension: A: PO: Initially 16 mg/d; *maint:* 8–32 mg/d in 1–2 divided doses; *max:* 32 mg/d	For hypertension and HF. May cause dizziness, hypotension, hyperkalemia, back pain, hyperbilirubinemia, rhinitis, pharyngitis, elevated hepatic enzymes, and infection. PB: 99%; t½: 9–12 h
Eprosartan	A: PO: Initially 600 mg/d; *maint:* 400–800 mg/d in 1–2 divided doses; *max:* 900 mg/d	For hypertension. May cause cough, fatigue, pharyngitis, rhinitis, dizziness, headache, chest pain, abdominal pain, and orthostatic hypotension. PB: 98%; t½: 5–9 h
Irbesartan	Hypertension: A: PO: Initially 150 mg/d; *maint:* 150–300 mg/d; *max:* 300 mg/d	For hypertension, diabetic nephropathy, and proteinuria. May cause dizziness, cough, fatigue, orthostatic hypotension, edema, anxiety, headache, chest pain, abdominal pain, dyspepsia, and diarrhea. PB: 90%; t½: 11–15 h

TABLE 42.3 Antihypertensives: Angiotensin-Converting Enzyme Inhibitors and Angiotensin II–Receptor Blockers—cont'd

Drug	Route and Dosage	Uses and Considerations
Losartan potassium	Hypertension: A: PO: Initially 50 mg/d; *maint:* 25–100 mg/d in 1–2 divided doses; *max:* 100 mg/d	For hypertension, diabetic nephropathy, and proteinuria. May cause dizziness, weakness, fatigue, headache, cough, orthostatic hypotension, edema, nasal congestion, pharyngitis, nausea, and infection. PB: 98%; t½: 2 h
Olmesartan medoxomil	A: PO: Initially 20 mg/d; for 2 wk, *maint:* 20–40 mg/d; *max:* 40 mg/d	For hypertension. May cause dizziness, headache, peripheral edema, orthostatic hypotension, hyperglycemia, sinusitis, pharyngitis, and rhinitis. PB: 99%; t½: 13 h
Telmisartan	Hypertension: A: PO: Initially 40 mg/d; *maint:* 20–80 mg/d; *max:* 80 mg/d	For hypertension and to prevent MI and CVA. May cause chest pain, orthostatic hypotension, sinusitis, dizziness, back pain, edema, cough, hyperkalemia, diarrhea, skin ulcer, and infection. PB: 99.5%; t½: 24 h
Valsartan	See Prototype Drug Chart: Valsartan	
Azilsartan	A: PO: Initially 40 mg/d; *maint:* 40–80 mg/d; *max:* 80 mg/d	For hypertension. May cause orthostatic hypotension, dizziness, weakness, fatigue, cough, muscle cramps, nausea, and diarrhea. PB: 99%; t½: 11 h
Nebivolol-valsartan	A: PO: 1 tab/d (5 mg nebivolol and 80 mg valsartan)	For hypertension. May cause dizziness, drowsiness, hypotension, hyperkalemia, syncope, vomiting, rash, pruritus, and erectile dysfunction. PB: nebivolol 98%, valsartan 95%; t½: nebivolol 12 h, valsartan 6 h
Aldosterone Receptor Antagonists		
Eplerenone	Hypertension: A: PO: 50 mg/d for 4 wk; may increase to 50 mg bid; *max:* 100 mg/d	For hypertension, HF, and AMI. May cause dizziness, bradycardia, fatigue, hyponatremia, hypertriglyceridemia, hypercholesterolemia, diarrhea, cough, hyperkalemia, hyperuricemia, and edema. PB: 50%; t½: 4–6 h
Direct Renin Inhibitors		
Aliskiren	A: PO: Initially 150 mg/d; *maint:* 150–300 mg/d; *max:* 300 mg/d	For hypertension. May cause dizziness, hypotension, hyperkalemia, peripheral edema, diarrhea, hyperuricemia, gout, pharyngitis, and cough. PB: UK; t½: 24 h

A, Adult; *ACE,* angiotensin-converting enzyme; *AMI,* acute myocardial infarction; *bid,* two times a day; *CVA,* cerebrovascular accident; *d,* day; *h,* hour; *HF,* heart failure; *maint,* maintenance; *max,* maximum; *MI,* myocardial infarction; *PB,* protein binding; *PO,* by mouth; *t½,* half-life; *tid,* three times a day; *UK,* unknown; *URI,* upper respiratory infection; *y,* year; *>,* greater than.

PROTOTYPE DRUG CHART

Valsartan

Drug Class	**Dosage**
Antihypertensive: Angiotensin II–receptor blocker	Hypertension: A: PO: Initially 80–160 mg/d; *maint:* 80–320 mg/d; *max:* 320 mg/d
Contraindications	**Drug-Lab-Food Interactions**
Hypersensitivity *Caution:* Renal and hepatic impairments, hypotension, heart failure, hypovolemia, hyperkalemia, older adults, Blacks, pregnancy, breastfeeding	Drug: Antihypertensives, diuretics, MAOIs, and alcohol may increase hypotensive effects; ACE inhibitors and aspirin may increase hyperkalemia and renal dysfunction; digoxin and NSAIDs may increase renal dysfunction; lithium may increase lithium toxicity. Lab: May increase AST, ALT, ALP, bilirubin, BUN, creatinine, Hct, Hgb
Pharmacokinetics	**Pharmacodynamics**
Absorption: Rapidly absorbed, 10%–35% in blood circulation Distribution: PB: 95% Metabolism: t½: 6 h Excretion: 13% in urine and 83% in bile/feces	PO: Onset: 2 h Peak: 6 h Duration: 24 h
Therapeutic Effects/Uses	
To treat hypertension and heart failure Mechanism of Action: Potent vasodilator that inhibits binding of angiotensin II.	
Side Effects	**Adverse Reactions**
Dizziness, drowsiness, cough, palpitations, blurred vision, headache, edema, nausea, diarrhea, abdominal and back pain, arthralgia, fatigue, muscle cramps, pharyngitis, erectile dysfunction	Orthostatic hypotension, chest pain, hyperkalemia, rhabdomyolysis, elevated hepatic enzymes *Life-threatening:* Renal dysfunction, neutropenia

A, Adult; *ACE,* angiotensin-converting enzyme; *ALP,* alkaline phosphatase; *ALT,* alanine aminotransferase; *AST,* aspartate aminotransferase; *BUN,* blood urea nitrogen; *d,* day; *h,* hour; *Hct,* hematocrit; *Hgb,* hemoglobin; *maint,* maintenance dose; *MAOI,* monoamine oxidase inhibitor; *max,* maximum; *NSAID,* nonsteroidal antiinflammatory drug; *PB,* protein binding; *PO,* by mouth; *t½,* half-life; *y,* years.

tablets, valsartan and hydrochlorothiazide tablets, and others should not cause serum potassium excess or loss. ARBs may be used as a first-line treatment for hypertension.

Prototype Drug Chart: Valsartan gives the pharmacologic data related to valsartan.

Pharmacokinetics. Valsartan is prescribed primarily to manage hypertension. The combination drug containing valsartan plus a low dose of hydrochlorothiazide is rapidly absorbed in the GI tract and undergoes first-pass metabolism in the liver to form active metabolites. It is highly protein bound at 95% and should not be given during pregnancy, especially during the second and third trimesters. The half-life is approximately 6 hours, and the drug is excreted in urine and feces.

Pharmacodynamics. Valsartan is a potent vasodilator. It blocks the binding of angiotensin II to the AT_1 receptors found in many tissues. Its peak time is approximately 6 hours, and it has a long duration of action (24 hours).

Like ACE inhibitors, ARBs are less effective for treating hypertension in African American patients. In addition, like ACE inhibitors, ARBs may cause angioedema. These agents can be taken with or without food and are suitable for patients with mild hepatic insufficiency.

Direct Renin Inhibitors

The first US Food and Drug Administration (FDA)-approved direct renin inhibitor for treating hypertension is aliskiren, which binds with renin and causes a reduction of angiotensin I, angiotensin II, and aldosterone levels (see Fig. 42.1). It is effective for mild and moderate hypertension. Aliskiren can be used alone or with another antihypertensive agent. It has an additive effect in reducing BP when combined with a thiazide diuretic or an ARB. This drug, when used as monotherapy, has not proven to be as effective in reducing BP in the African American population.

Calcium Channel Blockers

Slow calcium channels are found in the myocardium (heart muscle) and vascular smooth muscle (VSM) cells. Free calcium increases muscle contractility, peripheral resistance, and BP. Calcium channel blockers, also called *calcium antagonists* and *calcium blockers*, block the calcium channel in the VSM, promoting vasodilation. The large central arteries are not as sensitive to calcium blockers as coronary and cerebral arteries and the peripheral vessels. Calcium blockers are highly protein bound but have a short half-life. Slow-release preparations decrease the frequency of administration. Table 42.4 lists the calcium blockers in three groups: diphenylalkylamine (verapamil), benzothiazepine (diltiazem), and dihydropyridines (amlodipine and others).

Verapamil is used to treat chronic hypertension, angina pectoris, and cardiac dysrhythmias. Verapamil and diltiazem act on the arterioles and the heart. The dihydropyridines are the largest group of calcium channel blockers; most of these are used to control hypertension.

Nifedipine decreases BP in older adults and in those with low serum renin values. Nifedipine and verapamil are potent calcium blockers. In its immediate-release form (10- and 20-mg capsules), nifedipine has been associated with an increased incidence of profound hypotension, MI, and death, especially in older adults; therefore only extended-release preparations of nifedipine are recommended for chronic hypertension. For this reason, immediate-release nifedipine is usually prescribed for acute rises in BP only on an as-needed basis in the hospital setting. Like the vasodilators, calcium channel blockers can cause reflex tachycardia, although it is more prevalent with nifedipine.

Pharmacokinetics. Like other calcium blockers, amlodipine is highly protein bound. It is gradually absorbed via the GI tract. Because the half-life of amlodipine is longer than that of other calcium blockers, it is taken once a day.

Pharmacodynamics. Amlodipine may be used alone or with other antihypertensive drugs. Peripheral edema may occur because of its vasodilator effect, so persons with edema may need to take another type of antihypertensive drug. This drug has a long duration of action, so it is prescribed only once a day. Amlodipine may be combined with the ACE inhibitor benazepril (Lotrel).

Normally, beta blockers are not prescribed with calcium blockers, because both drugs decrease myocardium contractility. Calcium blockers lower BP better in African Americans than do drugs in other categories.

Side Effects and Adverse Reactions. The side effects and adverse reactions of calcium channel blockers include flushing, headache, dizziness, ankle edema, bradycardia, and AV block. Prototype Drug Chart: Amlodipine gives the pharmacologic data related to amlodipine.

TABLE 42.4 Antihypertensives: Calcium Channel Blockers

Drug	Route and Dosage	Uses and Considerations
Phenylalkylamines		
Verapamil	Hypertension: Regular release: A: PO: Initially 80 mg tid; *max:* 480 mg/d Older A: PO: Initially 40 mg tid; *max:* 480 mg/d Extended-release 12-h tablet: A: PO: Initially 180 mg/d in the morning; *maint:* 180–240 mg/d; *max:* 480 mg/d	For hypertension, angina, and dysrhythmia. May cause dizziness, headache, confusion, fatigue, orthostatic hypotension, bradycardia, weakness, blurred vision, peripheral edema, erectile dysfunction, nausea, and constipation. PB: 90%; t½: 2–10 h
Benzothiazepines		
Diltiazem hydrochloride	Hypertension: Extended release: A: PO: Initially 180–240 mg/d; *maint:* 120–540 mg/d; *max:* 540 mg/d	For hypertension, angina, and dysrhythmia. May cause headache, peripheral edema, dizziness, dyspepsia, bradycardia, hypotension, weakness, dyspnea, pharyngitis, rhinitis, infection, and fatigue. PB: 70%–80%; t½: 3.5–8 h
Dihydropyridines		
Amlodipine	See Prototype Drug Chart: Amlodipine	
Felodipine	A: PO: Initially 5 mg/d; *maint:* 2.5–10 mg/d; *max:* 10 mg/d Older A: PO: Initially 2.5 mg/d; *max:* 10 mg/d	For hypertension. May cause peripheral edema, palpitations, dizziness, infection, weakness, headache, hypotension, rash, and cough. PB: 99%; t½: 11–16 h

TABLE 42.4 Antihypertensives: Calcium Channel Blockers—cont'd

Drug	Route and Dosage	Uses and Considerations
Isradipine	Regular release: A: PO: Initially 2.5 mg bid; *maint:* 5–10 mg bid; *max:* 10 mg/d Extended release: A: PO: 5 mg/d; *max:* 20 mg/d	For hypertension. May cause headache, dizziness, palpitations, flushing, fatigue, hypotension, angina, tachycardia, abdominal pain, and peripheral edema. PB: 95%; t½: 8 h
Nicardipine hydrochloride	Hypertension: Regular release: A: PO: Initially 20 mg tid; *maint:* 20–40 mg tid; *max:* 120 mg/d Sustained release: A: PO: Initially 30 mg bid; *maint:* 30–60 mg bid; *max:* 120 mg/d A: IV: Initially 5 mg/h infusion; *max:* 15 mg/h	For hypertension and angina. May cause headache, dizziness, angina, orthostatic hypotension, palpitations, tachycardia, flushing, weakness, peripheral edema, nausea, and vomiting. PB: 95%; t½: 8.6 h
Nifedipine	Hypertension: Extended release: A: PO: 30–60 mg/d; *max:* 90 mg/d	For hypertension and angina. Common side effects include dizziness, headache, weakness, flushing, peripheral edema, palpitations, nausea, pyrosis, tremor, hypotension, muscle cramps, nasal congestion, cough, dyspnea, and fatigue. PB: 92%–98%; t½: 2–5 h
Nisoldipine	Extended release: A: PO: Initially 17 mg/d; *maint:* 17–34 mg/d; *max:* 34 mg/d Older A: PO: Initially 8.5 mg/d; *max:* 34 mg/d	For hypertension. May cause pharyngitis, sinusitis, headache, dizziness, flushing, orthostatic hypotension, palpitations, tachycardia, visual impairment, hypokalemia, and peripheral edema. PB: 99%; t½: 7–12 h

A, Adult; *bid,* twice a day; *CAD, coronary artery disease; d,* day; *h,* hour; *IV,* intravenous; *maint,* maintenance; *max,* maximum; *PB,* protein binding; *PO,* by mouth; *t½,* half-life; *tid,* three times a day; *y,* year; >, greater than.

📄 PROTOTYPE DRUG CHART

Amlodipine

Drug Class	**Dosage**
Antihypertensive: Calcium channel blocker	Hypertension: A: PO: Initially 5 mg/d; *maint:* 5–10 mg/d; *max:* 10 mg/d Older A: PO: 2.5 mg/d; *maint:* 2.5–10 mg/d; *max:* 10 mg/d

Contraindications	**Drug-Lab-Food Interactions**
Hypersensitivity *Caution:* Hepatic impairment, acute MI, coronary artery disease, older adults, pregnancy, breastfeeding	Drug: Antihypertensives may increase hypotensive effects; NSAIDs may increase renal dysfunction; hydrocodone and codeine may increase sedation; pseudoephedrine and phenylephrine decrease antihypertensive effects.

Pharmacokinetics	**Pharmacodynamics**
Absorption: Well absorbed Distribution: PB: 93% Metabolism: t½: 30–50 h Excretion: Excreted in urine	PO: Onset: UK Peak: 6–12 h Duration: 24 h

Therapeutic Effects/Uses

To treat hypertension and coronary artery disease.
Mechanism of Action: Inhibits influx of extracellular calcium across myocardial and vascular smooth muscle cell membranes, resulting in decreased myocardial contractility.

Side Effects	**Adverse Reactions**
Dizziness, drowsiness, anxiety, flushing, fatigue, weakness, syncope, peripheral edema, depression, visual impairment, paresthesia, diaphoresis, arthralgia, myalgia, muscle cramps, nausea, anorexia, abdominal pain, vomiting, diarrhea, constipation, nightmares, insomnia, weight loss/gain, rash, pruritus, erectile dysfunction	Orthostatic hypotension, bradycardia, chest pain, tachycardia, palpitations, dyspnea, hyperglycemia *Life-threatening:* Angioedema, dysrhythmia exacerbation, MI, thrombocytopenia

A, Adult; *d,* day; *h,* hour; *maint,* maintenance dose; *max,* maximum; *MI,* myocardial infarction; *NSAID,* nonsteroidal antiinflammatory drug; *PB,* protein binding; *PO,* by mouth; *t½,* half-life; *UK,* unknown.

CRITICAL THINKING CASE STUDY

A 72-year-old African American patient has heart failure and diabetes. Her vital signs are blood pressure 176/94, pulse 92, and respirations 30. Her medications include hydrochlorothiazide 50 mg/day, digoxin 0.125 mg/day, and atenolol 50 mg/day.

1. Why was hydrochlorothiazide prescribed for this patient? Explain the effects of hydrochlorothiazide on blood pressure.
2. Abnormal electrolytes and other laboratory test results may occur when taking hydrochlorothiazide. Would the following serum electrolyte and laboratory values be expected to *increase* or *decrease*?
   a. Sodium
   b. Potassium
   c. Calcium
   d. Magnesium
   e. Glucose
   f. Uric acid
3. Why should this patient's blood glucose level be monitored while she is taking hydrochlorothiazide?
4. What response does a health care provider need to keep in mind when prescribing antihypertensive agents? Explain your answer.
5. Atenolol is what type of antihypertensive? Would atenolol be effective in lowering this patient's blood pressure if given as the only antihypertensive drug? Explain your answer.
6. How effective is the combination of hydrochlorothiazide and atenolol for controlling this patient's blood pressure? Explain your answer.

7. When using a combination drug therapy to correct hypertension, would the dosage for each drug be the same? Explain your answer.
8. When abruptly discontinuing beta blockers for hypertension without the patient taking another antihypertensive, what might occur? Explain how adverse effects can be avoided.

This patient's blood glucose is 229. Her drugs for controlling hypertension are changed to prazosin 10 mg three times daily. Her cholesterol and LDL are elevated, and her serum potassium level is 3.2 mEq/L.

9. Why were this patient's hydrochlorothiazide and atenolol discontinued? Explain your answer.
10. What type of antihypertensive is prazosin? Explain the physiologic action of prazosin for lowering the blood pressure.
11. Does prazosin have an effect on the blood glucose level? What effect could prazosin have on this patient's abnormal lipid levels? Explain your answer.

This patient's ankles have become edematous. Hydrochlorothiazide is again prescribed.

12. Why was hydrochlorothiazide again added to the drug regimen?
13. Is the daily prazosin dose within the safe therapeutic prescribed range for this patient? Explain your answer. (You may refer to Prototype Drug Chart: Prazosin Hydrochloride.)
14. List the groups of antihypertensive drugs that can cause sodium and water retention.

REVIEW QUESTIONS

1. A patient's blood pressure is 130/84. The health care provider plans to suggest nonpharmacologic methods to lower blood pressure. Which should the nurse include in teaching? (Select all that apply.)
   a. Stress-reduction techniques
   b. An exercise program
   c. Salt restriction
   d. Smoking cessation
   e. A diet with increased protein
2. A patient has developed mild hypertension. The nurse acknowledges that the first-line drug for treating this patient's blood pressure might be which drug?
   a. Diuretic
   b. Alpha blocker
   c. Angiotensin-converting enzyme inhibitor
   d. Alpha/beta blocker
3. An African American patient has developed hypertension. The nurse is aware that which group(s) of antihypertensive drugs are *less effective* in African American patients?
   a. Diuretics
   b. Calcium channel blockers and vasodilators
   c. Beta blockers and angiotensin-converting enzyme inhibitors
   d. Alpha blockers
4. The nurse knows that which diuretic is most frequently combined with an antihypertensive drug?
   a. Chlorthalidone
   b. Hydrochlorothiazide
   c. Bendroflumethiazide
   d. A potassium-sparing diuretic

5. The nurse is administering a beta blocker to a patient. Which is the most important assessment to perform before administration?
   a. Urine output
   b. Apical pulse
   c. Potassium level
   d. Serum level of medication
6. Captopril has been prescribed for a patient. The nurse should teach the patient that the most commonly occurring side effect of an angiotensin-converting enzyme drug is which of the following?
   a. Nausea and vomiting
   b. Dizziness and headaches
   c. Upset stomach
   d. Constant, irritating cough
7. A patient is prescribed losartan. The nurse teaches the patient that an angiotensin II-receptor blocker acts by doing what?
   a. Inhibiting angiotensin-converting enzyme
   b. Blocking angiotensin II from angiotensin I receptors
   c. Preventing the release of angiotensin I
   d. Promoting the release of aldosterone
8. During an admission assessment, a patient states that she takes amlodipine. The nurse should inquire about which signs and symptoms to determine whether the patient has any common side effects of amlodipine? (Select all that apply.)
   a. Insomnia
   b. Dizziness
   c. Headache
   d. Angioedema
   e. Ankle edema
   f. Hacking cough

43

Anticoagulants, Antiplatelets, and Thrombolytics

http://evolve.elsevier.com/McCuistion/pharmacology

OBJECTIVES

- Compare the actions of anticoagulants, antiplatelets, and thrombolytics.
- Differentiate the side effects and adverse reactions of anticoagulants, antiplatelets, and thrombolytics.

- Apply the Clinical Judgment [Nursing Process], including patient teaching, for anticoagulants and thrombolytics.

OUTLINE

Various drugs are used to maintain or restore circulation. The three major groups of these drugs are (1) anticoagulants, (2) antiplatelets (antithrombotics), and (3) thrombolytics. The *anticoagulants* prevent the formation of clots that inhibit circulation. The *antiplatelets* prevent platelet aggregation, clumping together of platelets to form a clot. The *thrombolytics*, appropriately called *clot busters*, attack and dissolve blood clots that have already formed. Each of these three drug groups are discussed separately.

PATHOPHYSIOLOGY: THROMBUS FORMATION

Thrombosis is the formation of a clot in an arterial or venous vessel. The formation of an arterial thrombus could be caused by blood stasis (decreased circulation), platelet aggregation on the blood vessel wall, or blood coagulation. Arterial clots are usually made up of both white and red clots with the white clots, *platelets*, initiating the process, followed by fibrin formation and the trapping of red blood cells in the fibrin mesh. Blood clots found in the veins are from platelet aggregation with fibrin that attaches to red blood cells. Both types of thrombus can be dislodged from the vessel and become an *embolus*, a blood clot moving through the bloodstream.

Platelets do not usually stick together unless there is a break in the endothelial lining of a blood vessel. When platelets adhere to the broken surface of an endothelial lining, they synthesize thromboxane A_2, which is a product of prostaglandins and a potent stimulus for platelet aggregation, clumping of platelet cells. The platelet receptor protein that binds fibrinogen, *glycoprotein IIb/IIIa* (GP IIb/IIIa), also promotes platelet aggregation. Thromboxane A_2 and adenosine diphosphate (ADP) increase the activation of this receptor.

The thrombus inhibits blood flow, and the fibrin, platelets, and red blood cells (erythrocytes) surround the clot, building its size and structure. As the clot occludes the blood vessel, tissue ischemia occurs.

The venous thrombus usually develops because of slow blood flow, and the venous clot can form rapidly. Small pieces of the venous clot can detach and travel to the pulmonary artery and then to the lung. Inadequate oxygenation and gas exchange in the lungs is the end result.

Oral and parenteral anticoagulants, such as warfarin and heparin, act primarily to prevent venous thrombosis, whereas antiplatelet drugs act to prevent arterial thrombosis. However, both groups of drugs suppress thrombosis in general.

⚠ ANTICOAGULANTS

Anticoagulants are used to inhibit clot formation. Unlike thrombolytics, they do *not* dissolve clots that have already formed but rather act prophylactically to prevent new clots from forming. Anticoagulants are used in patients with venous and arterial disorders that put them at high risk for clot formation. Venous problems include deep venous thrombosis (DVT) and pulmonary embolism (PE), and arterial problems include coronary thrombosis, or myocardial infarction (MI); presence of artificial heart valves; and cerebrovascular accident (CVA), or stroke.

Heparin

Anticoagulants are administered orally or parenterally, both subcutaneously and by the intravenous (IV) route. Heparin, introduced in 1938, is a natural substance in the liver that prevents clot formation. It was first used in blood transfusions to prevent clotting. Heparin is

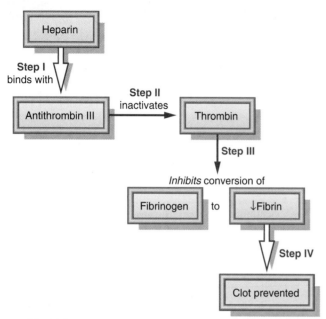

Fig. 43.1 Action of the parenteral anticoagulant heparin.

indicated for a rapid anticoagulant effect when a thrombosis occurs because of a DVT, PE, or an evolving stroke. Heparin is also used in open-heart surgery to prevent blood from clotting and in the critically ill patient with disseminated intravascular coagulation (DIC), which occurs when fibrin clots form within the vascular system. These clots consume proteins and platelets, depleting clotting factors and causing excess bleeding. However, the primary use of heparin is to prevent venous thrombosis, which can lead to PE or stroke.

Heparin combines with antithrombin III, which accelerates the anticoagulant cascade of reactions that prevents thrombosis formation. By inhibiting the action of thrombin, conversion of fibrinogen to fibrin does not occur, and the formation of a fibrin clot is prevented (Fig. 43.1).

Heparin is poorly absorbed through the gastrointestinal (GI) mucosa, and much is destroyed by heparinase, a liver enzyme. Because heparin is poorly absorbed orally, it is given subcutaneously for prophylaxis or by IV to treat acute thrombosis. It can be administered as an IV bolus or in IV fluid for continuous infusion. Heparin prolongs clotting time. Partial thromboplastin time (PTT) and activated partial thromboplastin time (aPTT) are laboratory tests used to detect deficiencies of certain clotting factors, and these tests are used to monitor heparin therapy. Heparin can decrease the platelet count, causing thrombocytopenia. If hemorrhage occurs during heparin therapy, the anticoagulant antagonist protamine sulfate is given by IV. Protamine sulfate can be an anticoagulant, but in the presence of heparin, it is an antagonist that reverses the action of heparin. Before discontinuing heparin, oral therapy with warfarin therapy is begun.

Low-Molecular-Weight Heparins

These derivatives of standard heparin were introduced to prevent venous thromboembolism. Studies have shown that by extracting only the low-molecular-weight fractions of standard heparin through depolymerization, the equivalent of anticoagulation can be achieved with a lower risk of bleeding. Low-molecular-weight heparins (LMWHs) produce more stable responses at recommended doses. As a result, frequent laboratory monitoring of aPTT is not required, because LMWH does not have the standard effect of heparin. Heparin prevents coagulation by combining with antithrombin III to inactivate factor Xa and thrombin. LMWH inactivates the Xa factor, but it is less able to inactivate thrombin.

The examples of LMWHs include enoxaparin and dalteparin.

The anticoagulant fondaparinux is a synthetically engineered antithrombotic designed to be effective as a once-daily subcutaneous injection. Categorized as a *selective factor Xa inhibitor*, fondaparinux is closely related in structure to heparin and LMWHs and is used for the same purposes.

These agents are most commonly prescribed to prevent DVT and acute PE after orthopedic or abdominal surgery. Hip and knee replacement anticoagulant therapy often includes enoxaparin, and abdominal surgery includes dalteparin. The drugs can be administered at home because aPTT monitoring is not necessary, whereas heparin must be given in the hospital. LMWHs are administered subcutaneously once or twice a day, depending on the drug or drug regimen, and they are available in prefilled syringes with attached needles. The patient or family member is taught how to administer the subcutaneous injection, which is usually given in the abdomen. Injection sites should be alternated with every dose. The average treatment period lasts 7 to 10 days. The LMWH is usually started in the hospital within 24 hours after surgery (Table 43.1).

The half-life of LMWHs is two to four times longer than that of heparin. Patients should be instructed not to take antiplatelet drugs such as aspirin while taking LMWHs or heparin. Bleeding because of LMWH use is less likely to occur than when heparin is given. LMWH overdose is rare; if bleeding occurs, protamine sulfate is the anticoagulant antagonist used. The dosage is 1 mg of protamine sulfate for every 100 units of unfractionated heparin or LMWH given to be neutralized.

Contraindications

The LMWHs are contraindicated for patients with strokes, peptic ulcers, and blood anomalies. These drugs should not be given to patients having eye, brain, or spinal surgery.

⚠ Direct Thrombin Inhibitors: Parenteral Anticoagulants II

Parenteral anticoagulants directly inhibit thrombin from converting fibrinogen to fibrin. These drugs differ from heparin-like anticoagulants. Argatroban and bivalirudin are given intravenously; bivalirudin binds with and inhibits free-flowing thrombin. Desirudin is administered subcutaneously, and dabigatran is an oral anticoagulant that does *not* require routine coagulation monitoring (see Table 43.1). These drugs are more expensive than the other anticoagulants.

Oral Anticoagulants

Oral anticoagulants inhibit hepatic synthesis of vitamin K, thus affecting the clotting factors II, VII, IX, and X. Warfarin is an oral anticoagulant synthesized from dicumarol. Warfarin is used mainly to prevent thromboembolic conditions such as thrombophlebitis, PE, and embolism formation caused by atrial fibrillation, which can lead to stroke. Oral anticoagulants prolong clotting time and are monitored by the prothrombin time (PT), a laboratory test that measures the time it takes blood to clot in the presence of certain clotting factors, which warfarin affects. This laboratory test is usually performed immediately before administering the next drug dose until the therapeutic level has been reached. Today, the international normalized ratio (INR) is the laboratory test most

❗ TABLE 43.1   Anticoagulants and Anticoagulant Antagonists

Drug	Route and Dosage	Uses and Considerations
Anticoagulants		
Heparins		
Heparin sodium	See Prototype Drug Chart: Heparin	
Low-Molecular-Weight Heparins (LMWHs)		
Dalteparin	DVT treatment: A: Subcut: 200 units/kg/d for 1 month, then 150 units/kg/d for months 2–6	For DVT and PE prophylaxis and treatment, prophylaxis of thrombosis, and unstable angina. May cause bleeding, hematoma, thrombocytopenia, elevated hepatic enzymes, hematuria, GI bleeding, and intracranial bleeding. PB: <10%; t½: 3–5 h
Enoxaparin sodium	DVT treatment: A: Subcut: 1 mg/kg q12h for 7 days	For prophylaxis of AMI, thrombosis, and unstable angina and for prophylaxis and treatment of PE and DVT. May cause bleeding, hematoma, fever, anemia, peripheral edema, and elevated liver enzymes. PB: UK; t½: 4.5–7 h
Oral Anticoagulants		
Warfarin	See Prototype Drug Chart: Warfarin Sodium	
Selective Factor Xa Inhibitors		
Fondaparinux	DVT treatment: A: Subcut: 5 mg/d if <50 kg, 7.5 mg if 50–100 kg, 10 mg if >100 mg for 5–9 d	For prophylaxis and treatment of DVT and PE. May cause anemia, bleeding, hypokalemia, infection, dizziness, confusion, headache, hematoma, intracranial bleeding, ocular hemorrhage, and insomnia. PB: 94%; t½: 18 h
Rivaroxaban	DVT treatment: A: PO: 15 mg bid for 21 d, then 20 mg/d; *max:* 30 mg/d	For prophylaxis and treatment of DVT, PE, stroke, and atrial fibrillation. May cause bleeding, GI bleeding, ocular hemorrhage, intracranial bleeding, abdominal and back pain, pruritus, and dyspepsia. PB: 92%–95%; t½: 5–9 h
Apixaban	DVT, PE: A: PO: 10 mg bid for 7 d, then 5 mg bid for 6 months; *max:* 10 mg/d	To prevent and treat DVT and PE and for prevention of atrial fibrillation. May cause hematoma, anemia, bleeding, epistaxis, hematuria, menorrhagia, hemoptysis, hematemesis, ocular hemorrhage, vaginal/GI/intracranial bleeding, and hypotension. PB: 87%; t½: 12 h
Edoxaban	DVT, PE: A: PO: After 5–10 d of initial therapy with parenteral anticoagulant may give 30 mg/d if ≤ 60 kg or 60 mg/d if >60 kg; *max:* 60 mg/d	For treatment of DVT, PE, and nonvalvular atrial fibrillation and stroke prophylaxis. May cause anemia, vaginal bleeding, elevated hepatic enzymes, epistaxis, GI bleeding, rash, intracranial bleeding, and hematuria. PB: 55%; t½: 10–14 h
Betrixaban	A: PO: 160 mg once, followed by 80 mg/d for 35–42 d; *maint:* 80 mg/d	For venous thromboembolism prophylaxis. May cause intracranial/ocular/GI bleeding, hematuria, hypokalemia, and constipation. PB: 60%; t½: 19–27 h
Direct-Acting Thrombin Inhibitors: Anticoagulants II (Intravenous)		
Argatroban	A: IV: Initially 2 mcg/kg/min infusion; adjust dose to maintain aPTT 1.5–3 times baseline; *max:* 10 mcg/kg/min	For PCI, HIT. May cause bleeding, hypotension, chest pain, dyspnea, rash, cough, back pain, nausea, vomiting, diarrhea, abdominal pain, hematuria, and headache. PB: 20%; t½: 39–51 min
Bivalirudin	PCI: A: IV bolus: 0.75 mg/kg; then IV infusion of 1.75 mg/kg/h throughout procedure	For thrombosis prophylaxis in PCI, unstable angina, and HIT. May cause back pain, bleeding, headache, nausea, hypo/hypertension, insomnia, anxiety, and bradycardia. PB: 0%; t½: 25 min
Desirudin	A: Subcut: 15 mg q12h for 9–12 d, give first dose 5–15 min before surgery	For DVT prophylaxis. May cause bleeding, hematoma, injection site reaction, phlebitis, and anemia. PB: 99%; t½: 2 h
Dabigatran	DVT: A: PO: 150 mg bid; *max:* 300 mg/d	For prevention of stroke and for prophylaxis and treatment of DVT, and PE. May cause bleeding, GI bleeding, headache, pharyngitis, epistaxis, nausea, vomiting, menorrhagia, pruritus, and edema. PB: 35%; t½: 12–17 h
Anticoagulant Antagonists		
Protamine sulfate	A: IV: Initially: 1 mg/100 units heparin to be neutralized; *max:* 100 mg in 2-h period	For heparin reversal. May cause hypotension, flushing, bradycardia, fatigue, bleeding, pulmonary edema, and dyspnea. PB: UK; t½: 7.4 min
Phytonadione	Vitamin K deficiency prevention: A: PO males: 120 mcg/d A: PO females: 90 mcg/d	For vitamin K deficiency, bleeding from warfarin toxicity. May cause anaphylaxis, dizziness, flushing, dysgeusia, dyspnea, hyperhidrosis, tachycardia, and hypotension. PB: UK; t½: UK

A, Adult; *AMI,* acute myocardial infarction; *aPTT,* activated partial thromboplastin time; *bid,* twice a day; *d,* day; *DVT,* deep vein thrombosis; *GI,* gastrointestinal; *h,* hour; *HIT,* heparin-induced thrombocytopenia; *IV,* intravenous; *max,* maximum; *min,* minute; *PB,* protein binding; *PCI,* percutaneous coronary intervention; *PE,* pulmonary embolism; *PO,* by mouth; *q12h,* every 12 hours; *subcut,* subcutaneous; *t½,* half-life; *UK,* unknown; *<,* less than.

frequently used to report PT results. It was introduced to account for variability in reported PTs from different laboratories. Reagents used in the PT test are compared with an international reference standard and reported as the INR; normal INR is 1.3 to 2. Patients on warfarin therapy are maintained at an INR of 2 to 3. The desired INR for patients who have a mechanical heart valve or recurrent systemic embolism is 2.5 to 3.5, but the desired level could be as high as 4.5.

Monitoring INR at regular intervals is required for the duration of drug therapy. Warfarin has a long half-life and very long duration. Drug accumulation can occur and can lead to external or internal bleeding, so the nurse must observe for petechiae, ecchymosis, tarry stools, and hematemesis and must teach the patient to do the same at home.

The antidote for warfarin overdose is vitamin K, but it takes 24 to 48 hours to be effective. Usually a low dose of oral vitamin K may be recommended for patients with an INR of 5.5. If excessive vitamin K is given, it may take warfarin 1 to 2 weeks before it can be effective again. For acute bleeding, fresh frozen plasma is indicated.

Table 43.1 describes pharmacologic data for anticoagulants and anticoagulant antagonists. Table 43.2 compares heparin and warfarin regarding action, uses, laboratory tests, and other considerations. Parenteral and oral anticoagulants (heparin and warfarin) are presented in Prototype Drug Chart: Heparin and Prototype Drug Chart: Warfarin Sodium.

Pharmacokinetics. Heparin is poorly absorbed through the GI mucosa, and much is destroyed by heparinase, a liver enzyme. Heparin is given parenterally, either subcutaneously for prophylactic anticoagulant therapy or by IV (bolus or continuous infusion) for an immediate response. Warfarin, an oral anticoagulant, is well absorbed through the GI mucosa; food will delay but not inhibit absorption.

The half-life of heparin is dose related; high doses prolong the half-life. The half-life of warfarin is 20 to 60 hours, in contrast to 30 to 150 minutes for heparin. Because warfarin has a long half-life and is highly protein bound, the drug can have cumulative effects. Bleeding can occur, especially if another highly protein-bound drug is administered together with warfarin. Kidney and liver disease prolong the half-life of both heparin and warfarin. Warfarin is metabolized to inactive metabolites excreted in urine and bile.

Pharmacodynamics. Heparin, administered for acute thromboembolic disorders, prevents thrombus formation and embolism. It has been effectively used to treat DIC, which causes multiple thrombi in small blood vessels. Warfarin is effective for long-term anticoagulant therapy. The PT level should be 1.5 to 2 times the reference value to be therapeutic, or INR should be 2.0 to 3.0. INR has effectively replaced the use of PT, because PT can vary from laboratory to laboratory and reagent to reagent. Higher INR levels (up to 3.5) are usually required for patients with prosthetic heart valves, cardiac valvular disease, and recurrent emboli. Heparin does not cross the placental barrier, unlike warfarin; warfarin use is not recommended during pregnancy.

IV heparin has a rapid onset; its peak time of action is reached in minutes, and its duration of action is short. After an IV heparin dose, the patient's clotting time will return to normal in 2 to 6 hours. Subcutaneous heparin is more slowly absorbed through the blood vessels in fatty tissue. Warfarin has a long onset of action, peak concentration, and duration of action, so drug accumulation may occur.

Side Effects and Adverse Reactions

Bleeding (hemorrhage) is the major adverse effect of warfarin. Patients should be monitored closely for signs of bleeding such as petechiae, ecchymosis, GI bleeding, ocular hemorrhage, and hematuria. Laboratory testing of PT or INR should be scheduled at recommended intervals.

Drug Interactions

Because warfarin is highly protein bound, it is affected by drug interactions. Aspirin, nonsteroidal antiinflammatory drugs (NSAIDs), other types of antiinflammatory drugs, sulfonamides, phenytoin, cimetidine, allopurinol, and oral hypoglycemic drugs for diabetes can displace warfarin from the protein-bound site and can cause more free-circulating anticoagulant. Numerous other drugs also increase the action of warfarin, and bleeding is likely to occur. Acetaminophen should be used instead of aspirin by patients taking warfarin. For frank bleeding resulting from excess free drug, parenteral vitamin K is given

TABLE 43.2 Comparison of Parenteral and Oral Anticoagulants

Factors to Consider	Heparin	Warfarin (Coumadin)
Methods of administration	Subcutaneously Intravenously	Primarily orally
Drug actions	Binds with antithrombin III, which inactivates thrombin and clotting factors, inhibiting fibrin formation	Inhibits hepatic synthesis of vitamin K, which decreases prothrombin and the clotting factors VII, IX, and X
Uses	Treatment of venous thrombosis, PE, thromboembolic complications (e.g., heart surgery, DIC)	Treatment of DVT, PE, TIA; prophylactic for cardiac valves
Contraindications/cautions	Hemophilia, peptic ulcer, severe (stage 3 or 4) hypertension, severe liver or renal disease, dissecting aneurysm	Hemophilia, peptic bleeding ulcer, blood dyscrasias, severe liver or kidney disease, AMI, alcoholism
Laboratory tests	PTT: 60–70 s Anticoagulant therapeutic level: 1.5–2 × control in seconds aPTT: 20–35 s Anticoagulant: aPTT: 30–85 s	PT: 11–15 s Anticoagulant therapeutic level: 1.25–2.5 × control in seconds INR: 1.3–2 Anticoagulant: INR 2–3 Prosthetic heart valves: INR up to 3.5
Side effects/adverse effects	Bleeding, hemorrhage, hematoma, severe hypotension	Bleeding, hemorrhage, GI bleeding, ecchymoses, hematuria
Antidote	Protamine sulfate	Phytonadione (vitamin K)

AMI, acute myocardial infarction; *aPTT,* activated partial thromboplastin time; *DIC,* disseminated intravascular coagulation; *DVT,* deep venous thrombosis; *GI,* gastrointestinal; *INR,* international normalized ratio; *PE,* pulmonary embolism; *PT,* prothrombin time; *PTT,* partial thromboplastin time; *s,* second; *TIA,* transient ischemic attack.

as a coagulant to decrease bleeding and promote clotting. However, caution must be used with this approach because the prothrombin can remain depressed for prolonged periods.

⚠️ Factor Xa Inhibitors

Factor Xa inhibitors include fondaparinux, given subcutaneously, and those given orally—rivaroxaban, apixaban, edoxaban, and betrixaban.

These drugs do not require routine coagulation monitoring and are given once or twice daily. Factor Xa inhibitors selectively block activity of clotting factor Xa to prevent clot formation. They are approved for the prevention of DVT and PE. The major adverse effect is bleeding. This drug category should not be given to patients weighing less than 50 kg because low body weight increases the risk for bleeding (see Table 43.1).

◎ CLINICAL JUDGMENT [NURSING PROCESS]

Anticoagulants: Warfarin and Heparin

Concept: Clotting
- A process in which blood is changed into a semisolid gel

Recognize Cues [Assessment]
- Obtain a history of abnormal clotting or health problems that affect clotting, such as severe alcoholism or severe liver or renal disease. Warfarin is contraindicated for patients with blood dyscrasias, peptic ulcer, cerebrovascular accident (CVA), hemophilia, or severe hypertension. Use with caution in patients with acute traumatic injury.
- Gather a drug history that includes a complementary and alternative therapy history of current drugs and products that the patient takes. Report if drug-drug or drug-herb interaction or other interaction with complementary and alternative therapy is probable. Warfarin is highly protein bound and can displace other highly protein-bound drugs, or warfarin could be displaced, which may result in bleeding.
- Develop a flowchart that lists prothrombin time (PT) or international normalized ratio (INR) and warfarin dosages. A baseline PT or INR should be obtained before warfarin is administered.

Analyze Cues and Prioritize Hypothesis [Patient Problems]
- Bleeding
- Tissue injury
- Dehydration

Generate Solutions [Planning]
- The patient will not have excessive bleeding.

Take Action [Nursing Interventions]
- Monitor vital signs. An increased pulse rate followed by a decreased systolic pressure can indicate a fluid volume deficit resulting from external or internal bleeding.
- ⚡ Monitor PT or INR for warfarin and activated partial thromboplastin time (aPTT) for heparin before administering anticoagulant. PT should be 1.25 to 2.5 times the control level, or INR should be 2 to 3, except for patients with prosthetic heart valves, in whom INR may be up to 3.5. Monitor platelet count because anticoagulants can decrease it.
- Examine the patient's mouth, nose (epistaxis), urine (hematuria), and skin (petechiae, purpura) for bleeding. Watch older adults closely for bleeding; their skin is thin, and capillary beds are fragile.
- Check stools periodically for occult blood.
- Keep anticoagulant antagonists available, protamine sulfate for heparin and vitamin K for warfarin, when the drug dose is increased or indications of frank bleeding are evident. Fresh frozen plasma may be needed for transfusion.

Patient Teaching
General
- Teach patients to inform their dentist when taking an anticoagulant. Contacting a health care provider may be necessary.
- Advise patients to use a soft toothbrush to prevent gums from bleeding.
- Warn patients to shave with an electric razor. Bleeding from shaving cuts may be difficult to control.
- Advise patients to have laboratory tests such as PT or INR performed as ordered by a health care provider. The warfarin dose is regulated according to INR derived from PT.
- Suggest that patients carry a medical identification card or wear a MedicAlert bracelet that lists the patient's name, telephone number, and the drug taken.
- Encourage patients *not* to smoke. Smoking increases drug metabolism, so warfarin dose may need to be increased. If a patient insists on smoking, notify the health care provider.
- Tell patients to check with a health care provider before taking over-the-counter (OTC) drugs. Aspirin should *not* be taken with warfarin because it intensifies warfarin's action, and bleeding is apt to occur. Suggest that patients use acetaminophen.
- Inform patients that many herbal products interact with anticoagulants and may increase bleeding. Closely monitor INR or PT.
- ⚡ Teach patients to control external hemorrhage from accidents or injuries by applying firm, direct pressure for at least 5 to 10 minutes with a clean, dry, absorbent material.

Side Effects
- Warn patients to report frank or occult bleeding such as petechiae, ecchymosis, purpura, tarry stools, bleeding gums, epistaxis, or expectoration of blood.

Diet
- Advise patients to avoid large amounts of green, leafy vegetables; broccoli; legumes; soybean oil (rich in vitamin K); coffee, tea, cola (caffeine); excessive alcohol; and certain herbs and nutritional supplements (coenzyme Q10) or to be very consistent with their intake. Coenzyme Q10, fish oils, substances high in vitamin K, St. John's wort, ginseng, and vitamin C may decrease the effectiveness of warfarin. Garlic, ginger, kava kava, green tea, chamomile tea, ginkgo biloba, and acute alcohol intoxication also decrease warfarin's effectiveness.

Evaluate Outcomes [Evaluation]
- Evaluate the effectiveness of drug therapy. The patient's PT or INR values are within the desired range, and the patient is free from significant side effects.

COMPLEMENTARY AND ALTERNATIVE THERAPIES

Anticoagulants: Warfarin and Heparin

- Dong quai, feverfew, garlic, ginger, meadowsweet, willow bark, chamomile tea, ginkgo, and bilberry may increase bleeding when taken with anticoagulants such as warfarin. Warfarin has an additive effect and increases the international normalized ratio (INR) and prothrombin time (PT).
- Excessive doses of anise may interfere with anticoagulants.
- Ginseng may decrease the effects of warfarin, thereby decreasing INR.
- Alfalfa may decrease anticoagulant activity.
- Goldenseal may decrease the effects of heparin and oral anticoagulants.
- Hawthorn increases the action of anticoagulants.
- Valerian and green tea may decrease the effects of warfarin.
- Cranberry may increase INR.

PROTOTYPE DRUG CHART

Warfarin Sodium

Drug Class	Dosage
Anticoagulant	DVT or PE: A: PO: 2–5 mg/d based on INR; *maint:* 2–10 mg/d; target INR 2–3

Contraindications	Drug-Lab-Food Interactions
Hematologic disorders, eclampsia, alcohol abuse, stroke, bleeding, head trauma, aneurysm, psychosis *Caution:* Diabetes mellitus, leukemia, anemia, thyroid disease, hepatic and renal impairment, peptic ulcer, atrial fibrillation, heart failure, cerebrovascular disease, breastfeeding	Increased effect with amiodarone, aspirin, NSAIDs, sulfonamides, thyroid drugs, allopurinol, histamine₂ blockers, oral hypoglycemics, metronidazole, miconazole, methyldopa, diuretics, oral antibiotics, vitamin E; decreased effect with barbiturates, laxatives, phenytoin, estrogens, vitamins C and K, oral contraceptives, rifampin Lab: May increase AST, ALT Food: Decrease diet rich in vitamin K

Pharmacokinetics	Pharmacodynamics
Absorption: PO: Well absorbed Distribution: PB: 97% Metabolism: t½: 20–60 h Excretion: In urine and bile	PO: Onset: 24–72 h Peak: 36–72 h, 5–7 d full effect Duration: 2–5 d

Therapeutic Effects/Uses

To prevent thrombosis associated with PE, MI, unstable angina, prosthetic heart valves, DVT, and PCI; to treat atrial fibrillation

Mechanism of Action: Inhibits hepatic synthesis of vitamin K clotting factors (II [prothrombin], VII, IX, and X) and anticoagulant proteins.

Side Effects	Adverse Reactions
Headache, alopecia, fever, weakness, priapism, petechiae, ecchymosis	Purple-toe syndrome, bone fracture, hypotension, chest pain, hematuria, ocular hemorrhage, intracranial/vaginal/GI bleeding *Life-threatening:* Hemorrhage

A, Adult; *ALT,* alanine transaminase; *aPTT,* activated partial thromboplastin time; *AST,* aspartate transaminase; *d,* day; *DIC,* disseminated intravascular coagulation; *DVT,* deep venous thrombosis; *GI,* gastrointestinal; *h,* hour; *HIT,* heparin-induced thrombocytopenia; *INR,* international normalized ratio; *IV,* intravenous; *maint,* maintenance; *MI,* myocardial infarction; *min,* minute; *NSAIDs,* nonsteroidal antiinflammatory drugs; *PB,* protein binding; *PCI,* percutaneous coronary intervention; *PE,* pulmonary embolism; *PO,* by mouth; *q,* every; *SSRI,* selective serotonin reuptake inhibitor; *subcut,* subcutaneous; *t½,* half-life; *UK,* unknown; *y,* years; *>,* greater than.

PROTOTYPE DRUG CHART

Heparin

Drug Class	Dosage
Anticoagulant	DVT or PE: A: IV: 80 units/kg bolus; *maint:* 18 units/kg/h infusion based on aPTT

Contraindications	Drug-Lab-Food Interactions
HIT, hypersensitivity *Caution:* Peptic ulcer, hepatic or renal disease, hemophilia, DIC, diverticulitis, head trauma, asthma, aneurysm, endocarditis, thrombocytopenia, older adults, pregnancy, breastfeeding	Increased effect with aspirin, NSAIDs, thrombolytics, probenecid, antibiotics, SSRIs; decreased effect with nitroglycerin, protamine sulfate

Pharmacokinetics	Pharmacodynamics
Absorption: Subcut or IV Distribution: PB: >80% Metabolism: t½: IV 30–150 min Excretion: Slowly in urine and reticuloendothelial system	Subcut: Onset: 20–30 min Peak: UK Duration: UK IV: Onset: Immediate Peak: 5–10 min Duration: 2–6 h

Therapeutic Effects/Uses

To prevent thromboembolism associated with PE, MI, unstable angina, prosthetic heart valves and PCI; and to treat DVT, DIC, and acute coronary syndrome.

Mechanism of Action: Inactivates thrombin, which prevents conversion of fibrinogen to fibrin.

Side Effects	Adverse Reactions
Itching, chills, headache, epistaxis, erythema, hematoma, hematemesis, hematuria, alopecia, elevated hepatic enzymes, nausea, vomiting, injection-site reaction, priapism	Bleeding, intracranial bleeding, ocular hemorrhage, anemia, bone fractures, osteoporosis, hyperkalemia, vitamin D deficiency, GI bleeding, hyperlipidemia, stroke, *Life-threatening:* Anaphylaxis, HIT, thrombocytopenia

A, Adult; *ALT,* alanine transaminase; *aPTT,* activated partial thromboplastin time; *AST,* aspartate transaminase; *d,* day; *DIC,* disseminated intravascular coagulation; *DVT,* deep venous thrombosis; *GI,* gastrointestinal; *h,* hour; *HIT,* heparin-induced thrombocytopenia; *INR,* international normalized ratio; *IV,* intravenous; *maint,* maintenance; *MI,* myocardial infarction; *min,* minute; *NSAIDs,* nonsteroidal antiinflammatory drugs; *PB,* protein binding; *PCI,* percutaneous coronary intervention; *PE,* pulmonary embolism; *PO,* by mouth; *q,* every; *SSRI,* selective serotonin reuptake inhibitor; *subcut,* subcutaneous; *t½,* half-life; *UK,* unknown; *y,* years; *>,* greater than.

Anticoagulant Antagonists

Bleeding occurs in about 10% of patients taking oral anticoagulants. Phytonadione, an antagonist of warfarin, is vitamin K₁ and is used for warfarin overdose or uncontrollable bleeding. Usually 5 to 10 mg of vitamin K₁ is given by slow intravenous infusion at once, and if it fails to control bleeding, fresh whole blood or fresh frozen plasma or platelets are generally given.

ANTIPLATELET DRUGS

Antiplatelets are used to prevent thrombosis in the arteries by suppressing platelet aggregation. Heparin and warfarin prevent thrombosis in the veins.

Antiplatelet drug therapy is mainly for prophylactic use in (1) prevention of MI or stroke for patients with a family history of these, (2) prevention of repeat MI or stroke, and (3) prevention of stroke for patients having transient ischemic attacks (TIAs).

Long-term, low-dose aspirin therapy has been found to be both an effective and inexpensive treatment for suppressing platelet aggregation. Aspirin inhibits cyclooxygenase (COX), an enzyme needed by platelets to synthesize thromboxane A_2 (TxA_2). For patients with a family history of stroke or MI, the recommended aspirin dose is 50 to 325 mg/day for stroke prophylaxis and 75 to 162 mg/day for MI prophylaxis. Because aspirin has prolonged antiplatelet activity, it should be discontinued at least 7 days before surgery.

Other antiplatelet drugs include anagrelide, clopidogrel, dipyridamole, prasugrel, ticagrelor, vorapaxar, cangrelor, abciximab, eptifibatide, and tirofiban. Clopidogrel and dipyridamole have effects similar to those of aspirin, but they are known as *adenosine diphosphate (ADP) antagonists,* and they affect platelet aggregation. Cilostazol inhibits platelet aggregation and is a vasodilator that may be used for intermittent claudication. Ticagrelor 90 mg twice a day is taken in conjunction with aspirin 75 to 100 mg in a maintenance regimen. Doses greater than 100 mg of aspirin should be avoided. Table 43.3 lists the antiplatelet drugs and their dosages, uses, and considerations.

TABLE 43.3   Antiplatelets

Drug	Route and Dosage	Uses and Considerations
Anagrelide hydrochloride	A: PO: Initially 0.5 mg qid or 1 mg bid for 1 wk; *maint:* 1.5–3 mg/d; *max:* 10 mg/d	For treatment of thrombocytosis, chronic myelogenous leukemia, and polycythemia vera. May cause headache, dizziness, palpitations, peripheral edema, weakness, flatulence, abdominal pain, nausea, diarrhea, anorexia, and dyspnea. PB: UK; t½: 1.5 h
Aspirin (ASA)	Thromboembolus prophylaxis: A: PO: 75–100 mg/d TDM: Salicylate toxicity is >300 mcg/mL	For prevention and treatment of stroke; MI, TIA, prosthetic heart valves, and thromboembolism prophylaxis. May cause abdominal pain, nausea, dyspepsia, gastritis, GI bleeding, intracranial bleeding, and epistaxis. PB: 20%–90%; t½: 3–10 h
Cilostazol	A: PO: 50–100 mg bid 30 min ac or 2 h pc; *max:* 200 mg/d	For claudication and PVD. Smoking may decrease serum levels. May cause headache, nausea, abdominal pain, diarrhea, nasopharyngitis, rhinitis, dizziness, infection, palpitations, and peripheral edema. PB: 95%–98%, t½: 11–13 h
Clopidogrel	See Prototype Drug Chart: Clopidogrel Bisulfate	
Dipyridamole	Thromboembolism prophylaxis: A: PO: 75–100 mg qid in combination with warfarin	For prevention of thromboembolism associated with prosthetic heart valves. May cause dizziness, headache, nausea, abdominal pain, dyspnea, flushing and chest pain. PB: 91%–99%; t½: 13.6 h
Prasugrel	A <75 y >60 kg: PO: Loading dose: 60 mg; *maint:* 10 mg/d in combination with 75–325 mg ASA A <75 y <60 kg: PO: Loading dose: 60 mg; *maint:* 5 mg/d in combination with 75–325 mg ASA A: >75 y: Not recommended except in high-risk individuals with a history of MI or diabetes	For thromboembolism prophylaxis. May cause headache, back pain, dizziness, bleeding, nausea, hypo/hypertension, dyspnea, hyperlipidemia, hypercholesterolemia and epistaxis. PB: 98%; t½: 2–15 h
Ticagrelor	A: PO: Loading dose: 180 mg with ASA 325 mg; begin maint in 12 h; *maint:* 90 mg bid with ASA 75–100 mg/d for 1 y, then 60 mg bid with ASA; *max:* 180 mg/d with 100 mg/d ASA	For thromboembolism prophylaxis. May cause headache, dizziness, bradycardia, bleeding, nausea, diarrhea, cough, hypo/hypertension, and dyspnea. PB: 99%; t½: 7 h
Vorapaxar	A: PO: 2.08 mg/d in combination with ASA and/or clopidogrel; *max:* 2.08 mg/d	A protease-activated receptor-1 antagonist for prevention of thrombosis, MI, PAD, and stroke. May cause bleeding, intracranial/GI bleeding, and anemia. PB: 99%; t½: 5–13 d
Cangrelor	A: IV: Initially 30 mcg/kg bolus before PCI, follow immediately with infusion of 4 mcg/kg/min for at least 2 h or duration of PCI, whichever is longer	For prevention of thrombosis in PCI and MI. May cause bleeding, dyspnea, hematoma, hematuria, and intracranial bleeding. PB: 97%; t½: 3–6 min
Combination of Antiplatelet Drugs		
Dipyridamole 200 mg and aspirin 25 mg	Stroke prevention: Extended release: A: PO: 1 cap bid in morning and evening; *max:* ASA 50 mg and dipyridamole 400 mg/d	For stroke prevention, ischemic stroke, and TIA. May cause headache, nausea, vomiting, diarrhea, abdominal pain, dyspepsia, fatigue, bleeding, and arthralgia. PB: ASA 20%–90%, dipyridamole 91%–99%; t½: ASA 3–10 h, dipyridamole 13.6 h
Aspirin (ASA) and omeprazole	A: PO: ASA 81 mg and omeprazole 40 mg/d or ASA 325 mg and omeprazole 40 mg/d	For prophylaxis of secondary cardiovascular and cerebrovascular events. May cause gastritis, nausea, diarrhea, anemia, blurred vision, bleeding, tinnitus, and hearing loss. PB: ASA 20%–90%, omeprazole 95%; t½: ASA 3–10 h, omeprazole 1 h

Continued

TABLE 43.3   Antiplatelets—cont'd

Drug	Route and Dosage	Uses and Considerations
Antiplatelets: Glycoprotein (GP) IIb/IIIa Receptor Antagonists		
Abciximab	A: IV bolus: 0.25 mg/kg given 10–60 min before PCI; follow with continuous infusion of 0.125 mcg/kg/min for 12 h; *max:* 10 mcg/min infusion; 0.25 mg/kg bolus	To prevent thrombosis in PCI, unstable angina, and AMI. May cause headache, dizziness, hypotension, bradycardia, bleeding, chest/back pain, nausea, vomiting, abdominal pain, and antibody formation. PB: UK; t½: 10–30 min
Eptifibatide	PCI: A: IV bolus: 180 mcg/kg, then 2 mcg/kg/min infusion until hospital discharge or 18–24 h; *max:* 15 mg/h infusion or 180 mcg/kg bolus	For prevention of thrombosis in PCI, unstable angina, and AMI. May cause hypotension, hematuria, and bleeding. PB: 25%; t½: 2.5 h
Tirofiban	A: IV: 25 mcg/kg bolus over 5 min followed by 0.15 mcg/kg/min infusion for 18 h	For unstable angina and AMI and to reduce thrombotic cardiovascular events. May cause dizziness, headache, hypotension, hyperhidrosis, bleeding, pelvic pain, edema, and bradycardia. PB: 35%; t½: 1.7–2 h

A, Adult; *ac,* before meals; *AMI,* acute myocardial infarction; *ASA,* acetylsalicylic acid (aspirin); *bid,* twice daily; *cap,* capsule; *d,* day; *ER,* extended release; *GI,* gastrointestinal; *h,* hour; *IV,* intravenous; *maint,* maintenance; *max,* maximum; *MI,* myocardial infarction; *min,* minute; *PAD,* peripheral artery disease; *PB,* protein binding; *pc,* after meals; *PCI,* percutaneous coronary intervention; *PO,* by mouth; *PVD,* peripheral vascular disease; *qd,* every day; *qid,* four times a day; *t½,* half-life; *TDM,* therapeutic drug monitoring; *TIA,* transient ischemic attack; *tid,* three times a day; *UK,* unknown; *wk,* week; *y,* years; *>,* greater than.

📄 PROTOTYPE DRUG CHART

Clopidogrel Bisulfate

Drug Class	**Dosage**
Antiplatelet	Thromboembolism prophylaxis in AMI: A: PO: LD: 300 mg and then 75 mg/d in combination with aspirin 75–325 mg/d

Contraindications	**Drug-Lab-Food Interactions**
Intracranial hemorrhage, GI bleeding *Caution:* Hepatic/renal disease, surgery, peptic ulcer, thrombotic thrombocytopenia purpura, trauma, older adults, pregnancy, breastfeeding	Drug: May increase bleeding when taken with NSAIDs, anticoagulants, omeprazole, antineoplastics, azole antifungals, SSRIs, and barbiturates; interferes with metabolism of phenytoin, warfarin, fluvastatin, tamoxifen, tolbutamide, NSAIDs, torsemide, calcium channel blockers, morphine, and amiodarone; increases effects of valsartan, rosuvastatin, glipizide, glyburide; effects are decreased with grapefruit juice. Lab: Prolongs bleeding time Herb: May increase bleeding when taken with ginger, garlic, ginkgo, feverfew, green tea

Pharmacokinetics	**Pharmacodynamics**
Absorption: Rapid Distribution: PB: 94%–98% Metabolism: t½: 6 h Excretion: 50% in urine and 50% in feces	PO: Onset: Initially 2 h for dose of 300–600 mg/d, 2 d for dose of 50–100 mg/d Peak: Initially 5–7 d, once established 30–60 min Duration: UK

Therapeutic Effects/Uses
To prevent thromboembolism associated with unstable angina, AMI, stroke, TIA Mechanism of Action: Inhibits platelet aggregation and prevents ADP from binding with the ADP platelet receptor

Side Effects	**Adverse Reactions**
Abdominal pain, dizziness, confusion, epistaxis, headaches, hematoma, dyspepsia, diarrhea, constipation, purpura, peripheral edema, rash, pruritus	Hypotension, hypertension, bronchospasm, bleeding, peptic ulcer, intracranial/GI bleeding *Life-threatening:* Agranulocytosis, aplastic anemia, thrombocytopenia, pancytopenia, hepatic failure, Stevens-Johnson syndrome

A, Adult; *ADP,* adenosine diphosphate; *AMI,* acute myocardial infarction; *d,* day; *GI,* gastrointestinal; *h,* hour; *LD,* loading dose; *MI,* myocardial infarction; *PB,* protein binding; *PO,* by mouth; *NSAID,* nonsteroidal antiinflammatory drug; *SSRI,* serotonin reuptake inhibitor; *t½,* half-life; *TIA,* transient ischemic attack; *UK,* unknown.

Clopidogrel is an antiplatelet drug frequently used after MI or stroke to prevent a second event. It may be prescribed singly or with aspirin. It has been stated that clopidogrel and aspirin are more effective in inhibiting platelet aggregation if used together than if used as separate antiplatelet therapies. Prototype Drug Chart: Clopidogrel Bisulfate lists the pharmacologic data for clopidogrel.

Pharmacokinetics. Clopidogrel is rapidly absorbed and has a high protein-binding power. Studies have not established a relationship between the concentration of the main metabolite and platelet aggregation. The half-life is 6 hours; it is usually prescribed once a day. Excretion of the drug metabolite occurs equally in the urine and in feces.

Pharmacodynamics. Clopidogrel prevents platelet aggregation by blocking the binding of ADP to the platelet ADP receptor. ADP-mediated activation of the GP IIb/IIIa complex inhibits platelet aggregation. Clopidogrel prolongs bleeding time; therefore it should be discontinued for 7 days preceding surgery. The onset of action and peak of clopidogrel is dependent on dosage. The drug should not be taken if the patient has a bleeding peptic ulcer, any active bleeding, or intracranial hemorrhage.

Abciximab, eptifibatide, and tirofiban are used primarily for acute coronary syndromes (unstable angina or non-Q-wave MI) and for preventing reocclusion of coronary arteries after percutaneous transluminal coronary angioplasty (PTCA). These drugs are usually given before and after PTCA. The drug of choice for angioplasty is abciximab. Abciximab, eptifibatide, and tirofiban block the binding of fibrinogen to the GP IIb/IIIa receptor on the platelet surface. They are called *platelet glycoprotein IIb/IIIa receptor antagonists*. After IV infusion, the antiplatelet effects at low levels for abciximab persist for up to 10 days; for eptifibatide and tirofiban, the antiplatelet effects last for 4 hours.

Complementary and alternative therapy products can interact with antiplatelet drugs.

COMPLEMENTARY AND ALTERNATIVE THERAPIES

Antiplatelets

Dong quai, feverfew, garlic, ginger, Korean ginseng, saw palmetto, and ginkgo biloba interfere with platelet aggregation. When these herbs are taken with an antiplatelet drug such as aspirin, increased bleeding may occur. Licorice may cause hypokalemia, which can potentiate drug toxicity. St. John's wort with clopidogrel may potentiate drug effects.

! THROMBOLYTICS

Thromboembolism, occlusion of an artery or vein caused by a thrombus or embolus, results in ischemia (deficient blood flow) that causes necrosis (death) of the tissue distal to the obstructed area. It takes approximately 1 to 2 weeks for the blood clot to disintegrate by natural fibrinolytic mechanisms. If a new thrombus or embolus can be dissolved more quickly, tissue necrosis is minimized, and blood flow to the area is reestablished faster. This is the basis for thrombolytic therapy.

Thrombolytics have been used since the early 1980s to promote the fibrinolytic mechanism (converting plasminogen to plasmin, which destroys the fibrin in the blood clot). The thrombus, or blood clot, disintegrates when a thrombolytic drug is administered as soon as possible after symptoms of an acute myocardial infarction (AMI), acute heart attack. Ideally, the thrombolytic should be administered within 3 to 4 hours or within 30 minutes after arriving at the hospital for treatment. However, benefits may be seen when administered within 12 hours after initial symptoms. Necrosis resulting from the blocked artery is prevented or minimized, and hospitalization time may be decreased. The need for cardiac bypass or coronary angioplasty can be evaluated soon after thrombolytic treatment. A thrombolytic drug should be administered within 3 hours of a thrombotic stroke. These drugs are also used for PE, DVT, noncoronary arterial occlusion from an acute thromboembolism, and thrombotic stroke.

Commonly used thrombolytics include alteplase, also known as *tissue plasminogen activator* (tPA), and tenecteplase (TNK tPA). Alteplase is clot specific and binds to the fibrin surface of a clot, promoting the conversion of plasminogen to plasmin. Plasmin, an enzyme, digests the fibrin in the clot. Plasmin also degrades fibrinogen, prothrombin, and other clotting factors. These drugs all induce fibrinolysis (fibrin breakdown). Prototype Drug Chart: Alteplase lists the pharmacologic data for alteplase.

Anticoagulants and antiplatelet drugs increase the risk of hemorrhage; therefore they should be avoided until the thrombolytic effect has passed. The health care provider needs to determine whether the patient has taken any of these drugs before seeking treatment.

Pharmacokinetics. The commercial preparation of alteplase is identical to natural human tissue plasminogen activator (tPA), the enzyme that converts plasminogen to plasmin. Alteplase is initially administered with 10% of dose as an IV bolus over 1 minute and 90% of dose is then infused over 60 minutes. A total dose of 90 mg is the

PROTOTYPE DRUG CHART

! Alteplase

Drug Class	Dosage
Thrombolytic agent	PE treatment: A: IV: 100 mg infusion over 2 h Ischemic CVA treatment: A: IV: 0.9 mg/kg (give 10% of dose as bolus over 1 min then 90% as an infusion over 1 h) within 3 h of symptom onset

Contraindications	Drug-Lab-Food Interactions
Intracranial bleeding, aneurysm, CVA, brain tumor, head trauma, thrombocytopenia, coagulopathy *Caution:* Atrial fibrillation, hepatic/renal disease, CABG, bleeding, peptic ulcer disease, diabetic retinopathy, older adults, pregnancy	Drug: Increased bleeding when taken with anticoagulants, NSAIDs, cefotetan, plicamycin, SNRIs, SSRIs, and cephalosporins; decreased effect when taken with aminocaproic acid, aprotinin Lab: Decrease in plasminogen, fibrinogen, hematocrit, and hemoglobin Complementary and Alternative Therapies: Increased bleeding with ginkgo biloba, garlic, feverfew, ginger, green tea, omega-3 fatty acids

Pharmacokinetics	Pharmacodynamics
Absorption: Direct IV Distribution: PB: UK Metabolism: t½: 30 min Excretion: Urine	A: IV: Onset: Immediate Peak: 5–10 min Duration: 1 h

Therapeutic Effects/Uses

To promote fibrinolysis associated with thrombosis in patients with AMI, PE, ischemic stroke, occluded IV catheter

Mechanism of Action: Alteplase promotes conversion of plasminogen to plasmin, an enzyme that digests the fibrin matrix of clots. Alteplase also initiates fibrinolysis.

Side Effects	Adverse Reactions
Epistaxis, infection, ecchymosis, nausea, vomiting, rash	Anaphylactoid reactions, laryngeal edema, angioedema; cholesterol microembolization, bleeding, hypo/hypertension, GI bleeding, MI, cerebral edema, rhabdomyolysis, bradycardia, tachycardia, heart failure, intracranial hemorrhage, seizures *Life-threatening:* Stroke; dysrhythmias; pulmonary edema, renal failure

A, Adult; *AMI*, acute myocardial infarction; *CABG*, coronary artery bypass graft; *CVA*, cerebrovascular accident; *GI*, gastrointestinal; *h*, hours; *IV*, intravenous; *MI*, myocardial infarction; *min*, minute; *NSAIDs*, nonsteroidal antiinflammatory drugs; *PB*, protein binding; *PE*, pulmonary embolism; *SNRI*, selective norepinephrine reuptake inhibitor; *SSRI*, selective serotonin reuptake inhibitor; *t½*, half-life; *UK*, unknown.

recommended maximum; a larger dose could result in risk for intracranial bleeding. Allergic reactions to alteplase occur less frequently than with other thrombolytics.

Pharmacodynamics. Alteplase is similar to natural human tissue plasminogen activator. It promotes thrombolysis by converting plasminogen to plasmin, which degrades fibrin, fibrinogen, and factors V, VIII, and XII. Peak action of alteplase occurs in 5 to 10 minutes. The duration of action is 1 hour.

Side Effects and Adverse Reactions

Allergic reactions can complicate thrombolytic therapy. Anaphylaxis (vascular collapse) occurs in less than 1% of patients receiving tenecteplase. Anaphylactoid reactions following alteplase and tenecteplase are severe and involve rash, laryngeal edema, angioedema, and anaphylactic shock. If the drugs are administered through an intracoronary catheter after MI, reperfusion dysrhythmia or hemorrhagic infarction at the myocardial necrotic area can result. The major complication of thrombolytic drugs is hemorrhage. The antithrombotic drug aminocaproic acid is used to stop bleeding by inhibiting plasminogen activation, which inhibits thrombolysis.

Table 43.4 lists the thrombolytic drugs and their dosages, uses, and considerations.

◎ CLINICAL JUDGMENT [NURSING PROCESS]
Thrombolytics

Concept: Clotting
- A process in which blood is changed into a semisolid gel

Recognize Cues [Assessment]
- Assess baseline vital signs for comparison with future values.
- Check baseline complete blood count (CBC), prothrombin time (PT), or international normalized ratio (INR) values before administration of thrombolytics.
- Obtain a medical and drug history. Contraindications for use of thrombolytics include recent cerebrovascular accident (CVA), active bleeding, severe hypertension, and anticoagulant therapy. Report if a patient takes aspirin or nonsteroidal antiinflammatory drugs (NSAIDs). Thrombolytics are contraindicated for patients with a recent history of traumatic injury, especially head injury.

Analyze Cues and Prioritize Hypothesis [Patient Problems]
- Bleeding
- Tissue injury
- Dehydration

Generate Solutions [Planning]
- The patient's vital signs will be within normal limits.
- The patient will be free of excessive bleeding.

Take Action [Nursing Interventions]
- Monitor vital signs. Increased pulse rate followed by decreased blood pressure usually indicates blood loss and impending shock. Record vital signs, and report changes.

- Observe for signs and symptoms of active bleeding from the mouth or rectum. Hemorrhage is a serious complication of thrombolytic treatment. Aminocaproic acid can be given as an intervention to stop bleeding.
- ⚡ Examine the patient for active bleeding for 24 hours after thrombolytic therapy has been discontinued: this should be done every 15 minutes for the first hour, then every 30 minutes until the eighth hour, and then hourly.
- ⚡ Observe for signs of allergic reaction to thrombolytics, such as itching, hives, flushing, fever, dyspnea, bronchospasm, hypotension, and/or cardiovascular collapse.
- Avoid administering aspirin or NSAIDs for pain or discomfort when the patient is receiving a thrombolytic. Acetaminophen can be substituted.
- Monitor the electrocardiogram (ECG) for presence of reperfusion dysrhythmias as the blood clot is dissolving; antidysrhythmic therapy may be indicated.
- Avoid venipuncture/arterial sticks.

Patient Teaching
General
- Explain thrombolytic treatment to patients and family. Be supportive.

Side Effects
- Advise patients to report any side effects such as lightheadedness, dizziness, palpitations, nausea, pruritus, or urticaria.

Evaluate Outcomes [Evaluation]
- Determine the effectiveness of drug therapy: the clot should have dissolved, vital signs should be stable with no signs or symptoms of active bleeding, and the patient should be pain free.

❗ TABLE 43.4 **Thrombolytics**

Drug	Route and Dosage	Uses and Considerations
Thrombolytics		
Tenecteplase	A: IV: 30–50 mg bolus over 5 s; administer within 30 min of arrival to hospital; *max:* 50 mg/dose	To promote fibrinolysis associated with coronary artery thrombosis and AMI. May cause bleeding, stroke, hematoma, epistaxis, and GI bleeding. PB: UK; t½: 90–130 min
Reteplase, r-PA	A: IV: 10 units over 2 min, follow in 30 min with second dose of 10 units; *max:* 20 units	For fibrinolytic therapy in AMI. Reteplae penetrates clots and activates plasminogen inside the clot, which may lead to a higher clot lysis rate. May cause bleeding, GI/intracranial bleeding, and purple-toe syndrome. PB: UK; t½: 13–16 min
Alteplase	See Prototype Drug Chart: Alteplase	
Hemostatics		
Aminocaproic acid	A: PO: LD: 5 g over first h; follow with 1–1.25 g/h for 8 h or until bleeding is controlled; *max:* 30 g/d A: IV: 4–5 g over first h, follow with 1 g/h for 8 h; or until bleeding controlled; *max:* 30 g/d	For bleeding due to hyperfibrinolysis. May cause hypotension, headache, dyspnea, edema, dizziness, bradycardia, vision impairment, and nausea, diarrhea. PB: UK; t½: 2 h

A, Adult; *AMI,* acute myocardial infarction; *d,* day; *GI,* gastrointestinal; *h,* hour; *IV,* intravenous; *LD,* loading dose; *max,* maximum; *min,* minutes; *PB,* protein binding; *PO,* by mouth; *s,* seconds; *t½,* half-life; *UK,* unknown.

CRITICAL THINKING CASE STUDY

A 57-year-old man has thrombophlebitis in the right lower leg. IV heparin, 5000 units by bolus, was given. After the IV bolus, heparin 5000 units given subcutaneously every 6 hours was prescribed. Other therapeutic means to decrease pain and alleviate swelling and redness were also prescribed, and an aPTT test was ordered.

1. Was the patient's heparin order within the safe daily dosage range?
2. What are the various methods for administering heparin?
3. Why was an aPTT test ordered? How would you determine whether the patient is within the desired range? Explain your answer.

After 5 days of heparin therapy, the patient was prescribed oral warfarin 5 mg daily. An INR test was ordered.

4. What is the pharmacologic action of warfarin? Is the warfarin dose within the safe daily dosage range? Explain your answer.
5. What are the half-life and protein binding for warfarin? If a patient takes a drug that is highly protein bound, would there be a drug interaction? Explain your answer.
6. Why was an INR ordered for the patient? What is the desired range?
7. What serious adverse reactions could result with prolonged use or large doses of warfarin?
8. What patient teaching interventions should the nurse include? List three interventions.
9. Months later, the patient has hematemesis. What nursing action should be taken?

REVIEW QUESTIONS

1. A patient is placed on heparin, and the nurse acknowledges that heparin is effective for preventing clot formation in patients who have which disorder(s)? (Select all that apply.)
   a. Coronary thrombosis
   b. Acute myocardial infarction
   c. Deep vein thrombosis
   d. Hemorrhagic stroke
   e. Disseminated intravascular coagulation
2. A patient who received heparin begins to bleed. The nurse anticipates that the health care provider will order which antidote?
   a. Protamine sulfate
   b. Phytonadione
   c. Aminocaproic acid
   d. Potassium chloride
3. A patient is prescribed enoxaparin. The nurse knows that low-molecular-weight heparin has what kind of half-life?
   a. A longer half-life than heparin
   b. A shorter half-life than heparin
   c. The same half-life as heparin
   d. A four-times shorter half-life than heparin
4. A patient had an orthopedic surgery and is prescribed enoxaparin. What would the nurse teach the patient and/or family members about this low-molecular-weight heparin before discharge?
   a. Visual demonstration of intramuscular heparin administration is recommended.
   b. Prothrombin time and international normalized ratio monitoring will be done weekly.
   c. Avoidance of green leafy vegetables is recommended.
   d. Watch for bleeding or excessive bruising.

5. A patient is being changed from an injectable anticoagulant to an oral anticoagulant. Which anticoagulant does the nurse realize is administered orally?
   a. Enoxaparin
   b. Warfarin
   c. Bivalirudin
   d. Dalteparin
   e. Tenecteplase
   f. Fondaparinux
6. A patient is taking warfarin 5 mg/day for atrial fibrillation. The patient's international normalized ratio is 3.8. The nurse would consider the international normalized ratio to be what?
   a. Within normal range
   b. Elevated range
   c. Low range
   d. Low-average range
7. Cilostazol is being prescribed for a patient with coronary artery disease. The nurse understands that which of the following is the major purpose for antiplatelet drug therapy?
   a. Dissolve the blood clot
   b. Decrease tissue necrosis
   c. Inhibit hepatic synthesis of vitamin K
   d. Suppress platelet aggregation

44

Antihyperlipidemics and Drugs to Improve Peripheral Blood Flow

http://evolve.elsevier.com/McCuistion/pharmacology

OBJECTIVES

- Describe the action of the two main drug groups: antihyperlipidemics and drugs that improve peripheral blood flow.
- Compare the side effects and adverse reactions of antihyperlipidemics.

- Differentiate the side effects and adverse reactions of peripheral vasodilators and blood viscosity reducer agents.
- Apply the Clinical Judgment [Nursing Process], including patient teaching, for antihyperlipidemics and blood viscosity reducer agents.

OUTLINE

Various drugs are used to maintain or decrease blood lipid concentrations and promote dilation of vessels. Drugs that lower blood lipids are called *antihyperlipidemics, antilipidemics, antilipemics,* and *hypolipidemics.* In this chapter, drugs used to lower lipoproteins are called antihyperlipidemics. Drugs that improve blood flow are called peripheral vasodilators, as they dilate vessels that have been narrowed by vasospasm, and blood viscosity reducer agents, which decrease viscosity of blood and increase erythrocyte flexibility.

LIPOPROTEINS

Lipids—cholesterol, triglycerides, and phospholipids—are bound in the inner shell of protein, a carrier that transports lipids in the bloodstream. When there is an excess of one or more lipids in the blood, the condition is known as hyperlipidemia or *hyperlipoproteinemia.* The four major categories of lipoprotein are high-density lipoprotein (HDL), low-density lipoprotein (LDL), very-low-density lipoprotein (VLDL), and chylomicrons. HDL, also known as "friendly" or "good" lipoprotein, is the smallest and densest lipoprotein, meaning that it contains more protein and less fat than the others. The function of HDL is to remove cholesterol from the bloodstream and deliver it to the liver for excretion in bile. LDL, the "bad" lipoprotein, contains 50% to 60% of cholesterol in the bloodstream. With an elevated LDL, the risk is greater for developing atherosclerotic plaques and heart disease. VLDL carries mostly triglycerides and less cholesterol. The chylomicrons are large particles that transport fatty acids and cholesterol to the liver. They are composed mostly of triglycerides.

Serum cholesterol and triglyceride measurements are frequently part of a regular physical examination or readmission evaluation and are used as baseline test results. If the levels are high, a 12- to 14-hour fasting lipid profile may be ordered. When cholesterol, triglycerides, and LDL are elevated, the patient is at increased risk for coronary artery disease (CAD). Table 44.1 lists the various serum lipids and their reference values (normal serum levels) according to risk classification.

APOLIPOPROTEINS

Apolipoproteins are within the lipoprotein shell and contain apolipoprotein (apo) A-1, B, and E. The major component of apoA-1 is HDL. The major component of apoB is LDL, which exists in two forms, apoB-100 and apoB-48. ApoB-100 has VLDL as well as LDL and is a better indicator of risk for CAD than LDL alone.

NONPHARMACOLOGIC METHODS OF CHOLESTEROL REDUCTION

Before drugs to lower LDL and raise HDL are prescribed, nondrug therapy should be initiated to decrease cholesterol. Saturated fats and cholesterol in the diet should be reduced. Total fat intake should be 30% or less of caloric intake, and cholesterol intake should be 300 mg/day or less. The patient should be advised to read labels on containers and buy appropriate foods. Patients should choose lean meats, especially chicken and fish.

In many cases, diet alone will not lower blood lipid levels. Because 75% to 85% of serum cholesterol is endogenously (internally) derived,

TABLE 44.1 Serum Lipid Values

Lipids	Desirable (mg/dL)	LEVEL OF RISK FOR CAD		
		Low Risk (mg/dL)	Moderate Risk (mg/dL)	High Risk (mg/dL)
Cholesterol	150–200	200	200–240	>240
Triglycerides	40–150	Values vary with age.	Values vary with age	>190
Lipoproteins				
LDL	<100	100–130	130–159	>160
HDL	>60	50–60	35–50	<35

CAD, Coronary artery disease; *HDL,* high-density lipoprotein; *LDL,* low-density lipoprotein; >, greater than; <, less than.

TABLE 44.2 Hyperlipidemia: Lipoprotein Phenotype

Type[a]	Major Lipids
I	Increased chylomicrons and increased triglycerides; uncommon
IIA	Increased low-density lipoprotein (LDL) and increased cholesterol; common
IIB	Increased very low-density lipoprotein (VLDL), increased LDL, increased cholesterol and triglycerides; very common
III	Moderately increased cholesterol and triglycerides; uncommon
IV	Increased VLDL and markedly increased triglycerides; very common
V	Increased chylomicrons, VLDL, and triglycerides; uncommon

[a]Types II and IV are commonly associated with coronary artery disease.

dietary modification alone will typically lower total cholesterol levels by only 10% to 30%. This and the fact that adherence to dietary restrictions is often short-lived explains why many patients do not respond to diet modification alone.

Exercise is an important aspect of the nonpharmacologic method to reduce cholesterol and increase HDL. For the older adult, exercise can be walking and bicycling. Smoking is another risk factor that should be eliminated. Smoking increases LDL cholesterol and decreases HDL.

If nonpharmacologic methods are ineffective for reducing LDL and VLDL cholesterol, and hyperlipidemia remains, antihyperlipidemic drugs are prescribed to lower blood lipid levels. It must be emphasized to the patient that dietary changes need to be made and an exercise program followed, even after drug therapy is initiated. The type of antihyperlipidemics ordered depends on the lipoprotein phenotype (Table 44.2).

ANTIHYPERLIPIDEMICS

Drugs that lower lipid levels include bile-acid sequestrants, fibrates (fibric acid), nicotinic acid, cholesterol absorption inhibitors, and hepatic 3-hydroxy-3-methylglutaryl-coenzyme A (HMG-CoA) reductase inhibitors, better known as *statins.* The statin drugs have fewer adverse effects and are well tolerated.

One of the first antihyperlipidemics, cholestyramine is a bile-acid sequestrant that reduces LDL cholesterol (LDL-C) levels by binding with bile acids in the intestine. It is effective against hyperlipidemia type II. This group may be used as an adjunct to the statins. The drug comes in a gritty powder that is mixed thoroughly in water or juice. Colestipol is another resin antihyperlipidemic similar to cholestyramine. Both are effective in lowering cholesterol. Colesevelam, another bile acid sequestrant similar to cholestyramine and colestipol,

is an agent that has fewer side effects (less constipation, flatulence, and cramping). Colesevelam also has less effect on the absorption of fat-soluble vitamins than the older agents and is usually the first-choice bile-acid sequestrant drug.

Gemfibrozil is a fibric acid derivative that is more effective for reducing triglyceride and VLDL levels than for reducing LDL. It is used primarily to reduce hyperlipidemia type IV, but it can also be used for type II hyperlipidemia. This drug is highly protein bound and should not be taken with anticoagulants because they compete for protein sites. The anticoagulant dose should be reduced during antihyperlipidemic therapy, and the international normalized ratio (INR) should be closely monitored. Fenofibrate has similar actions and some of the same side effects as gemfibrozil. If taken with warfarin, bleeding might occur. Both fenofibrate and gemfibrozil are highly protein bound.

Niacin (vitamin B$_3$) reduces VLDL and LDL. Niacin is actually very effective at lowering cholesterol levels, and its effect on the lipid profile is highly desirable. Because it has numerous side effects and large doses are required, as few as 20% of patients can initially tolerate niacin. However, with proper counseling, careful drug titration, and concomitant use of aspirin, this number can be increased to as much as 60% to 70%. Niacin is only recommended in specific clinical situations such as triglyceride levels over 500 mg/dL or if intolerant to other treatment.

Ezetimibe is a cholesterol absorption inhibitor that acts on the cells in the small intestine to inhibit cholesterol absorption. It decreases cholesterol from dietary absorption, reducing serum cholesterol, LDL, triglycerides, and apoB levels. Ezetimibe causes only a small increase in HDL. It must be combined with a statin (e.g., simvastatin) for optimum effect.

Statins

The statin drugs inhibit the enzyme HMG-CoA reductase in cholesterol biosynthesis; thus statins are called *HMG-CoA reductase inhibitors.* By inhibiting cholesterol synthesis in the liver, this group of antihyperlipidemics decreases the concentration of cholesterol, decreases LDL, and slightly increases HDL cholesterol. Reduction of LDL cholesterol may be seen as early as 2 weeks after initiating therapy. The statin group has been useful in decreasing CAD and reducing mortality rates.

Numerous statins have been approved since statins were first introduced. The present group of statins includes atorvastatin calcium, fluvastatin, lovastatin, pravastatin sodium, simvastatin, pitavastatin, and rosuvastatin. Lovastatin was the first statin used to decrease cholesterol. It is effective for lowering LDL (hyperlipidemia type II) within several weeks. Gastrointestinal (GI) disturbances, headaches, muscle cramps, and fatigue are early complaints. With all statins, serum liver enzymes should be monitored, and an annual eye examination is needed because cataract formation may result. The patient should report immediately any muscle aches or weakness, which can lead to rhabdomyolysis, a muscle disintegration that can become fatal.

The statins have actions in decreasing serum cholesterol, LDL, VLDL, and triglycerides, and they slightly elevate HDL. Atorvastatin, lovastatin, rosuvastatin, and simvastatin are more effective at lowering LDL than the other statins. Rosuvastatin and atorvastatin are at the top of the list of most prescribed drugs in the United States.

The statin drugs can be combined with other drugs to decrease blood pressure and blood clotting and to enhance the antihyperlipidemic effect. Examples are atorvastatin and amlodipine; and simvastatin and ezetimibe. Table 44.3 lists these combination drugs and their dosages, uses, and considerations.

If antihyperlipidemic therapy is withdrawn, cholesterol and LDL levels return to pretreatment levels. The patient taking an antihyperlipidemic drug should understand that antihyperlipidemic therapy is a lifetime commitment for maintaining a decrease in serum lipid levels. Abruptly stopping the statin drug could cause a threefold rebound effect that may cause death from acute myocardial infarction (AMI).

Laboratory Tests

Reference values for homocysteine, an amino acid, are 4 to 17 mmol/L (fasting). Homocysteine is a by-product of protein and is found in eggs, chicken, beef, and cheddar cheese. A high level of homocysteine has been linked to cardiovascular disease, stroke, and Alzheimer disease. It may also promote blood clotting, and it has been stated that an increase in serum homocysteine can damage the inner lining of blood vessels and promote a thickening and loss of flexibility in the vessel. Three vitamins that can lower serum homocysteine levels are vitamin B_6 (pyridoxine), vitamin B_{12} (cyanocobalamin), and folic acid.

High-sensitivity C-reactive protein (hsCRP) low risk is less than 1 mg/L, moderate risk is 1 to 3 mg/L, and high risk is greater than 3 mg/L. The standard C-reactive protein (CRP) is produced in the liver in response to tissue injury and inflammation. The hsCRP is a highly sensitive test for detecting the inflammatory protein that can be associated with cardiovascular and peripheral vascular disease. This test is frequently ordered along with cholesterol screening. Approximately one-third of persons who have had a heart attack have normal cholesterol levels and normal blood pressure. A positive hsCRP test can indicate that the patient is at high risk for CAD, making it a valuable test for predicting CAD. This test can detect an inflammatory process caused by the buildup of atherosclerotic plaque in the arterial system, particularly the coronary arteries.

Prototype Drug Chart: Atorvastatin lists the pharmacologic data for this frequently prescribed antihyperlipidemic.

Pharmacokinetics. Atorvastatin decreases LDL by 43% to 60% at an average dose of 10 to 80 mg. It is highly protein bound at 98%, so it usually is prescribed as a once-daily dose. Atorvastatin has a half-life of 14 hours.

Pharmacodynamics. The positive effect of lowering lipids with atorvastatin is seen in about 3 to 5 days. The peak time after a dose of atorvastatin is 1 to 2 hours; however, it takes 2 to 4 weeks to achieve therapeutic effect. Atorvastatin may be taken without regard to meals, but grapefruit juice should be avoided as it could cause an increase in drug concentration. When the patient is taking high doses of atorvastatin or any other statin, myopathy and rhabdomyolysis—disintegration of striated muscle fibers—may occur. If the patient complains of muscle pain or tenderness, it should be reported immediately.

Side Effects and Adverse Reactions

Side effects and adverse reactions of cholestyramine include constipation and peptic ulcer. Constipation can be decreased or alleviated by increasing intake of fluids and foods high in fiber. Early signs of peptic ulcer are nausea and abdominal discomfort, followed later by abdominal pain and distension. To avoid GI discomfort, the drug must be taken with and followed by sufficient fluids.

The many side effects of niacin—which include GI disturbances (nausea, vomiting, and diarrhea), flushing of the skin, abnormal liver function (elevated serum liver enzymes), hyperglycemia, and hyperuricemia—decrease its usefulness. However, as mentioned, aspirin and careful drug titration can reduce side effects to a manageable level in most patients.

The statin drugs can cause a dose-related increase in liver enzyme levels. Serum liver enzyme levels (alkaline phosphatase [ALP], alanine aminotransferase [ALT], gamma-glutamyl transferase [GGT]) should be monitored. Baseline liver enzyme studies should be obtained before initiating statin therapy. A slight transient increase in serum liver enzyme levels may be within normal range for the patient, but it should be rechecked in 1 week or so. Patients with acute hepatic disorders should not take a statin drug.

The serious skeletal muscle adverse effect, rhabdomyolysis, has been reported with use of the statin drug class, although it is rare. Patients should be advised to promptly report to the health care provider any unexplained muscle tenderness or weakness, especially if accompanied by fever or malaise. Table 44.3 lists the pharmacologic data for antihyperlipidemics.

❀ COMPLEMENTARY AND ALTERNATIVE THERAPIES

Statins

Black cohosh may potentiate an increase in liver enzymes.
Chinese skullcap may increase drug levels of rosuvastatin.
Cranberry may increase side effects of simvastatin.
Ginkgo biloba may increase drug levels of statins.
Green tea may increase side effects of statins.
St. John's wort may decrease effect and drug levels of statins.

DRUGS TO IMPROVE PERIPHERAL BLOOD FLOW

A common problem in older adults is peripheral arterial disease (PAD), also called *peripheral vascular disease* (PVD). It is characterized by numbness and coolness of the extremities, claudication (pain and weakness of a limb when walking but no symptoms at rest), and possible leg ulcers. The primary cause is arteriosclerosis and hyperlipidemia, resulting in atherosclerosis, after which the arteries become occluded.

Peripheral vasodilators increase blood flow to the extremities. They are used in peripheral vascular disorders of venous and arterial vessels. They are more effective for disorders that result from vasospasm (Raynaud disease) than from vessel occlusion or arteriosclerosis (arteriosclerosis obliterans, thromboangiitis obliterans [Buerger disease]). In Raynaud disease, cold exposure or emotional upset can trigger vasospasm of the toes and fingers; these patients have benefited from vasodilators. Patients with diabetes mellitus are more likely to have PAD by two to four times the usual rate and are at risk of intermittent claudication.

Individuals with PAD who are treated with HMG-CoA reductase inhibitors (statins) for dyslipidemia may see an improvement in intermittent claudication symptoms as well as a decrease in serum lipids. Also, patients with PAD who are hypertensive see improvement for both conditions when taking the antihypertensive drug ramipril, an angiotensin-converting enzyme (ACE) inhibitor. The alpha blocker prazosin and the calcium channel blocker nifedipine have been used as peripheral vasodilators. The antiplatelet drugs clopidogrel and aspirin

TABLE 44.3 Antihyperlipidemics

Generic	Route and Dosage	Uses and Considerations
Bile-Acid Sequestrants		
Cholestyramine	A: PO: Initially 4 g qd/bid before meals; mix powder in 60–180 mL of fluid; *maint:* 4–16 g daily in 2 divided doses; *max:* 24 g daily	For hypercholesterolemia. May cause anorexia, nausea, vomiting, diarrhea, constipation, steatorrhea, abdominal pain, eructation, flatulence, osteoporosis, peptic ulcer, and GI bleeding. PB: UK; t½: UK
Colesevelam	A: PO: 1.875 g bid; *max:* 3.75 g/d	For hypercholesterolemia. May cause headache, dyspepsia, constipation, hypertension, weakness, nausea, influenza, hypoglycemia, and hypertriglyceridemia. PB: UK; t½: UK
Colestipol hydrochloride	A: PO: Initially 2 g tablets qd or bid, may increase at 1- to 2-month intervals; *max:* 16 g daily	For hypercholesterolemia. May cause nausea, vomiting, diarrhea, constipation, cholelithiasis, peptic ulcer, and GI bleeding. PB: UK; t½: UK
Fibrates (Fibric Acid)		
Fenofibrate	Lipofen capsules: A: PO: 50–150 mg daily with food; *max:* 150 mg daily	For hypercholesterolemia and hypertriglyceridemia. May cause dizziness, headache, weakness, nausea, diarrhea, constipation, abdominal pain, cholelithiasis, back pain, and elevated hepatic enzymes. PB: 99%; t½: 20 h
Gemfibrozil	A: PO: 600 mg bid 30 min before morning and evening meals; *max:* 1200 mg daily	For hyperlipoproteinemia and hypertriglyceridemia. May cause dizziness, headache, elevated hepatic enzymes, fatigue, nausea, vomiting, dyspepsia, abdominal pain, cholelithiasis, constipation, and diarrhea. PB: 95%; t½: 1.5 h
Niacin		
Niacin	Regular release: A: PO: Initially 250 mg qd after evening meal; may increase q4–7d; *max:* 6 g qd Sustained release: A: PO: 1–2 g/d in 2–3 divided doses; *max:* 2 g/d	For hypercholesterolemia. May cause flushing, hypotension, dizziness, headache, cough, pruritus, nausea, vomiting, diarrhea, hyperglycemia, hyperuricemia, rash, edema, and weakness. PB: <20%; t½: 20–48 min
Cholesterol Absorption Inhibitors		
Ezetimibe	A: PO: 10 mg daily; *max:* 10 mg daily	For hypercholesterolemia. May cause diarrhea, arthralgia, abdominal and back pain, fatigue, infection, pharyngitis, elevated hepatic enzymes, cholelithiasis, and myalgia. PB: 90%; t½: 22 h
Statins (HMG-CoA Reductase Inhibitors)		
Atorvastatin calcium	See Prototype Drug Chart: Atorvastatin	
Fluvastatin sodium	Regular release: A: PO: Initially 20–40 mg daily; *maint:* 20–80 mg daily; *max:* 80 mg qd Extended release: A: PO: 20–80 mg daily; *max:* 80 mg daily	For hypercholesterolemia. May cause headache, nausea, abdominal pain, dyspepsia, diarrhea, hypertension, myalgia, peripheral edema, influenza, arthralgia, constipation, and elevated hepatic enzymes. PB: 98%; t½: Immediate release 2.5–2.7 h, extended release 9 h
Lovastatin	Immediate release: A: PO: Initially 10–20 mg qd with evening meal; *max:* 80 mg qd Extended release: A: PO: 20–60 mg qd at bedtime; *max:* 60 mg qd	For hypercholesterolemia. May cause headache, sinusitis, infection, arthralgia, nausea, abdominal pain, diarrhea, constipation, flatulence, influenza, weakness, back pain, and myalgia. PB: 95%; t½: 1.1–1.7 h
Pravastatin sodium	A: PO: Initially 40 mg daily; *maint:* 10–80 mg daily; *max:* 80 mg daily	For hypercholesterolemia. May cause headache, dizziness, dyspepsia, flatulence, nausea, vomiting, diarrhea, fatigue, and muscular skeletal pain. PB: 50%; t½: 2–3 h
Rosuvastatin	A: PO: 5–10 mg qd; *maint:* 5–40 mg/d; *max:* 40 mg qd	For hypercholesterolemia. May cause dizziness, headache, nausea, constipation, diarrhea, abdominal pain, arthralgia, myalgia, and dyspepsia. PB: 88%; t½: 20 h
Simvastatin	A: PO: Initially 10–20 mg qd at hs; *maint:* 5–40 mg daily in evening; *max:* 40 mg daily	For hypercholesterolemia. May cause headache, edema, insomnia, nausea, myalgia, abdominal pain, constipation, atrial fibrillation, and infection. PB: 95%; t½: 1.9 h
Pitavastatin	A: PO: Initially 2 mg qd; *max:* 4 mg qd	For hypercholesterolemia, hyperlipoproteinemia, and hypertriglyceridemia. May cause headache, myalgia, back pain, constipation, diarrhea, arthralgia, and abdominal pain. PB: 99%; t½: 12 h
Miscellaneous Antilipemics		
Icosapent ethyl	A: PO: 2 g q12h; *max:* 4 g daily with food	For hypertriglyceridemia. May cause arthralgia, bleeding, peripheral edema, gout, musculoskeletal pain, constipation, and atrial fibrillation/flutter. PB: 99%; t½: 89 h

Continued

TABLE 44.3   Antihyperlipidemics—cont'd

Generic	Route and Dosage	Uses and Considerations
Lomitapide	A: PO: Initially 5 mg daily 2 h after evening meal, may increase to 10 mg in 2 wk; *maint:* 10–60 mg daily; *max:* 60 mg daily	For hypercholesterolemia. May cause dizziness, fatigue, back pain, influenza, chest pain, elevated hepatic enzymes, dyspepsia, nausea, vomiting, diarrhea, constipation, abdominal pain, GERD, steatosis, weight loss, flatulence, and pharyngitis. PB: 99.8%; t½: 39.7 h
Mipomersen	A: Subcut: 200 mg/wk; *max:* 200 mg/wk	For hypercholesterolemia. May cause headache, fatigue, nausea, influenza, injection site reaction/skin discoloration, hematoma, antibody formation, pruritus, erythema, steatosis, elevated hepatic enzymes, and proteinuria. PB: 90%; t½: 1–2 mo
Alirocumab	A: Subcut: Initially 75 mg q2wk; *max:* 150 mg q2wk	For hypercholesterolemia and hyperlipidemia. May cause myalgia, diarrhea, antibody formation, infection, injection site reaction, nasopharyngitis, chest pain, and influenza. PB: UK; t½: 17–20 d
Evolocumab	A: Subcut: 140 mg q2wk or 420 mg q1mo; *max:* 420 mg/mo	For hypercholesterolemia. May cause dizziness, headache, hyperglycemia, infection, arthralgia, myalgia, diarrhea, nasopharyngitis, hypertension, influenza, sinusitis, cough, back pain, musculoskeletal pain, and injection site reaction. PB: UK; t½: 11–17 d
Bempedoic acid	A: PO: 180 mg/d; *max:* 180 mg/d	For hypercholesterolemia. May cause back/abdominal pain, muscle cramps, infection, hyperuricemia, leukopenia, and thrombocytosis. PB: 99%; t½: 10–32 h
Evinacumab	A: IV: 15 mg/kg over 60 min q4wk; *max:* 15 mg/kg q4wk	For hypercholesterolemia. May cause pharyngitis, rhinorrhea, nasal congestion, infusion-related reactions, dizziness, weakness, abdominal pain, nausea, and constipation. PB: UK; t½: UK
Combination Antihyperlipidemic Drugs		
Amlodipine and atorvastatin	A: PO: Initially 5–10 mg amlodipine and 10–20 mg atorvastatin daily; *maint:* 10 mg amlodipine and 10–80 mg atorvastatin daily; *max:* 10 mg amlodipine and 80 mg atorvastatin daily Older A: PO: 2.5 mg amlodipine and 10–20 mg atorvastatin; *max:* 10 mg amlodipine and 80 mg atorvastatin	For hypercholesterolemia, hyperlipoproteinemia, and hypertriglyceridemia. May cause headache, fatigue, nasopharyngitis, gynecomastia, dyspepsia, nausea, diarrhea, arthralgia, palpitations, and edema. PB: amlodipine 93%, atorvastatin 98%; t½: amlodipine 30–50 h, atorvastatin 14 h
Ezetimibe and simvastatin	A: PO: Initially 10 mg ezetimibe and 10–20 mg simvastatin qd at hs; *maint:* 10 mg ezetimibe and 40 mg simvastatin daily; *max:* 10 mg ezetimibe and 40 mg simvastatin daily	For hypercholesterolemia and hyperlipoproteinemia. May cause headache, diarrhea, myalgia, infection, influenza, musculoskeletal pain, and elevated hepatic enzymes. PB: ezetimibe 90%, simvastatin 95%; t½: ezetimibe 22 h, simvastatin 1.9 h

A, Adult; *ac,* before meals; *bid,* twice a day; *d,* day; *GERD,* gastroesophageal reflux disease; *GI,* gastrointestinal; *h,* hour; *HMG-CoA,* 3-hydroxy-3-methylglutaryl-coenzyme A; *maint,* maintenance; *max,* maximum; *min,* minute; *mo,* months; *NA,* not applicable; *PB,* protein binding; *PO,* by mouth; *q,* every; *subcut,* subcutaneously; *t½,* half-life; *tab,* tablet; *tid,* three times a day; *UK,* unknown; *URI,* upper respiratory infection; *UTI,* urinary tract infection; *wk,* weeks; *y,* year; <, less than; >, greater than.

have been used to decrease PAD symptoms. Another antiplatelet drug, cilostazol, has been approved by the US Food and Drug Administration (FDA) for treating intermittent claudication. It decreases arterial thrombi. Ginkgo biloba, taken with an antiplatelet drug, has been used to treat intermittent claudication because of its vasodilating and antioxidant effects, although this product has not been approved by the FDA. Most of the drugs used for treating PAD do not cure the health problem, but they can aid in relieving PAD symptoms.

 COMPLEMENTARY AND ALTERNATIVE THERAPIES

Cilostazol
Licorice may cause hypokalemia, which can potentiate drug toxicity.

Cilostazol

Cilostazol is an antiplatelet drug that has a dual purpose of inhibiting platelet aggregation as well as causing vasodilation to treat intermittent claudication. Prototype Drug Chart: Cilostazol lists the pharmacologic data for cilostazol.

Pharmacokinetics. Cilostazol is a direct-acting vasodilator that is absorbed from the GI tract. It is highly protein bound at 95% to 98% and has a half-life of 11 to 13 hours and is usually taken two times a day.

Pharmacodynamics. Cilostazol causes arterial vasodilation, especially within the femoral vasculature. Common adverse effects include headache, diarrhea, and abnormal stools. This drug has an onset of action within 2 to 12 weeks.

Side Effects and Adverse Reactions

Dizziness, tachycardia, palpitations, orthostatic hypotension, nausea, vomiting, and diarrhea may occur with cilostazol. The effectiveness of peripheral vasodilators in increasing blood flow by vasodilation is questionable in the presence of arteriosclerosis. These drugs may decrease some of the symptoms of cerebrovascular insufficiency. Table 44.4 lists the peripheral vasodilators and their dosages, uses, and considerations.

Pentoxifylline

Pentoxifylline, classified as a *hemorrheologic agent or blood viscosity reducer agent,* improves microcirculation and tissue perfusion by decreasing blood viscosity and improving the flexibility of erythrocytes, thus increasing tissue oxygenation. It inhibits aggregation of

PROTOTYPE DRUG CHART

Atorvastatin

Drug Class	Dosage
Antihyperlipidemic: HMG-CoA reductase inhibitor	A: PO: Initially 10–20 mg qd; *maint:* 10–80 mg qd; *max:* 80 mg qd
Contraindications	**Drug-Lab-Food Interactions**
Hepatic disease/encephalopathy, cholestasis, pregnancy, breastfeeding *Caution:* Alcohol use disorder, diabetes mellitus, seizures, renal impairment, stroke, hypotension, hypothyroidism, electrolyte imbalance, rhabdomyolysis, older adults	Drug: Decreased effect with antacids, phenytoin, and propranolol; may increase digoxin level, oral contraceptive efficacy; increased drug effects with macrolide antibiotics and antifungals
Pharmacokinetics	**Pharmacodynamics**
Absorption: Rapid Distribution: PB: 98% Metabolism: t½: 14–30 h Excretion: Primarily in feces	PO: Onset: UK Peak: 1–2 h Duration: UK
Therapeutic Effects/Uses	
To decrease cholesterol levels and serum lipids, especially LDL and triglycerides; for treatment of atherosclerosis, hypercholesterolemia, hyperlipoproteinemia, and hypertriglyceridemia Mechanism of Action: Inhibits HMG-CoA reductase, the enzyme necessary for hepatic production of cholesterol.	
Side Effects	**Adverse Reactions**
Dizziness, insomnia, memory impairment, flushing, nightmares, blurred vision, weakness, myalgia, dyspepsia, nausea, diarrhea, flatulence, abdominal pain, peripheral neuropathy	Rhabdomyolysis (rare), tendon rupture hyperglycemia, diabetes mellitus, *Life-threatening:* Hepatic/renal failure, stroke, leukopenia, hemolytic anemia, thrombocytopenia

A, Adult; *d*, day; *h*, hour; *HMG-CoA*, 3-hydroxy-3-methyl glutaryl-coenzyme A; *LDL*, low-density lipoprotein; *maint*, maintenance; *max*, maximum dosage; *PB*, protein binding; *PO*, by mouth; *t½*, half-life; *UK*, unknown.

◎ CLINICAL JUDGMENT [NURSING PROCESS]

Antihyperlipidemics

Concept: Perfusion
- The passage of blood flow through the arteries and capillaries that deliver oxygen and nutrients to body cells

Recognize Cues [Assessment]
- Assess vital signs and baseline serum chemistry values (cholesterol, triglycerides, aspartate aminotransferase [AST], alanine aminotransferase [ALT], and creatine phosphokinase [CPK]).
- Obtain a medical history. Statin drugs are contraindicated for patients with liver disorders and in pregnant patients.

Analyze Cues and Prioritize Hypothesis [Patient Problems]
- Hyperglycemia
- Vomiting
- Ischemia
- Nausea
- Decreased visual acuity

Generate Solutions [Planning]
- The patient's cholesterol level will be less than 200 mg/dL in 6 to 8 weeks.
- The patient will choose foods from a list that are low in fat, cholesterol, and complex sugars.

Take Action [Nursing Interventions]
- Monitor the patient's blood lipid levels—cholesterol, triglycerides, low-density lipoprotein (LDL), and high-density lipoprotein (HDL)—every 6 to 8 weeks

for the first 6 months after statin therapy, then every 3 to 6 months. For a lipid-level profile, the patient should fast for 12 to 14 hours. The desired values are less than 200 mg/dL for cholesterol; less than 150 mg/dL for triglycerides, although this can vary; less than 100 mg/dL for LDL; and more than 60 mg/dL for HDL. Cholesterol levels higher than 240 mg/dL, LDL levels higher than 160 mg/dL, and HDL levels below 35 mg/dL can lead to severe cardiovascular events or cerebrovascular accident (CVA).
- Monitor laboratory tests for liver function (ALT, alkaline phosphatase [ALP], and gamma-glutamyl transferase [GGT]). Antihyperlipidemic drugs can cause liver disorders.
- Observe for signs and symptoms of gastrointestinal (GI) upset. Taking the drug with sufficient water or with meals may alleviate some of the discomfort.

Patient Teaching
General
- Emphasize the need to comply with the drug regimen to lower blood lipids.
- Inform patients that it may take several weeks before blood lipid levels decline.
- Explain that laboratory tests for blood lipids—cholesterol, triglycerides, LDL, and HDL—are usually ordered every 3 to 6 months.
- Advise patients to have serum liver enzymes monitored as indicated by their health care provider. Lovastatin, pravastatin, and simvastatin are contraindicated in acute hepatic disease and pregnancy.
- Instruct patients to have an annual eye examination and to report changes in visual acuity.

Continued

CLINICAL JUDGMENT [NURSING PROCESS]—CONT'D

Antihyperlipidemics

- Advise patients taking gemfibrozil that the drug may increase their risk for bleeding if they are also taking an oral anticoagulant, so bleeding should be reported. Drug dosage can be changed, or another antihyperlipidemic may be ordered.
- Instruct patients to take nicotinic acid with meals to decrease GI discomfort.

Self-Administration

- Teach patients to mix cholestyramine/colestipol powder well in water or juice.

Side Effects of Cholestyramine, Colestipol, and Niacin

- Advise patients that constipation may occur with cholestyramine and colestipol. Increasing fluid intake and food bulk should help alleviate the problem.
- Explain to patients that flushing is common with niacin and should decrease with continued use of the drug. Usually the drug is started at a low dose.
- Advise patients that large doses of niacin can cause vasodilation and produce dizziness and faintness (syncope).

Side Effects of Ezetimibe

- Explain to patients that ezetimibe may cause headaches and GI upset. If it continues, notify the health care provider.

Side Effects of Statins

- Explain to patients that serum liver enzyme levels are periodically monitored.
- ⚡ Encourage patients to promptly report any unexplained muscle tenderness or weakness that may be caused by rhabdomyolysis.
- ⚡ Caution patients not to abruptly stop taking their statin drug because a serious rebound effect might occur that could lead to acute myocardial infarction (AMI) and possible death. Before stopping a statin, the patient should talk to his or her health care provider.

Diet

- Explain to patients that GI discomfort is a common problem with most antihyperlipidemics. Suggest increasing fluid intake when taking the medication.
- Encourage patients to consume foods that are low in animal fats, cholesterol, and complex sugars. Lovastatin and other antihyperlipidemics are adjuncts to, not substitutes for, a low-fat diet.

Evaluate Outcomes [Evaluation]

- Evaluate effectiveness of the antihyperlipidemic drug. The patient's cholesterol level should be within the desired range.
- Determine that the patient is maintaining a low-fat, low-cholesterol diet.

📄 PROTOTYPE DRUG CHART

Cilostazol

Drug Class	Dosage
Direct-acting vasodilator	A: PO: 50–100 mg q12h 30 min before or 2 h after morning and evening meals with full glass of water; do not administer with grapefruit juice; *max:* 200 mg qd
Contraindications	**Drug-Lab-Food Interactions**
Heart failure, hypersensitivity, bleeding disorders *Caution:* Hepatic and renal disease, tobacco smokers, cardiovascular disease, dysrhythmias, pregnancy, breastfeeding, older adults	Drug: Increased effects with aspirin, cimetidine, clarithromycin, erythromycin, enoxaparin, ticlopidine, warfarin Food: Grapefruit and green tea will increase levels; ginger and ginkgo biloba may prolong bleeding time; St. John's wort will decrease effect.
Pharmacokinetics	**Pharmacodynamics**
Absorption: PO: Readily absorbed Distribution: PB: 95%–98% Metabolism: t½: 11–13 h Excretion: In urine (74%), feces (20%)	PO: Onset: 2–12 wk Peak: UK Duration: UK
Therapeutic Effects/Uses	
To treat peripheral vascular disease and claudication Mechanism of Action: Acts directly to inhibit platelet aggregation and cause vasodilation, especially in femoral vasculature.	
Side Effects	**Adverse Reactions**
Dizziness, headache, nasopharyngitis, rhinitis, cough, dyspepsia, myalgia, flushing, nausea, vomiting, flatulence, diarrhea, melena, back and abdominal pain, peripheral edema, infection, influenza, cholelithiasis	Tachycardia, palpitations, angina, HF, MI, hypo/hypertension, peptic ulcer, gout, diabetes mellitus, elevated hepatic enzymes *Life-threatening:* Thrombocytopenia, leukopenia, aplastic anemia, agranulocytosis, dysrhythmias, Stevens-Johnson syndrome

A, Adult; *h,* hour; *max,* maximum dosage; *min,* minutes; *PB,* protein binding; *PO,* by mouth; *q,* every; *t½,* half-life; *UK,* unknown; *wk,* weeks.

TABLE 44.4   Peripheral Vasodilators and Blood Viscosity Reducer Agent

Generic	Route and Dosage	Uses and Considerations
Direct-Acting Vasodilator		
Cilostazol	See Prototype Drug Chart: Cilostazol	
Blood Viscosity Reducer Agent		
Pentoxifylline	A: PO: 400 mg tid with meals; *max:* 1200 mg daily	For claudication. May cause blurred vision, confusion, nausea, vomiting, constipation, cholestasis, tachycardia, edema, and hypotension. PB: UK; t½: 0.4–0.8 h

A, Adult; *max,* maximum; *PB,* protein binding; *PO,* by mouth; *t½,* half-life; *tid,* three times a day; *UK,* unknown.

◎ CLINICAL JUDGMENT [NURSING PROCESS]

Peripheral Vasodilator: Cilostazol

Concept: Perfusion
- The passage of blood flow through arteries and capillaries that deliver oxygen and nutrients to body cells

Recognize Cues [Assessment]
- Obtain baseline vital signs for future comparison.
- Assess for signs of inadequate blood flow to the extremities: pallor, coldness of extremities, and pain.

Analyze Cues and Prioritize Hypothesis [Patient Problems]
- Hyperglycemia
- Hypotension
- Ischemia
- Discomfort
- Decreased visual acuity

Generate Solutions [Planning]
- The patient's legs will be warm and pink.
- The patient will report that pain has decreased.

Take Action [Nursing Interventions]
- Monitor vital signs, especially blood pressure and heart rate. Tachycardia and orthostatic hypotension can be problematic with peripheral vasodilators.

Patient Teaching
General
- Inform patients that a desired therapeutic response may take 1.5 to 3 months.
- Advise patients not to smoke because smoking increases vasospasm.
- Instruct patients to use aspirin or aspirin-like compounds only with the health care provider's approval. Salicylates help prevent platelet aggregation.

Side Effects
- Encourage patients to change position slowly but frequently to avoid orthostatic hypotension. Orthostatic hypotension is common when taking high doses of a vasodilator.
- Instruct patients to report side effects of cilostazol, such as flushing, headaches, and dizziness.

Diet
- Suggest that patients with gastrointestinal (GI) disturbances take cilostazol with meals.
- Advise patients not to ingest alcohol with a vasodilator because it may cause a hypotensive reaction.

Evaluate Outcomes [Evaluation]
- Evaluate effectiveness of cilostazol therapy; blood flow is increased in extremities, and pain has subsided.
- The patient should experience no side effects from the prescribed drug.

platelets and red blood cells, and because it decreases blood viscosity, it helps increase flow through peripheral vessels. A derivative of the xanthine group, pentoxifylline has been approved by the FDA for patients with intermittent claudication, and it has been prescribed for those with Buerger disease resulting from arterial occlusions. However, in one research study, pentoxifylline was not determined to be more effective than a placebo.

Reactions to an overdose of pentoxifylline include tachycardia, hypotension, and blurred vision. The drug should be taken with food, and the patient should avoid smoking because nicotine increases vasoconstriction. Patients taking an antihypertensive drug along with pentoxifylline may need to have the antihypertensive dosage decreased to avoid side effects. The most common side effects of pentoxifylline are nausea and vomiting.

■ CRITICAL THINKING CASE STUDY

The patient had a myocardial infarction (MI) 3 years ago. He was prescribed gemfibrozil 600 mg twice daily before meals, but his cholesterol remained between 220 and 240 mg/dL, and his LDL was 140 mg/dL. His anticholesterol drug was changed to simvastatin 20 mg/day in the evening.
1. How does simvastatin differ from gemfibrozil?
2. Why do you think the patient's cholesterol drug, gemfibrozil, was changed to simvastatin?
3. While the patient is taking simvastatin, which group of serum levels should be monitored?

4. How long after taking simvastatin should the patient's cholesterol and lipoproteins be checked?
5. What is the maximum dose for simvastatin?
6. The patient complains of muscle pain and muscle weakness. What might this indicate?
7. Could the patient receive both gemfibrozil and simvastatin? Explain your answer.
8. The patient is on vacation and does not have enough simvastatin tablets. What should he do?

REVIEW QUESTIONS

1. A patient has a serum cholesterol level of 265 mg/dL, a triglyceride level of 235 mg/dL, and a low-density lipoprotein of 180 mg/dL. What do these serum levels indicate?
   a. Hypolipidemia
   b. Normolipidemia
   c. Hyperlipidemia
   d. Alipidemia

2 The nurse knows that a patient's total cholesterol level should be within which range?
   a. 150 to 200 mg/dL
   b. 200 to 225 mg/dL
   c. 225 to 250 mg/dL
   d. Greater than 250 mg/dL

3. A patient has a low-density lipoprotein of 175 mg/dL and a high-density lipoprotein of 30 mg/dL. What teaching should the nurse implement for this patient?
   a. Discuss medications ordered, dietary changes, and exercise.
   b. No changes in lifestyle are needed; continue with the current plan.
   c. Discuss how to have fat intake be 40% of caloric intake.
   d. Begin keeping a food diary, and schedule laboratory work to be repeated in 6 months.

4. Which laboratory test value does the nurse realize can contribute to the development of cardiovascular disease and stroke?
   a. Decreased antidiuretic hormone
   b. Increased homocysteine level
   c. Decreased triglycerides
   d. Increased high-density lipoprotein level

5. A patient is taking lovastatin. Which serum level is most important for the nurse to monitor?
   a. Blood urea nitrogen
   b. Complete blood count
   c. Cardiac enzymes
   d. Hepatic enzymes

6. For what severe skeletal muscle adverse reaction should the nurse observe in a patient taking rosuvastatin?
   a. Myasthenia gravis
   b. Rhabdomyolysis
   c. Dyskinesia
   d. Agranulocytosis

7. A patient is taking ezetimibe and asks the nurse how it works. The nurse should explain that ezetimibe does what?
   a. Inhibits absorption of dietary cholesterol in the intestines
   b. Binds with bile acids in the intestines to reduce low-density lipoprotein levels
   c. Inhibits 3-hydroxy-3-methylglutaryl-coenzyme A reductase, which is necessary for cholesterol production in the liver
   d. Forms insoluble complexes and reduces circulating cholesterol in the blood

8. A patient is diagnosed with peripheral arterial disease. He is prescribed pentoxifylline. What does the nurse realize are the effects of pentoxifylline? (Select all that apply.)
   a. May lead to hypertension and bradycardia
   b. Improves microcirculation and tissue perfusion
   c. Decreases blood viscosity and improves flexibility of erythrocytes
   d. Alleviates intermittent claudication
   e. Commonly causes an adverse effect of rhabdomyolysis
   f. Allows vasodilation of arteries in skeletal muscles

45

Gastrointestinal Tract Disorders

http://evolve.elsevier.com/McCuistion/pharmacology

OBJECTIVES

- Compare the pharmacological treatment of vomiting, diarrhea, and constipation.
- Differentiate the actions and side effects of antiemetics, emetics, antidiarrheals, and laxatives.

- Apply the Clinical Judgment [Nursing Process] for the patient taking antiemetics, antidiarrheals, and laxatives.
- Differentiate contraindications to the use of antiemetics, emetics, antidiarrheals, and laxatives.

OUTLINE

OVERVIEW OF THE GASTROINTESTINAL SYSTEM

The gastrointestinal (GI) system, or GI tract, comprises the alimentary canal and the digestive tract, and begins at the oral cavity and ends at the anus. Major structures of the GI system are (1) the oral cavity (mouth, tongue, and pharynx), (2) the esophagus, (3) the stomach, (4) the small intestine (duodenum, jejunum, and ileum), (5) the large intestine (cecum, colon, and rectum), and (6) the anus. The accessory organs and glands that contribute to the digestive process are (1) the salivary glands, (2) the pancreas, (3) the gallbladder, and (4) the liver (Fig. 45.1). The main functions of the GI system are digestion of food particles and absorption of the digestive contents—nutrients, electrolytes, minerals, and fluids—into the circulatory system for cellular use. Digestion and absorption take place in the small intestine and, to a lesser extent, in the stomach. Undigested material passes through the lower intestinal tract with the aid of peristalsis to the rectum and anus, where it is excreted as feces, or stool.

Oral Cavity

The oral cavity, or mouth, starts the digestive process by (1) breaking up food into smaller particles; (2) adding saliva, which contains the enzyme amylase for digesting starch (the beginning of the digestive process); and (3) swallowing, a voluntary movement of food that becomes involuntary (peristalsis) in the esophagus, stomach, and intestines. Swallowing occurs in the pharynx (throat), which connects the mouth and esophagus.

Esophagus

The esophagus, a tube that extends from the pharynx to the stomach, is composed of striated muscle in its upper portion and smooth muscle in its lower portion. The inner lining of the esophagus is a mucous membrane that secretes mucus. The peristaltic process of contraction begins in the esophagus and ends in the lower large intestine. There are two sphincters, the *superior esophageal (hyperpharyngeal) sphincter* and the *lower esophageal sphincter*. The lower esophageal sphincter prevents gastric reflux into the esophagus, a condition called *reflux esophagitis*.

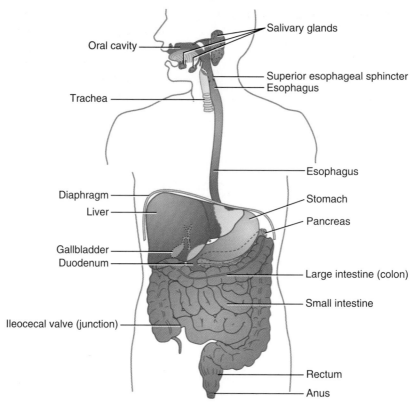

Fig. 45.1 The gastrointestinal system and alimentary canal.

Stomach

The stomach is a hollow organ that lies between the esophagus and the intestine. The body of the stomach has lesser and greater curvatures. It can hold 1000 to 2000 mL of gastric contents and empties in 2 to 6 hours (average is 3 to 4 hours), depending on gastric content and motility. Two sphincters—the *cardiac sphincter,* which lies at the upper opening of the stomach, and the *pyloric sphincter,* located at the lower portion of the stomach or the head of the duodenum—regulate the entrance of food into the stomach.

The interior lining of the stomach has mucosal folds that contain glands that secrete gastric juices. The four types of cells in the stomach mucosa that secrete these juices are (1) *chief cells,* which secrete the proenzyme pepsinogen (pepsin); (2) *parietal cells,* which secrete hydrochloric acid (HCl); (3) *gastrin-producing cells,* which secrete gastrin, a hormone that regulates enzyme release during digestion; and (4) *mucus-producing cells* that release mucus to protect the stomach lining, which extends into the duodenum.

Small Intestine

The small intestine begins at the pyloric sphincter of the stomach and extends to the ileocecal valve at the cecum. Most drug absorption occurs in the duodenum, but lipid-soluble drugs and alcohol are absorbed from the stomach. The lower digestive process begins in the stomach, but most of the digestive contents are absorbed from the small intestine. The duodenum releases the hormone secretin, which suppresses gastric acid secretion and causes the intestinal juices to have a higher pH than the gastric juices. The intestinal cells also release the hormone cholecystokinin, which in turn stimulates the release of pancreatic enzymes and the contraction of the gallbladder to release bile into the duodenum. Hormones, bile, and pancreatic enzymes (trypsin, chymotrypsin, lipase, and amylase) complete the digestion of carbohydrates, protein, and fat in preparation for absorption.

Large Intestine

The large intestine accepts undigested material from the small intestine, absorbs water, secretes mucus, and with peristaltic contractions moves the remaining intestinal contents to the rectum for elimination. Defecation completes the process.

DRUGS FOR GASTROINTESTINAL DISORDERS

Vomiting, diarrhea, and constipation are GI problems that frequently require drug intervention. This chapter describes the antiemetics used to control vomiting. This chapter also discusses emetics used to eliminate ingested toxins and drugs, antidiarrheal drugs, and laxatives. The nursing process is considered in relation to each of these drug groups.

Drug groups used to correct or control vomiting, diarrhea, and constipation are antiemetics, emetics, antidiarrheals, and laxatives. Each of these drug groups is discussed separately. Drugs used to treat peptic ulcers are discussed in Chapter 43.

VOMITING

Vomiting (emesis), the expulsion of gastric contents, has a multitude of causes, including motion sickness, viral and bacterial infection, food intolerance, surgery, pregnancy, pain, shock, effects of selected drugs (e.g., antineoplastics, antibiotics), radiation, and disturbances of the middle ear that affect equilibrium. Nausea, a queasy sensation, may or may not precede the expulsion. The cause of the vomiting must be identified. Antiemetics can mask the underlying cause of vomiting and should not be used until the cause has been determined, unless the vomiting is so severe as to cause dehydration and electrolyte imbalance.

Two major cerebral centers—the chemoreceptor trigger zone (CTZ), which lies near the medulla, and the vomiting center in the medulla—cause vomiting when stimulated (Fig. 45.2). The CTZ receives most of the impulses from drugs, toxins, and the vestibular center in the ear and transmits them to the vomiting center. The neurotransmitter dopamine stimulates the CTZ, which in turn stimulates the vomiting center. Levodopa, a drug with dopamine-like properties, can cause vomiting by stimulating the CTZ. Some sensory impulses—such as odor, smell, taste, and gastric mucosal irritation—are transmitted directly to the vomiting center. The neurotransmitter acetylcholine is also a vomiting stimulant. When the vomiting center is stimulated, the motor neuron responds by causing contraction of the diaphragm, the anterior abdominal muscles, and the stomach. The glottis closes, the abdominal wall moves upward, and vomiting occurs.

Nonpharmacologic measures should be used first when nausea and vomiting occur. If the nonpharmacologic measures are not effective, antiemetics are combined with nonpharmacologic measures. The two major groups of antiemetics are *nonprescription* (antihistamines, bismuth subsalicylate, and phosphorated carbohydrate solution) and *prescription* (antihistamines, dopamine antagonists, serotonin antagonists, cannabinoids, and miscellaneous antiemetics).

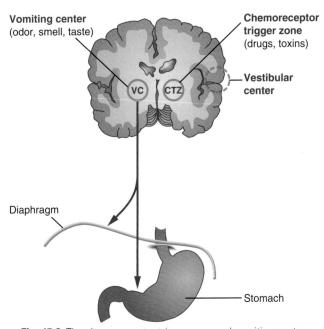

Fig. 45.2 The chemoreceptor trigger zone and vomiting center.

Nonpharmacologic Measures

The nonpharmacologic methods of decreasing nausea and vomiting include administration of weak tea, flat soda, gelatin, Gatorade, and Pedialyte (for use in children). Crackers and dry toast may be helpful. When dehydration becomes severe, intravenous (IV) fluids are needed to restore body fluid balance.

Nonprescription Antiemetics

Nonprescription antiemetics (antivomiting agents) can be purchased as over-the-counter (OTC) drugs. These drugs are frequently used to prevent motion sickness but have minimal effect on controlling severe vomiting resulting from anticancer agents (antineoplastics), radiation, and toxins. To prevent motion sickness, the antiemetic should be taken 30 minutes before travel. These drugs are not effective in relieving motion sickness if taken after vomiting has occurred.

Selected antihistamine antiemetics—such as dimenhydrinate, cyclizine hydrochloride, meclizine hydrochloride, and diphenhydramine hydrochloride—can be purchased without a prescription to prevent nausea, vomiting, and dizziness (vertigo) caused by motion. These drugs inhibit vestibular stimulation in the middle ear. Diphenhydramine is also used to prevent or alleviate allergic reactions to drugs, insects, and food by acting as an antagonist to histamine$_1$ (H$_1$) receptors.

The side effects of antihistamine antiemetics are similar to those of anticholinergics and include drowsiness, dry mouth, and constipation. Table 45.1 lists the nonprescription antiemetics used for vomiting caused by motion sickness. Diphenhydramine characteristics are explained in Prototype Drug Chart: Diphenhydramine in Chapter 35.

Several nonprescription drugs, such as bismuth subsalicylate, act directly on the gastric mucosa to suppress vomiting. They are marketed in liquid and chewable tablet forms and can be taken for gastric discomfort or diarrhea. Phosphorated carbohydrate solution, a hyperosmolar carbohydrate, decreases nausea and vomiting by changing the gastric pH; it may also decrease smooth-muscle contraction of the stomach. Its effectiveness as an antiemetic has not been verified. Patients with diabetes mellitus should avoid this drug because of its high sugar content.

Antiemetics that were once frequently used for the treatment of nausea and vomiting during pregnancy are no longer recommended because they may cause harm to the fetus. Instead, nonpharmacologic methods are used when possible to alleviate nausea and vomiting during pregnancy. Ginger and red raspberry leaf tea have been used effectively but are not regulated by the US Food and Drug Administration (FDA). When antiemetics are necessary, a

TABLE 45.1   Nonprescription Antiemetics: Antihistamine

Drug	Route and Dosage	Uses and Considerations
Motion Sickness		
Cyclizine hydrochloride	A: PO: 50 mg tablet q4–6h, 30 min before travel; *max:* 200 mg/d	For prevention and treatment of nausea, vomiting, and dizziness associated with motion sickness. Avoid concurrent alcohol use. May cause drowsiness, blurred vision, fatigue, dry mouth, anorexia, constipation, and nasal dryness. PB: UK; t½: 13 h
Dimenhydrinate	A: PO: Initially 50 mg 30–60 min before travel or activity; *maint:* 50–100 mg q4–6h PRN; *max:* 400 mg/d A: IM/IV: 50–100 mg q4h PRN; *max:* 400 mg/d	To prevent and treat motion sickness, dizziness, nausea, and vomiting. May cause drowsiness, dizziness, headache, restlessness, blurred vision, anorexia, dry mouth, insomnia, and tachycardia. PB: 78%; t½: 3.5 h
Meclizine hydrochloride	Motion sickness: A: PO: 25–50 mg 1 h before travel; may repeat q24h PRN; *max:* 50 mg/d Vertigo: A: PO: 25–100 mg/d in divided doses; *max:* 100 mg/d	For prevention and treatment of nausea, vomiting, and dizziness due to motion sickness and vertigo associated with a vestibular disorder. May cause drowsiness, headache, ataxia, fatigue, blurred vision, anorexia, and dry mouth. PB: UK; t½: 5–6 h

A, Adult; *d,* day; *h,* hour; *maint,* maintenance dose; *max,* maximum; *min,* minute; *PB,* protein binding; *PO,* by mouth; *PRN,* as needed; *q,* every; *t½,* half-life; *UK,* unknown; *y,* year; *>,* greater than.

delayed-release combination of pyridoxine and doxylamine is usually preferred. If vomiting becomes severe and threatens the well-being of the mother and fetus, an antiemetic such as promethazine or metoclopramide can be administered. Other antiemetics may be prescribed cautiously.

Prescription Antiemetics

Common prescription antiemetics are classified into the following groups: (1) antihistamines, (2) anticholinergics, (3) dopamine antagonists, (4) benzodiazepines, (5) serotonin antagonists, (6) glucocorticoids, (7) cannabinoids (for patients with certain diagnoses, such as cancer), and (8) miscellaneous. Many of these drugs act as antagonists to dopamine, histamine, serotonin, and acetylcholine, which are associated with vomiting. Antihistamines and anticholinergics act primarily on the vomiting center; they also act by decreasing stimulation of the CTZ and vestibular pathways. The cannabinoids act on the cerebral cortex. Phenothiazines, the miscellaneous antiemetics (e.g., metoclopramide), and trimethobenzamide act on the CTZ. Drug combination therapy is commonly used to manage chemotherapy-induced nausea and vomiting. Lorazepam, glucocorticoids, and serotonin (5-HT$_3$)-receptor antagonists are quite effective in combination therapy. Lorazepam, haloperidol, and glucocorticoids are not approved by the FDA as antiemetics but are extremely effective when combined for this unlabeled use.

Antihistamines and Anticholinergics

Only a few prescription antihistamines and anticholinergics are used in the treatment of nausea and vomiting. Table 45.2 lists these drugs and their dosages, uses, and considerations.

Side Effects and Adverse Reactions. Side effects include drowsiness, which can be a major problem; dry mouth; blurred vision caused by pupillary dilation; tachycardia (with anticholinergic use); and constipation. These drugs should *not* be used by patients with glaucoma.

Dopamine Antagonists

These agents suppress emesis by blocking dopamine (D$_2$) receptors in the CTZ. The categories of dopamine antagonists include phenothiazines, butyrophenones, and benzodiazepines. Common side effects of dopamine antagonists are extrapyramidal symptoms, or extrapyramidal syndrome (EPS), caused by blocking dopamine receptors, and hypotension. See Chapter 22 for a more detailed description of EPS and phenothiazines.

Phenothiazine Antiemetics

Selected piperazine phenothiazines are used to treat nausea and vomiting resulting from surgery, anesthetics, chemotherapy, and radiation sickness. They act by inhibiting the CTZ. When used in patients with cancer, these drugs are commonly given the night before treatment, the day of treatment, and for 24 hours after treatment. Not all phenothiazines are effective antiemetic agents. When prescribed for vomiting, the drug dosage is usually smaller than is used for psychiatric disorders.

Chlorpromazine and prochlorperazine edisylate were the first phenothiazines used for both psychosis and vomiting. Promethazine, a phenothiazine introduced as an antihistamine in the 1940s, has a sedative effect and can also be used for motion sickness and management of nausea and vomiting.

⚠ When promethazine is administered intravenously, it is a high-alert medication that may cause significant harm to the patient if given incorrectly. Prototype Drug Chart: Promethazine Hydrochloride lists the pharmacological data for promethazine.

Pharmacokinetics. Promethazine is readily absorbed in the GI tract. It has 80% to 93% protein-binding capacity. Promethazine is metabolized by the liver and is excreted in urine and feces.

Pharmacodynamics. Promethazine blocks H$_1$-receptor sites on effector cells and impedes histamine-mediated responses. The onset of action of oral promethazine is 15 to 60 minutes, and onset with intramuscular (IM) administration is 20 minutes. The duration of action is from 4 to 6 hours. The onset of action of IV promethazine is 3 to 5 minutes; the duration of action is the same as for the oral preparation.

Drug and Laboratory Interactions. Central nervous system (CNS) depression increases when promethazine is taken with alcohol, narcotics, sedative-hypnotics, and general anesthetics. Anticholinergic effects increase when promethazine is combined with antihistamines, anticholinergics such as atropine, and other phenothiazines. Promethazine may interfere with urinary pregnancy tests, producing false results.

Side Effects and Adverse Reactions. Phenothiazines have antihistamine and anticholinergic properties. The side effects of phenothiazine antiemetics are moderate sedation, hypotension, extrapyramidal symptoms, CNS effects (restlessness, weakness, dystonic reactions, agitation), and mild anticholinergic symptoms (dry mouth, urinary retention, and constipation). Because the dose is lower for vomiting than for psychosis, the side effects are not so severe. Promethazine is relatively free of extrapyramidal symptoms at antiemetic doses. Table 45.2 lists the pharmacological data for phenothiazines and other prescription antiemetics.

Butyrophenones

Droperidol, like phenothiazines, block the D$_2$ receptors in the CTZ. They are used to treat postoperative nausea and the vomiting and emesis associated with toxins, cancer chemotherapy, and radiation therapy. Like phenothiazines, droperidol is likely to cause extrapyramidal symptoms if used for an extended time. Hypotension may result; therefore blood pressure should be monitored.

Benzodiazepines

Select benzodiazepines indirectly control nausea and vomiting that may occur with cancer chemotherapy. Lorazepam is the drug of choice. Previously, diazepam was the preferred benzodiazepine, but lorazepam effectively provides emesis control, sedation, anxiety reduction, and amnesia when used in combination with a glucocorticoid and serotonin (5-HT$_3$)-receptor antagonist.

Serotonin-Receptor Antagonists

Serotonin antagonists suppress nausea and vomiting by blocking the serotonin (5-HT$_3$) receptors in the CTZ and blocking the afferent vagal nerve terminals in the upper GI tract.

Serotonin antagonists—ondansetron, granisetron, dolasetron, and palonosetron—are the most effective of all antiemetics in suppressing nausea and vomiting caused by cancer chemotherapy–induced emesis or emetogenic anticancer drugs. Ondansetron (the first serotonin antagonist), granisetron, and dolasetron do *not* block the dopamine receptors; therefore they do not cause extrapyramidal symptoms as do the phenothiazine antiemetics. These drugs can be administered orally and intravenously. They are also effective in preventing nausea and vomiting before and after surgery. Common side effects include headache, dizziness, hypotension, palpitations, constipation, edema, and fatigue.

Glucocorticoids (Corticosteroids)

Dexamethasone and methylprednisolone are two agents that are effective in suppressing emesis associated with cancer chemotherapy.

TABLE 45.2 Prescription Antiemetics

Drug	Route and Dosage	Uses and Considerations
Prescription Antihistamines		
Hydroxyzine	Postoperative nausea/vomiting: A: IM: 25–100 mg single dose; *max:* 600 mg/d	For postoperative nausea and vomiting, pruritus, vertigo, anxiety, agitation, and sedation induction. Give deep in large muscle. May cause drowsiness, dizziness, fatigue, ataxia, headache, blurred vision, dry mouth, urinary retention, and constipation. PB: UK; t½: 14–25 h
Anticholinergics		
Scopolamine	Motion sickness: A: Transdermal patch: 1 mg patch; apply patch to a hairless area behind the ear at least 4 h before travel and q3d PRN	For nausea and vomiting, motion sickness, and procedural sedation. May cause dizziness, drowsiness, fatigue, headache, blurred vision, dry conjunctiva/cornea of eye, dilated pupils, visual impairment, agitation, confusion, restlessness, orthostatic hypotension, dry mouth, and constipation. Alternate ears if using for longer than 3 d, wash hands after applying patch, and wear no more than one patch at a time. PB: UK; t½: 8 h
Dopamine Antagonists		
Phenothiazines		
Prochlorperazine maleate	Nausea and vomiting: A: PO/IM/IV: 5–10 mg tid/qid PRN (give deep in the muscle); *max:* 40 mg/d SR: 10–15 mg q12h PR: 25 mg bid; *max:* 50 mg/d	For nausea, vomiting, schizophrenia, and anxiety. May cause drowsiness, dizziness, headache, insomnia, blurred vision, dry mouth, EPS, erectile/ejaculatory dysfunction, and constipation. Not approved for patients with dementia-related psychosis. PB: 91%–99%; t½: 6–22 h
Promethazine	See Prototype Drug Chart: Promethazine Hydrochloride	
Chlorpromazine	Nausea: A: PO: 10–25 mg q4–6h PRN A: IM: Initially 25 mg then, if tolerated, may give 25–50 mg q3–4h PRN	For nausea and vomiting, hiccups, and schizophrenia. May cause drowsiness, dizziness, weight gain, dry mouth, photosensitivity, constipation, and skin hyperpigmentation. PB: 90%–99%; t½: 2–30 h
Butyrophenones		
Droperidol	Postoperative nausea and vomiting: A: IM/IV: Initially 0.625–2.5 mg, may then give 1.25 mg if needed; *max:* 2.5 mg/initial dose	For prevention and treatment of postoperative nausea and vomiting and sedation induction. May cause hypo/hypertension, tachycardia, dizziness, drowsiness, anxiety, restlessness, dysrhythmias, and EPS. PB: 85%–90%: t½: 2 h
Benzodiazepines		
Lorazepam	Chemo-induced nausea/vomiting: A: IV: 0.025 mg/kg 45 min before chemo	For prevention of chemo-induced nausea and vomiting and for anxiety, insomnia, procedural sedation, and status epilepticus. May cause dizziness, drowsiness, ataxia, confusion, injection site reaction, constipation, weakness, hypotension, restlessness, headache, and erythema. PB: 85%; t½: 12–14 h
Benzamides		
Amisulpride	A: IV: 10 mg in single dose over 1–2 min; *max:* 10 mg/dose	For postoperative nausea and vomiting. May cause chills, drowsiness, injection site reaction, hypotension, and hypokalemia. PB: 25%–30%; t½: 4–5 h
Serotonin (5-HT₃) Receptor Antagonists		
Granisetron	Chemotherapy-induced nausea/vomiting: A: PO: 1 mg bid (1 h before and 12 h after chemo); *max:* 2 mg/d A: IV: 10 mcg/kg 30 min before chemo; *max:* 40 mcg/kg A: Transdermal patch: Apply 1 patch (3.1 mg/24 h) at least 24–48 h before chemo; remove patch no sooner than 24 h after chemo completion	For prevention and treatment of radiation- and chemo-induced nausea and vomiting. May cause dizziness, headache, weakness, hematoma, fatigue, anorexia, dyspepsia, nausea, vomiting, abdominal pain, diarrhea, constipation, leukopenia, and injection site reaction. PB: 65%; t½: 6.23 h PO, 5–7.7 h IV
Ondansetron hydrochloride	A: PO: 8 mg 30 min before chemo; may repeat in 8 h, then q12h for 1–2 d after chemo; *max:* 24 mg/d A: IV: 0.15 mg/kg (150 mcg/kg) 30 min before chemo, infused over 15 min, then q4h × 2	For postoperative and chemo- and radiation-induced nausea and vomiting. May cause dizziness, drowsiness, agitation, headache, fatigue, malaise, diarrhea, hypotension, urinary retention, fever, and constipation. PB: 70%–76%; t½: 3.1–5.8 h
Palonosetron	Postoperative nausea/vomiting: A: IV: 0.075 mg over 10 s before induction as a single dose; *max:* 0.25 mg/single dose	To prevent postoperative and chemo-induced nausea and vomiting. May cause headache, dizziness, hypotension, flatulence, constipation, diarrhea, and urinary retention. PB: 62%; t½: 40 h
Dolasetron	A: PO: 100 mg within 1 h before chemo A: IV: 12.5 mg as single dose	For nausea and vomiting. May cause headache, dizziness, hypotension, diarrhea, fatigue, and fever. PB: 69%–77%; t½: <10 min

Continued

TABLE 45.2 Prescription Antiemetics—cont'd

Drug	Route and Dosage	Uses and Considerations
Cannabinoids		
Dronabinol CSS III	Chemotherapy-induced nausea: A: PO: 5 mg/m² capsules 1–3 h before chemo, then q2–4h after; *max:* 15 mg/m²/dose or 6 doses/d	For anorexia and chemo-induced nausea and vomiting. May cause drowsiness, dizziness, impaired cognition, euphoria, dysphoria, paranoia, emotional lability, nausea, vomiting, and abdominal pain. PB: 97%; t½: 25–36 h
Miscellaneous		
Metoclopramide hydrochloride	Postoperative nausea/vomiting: A: IM/IV: 10–20 mg at end of surgery, may repeat q4–6h	For prevention and treatment of postoperative and chemo-induced nausea and vomiting, diabetic gastroparesis, and GERD. Avoid alcohol and CNS depressants. May cause drowsiness, dizziness, dysgeusia, fatigue, restlessness, headache, nausea, and vomiting. PB: 30%; t½: 2.5–6 h
Trimethobenzamide hydrochloride	A: PO: 300 mg tid/qid PRN; *max:* 1200 mg/d A: IM: 200 mg tid/qid PRN; *max:* 800 mg/d	For nausea and vomiting. Avoid with CNS depressants and if sensitive to benzocaine or similar local anesthetics. May cause drowsiness, dizziness, headache, hypotension, blurred vision, injection site reaction, EPS, and diarrhea. PB: UK; t½: 7–9 h
Aprepitant	Chemo-induced nausea/vomiting: A: PO: Day 1, give 125 mg 1 h before chemo; Days 2 and 3, give 80 mg 1 h before chemo or, if no chemo is scheduled, give in the morning	For prevention of postoperative and chemo-induced nausea and vomiting. May cause dizziness, fatigue, headache, weakness, hiccups, cough, abdominal pain, dyspepsia, and diarrhea. PB: 95%; t½: 9–13 h
Netupitant and palonosetron	A: PO: 1 capsule (netupitant 300 mg/palonosetron 0.5 mg) 1 h before chemo A: IV: 1 vial (netupitant 235 mg palonosetron 0.25 mg) 30 min before chemo, give over 30 min	For prevention of chemo-induced nausea and vomiting. May cause headache, weakness, fatigue, dyspepsia, erythema, and constipation. PB: palonosetron 62%, netupitant 99.5%; t½: palonosetron 40 h, netupitant 51–109 h
Rolapitant	A: PO: 180 mg day 1, 1–2 h and 30 min before chemo A: IV: 166.5 mg over 30 min 1–2 h before chemo and 30 min before chemo on day 1, repeat q2wk prior to chemo	For prevention of chemo-induced nausea and vomiting. May cause dizziness, anorexia, abdominal pain, dyspepsia, infusion site reactions, hiccups, stomatitis, neutropenia, and infections. PB: 99.8%; t½: 169–205 h

A, Adult; *bid,* twice a day; *CNS,* central nervous system; *CSS,* Controlled Substances Schedule; *d,* day; *EPS,* extrapyramidal symptoms; *GERD,* gastroesophageal reflux disease; *GI,* gastrointestinal; *h,* hour; *IBS,* irritable bowel syndrome; *IM,* intramuscular; *IV,* intravenous; *max,* maximum; *min,* minute; *mo,* month; *PB,* protein binding; *PO,* by mouth; *PR,* per rectum; *PRN,* as needed; *q,* every; *qid,* four times a day; *s,* second; *SR,* sustained release; *t½,* half-life; *tid,* three times a day; *UK,* unknown; *UTI,* urinary tract infection; *y,* year; *>,* greater than.

📄 PROTOTYPE DRUG CHART

❗ *Promethazine Hydrochloride*

Drug Class	**Dosage**
Antiemetic: Phenothiazine	Nausea/vomiting: A: PO/PR/IM/IV: 12.5–25 mg q4–6h PRN; *max:* 100 mg/d

Contraindications	**Drug-Lab-Food Interactions**
Hypersensitivity, asthma, coma *Caution:* Glaucoma, GI obstruction, bone marrow depression, hepatic disease, COPD, dehydration, diabetes mellitus, bradycardia, hypocalcemia, hypokalemia, hypomagnesemia, older adults, breastfeeding	Drug: Increases CNS depression and anticholinergic effects when taken with alcohol and other CNS depressants; lowers seizure threshold with phenytoin and tramadol Lab: False pregnancy test

Pharmacokinetics	**Pharmacodynamics**
Absorption: PO: Easily absorbed from GI tract Distribution: PB: 80%–93% Metabolism: t½: 10–14 h Excretion: In urine and feces	PO: Onset: 15–60 min Peak: UK; duration: 4–6 h IM: Onset: 20 min Peak: UK; duration: 4–6 h IV: Onset: 3–5 min Peak: UK; duration: 4–6 h PR: Onset: 15–60 min Peak: UK; duration: 4–6 h

Therapeutic Effects/Uses

To treat and prevent motion sickness, nausea, vomiting, and sedation induction
Mechanism of Action: Blocks H₁ receptor sites and inhibits CTZ.

Side Effects	**Adverse Reactions**
Drowsiness, dizziness, confusion, agitation, insomnia, dry mouth, constipation, blurred vision, excitability, photosensitivity, fatigue, urinary retention, injection site reaction, skin hyperpigmentation, erectile/ejaculation dysfunction	Extrapyramidal syndrome, seizures, dyspnea, hypo/hypertension *Life-threatening:* Agranulocytosis, leukopenia, thrombocytopenia, NMS, respiratory depression

A, Adult; *CNS,* central nervous system; *COPD,* chronic obstructive pulmonary disorder; *CTZ,* chemoreceptor trigger zone; *d,* day; *GI,* gastrointestinal; *h,* hour; *H₁,* histamine 1; *IM,* intramuscular; *IV,* intravenous; *max,* maximum; *min,* minute; *NMS,* neuroleptic malignant syndrome; *PB,* protein binding; *PO,* by mouth; *PR,* per rectum; *PRN,* as needed; *q4–6h,* every 4 to 6 hours; *t½,* half-life; *UK,* unknown; *y,* year; *>,* greater than.

Because these glucocorticoids are administered intravenously and for only a short while, side effects normally associated with glucocorticoids are minimized. Glucocorticoids are discussed in Chapter 46.

Cannabinoids

Cannabinoids, the active ingredients in cannabis, were approved for clinical use in 1985 to alleviate nausea and vomiting resulting from cancer treatment. These agents may be prescribed for patients receiving chemotherapy who do not respond to or are unable to take other antiemetics. They are contraindicated for patients with psychiatric disorders. Cannabinoids can be used as an appetite stimulant for patients with acquired immunodeficiency syndrome (AIDS). The cannabinoid dronabinol is described in Table 45.2.

Side Effects and Adverse Reactions. Side effects that can occur as a result of cannabinoid use include mood changes, euphoria, drowsiness, dizziness, headaches, depersonalization, nightmares, confusion, incoordination, memory lapse, dry mouth, orthostatic hypotension or hypertension, and tachycardia. Less common symptoms are depression, anxiety, and manic psychosis.

Miscellaneous Antiemetics

Trimethobenzamide. Trimethobenzamide is in the class of miscellaneous antiemetics because it does not act strictly as an antihistamine, anticholinergic, or phenothiazine. The drug suppresses impulses to the CTZ.

Metoclopramide. Metoclopramide suppresses emesis by blocking the dopamine receptors in the CTZ. It is used in the treatment of postoperative emesis, cancer chemotherapy, and radiation therapy. High doses can cause sedation and fatigue. With this agent, the occurrence of extrapyramidal symptoms is more prevalent in children than in adults. Metoclopramide should not be given if the patient has GI obstruction, hemorrhage, or perforation.

Side Effects and Adverse Reactions. The side effects and adverse reactions of the miscellaneous antiemetics are drowsiness, fatigue, headache and anticholinergic symptoms such as dry mouth, increased heart rate, urine retention, constipation, and blurred vision. Trimethobenzamide can cause hypotension, blurred vision, and extrapyramidal symptoms that include abnormal involuntary movements, postural disturbances, and alterations in muscle tone.

Table 45.2 lists pharmacological data for the miscellaneous antiemetics along with other prescription antiemetics.

⚡ PATIENT SAFETY

Do not Confuse...
- **Antivert**, an antiemetic, with **Axert**, an antimigraine drug
- **Lorazepam**, which controls nausea and vomiting, with **alprazolam**, an anxiolytic
- **Hydroxyzine**, an antiemetic, with **hydralazine**, an antihypertensive drug

---

◎ CLINICAL JUDGMENT [NURSING PROCESS]

Antiemetics

Concept: Fluid and Electrolyte Imbalance
- The maintenance of correct electrolyte concentrations and fluid balance in body compartments

Recognize Cues [Assessment]
- Determine a history of the onset, frequency, and amount of vomiting and contents of the vomitus. If appropriate, elicit from the patient possible causative factors such as food (e.g., seafood, mayonnaise, pregnancy, exposure to virus).
- Obtain a history of present health problems. Patients with glaucoma should avoid many of the antiemetics.
- Record vital signs for abnormalities and for future comparisons.
- Assess urinalysis before and during therapy.
- Assess the patient for dehydration due to excess fluid loss from vomiting.

Analyze Cues and Prioritize Hypothesis [Patient Problems]
- Hypotension
- Vomiting
- Hypokalemia
- Hyponatremia
- Dehydration
- Nausea
- Discomfort

Generate Solutions [Planning]
- The patient will state they will adhere to the treatment regimen to alleviate vomiting.
- The patient will report that vomiting has decreased in frequency.
- The patient will retain small amounts of food and fluid.

Take Action [Nursing Interventions]
- Check vital signs. If vomiting is severe, dehydration may occur, and shock-like symptoms may be present.

- Monitor bowel sounds for hypoactivity or hyperactivity.
- Provide mouth care after vomiting. Encourage patients to maintain oral hygiene.

Patient Teaching
General
- Instruct patients to store drugs in airtight, light-resistant containers if required.
- Tell patients to avoid over-the-counter (OTC) preparations.
- Warn patients not to consume alcohol while taking antiemetics. Alcohol can intensify the sedative effect.
- ⚡ Advise pregnant patients to avoid antiemetics during the first trimester because of possible teratogenic effects on the fetus. Encourage these patients to seek medical advice about OTC and prescription antiemetics.

Side Effects
- Tell the patient to report sore throat, fever, and mouth sores; notify the health care provider and have blood drawn for a complete blood count (CBC).
- ⚡ Alert patients to avoid driving a motor vehicle or engaging in dangerous activities because drowsiness is common with antiemetics. If drowsiness becomes a problem, a decrease in dosage may be indicated.
- Caution patients with hepatic disorders to seek medical advice before taking phenothiazines. Instruct patients to report dizziness.
- Suggest to patients nonpharmacologic methods of alleviating nausea and vomiting such as flat soda, weak tea, crackers, and dry toast.

Evaluate Outcomes [Evaluation]
- Evaluate the effectiveness of nonpharmacologic methods and antiemetics by noting the absence of vomiting. Identify any side effects that may result from drugs.

TABLE 45.3   Adsorbents

Drug	Route and Dosage	Uses and Considerations
Adsorbents		
Charcoal, activated	A: PO: 50–100 g in 6–8 oz of water q4–6h PRN	Promotes absorption of poison/toxic/overdose substances. Administer within 30 min of ingesting substance. May cause tongue/dental discoloration, abdominal pain, diarrhea, stool discoloration, and constipation. PB: NA; t½: NA

A, Adult; *min,* minute; *NA,* not applicable; *PB,* protein binding; *PO,* by mouth; *PRN,* as necessary; *q4–6h,* every 4 to 6 hours; *t½,* half-life; *UK,* unknown; *y,* year; <, less than.

EMETICS

Emetics are drugs used to induce vomiting. When an individual has consumed certain toxic substances, induced vomiting (emesis) may be indicated to expel the substance before absorption occurs. Vomiting can be induced in a number of ways without using drugs, such as putting a finger in the back of the throat.

Vomiting should not be induced if caustic substances such as ammonia, chlorine bleach, lye, toilet cleaners, or battery acid have been ingested. Regurgitating these substances can cause additional injury to the esophagus. To prevent aspiration, vomiting should also be avoided if petroleum distillates are ingested; these include gasoline, kerosene, paint thinners, and lighter fluid. Activated charcoal is given or gastric lavage is done when emesis is contraindicated (Table 45.3).

DIARRHEA

Diarrhea, frequent liquid stool, is a symptom of an intestinal disorder. Causes include (1) foods (spicy, spoiled), (2) fecal impaction, (3) bacteria *(Escherichia coli, Salmonella)* or viruses (parvovirus, rotavirus), (4) toxins, (5) drug reactions, (6) laxative abuse, (7) malabsorption syndrome caused by lack of digestive enzymes, (8) stress and anxiety, (9) bowel tumor, and (10) inflammatory bowel disease such as ulcerative colitis or Crohn disease. Diarrhea can be mild to severe. Antidiarrheals should not be used for more than 2 days and should not be used if fever is present.

Because intestinal fluids are rich in water, sodium, potassium, and bicarbonate, diarrhea can cause minor or severe dehydration and electrolyte imbalances. The loss of bicarbonate places the patient at risk for developing metabolic acidosis. Patients with diarrhea should avoid milk products and foods rich in fat. Diarrhea can develop very quickly and can be life-threatening to young patients and older adults, who may not be able to compensate for the fluid and electrolyte losses.

Nonpharmacologic Measures

The cause of diarrhea should be identified. Nonpharmacologic treatment for diarrhea is recommended until the underlying cause can be determined. This includes use of clear liquids and oral solutions such as Gatorade (for adults) and Pedialyte or Rehydralyte (for children) and IV electrolyte solutions. Antidiarrheal drugs are frequently used in combination with nonpharmacologic treatment.

Travelers' Diarrhea

Travelers' diarrhea, also called *acute diarrhea,* is usually caused by *E. coli.* It ordinarily lasts less than 2 days; however, if it becomes severe, fluoroquinolone antibiotics are usually prescribed. Loperamide may be used to slow peristalsis and decrease the frequency of defecation, but it can also slow the exit of the organism from the GI tract. Travelers' diarrhea can be reduced by drinking bottled water, washing fruit, and eating cooked vegetables. Meats should be cooked until well-done.

Antidiarrheals

There are various antidiarrheals for treating diarrhea and decreasing hypermotility (increased peristalsis). Usually, an underlying cause of the diarrhea needs to be corrected as well. The antidiarrheals are classified as (1) opiates and opiate-related agents, (2) adsorbents, and (3) miscellaneous antidiarrheals.

Opiates and Opiate-Related Agents

Opiates decrease intestinal motility, thereby decreasing peristalsis. Constipation is a common side effect of opium preparations. Codeine is an example. Opiates are frequently combined with other antidiarrheal agents. Opium antidiarrheals can cause CNS depression when taken with alcohol, sedatives, or tranquilizers. The duration of action of opiates is approximately 2 hours.

Diphenoxylate with atropine is an opiate that has less potential for causing drug dependence than other opiates such as codeine. Difenoxin is an active metabolite of diphenoxylate, but it is more potent than diphenoxylate. Both drugs are combined with atropine to decrease abdominal cramping, intestinal motility, and hypersecretion. Diphenoxylate with atropine is frequently prescribed for travelers' diarrhea, and difenoxin with atropine is prescribed to treat nonspecific and chronic diarrhea. With prolonged use of these drugs, physical dependence may occur. Diphenoxylate antidiarrheal products are approximately 50% atropine, which will discourage drug abuse. Drugs with atropine are contraindicated in glaucoma. Prototype Drug Chart: Diphenoxylate With Atropine lists the pharmacological data for diphenoxylate with atropine.

Loperamide is structurally related to diphenoxylate but causes less CNS depression than diphenoxylate and difenoxin. It can be purchased as an OTC drug, and it protects against diarrhea, reduces fecal volume, and decreases intestinal fluid and electrolyte losses.

Patients with severe hepatic impairment should not take products that contain diphenoxylate, difenoxin, or loperamide. Children and older adults who take diphenoxylate are more susceptible to respiratory depression than are other age groups.

Pharmacokinetics. Diphenoxylate with atropine is well absorbed from the GI tract. The diphenoxylate is metabolized by the liver mainly as metabolites. There are two half-lives: 3 hours for diphenoxylate and 3 to 14 hours for the diphenoxylate metabolites. The drug is excreted in the feces and urine.

Pharmacodynamics. Diphenoxylate with atropine is an opium agonist with anticholinergic properties (atropine) that decreases GI motility (peristalsis). It has a moderate onset of action of 45 to 60 minutes, and the duration of action is 3 to 4 hours. Many side effects are caused by the anticholinergic atropine. Patients with severe glaucoma should take another antidiarrheal that does not have an anticholinergic effect. If this drug is taken with alcohol, narcotics, or sedative-hypnotics, CNS depression can occur.

PROTOTYPE DRUG CHART

Diphenoxylate With Atropine

Drug Class	Dosage
Antidiarrheal CSS V	A: PO: Initially 2 tablets (diphenoxylate 2.5 mg, atropine 0.025 mg each tablet) qid; *max*: 8 tablets/d

Contraindications	Drug-Lab-Food Interactions
Severe diarrhea due to pseudomembranous colitis, infection, jaundice, glaucoma, children *Caution:* Hepatic disease, electrolyte imbalance, dehydration, ulcerative colitis, substance abuse, older adults, breastfeeding	Drug: Increased CNS depression with alcohol, antihistamines, opioids, sedative-hypnotics; MAOIs may enhance hypertensive crisis Lab: Increased serum liver enzymes, amylase

Pharmacokinetics	Pharmacodynamics
Absorption: PO: Well absorbed Distribution: PB: UK Metabolism: t½: 3–14 h Excretion: In feces and urine	PO: Onset: 45–60 min Peak: 2 h Duration: 3–4 h

Therapeutic Effects/Uses	
To treat diarrhea by slowing intestinal motility Mechanism of Action: Inhibits gastric motility by exerting effect on smooth muscle cells of GI tract.	

Side Effects	Adverse Reactions
Drowsiness, dizziness, euphoria, headache, restlessness, abdominal pain, nausea, vomiting, constipation, dry mouth, anorexia	Angioedema, pancreatitis *Life-threatening:* Ileus, toxic megacolon, anaphylaxis, respiratory depression

A, Adult; *CNS*, central nervous system; *CSS*, Controlled Substances Schedule; *d*, day; *GI*, gastrointestinal; *h*, hour; *MAOI*, monoamine oxidase inhibitor; *max*, maximum; *min*, minute; *PB*, protein binding; *PO*, by mouth; *PRN*, as necessary; *qid*, four times a day; *t½*, half-life; *tid*, three times a day; *UK*, unknown; *y*, year; *<*, less than.

CLINICAL JUDGMENT [NURSING PROCESS]

Antidiarrheals

Concept: Fluid and Electrolyte Imbalance
- The maintenance of correct electrolyte concentrations and fluid balance in body compartments

Recognize Cues [Assessment]
- Obtain a history of any viral or bacterial infection, drugs taken, and foods ingested that could be contributing factors to diarrhea. Many antidiarrheals are contraindicated if the patient has liver disease, narcotic dependence, ulcerative colitis, or glaucoma.
- Check vital signs to provide a baseline for future comparisons and to determine body fluid and electrolyte losses.
- Determine frequency and consistency of bowel movements.
- Assess bowel sounds. Hyperactive sounds can indicate increased intestinal motility.
- Report if a patient has a narcotic drug history. If opiate or opiate-related antidiarrheals are given, drug misuse or abuse may occur.

Analyze Cues and Prioritize Hypothesis [Patient Problems]
- Hypotension
- Vomiting
- Hypokalemia
- Hyponatremia
- Dehydration
- Nausea
- Discomfort

Generate Solutions [Planning]
- The patient will report having bowel movements that are formed.
- The patient will drink an adequate amount of fluids.

Take Action [Nursing Interventions]
- Record vital signs. Report tachycardia or systolic blood pressure decreases of 10 to 15 mm Hg. Monitor respirations. Opiates and opiate-related drugs can cause central nervous system (CNS) depression.
- Monitor frequency of bowel movements and bowel sounds. Notify a health care provider if intestinal hypoactivity occurs when taking a drug.
- ⚡ Check for signs and symptoms of dehydration resulting from persistent diarrhea. Fluid replacement may be necessary. With prolonged diarrhea, check serum electrolytes.
- Administer antidiarrheals cautiously to pregnant patients and those with glaucoma, liver disorders, or ulcerative colitis.
- ⚡ Recognize that a drug may need to be withheld if diarrhea continues for more than 48 hours or acute abdominal pain develops.

Patient Teaching
- Instruct patients not to take sedatives, tranquilizers, or other narcotics with antidiarrheal drugs. CNS depression may occur.
- Tell patients to avoid over-the-counter (OTC) preparations; they may contain alcohol and can promote liver damage, and concurrent use with loratadine and loperamide may lead to significant interaction.
- Counsel patients to take drugs only as prescribed. Advise that drugs may be habit-forming and that they should not exceed the recommended dose.
- Encourage patients to drink clear liquids.
- Advise patients not to ingest fried foods or milk products until diarrhea has stopped.
- Teach patients that constipation can result from overuse of antidiarrheal drugs.

Evaluate Outcomes [Evaluation]
- Evaluate the effectiveness of the drug; diarrhea has stopped.
- Monitor long-term use of opiates and opiate-related drugs for possible abuse and physical dependence.
- Continue to monitor vital signs and report abnormal changes.

TABLE 45.4 Antidiarrheals: Opiates and Opiate-Related Agents, Adsorbents, and Miscellaneous Agents

Drug	Route and Dosage	Uses and Considerations
Opiates and Opiate-Related Agents		
Difenoxin and atropine CSS IV	A: PO: Initially 2 tablets (difenoxin 1 mg, atropine 0.025 mg each tablet), then 1 tablet after each loose stool; *max:* 8 tablets/d	For diarrhea. Avoid use in patients with narrow-angle glaucoma. May cause dizziness, drowsiness, blurred vision, headache, fatigue, flushing, dry mouth, anorexia, nausea, vomiting, constipation, tachycardia, toxic megacolon, and urinary retention. PB: UK; t½: UK
Diphenoxylate and atropine CSS V	See Prototype Drug Chart: Diphenoxylate With Atropine	
Loperamide hydrochloride	A: PO: Initially 4 mg, then 2 mg after each unformed stool; *max:* 16 mg/d	For diarrhea. May cause drowsiness, dizziness, dry mouth, fatigue, headache, nausea, abdominal cramps, constipation, flatulence, vomiting, toxic megacolon, and urinary retention. PB: 97%; t½: 10.8 h
Adsorbents		
Bismuth subsalicylate	A: PO: 2 tab (524 mg) q30–60min PRN; *max:* 8 doses/d	For nausea, diarrhea, dyspepsia, and pyrosis. May cause dizziness, anxiety, drowsiness, headache, confusion, tinnitus, abdominal pain, constipation, tongue discoloration, hearing loss, and stool discoloration. PB: 90%; t½: bismuth 21–72 d, salicylate 2–5 h
Miscellaneous		
Crofelemer	A: PO: 125 mg bid; *max:* 250 mg/d	For diarrhea in patients with HIV/AIDS. May cause flatulence, nausea, cough, abdominal pain, constipation, arthralgia, dry mouth, infection, back pain, and hyperbilirubinemia. PB: UK; t½: UK
Eluxadoline	A: PO: 75–100 mg bid; *max:* 200 mg/d	For treatment of IBS with diarrhea. May cause dizziness, drowsiness, euphoria, nausea, vomiting, abdominal pain, constipation, infection, and pharyngitis. PB: 81%; t½: 3.7–6 h
Rifaximin	Travelers' diarrhea: A: PO: 200 mg tid for 3 d; *max:* 600 mg/d	For treatment of IBS, travelers' diarrhea, and hepatic encephalopathy. May cause dizziness, headache, fatigue, nausea, abdominal pain, ascites, pruritus, arthralgia, anemia, and peripheral edema. PB: 67.5%; t½: 5.63–6.08 h
Rifamycin	A: PO: 388 mg bid for 3 d; *max:* 776 mg/d	For travelers' diarrhea. May cause headache, dyspepsia, abdominal pain, constipation, and CDAD. PB: 80%; t½: UK

A, Adult; *AIDS,* acquired immunodeficiency syndrome; *bid,* twice a day; *CDAD, Clostridium difficile*–associated diarrhea; *CNS,* central nervous system; *CSS,* Controlled Substances Schedule; *d,* day; *GI,* gastrointestinal; *h,* hour; *HIV,* human immunodeficiency virus; *IBS,* irritable bowel syndrome; *max,* maximum; *min,* minute; *PB,* protein binding; *PO,* by mouth; *PRN,* as needed; *q,* every *qid,* four times a day; *t½,* half-life; *tab,* tablet; *tid,* three times a day; *UK,* unknown; *y,* year; *>,* greater than.

Adsorbents

Adsorbents act by coating the wall of the GI tract and adsorbing bacteria or toxins that cause diarrhea. Adsorbent antidiarrheals include kaolin and pectin. These agents are combined as a mild or moderate antidiarrheal that can be purchased without a prescription and used in combination with other antidiarrheals. Bismuth subsalicylate is considered an adsorbent because it adsorbs bacterial toxins. Bismuth subsalicylate is an OTC drug commonly used to treat travelers' diarrhea, and it can also be used as an antacid for gastric discomfort. Side effects include dizziness, drowsiness, headache, tongue and stool discoloration, and anxiety. Colestipol and cholestyramine are prescription drugs that have been used to treat diarrhea due to excess bile acids in the colon. They are effective, although they have not been approved by the FDA for this purpose. Table 45.4 lists the pharmacological data for antidiarrheal adsorbents.

Miscellaneous Antidiarrheals

Various miscellaneous antidiarrheals are prescribed to control diarrhea. This group includes rifaximin. Side effects include dizziness, nausea, dry mouth, flatulence, constipation, and fatigue. Table 45.4 includes these other antidiarrheals.

CONSTIPATION

Constipation, the accumulation of hard fecal material in the large intestine, is a relatively common complaint and a major problem for older adults. Insufficient water intake and poor dietary habits are contributing factors. Other causes include (1) fecal impaction, (2) bowel obstruction, (3) chronic laxative use, (4) neurological disorders (paraplegia), (5) ignoring the urge to defecate, (6) lack of exercise, and (7) select drugs such as anticholinergics, narcotics, and certain antacids.

Nonpharmacologic Measures

Nonpharmacologic management includes diet (high fiber), water, exercise, and routine bowel habits. A "normal" number of bowel movements ranges between one and three per day to three per week. What is normal varies from person to person; the nurse should determine what normal bowel habits are for each patient. At times a laxative may be needed, but the patient should also use nonpharmacologic measures to prevent constipation.

Laxatives

Laxatives and cathartics are used to eliminate fecal matter. Laxatives promote a soft stool, cathartics result in a soft to watery stool with some cramping, and frequently dosage determines whether a drug acts as a laxative or cathartic. Because these terms are often used interchangeably, *laxative* will cover both classes in this chapter. Purgatives are harsh cathartics that cause a watery stool with abdominal cramping. There are four types of laxatives: (1) osmotics (saline), (2) stimulants (contact or irritants), (3) bulk-forming, and (4) emollients (stool softeners).

Laxatives should be avoided if there is any question that the patient may have intestinal obstruction, if abdominal pain is severe, or if symptoms of appendicitis, ulcerative colitis, or diverticulitis are present. Most laxatives stimulate peristalsis. Laxative abuse from chronic use is a common problem, especially in older adults. Laxative dependence can become a problem, so patient teaching is an important nursing responsibility.

Osmotic (Saline) Laxatives

Osmotics, hyperosmolar laxatives, include salts or saline products, lactulose, and glycerin. Saline products consist of sodium or magnesium, and a small amount is systemically absorbed. Serum electrolytes should be monitored to avoid electrolyte imbalance. Hyperosmolar salts pull water into the colon and increase water in the feces to increase bulk, which stimulates peristalsis. Saline cathartics cause a semiformed to watery stool according to low or high doses. Good renal function is needed to excrete any excess salts. Saline cathartics are contraindicated for patients with heart failure.

Osmotic laxatives contain electrolyte salts, including (1) sodium salts (sodium phosphate or Phospho-Soda, sodium biphosphate) and (2) magnesium salts (magnesium hydroxide [Milk of Magnesia], magnesium citrate). High doses of salt laxatives are used for bowel preparation for diagnostic and surgical procedures. Another laxative used for bowel preparation is polyethylene glycol (PEG) with electrolytes. With PEG, however, a large volume of solution—approximately 3 to 4 L over 3 hours—must be ingested. Patients may be advised to keep PEG refrigerated to make it more palatable. The positive aspect is that the solution is an isotonic, nonabsorbable osmotic substance that contains sodium salts and potassium chloride; thus it can be used by patients with renal impairment or cardiac disorders.

Lactulose, another saline laxative that is not absorbed, draws water into the intestines to form a soft stool. It decreases the serum ammonia level and is useful in liver diseases, such as cirrhosis. Glycerin acts like lactulose, increasing water in the feces in the large intestine. The bulk that results from the increased water in the feces stimulates peristalsis and defecation.

Side Effects and Adverse Reactions. Adequate renal function is needed to excrete excess magnesium. Patients who have renal insufficiency should avoid magnesium salts. Hypermagnesemia can result from continuous use of magnesium salts, causing symptoms such as drowsiness, weakness, paralysis, complete heart block, hypotension, flush, and respiratory depression.

The side effects of excess lactulose use include flatulence, diarrhea, abdominal cramps, nausea, and vomiting. Patients who have diabetes mellitus should avoid lactulose because it contains glucose and fructose.

Stimulant (Contact) Laxatives

Stimulant (contact or irritant) laxatives increase peristalsis by irritating sensory nerve endings in the intestinal mucosa. Types include those that contain bisacodyl, senna, and castor oil (purgative). Bisacodyl is the most frequently used and abused laxative and can be purchased OTC. Bisacodyl and several others of these drugs are used to empty the bowel before diagnostic tests (barium enema). Prototype Drug Chart: Bisacodyl lists the pharmacological data for the stimulant laxative bisacodyl.

Castor oil is a harsh laxative (purgative) that acts on the small bowel and produces a watery stool. The action is quick, within 2 to 6 hours, so the laxative should not be taken at bedtime. Castor oil is not FDA approved to correct constipation; rather, it is used mainly for bowel preparation.

Pharmacokinetics. The contact laxative bisacodyl is minimally absorbed from the GI tract. It is excreted in feces, but because of the small amount of bisacodyl absorption, a portion is excreted in urine.

Pharmacodynamics. Bisacodyl promotes defecation by irritating the colon, causing defecation; psyllium compounds increase fecal bulk and peristalsis. The onset of action of oral bisacodyl occurs within 6 to 8 hours, and with the suppository (rectal administration), it occurs within 15 to 60 minutes.

Side Effects and Adverse Reactions. Side effects include dizziness, nausea, abdominal cramps, weakness, and reddish-brown urine caused by excretion of phenolphthalein, senna, or cascara.

With excessive and chronic use of bisacodyl, fluid and electrolyte imbalances—especially of potassium and calcium—are likely to occur. Systemic effects occur infrequently because absorption of bisacodyl is minimal. Mild cramping and diarrhea are side effects of bisacodyl.

Castor oil should not be used in early pregnancy because it stimulates uterine contractions, and spontaneous abortion may result. Prolonged use of senna can damage nerves, which may result in loss of intestinal muscular tone. Table 45.5 lists the osmotic and stimulant laxatives with their dosages, uses, and considerations.

Bulk-Forming Laxatives

Bulk-forming laxatives are natural fibrous substances that promote large, soft stools by absorbing water into the intestine, increasing fecal bulk and peristalsis. These agents are nonabsorbable. Defecation usually occurs within 8 to 24 hours; however, it may take up to 3 days after drug therapy is started for the stool to be soft and well formed. Powdered bulk-forming laxatives, which sometimes come in flavored and sugar-free forms, should be mixed in a glass of water or juice, stirred, drunk immediately, and followed by a half to a full glass of water. Insufficient fluid intake can cause the drug to solidify in the GI tract, which can result in intestinal obstruction. This group of laxatives does not cause laxative dependence and may be used by patients with diverticulosis, irritable bowel syndrome (IBS), and ileostomy and colostomy.

Polycarbophil, polyethylene glycol, methylcellulose, and psyllium are examples of bulk-forming laxatives. Patients with hypercalcemia should avoid calcium polycarbophil because of the significant amount of calcium in the drug. Prototype Drug Chart: Psyllium lists the pharmacological data for the bulk-forming laxative psyllium.

Pharmacokinetics. The bulk-forming laxative psyllium is a nondigestible and nonabsorbent substance that becomes a viscous solution when mixed with water. Because it is not absorbed, there is no protein binding or half-life for the drug. Psyllium is excreted in the feces.

Pharmacodynamics. The onset of action for psyllium is 12 to 72 hours. Peak action is 1 to 3 days. The duration of action is unknown.

📄 **PROTOTYPE DRUG CHART**

Bisacodyl

Drug Class	Dosage
Laxative: Stimulant	A: PO: 5–15 mg/d single dose; *max:* 15 mg/d A: supp PR: 10 mg/d

Contraindications	Drug-Lab-Food Interactions
Hypersensitivity, GI bleeding *Caution:* Diarrhea, diverticulitis, electrolyte imbalance, ulcerative colitis, fecal impaction, GI obstruction, appendicitis, abdominal pain, vomiting, pregnancy, breastfeeding	Drug: Decreased effect with antacids, histamine$_2$ blockers, proton pump inhibitors Food: Milk

Pharmacokinetics	Pharmacodynamics
Absorption: Minimal (5%–15%) Distribution: PB: UK Metabolism: t½: UK Excretion: In bile and urine	PO: Onset: 6–8 h Peak: N/A Duration: N/A PR: Onset: 15–60 min Peak: N/A Duration: N/A

Therapeutic Effects/Uses	
Bowel preparation, prevention and short-term treatment for constipation Mechanism of Action: Increases peristalsis by direct effect on smooth muscle of intestine.	

Side Effects	Adverse Reactions
Proctitis, nausea, vomiting, abdominal cramps, diarrhea, rectal irritation	Dependence, hypokalemia

A, Adult; *d,* day; *GI,* gastrointestinal; *h,* hour; *max,* maximum; *min,* minute; *N/A,* not applicable; *PB,* protein binding; *PO,* by mouth; *PR,* per rectum; *supp,* suppository; *t½,* half-life; *UK,* unknown; *y,* year; *>,* greater than.

TABLE 45.5   Laxatives: Osmotics (Saline), Stimulants, and Selective Chloride Channel Activators

Drug	Route and Dosage	Uses and Considerations
Osmotics: Saline		
Glycerin	A: PR: 1 supp, retain 15 min	For constipation. Use with caution in patients with intestinal obstruction, appendicitis, undiagnosed abdominal pain. May cause dizziness, nausea, diarrhea, abdominal cramps, perianal irritation, tenesmus, and rectal bleeding/irritation. PB: UK; t½: UK
Lactulose	Constipation: A: PO: 15–30 mL/d, may increase to 60 mL/d PRN	For constipation and hepatic encephalopathy. May cause flatulence, eructation, nausea, vomiting, diarrhea, abdominal pain, metabolic acidosis, hypokalemia, and hypernatremia. PB: UK; t½: UK
Magnesium citrate	Constipation: A: PO: 150–300 mL in single or divided dose	For constipation and bowel preparation. May cause drowsiness, nausea, vomiting, diarrhea, abdominal cramps, flatulence, hypermagnesemia, and dehydration. PB: UK; t½: UK
Magnesium hydroxide	A: PO: 15–60 mL, preferably at bedtime	For constipation, dyspepsia, and pyrosis. Take with a glass of water. May cause chalky taste, nausea, vomiting, diarrhea, dehydration, and hypermagnesemia. PB: UK; t½: UK
Lactitol	A: PO: 20 g/d; *max:* 20 g/d	For chronic constipation. May cause flatulence, abdominal pain, diarrhea, infection, rash, pruritus, and hypertension. PB: UK; t½: 2.4 h
Polyethylene glycol	A: PO: 17 g (1 Tbsp) in 4–8 oz water qd; *max:* 34 g/d	For constipation and bowel preparation. May cause nausea, flatulence, diarrhea, abdominal cramps, and fecal incontinence. PB: NA; t½: NA
Stimulants		
Bisacodyl	See Prototype Drug Chart: Bisacodyl	
Senna	Constipation: A: PO: 1–2 tab or 10–15 mL syrup with full glass of water at bedtime; *max:* 4 tab bid or 15 mL bid	For constipation and bowel preparation. May cause nausea, vomiting, diarrhea, and abdominal cramps. Prolonged use may cause fluid and electrolyte imbalances. PB: UK; t½: UK
Selective Chloride Channel Activator		
Lubiprostone	A: PO: 24 mcg bid with food and water; *max:* 48 mcg/d	For treatment of constipation, IBS, and opioid-induced constipation. May cause headache, peripheral edema, fatigue, dizziness, nausea, diarrhea, abdominal pain, and flatulence. PB: 94%; t½: 0.9–1.4 h

TABLE 45.5 Laxatives: Osmotics (Saline), Stimulants, and Selective Chloride Channel Activators—cont'd

Drug	Route and Dosage	Uses and Considerations
Miscellaneous		
Linaclotide	Constipation: A: PO: 145 mcg/d on empty stomach at least 30 min before first meal; *max:* 290 mcg/d	For constipation and IBS. May cause headache, flatulence, abdominal pain, diarrhea, hypokalemia, hyponatremia, infection, and hypotension. PB: UK; t½: UK
Naloxegol	A: PO: 12.5–25 mg/d on empty stomach 1 h before first meal; *max:* 25 mg/d	For opiate agonist–induced constipation. May cause headache, flatulence, nausea, vomiting, diarrhea, abdominal pain, and hyperhidrosis. PB: 4.2%; t½: 6–11 h
Naldemedine	A: PO: 0.2 mg/d	For opiate agonist–induced constipation. May cause abdominal pain, nausea, vomiting, and diarrhea. PB: 93%–94%; t½: 11 h
Methylnaltrexone	A: PO: 450 mg/d in the morning A: Subcut: 8–12 mg qod PRN or 0.15 mg/kg qod PRN	For opioid induced constipation. May cause headache, dizziness, nausea, vomiting, diarrhea, abdominal pain flatulence, and hyperhidrosis. PB: 11–15%; t½: 15 h
Prucalopride	A: PO: 2 mg/d	For chronic idiopathic constipation. May cause headache, dizziness, nausea, vomiting, diarrhea, flatulence, and abdominal pain. PB: 30%; t½: 24 h
Tenapanor	A: PO: 50 mg bid before breakfast and dinner; *max:* 100 mg/d	For IBS with constipation. May cause dizziness, flatulence, abdominal pain, diarrhea, dehydration, hyperkalemia, and GI bleeding. PB: UK; t½: UK

A, Adult; *bid,* twice a day; *d,* day; *h,* hour; *IBS,* irritable bowel syndrome; *max,* maximum; *min,* minute; *PB,* protein binding; *PO,* by mouth; *PR,* per rectum; *PRN,* as needed; *qod,* every other day; *supp,* suppository; *t½,* half-life; *tab,* tablet; *UK,* unknown; *URI,* upper respiratory infection; *y,* year; *>,* greater than; *<,* less than.

Side Effects and Adverse Reactions. Bulk-forming laxatives are not systemically absorbed, so there is no systemic effect. If bulk-forming laxatives are excessively used, nausea, vomiting, flatulence, or diarrhea may occur. Abdominal cramps may occur if the drug is used in dry form.

Chloride Channel Activators

Selective chloride channel activators are used to treat idiopathic constipation in adults. The first drug in this category is lubiprostone, manufactured by Sucampo Pharmaceuticals. Lubiprostone activates chloride channels in the lining of the small intestine, leading to an increase in intestinal fluid secretion and motility. By enhancing the passage of stool, lubiprostone relieves constipation and accompanying symptoms of abdominal discomfort, pain, and bloating. Lubiprostone is contraindicated for patients with a history of mechanical GI obstruction, Crohn disease, diverticulitis, and severe diarrhea. Adverse effects of lubiprostone include nausea that seems to be dose dependent, diarrhea, headache, abdominal distension, and flatulence.

Emollients (Stool Softeners)

Emollients are lubricants and stool softeners (surface-acting or wetting drugs) used to prevent constipation. These drugs decrease straining during defecation. Lubricants such as mineral oil increase water retention in the stool. Mineral oil absorbs the essential fat-soluble vitamins A, D, E, and K. Some of the minerals can be absorbed into the lymphatic system.

Stool softeners work by lowering surface tension and promoting water accumulation in the intestine and stool. They are frequently prescribed for patients after myocardial infarction or surgery. They are also given before administration of other laxatives in treating fecal impaction. Docusate calcium, docusate sodium, and docusate sodium with senna are examples of stool softeners.

Side Effects and Adverse Reactions. Side effects of mineral oil include nausea, vomiting, diarrhea, and abdominal cramping.

📄 PROTOTYPE DRUG CHART

Psyllium

Drug Class	Dosage
Laxative: Bulk forming	A: PO: 1 rounded tsp in 8 oz water followed by 8 oz water 1–3 times/d

Contraindications	Drug-Lab-Food Interactions
Hypersensitivity, GI bleeding, dysphagia *Caution:* GI obstruction, abdominal pain, appendicitis, older As	Drug: Decreased absorption of oral anticoagulants, aspirin, and digoxin

Pharmacokinetics	Pharmacodynamics
Absorption: Not absorbed Distribution: PB: N/A Metabolism: t½: N/A Excretion: In feces	PO: Onset: 12–72 h Peak: 1–3 d Duration: UK

Therapeutic Effects/Uses

To control constipation
Mechanism of Action: Acts as a bulk-forming laxative by drawing water into the intestine.

Side Effects	Adverse Reactions
Nausea, vomiting, abdominal cramps, flatulence	GI obstruction *Life-threatening:* Bronchospasm, anaphylaxis

A, Adult; *d,* day; *GI,* gastrointestinal; *h,* hour; *N/A,* not applicable; *PB,* protein binding; *PO,* by mouth; *t½,* half-life; *tsp,* teaspoon; *UK,* unknown; *y,* year; *>,* greater than.

This laxative is not indicated for children, older adults, or patients with debilitating diseases because they might aspirate the mineral oil, resulting in lipid pneumonia. The docusate group of drugs may cause mild cramping.

Contraindications. Contraindications to the use of laxatives include pregnancy and inflammatory disorders of the GI tract such as appendicitis, ulcerative colitis, undiagnosed severe pain that could be caused by inflammation within the intestine (diverticulitis, appendicitis), along with spastic colon or bowel obstruction. Laxatives are contraindicated when any of these conditions is suspected. Table 45.6 lists the laxatives and their dosages, uses, and considerations.

TABLE 45.6 Laxatives: Bulk Forming, Emollients, and Evacuants

Drug	Route and Dosage	Uses and Considerations
Bulk Forming		
Polycarbophil	A: PO: 1250 mg qd–qid PRN; *max.* 5000 mg/d	For constipation and IBS, administer with a full glass of water. May cause dizziness, drowsiness, anorexia, nausea, vomiting, flatulence, abdominal cramps, and diarrhea. PB: NA; t½: NA
Methylcellulose	A: PO: 2 g powder (1 heaping Tbsp) 1–3 times/d in 8–10 oz of water or 2 caplets up to 6 times/d; *max*: 3 doses/d or 12 caplets/d	For constipation. Take immediately after mixing in water. May cause nausea, vomiting, diarrhea, abdominal cramps, and GI obstruction. PB: NA; t½: NA
Psyllium hydrophilic mucilloid	See Prototype Drug Chart: Psyllium	
Stool Softeners		
Docusate calcium; docusate sodium	Docusate calcium: A: PO: 240 mg/d Docusate sodium: A: PO: 50–360 mg/d	For constipation. May cause throat irritation, diarrhea, and abdominal cramps. PB: NA; t½: NA
Docusate sodium with senna	A: PO: 2–4 tabs/d	For constipation. May cause urine discoloration, hypokalemia, flatulence, nausea, vomiting, abdominal cramps, and diarrhea. PB: NA; t½: NA
Emollient: Lubricant		
Mineral oil	A: PO: 30–90 mL/d	For constipation and fecal impaction. May be useful for those with cardiac disorders and after anorectal surgery. Avoid prolonged use because vitamins A, D, E, and K may be lost; may cause dizziness, weakness, nausea, diarrhea, abdominal cramps, fecal urgency/incontinence, and skin irritation, PB: NA; t½: NA
Evacuant/Bowel Preparation		
Polyethylene glycol–electrolyte solution	A: PO: 240 mL q10–15min for total of 4 L	For constipation and bowel preparation. May cause chills, polydipsia, dizziness, headache, malaise, vomiting, dyspepsia, nausea, abdominal cramps, diarrhea, and fecal urgency/incontinence. PB: NA; t½: NA

A, Adult; *d*, day; *GI*, gastrointestinal; *IBS*, irritable bowel syndrome; *max*, maximum; *NA*, not applicable; *PB*, protein binding; *PO*, by mouth; *q10–15 min*, every 10 to 15 minutes; *qd*, every day; *t½*, half-life; *tab*, tablet; *Tbsp*, tablespoon; *UK*, unknown; *y*, year; *>*, greater than.

CLINICAL JUDGMENT [NURSING PROCESS]

Laxative: Stimulant

Concept: Elimination
- The excretion of waste products through the intestinal tract and the expelling of stool by means of intestinal smooth muscle contraction

Recognize Cues [Assessment]
- Obtain a history of constipation and possible causes (insufficient water or fluid intake, diet deficient in bulk or fiber, inactivity), frequency and consistency of stools, and general health status.
- Record baseline vital signs for identification of abnormalities and for future comparisons.
- Evaluate renal function.
- Assess electrolyte balance of patients who frequently use laxatives.

Analyze Cues and Prioritize Hypothesis [Patient Problems]
- Discomfort
- Constipation
- Fatigue
- Reduced intestinal motility

Generate Solutions [Planning]
- The patient will report a normal bowel elimination pattern.
- The patient will exercise, eat foods high in fiber, and have adequate fluid intake to avoid constipation.

Take Action [Nursing Interventions]
- Monitor fluid intake and output.
- Note signs and symptoms of fluid and electrolyte imbalances that may result from watery stools. Habitual use of laxatives can cause fluid volume deficit, electrolyte losses, and loss of the urge to defecate.

Patient Teaching
General
- Encourage patients to increase water intake (if not contraindicated), which will decrease hard, dry stools.
- ⚡ Advise patients to avoid overuse of laxatives, which can lead to fluid and electrolyte imbalances and drug dependence. Suggest exercise to help increase peristalsis.
- Teach patients not to chew tablets but to swallow them whole.
- Direct patients to store suppositories at less than 86°F (30°C).
- Counsel patients to take drugs only with water to increase absorption.
- Educate patients not to take the drug within 1 hour of any other drug.
- Warn patients that the drug is not for long-term use; bowel tone may be lost.
- Encourage patients to time administration of the drug so as not to interfere with activities or sleep.

Side Effects
- Advise patients to discontinue use if rectal bleeding, nausea, vomiting, or cramping occurs.

Diet
- Inform patients to consume foods high in fiber such as bran, whole grains, and fruits.

Evaluate Outcomes [Evaluation]
- Determine the effectiveness of nonpharmacologic methods for alleviating constipation.
- Evaluate the patient's use of laxatives in managing constipation. Identify laxative abuse.

CLINICAL JUDGMENT [NURSING PROCESS]

Laxative: Bulk Forming

Concept: Elimination
- The excretion of waste products through the intestinal tract and the expelling of stool by means of intestinal smooth muscle contraction

Recognize Cues [Assessment]
- Obtain a history of constipation and possible causes (insufficient water or fluid intake, diet deficient in bulk or fiber, inactivity), frequency and consistency of stools, and general health status.
- Record baseline vital signs for identification of abnormalities and for future comparisons.
- Assess renal function, urine output, blood urea nitrogen (BUN), and serum creatinine.

Analyze Cues and Prioritize Hypothesis [Patient Problems]
- Discomfort
- Constipation
- Fatigue
- Reduced intestinal motility

Generate Solutions [Planning]
- The patient will report a normal bowel elimination pattern.
- The patient will exercise, eat foods high in fiber, and have adequate fluid intake to avoid constipation.

Take Action [Nursing Interventions]
- ⚡ Check fluid intake and output. Note signs and symptoms of fluid and electrolyte imbalances that may result from watery stools. Habitual use of laxatives can cause fluid volume deficit and electrolyte losses.
- Monitor bowel sounds.
- Identify the cause of constipation.
- Avoid inhalation of psyllium dust.

Patient Teaching
General
- Teach patients to mix the agent with water immediately before use to avoid gastrointestinal (GI) obstruction.
- Advise patients *not* to swallow the agent in dry form.
- Counsel patients to avoid overuse of laxatives, which can lead to fluid and electrolyte imbalances and laxative dependence. Suggest exercise to help increase peristalsis.
- ⚡ Advise patients to avoid inhaling psyllium dust; it may cause watery eyes, runny nose, and wheezing.

Side Effects
- Encourage patients to discontinue use if nausea, vomiting, cramping, or rectal bleeding occurs.

Diet
- ⚡ Instruct patients to mix the drug in 8 to 10 oz of water and to stir and drink it immediately. At least one glass of extra water should follow. Insufficient water can cause the drug to solidify, which can lead to dry, hard stools; fecal impaction; and esophageal obstruction.
- Encourage patients to increase foods rich in fiber such as bran, grains, vegetables, and fruits.
- Advise patients to increase water intake to at least 8 oz of fluids per day, which will decrease hard, dry stools.

Evaluate Outcomes [Evaluation]
- Determine the effectiveness of nonpharmacologic methods for alleviating constipation.
- Evaluate patients' use of laxatives in managing constipation.
- Identify laxative abuse.

CRITICAL THINKING CASE STUDY

A 34-year-old woman has been vomiting for 48 hours. In the past 12 hours, the patient has had vomiting and diarrhea. Prochlorperazine 10 mg was administered intramuscularly.

1. What nonpharmacologic measures should the nurse suggest when vomiting occurs?
2. Why was the patient given prochlorperazine intramuscularly and not orally or rectally?
3. What electrolyte imbalances may occur as a result of vomiting and diarrhea? Explain how they can be replaced.
4. What are the side effects of prochlorperazine?

5. Could a serotonin antagonist be given to the patient instead of prochlorperazine? Explain your answer.

The patient was prescribed difenoxin with atropine 2 tablets initially, then 1 tablet after each loose stool.

6. Is the diphenoxylate with atropine dosage for the patient within the normal prescribed range?
7. What clinical conditions are contraindicated for the use of difenoxin with atropine?
8. What are some combination drugs that may be prescribed to control diarrhea? Give their advantages and disadvantages.

REVIEW QUESTIONS

1. A patient complains of constipation and requires a laxative. In providing teaching for this patient, the nurse reviews the common causes of constipation, including which cause?
   a. Motion sickness
   b. Poor dietary habits
   c. Food intolerance
   d. Bacteria (Escherichia coli)
2. A patient with nausea is taking ondansetron. She asks the nurse how this drug works. The nurse is aware that this medication has which action?
   a. Enhances histamine[1] receptor sites
   b. Blocks serotonin receptors in the chemoreceptor trigger zone
   c. Blocks dopamine receptors in the chemoreceptor trigger zone
   d. Stimulates anticholinergic receptor sites
3. A patient who has constipation is prescribed a bisacodyl suppository. Which explanation will the nurse use to explain the action of bisacodyl?
   a. Acts on smooth intestinal muscle to gently increase peristalsis
   b. Absorbs water into the intestines to increase bulk and peristalsis
   c. Lowers surface tension and increases water accumulation in the intestines
   d. Pulls salts into the colon and increases water in the feces to increase bulk

4. A patient is using scopolamine to prevent motion sickness. About which common side effect should the nurse teach the patient?
   a. Diarrhea
   b. Vomiting
   c. Insomnia
   d. Dry mouth
5. When metoclopramide is given for nausea, the nurse plans to caution the patient to avoid which substance?
   a. Milk
   b. Coffee
   c. Alcohol
   d. Carbonated beverages
6. The nurse is administering difenoxin with atropine to a patient. Which should be included in the patient teaching regarding this medication? (Select all that apply.)
   a. Caution the patient to avoid laxative abuse.
   b. Record the frequency of bowel movements.
   c. Caution the patient against taking sedatives concurrently.
   d. Encourage the patient to increase fluids.
   e. Instruct the patient to avoid this drug if he or she has narrow-angle glaucoma.
   f. Teach the patient that the drug acts by drawing water into the intestine.

46

Antiulcer Drugs

http://evolve.elsevier.com/McCuistion/pharmacology

OBJECTIVES

- Explain the predisposing factors for peptic ulcers.
- Differentiate between peptic ulcer, gastric ulcer, duodenal ulcer, and gastroesophageal reflux disease (GERD).
- Compare the actions of the seven groups of antiulcer drugs used in the treatment of peptic ulcer: tranquilizers, anticholinergics, antacids, histamine$_2$ blockers, proton pump inhibitors, pepsin inhibitors, and prostaglandin analogues.

- Plan patient teaching for anticholinergic, antacid, and histamine$_2$ blocker drug groups.
- Differentiate among the side effects of anticholinergics and systemic and nonsystemic antacids.
- Apply the Clinical Judgment [Nursing Process], including teaching, to antiulcer drugs.

OUTLINE

This chapter discusses drugs used to prevent and treat peptic ulcers, both gastric and duodenal. These drugs include tranquilizers, anticholinergics, antacids, histamine$_2$ blockers, proton pump inhibitors (PPIs), a pepsin inhibitor, and a prostaglandin analogue antiulcer drug.

Peptic ulcer is a broad term for an ulcer or erosion that occurs in the esophagus, stomach, or duodenum within the upper gastrointestinal (GI) tract. Ulcers are more specifically named according to the site of involvement: esophageal, gastric, or duodenal. Duodenal ulcers occur 10 times more frequently than gastric and esophageal ulcers. The release of hydrochloric acid (HCl) from the parietal cells of the stomach is influenced by histamine, gastrin, and acetylcholine. Peptic ulcers occur when there is a hypersecretion of HCl and pepsin, which erode the GI mucosal lining.

The gastric secretions in the stomach strive to maintain a pH of 2 to 5. Pepsin, a digestive enzyme, is activated at a pH of 2, and the acid-pepsin complex of gastric secretions can cause mucosal damage. If the pH of gastric secretions increases to 5, the activity of pepsin declines. The gastric mucosal barrier (GMB) is a thick, viscous, mucous material that provides a barrier between the mucosal lining and acidic gastric secretions. The GMB maintains the integrity of the gastric mucosal lining and is a defense against corrosive substances. The two sphincter muscles—the *cardiac,* located at the upper portion of the stomach, and the *pyloric,* located at the lower portion of the stomach—act as barriers to prevent reflux of acid into the esophagus and duodenum. Fig. 46.1 shows common sites of peptic ulcers.

An esophageal ulcer results from reflux of acidic gastric secretions into the esophagus as a result of a defective or incompetent cardiac sphincter. A gastric ulcer frequently occurs because of a breakdown of the GMB. A duodenal ulcer is caused by hypersecretion of acid from the stomach passing into the duodenum because of (1) insufficient buffers to neutralize gastric acid in the stomach, (2) a defective or incompetent pyloric sphincter, or (3) hypermotility of the stomach. Gastroesophageal reflux disease (GERD) is inflammation or erosion of the esophageal mucosa caused by a reflux of gastric acid content from the stomach into the esophagus.

PREDISPOSING FACTORS IN PEPTIC ULCER DISEASE

The nurse needs to assist the patient in identifying possible causes of the ulcer and to teach ways to alleviate it. Predisposing factors include mechanical disturbances, genetic influences, bacterial organisms,

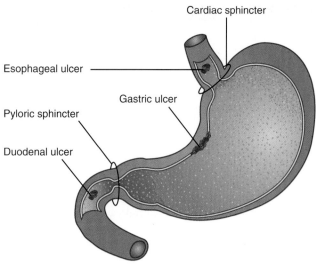

Fig. 46.1 Common sites of peptic ulcers.

TABLE 46.1 Predisposing Factors for Peptic Ulcer Disease

Predisposing Factors	Effects
Mechanical disturbances	Hypersecretion of acid and pepsin; inadequate GMB mucous secretion; impaired GMB resistance; hypermotility of the stomach; incompetent (defective) cardiac or pyloric sphincter
Genetic influences	Increased number of parietal cells in the stomach; susceptibility of mucosal lining to acid penetration; susceptibility to excess acetylcholine and histamine; excess hydrochloric acid caused by external stimuli
Environmental influences	Foods and liquids containing caffeine; fatty, fried, and highly spiced foods; alcohol; nicotine, especially from cigarette smoking; stressful situations; pregnancy; massive trauma; major surgery
Helicobacter pylori	A gram-negative bacterium, *H. pylori*, infects gastric mucosa and can cause gastritis, gastric ulcer, and duodenal ulcer. If not eradicated, peptic ulcer may return as frequently as every year. *H. pylori* can lead to atrophic gastritis in some patients. Serology and special breath tests can detect the presence of *H. pylori*.
Drugs	NSAIDs, including aspirin and aspirin compounds, ibuprofen, and indomethacin; corticosteroids; potassium salts; antineoplastic drugs

GMB, Gastric mucosal barrier; *NSAIDs*, nonsteroidal antiinflammatory drugs.

environmental factors, and certain drugs. Healing of an ulcer takes 4 to 8 weeks. Complications can occur as the result of scar tissue. Table 46.1 lists the predisposing factors for peptic ulcers and their effects.

The classic symptom of peptic ulcers is gnawing, aching pain. With a gastric ulcer, pain occurs 30 minutes to 1.5 hours after eating, and with a duodenal ulcer, pain occurs 2 to 3 hours after eating. Small, frequent meals of nonirritating foods decrease the pain. With treatment, pain usually subsides in 10 days; however, the healing process may take 1 to 2 months.

A **stress ulcer** usually follows a critical situation such as extensive trauma, such as burns, or major surgery (e.g., cardiac surgery). Prophylactic use of antiulcer drugs decreases the incidence of stress ulcers.

Helicobacter pylori

Helicobacter pylori, a gram-negative bacillus, is linked with the development of peptic ulcer and is known to cause gastritis, gastric ulcer, and duodenal ulcer. When a peptic ulcer recurs after antiulcer therapy, and the ulcer is not caused by nonsteroidal antiinflammatory drugs (NSAIDs) such as aspirin or ibuprofen, the patient should be tested for the presence of *H. pylori*, which may have infected the gastric mucosa. In the past, endoscopy and a biopsy of the gastric antrum were needed to check for *H. pylori*. Currently, a noninvasive breath test—the Meretek UBT (urea breath test)—can detect *H. pylori*. This test consists of drinking a liquid containing 13C urea and breathing into a container. If *H. pylori* is present, the bacterial urease hydrolyzes the urea, releasing $13CO_2$, which is detected by a spectrometer. This test is 90% to 95% effective for detecting *H. pylori* and also notes progress in treatment. In addition, a blood test may be performed to check for antibodies to *H. pylori,* and a stool test may be done to check for antigens to determine whether the immune system has been triggered to fight *H. pylori*.

There are various protocols for treating *H. pylori* infection, but antibacterial agents are the treatment of choice. The use of only one antibacterial agent is not effective for eradicating *H. pylori* because the bacterium can readily become resistant to that drug. Treatment to eradicate this bacterial infection includes using a dual-, triple-, or quadruple-drug therapy program in a variety of drug combinations— such as with amoxicillin, tetracycline, clarithromycin, omeprazole, lansoprazole, metronidazole, or bismuth subsalicylate—on a 7- to 14-day treatment plan. The combination of drugs differs for each patient according to the patient's drug tolerance. A common treatment protocol is the triple therapy of metronidazole (or amoxicillin), omeprazole (or lansoprazole), and clarithromycin (MOC). The drug regimen eradicates more than 90% of peptic ulcers caused by *H. pylori*.

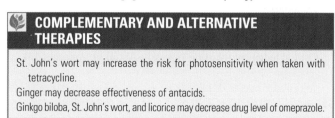

COMPLEMENTARY AND ALTERNATIVE THERAPIES

St. John's wort may increase the risk for photosensitivity when taken with tetracycline.

Ginger may decrease effectiveness of antacids.

Ginkgo biloba, St. John's wort, and licorice may decrease drug level of omeprazole.

One of the PPIs, such as omeprazole or lansoprazole, is frequently used as a component of combination drug therapy because each suppresses acid secretion by inhibiting the enzyme hydrogen or potassium adenosine triphosphatase (ATPase), which makes gastric acid. These agents block the final steps of acid production. If triple therapy fails to eradicate *H. pylori*, quadruple therapy using two antibiotics, a PPI, and a bismuth or histamine$_2$ (H$_2$) blocker is recommended. After completion of the treatment regimen, 6 weeks of standard acid suppression— such as H$_2$ blocker therapy—is recommended. Table 46.2 lists agents used to treat *H. pylori* with their dosages, uses, and considerations. Antibiotics are discussed in more detail in Chapter 26.

Gastroesophageal Reflux Disease

GERD, also called *reflux esophagitis,* is an inflammation of the esophageal mucosa caused by reflux of gastric acid content into the esophagus. Its main cause is an incompetent lower esophageal sphincter. Smoking tends to accelerate the disease process.

Medical treatment for GERD is similar to the treatment for peptic ulcers. This includes use of the common antiulcer drugs to neutralize gastric contents and reduce gastric acid secretion. Drugs used in treatment include H$_2$ blockers such as famotidine and PPIs such as omeprazole, lansoprazole, rabeprazole, pantoprazole, or esomeprazole. A

TABLE 46.2   Pharmacological Agents Used to Treat *Helicobacter pylori* Infection

Drug	Route and Dosage	Uses and Considerations
Antiinfective Agents		
Metronidazole hydrochloride	A: PO: 500 mg tid	To treat numerous organisms, including *H. pylori;* used in combination with other drugs to treat *H. pylori*
Amoxicillin	A: PO: 1000 mg bid	Used in triple- or quadruple-drug therapy for *H. pylori*
Clarithromycin	A: PO: 500 mg bid	Used in dual- and triple-drug therapy for *H. pylori*
Tetracycline	A: PO: 500 mg qid	Used in triple- and quadruple-drug therapy for *H. pylori*
Proton Pump Inhibitors (PPIs)		
Omeprazole	A: PO: 40 mg/d	Used in dual-, triple-, and quadruple-drug therapy for *H. pylori*
Lansoprazole	A: PO: 30 mg tid	Used in dual- and triple-drug therapy for *H. pylori*
Esomeprazole	A: PO: 40–80 mg/d	Used in therapy for *H. pylori*
Pantoprazole	A: PO: 40–80 mg bid	Used in therapy for *H. pylori*
Rabeprazole	A: PO: 20–40 mg bid	Used in therapy for *H. pylori*

A, Adult; *bid,* twice a day; *d,* day; *PO,* by mouth; *qid,* four times a day.

PPI relieves symptoms faster and maintains healing better than an H₂ blocker. Once the strictures are relieved by dilation, they are less likely to recur if the patient was taking PPIs rather than an H₂ blocker.

Effective management of GERD keeps the esophageal mucosa healed and the patient free from symptoms, but GERD is a chronic disorder that requires continuous care.

NONPHARMACOLOGIC MEASURES FOR MANAGING PEPTIC ULCER AND GASTROESOPHAGEAL REFLUX DISEASE

Nonpharmacologic measures, along with drug therapy, are an important part of treatment for a GI disorder. Once the GI problem is resolved, the patient should continue to follow nonpharmacologic measures to avoid recurrence of the condition.

Avoiding tobacco and alcohol can decrease gastric secretions. With GERD, nicotine relaxes the lower esophageal sphincter, permitting gastric acid reflux. Obesity enhances GERD, so weight loss is helpful in decreasing symptoms. The patient should avoid hot, spicy, and greasy foods, which could aggravate the gastric problem. Certain drugs like NSAIDs, which include aspirin, should be taken with food or in a decreased dosage. Glucocorticoids can cause gastric ulceration and should be taken with food.

To relieve symptoms of GERD, the patient should raise the head of the bed, not eat before bedtime, and wear loose-fitting clothing.

⚡ PATIENT SAFETY

Do Not Confuse...
- **Zantac**, an H₂ blocker, with **Xanax**, an anxiolytic

ANTIULCER DRUGS

The seven groups of antiulcer agents are (1) tranquilizers, which decrease vagal activity; (2) anticholinergics, which decrease acetylcholine by blocking the cholinergic receptors; (3) antacids, which neutralize gastric acid; (4) H₂ blockers, which block the H₂ receptor; (5) PPIs, which inhibit gastric acid secretion, regardless of acetylcholine

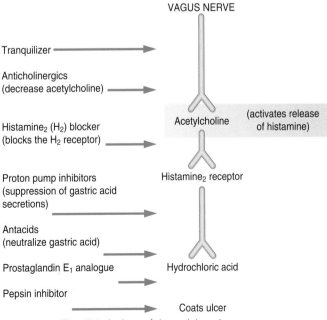

Fig. 46.2 Actions of the antiulcer drug groups.

TABLE 46.3   Antiulcer Drugs: Anticholinergics

Drug	Route and Dosage: Initially	Uses and Considerations
Glycopyrrolate	Ulcer: A: PO: 1–2 mg bid/tid; *max:* 6 mg/d A: IM/IV: 100–200 mcg q4h PRN; *max:* 0.2 mg/dose	For gastric and duodenal ulcers, bradycardia, and aspiration prophylaxis. May cause headache, dyspnea, sinusitis, dry mouth, infection, flushing, nausea, vomiting, weakness, erectile dysfunction, urinary retention, and constipation. PB: UK; t½: 0.5–3 h
Propantheline	A: PO: 15 mg tid 30 min ac and 30 mg at bedtime	For peptic ulcers. May cause headache, dizziness, blurred vision, weakness, flushing, dry mouth, nausea, vomiting, constipation, and urinary retention. PB: UK; t½: 1.6 h
Chlordiazepoxide and clidinium bromide	Peptic ulcer: A: PO: 1–2 capsules (5 mg chlordiazepoxide, 2.5 mg clidinium each capsule) tid/qid 30–60 min ac and at bedtime; *max:* 8 capsules/d Older A: Initially 1 capsule bid	For peptic ulcer disease and IBS. May cause agitation, confusion, blurred vision, drowsiness, dizziness, ataxia, headache, dry mouth, nausea, vomiting, constipation, urinary retention, and weakness. PB: chlordiazepoxide 96%, clidinium UK; t½: chlordiazepoxide 5–100 h, clidinium 2.4–20 h

A, Adult; *ac,* before meals; *bid,* twice a day; *cap,* capsule; *d,* day; *h,* hour; *IBS,* irritable bowel syndrome; *IM,* intramuscular; *IV,* intravenous; *max,* maximum; *min,* minutes; *PB,* protein binding; *PO,* by mouth; *q4h,* every 4 hours; *qid,* four times a day; *t½,* half-life; *tid,* three times a day; *UK,* unknown; *y,* years; *>,* greater than.

or histamine release; (6) the pepsin inhibitor sucralfate; and (7) the prostaglandin E_1 analogue misoprostol, which inhibits gastric acid secretion and protects the mucosa. Currently, tranquilizers and anticholinergics are used infrequently due to potential adverse effects and much more effective drugs on the market. Fig. 46.2 shows the action of the antiulcer drug groups, each of which is discussed separately.

Tranquilizers

Tranquilizers have minimal effect in preventing and treating ulcers; however, they reduce vagal stimulation and decrease anxiety. A combination of the anxiolytic chlordiazepoxide and the anticholinergic clidinium bromide may be used in the treatment of ulcers. Adverse effects may include edema, ataxia, confusion, and agranulocytosis.

Anticholinergics

Anticholinergics (antimuscarinics, parasympatholytics) and antacids were the drugs of choice for peptic ulcers for many years. However, anticholinergic use declined with the introduction of H_2 blockers in 1975. These drugs relieve pain by decreasing GI motility and secretion. They act by inhibiting acetylcholine and blocking histamine and HCl. Anticholinergics delay gastric emptying time, so they are used more frequently for duodenal ulcers than for gastric ulcers. The anticholinergic propantheline bromide inhibits gastric secretions in the treatment of peptic ulcers.

Anticholinergics should be taken 30 minutes to 1 hour before meals and at least 2 hours after the evening meal for the bedtime dose to decrease acid secretion that occurs with eating. Antacids can slow the absorption of anticholinergics and therefore should be taken 2 hours after anticholinergic administration.

Table 46.3 lists selected anticholinergic drugs used to treat peptic ulcer. Anticholinergics should be used as adjunctive therapy and not as the only antiulcer drug. Anticholinergics are discussed in more detail in Chapter 16.

Side Effects and Adverse Reactions. Anticholinergics have many side effects, including dry mouth, decreased secretions, headache, blurred vision, drowsiness, dizziness, asthenia, palpitations, erectile dysfunction, urinary retention, and constipation. Because anticholinergics decrease GI motility, gastric emptying time is delayed, which can stimulate gastric secretions and aggravate the ulceration.

Antacids

Antacids promote ulcer healing by neutralizing HCl and reducing pepsin activity; they do not coat the ulcer. There are two types of antacids: those that have a *systemic* effect and those that have a *nonsystemic* effect.

📄 **PROTOTYPE DRUG CHART**

Aluminum Hydroxide

Drug Class	Dosage
Antiulcer: Antacid	Hyperacidity: A: PO: 40–60 mL (80–140 mEq) q3–6h or 1–3 h pc and at bedtime

Contraindications	Drug-Lab-Food Interactions
Hypersensitivity to aluminum products *Caution:* Diarrhea, hepatic/renal disease, hypophosphatemia, dehydration, GI bleeding/obstruction, older adults, children, pregnancy	Drug: Decreased effects with tetracycline, phenothiazine, isoniazid, phenytoin, digitalis, quinidine, amphetamines, fluoroquinolones, and captopril; may increase effects of benzodiazepines, glipizide, and glyburide Lab: Increased urine pH

Pharmacokinetics	Pharmacodynamics
Absorption: PO: Small amount absorbed Distribution: PB: UK Metabolism: t½: UK Excretion: In feces; small amount in urine	PO: Onset: 15–30 min Peak: 0.5 h Duration: 1–3 h

Therapeutic Effects/Uses

To treat hyperacidity, gastric and duodenal ulcer, and reflux esophagitis; to reduce hyperphosphatemia

Mechanism of Action: Neutralizes gastric acidity.

Side Effects	Adverse Reactions
Anorexia, constipation, weakness, impaired cognition	Hypophosphatemia, hypercalcemia, osteoporosis, nephrolithiasis, and GI obstruction.

A, Adult; *GI,* gastrointestinal; *h,* hour; *min,* minute; *PB,* protein binding; *PO,* by mouth; *t½,* half-life; *UK,* unknown.

TABLE 46.4 Antiulcer Drugs: Antacids

Drug	Route and Dosage	Uses and Considerations
Aluminum hydroxide	See Prototype Drug Chart: Aluminum Hydroxide	
Calcium carbonate	Dyspepsia: A: PO: 1000–3000 mg may repeat PRN; *max:* 7500 mg/d up to 2 weeks	To treat pyrosis, dyspepsia, hypocalcemia, and hyperphosphatemia and for osteoporosis prophylaxis. May cause hypercalcemia, hypophosphatemia, nausea, vomiting, constipation, flatulence, headache, and metabolic alkalosis. PB: 40%; t½: UK
Calcium carbonate and magnesium hydroxide	Regular strength: A: PO: Chew 2–4 tabs PRN; *max:* 12 tabs/d	To treat pyrosis and dyspepsia. May cause metabolic alkalosis, hypermagnesemia, hypercalcemia, hypophosphatemia, eructation, flatulence, gastric hypersecretion, nausea, vomiting, and constipation. PB: 40%; t½: UK
Magnesium hydroxide and aluminum hydroxide	A: PO: 10–20 mL qid; *max:* 80 mL/d	To treat gastric and duodenal ulcers, dyspepsia, pyrosis, and GERD. May cause weakness, anorexia, nausea, vomiting, constipation, hypercalcemia, hypermagnesemia, and hypophosphatemia. PB: UK; t½: UK
Magnesium hydroxide 200 mg and aluminum hydroxide 200 mg with simethicone 25 mg	A: PO: 10–20 mL or 2–4 tsp between meals and at bedtime Extra strength: A: PO: 1–2 tabs between meals and at bedtime	To treat dyspepsia, pyrosis, and flatulence. May cause hypercalcemia, hypermagnesemia, hypophosphatemia, anorexia, nausea, vomiting, constipation, diarrhea, and weakness. PB: UK; t½: UK
Magnesium trisilicate with aluminum hydroxide	A: PO: 2–4 tab (magnesium hydroxide 14.2 mg and aluminum hydroxide 80 mg) qid; *max:* 16 tab/d	To treat dyspepsia, pyrosis, and GERD. May cause hypermagnesemia, hypercalcemia, hypophosphatemia, anorexia, nausea, vomiting, constipation, and weakness. PB: UK; t½: UK
Sodium bicarbonate	Dyspepsia: A: PO: 300 mg–2 g 1–4 times/d	To treat dyspepsia, pyrosis, hyperkalemia, and metabolic acidosis. Rarely used for peptic ulcer disease because it can be absorbed and affect systemic acid-base balance. May cause flatulence, gastric distension, peripheral edema, hypernatremia, metabolic alkalosis, and tremor. PB: UK; t½: UK

A, Adult; *d,* day; *GERD,* gastroesophageal reflux disease; *GI,* gastrointestinal; *max,* maximum; *PB,* protein binding; *PO,* by mouth; *PRN,* as needed, *qid,* four times a day; *t½,* half-life; *tab,* tablet; *UK,* unknown; *y,* years; >, greater than.

Sodium bicarbonate, a systemically absorbed antacid, was one of the first antiulcer drugs. Because it has many side effects (sodium excess, causing hypernatremia and water retention; metabolic alkalosis caused by excess bicarbonate; and acid rebound [excess acid secretion]), sodium bicarbonate is seldom used to treat peptic ulcers.

Calcium carbonate is most effective in neutralizing acid; however, one-third to one-half of the drug can be systemically absorbed and can cause acid rebound. Hypercalcemia and Burnett syndrome, formerly called *milk-alkali syndrome,* can result from excessive use of calcium carbonate. Burnett syndrome is intensified if milk products are ingested with calcium carbonate. It is identified by the presence of alkalosis, hypercalcemia, and, in severe cases, crystalluria and renal failure.

The nonsystemic antacids are composed of alkaline salts such as aluminum (aluminum hydroxide) and magnesium (magnesium hydroxide, magnesium trisilicate). A small degree of systemic absorption occurs with these drugs, mainly of aluminum. Magnesium hydroxidehas greater neutralizing power than aluminum hydroxide. Magnesium compounds can cause diarrhea, and aluminum and calcium compounds can cause constipation with long-term use. A combination of magnesium and aluminum salts neutralizes gastric acid without causing severe diarrhea or constipation. Simethicone, an antigas agent, is found in many antacids. Prototype Drug Chart: Aluminum Hydroxide lists the pharmacological data for aluminum hydroxide antacids.

Pharmacokinetics. Aluminum hydroxide was one of the first antacids used to neutralize HCl. Aluminum products are frequently used to lower high serum phosphate (hyperphosphatemia). Because aluminum hydroxide alone can cause constipation, and magnesium products alone can cause diarrhea, combination drugs such as aluminum hydroxide and magnesium hydroxide have become popular because they decrease these side effects. Only a small amount of aluminum hydroxide is absorbed from the GI tract. It is primarily bound to phosphate and excreted in the feces. The small portion that is absorbed is excreted in the urine.

Pharmacodynamics. Aluminum hydroxide neutralizes gastric acid, including HCl, and increases the pH of gastric secretions; an elevated pH inactivates pepsin. The onset of action is fairly rapid, but the duration of action varies, depending on whether the antacid is taken with or without food. If the antacid is taken after a meal, the duration of action may be up to 3 hours because food delays gastric emptying time. Frequent dosing may be necessary if the antacid is given during a fasting state or early in the course of treatment.

The ideal dosing interval for antacids is 1 to 3 hours after meals (maximum acid secretion occurs after eating) and at bedtime. Antacids taken on an empty stomach are effective for 30 to 60 minutes before passing into the duodenum. Chewable tablets should be followed by water. Liquid antacids should also be taken with water (2 to 4 oz) to ensure that the drug reaches the stomach; however, no more than 4 ounces of water should be taken because water quickens gastric emptying time. Antacids should not be administered with other oral medications as there are numerous drug interactions.

Antacids that contain magnesium salts are contraindicated in patients with impaired renal function because of the risk for hypermagnesemia. Magnesium is primarily excreted by the kidneys; however, hypermagnesemia is usually not a problem unless a patient with renal insufficiency is ingesting magnesium. Prolonged use of aluminum hydroxides can cause hypophosphatemia (low serum phosphate), osteoporosis, nephrolithiasis, and osteomalacia. If hyperphosphatemia occurs because of poor renal function, aluminum hydroxide can be given to decrease the phosphate level. In patients with renal

◎ CLINICAL JUDGMENT [NURSING PROCESS]

Antiulcer: Antacids

Concept: Pain
- An unpleasant feeling of discomfort usually associated with tissue damage

Recognize Cues [Assessment]
- Evaluate patient pain, including the type, duration, severity, and frequency.
- Check renal function.
- Assess for fluid and electrolyte imbalances, especially serum phosphate and calcium levels.
- Obtain a drug history and report probable drug-drug interactions.

Analyze Cues and Prioritize Hypothesis [Patient Problems]
- Acute pain
- Injury
- Gastric irritation
- Nausea
- Discomfort

Generate Solutions [Planning]
- The patient will report that abdominal pain has decreased after 1 to 2 weeks of antiulcer drug management.

Take Action [Nursing Interventions]
- Avoid administering antacids with other oral drugs because antacids can delay their absorption. Do not give an antacid with tetracycline, digoxin, or quinidine because it binds with and inactivates most of the drug. Antacids are not given with any other medications.
- Shake suspensions well before administering and follow them with water.
- Monitor electrolytes and urinary pH, calcium, and phosphate levels.

Patient Teaching
General
- ⚡ Teach patients to report pain, coughing, or vomiting of blood.

- Encourage patients to drink 2 oz of water after taking an antacid to ensure that the drug reaches the stomach.
- Direct patients to take antacids 1 to 3 hours after meals and at bedtime. Instruct patients not to take antacids at mealtime; they slow gastric emptying time, causing increased gastrointestinal (GI) activity and gastric secretions.
- Advise patients to notify a health care provider if constipation or diarrhea occurs; the antacid may have to be changed. Self-treatment should be avoided.
- ⚡ Warn that taking an unlimited amount of the antacid is contraindicated.
- Warn patients to avoid taking antacids with milk or foods high in vitamin D.
- Advise patients to avoid taking antacids with other oral medications because they may interfere with absorption.
- Guide patients on a sodium-restricted diet to check antacid labels for sodium content.
- Alert patients to consult with a health care provider before taking self-prescribed antacids for longer than 2 weeks.
- Inform patients on the use of relaxation techniques.

Self-Administration
- Teach patients how to take antacids correctly. Chewable tablets must be thoroughly chewed and followed with water. With liquid antacids, patients should follow the antacid with 2 to 4 oz of water. Increased amounts of water with antacids increases gastric emptying time.

Side Effects
- Direct patients to avoid foods and beverages that can cause gastric irritation (high-fat or spicy meals; caffeine-containing coffee and soda; alcohol).
- Explain to patients that stools may become speckled or white.

Evaluate Outcomes [Evaluation]
- Determine the effectiveness of the antiulcer treatment and the presence of side effects. The patient should be free of pain, and healing should progress.

---

insufficiency, aluminum salt ingestion can cause encephalopathy from accumulation of aluminum in the brain. Table 46.4 lists the antacids and their dosages, uses, and considerations.

Histamine$_2$ Blockers

The histamine$_2$ (H2) receptor antagonists, or H$_2$ blockers, are popular drugs used in the treatment of gastric and duodenal ulcers. Histamine$_2$ blockers prevent acid reflux in the esophagus (reflux esophagitis). These drugs block the H$_2$ receptors of the parietal cells in the stomach, thus reducing gastric acid secretion and concentration. Antihistamines used to treat allergic conditions act against histamine$_1$ (H$_1$); they are not the same as H$_2$ blockers.

The first H$_2$ blocker was cimetidine, introduced in 1975. Cimetidine, which has a short half-life and a short duration of action, blocks about 70% of acid secretion for 4 hours. Good kidney function is necessary because approximately 50% to 80% of the drug is excreted unchanged in the urine. In patients with renal insufficiency, the dose and frequency may need to be reduced. Antacids can be given 1 hour before or after cimetidine as part of an antiulcer drug regimen; however, if they are given at the same time, the effectiveness of the H$_2$ blocker is decreased.

Two H$_2$ blockers—famotidine and nizatidine—are more potent than cimetidine. In addition to blocking gastric acid secretions, they promote healing of the ulcer by eliminating its cause. Their duration

of action is longer, decreasing the frequency of dosing, and they have fewer side effects and fewer drug interactions than cimetidine. Prototype Drug Chart: Famotidine lists the pharmacological data for famotidine, which is a frequently prescribed H$_2$ blocker.

Pharmacokinetics. Famotidine is rapidly absorbed and reaches its peak concentration after a single dose in 1 to 3 hours. Famotidine has a low protein-binding power and a short half-life. A dose of famotidine is 30% to 35% metabolized by the liver. Approximately 65% to 70% is excreted in the urine.

Pharmacodynamics. Famotidine inhibits binding of H$_2$ receptors on the gastric membrane of parietal cells, thereby reducing gastric acid secretions. The drug is effective in treating gastric and duodenal ulcers and can be used prophylactically. Famotidine is also useful in relieving symptoms of pyrosis, dyspepsia, GERD, and Zollinger-Ellison syndrome.

Famotidine has a similar onset of action of 1 hour and a longer duration of action (up to 12 hours) than cimetidine. Because the duration of action of cimetidine is only 4 to 5 hours, it is frequently given two to four times a day.

Famotidine is 50% to 80% more potent than cimetidine. It is indicated for short-term use (4 to 8 weeks) for duodenal ulcer and for Zollinger-Ellison syndrome.

Nizatidine is an H$_2$ blocker that can relieve nocturnal gastric acid secretion for 12 hours. This drug is similar to famotidine, and none

PROTOTYPE DRUG CHART

Famotidine

Drug Class	Dosage
Antiulcer: Histamine$_2$ blocker	Peptic ulcer: A: PO: 40 mg at bedtime for 4–8 wk A: IV: 20 mg q12h

Contraindications	Drug-Lab-Food Interactions
Hypersensitivity *Caution:* Pregnancy, breastfeeding, infection, tobacco smoking, vitamin B$_{12}$ deficiency, renal/hepatic disease, older adults, children	Drug: Decreased absorption of iron; decreased effects of ketoconazole, naproxen, pseudoephedrine; increased action of metformin Lab: Increased serum alkaline phosphatase

Pharmacokinetics	Pharmacodynamics
Absorption: PO: Well absorbed, 50% Distribution: PB: 15%–20% Metabolism: t½: 2.5–3.5 h Excretion: In urine and feces	PO: Onset: 1 h Peak: 1–3 h Duration: 10–12 h IV: Onset: 10–15 min Peak: 30 min Duration: 10–12 h

Therapeutic Effects/Uses

To prevent and treat gastric and duodenal ulcers, pyrosis, dyspepsia, esophagitis, GERD, and Zollinger-Ellison syndrome
Mechanism of Action: Inhibits gastric acid secretion by inhibiting histamine$_2$ receptors in parietal cells.

Side Effects	Adverse Reactions
Headache, dizziness, drowsiness, confusion, agitation, insomnia, nausea, vomiting, diarrhea, constipation, depression, rash, fatigue, arthralgia, muscle cramps, weakness, erectile dysfunction	Palpitations, gynecomastia, vitamin B$_{12}$ deficiency *Life-threatening:* Anaphylactoid reactions, agranulocytosis, leukopenia, thrombocytopenia, pancytopenia, dysrhythmia, bronchospasm

A, Adult; *d,* day; *GERD,* gastroesophageal reflux disease; *h,* hour; *IM,* intramuscular; *IV,* intravenous; *max,* maximum; *min,* minute; *PB,* protein binding; *PO,* by mouth; *q12h,* every 12 hours; *t½,* half-life.

TABLE 46.5 Antiulcer Drugs: Histamine$_2$ Blockers

Drug	Route and Dosage	Uses and Considerations
Cimetidine	Peptic ulcer: A: PO: 800 mg/d at bedtime or 400 mg bid or 300 mg qid with meals and hs for 8–12 weeks; max: 1200 mg/d A: IV/IM: 300 mg q6h	To treat peptic ulcers, GERD, pyrosis, and dyspepsia. May cause headache, dizziness, diarrhea, drowsiness, agitation, gynecomastia, and erectile dysfunction. PB: 20%; t½: 2 h
Famotidine	See Prototype Drug Chart: Famotidine	
Nizatidine	Peptic ulcers: A: PO: 150 mg q12h or 300 mg at bedtime for 8 weeks; *max:* 300 mg/d	To treat peptic ulcers, dyspepsia, *H. pylori* infection, pyrosis, and GERD. May cause dizziness, cough, irritability, headache, fever, rhinitis, nasal congestion, vomiting, diarrhea, vitamin B$_{12}$ deficiency, and erectile dysfunction. PB: 35%; t½: 1–2 h

A, Adult; *ac,* before meals; *bid,* twice daily; *d,* day; *GERD,* gastroesophageal reflux disease; *h,* hour; *IM,* intramuscular; *IV,* intravenous; *max,* maximum; *min,* minute; *PB,* protein binding; *PO,* by mouth; *q,* every; *t½,* half-life; *y,* years; *>,* greater than; *<,* less than.

of these agents suppresses the metabolism of other drugs. To prevent recurrence of duodenal ulcers, administer nizatidine 150 mg twice a day at bedtime or famotidine 40 mg once a day at bedtime. Both nizatidine and famotidine have low protein-binding capacities and similar half-lives.

Table 46.5 lists the H$_2$ blockers and their dosages, uses, and considerations.

Side Effects and Adverse Reactions. Side effects and adverse reactions of H$_2$ blockers include headache, agitation, dizziness, nausea, vomiting, constipation or diarrhea, pruritus, skin rash, vitamin B$_{12}$ deficiency, erectile dysfunction, and blood dyscrasias. Famotidine has fewer side effects than cimetidine.

Drug and Laboratory Interactions. Cimetidine interacts with many drugs. By inhibiting hepatic drug metabolism, it enhances the effects

CLINICAL JUDGMENT [NURSING PROCESS]

Antiulcer: Histamine₂ Blocker

Concept: Pain
- An unpleasant feeling of discomfort usually associated with tissue damage

Recognize Cues [Assessment]
- Determine the patient's pain, including the type, duration, severity, frequency, and location.
- Evaluate gastrointestinal (GI) complaints.
- Check mental status.
- Assess fluid and electrolyte imbalances, including intake and output.
- Monitor gastric pH (>5 is desired), blood urea nitrogen (BUN), and creatinine.
- Determine a drug history and report probable drug-drug interactions.

Analyze Cues and Prioritize Hypothesis [Patient Problems]
- Acute pain
- Injury
- Gastric irritation
- Discomfort

Generate Solutions [Planning]
- The patient will report that abdominal pain has decreased after 1 to 2 weeks of drug therapy.

Take Action [Nursing Interventions]
- ⚡ Be alert that older adults have less gastric acid and need reduced doses of the drug. Metabolic acidosis must be prevented.

Patient Teaching
General
- ⚡ Teach patients to report pain, coughing, or vomiting of blood.
- Advise patients to avoid smoking because it can hamper the effectiveness of the drug.
- Remind patients that the drug must be taken exactly as prescribed to be effective.
- Direct patients to separate famotidine and iron dosage by at least 1 hour.
- ⚡ Warn patients not to drive a motor vehicle or engage in dangerous activities until stabilized on the drug.
- Tell patients that drug-induced erectile dysfunction is reversible.
- Educate patients in the use of relaxation techniques to decrease anxiety.

Diet
- Teach patients to eat foods high in vitamin B₁₂ to avoid deficiency from drug therapy.
- Alert patients to avoid foods and liquids that cause gastric irritation, such as caffeine-containing beverages, alcohol, and spices.

Evaluate Outcomes [Evaluation]
- Determine the effectiveness of drug therapy and the presence of any side effects or adverse reactions. The patient should be free of pain, and healing should progress.

of oral anticoagulants, theophylline, caffeine, phenytoin, diazepam, propranolol, phenobarbital, and calcium channel blockers. Cimetidine can cause an increase in blood urea nitrogen (BUN), serum creatinine, and serum alkaline phosphatase. Cimetidine should not be taken with iron because its H₂-blocking action could be decreased.

Proton Pump Inhibitors (Gastric Acid Secretion Inhibitors, Gastric Acid Pump Inhibitors)

PPIs suppress gastric acid secretion by inhibiting the hydrogen/potassium ATPase enzyme system located in the gastric parietal cells. They tend to inhibit gastric acid secretion up to 90% more than the H₂ blockers (histamine antagonists). These agents block the final step of acid production.

Omeprazole was the first PPI marketed, followed by lansoprazole, rabeprazole, pantoprazole, esomeprazole, and dexlansoprazole, a delayed-release oral capsule. These agents are effective in suppressing gastric acid secretions and are used to treat peptic ulcers and GERD. With lansoprazole, ulcer relief usually occurs in 1 week. Rabeprazole is more effective in treating duodenal ulcers than gastric ulcers, but it is most effective for treating GERD and hypersecretory disease (Zollinger-Ellison syndrome). Pantoprazole is prescribed to treat short-term erosive GERD. Intravenous (IV) pantoprazole is also reported as effective in treating Zollinger-Ellison syndrome. Esomeprazole has the highest success rate for healing erosive GERD, more so than omeprazole. Omeprazole promotes irreversible hydrogen or potassium ATPase inhibition until new enzyme is synthesized, which could take days, whereas rabeprazole causes reversible ATPase inhibition. Dexlansoprazole is prescribed to treat erosive esophagitis and symptomatic nonerosive GERD.

All PPIs in large doses can be combined with antibiotics to treat *H. pylori*. Prototype Drug Chart: Pantoprazole lists the pharmacological data for pantoprazole.

⚡ **PATIENT SAFETY**

Do Not Confuse...
- **Protonix**, a PPI, with **Lotronex**, a serotonin 5-HT₃ receptor antagonist used for irritable bowel syndrome
- **AcipHex**, a PPI, with **Aricept**, an Alzheimer drug
- **Nexium**, a PPI, with **Nexavar**, a biologic response modifier
- **Rabeprazole**, a PPI, with **aripiprazole**, an atypical antipsychotic
- **Misoprostol**, an antiulcer agent, with **mifepristone**, a postcoital contraceptive agent

Two combination medications involving PPIs are omeprazole with sodium bicarbonate and esomeprazole with naproxen. These combinations are used to treat GERD, erosive esophagitis, and gastric or duodenal ulcers.

Pharmacokinetics and Pharmacodynamics. The duration of action for pantoprazole is 24 hours. This drug has a half-life of 1 to 10 hours and is highly protein bound (99%). PPIs should usually be taken before meals. Caution should be used in patients with hepatic impairment, and liver enzymes should be monitored. Possible side effects include headache, dizziness, diarrhea or constipation, abdominal pain, vitamin B₁₂ deficiency, and hypomagnesemia. Prolonged use of PPIs may increase the risk for cancer, although this has only been proven in mice, not humans.

PROTOTYPE DRUG CHART
Pantoprazole

Drug Class	Dosage
Antiulcer: Proton pump inhibitor	GERD: A: PO/IV: 40 mg/d 1 h before first meal of day for 8–16 wk PO and for 7–10 d IV

Contraindications	Drug-Lab-Food Interactions
Hypersensitivity *Caution:* Hepatic impairment, pregnancy, breastfeeding, diarrhea, bone fractures, osteoporosis, older adults	Drug: May interfere with absorption of ampicillin, ketoconazole, digoxin; statins increase PPI absorption and bioavailability; thiazide, loop, and potassium-sparing diuretics; beta blockers, ACE inhibitors, and ARBs may lead to hypomagnesemia. Food: Food decreases peak levels. Herb: St. John's wort decreases drug levels

Pharmacokinetics	Pharmacodynamics
Absorption: Rapidly absorbed in GI tract Distribution: PB: 99% Metabolism: t½: 1–10 h Excretion: Primarily in urine, also in bile and feces	PO: Onset: 2.5 h Peak: 2.5 h Duration: 24 hIV: Onset: 15–30 min Peak: UKDuration: 24 h

Therapeutic Effects/Uses
To treat duodenal ulcers, GERD, esophagitis, dyspepsia, pyrosis, *Helicobacter pylori* infection, and Zollinger-Ellison syndrome and to prevent NSAID-induced ulcers
Mechanism of Action: Suppresses gastric acid secretion by inhibiting hydrogen/potassium ATPase enzyme in gastric parietal cells.

Side Effects	Adverse Reactions
Headache, dizziness, drowsiness, depression, blurred vision, fatigue, dry mouth, nausea, vomiting, flatulence, constipation, diarrhea, abdominal pain, edema, weakness, arthralgia, myalgia, vitamin B_{12} deficiency	GI bleeding, anemia, hypomagnesemia, hypertriglyceridemia, hyperbilirubinemia, hyponatremia, bone fractures, tachycardia, palpitations, angioedema *Life-threatening:* Leukopenia, agranulocytosis, pancytopenia, thrombocytopenia, dysrhythmia, CDAD, Stevens-Johnson syndrome, hepatic failure

A, Adult; *ALT*, alanine aminotransferase; *AST*, aspartate aminotransferase; *ATP*, adenosine triphosphate; *CDAD, Clostridium difficile*–associated disease; *d*, day; *GERD*, gastroesophageal reflux disease; *GI*, gastrointestinal; *h*, hour; *NSAID*, nonsteroidal antiinflammatory drug; *PB*, protein binding; *PO*, by mouth; *PPI*, proton pump inhibitor; *t½*, half-life; *y*, years; *>*, greater than.

TABLE 46.6 Antiulcer Drugs: Proton Pump Inhibitors, Pepsin Inhibitors, and Prostaglandin Analogues

Drug	Route and Dosage	Uses and Considerations
Proton Pump Inhibitors (Gastric Acid Secretion Inhibitors)		
Esomeprazole	GERD: A: PO: 20 mg qd 1 h before first meal of the day; *max:* 40 mg/d	For GERD, dyspepsia, *Helicobacter pylori* infection, pyrosis, Zollinger-Ellison syndrome, and NSAID-induced ulcer prophylaxis. May cause headache, dry mouth, abdominal pain, dyspepsia, nausea, diarrhea, GI bleeding, constipation, and flatulence. PB: 97%; t½: 1.5 h
Lansoprazole	Peptic ulcer: A: PO: 15–30 mg/d 30–60 min ac; *max:* 30 mg/d	To treat peptic ulcers, GERD, dyspepsia, *Helicobacter pylori* infection, pyrosis, and Zollinger-Ellison syndrome, and for NSAID-induced ulcer prophylaxis. May cause headache, dizziness, abdominal pain, nausea, diarrhea, constipation, rash, vitamin B_{12} deficiency, and hypomagnesemia. PB: 97%; t½: 1.5 h
Omeprazole	Peptic ulcer: Delayed release: A: PO: 20–40 mg/d for 4–8 wk; *max:* 40 mg/d	To treat peptic ulcer, GERD, dyspepsia, pyrosis, Zollinger-Ellison syndrome, and *H. pylori* infection. May cause headache, dizziness, nausea, vomiting, diarrhea, abdominal pain, flatulence, constipation, and weakness. PB: 95%; t½: 30–60 min
Pantoprazole	See Prototype Drug Chart: Pantoprazole	
Rabeprazole	Duodenal ulcer: A: PO: 20 mg/d in morning up to 4 wk; *max:* 40 mg/d	For duodenal ulcer, GERD, Zollinger-Ellison syndrome, esophagitis, and *H. pylori* infection. May cause headache, dizziness, nausea, diarrhea, abdominal pain, flatulence, vomiting, vitamin B_{12} deficiency, and hypomagnesemia. PB: 96.3%; t½: 1–2 h

Continued

TABLE 46.6 Antiulcer Drugs: Proton Pump Inhibitors, Pepsin Inhibitors, and Prostaglandin Analogues—cont'd

Drug	Route and Dosage	Uses and Considerations
Dexlansoprazole	GERD: Delayed release: A: PO: 30–60 mg/d for up to 4–8 wk; *max:* 60 mg/d	For esophagitis, pyrosis, and GERD. May cause nausea, abdominal pain, diarrhea, vitamin B_{12} deficiency, hypomagnesemia, hyponatremia. PB: 96.1%–98.8%; t½: 1–2 h
Pepsin Inhibitor		
Sucralfate	See Prototype Drug Chart: Sucralfate	
Prostaglandin Analogue		
Misoprostol	A: PO: 100–200 mcg qid with meals and at bedtime; *max:* 800 mcg/d	For prevention of NSAID-induced ulcer. May be taken during NSAID therapy, including with aspirin. May cause headache, nausea, vomiting, flatulence, diarrhea, abdominal pain, chills, shivering, and hyperthermia. PB: <90%; t½: UK
Combinations		
Omeprazole 20 mg and sodium bicarbonate 1100 mg	GERD: A: PO: 1 capsule (omeprazole 20 mg, sodium bicarbonate 1100 mg)/d for 4–8 wk	To treat peptic ulcers, GERD, esophagitis, and pyrosis and to prevent stress gastritis. May cause headache, abdominal pain, flatulence, nausea, vomiting, constipation, and diarrhea. PB: omeprazole 95%, sodium bicarbonate UK; t½: omeprazole 60 min, sodium bicarbonate UK
Esomeprazole and naproxen	A: PO: 1 tablet (esomeprazole 20 mg and naproxen 375 mg or esomeprazole 20 mg and naproxen 500 mg) bid; *max:* esomeprazole 40 mg/d and naproxen 1000 mg/d	To prevent NSAID-associated gastric ulcers. May cause headache, dizziness, drowsiness, ecchymosis, pyrosis, nausea, gastritis, palpitations, and purpura. PB: esomeprazole 97%, naproxen 99%; t½: esomeprazole 1.2–1.5 h, naproxen 12–17 h

A, Adult; *ac,* before meals; *bid,* two times a day; *d,* day; *GERD,* gastroesophageal reflux disease; *GI,* gastrointestinal; *h,* hour; *IV,* intravenous; *max,* maximum; *min,* minute; *NSAID,* nonsteroidal antiinflammatory drug; *PB,* protein binding; *PO,* by mouth; *qid,* four times a day; *t½,* half-life; *UK,* unknown; *wk,* week; *y,* year; *>,* greater than.

Table 46.6 lists the PPIs and their dosages, uses, and considerations.

Drug Interactions. PPIs can enhance the action of digoxin, oral anticoagulants, certain benzodiazepines, and phenytoin because they interfere with liver metabolism of these drugs.

Pepsin Inhibitors (Mucosal Protective Drugs)

Sucralfate, a complex of sulfated sucrose and aluminum hydroxide, is classified as a pepsin inhibitor, or *mucosal protective drug.* It is nonabsorbable and combines with protein to form a viscous substance that covers the ulcer and protects it from acid and pepsin. This drug does not neutralize acid or decrease acid secretions.

The dosage of sucralfate is 1 g, usually four times a day, before meals and at bedtime. If antacids are added to decrease pain, they should be given either 30 minutes before or 30 minutes after the administration of sucralfate. Because sucralfate is not systemically absorbed, side effects are few; however, it can cause dry mouth, headache, drowsiness, dizziness, and constipation. If the drug is stored at room temperature in an airtight container, it will remain stable for up to 2 years. Prototype Drug Chart: Sucralfate lists the pharmacological data for sucralfate.

Pharmacokinetics. Less than 5% of sucralfate is absorbed by the GI tract. It has a half-life of 6 to 20 hours, and 90% of the drug is excreted in feces within 48 hours. However, any drug that is absorbed systemically is excreted primarily in the urine.

Pharmacodynamics. Sucralfate promotes healing by adhering to the ulcer surface. Onset of action occurs within 1 to 2 hours and duration of action is usually 6 hours. Sucralfate decreases the absorption of tetracycline, phenytoin, fat-soluble vitamins, and the antibacterial agents ciprofloxacin and norfloxacin. Antacids decrease the effects of sucralfate.

PROTOTYPE DRUG CHART

Sucralfate

Drug Class	Dosage
Antiulcer: Pepsin inhibitor	Peptic ulcer: A: PO: 1 g qid 1 h before meals and at bedtime for 4–8 weeks

Contraindications	Drug-Lab-Food Interactions
Hypersensitivity *Caution:* Renal impairment, diabetes mellitus, dysphagia, pregnancy, breastfeeding, older adults	Drug: Decreased effects with tetracycline, phenytoin, digoxin; altered absorption with fluoroquinolones, antacids, ketoconazole, furosemide, lansoprazole, thyroid hormones

Pharmacokinetics	Pharmacodynamics
Absorption: PO: Minimal absorption (<5%) Distribution: PB: UK Metabolism: t½: 6–20 h Excretion: In urine	PO: Onset: 1–2 h Peak: UK Duration: 6 h

Therapeutic Effects/Uses

To prevent gastric mucosal injury from drug-induced ulcers (aspirin, NSAIDs); to treat duodenal ulcers
Mechanism of Action: In combination with gastric acid, forms a protective covering on the ulcer surface.

Side Effects	Adverse Reactions
Dizziness, drowsiness, headache, nausea, vomiting, flatulence, constipation, dry mouth, rash, pruritus	Hyperglycemia, hypophosphatemia, angioedema

A, Adult; *h*, hour; *NSAID*, nonsteroidal antiinflammatory drug; *PB*, protein binding; *PO*, by mouth; *qid*, four times a day; *t½*, half-life; *UK*, unknown; <, less than.

CLINICAL JUDGMENT [NURSING PROCESS]

Antiulcer: Pepsin Inhibitors

Concept: Pain
- An unpleasant feeling of discomfort usually associated with tissue damage

Recognize Cues [Assessment]
- Evaluate the patient's pain, including the type, duration, severity, and frequency. Ulcer pain usually occurs after meals and during the night.
- Determine the patient's renal function. Report urine output of less than 600 mL/day or less than 30 mL/h.
- Assess for fluid and electrolyte imbalances.
- Measure gastric pH (>5 is desired).

Analyze Cues and Prioritize Hypothesis [Patient Planning]
- Acute pain
- Injury
- Gastric irritation
- Discomfort

Generate Solutions [Planning]
- The patient will report relief of abdominal pain after 1 to 2 weeks of antiulcer drug management.

Take Action [Nursing Interventions]
- Administer drug on an empty stomach.
- Administer antacid 30 minutes before or 30 minutes after sucralfate. Allow 1 to 2 hours to elapse between sucralfate and other prescribed drugs; sucralfate binds with certain drugs (e.g., tetracycline, phenytoin), reducing their effect.

Patient Teaching
General
- Advise patients to take the prescribed drug exactly as ordered. Therapy usually requires 4 to 8 weeks for optimal ulcer healing. Advise patients to continue to take the drug even if they are feeling better.
- Increase fluids, dietary bulk, and exercise to prevent constipation.
- Educate patients in use of relaxation techniques.
- Monitor for severe, persistent constipation.
- Emphasize the need for follow-up medical care.
- Emphasize cessation of smoking as indicated.

Side Effects
- ⚡ Direct patients to report pain, coughing, or vomiting of blood.

Diet
- Teach patients to avoid liquids and foods that can cause gastric irritation, such as caffeine-containing beverages, alcohol, certain fats, and spices.

Evaluate Outcomes [Evaluation]
- Determine the effectiveness of the antiulcer treatment and the presence of any side effects. The patient should be free of pain, and healing should progress.

Prostaglandin Analogue Antiulcer Drug

Misoprostol, a synthetic prostaglandin analogue, is a drug used to prevent and treat peptic ulcer. It appears to suppress gastric acid secretion and to increase cytoprotective mucus in the GI tract. It causes a moderate decrease in pepsin secretion. Misoprostol is considered as effective as cimetidine. Patients who complain of gastric distress from NSAIDs such as aspirin or indomethacin prescribed for long-term therapy can benefit from misoprostol. When a patient takes high doses of NSAIDs, misoprostol is frequently recommended for the duration of the NSAID therapy. Misoprostol is contraindicated during pregnancy and for women of childbearing age. Side effects include headache, abdominal pain, nausea, vomiting, flatulence, diarrhea, and constipation.

Table 46.6 lists the pharmacological data for the PPIs, pepsin inhibitors, and a prostaglandin analogue.

CRITICAL THINKING CASE STUDY

A 48-year-old patient complains of a gnawing, aching pain in the abdominal area that usually occurs several hours after eating. He says that over-the-counter antacids help somewhat, but the pain has recently intensified. Diagnostic tests indicate that he has a duodenal ulcer.

1. Differentiate between peptic ulcer, gastric ulcer, and duodenal ulcer. Explain your answer.
2. What are the predisposing factors related to peptic ulcers? What additional information do you need from the patient?
3. What nonpharmacologic measures can you suggest to alleviate symptoms related to peptic ulcer?

The health care provider prescribed aluminum hydroxide and magnesium hydroxide 20 mL to be taken 2 hours after meals and famotidine 40 mg per day. The dose of magnesium hydroxide and aluminum hydroxide with simethicone is to be taken either 1 hour before or 1 hour after the famotidine.

4. The patient asks the nurse the purposes for magnesium hydroxide and aluminum hydroxide with famotidine. What is the nurse's best response?

5. In what ways are famotidine and cimetidine the same, and how do they differ? Explain your answer.
6. As part of patient teaching, the nurse discusses side effects of famotidine with the patient. What is the most effective way to present this information? Develop a plan.

The patient states that he drinks beer at lunch and has two gin and tonics in the afternoon. He states that the drinks help him relax.

7. What nursing intervention should be taken in regard to the patient's alcohol intake and smoking?
8. What foods should he avoid?

A week later the patient states that he discontinued the prescribed medications because he "felt better." However, the pain recurred, and he asked whether he should resume taking the medications.

9. What is the nurse's best response? What should be included in the patient teaching?

REVIEW QUESTIONS

1. A patient is diagnosed with peptic ulcer disease. The nurse realizes that which of these is a predisposing factor for this condition?
   a. *Helicobacter pylori*
   b. Hyposecretion of pepsin
   c. Decreased hydrochloric acid
   d. *Escherichia coli*
2. A student nurse is preparing to administer sucralfate to a patient. Which statement by the student nurse demonstrates understanding of sucralfate's mechanism of action?
   a. Sucralfate neutralizes gastric acidity.
   b. Gastric acid secretion is decreased by inhibiting histamine at histamine$_2$ receptors in parietal cells.
   c. Gastric acid secretion is suppressed by inhibiting the hydrogen/potassium adenosine triphosphatase enzyme.
   d. Sucralfate combines with protein to form a viscous substance that forms a protective covering over the ulcer.
3. A patient is taking famotidine. What information should the nurse teach the patient about this drug? (Select all that apply.)
   a. The drug should be administered for 4 to 8 weeks.
   b. The drug must be administered 30 minutes before meals.
   c. The drug must be administered separately from iron by at least 1 hour.
   d. The drug must always be administered with magnesium hydroxide.
   e. Smoking should be avoided while taking this drug.
   f. Foods high in vitamin B$_{12}$ should be increased in the diet.

4. When a patient complains of pain accompanying a peptic ulcer, why should the nurse give an antacid?
   a. Antacids decrease gastrointestinal motility.
   b. Antacids decrease gastric acid secretion.
   c. Antacids strengthen the lower esophageal sphincter's action.
   d. Antacids neutralize hydrochloric acid and reduce pepsin activity.
5. A patient is taking famotidine to inhibit gastric secretions. Which side effects of famotidine will the nurse teach the patient? (Select all that apply.)
   a. Dizziness
   b. Headaches
   c. Hypokalemia
   d. Hyperkalemia
   e. Blurred vision
   f. Erectile dysfunction
6. The patient is taking esomeprazole for erosive gastroesophageal reflux disease. Which should the nurse include in patient teaching?
   a. Take the medication daily with breakfast.
   b. Healing should occur in 1 week.
   c. This medication decreases stomach acid secretion.
   d. A blood test to check kidney function should be done.

47

Eye and Ear Disorders

http://evolve.elsevier.com/McCuistion/pharmacology

OBJECTIVES

- Describe the drug groups commonly used for disorders of the eye and ear.
- Discuss the mechanisms of action, routes, side effects and adverse reactions, and contraindications for selected drugs in each group.
- Discuss the Clinical Judgment [Nursing Process] related to drugs used in treating and managing disorders of the eye and ear.
- Identify patient teaching needed for eye and ear drugs.

OUTLINE

OVERVIEW OF THE EYE

Protected within the orbits of the skull, the eyeballs are controlled by the third, fourth, and sixth cranial nerves and are connected to six extraocular muscles. The eye has three layers: (1) the cornea and sclera; (2) the choroid, iris, and ciliary body; and (3) the retina. Fig. 47.1 illustrates the basic structures of the eye.

The cornea, the anterior covering of the eye, is transparent and allows light to enter the eye. It has no blood vessels and receives nutrition from the aqueous humor. An abraded cornea is susceptible to infection. Loss of corneal transparency is usually caused by increased intraocular pressure (IOP).

The sclera is the opaque, white fibrous envelope of the eye. Within the sclera are the posterior and anterior chambers. The posterior chamber has a blind spot around the optic nerve that is insensitive to light. The lens is held in place by ligaments and separates these two chambers. The normally transparent lens focuses light on the retina by changing its shape through a process called accommodation.

The anterior chamber, filled with aqueous humor secreted by the ciliary body, lies in front of the lens. The fluid flows into the anterior chamber through a space between the lens and iris. The excess fluid drains into the canal of Schlemm. An increase in IOP, resulting in glaucoma, occurs with increased production or decreased drainage of aqueous humor.

The choroid, iris, and ciliary body—the thickened part of the vascular covering of the eye that provides attachment to ligaments and support to the lens—constitute the second layer. The choroid absorbs light, and the iris surrounds the pupil and gives the eye its color. By dilating and constricting, the iris controls the quantity of light that reaches the lens.

The retina, the third layer, consists of nerves, rods, and cones that serve as visual sensory receptors. The retina is connected to the brain via the optic nerve.

The eyebrows, eyelashes, eyelids, tears, and corneal and conjunctival reflexes all serve to protect the eye. Bilateral blinking occurs every few seconds during waking hours to keep the eye moist and free of foreign material.

DRUGS FOR DISORDERS OF THE EYE

Problems associated with eye eyes may occur as a result of injuries, infections, or specific noninfectious eye disorders, such as glaucoma and macular degeneration. Most drugs used to treat these conditions are topical medications in formulations developed specifically for eyes. Drugs designed to be applied to the eyes are known as ocular or ophthalmic drugs.

Diagnostic Stains

Diagnostic stains (Table 47.1) are frequently used to locate extraocular lesions or foreign objects, evaluate dry eyes, or evaluate extraocular changes. Stains may be combined with local anesthetics to allow examination that is more thorough by alleviating pain associated with the examination. Patients should be informed that these drugs will cause discoloring of the external eye but will dissipate over several hours; they may also stain nasal secretions if the lacrimal ducts (tear ducts) are patent, and they discolor soft contact lenses. Contact lenses should be removed before administration, and the eye should be rinsed with sterile normal saline solution after the procedure. Contact lenses can be replaced after 1 hour.

Topical Anesthetics

Topical anesthetics are used in selected aspects of a comprehensive eye examination and in a variety of ophthalmic procedures. Ophthalmic

anesthetics act by locally blocking the pain signals at the eye's nerve endings. The two most common topical ophthalmic anesthetics are proparacaine hydrochloride (HCl) and tetracaine HCl. Both medications, available in solutions, are administered as drops. Ophthalmic anesthetics should be administered by a trained clinician.

Corneal anesthesia usually starts occurring within 15 seconds and lasts about 15 minutes. The blink reflex is temporarily lost; therefore the corneal epithelium may become dry. Protecting the eye from irritating chemicals, foreign bodies, and corneal scratches is important. The patient must be instructed that the affected eye will be insensitive to touch and to not rub, touch, or wipe the affected eye. Contact lenses may be reinserted after the anesthetic has completely worn off, usually after 20 minutes.

Antiinfectives

Antiinfectives (Table 47.2) are frequently used for eye infections. Conjunctivitis, an inflammation of the membrane (conjunctiva) covering the eye and inner eyelids, is the most common eye condition. Conjunctivitis is also called "pink eye" and can occur because of bacteria, viruses, and allergens. Bacterial conjunctivitis usually requires antiinfective therapy to either kill or inhibit the spread of bacteria. Some ocular viral infections (e.g., cytomegalovirus [CMV] and herpes simplex virus [HSV]) may require antiviral therapy. Examples of other ocular conditions caused by pathogens treated with ophthalmic antiinfective drugs include the following:

- Blepharitis, infection of the margins of the eyelid
- Chalazion, infection of the meibomian glands of the eyelids that may produce cysts, causing blockage of the ducts
- Bacterial and fungal endophthalmitis, infection and inflammation of structures of the inner eye
- Hordeolum, a local infection of eyelash follicles and glands on lid margins, also known as a *stye*
- Infectious keratitis, corneal infection and inflammation
- Infectious uveitis, infection of the vascular layer of the eye (ciliary body, choroid, and iris)

Before administering ophthalmic antiinfectives, the nurse should screen the patient for previous allergic reactions. Noninfectious conjunctivitis and local skin and eye irritation are possible side effects of ophthalmic antiinfective drugs.

Antiinflammatories

Inflammatory conditions of the eye not related to infectious pathogens often require treatment with antiinflammatory drugs (Table 47.3). If the inflammation is secondary to a bacterial or fungal infection, an antibiotic or antifungal agent is included in the medication regimen. Some ocular antiinflammatories are combined with antibacterials. Many antiinflammatories are not appropriate in patients with ocular viral infections.

Inflammation associated with keratoconjunctivitis sicca, causing lymphocytes to damage the lacrimal gland, results in fibrosis and loss of tear production; this can lead to xerophthalmia (dry eyes). Immunomodulators, such as cyclosporine ophthalmic emulsion, is an immunosuppressant that relieves xerophthalmia by a mechanism that is different from over-the-counter (OTC) lubricants. Ophthalmic cyclosporine acts as a partial immunomodulatory that causes apoptosis of lymphocytes and allows tear production to resume.

Ophthalmic nonsteroidal antiinflammatory drugs (NSAIDs) such as diclofenac sodium and ketorolac tromethamine inhibit miosis by preventing the formation of ocular prostaglandins. Most of these drugs are used for management or prevention of ocular inflammation before and after eye surgery. Unlike corticosteroids, NSAIDs do not affect intraocular pressure (IOP; further discussed in Glaucoma and Ocular Hypertension Drugs). However, ocular NSAIDs can increase

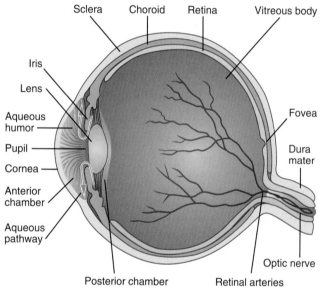

Sclera Choroid Retina Vitreous body

Iris

Lens

Aqueous humor

Pupil

Cornea

Anterior chamber

Aqueous pathway

Fovea

Dura mater

Optic nerve

Posterior chamber Retinal arteries

Fig. 47.1 Basic structures of the eye.

TABLE 47.1 Diagnostic Stains for Eye Disorders

Diagnostic Aid	Purpose
Fluorescein sodium, ophthalmic	Stains the anterior segment of the eye to visualize the anterior ocular surface for defects and for contact lens fitting. When viewed through the cobalt blue filter of the ophthalmoscope or under a Wood lamp, corneal scratches and lesions fluoresce a bright yellow green.
Rose bengal, ophthalmic	Stains the anterior segment of the eye to visualize defects or dry eye. Defective and normal cells are stained a pink-violet color. Staining of normal cells and stinging and mild tissue toxicity limit use.
Lissamine green	Stains the anterior segment of the eye to visualize defects and dry eyes. Defective cells are stained green.

TABLE 47.2 Ophthalmic Antiinfectives

Generic	Route and Dosage[a]	Uses and Considerations
Antibacterials		
Ciprofloxacin HCl, 0.3% ophthalmic solution and ointment	Bacterial conjunctivitis: Sol: A: 1–2 gtt q2h while awake for 2 d, then q4h while awake for 5 d Bacterial conjunctivitis: Oint: A: ½-inch ribbon tid for 2 d, then ½-inch ribbon bid for 5 d Corneal ulcer: Sol: A: Day 1: 2 gtt q15min for 6 h, then 2 gtt q30min Day 2: 2 gtt q1h Days 3–14: 2 gtt q4h	For bacterial conjunctivitis and corneal ulceration.
Gentamicin sulfate, 0.3% ophthalmic solution and ointment	Sol 0.3%: A: 1–2 gtt q4h; may increase to 2 gtt q1h for severe infections Oint 0.3%: A: ½-inch ribbon 2–3 times daily	For blepharitis, blepharoconjunctivitis, bacterial conjunctivitis, corneal ulcer, dacryocystitis, keratitis, keratoconjunctivitis, acute meibomianitis, and bacterial and fungal corneal lesion/abrasion. May cause ototoxicity (of the eighth cranial nerve) that could be permanent.
Levofloxacin, 0.5% ophthalmic solution	A: 1–2 gtt q2h; max: 8 doses/d for 1–2 d, then q4h; *max:* 4 doses/d for 5 d	For bacterial conjunctivitis and corneal ulcers. (Systemic therapy is required for treatment of hordeolum, dacryocystitis, and meibomianitis.)
Neomycin, polymyxin B sulfate, bacitracin; ophthalmic	Oint: A: ½-inch ribbon q3–4h for 7–10 d Max dose: 8 applications/d for 10 d	For bacterial conjunctivitis, blepharitis, blepharoconjunctivitis, keratitis, and keratoconjunctivitis. A triple antibiotic is effective against many gram-positive and -negative microorganisms.
Ofloxacin, 0.3% ophthalmic solution	Bacterial conjunctivitis: A: 1–2 gtt q2–4h while awake for 2 d, then 1–2 gtt qid for 5 d Bacterial corneal ulcer: A: 1–2 gtt q30min while awake and q4–6h after retiring; days 3–6: 1–2 gtt q1h while awake; days 7–9: 1–2 gtt qid	For bacterial conjunctivitis, bacterial corneal ulcer.
Sulfacetamide, 10% ophthalmic solution and ointment	Sol: A: 1–2 gtt q1–3h while awake, less frequently at night Oint: A: Small ribbon 4 times during the day and at bedtime	For chlamydial conjunctivitis, corneal ulcer, and other superficial ophthalmic infections; not effective against fungal, viral, or all types of bacterial infection. Continued use may result in nonsusceptible microorganism overgrowth. Ointment may be applied at night with the ophthalmic solution. Ophthalmic sulfonamides are incompatible with preparations that contain silver salts (e.g., silver nitrate). Ointment may delay corneal wound healing. Purulent exudates that contain PABA can inactivate the drug's antibacterial activity.
Tobramycin, 0.3% ophthalmic solution and ointment	Sol: A: 1–2 gtt q4h; for severe infection, apply 2 gtt hourly until improvement is seen, then decrease frequency. Oint: A: Thin strip q8–12h. For severe infections, apply q3–4h	For superficial external ocular infections. Tobramycin may delay healing of corneal abrasion or lesions.
Antifungals		
Natamycin, 5% ophthalmic suspension	A: 1 gtt q1–2h for 3–4 d, then 1 gtt q3–4h for 14–21 d; *max:* 24 gtt/d	For external ocular fungal infections. Drops possess no antibacterial or antiviral activity, and prolonged treatment may result in bacterial or viral infection. Patients allergic to cheese may have sensitivity to natamycin.
Antivirals		
Trifluridine, 1% ophthalmic solution	A: 1 gtt q2h while awake; *max:* 9 gtt/d until corneal ulcer is re-epithelialized, then 1 gtt q4h for 7 d; max: 21-d treatment	For herpetic ophthalmic infections and keratoconjunctivitis caused by HSV-1 and HSV-2. Treatment longer than 21 d can result in ocular toxicity.

A, Adult; *bid*, twice a day; *d*, day; *HSV*, herpes simplex virus; *gtt*, drops; *h*, hour; *HCl*, hydrochloride; *max*, maximum; *min*, minute; *mo*, months; *Oint*, ointment; *PABA*, para-aminobenzoic acid; *q*, every; *qid*, four times a day; *sol*, solution; *tid*, three times a day; *y*, year; *>*, greater than; *≥*, greater than or equal to.

[a]To minimize systemic absorption, gently apply pressure on inner canthus.

TABLE 47.3   Ophthalmic Antiinflammatories

Generic	Route and Dosage	Uses and Considerations
Immunosuppressants		
Cyclosporine, 0.05% ophthalmic emulsion	A: 1 gtt q12h	For xerophthalmia due to ocular inflammation associated with keratoconjunctivitis sicca. Artificial tears may be used concomitantly with cyclosporine ocular drops, allowing 15 min between the products. Absolute contraindication: Patients with active ocular infection. Emulsion must be thoroughly mixed by inverting the bottle a few times to obtain a uniform, white, opaque emulsion before using.
Nonsteroidal Antiinflammatory Drugs (NSAIDs)		
Diclofenac sodium, 0.1% ophthalmic solution	24 h after cataract surgery: A: 1 gtt qid for 2 wk Corneal refractive surgery: A: 1–2 gtt within 1 h of surgery, then 1–2 gtt q15min after surgery, then qid 4–6 h after surgery for up to 3 d	For postoperative inflammation after cataract surgery and ocular pain/photophobia after corneal refractive surgery. Use a separate bottle for each eye. May increase ocular bleeding and delay healing.
Flurbiprofen sodium, 0.03% ophthalmic solution	A: 1 gtt q30min starting 2 h before surgery for a total dose of 4 gtt	For prevention of intraoperative miosis. If eye involvement is bilateral, one bottle per eye should be used to avoid cross-contamination. May increase ocular bleeding and delay healing. Concomitant use with ocular corticosteroid can cause corneal erosion.
Ketorolac tromethamine, ophthalmic solution	Allergic conjunctivitis: Sol 0.5%: A: 1 gtt qid After cataract surgery: Sol 0.5%: A: 1 gtt qid for 2 wk Sol 0.45%: A: 1 gtt bid 1 d before surgery; continue on day of surgery and for 2 wk After corneal refractive surgery: Sol 0.4%: A: 1 gtt qid for 4 d	For relief of ocular itching due to allergic conjunctivitis, postoperative inflammation after cataract surgery, and postoperative corneal refractive surgery. Use separate bottle for each eye to prevent cross-contamination. Ocular NSAIDs may result in keratitis; use for longer than 14 d postoperatively may cause corneal adverse events. May increase ocular bleeding and delay healing.
Corticosteroids		
Dexamethasone, 0.1% ophthalmic solution	A: 1–2 gtt q1h while awake and q2h at night; taper to q4h	For corticosteroid-responsive ocular disorders (e.g., allergic conjunctivitis, herpes zoster ocular infection, optic neuritis, corneal injury). Can cause increased IOP, which is reversible. Can also cause optic neuritis and visual defects.
Loteprednol etabonate, 0.2% and 0.5% ophthalmic suspension; 0.5% ophthalmic gel and ointment	Allergic conjunctivitis: Susp 0.2%: A: 1 gtt qid Steroid-responsive disorders: Susp 0.5%: A: 1–2 gtt qid; may increase to 1 gtt qh if needed 24 h after ocular surgery: Susp/gel 0.5%: 1–2 gtt qid for 2 wk or Oint 0.5%: ½-inch qid for 2 wk 24 h after ocular surgery for postoperative pain: Oint 0.5%: ½-inch qid for 2 wk or Gel 0.5%: 1–2 gtt qid for 2 wk	For allergic conjunctivitis, steroid-responsive ophthalmic disorders including iritis, keratitis, ocular pain, and postoperative ocular inflammation Do not discontinue prematurely; ophthalmologic examination should be done after 14 d of therapy.
Prednisolone sodium phosphate 1% ophthalmic solution	Dosage must be individualized and is variable depending on nature and severity. A: 1–2 gtt qh while awake, q2h during the night; *maint:* 1 gtt q4–6h; taper as indicated	For corticosteroid-responsive ocular disorders (e.g., allergic conjunctivitis, herpes zoster ocular infection, optic neuritis, corneal injury, postoperative ocular inflammation). Can mask other infections. May delay healing. Contraindication: Most cornea and conjunctiva viral infection, unless appropriate antiviral therapy is co-administered, and ocular fungal infection.
Ophthalmic Antibacterial and Corticosteroid Combinations		
Refer to individual drug information for general considerations.		
Neomycin sulfate/polymyxin B sulfate/dexamethasone, ophthalmic suspension and ointment	Severe disease: Susp: A: 1–2 gtt q1h Mild disease: Susp: A/C ≥2 y: 1–2 gtt q4–6h, taper gradually; *max:* 48 gtt/d Oint: A: ½-inch ribbon tid/qid; *max:* ½-inch oint qid	For external ocular inflammation and abrasion

TABLE 47.3 Ophthalmic Antiinflammatories—cont'd

Generic	Route and Dosage	Uses and Considerations
Gentamicin sulfate/ prednisolone acetate, ophthalmic suspension and ointment	Susp: A: 1 gtt bid–qid; *max:* 24 gtt/d Oint: A: ½-inch qd–tid; *max:* ½-inch tid	For external ocular inflammation and abrasion
Tobramycin/dexamethasone, ophthalmic suspension and ointment	Susp: A: 1–2 gtt q4–6h Oint: A: ½-inch ribbon q6–8h	External ocular inflammation and abrasion
Ophthalmic Allergy Treatment Drugs		
Azelastine HCl, 0.05% ophthalmic solution	A: 1 gtt bid	For ocular pruritus due to allergic conjunctivitis. Drug can cause cephalgia, fatigue, dysgeusia, conjunctivitis, abnormal vision, and xerophthalmia.
Cromolyn sodium, 4% ophthalmic solution	A: 1–2 gtt 4–6 times/d at regular intervals	For allergic conjunctivitis. Transient ocular irritation may occur during therapy.
Emedastine difumarate, ophthalmic solution	A: 1 gtt up to 4 times/d; *max:* 4 gtt/d	For ocular pruritus due to allergic conjunctivitis. Cephalgia may occur along with asthenia, blurred vision, dysgeusia, and ocular irritation. *Do not confuse* emedastine with epinastine.
Epinastine, 0.05% ophthalmic solution	A: 1 gtt bid	For ocular pruritus due to allergic conjunctivitis. Does not cross the blood-brain barrier. May cause ocular irritation and worsen pruritus. Continue treatment through period of allergen exposure, even when symptoms are absent. *Do not confuse* epinastine with emedastine.
Ketotifen fumarate	A: 1 gtt q8–12h	For ocular pruritus due to allergic conjunctivitis. Cephalgia and rhinitis may occur.
Olopatadine HCl, 0.2% ophthalmic solution	A: 1 gtt bid at an interval of 6–8 h	For allergic conjunctivitis. Cephalgia or dysgeusia may occur during therapy. Use until offending allergen is terminated.

A, Adult; *bid,* twice daily; *d,* day; *gtt,* drops; *h,* hour; *HCl,* hydrochloride; *IOP,* intraocular pressure; *maint,* maintenance; *max,* maximum; *min,* minute; *oint,* ointment; *q,* every; *qid,* four times daily; *sol,* solution; *susp,* suspension; *tid,* thrice daily; *wk,* week; *y,* year; >, greater than; ≥, greater than or equal to.

bleeding tendencies and delay corneal healing. Topical NSAIDs are not expected to increase cardiovascular risk, hepatic reactions, or other systemic adverse effects; however, ocular NSAIDs can cause bleeding of ocular tissues.

Ophthalmic corticosteroids such as dexamethasone and predniso-lone acetate are another type of antiinflammatory. Corticosteroids are used to treat a number of eye conditions, such as allergic conjunctivitis, herpes zoster keratitis (not herpes simplex keratitis), corneal abrasion, postoperative ocular inflammation, and optic neuritis. ⚡ Ocular corticosteroids can mask infections and delay healing, and are contra-indicated in persons with untreated ocular infections. Corticosteroids can worsen glaucoma by reducing the outflow of aqueous humor and increasing IOP; the effects are usually reversible upon discontinuation of the drug. Prolonged use can cause open-angle glaucoma, ocular nerve damage, or visual defects. Refer to Chapter 24 for more informa-tion on corticosteroids.

When allergies are the cause of eye inflammation, ophthalmic drugs are commonly prescribed to treat the underlying cause. These allergy drugs contain antihistamines and mast cell stabilizers. Antihistamines block histamine from activating histamine receptors in the tissues. Degranulation of mast cells releases histamine and other inflammatory mediators; mast cell stabilizers prevent mast cells from degranulating. Ocular sensations that include burning, stinging, and blurred vision are common adverse effects reported. Other adverse effects include cephalgia, dysgeusia, and rhinitis.

Decongestants

Eye inflammation typically presents with redness due to vascular congestion of the conjunctiva. Ophthalmic decongestants such as phenylephrine, naphazoline, and tetrahydrozoline stimulate alpha-adrenergic receptors in the arterioles of the conjunctiva, vasoconstrict-ing (narrowing) the blood vessels and thereby decreasing congestion. Many ocular decongestants are available without prescription. If these are absorbed in significant amounts, their sympathetic nervous system effects may pose problems for patients with increased IOP and hyper-tension. ⚡ Ocular decongestants are contraindicated in patients with angle-closure glaucoma because these drugs may contribute to acute angle closure, a medical emergency.

Lubricants

Eye lubricants moisten eyes to alleviate discomfort such as the burn-ing and irritation associated with xerophthalmia. They are also used to moisten contact lenses and artificial eyes. During anesthesia and in acute or chronic central nervous system (CNS) disorders that result in unconsciousness or decreased blinking, lubricants keep eyes moist and maintain the integrity of the epithelial surface of the eye.

Many brands and forms of ocular lubricants (artificial tears) are available OTC without a prescription. Although these agents are typi-cally safe, the nurse must be alert to potential allergic reactions to pre-servatives found in lubricants.

Glaucoma and Ocular Hypertension Drugs

In the anterior chamber of the eye, aqueous humor, a clear fluid, flows continuously in and out of the chamber. As aqueous humor is formed, excess fluid drains through the trabecular meshwork structure of the eye and out the canal of Schlemm, with a much smaller fraction of the fluid exiting through the uveoscleral structure at the root of the iris (Fig. 47.2A). Overproduction of the fluid or improper drainage causes

Normal flow of aqueous humor

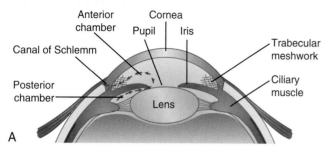

A

Open-angle glaucoma

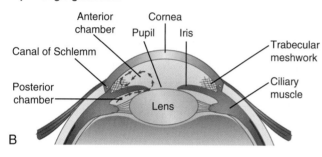

B

Angle-closure glaucoma

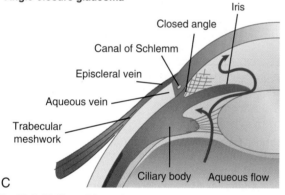

C

Fig. 47.2 (A) Normal flow of aqueous humor. (B) Open-angle glaucoma. (C) Angle-closure glaucoma.

IOP to increase, and this buildup of pressure can damage the optic nerve and result in glaucoma. Without treatment, permanent vision loss can occur.

There are two types of glaucoma, open-angle and angle-closure. In open-angle glaucoma, the trabecular network is open but becomes clogged (see Fig. 47.2B). Over time, as blockage of the trabecular network worsens, the IOP gradually increases, which damages the optic nerve.

In angle-closure glaucoma, also known as *closed-angle* or *narrow-angle glaucoma*, the iris is situated close to the drainage angle blocking the trabecular network (see Fig. 47.2C). Because the excess aqueous humor cannot drain, it builds up within the eye and increases IOP. When the drainage angle is completely blocked, eye pressure increases quickly, and the vision becomes suddenly blurred; this is a medical emergency and must be treated immediately. Management of angle-closure glaucoma is often surgical; however, pharmacologic management is sometimes indicated. ⚡ Anticholinergic drugs (see Chapter 16) can cause mydriasis and can worsen angle-closure glaucoma.

Glaucoma is further classified as either primary or secondary. Primary glaucoma occurs because of a pathologic change within the eye that happens without a known cause. Primary open-angle glaucoma (POAG), the most common type of glaucoma, is a chronic condition that develops slowly over time as the trabecular meshwork becomes clogged for unknown reasons. Secondary glaucoma occurs in response to a known cause such as injury, disease, or medication. Although a number of drugs can increase the risk of secondary glaucoma, those that cause pupillary dilation are particularly problematic because they give the iris more flexibility to move toward the drainage angle, blocking the trabecular meshwork. People who are at risk for glaucoma should avoid decongestants. Certain herbal preparations (e.g., goldenseal, ephedra, and bitter orange) can also create problems when given to patients who have glaucoma.

⚡ PATIENT SAFETY

Herbs that should be avoided in patients with glaucoma include bitter orange, blood root, celandine, coffee, corkwood, ephedra, goldenseal, and jimson weed. Because all herbs have inherent risks, it is important to receive approval from the patient's health care provider before recommending herbal preparations.

Until recently, drugs for glaucoma (Table 47.4) belonged to one of six drug categories: (1) prostaglandin analogues, (2) beta-adrenergic blockers, (3) alpha-adrenergic agonists, (4) cholinergic agents, (5) carbonic anhydrase inhibitors (CAIs), or (6) systemic hyperosmotic drugs. A seventh class, rho kinase inhibitor (netarsudil ophthalmic), is indicated to reduce ocular pressure in patients with open-angle glaucoma by increasing aqueous humor outflow. Prostaglandin analogues and beta-adrenergic blockers are typically first-line therapy, followed by alpha-adrenergic agonists. Each category acts in different ways to decrease IOP. Even though damage due to glaucoma cannot be reversed, treatments may prevent further damage.

Prostaglandin Analogues

Prostaglandin analogues are first-line drugs used primarily in the treatment of open-angle glaucoma and ocular hypertension. These drugs decrease IOP by improving trabecular outflow and by increasing the uveoscleral pathway, which is an alternate pathway of aqueous humor outflow. Examples of prostaglandin analogues include bimatoprost, latanoprost (Prototype Drug Chart: Latanoprost), tafluprost, and travoprost. Prostaglandin analogues are taken at bedtime.

Side Effects and Adverse Reactions. Prostaglandin analogues used for glaucoma have unique side effects. These drugs gradually change the color of the iris by increasing brown pigmentation. This effect is most noticeable in individuals with green-brown and yellow-brown irises, and it may be permanent. Darkening of the eyelids may also occur. Another side effect is the development of eyelash hypertrichosis, which is a growth in the number, length, thickness, and pigmentation of eyelashes. Patients may also develop macular edema, blurred vision, redness of the conjunctiva, and itching or stinging of the eye. Systemic effects such as bronchospasm, dizziness, dyspnea, and myalgia are rare. Prostaglandin analogues are generally better tolerated than alternative drugs for glaucoma.

Cholinergic Agents

Ophthalmic cholinergic agents cause miosis, a constriction of the pupil and contraction of the ciliary muscle. These actions result in a widening of the trabecular meshwork to improve outflow of excess aqueous humor. Additionally, as the pupil constricts, it straightens the iris, thus opening or widening the drainage angle to relieve angle-closure glaucoma. The two types of cholinergics are cholinergic agonists and cholinesterase inhibitors. Although their outcomes are similar, cholinergic

TABLE 47.4 Glaucoma Drugs

Generic	Route and Dosage	Uses and Considerations
Beta-Adrenergic Blockers		
Betaxolol HCl, 0.5% ophthalmic solution or 0.25% suspension	Sol: A: 1–2 gtt q12h Susp: A: 1 gtt q12h	Selective beta blocker for chronic open-angle glaucoma and ocular hypertension (increased IOP). The ophthalmic drug has not been shown to have significant effects on heart rate, blood pressure, or pulmonary function; however, such preparations can be absorbed systemically with the same adverse reactions and drug interactions. May have additive effects in patients receiving oral beta blockers. Absolute contraindications: AV block, bradycardia, cardiogenic shock, HF
Carteolol HCl, 1% ophthalmic solution	A: 1 gtt q12h	Nonselective beta blocker for chronic open-angle glaucoma or ocular hypertension. Conjunctival hyperemia and eye irritation may occur. Absolute contraindications: AV block, bradycardia, cardiogenic shock, HF
Levobunolol HCl, 0.25% or 0.5% ophthalmic solution	A: 1–2 gtt of 0.25% bid or 1–2 gtt of 0.5% once daily	Nonselective beta blocker for increased IOP for open-angle glaucoma or ocular hypertension; to be used with topical miotics. Ocular irritation, dizziness, fatigue, and depression may occur. Absolute contraindications: Asthma, AV block, bradycardia, cardiogenic shock, COPD, HF, sick sinus syndrome, sulfite hypersensitivity
Timolol hemihydrate or maleate, 0.25% or 0.5% ophthalmic solution or gel-forming solution	See Prototype Drug Chart: Timolol	
Carbonic Anhydrase Inhibitors		
Acetazolamide	Regular release: A: PO: 250 mg qd-qid; *max:* 1 g/d Extended release: A: PO: 500 mg bid; *max:* 1 g/d A: IV: 500 mg for acute increased IOP or patients unable to take oral dosage; may repeat in 2–4 h Geriatrics: With all formulations, consider dose reduction.	Adjunctive treatment of glaucoma; reduces IOP. Must be administered systemically; penetration is poor when administered topically to the cornea. Volume loss may cause dehydration and postural hypotension. Electrolyte imbalance may occur. Adverse GI effects (e.g., dysgeusia, xerostomia, anorexia) may occur. Drug may be given without regard to food. Absolute contraindications: Acidosis, metabolic acidosis, angle-closure glaucoma, adrenal insufficiency, hepatic disease, or renal failure; hyperchloremia, hypokalemia, hyponatremia, anuria
Brinzolamide, 1% ophthalmic suspension	A: 1 gtt tid	For increased IOP due to ocular hypertension or open-angle glaucoma. Corneal edema may occur with low endothelial cell counts. With ocular administration, drug is absorbed systemically. Must be shaken well before each use. Absolute contraindication: Sulfonamide hypersensitivity (contains sulfonamide derivative)
Dorzolamide, 2% ophthalmic solution	A: 1 gtt tid	For increased IOP due to ocular hypertension or open-angle glaucoma. It is not recommended to topically administer CAIs concomitantly with oral CAIs.
Combination Drugs for Glaucoma		
Refer to individual drug information for general considerations.		
Timolol maleate/dorzolamide	A: 1 gtt bid	Timolol is a nonselective beta blocker and dorzolamide is a carbonic anhydrase II inhibitor.
Brimonidine/timolol maleate	A: 1 gtt q12h	Brimonidine is a selective alpha-agonist and timolol is a nonselective beta blocker.
Prostaglandin Analogues		
Latanoprost, 0.005% ophthalmic solution	See Prototype Drug Chart: Latanoprost	
Bimatoprost, 0.03% ophthalmic solution	A: 1 gtt at bedtime	For increased IOP due to ocular hypertension or open-angle glaucoma. Macular edema, iritis, and cataracts may occur.
Travoprost, 0.004% ophthalmic solution	A: 1 gtt at bedtime	For increased IOP due to ocular hypertension or open-angle glaucoma. Macular edema or keratitis may occur.
Tafluprost, 0.0015% ophthalmic solution	A: 1 gtt every evening	For increased IOP due to ocular hypertension or open-angle glaucoma. Drug may cause macular edema or uveitis/iritis.
RHO Kinase Inhibitors		
Netarsudil ophthalmic 0.02% sol	A: 1 gtt every evening	For increased IOP due to open-angle glaucoma or ocular hypertension. Drug may cause keratitis, ocular pain, erythema, and vision changes.

A, Adult; *AV,* atrioventricular; *bid,* twice daily; *CAI,* carbonic anhydrase inhibitor; *COPD,* chronic obstructive pulmonary disease; *d,* day; *GI,* gastrointestinal; *gtt,* drop; *h,* hour; *HCl,* hydrochloride; *HF,* heart failure; *IOP,* intraocular pressure; *IV,* intravenously; *max,* maximum; *N,* newborn; *PO,* by mouth; *q,* every; *qid,* four times daily; *Sol,* solution; *Susp,* suspension; *tid,* thrice daily; *wk,* weeks; *y,* year; ≥, greater than or equal to.

PROTOTYPE DRUG CHART

Timolol

Drug Class	Dosage
Nonselective beta blocker	Sol: 1 gtt of 0.25% bid; may increase to 1 gtt of 0.5% bid and titrate down to once daily dosing.
	Gel: 1 gtt of 0.25% once daily; may increase to 1 gtt of 0.5% once daily.

Contraindications	Drug-Lab-Food Interactions
Absolute contraindications: COPD and RAD, AV block, bradycardia, cardiogenic shock, and heart failure. Caution against abrupt discontinuation.	Drugs: Ophthalmic timolol can be absorbed systemically; therefore drug-drug interactions are similar to other formulations. See Chapter 15 for more general drug-drug interactions with beta blockers. Some herbal agents may lower vascular resistance (e.g., hawthorn *[Crataegus laevigata]* and ephedra [Ma-huang]).

Pharmacokinetics	Pharmacodynamics
Absorption: Systemic absorption can occur.	Onset: 30 min
Distribution: UK	Peak: 1–2 h
Metabolism: Hepatic; $t\frac{1}{2}$: 4 h	Duration: <24 h
Excretion: Primarily in urine	

Therapeutic Effects/Uses
Reduction of IOP in open-angle glaucoma or ocular hypertension
Mechanism of Action: Nonselectively antagonizes beta$_1$- and beta$_2$-adrenergic receptors, reducing IOP without affecting visual acuity, pupil size, or accommodation.

Side Effects	Adverse Reactions
Adverse effects for ocular timolol are the same as for the oral drug. See Chapter 15 for more information on timolol and other nonselective beta blockers.	See Chapter 15 for more information on beta blockers.

AV, Atrioventricular; *bid*, twice daily; *COPD*, chronic obstructive pulmonary disease; *gtt*, drop; *h*, hour; *IOP*, intraocular pressure; *min*, minute; *RAD*, respiratory airway disease; *Sol*, solution; *t½*, half-life; *UK*, unknown; <, less than.

agonists and cholinesterase inhibitors differ in their mechanism of action.

Cholinergic agonists are direct-acting cholinergics that directly stimulate cholinergic receptors. As a result, these drugs have the same action as the parasympathetic neurotransmitter acetylcholine. Pilocarpine is an example of a cholinergic agonist.

Cholinesterase inhibitors such as echothiophate are indirect-acting cholinergics, which inactivate the enzyme cholinesterase that typically breaks down acetylcholine. By inhibiting enzymatic destruction of acetylcholine, more acetylcholine is available to stimulate cholinergic receptors in the eye.

Side Effects and Adverse Reactions. Systemic absorption of cholinesterase inhibitors through the conjunctiva and lacrimal duct can produce systemic parasympathomimetic effects that include cardiac irregularities, diarrhea, hyperhidrosis, respiratory depression, and urinary incontinence. Other adverse effects from cholinesterase inhibitors include iritis, uveitis, and retinal detachment in addition to common complaints such as ocular irritation and pain, lacrimation, myopia with blurred vision, and paradoxical ocular hypertension. Systemic effects from cholinergic agonists are rare; ocular adverse effects are similar to those of the cholinesterase inhibitors. Cholinergic agonists and cholinesterase inhibitors are contraindicated for use in persons with angle-closure glaucoma.

Figs. 47.2B and 47.2C illustrate increased IOP resulting in open-angle and angle-closure glaucoma. Refer to Chapter 16 for more information on cholinergic drugs.

Beta-Adrenergic Blockers

Selective and nonselective beta-adrenergic blockers and beta blockers are first-line drugs used in the treatment of glaucoma.

Beta-adrenergic blockers decrease IOP by decreasing the production of aqueous humor. Examples of ophthalmic nonselective beta-adrenergic blockers include carteolol, levobunolol, and timolol (Prototype Drug Chart: Timolol). Selective ocular beta blockers include betaxolol.

Side Effects and Adverse Reactions. In the eye, beta-adrenergic blockers (beta blockers) may cause some eye discomfort, which is possible with most eye medications. Some types cause miosis. Because the pupil does not dilate adequately in dark environments, patients taking these drugs may experience vision problems at night.

Although ophthalmic drugs do not typically enter the general circulation in large amounts, it can occur to the extent that systemic effects occur. ⚡ Ophthalmic beta-adrenergic blockers can slow the heart rate, which can worsen bradycardia, atrioventricular (AV) heart block, and heart failure. Also, these drugs can prevent adequate bronchodilation in patients who have asthma and other obstructive pulmonary diseases. See Chapter 15 for more information on beta-adrenergic blockers.

Alpha-Adrenergic Agonists

Ophthalmic alpha-adrenergic agonists such as apraclonidine and brimonidine control or prevent elevation of IOP postsurgically by decreasing production and improving outflow of aqueous humor. The major site of action is in the ciliary body. ⚠ Absolute contraindications for alpha-adrenergic agonists include persons on monoamine oxidase inhibitor (MAOI) therapy. No specific drug interactions with systemic and ophthalmic drugs were noted; however, caution is advised when using these drugs with other alpha blockers, tricyclic antidepressants (TCAs), and CNS depressants.

📄 PROTOTYPE DRUG CHART

Latanoprost

Drug Class	Dosage
Prostaglandin analogue	1 gtt q evening in affected eye(s)

Contraindications	Drug-Lab-Food Interactions
Latanoprost is indicated only for open-angle glaucoma or ocular hypertension. No absolute contraindications exist, but use caution in patients with a torn or absent lens, intraocular inflammation, or risk of macular edema. Drug is absorbed by soft contact lenses, so advise patients with these to use alternate means of vision correction. *Caution:* Patients with history of diabetic retinopathy who took latanoprost experienced retinal detachment, retinal embolus, and vitreous hemorrhage. This may or may not be related to the latanoprost, but caution is urged.	Drugs: Concomitant administration with eyedrops containing thimerosal causes latanoprost to precipitate out of solution; latanoprost- and thimerosal-containing ophthalmic preparations should be administered at least 5 min apart. Bromfenac ophthalmic solution, an NSAID, may reduce latanoprost's ability to lower IOP. Bimatoprost ophthalmic solution to promote growth of eyelashes may decrease the ability of latanoprost to lower IOP. Combining latanoprost with other prostaglandin analogues is not recommended; combination may decrease the IOP-lowering effects or cause a paradoxical increase in IOP.

Pharmacokinetics	Pharmacodynamics
Absorption: Through the cornea and hydrolyzed to its active form Distribution: 0.16 ± 0.02 L/kg. Primary measurable concentration is in the eye; levels are often undetectable in serum. Metabolism: Hepatic; $t\frac{1}{2}$: 17 min Excretion: Primarily in urine (88%)	Onset: 3–4 h Peak: 8–12 h Duration: 24 h

Therapeutic Effects/Uses
Reduction of IOP in open-angle glaucoma or ocular hypertension   Mechanism of Action: Prostaglandin FP receptor selective agonist increases aqueous humor outflow.

Side Effects	Adverse Reactions
Ophthalmic effects: Blurred vision, burning/stinging/pruritus/redness, brown pigmentation of iris; increased number/length/thickness and darkening of eyelashes; foreign body sensation, punctate epithelial keratopathy, photophobia, lid edema/erythema/discomfort/crusting	Eye pain, eye infection, loss of vision, dizziness, dyspnea

gtt, Drop; *h*, hour; *IOP*, intraocular pressure; *min*, minutes; *NSAID*, nonsteroidal antiinflammatory drug; *q*, every; *t½*, half-life.

Side Effects and Adverse Reactions. Apraclonidine and brimonidine have minimal, if any, systemic effects. Because of the relative safety of alpha$_2$-adrenergic agonists, they are often used when ophthalmic beta-adrenergic antagonists are contraindicated. The most common effects of topical administration are burning, stinging, blurred vision, and headache. Serious reactions include corneal erosion, keratitis, arrhythmias, and asthma.

Carbonic Anhydrase Inhibitors

Carbonic anhydrase inhibitors (CAIs) decrease IOP by decreasing the production of aqueous humor. These drugs, initially developed as diuretics, are sometimes used for adjunctive treatment of glaucoma. They are indicated for both open-angle and acute angle-closure glaucoma. CAIs are not as effective as other drugs for glaucoma, and they carry a greater risk of adverse effects. For these reasons, they are generally added to a therapeutic regimen only after other treatment options have been exhausted. Both topical (e.g., brinzolamide, dorzolamide) and systemic (e.g., acetazolamide) formulations are available.

Side Effects and Adverse Reactions. Adverse effects of CAIs, particularly with the systemic forms, include CNS effects such as lethargy, drowsiness, headache, seizures, paresthesias, and mental status changes. Gastrointestinal (GI) effects such as nausea, vomiting, diarrhea, dysgeusia, and anorexia may occur. Because CAIs have diuretic effects, polyuria and increased thirst are common, and fluid and electrolyte disturbances may occur as a result. CAIs may promote hyperuricemia, which may precipitate gout attacks, and they may also worsen liver disease, resulting in hepatic encephalopathy and even hepatic necrosis. Because they are sulfonamides, they should not be given to patients who have experienced allergic reactions to other sulfonamide drugs.

Mydriatics and Cycloplegics

Mydriatics dilate the pupils, and cycloplegics paralyze the muscles of accommodation; both are used in diagnostic procedures and ophthalmic surgery.

Anticholinergics actively block acetylcholine from attaching to cholinergic receptors, resulting in both dilation of the pupils and paralysis of the muscles of accommodation. This is accomplished by blocking the response of sphincter muscles that normally constrict the pupil when cholinergic receptors are stimulated. Commonly prescribed anticholinergics for mydriasis and cycloplegic refraction include atropine

CLINICAL JUDGMENT [NURSING PROCESS]

Glaucoma and Ocular Hypertension Drugs

Concept: Sensory Perception
- Receiving and interpreting various stimuli (vision) for functional nervous system pathways to the brain

Recognize Cues [Assessment]
- Conduct a detailed current medication history that includes prescriptions, over-the-counter (OTC) medicines, antacids, dietary supplements, vitamins, and herbal supplements.
- Obtain a list of drug and food allergies and compare to the prescribed drugs to determine any drug-drug and drug-supplement interactions.
- Obtain baseline information about physical status that includes height, weight, vital signs, cardiopulmonary assessment, intake and output, skin assessment, nutritional status, and any underlying diseases.
- Check baseline visual acuity and intraocular pressure (IOP) measurements.
- ⚡ Assess for contraindications for glaucoma drugs, such as respiratory or cardiac disorders, angle-closure glaucoma, hypertension, acute ocular infection, immunosuppression, and hepatic or renal disorders.

Analyze Cues and Prioritize Hypothesis [Patient Problems]
- Decreased visual acuity related to disease progression
- Reduced sensory perception, vision related to disease progression, and drug-induced visual changes
- Potential for social isolation

Generate Solutions [Planning]
- The patient/caregiver will verbalize understanding for the drug therapy and identify when to notify the clinician.
- The patient will take medications in dose and at times prescribed.
- The patient will demonstrate the proper method of ophthalmic drug administration.
- The patient will avoid contaminating the tip of the tube or dropper.
- The patient will maintain an IOP within the target range.
- The patient will remain free of ocular infection during therapy.

Take Action [Nursing Interventions]
- Monitor for significant alterations in patient status.
- ⚡ Monitor patients for xerostomia, dehydration, fluid overload, blood dyscrasias, electrolyte imbalances, blurred vision, dyspnea, bradycardia or tachycardia, hypertension, and pulmonary changes.

Patient Teaching
General
- Advise patients to never stop medication suddenly.
- Advise patients to avoid driving or operating machinery while vision is impaired.
- Explain the importance of follow-up appointments for subsequent ophthalmologic examination and reevaluation of IOP.
- Counsel patients with glaucoma to avoid drugs with the potential to increase IOP, such as decongestants, anticholinergics, and corticosteroids.
- Instruct patients to put in eyedrops first before any ophthalmic ointment (if prescribed).
- Instruct patients to wait at least 5 minutes between different ophthalmic medications.
- Teach patients/caregivers not to touch the tip of the tube or eyedropper to the eye, finger, or any other object.
- See Chapter 10 for more information on ocular drug administration.

Side Effects
- Explain to patients/caregivers when to notify the clinician (e.g., with fever, wheezing, weight gain, sudden vision changes, or high blood pressure).

Evaluate Outcomes [Evaluation]
- Evaluate patient and family knowledge of purpose and administration of medications.
- Evaluate effectiveness of drug therapy. IOP should be reduced from baseline measurements.
- Evaluate for alleviation or decrease in adverse effects after interventions targeted to unwanted effects of glaucoma therapy.

---

sulfate, cyclopentolate hydrochloride, homatropine hydrobromide, phenylephrine hydrochloride, and tropicamide. An ophthalmic alpha-receptor antagonist, dapiprazole, is available to reverse drug-induced mydriasis with phenylephrine.

Side Effects and Adverse Reactions. Side effects of topical anticholinergics include xerophthalmia (dry eyes), photophobia (sensitivity to light), and blurred vision. Although uncommon with topical use, systemic effects are typical of all anticholinergic drugs and include xerostomia, cephalgia, and constipation. Serious systemic effects include increased IOP, psychosis, seizures, hypotension, tachycardia, cardiovascular collapse, respiratory depression, and muscle rigidity. These drugs are contraindicated in patients with angle-closure glaucoma because the paralyzed iris may block the

⚡ PATIENT SAFETY

Do not Confuse...
- **Oral** alpha-adrenergic or beta blockers with **ophthalmic** preparations
- **Ocular** with **otic**
- **Prednisone** with **prednisolone** ophthalmic
- **Ophthalmic** solutions with **otic** or other topical solutions of the same name (e.g., Cortisporin *ophthalmic* solution with Cortisporin *otic* solution)

outlet for outflow of aqueous humor (see Fig. 47.2C). Table 47.5 lists selected mydriatics and cycloplegics along with their dosages, uses, and considerations.

Drugs for Macular Degeneration

Age-related macular degeneration (AMD) is a leading cause of vision loss in older adults. AMD is a deterioration of the macula, which is the part of the eye responsible for sharp central vision; damage to the macula blurs central vision in the affected eye. Two forms of AMD include wet (neovascular or exudative), which progresses quite rapidly, and dry (atrophic), which slowly destroys vision over a period of years.

Dry AMD is more common and occurs in response to the deposit of extracellular material, called drusen, under the retina. This is coupled with thinning of the retina, which eventually stops functioning properly. Vision loss occurs gradually. Occasionally, dry AMD will progress to wet AMD.

There is no known treatment or medication for dry AMD. An effective drug has not been identified to treat dry AMD, but several drugs are currently in the trial stages. Some studies suggest that antioxidants, such as vitamins C and E, and zinc supplements may have a role in preventing or slowing progression of dry AMD. A healthy diet of dark leafy greens, yellow fruits, vegetables, and fish has also shown to be beneficial to those with AMD.

TABLE 47.5 Mydriatics and Cycloplegics

Generic	Route and Dosage	Uses and Considerations
Atropine sulfate, 1% ophthalmic solution or ointment	Cycloplegic refraction: A: 1–2 gtt of sol or 0.3–0.5 cm ribbon of oint up to 3 times daily for 14 d; start 1 h before procedure. Iritis/uveitis: A: 1–2 gtt of sol or 0.3–0.5 cm ribbon of oint up to 3 times daily	For cycloplegic refraction, especially in children, and uveitis/iritis. Atropine antagonizes acetylcholine receptors and inhibits cholinergic effects. The most potent cycloplegic, atropine, may cause seizures, arrhythmias, hypotension, respiratory depression, and hallucinations. Contraindications: Glaucoma, tachycardia
Cyclopentolate HCl, 0.5%, 1%, 2% ophthalmic solution	A: 1–2 gtt × 1; may repeat × 1 in 5–10 min	For cycloplegia and mydriasis induction
Homatropine hydrobromide, 2% and 5% solution	Mydriasis and cycloplegia: A: 1–2 gtt before procedure; may repeat × 1 in 5–10 min Uveitis: A: 1–2 gtt q3–4h	For mydriasis and cycloplegia for eye examination and uveitis. Homatropine is similar to atropine but onset is faster and duration is shorter. Do not use 5% sol in children.
Phenylephrine HCl, 2.5% and 10% ophthalmic solution	Acute glaucoma: A: 1 gtt. Repeat as necessary. Use with miotic drugs to improve visual acuity Mydriasis induction: A: 1 gtt 15–30 min before procedure, may repeat at 3–5 min intervals; *max:* 3 gtt/eye Uveitis: A: 1 gtt of 2.5% up to 3 times for 2 d or 1 gtt of 10% once a day for up to 2 d	For treatment of acute open-angle glaucoma and for mydriasis induction and pupillary dilation in uveitis for examination. Do not use 10% sol in neonates and children.
Tropicamide	Refraction: A: 1%: 1–2 gtt; repeat in 5 min Fundus examination: 0.5%: 1–2 gtt 15–20 min before examination	Mydriasis and cycloplegia for eye examination

A, Adult; *d*, day; *gtt*, drop; *h*, hour; *HCl*, hydrochloride; *max*, maximum dosage; *min*, minute; *oint*, ointment; *q*, every; *sol*, solution.

Wet or exudative AMD is associated with the growth of abnormal blood vessels behind the retina. Leakage of fluid from these vessels collects behind the retina and shifts the macula from its normal position. Wet macular degeneration accounts for 10% of AMD cases; however, it causes greater destruction and is responsible for 80% of cases in which patients suffer severe vision loss or become legally blind.

Pharmacologic management of wet AMD targets vascular endothelial growth factor (VEGF), a substance that plays a role in the formation of abnormal vessels in the eye. These VEGF inhibitors are intravitreal drugs that are injected into the eye by an ophthalmologist and include ranibizumab, pegaptanib, and aflibercept. Other VEGF inhibitors, such as bevacizumab, are still being investigated. Intravitreal VEGF is contraindicated in persons with ocular infections.

Drugs for Inherited Retinal Dystrophies

Inherited retinal dystrophy (IRD) is a group of severe and progressive disorders leading to blindness among young people. Until recently, no cure or treatment was available. With the emergence of gene therapy, the US Food and Drug Administration (FDA) approved the first gene therapy (voretigene neparvovec-rzyl) for retinal dystrophy in late 2017. Ophthalmic gene therapy uses a vector, a modified virus, to deliver a normal copy of the gene encoding human retinal pigment epithelial 65 KDa protein (RPE65) to retinal cells to restore the visual cycle. Voretigene neparvovec-rzyl is administered subretinally in each eye at least 6 days apart. Side effects include vision decline, eye infections, bleeding in the retina, increased IOP, and formation of cataracts, among others.

Administration of Eyedrops and Ointments

Techniques for administering eyedrops and ophthalmic ointments are described in Chapter 10. Patients who wear contact lenses should be knowledgeable about products associated with the lenses. Wearing contact lenses is usually discouraged; however, if contact lenses must be worn, patients should wait at least 15 minutes after instilling ocular drugs before reinserting the contact lenses.

Patients With Eye Disorders: General Suggestions for Teaching

- Listen to patient concerns. Eye disorders that carry the possibility of blindness promote high anxiety in patients.
- Provide patient education regarding expected drug effect, dosage, and side effects, and when to notify the health care provider.
- Use lay terms rather than medical terminology when providing education.
- Provide written instructions for confused or forgetful patients.
- When developing patient education materials, write them at a fifth- to eighth-grade reading level; use a large, easily read font; and give instructions in the patient's primary language.
- Supplement written instructions with images or pictograms to clarify.
- Instruct patients or family members that one drop of eye medication is the preferred amount with prescriptions written for one to two drops; the conjunctival sac of the lower lid typically holds the volume of one drop without overflowing. The second drop may cause overflow, have a greater chance of systemic toxicity, and have an increased cost of treatment.

- If a second topical medication is ordered to be given at the same time, instruct patients to wait at least 5 minutes before instilling the second medication.
- Instruct patients or family members on proper administration of eyedrops or ointment. Teach them how to maintain sterile technique and prevent dropper contamination.
- Ask patients for a return demonstration of any procedure to ensure their ability to carry it out properly and to determine whether additional teaching is needed.
- Advise patients that ointments will diminish vision for a short period due to the film coating the eye. Advise them to avoid potential safety hazards during this time.
- Instruct patients to store drugs away from heat.
- Counsel patients not to stop any medication suddenly without prior approval from the prescribing health care provider.
- Advise patients to check labels on OTC drugs with a pharmacist.
- Instruct patients to carry an identification card or wear a medical alert bracelet at all times if they are allergic to any medications.
- Encourage patients to keep health care appointments. Recommend that patients bring a list of questions about their condition or medications.
- Tailor instructions for patients who wear contact lenses. Notify them of any special procedures that need to be done with use of contact lenses and the various ophthalmic medications. Advise patients to avoid wearing contact lenses in the presence of eye infections.

OVERVIEW OF THE EAR

The ear is divided into the external, middle, and inner ear. Fig. 47.3 illustrates the basic structures of the ear.

The external ear consists of the pinna and the external auditory canal. The external auditory canal transmits sound to the tympanic membrane (TM; eardrum), a transparent partition between the external and middle ear. The eardrum in turn transmits sound to the bones of the middle ear; it also serves a protective function.

The middle ear, an air-filled cavity, contains three auditory ossicles—the malleus, incus, and stapes—that transmit sound waves to the inner ear. The tip of the malleus is attached to the eardrum; its head is attached to the incus, which is attached to the stapes. The eustachian tube provides a direct connection to the nasopharynx and equalizes

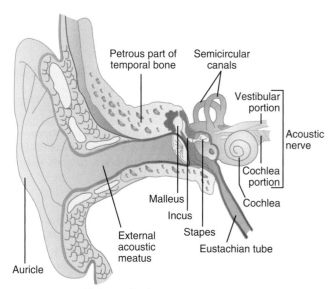

Fig. 47.3 Basic structures of the ear.

air pressure on both sides of the eardrum to prevent it from rupturing. Swallowing, yawning, and chewing gum help the eustachian tube relieve pressure changes during airplane flights.

The inner ear is a series of labyrinths (canals) that consist of a bony section and a membranous section. The vestibule, cochlea, and semicircular canals make up the bony labyrinth. The vestibular area is responsible for maintaining equilibrium and balance. The cochlea is the principal hearing organ.

Professional evaluation of ear problems is essential, because hearing loss can result from untreated disorders. External ear disorders can be treated with OTC products, whereas prescription drugs are required to treat middle ear disorders.

DRUGS FOR DISORDERS OF THE EAR

Antiinfectives

Common ear conditions that require antibacterial drugs are acute otitis media (AOM) and acute otitis externa (AOE), commonly known as *swimmer's ear*. AOM occurs more often in children, and *Streptococcus pneumoniae* is the most common pathogen, followed by *Haemophilus influenzae* and *Moraxella catarrhalis*. AOM may also be caused by other microorganisms, such as viruses.

Risk factors for the development of AOM include age younger than 2 years, attending day care centers, and exposure to environmental pollutants such as tobacco smoke. A significant decline in AOM has occurred since the pneumococcal conjugate vaccine (PCV) was introduced in 2000. Because it provides immunization against *S. pneumoniae*, families should be urged to have children receive the scheduled PCV13 as a prophylactic measure against AOM as well as against the other more serious conditions that this vaccine prevents.

AOM is usually related to a dysfunction of the eustachian tube, especially after an upper respiratory infection from a virus. The TM is usually bulging, and patients complain of otalgia (ear pain). Other symptoms may include fever and irritability.

Oral amoxicillin is usually the drug of choice when antibiotics are indicated for AOM. The recommended dosage for children 6 months and older is 80 to 90 mg/kg every 12 hours for 7 to 10 days depending on the severity of the condition and the age of the patient. The dosage for adults is 500 to 875 mg every 8 to 12 hours, depending on the severity. Azithromycin and clarithromycin are often ordered if the patient is severely allergic to penicillin. For more mild penicillin allergies, a cephalosporin may be ordered; however, the nurse should be alert to any signs or symptoms of penicillin-cephalosporin cross-sensitivity. For otalgia, topical analgesics such as benzocaine are usually used, especially at bedtime.

Otitis externa (OE) is an infection of the external auditory canal that occurs when excess moisture and breaks in the epithelium allow some pathogen, usually bacterial or fungal, to invade the tissues. The cerumen is lipid rich and hydrophobic (repels water), and it protects the skin from water penetration. However, excessive cerumen can obstruct the canal and can trap water. Trapped moisture in the canal elevates the pH and removes the protective cerumen, allowing pathogens a warm, dark, moist area in which to grow. Like many areas of the body, the external canal contains normal bacterial flora that protect the ear; however, when protective mechanisms fail, a pathogenic flora results. *Pseudomonas aeruginosa* and *Staphylococcus aureus* are the pathogens most often responsible. Fever, otalgia, lymphadenopathy, and swelling can occur. Treatment is usually with topical antibacterial or antifungal drugs, depending on the source of the infection. These are often prescribed as a combination product that contains an antiinflammatory (corticosteroid) drug. An analgesic may also be needed.

If the external ear canal (EAC) becomes so swollen that eardrops cannot reach the inner recesses of the EAC, a wick is usually used (Fig. 47.4). A wick is a thin cylinder composed of highly compressed absorbable material inserted into the edematous canal, and eardrops are applied to the exposed tip of the wick. Sufficient drops should be administered to keep the wick moist, which pulls the medication down the length of the wick as the moisture is absorbed, exposing the tissues along the EAC to medication. Wicks should be replaced every 24 to 48 hours. Once the swelling resolves, the wick will fall out, or it can be manually removed.

Oral antibiotics are rarely needed; however, when associated with otitis media or systemic illness, oral drugs are needed. Additionally, if patients are immunosuppressed, oral antibiotics are warranted.

⚡ Patency of the TM presents a special concern when eardrops are used. This is especially true when an edematous EAC prevents adequate visualization of the TM. Topical antibiotics such as neomycin

and polymyxin B with hydrocortisone are very effective in treating OE because polymyxin B is effective against *P. aeruginosa*, and neomycin is effective against *S. aureus*. However, if this drug combination is given to a patient with a perforated TM, the risk of ototoxicity is significant. Chloramphenicol is another drug for OE but is contraindicated with a perforated TM. Fluoroquinolones, on the other hand, are effective against both organisms and are safe to use when the TM is incompetent; therefore they are usually the first drug chosen when prescribing treatment for OE. When OE is caused by the growth of fungi, restoring an acidic environment with an acidifying solution such as acetic acid is usually sufficient. A topical antifungal otic solution such as clotrimazole is typically used if the fungal infection is severe.

Side Effects and Adverse Reactions. The most common side effects of otic antimicrobials are burning and stinging, but ototoxicity can occur with aminoglycoside antibiotics. Chloramphenicol may cause bone marrow suppression and can result in decreased erythrocytes, leukocytes, and platelets. Opportunistic overgrowth of nonsusceptible organisms may occur with any of these drugs. Hypersensitivity is a contraindication.

Table 47.6 lists selected antiinfectives used to treat ear disorders and their dosages, uses, and considerations.

Antihistamines and Decongestants

For years, antihistamines and decongestants were thought to reduce middle-ear congestion and eustachian tube dysfunction associated with otitis media with effusion (OME), a noninfectious collection of fluid in the middle ear. The rationale was that these drugs would reduce edema of the eustachian tube, which would promote drainage from the middle ear.

In 2006 a landmark Cochrane review of the medical literature concluded that antihistamines and decongestants were not as effective as once assumed and that the risks of adverse effects outweighed the benefits. Shortly thereafter, the American Academy of Pediatrics recommended against their use for ear conditions in young children. A 2012 report by the Agency for Healthcare Research and Quality (AHRQ) states that "the effects on multiple short- and long-term outcomes repeatedly demonstrated no benefit for use of these medications over placebo for treating OME.... The reviewed studies found evidence of

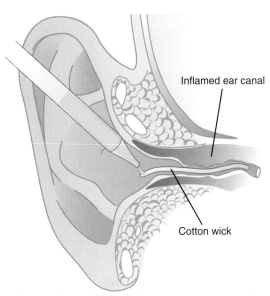

Fig. 47.4 Ear wick inserted into an edematous canal.

Labels: Inflamed ear canal; Cotton wick

TABLE 47.6 Otic Antiinfectives

Generic	Route and Dosage	Uses and Considerations
Topical (Otic)		
General considerations: To minimize dizziness upon administration, warm the container between the hands for at least 1 minute before use. After administration, maintain patient position for at least 1 minute.		
Acetic acid, 2% otic solution	A: 4–6 gtt q2–3h After administration to affected ear, maintain administration position for 5 min	For bacterial or fungal infection of the external ear canal (acute diffuse otitis externa). Solution is concentrated and is a highly corrosive irritant; it must be diluted before use. Systemic absorption is unlikely. Absolute contraindications: Perforated TM
Ciprofloxacin otic, 0.2% otic solution	OE due to *Pseudomonas aeruginosa* or *Staphylococcus aureus*: A: 0.5 mg (one 0.25-mL single-use container): Instill contents q12h for 7 d; max: 1 mg/d	For bacterial infection (OE). Use caution treating *Pseudomonas aeruginosa* or *Staphylococcus aureus*; resistant strains have been noted. Otic route should not result in clinically significant plasma concentration. Absolute contraindication: Quinolone hypersensitivity
Ofloxacin 0.3% otic solution	OE: A: 10 gtt once daily for 7 d Chronic OM: A: 10 gtt bid for 14 d	For OE due to *Escherichia coli*, *P. aeruginosa*, or *S. aureus*; chronic OM with perforated TM due to *P. aeruginosa*, *S. aureus*, or *Proteus mirabilis*; acute OM with tympanostomy tubes due to *Haemophilus influenzae*, *Moraxella catarrhalis*, *P. aeruginosa*, *S. aureus*, or *Streptococcus pneumoniae*. GI effects (dysgeusia, nausea, vomiting) and otic effects (otalgia, otorrhagia, tinnitus) may occur with otic ofloxacin.

A, Adult; *bid*, twice daily; *d*, day; *GI*, gastrointestinal; *gtt*, drops; *h*, hour; *max*, maximum dosage; *min*, minute; *OE*, otitis externa; *OM*, otitis media; *q*, every; *TM*, tympanic membrane; *y*, year; >, greater than; ≥, greater than or equal to.

◎ CLINICAL JUDGMENT [NURSING PROCESS]

Topical Antiinfectives: Ear Conditions

Concept: Sensory Perception
- Receiving and interpreting various stimuli (auditory) for functional nervous system pathways to the brain

Recognize Cues [Assessment]
- Conduct a detailed medication history that includes current prescriptions, over-the-counter (OTC) medicines, antacids, dietary supplements, vitamins, and herbal supplements.
- Obtain a list of drug and food allergies.
- Record otoscopic examination findings for future comparisons.
- Check audiometry and tympanometry, and perform other testing as indicated.
- Assess for conditions in which selected antiinfectives are contraindicated or relatively contraindicated.

Analyze Cues and Prioritize Hypothesis [Patient Problems]
- Reduced sensory perception related to inflammation and/or medication
- Auditory pain related to inflammation

Generate Solutions [Planning]
- The patient will verbalize understanding of the therapy.
- The patient will be free from ear infection after completion of the drug regimen.
- The patient will report a tolerable pain level.
- The patient will report any adverse drug effects.

Take Action [Nursing Interventions]
- Complete culture and sensitivity testing, if ordered, before starting drug therapy.
- Ensure tympanic membrane (TM) patency before administering eardrops other than fluoroquinolones.

- Provide relief of associated pain, if present.
- Monitor for significant alterations in patient status.
- Assess for the development of superinfections.

Patient Teaching
General
- Instruct patients to complete the entire course of medication (usually 10 to 14 days) and not to stop medication when the ear feels better.
- Instruct patients who are prone to otitis externa (OE) on prevention of OE. The Centers for Disease Control and Prevention recommend the following:
  - Keep water out of ears by using custom-fitted earplugs.
  - If water enters the ear, tilt the ear downward to allow water to drain out. Pull the ear in different directions to enhance water drainage.
  - Use a portable hair dryer to facilitate drying.
- Instruct the patient to wear a MedicAlert bracelet at all times if allergic to any medications.
- See Chapter 10 for information on the administration of eardrops.

Side Effects
- Inform patient to report any ringing of the ears.
- Instruct patient to report signs and symptoms of infection, such as fever or chills.

Evaluate Outcomes [Evaluation]
- Evaluate patient and family knowledge of the drug regimen.
- Determine the effectiveness of the drug therapy.
- Inquire regarding alleviation of side effects.

---

increased side effects and harms with use of these medications." Unfortunately, many patients are not aware of these findings and may continue to take these drugs.

The importance of the nurse's role in educating patients regarding this concern cannot be overstated. Numerous OTC antihistamine-decongestant medications are readily available to unknowing patients. Examples of antihistamines include chlorphenamine, clemastine, diphenhydramine, and many others. Examples of decongestants are phenylephrine and pseudoephedrine. (Pseudoephedrine requires a prescription in some states.) Of even greater concern is that most of these are available as combination products that contain both an antihistamine and a decongestant. (See Chapter 38 for a discussion of upper respiratory drugs.)

Cerumenolytics

Cerumen, or earwax, is produced by glands in the outer half of the EAC. Usually cerumen moves to the EAC by itself and is washed away; however, sometimes it accumulates due to overproduction or narrowing of the EAC. In these instances, cerumen can harden in the EAC, creating impaction that can lead to pain, itching, tinnitus, and hearing loss.

Cerumenolytics are topical otic agents that soften or break up the cerumen so that it can be removed. Preparations for cerumenolytics include water-based, oil-based, and nonwater-, nonoil-based products. Water-based products provide hydration to the dried cerumen, allowing it to disintegrate. Oil-based solutions lubricate and soften the cerumen but do not disintegrate it. An example is carbamide peroxide, which is available OTC. Patients may also elect to use regular mineral oil to soften the wax or prevent cerumen

impaction. Generally, 2 to 5 drops applied twice a day for 4 days is sufficient.

Administration of Ear Medications

Ear medications are usually contained in a liquid vehicle for ease of administration. Guidelines for the administration of eardrops are provided in Chapter 10.

Sometimes cerumenolytics alone are insufficient. In these instances, ear irrigation can be used to flush the cerumen deposits out of the ear canal. Irrigation is best accomplished when direct visualization of the TM is possible, and it must be done gently to avoid damage to the TM. It is also important to warm the water to prevent nausea and vomiting.

Frequently used irrigating solutions include hydrogen peroxide 3% in a 1:1 solution with warm water, normal saline, or acetic acid (vinegar) mixed with warm water. Contraindications to irrigation include perforation of the TM and prior hypersensitivity.

Patients With Ear Disorders: General Suggestions for Teaching

- Instruct patients to not insert any foreign objects into the ear canal.
- Instruct patients to keep drugs away from heat.
- Provide education regarding the expected drug effect, dosage, and side effects, and when to notify the health care provider.
- Teach patients about OTC drug concerns, particularly with antihistamines and decongestants. OTC drugs may interact with prescribed drugs and may have risks that outweigh any drug benefit.
- Advise patients to contact their health care provider before using OTC drugs or herbal preparations to treat ear disorders.
- Encourage patients to keep follow-up appointments.

CRITICAL THINKING SINGLE EPISODE CASE STUDY

SLO/Objective: Prioritize appropriate actions for patients receiving eye medications

NGN Item Type: Cloze

Cognitive Skills: Generate Solutions

A 70-year-old female with a history of glaucoma complains of shortness of breath, dizziness, and weakness shortly after the nurse instilled latanoprost 0.005% and timolol 0.25% ophthalmic solution. Other patient data include:

- Blood pressure 100/62 mm Hg
- WBC 5000/mm^3
- Hemoglobin 12 g/dL
- Platelets 159,000/mm^3
- Heart rate 64 beats per minute (irregular)
- Respiratory rate 18 breaths per minute
- Serum sodium 138 mEq/L
- Serum potassium 4.8 mEq/L
- BUN 13 mg/dL
- Creatinine 0.9 mg/dL
- ALT 13 IU/L
- AST 53 IU/L

Choose the *most likely* options for the information missing from the statements below by selecting from the list of options provided.

The patient most likely is experiencing side effects from her eye drops, and the nurse would further review the patient's medical record for any history of _____1_____, _____1_____, _____1_____, or _____1_____. The nurse notifies the prescriber and continues to monitor the patient's _____2_____, _____2_____, _____2_____, and _____2_____. The nurse explains to the patient to notify the nurse if she experiences _____3_____, _____3_____, _____3_____, or _____3_____.

Option 1	Option 2	Option 3
Cardiac disorders	Visual acuity	Difficulty breathing
Renal disorders	Lung sounds	Polyuria
Hypertension	Vital signs	Cephalgia
Angle-closure glaucoma	Bowel habits	Chest discomforts
Immunosuppression	Cardiac rhythms	Constipation
Respiratory disorders	Electrolytes	Blurry vision

Answers:

The patient most likely is experiencing side effects from her eye drops, and the nurse would further review the patient's medical record for any history of **cardiac disorders, hypertension, angle-closure glaucoma,** or **respiratory disorders**. The nurse notifies the prescriber and continues to monitor the patient's **visual acuity, lung sounds, vital signs,** and **cardiac rhythms**. The nurse explains to the patient to notify the nurse if she experiences **difficulty breathing, cephalgia, chest discomfort,** or **blurry vision.**

Rationale:

Latanoprost is a prostaglandin analogue. While there are no absolute contraindications for this drug, caution is advised for persons with history of diabetic retinopathy, as there is a possible increased risk for retinal detachment, retinal embolus, or vitreous hemorrhage. Ocular examination and visual acuity should be assessed to determine potential complications. However, timolol is a nonselective beta antagonist that can cause respiratory and cardiac events. Absolute contraindications include persons with chronic obstructive or restrictive lung disease or those who have heart failure, atrioventricular (AV) block, or bradycardia. Because timolol nonselectively blocks beta receptors, preexisting AV blocks can worsen, new AV blocks can occur, cardiac workload can decrease, or bradycardia can occur. Even though timolol is administered topically to the eye, enough of the drug can enter the systemic circulation to produce beta-adrenergic blocking events, such as hypotension, bradycardia, and bronchospasms. The patient's blood pressure is 100/62 mm Hg and heart rate is 64 beats per minute. While these numbers are within normal parameters, they could be abnormally low for the patient, which could result in the patient's symptoms of shortness of breath, dizziness, and weakness. Timolol can worsen heart failure. The nurse would notify the prescriber to possibly hold timolol and continue monitoring patient's vital signs, assessing visual acuity, assessing lung sounds, and monitoring cardiac rhythms. If the blood pressure, heart rate, and arrhythmia continue to worsen, the patient would most likely require vasopressors. If the patient develops adventitious lung sounds, heart failure may occur. The patient should be instructed to notify the nurse immediately if she experiences continued or worsening difficulty breathing, cephalgia, chest discomfort, and/or blurry vision. Cephalgia, chest pain, and blurry vision can occur due to continued decreased tissue perfusion.

Reference:

Wang, Z., Denys, I., Chen, F., Cai, L., Wang, X., Kapusta, D.R., Lv, Y., & Gao, J. (2019). Complete atrioventricular block due to timolol eye drops: A case report and literature review. *BMC Pharmacology and Toxicology, 20*(73). doi: 10.1186/s40360-019-0370-2.

REVIEW QUESTIONS

1. A patient is taking oral acetazolamide, a carbonic anhydrase inhibitor, to decrease intraocular pressure. When providing drug education, which side effect would the nurse advise the patient to anticipate?
   a. Increased weight
   b. Light sensitivity
   c. Burning or stinging of the eyes
   d. Increased urine output

2. Which drug is most useful to prevent and treat cerumen impaction?
   a. Hydrogen peroxide
   b. Rubbing alcohol
   c. Charcoal
   d. Clove oil

3. The ophthalmologist asks the nurse to prepare to assist in the administration of tetracaine, fluorescein stain, and atropine for a diagnostic eye examination. Before assisting in the procedure, it is most important for the nurse to inform the ophthalmologist if the patient has a history of which condition?
   a. Cataracts
   b. Angle-closure glaucoma
   c. Open-angle glaucoma
   d. Macular degeneration

4. The nurse has a patient demonstrate self-administration of eyedrops. Place the steps in the order in which the patient will perform them.
   a. Pull the lower lid away from the eye so that a pouch is formed.
   b. Gently shake the bottle to evenly distribute the drug.
   c. Press a finger against the inner corner of the eye for 2 to 3 minutes.
   d. Remove the cap.
   e. Tilt the head backward and look upward.
   f. Place the dropper just above the pouch without touching the tip to the eye or finger.
   g. Wash hands.
   h. Gently squeeze one drop of medicine into the pouch.
5. When collecting a medication history from a patient with primary open-angle glaucoma, the nurse identifies several drugs that could exacerbate glaucoma. Which drug poses a priority concern for this particular patient?
   a. Cyclobenzaprine, an antispasmodic
   b. Oxymetazoline, a decongestant
   c. Prednisone, a corticosteroid
   d. Sulfamethoxazole-trimethoprim, a sulfonamide-antibiotic combination
6. The nurse asks a parent to demonstrate administration of eardrops on a toddler. Which steps by the parent indicate the need for additional education? (Select all that apply.)
   a. Position with the affected ear upward.
   b. Pull the ear backward and upward.
   c. Instill one drop of medication at a time allowing 3 to 5 minutes between each drop.
   d. Apply gentle pressure to the flap (tragus) over the ear canal.
   e. Keep the ear positioned upward for 5 minutes.

48

Dermatologic Disorders

OBJECTIVES

- Describe nonpharmacologic measures used to treat mild acne vulgaris.
- Describe at least three drugs that can cause drug-induced dermatitis and their characteristic symptoms.

- Compare the topical antibacterial drugs used to prevent and treat burn tissue infection.
- Discuss the Clinical Judgment [Nursing Process], including teaching, related to commonly used drugs for acne vulgaris, psoriasis, and burns.

OUTLINE

OVERVIEW OF THE SKIN

Skin, the largest organ of the body, consists of two major layers: the *epidermis* is the outer layer of skin, and the *dermis* is the layer beneath the epidermis. The functions of the skin include (1) protecting the body from the environment, (2) aiding in body temperature control, and (3) preventing body fluid loss.

The epidermis has four layers: (1) the basal layer, or *stratum germinativum,* the deepest layer lying over the dermis; (2) the spinous layer, or *stratum spinosum;* (3) the granular layer, or *stratum granulosum;* and (4) the cornified layer, or *stratum corneum,* the outer layer of the epidermis.

The dermis has two layers: the *papillary layer* lies next to the epidermis, and the *reticular layer* is the deeper layer of the dermis. The dermal layers consist of fibroblasts, collagen fibers, and elastic fibers. The collagen and elastic fibers give the skin its strength and elasticity. Within the dermal layer are sweat glands, hair follicles, sebaceous glands, blood vessels, and sensory nerve terminals. Fig. 48.1 shows the layers of the skin.

The subcutaneous tissue, primarily fatty tissue, lies under the dermis. Besides fatty cells, subcutaneous tissue contains blood and lymphatic vessels, nerve fibers, and elastic fibers. It supports and protects the dermis.

Numerous skin lesions and eruptions require mild to aggressive drug therapy. Skin disorders include acne vulgaris, psoriasis, eczema dermatitis, contact dermatitis, drug-induced dermatitis, rosacea, and burn infection. Skin eruptions may result from viruses, such as herpes simplex and zoster; fungi (e.g., tinea pedis [athlete's foot], tinea capitis [ringworm]); and bacteria.

Skin lesions may appear as macules (flat and nonpalpable, usually less than 10 mm in diameter with varying colors), papules (raised and palpable, less than 10 mm in diameter), vesicles (clear, fluid-filled blisters smaller than 10 mm in diameter), or plaques (palpable lesions that are depressed or elevated compared with the skin surface and greater than 10 mm in diameter). Treatments for skin eruptions include topical creams, ointments, pastes, gels, lotions, and solutions. Selected skin disorders and their drug therapy regimens are discussed separately. Treatment information can be found at the American Academy of Dermatology (AAD) website at https://www.aad.org.

ACNE VULGARIS

Acne is the most common skin disorder in the United States. Acne is more prevalent among adolescents, but adults and children can also develop acne. Acne vulgaris is the formation of papules, nodules, and

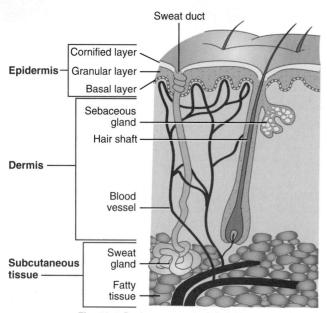

Fig. 48.1 Basic structures of the skin.

cysts on the face, neck, shoulders, and back that results not from dirt but from keratin plugs at the base of the pilosebaceous oil glands near the hair follicles. The keratin plugs trap normal skin flora, including bacteria commonly found on the skin; the primary bacterium is *Propionibacterium acnes*. Bacteria start proliferating, which causes inflammation and irritation. During adolescence, production of androgens and sebum—an oily skin lubricant—are increased. The sebum combines with keratin, a protein that is part of the skin, to form a plug that results in acne. Comedones are types of noninflammatory acne lesions that may be open (blackheads) or closed (whiteheads). Open comedones are dilated hair follicle openings that allow oxidation of the debris within the follicle; closed comedones are small, plugged hair follicles. As with other forms of acne, comedones are not a result of poor hygiene. All forms of acne should be treated to prevent lifelong scars. Acne can be treated nonpharmacologically and pharmacologically. Table 48.1 lists the drugs commonly used to control acne vulgaris along with their dosages, uses, and considerations.

Nonpharmacologic Approach

Nonpharmacologic measures should be tried before drug therapy is initiated. A prescribed or suggested cleansing agent, such as antibacterial soap, is necessary for all types of acne. The skin should be gently cleansed twice daily, but vigorous scrubbing should be avoided. Overscrubbing and overwashing can irritate the skin, worsening the acne and possibly causing an infection. The American Osteopathic College of Dermatology recommends *not* using abrasive cleaners. In addition to facial hygiene, shampooing hair to decrease the oiliness may help with acne. Keeping hair away from the face has also been shown to decrease acne. Cosmetics should be water based because oil-based products can increase the clogging of skin pores. A well-balanced diet low in fat and sugar is recommended, and excessive carbohydrates should be avoided. Decreasing emotional stress and increasing emotional support are also suggested. If drug therapy is necessary, nonpharmacologic measures should be maintained as well.

Pharmacologic Treatment

Acne is not curable, but it is manageable. Acne medications may help decrease scar formation related to acne. The best course for patients

with acne is to see a dermatologist who can prescribe treatment specific to the individual; therefore the course of therapy will vary according to the severity and extent of the acne.

Topical Antiacne Drugs

Mild acne is generally treated with topical drugs that treat existing acne and prevent new eruptions. Commonly used topical therapies for mild acne include benzoyl peroxide (BP), retinoids, salicylic acid, antibiotics, or combinations of these in addition to gentle cleansing.

BP is an antibacterial medicine that kills *P. acnes*, the predominant organism in sebaceous follicles and comedones. BP releases free radical oxygen species that oxidize bacterial proteins. When included as an adjunct to an antibiotic regimen, control of acne is enhanced. Resolution of acne usually occurs within 4 to 6 weeks. BP is applied as a cream, lotion, or gel once or twice a day and can be left on or washed off. Washing BP off may be better tolerated in patients with sensitive skin.

Topical retinoids such as tretinoin, adapalene, and tazarotene are derivatives of vitamin A and are used for mild to moderate acne that alters keratinization. They are the mainstay of topical therapy because of their comedolytic activities, and they also have antiinflammatory properties. Retinoids alter the intracrine and paracrine mediators of cell differentiation and proliferation, apoptosis, and reproduction, thereby modifying gene expression, subsequent protein synthesis, and epithelial cell growth. Retinoids prevent horny cell cohesion, or keratolysis, and increase epithelial cell turnover. They do *not* affect microorganisms in acne and sebum production. Topical retinoids are appropriate for all types of acne when used in combination with other antiacne therapy. They also allow maintenance of acne clearance after discontinuing oral antibiotics. Of the retinoids, tazarotene is contraindicated with pregnancy. Retinoids should *not* be used before or after extended sun exposure or sunburn because they can increase the risk of sunburn and intensify existing sunburn.

Another antiacne topical drug, azelaic acid, has antibacterial, antiinflammatory, and mild comedolytic actions. Azelaic acid is as effective as BP and tretinoin combined. Salicylic acid is also a comedolytic treatment that is available over the counter (OTC) in various strengths. However, the efficacy of salicylic acid is still unknown. Topical treatments with retinoids, azelaic acid, and salicylic acid can cause burning, pruritus, and erythema after several applications; however, they are less common with azelaic acid.

Moderate to severe acne may require a stronger concentration of BP, and topical antibiotics, such as tetracycline, erythromycin, and clindamycin, may be added to the treatment regimen. Erythromycin and clindamycin are the recommended topical antibiotics for acne therapy; however, erythromycin has reduced efficacy compared with clindamycin. Topical antibiotics accumulate in the hair follicle and have both antiinflammatory and antibacterial effects. Topical antibiotics as monotherapy are *not* recommended due to the development of antibiotic resistance. Severe, painful acne may be treated with steroid injection.

Systemic Antiacne Drugs

For severe acne, adjunctive treatment is usually warranted with oral antibiotics (e.g., doxycycline and minocycline [drugs of choice], tetracycline, amoxicillin) in addition to topical corticosteroids (Box 48.1). Tetracycline antibiotics, however, should not be used among the very young and among pregnant patients; drugs of the tetracycline class may cause dental discoloration to the developing teeth and have teratogenic effects on the fetus. Instead, amoxicillin or another nontetracycline drug may be given for severe acne. See Chapter 26 for more information on antibacterials.

TABLE 48.1 Drugs for Acne Vulgaris and Psoriasis

Generic	Route and Dosage	Uses and Considerations
ACNE VULGARIS		
Systemic Preparations		
Tetracycline hydrochloride	A: PO: Initially, 125–250 mg q6h for 1–2 wk, then decrease slowly to 125–500 mg daily or every other day	For moderate to severe inflammatory acne vulgaris concomitantly with topical retinoid and benzoyl peroxide (BP). Best on an empty stomach (1 h before or 2 h after meal/milk). To reduce risk of esophageal irritation or ulceration, take with plenty of water and do not take at bedtime; not for patients with esophageal disorders. Permanent discoloration during tooth development and enamel hypoplasia may occur. See Chapter 26 for other considerations.
Minocycline hydrochloride	Severe acne: A: IV/PO: 200 mg for 1 dose, then 100 mg q12h Nonnodular moderate to severe acne: A: PO: 1 mg/kg extended-release capsule/tablets once daily for 12 wk	For adjunctive treatment of moderate to severe inflammatory acne; monotherapy should be avoided. Drug considerations are similar to those of tetracycline.
Doxycycline	A: weighing ≥45 kg: PO: 100 mg q12h on day 1, then 100 mg once daily	Adjunctive treatment for severe acne; monotherapy should be avoided. Drug considerations are similar to those of tetracycline.
Isotretinoin	A: PO: 0.5–1 mg/kg/d in 2 divided doses Take with meals to increase bioavailability Patient may repeat the course at least 8 wk after completion of the prior course	For moderate to severe nodular acne unresponsive to conventional treatment, including antibiotics. Vitamin A derivative; reverses sebum production by reducing the size of sebaceous glands. Unlike vitamin A, isotretinoin does not accumulate in the liver. Adverse effects relate to toxicity to cardiovascular, endocrine, hematologic, GI, hepatic, musculoskeletal, respiratory, ocular, and otic systems. Interacts with tetracycline, vitamin A, methotrexate, contraceptives, and alcohol. Baseline hepatic function, lipid panel, and pregnancy tests must be obtained. Women of childbearing age must have a pregnancy test every 30 days.
Amoxicillin	A: PO: 250 mg bid up to 500 mg tid	Adjunctive treatment for acne, especially during pregnancy. Shake suspension well before each administration. Suspension may be added to formula, milk, and other liquids. For other considerations and uses, see Chapter 26.
Topical Preparations		
General considerations: When using multiple topical products for acne, apply each product at different times throughout the day to decrease skin irritation. Common side effects of topical drugs include xerosis of skin, erythema, and pruritus. Avoid eyes, mouth, and mucous membranes when using topical antiacne preparations.		
Keratolytic Agents		
Azelaic acid	A: Apply a thin layer to the affected area twice daily, morning and evening	For mild to moderate inflammatory acne; has antimicrobial effect against *Propionibacterium acnes* and *Staphylococcus epidermidis* and an antikeratinizing effect on the follicular epidermis. May cause hypopigmentation in patients with dark complexions.
Benzoyl peroxide	A: 2.5%, 5%, or 10% gel, wash, or cream: 1–4 times/d	First-line therapy for mild to moderate inflammatory and noninflammatory acne lesions. Promotes keratolysis, removal of the horny layer of epidermis, resulting in drying and desquamative actions. Can be used concomitantly with other antiacne therapies.
Salicylic acid	A: 0.5%–6% cream, gel, and shampoo 1–3 times/d; if erythema or peeling occurs, reduce application	For mild to moderate acne; promotes desquamation of the horny layer of skin. Monitor for salicylic toxicity; use of salicylic acid in children with viral infections is not recommended due to increased risk for Reye syndrome.
Antibiotics		
General considerations: Antibiotics may be given concurrently with benzoyl peroxide.		
Erythromycin	A: 2% solution, pledget, or gel 1–2 times/d	For mild to moderate inflammatory acne
Clindamycin	A: 1% gel, lotion, solution, or pledget: Apply twice daily to the affected area 1% foam: Apply once daily	For moderate acne. May cause colitis, dermatitis, folliculitis, pruritus, erythema, dry skin, and peeling. Dispense foam into cap or onto a cool surface to prevent premature melting. Shake other formulations well before use. Can have neuromuscular blocking action; use cautiously with opiate agonists; monitor for any CNS depression (e.g., bradypnea, weakness, paralysis).
Vitamin A Derivatives		
General considerations: Topical vitamin A derivatives may be used concurrently with benzoyl peroxide and other antiacne therapies.		

Continued

TABLE 48.1   Drugs for Acne Vulgaris and Psoriasis—cont'd

Generic	Route and Dosage	Uses and Considerations
ACNE VULGARIS		
Tretinoin	A: Apply a thin layer to the affected area once daily at bedtime	For mild to moderate acne. Cleanse area first, pat dry, and wait 20–30 min before applying. Wash hands immediately after applying. Caution in patients with fish allergies.
Adapalene	A: 0.1% lotion or gel, 0.3% gel: Apply once daily at bedtime after washing the face with nonmedicated soap	For mild to moderate acne, adapalene causes less skin irritation than tretinoin.
Tazarotene	A: 0.1% cream, gel, or foam: Apply a thin film once daily in the evening	For mild to moderate acne; can also be used for psoriasis. Photosensitivity can occur; avoid unnecessary environmental exposures. May use a moisturizer as needed.
Oral Contraceptives		
Ethinyl estradiol/norethindrone acetate/ferrous fumarate	A: PO: 1 pill every day at the same time for 21 d followed by 1 wk of no tablets	For the treatment of acne vulgaris. See Chapter 52 for more information on drug uses and considerations.
Ethinyl estradiol/norgestimate	A: PO: 1 tab at the same time each day	For the treatment of acne vulgaris. See Chapter 52 for more information on drug uses and considerations.
PSORIASIS		
Systemic Preparations		
Methoxsalen	A: PO: 10–70 mg 2–3 times weekly, according to body weight. Administer 2 h before exposure to therapeutic UV rays	Systemic antimetabolite for severe psoriasis not responsive to other therapy. Soft and hard gelatin capsules are *not* interchangeable. Separate doses by at least 48 h. Administer with food or milk. Contraindicated in patients with history of or current invasive cutaneous carcinoma or melanoma. Avoid sunlight during drug therapy; sunlight could cause severe burning and blistering.
Acitretin	A: PO: 25–50 mg/d with main meal. Trials found that 25 mg/d for treatment of psoriasis vulgaris is similar in efficacy to 50 mg/d with fewer and less severe adverse clinical and laboratory events	Retinoid for recalcitrant psoriasis. May take up to 6 mo for maximal response to treatment. May be given concurrently with phototherapy. Give with food for increased bioavailability.
Topical Preparations		
Anthralin	A: Apply sparingly to lesions once daily and leave on up to 30 min. Rinse thoroughly with cool to lukewarm water, then wash with soap	For stable plaque psoriasis. May stain clothing, skin, and hair.
Calcipotriene	A: Apply up to twice daily	Vitamin D analogue for chronic plaque psoriasis. More effective when used with a topical corticosteroid. Do not exceed 100 g/wk. Excess use may increase serum calcium level. Contraindicated in persons with hypercalcemia. Avoid UV rays.
Clobetasol propionate	A/C ≥12 y: Cream, gel, foam, or ointment: Apply a thin layer twice daily A/C ≥16 y: Emollient cream *only*: Apply a thin layer twice daily A: Spray and lotion: Apply twice daily	Super-high-potency corticosteroid for moderate to severe plaque psoriasis. [!] Do not use occlusive dressings. With any formulation, do not exceed 50 g/wk. Reassess lesions after 2 wk of treatment. Contraindicated for application to the axilla, face, or groin.
Coal tar	A: Foam, lotion, suspension, or shampoo: Apply up to 4 times daily, depending on formulation	For mild to moderate psoriasis. No maximum dosage. Wash affected area to remove loose psoriatic scales for better penetration. Allow skin to air dry after treatment. May stain clothing, skin, and hair. Do not use on inflamed, broken, or infected skin due to increased risk of systemic absorption. UV rays should be avoided for 24 h after treatment.
Tazarotene	A: Cream: Apply to affected areas once daily in the evening A: Gel: Apply once daily in the evening	For stable plaque psoriasis. Can also be used for acne vulgaris. May use with skin emollients, but apply at least 1 h before tazarotene. Avoid application to unaffected skin due to increased systemic absorption.

TABLE 48.1	**Drugs for Acne Vulgaris and Psoriasis—cont'd**	
Generic	**Route and Dosage**	**Uses and Considerations**
	PSORIASIS	

! Biologic Agents

General considerations: Before initiating therapy, patients must be tested for active infections (e.g., TB, HBV). Rotate injection sites; subsequent injections should be at least 1 inch from previous injection sites. Do not inject in areas that are bruised, red, tender, or hard.

Generic	Route and Dosage	Uses and Considerations
Adalimumab	Psoriasis: A: Subcut: Start with 80 mg on week 1, then 40 mg on week 2, then 40 mg every other week Psoriatic arthritis: A: Subcut: 40 mg every other week	A TNF-α MAb for moderate to severe chronic plaque psoriasis and psoriatic arthritis when other systemic therapy is not appropriate. Rotate injections on the front of thighs and abdomen. Subsequent injections should be at least an inch away from previous injection sites.
Etanercept	Psoriatic arthritis: A: Subcut: 50 mg/wk up to twice weekly Psoriasis: Start with 50 mg twice weekly 3–4 d apart for 3 mo; then 50 mg/wk	TNF inhibitor for moderate to severe psoriasis. May be administered in an outpatient setting; teach patient or caregiver thoroughly on proper administration. Do not inject directly into scaly patches or lesions. Contraindicated in persons with sepsis.
Infliximab	A: IV: 5 mg/kg given at weeks 0, 2, and 6 and then every 8 wk	Chimeric MAb for chronic severe psoriasis and psoriatic arthritis. Infuse over at least 2 h with appropriate filter. *Absolute contraindications:* Heart failure, murine protein hypersensitivity. Black box warning includes infection (viral, fungal, bacterial) and neoplastic disease.
Ustekinumab	Based on weight: A >100 kg: Subcut: 90 mg, repeat 4 wk later, then 90 mg q12wk starting at wk 16 A ≤100 kg: Subcut: 45 mg, repeat in 4 wk, then q12wk starting at wk 16	IL-12 and IL-23 antagonists for moderate to severe plaque psoriasis for patients receiving phototherapy or systemic therapy for psoriatic arthritis.

A, Adult; *bid,* twice daily; *CNS,* central nervous system; *d,* day; *GI,* gastrointestinal; *h,* hour; *HBV,* hepatitis B virus; *IL,* interleukin; *IV,* intravenous; *MAb,* monoclonal antibody; *min,* minutes; *mo,* month; *PO,* by mouth; *q,* every; *Subcut,* subcutaneous; *tab,* tablet; *TB,* tuberculosis; *tid,* three times daily; *TNF,* tumor necrosis factor; *UV,* ultraviolet; *wk,* week; *y,* year; >, greater than; <, less than; ≥, greater than or equal to; ≤, less than or equal to.

Isotretinoin, a derivative of vitamin A taken orally, is used for treatment of severe cystic acne that is not responsive to conventional therapy. It decreases sebum formation and secretion and has antiinflammatory and antikeratinizing (keratolytic) effects, decreasing lesions and scars due to acne. Additional benefits of isotretinoin include a decrease in anxiety and depression. The typical patient takes this drug for 4 to 6 months. Adverse reactions may occur that are dose dependent; these include cheilitis, dizziness, cephalgia, conjunctivitis, skin irritation, pruritus, epistaxis, myalgia, arthralgia, temporary hair thinning, photosensitivity, depression, and suicidal thoughts. Usually, one course of treatment with isotretinoin controls severe acne. Because isotretinoin is a derivative of vitamin A, patients should not take vitamin A concomitantly. Using vitamin A or tetracycline with isotretinoin may increase its adverse effects. Baseline blood tests—liver function tests (LFTs), serum lipid panel, and pregnancy tests among female patients of childbearing age—are required before initiating isotretinoin therapy and at intervals throughout therapy. **!** Isotretinoin must *not* be used during pregnancy; it is a known teratogen. Additional cautions associated with isotretinoin are to not breastfeed or to give blood during or for 1 month after therapy; patients should not take other medications or herbal products without first consulting their health care provider, drive at night without knowing the effect of isotretinoin on night vision, or have cosmetic procedures to smooth skin. The patient should be instructed to avoid excessively vigorous activity and to contact the health care provider and stop taking isotretinoin if they experience muscle weakness, which may be an indication of serious muscle damage.

! Because of isotretinoin's powerful teratogenicity, a risk management system to prevent isotretinoin-related teratogenicity was implemented. iPLEDGE is the third risk management program to prevent exposure to isotretinoin during pregnancy. Before starting isotretinoin therapy, both males and females must enroll in the iPLEDGE risk management program and adhere to it. The program was created to ensure patients who receive isotretinoin use two forms of contraception, that no patient is pregnant when treatment is initiated, and that no patient becomes pregnant while taking the drug or for at least 1 month after completing a course of isotretinoin. This comprehensive program also has rules for the health care provider, patient, pharmacist, and wholesaler. Further information can be found at https://www.ipledgeprogram.com.

PSORIASIS

Psoriasis is a multisystem disease with predominant skin and joint disorders. According to the AAD, it affects nearly 3.2% of the population; of those affected, 80% have mild to moderate disease. A majority of the manifestations are exhibited as chronic skin inflammation characterized by scaly, erythematous plaques or scales. These plaques may be painful and are often pruritic, at times causing significant quality-of-life issues. They can appear on the scalp, elbows, palms, knees, and soles of the feet. Psoriasis is a chronic disease, and the manifestations wax and wane. Of the different forms of psoriasis, plaque psoriasis is the most common form. Approximately 25% to 30% of people with psoriasis have joint psoriatic arthritis. Depending on the severity of the disease,

BOX 48.1   Topical Corticosteroids

Very High Potency
Betamethasone dipropionate, augmented 0.05% (ointment)
Clobetasol propionate 0.05%
Diflorasone diacetate 0.05% (ointment)
Halobetasol propionate 0.05%

High Potency
Amcinonide 0.1%
Betamethasone dipropionate, augmented 0.05% (cream)
Desoximetasone 0.25% (cream, ointment) and 0.05% (gel)
Diflorasone diacetate 0.05% (cream)
Fluocinonide 0.05%
Halcinonide 0.1%
Triamcinolone acetonide 0.5%

Medium Potency
Betamethasone valerate 0.1%
Fluocinolone acetonide 0.025% (cream, ointment)
Flurandrenolide 0.05%
Fluticasone propionate 0.05% (cream) and 0.005% (ointment)
Mometasone furoate 0.1%
Triamcinolone acetonide 0.1% (cream, ointment)

Low-Medium Potency
Hydrocortisone butyrate 0.1%
Hydrocortisone probutate 0.1%
Hydrocortisone valerate 0.2%
Prednicarbate 0.1%

Low Potency
Alclometasone dipropionate 0.05%
Fluocinolone acetonide 0.01% (cream, solution)

Lowest Potency
Dexamethasone 0.1%
Hydrocortisone base or acetate 0.25%, 0.5%, 1%

recommendations for the treatment of psoriasis include topical and systemic treatments and/or phototherapy. Table 48.1 lists some drugs, dosages, uses, and considerations for psoriasis. Table 48.2 lists current treatment modalities for psoriasis and psoriatic arthritis.

Topical Drugs

Vehicles for topical preparations are many and may include ointments, creams, lotions, solutions, gels, foams, and tape, among others. More than one topical medication may be used concomitantly to increase the effectiveness of each drug. If more than one topical drug is used, patients need to be instructed to apply each drug at separate times throughout the day. Topical drugs for psoriasis include corticosteroids, vitamin D analogues, tazarotene, calcineurin inhibitors (e.g., tacrolimus and pimecrolimus), salicylic acid, anthralin, and coal tar.

Topical corticosteroids are the principal treatment for the majority of patients. Corticosteroids are available in a variety of vehicles that are sold OTC or by prescription; differing levels of potency are also available such that the weakest formula (e.g., 1% hydrocortisone) is available OTC and the strongest (e.g., clobetasol propionate) is by prescription (see Box 48.1). Corticosteroids are classified according to their potency, class 1 to class 7, in which class 1 is the strongest (superpotent). The lower-potency topical steroids are reserved for sensitive skin (e.g., face, intertriginous areas, thin skin areas, in infants and older adults). Patients with thick skin and those with scales or plaques often require the highest-potency steroids. ⚡ The usual length of treatment for most topical steroids is 4 weeks; otherwise, adverse effects that include cutaneous side effects and systemic absorption may occur. Tapering topical steroids after clinical response is recommended by the AAD. Cutaneous side effects include skin atrophy, telangiectasia, striae distensae, acne, folliculitis, and purpura. Other effects include worsening of existing or preexisting skin conditions (dermatoses) and fungal infections (tineas). Worsening of psoriasis can also occur (rebound effect) with the use of topical corticosteroids. Even though systemic side effects are fewer than cutaneous side effects with topical steroids, these can still occur. Systemic effects usually occur with the highest-potency preparation used over a large surface for a prolonged period. Examples of systemic side effects include Cushing syndrome, cataracts, glaucoma, and suppression of the hypothalamic-pituitary-adrenal (HPA) axis, which can cause growth retardation.

TABLE 48.2   Current Approved Treatment Modalities for Psoriasis and Psoriatic Arthritis

Biologics	Topical Treatments	Systemic Treatments	Phototherapy and Photochemotherapy
Adalimumab	Anthralin	Acitretin	Broadband and narrowband B
Certolizumab	Coal tar	Apremilast	Excimer laser therapy
Etanercept	Corticosteroids	Cyclosporine	Oral PUVA therapy
Infliximab	Emollients	Fumaric acid esters	Topical PUVA therapy
Guselkumab	Pimecrolimus	Methotrexate	
Ixekizumab	Salicylic acid	Retinoids	
Secukinumab	Tacrolimus	Sulfasalazine	
Tildrakizumab	Tazarotene		
Ustekinumab	Vitamin D analogues		
	Combination therapy of all previously mentioned		

PUVA, Psoralen and ultraviolet A; *TNF*, tumor necrosis factor.
Data from American Academy of Dermatology. (2020). *Psoriasis clinical guideline.* Retrieved from https://www.aad.org/member/clinical-quality/guidelines/psoriasis.

⚡ TABLE 48.3 Methotrexate Drug Interactions

NSAIDs	Antibiotics	Others
Salicylates	Trimethoprim-sulfamethoxazole	Acitretin
Naproxen		Barbiturates
Ibuprofen	Sulfonamides	Ethanol
Indomethacin	Penicillins	Vaccines with live virus
Phenylbutazone	Minocycline	Phenytoin
	Ciprofloxacin	Sulfonylureas
		Theophylline

NSAIDs, Nonsteroidal antiinflammatory drugs.
From Medscape (2021). *Methotrexate.* Retrieved from https://reference.medscape.com/drug/trexall-otrexup-methotrexate-343201#3.

Synthetic vitamin D analogues (e.g., calcipotriene) bind to vitamin D receptors, enhancing the differentiation of keratinocytes while inhibiting their proliferation. Calcipotriene is available in solution, foam, and cream and is usually combined with topical corticosteroids to increase clinical response. Local side effects include burning, pruritus, edema, peeling, dryness, and erythema. Systemic side effects usually occur due to overapplication and include hypercalcemia and suppression of parathyroid hormone. Patients need to be instructed to avoid ultraviolet (UV) light because UVA inactivates calcipotriene.

Topical tazarotene, a retinoid, normalizes abnormal keratinocyte differentiation and decreases hyperproliferation and inflammation. Tazarotene may be used concurrently with moisturizers and topical corticosteroids. Common side effects include local irritation. Tazarotene is a teratogen; therefore its use is contraindicated during pregnancy.

Topical calcineurin inhibitors (CIs) such as tacrolimus and pimecrolimus block the synthesis of proinflammatory cytokines, a major pathogenesis of psoriasis. Common side effects include burning and pruritus of the skin, which appears to increase when applied immediately after bathing. Topical tacrolimus and pimecrolimus are not approved for infants and children younger than 2 years. Increased susceptibility to infection can occur with the use of topical CIs, including reactivation of latent viral infection.

Other topical preparations include salicylic acid, anthralin, and coal tar. Salicylic acid is a keratolytic agent that loosens psoriatic plaques. Like other salicylate drugs, topical salicylates may be absorbed systemically and cause toxicity; therefore topical salicylic acid should not be used by children due to the risk of Reye syndrome. Anthralin normalizes keratinocyte differentiation and is commonly used for short, contact therapy. Common side effects include skin irritation and staining of adjoining skin, nails, and clothing. Coal tar products are available in shampoos, lotions, creams, and bath solutions. They have an unpleasant odor and can cause burning and stinging, so they are rarely used.

UVA may be used to suppress mitotic (cell division) activity. Photochemotherapy, a combination of UV radiation and the psoralen derivative methoxsalen (a photosensitive drug), is used to decrease proliferation of epidermal cells. This type of therapy is called psoralen and ultraviolet A (PUVA), which permits lower doses of methoxsalen and UVA to be given. Common side effects of PUVA include erythema, pruritus, xerosis, irregular pigmentation, and gastrointestinal (GI) symptoms such as nausea and vomiting. Other toxicities include blisters, melanonychia, hypertrichosis, and squamous cell carcinoma (SCC). PUVA is contraindicated in patients with known lupus erythematosus, xeroderma pigmentosum, and porphyria. A topical preparation of methoxsalen must be administered only by a trained clinician.

Systemic Drugs

Traditional systemic drugs for psoriasis (e.g., methotrexate, cyclosporine, acitretin) are commonly used for refractory psoriasis. Biologic response modifiers (BRMs) also have a role in the treatment of psoriasis without the toxicity of traditional systemic treatment to the liver, kidneys, and bone marrow; furthermore, BRMs are not teratogenic.

A folate antimetabolite, ⚠ methotrexate is a systemic drug that slows high growth fraction. It is prescribed to decrease the acceleration of epidermal cell growth in severe psoriasis. However, methotrexate can cause toxicity to the liver (hepatic fibrosis and cirrhosis), blood (myelosuppression), and lungs (pulmonary fibrosis). Other common adverse effects include nausea, anorexia, stomatitis, and fatigue. It is considered teratogenic and is contraindicated in women of childbearing age who are trying to conceive. Methotrexate has numerous drug-drug interactions, thereby increasing the risk of methotrexate toxicity (Table 48.3 lists some of the drugs that interact with methotrexate). Before methotrexate administration is initiated, a careful history, physical and laboratory tests (e.g., complete blood count [CBC], creatinine, LFTs, protein status, bilirubin, screening for latent tuberculosis [TB] infections), and chest radiograph must be obtained. During treatment, ongoing studies include CBC and renal and hepatic function tests. Methotrexate has been used in combination with approved BRMs for psoriasis. See Chapter 35 for more nursing considerations with antimetabolites.

Cyclosporine, a cyclic polypeptide immunosuppressive drug, is the most effective systemic preparation for psoriasis. It inhibits T-cell activation and has minimal toxicities in otherwise healthy patients. It must be administered on a consistent schedule with regard to time of day and in relation to meals to decrease serum level variations. As with other immunosuppressive drugs, patients must be assessed for active infections before initiating therapy. Patients must also be monitored for nephrotoxicity and hypertension. Other common side effects include hypertrichosis (darkening of hair), cephalgia, paresthesia, myalgia, arthralgia, asthenia, and fatigue.

Acitretin, a vitamin A derivative, is the least effective drug as monotherapy and is usually used concurrently with phototherapy. It is more effective with pustular psoriasis, and clinical response is dose dependent. Adverse effects include mucocutaneous effects, erythematous scaly patches with superficial fissures, and periungual pyogenic granulomas. Noncutaneous adverse effects include hyperlipidemia, pancreatitis, elevated transaminases, and pseudotumor cerebri–like symptoms. Its use is contraindicated with pregnancy.

High-cost BRMs are helpful in the management of psoriasis in patients who are refractory to ultraviolet B (UVB) phototherapy who need improved control. Drugs approved by the US Food and Drug Administration (FDA) include tumor necrosis factor (TNF) inhibitors (e.g., etanercept, infliximab, adalimumab) and interleukin antagonists (e.g., ustekinumab). All TNF inhibitors have a risk of severe opportunistic infection. TB and hepatitis B virus (HBV) testing should be conducted on all patients before administering TNF inhibitors. Caution is advised when administering drug to patients with a history of congestive heart failure. These biologic agents are expensive but tend to have fewer side effects with comparable efficacy to traditional systemic treatments. TNF inhibitors are contraindicated in patients with active infections or demyelinating disease (e.g., multiple sclerosis). Adalimumab is the first fully human TNF-inhibitor monoclonal antibody (mAb). Infliximab is a chimeric mAb, and ustekinumab is a human immunoglobulin G (IgG) monoclonal antibody. New mAbs include brodalumab, guselkumab, and tildrakizumab. More information on mAbs can be found in Chapter 36. Etanercept is a soluble recombinant human TNF-α inhibitor. Table 48.1 lists the drugs, including biologics, that are currently being used to control psoriasis.

◎ CLINICAL JUDGMENT [NURSING PROCESS]

Acne Vulgaris and Psoriasis

Concept: Tissue Integrity
- The ability for the body tissues to repair itself

Recognize Cues [Assessment]
- Obtain a history from the patient in regard to the onset of skin lesions. Note if there is a familial history.
- Assess the patient's skin eruptions. Describe lesions, locations (body surface area [BSA]), and drainage, if present.
- Obtain cultures of purulent, draining skin lesions.
- Determine baseline vital signs and weight. Report any elevation in temperature.
- Obtain baseline laboratory values (complete blood count [CBC], lipid panel, renal function, and hepatic function).
- Obtain chest radiograph, electrocardiography (ECG), and, if applicable, conduct pregnancy, tuberculosis (TB), and hepatitis B virus (HBV) tests.
- Assess the psychological effects of skin lesions and any changes in perception of body image.
- Assess the effects of skin lesions on quality of life.

Analyze Cues and Prioritize Hypothesis [Patient Problems]
- Skin tissue injury related to disease process
- Sun-exposed skin rash related to side effects of drugs
- Need for teaching related to complex skin regimen
- Potential for decreased self-esteem

Generate Solutions [Planning]
- The patient will have increased knowledge of management of the skin condition.
- The patient will verbalize the need for two methods of contraception during the required period.
- The patient will verbalize lesions have diminished after drug therapy and skin care.
- The patient will be free from infection during therapy.
- The patient will report improved body image.

Take Action [Nursing Interventions]
- Establish rapport; the patient may be embarrassed.
- Apply topical medications to skin lesions using aseptic technique.
- Monitor vital signs and perform required diagnostic tests. Report abnormal findings.
- During drug therapy, check lesion sites for improvement, and monitor for adverse reactions to drug therapy.
- Listen to the patient's body image concerns and provide community resources if applicable.

Patient Teaching
General
- Advise patients not to use harsh cleansers. Instruct them to gently cleanse the skin several times a day and pat dry. Allow to dry for 20 to 30 minutes before applying product.
- Teach patients to apply topical drugs using clean technique.
- Instruct patients to notify their health care provider if pregnant or if there is a possibility of pregnancy. Many drugs used to treat acne and psoriasis are teratogenic.
- Advise patients to keep health care appointments and to have diagnostic tests performed as prescribed.

Side Effects
- Inform patients about side effects and adverse reactions associated with drugs.
- Advise patients to report abnormal findings immediately.

Evaluate Outcomes [Evaluation]
- Evaluate the patient's knowledge of management of the condition.
- Evaluate the effectiveness of drug therapy. If improvement is not apparent, the drug therapy and skin care regimen may need to be changed.
- Be aware of the different time periods for improvement with various drug therapies.

VERRUCA VULGARIS (WARTS)

The common wart is a hard, horny nodule that may appear anywhere on the body, particularly on the hands and feet. Warts occur when the top layer of the skin becomes infected with human papillomavirus (HPV). Warts may be benign lesions, or they may be precursors to cancerous lesions. Warts are contagious and can be spread by contact. Most warts do not require treatment, but they may be removed by cryotherapy (freezing), electrodessication, or surgical excision. Other treatments include using chemical peels with salicylic acid, tretinoin, and glycolic acid; injection of anticancer drugs, such as bleomycin; or immunotherapy, such as diphencyprone (DCP). Salicylic acid promotes desquamation. It can be absorbed through the skin, and salicylism (toxicity) could occur. Podophyllum resin is indicated mainly for venereal warts and is not as effective against the common wart. This drug also can be absorbed through the skin; toxic symptoms such as peripheral neuropathy, blood dyscrasias, and kidney impairment may result if a large area is treated. Podophyllum could cause teratogenic effects; therefore it should not be used during pregnancy. Imiquimod and podofilox may be prescribed as alternative agents for podophyllin, and both may be used for topical treatment of external genital and perianal warts. Bleomycin injections are also used for warts. Side effects of bleomycin injection include nail loss if given for warts on the fingers.

Immunotherapy uses the patient's own immune system to fight the warts by causing an allergic reaction to the treated warts, which may cause the warts to disappear.

Cantharidin is used to remove the common wart. For treatment, cantharidin is applied to the wart and allowed to dry, and then the wart is covered with nonporous tape for 24 to 48 hours. Occlusion allows a blister to form beneath the wart, where live viruses are located. A follow-up visit at 2 weeks will allow the hyperkeratosis to be debrided. If verruca is noted after debridement, the procedure may be repeated. Side effects include a tingling or burning sensation at the application site.

Many OTC agents are used to remove warts. The efficacy of some of these is questionable; however, some that contain chemical compounds such as salicylic acid may be effective.

DRUG-INDUCED DERMATITIS

An adverse reaction to drug therapy may result in skin lesions that vary from a rash, urticaria, papules, and vesicles to life-threatening skin eruptions such as erythema multiforme (red blisters over a large portion of the body), Stevens-Johnson syndrome (large blisters in the oral and anogenital mucosa, pharynx, eyes, and viscera), and toxic epidermal necrolysis (widespread detachment of the epidermis from underlying skin layers). A hypersensitive reaction to a drug is caused by the formation of sensitizing lymphocytes. If multiple drug therapy is used, the last drug given may be the cause of the hypersensitivity and skin eruptions. The usual skin reaction is a rash, which may take several hours or a day to appear, and urticaria (hives), which usually takes a few minutes to appear. Certain drugs, such as penicillin, are known to cause hypersensitivity.

Other drug-induced dermatitides include discoid lupus erythematosus and exfoliative dermatitis. Hydralazine hydrochloride (e.g., isoniazid, phenothiazines, anticonvulsants, and antidysrhythmics such as procainamide) may cause lupus-like symptoms. If lupus symptoms occur, the drug should be discontinued. Certain antibacterials and anticonvulsants may cause exfoliative dermatitis, resulting in erythema of the skin, itching, desquamation of large areas of the skin, and loss of body hair (e.g., sulfa antibiotics are one cause of toxic epidermal necrolysis).

CONTACT DERMATITIS

Contact dermatitis is a common form of eczema that results when skin is exposed to irritants (irritant contact dermatitis) or allergens (allergic contact dermatitis). Frequent contact with water (hand washing) can cause irritant contact dermatitis that usually starts with dry, cracked hands that sometimes develop pruritus and bleeding. Lips can also develop irritant contact dermatitis due to continuous licking of the lips. Other irritants include bleach, pepper spray, foods, and soap.

Allergic contact dermatitis is due to exposure to allergens. Examples of such allergens include poison ivy, sumac, and oak; nickel; makeup; jewelry; and latex gloves. Allergic contact dermatitis is considered a delayed hypersensitivity reaction. It may take hours to weeks for skin to develop manifestations, especially if it is a first-time exposure. Manifestations include skin rash with pruritus, swelling, burning, stinging, blistering, oozing, or scaling at the affected skin sites.

Nonpharmacologic treatments include avoiding direct contact with the causative irritant or allergen. Protective gloves or clothing may be necessary if the chemical is associated with work; skin that has been in contact with the irritant should be immediately cleansed and dried. Skin moisturizers, antihistamines (e.g., diphenhydramine), and/or topical corticosteroids may be used, depending on the severity of the dermatitis. Oatmeal baths can also relieve discomfort. Patch testing may be needed to determine the causal factor. Treatment may consist of wet dressings containing Burow's solution (aluminum acetate); lotions that contain zinc oxide, such as calamine; calcium hydroxide solution; and glycerin. Calamine lotion is primarily used for plant irritations. If itching persists, an oral antihistamine (e.g., diphenhydramine) may be used. Topical antipruritics should not be applied to open wounds or mucous membranes (e.g., eyes, mouth, or genital area). Other antipruritic treatments include baths of oatmeal and applications of corticosteroid ointments, creams, or gels.

Topical corticosteroids can alleviate dermatitis but can be systemically absorbed into the circulation. The amount and rate of absorption depend on the vehicle (cream, lotion, or ointment), drug concentration, drug composition, and skin area to which the steroid is applied. Absorption is greater where the skin is more permeable, such as the face, scalp, eyelids, neck, axilla, and genital area. Side effects and adverse reactions may occur with prolonged use of the topical drug or if the drug is continuously covered with a dressing. Prolonged use of a topical steroid can cause thinning of the skin with atrophy of the epidermis and dermis and purpura from small-vessel eruptions; therefore prolonged use is discouraged.

IMPETIGO

Impetigo, an infection of the skin that is usually due to *Streptococcus* or *Staphylococcus* species, is most commonly seen in children 2 to 5 years old. Topical therapies are used in the treatment of mild and moderate infection, and oral drugs are used for severe infection. The two drugs of choice are mupirocin and retapamulin. The lesions should be soaked to facilitate the removal of crusts, and the topical antibiotic should be applied at the base of the lesion. With multiple lesions and ineffective topical therapy, oral antibiotics are needed.

ROSACEA

Rosacea is a common skin disorder, presented usually with rashes. Other signs and symptoms can include flushing, visible blood vessels, swelling, and acne-like breakouts. Other people may present with thick skin and course texture. Treatments for rosacea are geared toward avoiding triggers that exacerbate rosacea, limiting UV exposures with the use of a broad-spectrum sunblock, and using mild skin products. For rosacea with acne-like breakouts, azelaic acid, metronidazole, sodium sulfacetamide/sulfur, and retinoid may be used. Other treatments include antibacterials such as tetracycline and isotretinoin.

HAIR LOSS AND BALDNESS

Hair loss, or alopecia, occurs when the hair shaft is lost and the hair follicle cannot regenerate. Permanent hair loss is associated with a familial history and occurs during the aging process, earlier in some individuals than others. Also known to cause alopecia are some drugs, which include anticancer agents, sulfonamides, anticonvulsants, aminoglycosides, and some nonsteroidal antiinflammatory drugs (NSAIDs) such as indomethacin. Severe febrile illnesses, pregnancy, myxedema (a condition resulting from hypothyroidism), and cancer therapies are some of the health conditions that contribute to temporary hair loss.

Minoxidil solution has been approved by the FDA for treating hair loss in men and women. A 5% solution is approved for men, 2% for women. The exact mechanism of action to stimulate hair growth is not known. Hair regrowth is usually seen after several months of use, but a few months after discontinuation, hair loss resumes. Minoxidil is available OTC in the form of a solution or foam. Systemic absorption of minoxidil is minimal, so adverse reactions seldom occur. Occasionally, headaches and a slight decrease in systolic blood pressure occur.

Finasteride (1 mg) is an oral drug used for alopecia in males. For growing hair, finasteride is effective in 50% of men. It has been reported that it is relatively ineffective in growing hair in older men, even with an increased dose. Like minoxidil, clinical response is not seen until the drug has been used daily for 3 months or longer; discontinuing the drug leads to hair loss within 12 months. Finasteride is contraindicated in pregnancy and pregnant women should not handle the drug. Side effects include decreased libido, impotence, and ejaculation disorder.

SUNSCREENS

Sunscreens are primarily used to block UV rays that cause sunburn, but they also protect against certain types of keratosis, skin cancer, premature aging, cold sores and fever blisters, and UV photosensitivity reactions. There are two types of sunscreens: chemical blockers and physical blockers. *Chemical blockers* (e.g., oxybenzone and ecamsule) absorb UV radiation and are effective against UVA radiation, and *physical blockers* (e.g., titanium dioxide and zinc oxide) reflect or scatter UV radiation and are effective against both UVA and UVB radiation. UVB radiation is the primary cause of sunburn and skin cancer, whereas

TABLE 48.4 Degree and Tissue Depth of Burns

Type	Degree	Depth	Characteristics
Superficial epidermal	First	Outer layer of skin; epidermis (e.g., sunburn without blisters)	Erythema, edema, pain
Partial or full-thickness superficial	Second	Epidermis, upper layers of dermis; blisters may be present	Partial: Wound is pink and blanches; erythema is present and burn is painful and wet appearing. Full: Blanching is sluggish or absent; burn is red/white and dry in appearance; pain may be present but will be diminished.
Full-thickness	Third	All layers extending into the subcutaneous tissues	Skin can appear black or white and dry and is leathery in texture; area will not blanch, and no pain is experienced.

TABLE 48.5 Topical Antiinfectives: Burns

Generic (Brand)	Route and Dosage	Uses and Considerations
Mafenide acetate	See Prototype Drug Chart: Mafenide Acetate	
Silver sulfadiazine	A: 1% Cream: Apply twice daily to a thickness of 1.6 mm	To prevent and treat infection of second- and third-degree burns. Ten percent of drug is absorbed. Excessive use or extensive application area may cause sulfa crystals (crystalluria).

A, Adult; *mm*, millimeter.

UVA is responsible for loss of elasticity (wrinkling) and collagen damage of the skin. UVA radiation also contributes to skin cancer and penetrates the skin at a deeper level than UVB, thereby causing damage to deeper skin structures. Broad-spectrum sunscreen protects from both UVA and UVB radiation. The FDA passed a ruling that sunscreen with a sun protection factor (SPF) of less than 15 can denote that it prevents sunburn, and an SPF of 15 and above can reduce the risk of skin cancer and early skin aging if used as directed with other sun-protection measures such as wearing sun-blocking clothing, limiting sun exposure between 10 a.m. and 2 p.m., and reapplying sunscreen at least every 2 hours. The American Academy of Dermatology recommends water-resistant sunscreen with an SPF 30 or higher. Sunscreen with an SPF 30 blocks 97% of UVB rays. Common side effects of sunscreens include cutaneous reactions (e.g., erythema, pruritus, folliculitis, contact dermatitis, and acne vulgaris).

BURNS AND BURN PREPARATIONS

Burns from heat (*thermal burns,* the most common kind of burn injury), electricity (*electrical burns*), and chemical agents (*chemical burns*) can all cause skin lesions. Burns are classified according to degree and depth of the tissue injury (Table 48.4). Burns need immediate attention, regardless of the degree and depth of tissue injury. For minor burns, a cool, wet compress is applied to prevent further tissue damage caused by heat. After the affected area is cooled off, it should be cleansed gently with soap and water; intact blisters should not be opened. After cleaning the area, apply a thin layer of ointment, such as aloe vera or petroleum jelly. A thin layer of antibiotic ointment (e.g., bacitracin, neomycin sulfate, polymyxin B sulfate) can be applied to affected areas one to three times daily if the area becomes infected.

Persons with burns that involve the dermis and subcutaneous tissue should seek medical help immediately at a health care facility.

Persons with extensive second-degree burns and beyond are at risk of dehydration through interstitial fluid loss and are vulnerable to infection and sepsis. Dehydration can cause hypovolemic shock. Primary attention should be to the airway, breathing, and circulation (ABC). Intravenous (IV) fluid therapy should be started immediately, and an analgesic is given for pain. For extensive burns, the amount of fluids should be determined by calculating the percentage of the person's body surface area that was burned. The most common formulation to determine the degree of injury is the Wallace Rule of Nines. The Parkland formula can help determine the amount of fluid needed in the first 24 hours for persons with critical burn injury. Burn areas are kept clean, and any necrotic tissue is debrided. Broad-spectrum topical antiinfectives effective against many gram-positive and gram-negative organisms and fungi are applied to burn areas to prevent infection. Examples of these antiinfectives include mafenide acetate, silver sulfadiazine, and silver nitrate 0.5% solution. Table 48.5 lists selected topical medications for burns along with their dosages, uses, and considerations. Prototype Drug Chart: Mafenide Acetate lists the pharmacologic data for the antibacterial drug mafenide acetate.

Silver Sulfadiazine

Silver sulfadiazine is a common antiinfective used to prevent and treat infections in second- and third-degree burns and it is not absorbed through the skin. It is applied at least twice daily. Silver sulfadiazine possesses activity against both gram-negative and gram-positive organisms and fungi. Unlike mafenide, it is not a carbonic anhydrase inhibitor. Sulfadiazine is metabolized by the liver and is excreted in the urine. It is contraindicated in near-term pregnancy and among neonates and infants younger than 2 months. Side effects and adverse reactions may include photosensitivity, skin discoloration, burning sensation, rashes, erythema multiforme, skin necrosis, and leukopenia.

PROTOTYPE DRUG CHART

Mafenide Acetate

Drug Class	Dosage
Topical antiinfective	A: Cream: Apply a layer of 1.6 mm thickness evenly to the affected area once or twice daily; reapply PRN. Be sure burn is covered with cream at all times. A: Sol: Apply to dressing-covered graft site every 4 h or as needed to maintain wet dressing.

Contraindications	Drug-Lab-Food Interactions
Hypersensitivity, inhalation injury *Caution:* Renal failure, acid-base imbalance, or hypersensitivity to other sulfonamides/sulfites	No significant drug interactions; caution when using other carbonic anhydrase inhibitors due to increased risk of metabolic acidosis.

Pharmacokinetics	Pharmacodynamics
Absorption: Diffuses through devascularized areas with variable systemic absorption Distribution: PB: UK Metabolism: t½: UK Excretion: In urine	Onset: On contact Peak: 2 h Duration: 4 h

Therapeutic Effects/Uses

Synthetic sulfonamide antibiotics are indicated as an adjunctive treatment for second- and third-degree burns and it is not absorbed through the skin, to prevent organism invasion of burned tissue areas, and to treat burn infections.

Mechanism of Action: Bacteriostatic activity against many gram-negative and gram-positive bacteria, including *Pseudomonas aeruginosa* and other anaerobic strains.

Side Effects	Adverse Reactions
Rash, burning sensation, urticaria, pruritus, swelling, erythema	Metabolic acidosis, respiratory alkalosis, blistering, superinfection (e.g., fungal) *Life-threatening:* Bone marrow suppression, fatal hemolytic anemia

A, Adult; *h,* hour; *mm,* millimeter; *mo,* month; *PB,* protein binding; *PRN,* as needed; *sol,* solution; *t½,* half-life; *UK,* unknown; *>,* greater than; *≥,* greater than or equal to.

CLINICAL JUDGMENT [NURSING PROCESS]

Topical Antiinfectives: Burns

Concept: Tissue Integrity
- The ability of the body tissue to repair itself

Recognize Cues [Assessment]
- Determine the stability of the patient by assessing airway, breathing, and circulation.
- Determine fluid status. Report signs and symptoms of hypovolemia or hypervolemia.
- Check the patient's vital signs. Report abnormal findings, such as elevated temperature.
- Assess burned tissue for signs of infection such as foul odor, purulent drainage, erythema, and heat.
- Culture the purulent wound.

Analyze Cues and Prioritize Hypothesis [Patient Problems]
- Decreased potential for fluid volume and potential for imbalanced perfusion
- Potential for infection
- Acute pain related to thermal injury
- Deficient knowledge related to management of burns

Generate Solutions [Planning]
- The patient will remain hemodynamically stable.
- The patient will remain free from infection.
- The patient will report decreased or tolerable pain level.
- The patient will remain hydrated.

Take Action [Nursing Interventions]
- Monitor the patient for any cardiopulmonary difficulties, vital signs, or infection.
- Administer prescribed analgesia before treatment, if needed.
- Cleanse burned tissue sites using aseptic technique.
- Apply topical antibacterial drugs and dressings with sterile technique.
- Maintain the patient's fluid balance and renal function.
- Monitor the patient for side effects and adverse reactions to topical drugs.
- Closely monitor the patient's acid-base balance, especially in the presence of pulmonary or renal dysfunction.
- Store drugs in a dry place at room temperature.

Patient Teaching
- Instruct the patient and family about pain management, medications used to treat burns, and signs of complications from burns, such as fluid excess or deficit.
- Teach the patient and family how to apply a topical agent and dressings to burned areas.
- Teach the patient and family about signs and symptoms of infection and to report them promptly to the health care provider.

Evaluate Outcomes [Evaluation]
- Evaluate patient's cardiopulmonary status, ensuring breathing and circulation is stable.
- Evaluate patient and family knowledge of burn management.
- Evaluate the effectiveness of treatment interventions to burned tissue areas by determining whether healing is proceeding and sites are free from infection.

CRITICAL THINKING CASE STUDY

A 15-year-old female patient complains about blackheads and large, raised acne with surrounding erythema on her face. She seeks help from a health care provider.

1. To assist in identifying her skin problem, what would the health history and assessment include?

2. Which nonpharmacologic measures might the nurse discuss with the patient in caring for her skin condition?

The patient's skin disorder does not improve. Her health care provider says she has acne vulgaris and has prescribed benzoyl peroxide and oral tetracycline.

3. The patient asks the nurse how to use benzoyl peroxide. What would the explanation of the method and frequency for use of benzoyl peroxide include?

4. What would be included in the patient teaching related to the use of oral tetracycline?

5. What other drugs for acne might the patient use? Explain their uses and side effects.

6. The patient asks if she will have to remain on benzoyl peroxide and oral tetracycline for the rest of her life. What is the nurse's best response or course of action? Explain your answer.

REVIEW QUESTIONS

1. A patient being seen for skin concerns asks, "What do keratolytic drugs remove?" Which response would be best by the nurse?
   a. A horny layer of dermis
   b. A horny layer of epidermis
   c. Erythematous lesions
   d. Hair follicles

2. A patient is to begin therapy with isotretinoin and asks, "What do I have to remember to do while taking this medicine?" How would the nurse respond? (Select all that apply.)
   a. Avoid sunlight.
   b. Monitor your weight.
   c. Keep appointments for laboratory tests.
   d. Use two forms of contraceptives.
   e. Always take the drug with food.

3. The nurse is doing health teaching with a patient who has psoriasis. Which nursing implication is a priority for a patient on infliximab to treat psoriasis?
   a. Monitor weight daily.
   b. Monitor electrolytes.
   c. Monitor urine output.
   d. Monitor complete blood count.

4. A 55-year-old patient is concerned about hair loss. The nurse expects that the patient's baldness may be treated with which drug?
   a. Dexamethasone
   b. Para-aminobenzoic acid
   c. Mupirocin
   d. Finasteride

5. The nurse reviews the patient's medication history. Based on the patient's prolonged use of topical corticosteroids, which assessment will the nurse include? (Select all that apply.)
   a. Weight gain
   b. Thinning of the skin
   c. Erythematous lesions
   d. Purpura
   e. Urinary retention

6. A 20-year-old female comes to the clinic for follow-up related to isotretinoin use. Which information from the iPLEDGE program would the nurse provide to the patient? (Select all that apply.)
   a. One method of contraception must be used throughout treatment.
   b. A review of iPLEDGE educational materials.
   c. A negative pregnancy test is required before each monthly refill.
   d. Informed consent is not required.
   e. A prescription for a 60-day supply of drug is to be given.

7. The school nurse prepares a program for junior high school students on sun safety. Which information would the nurse include? (Select all that apply.)
   a. Sunscreen products should contain information about ultraviolet A and B sun protection that includes the sun protection factor.
   b. Ultraviolet B radiation is greatest between 10 a.m. and 2 p.m.
   c. Clouds block radiation, so sunscreen is not needed on cloudy days.
   d. The sun protection factor (SPF) should be at least 30 in sunscreen products.
   e. Sunscreen is to be applied once daily.

8. A patient is receiving etanercept. Which nursing intervention is appropriate for this patient? (Select all that apply.)
   a. Drug is administered topically.
   b. Tuberculin test is required before the start of therapy.
   c. Monitor for injection site reaction.
   d. Monitor for seizures.
   e. Monitor for heart failure.

9. The nurse is teaching the patient about clobetasol. Which information would to be included in the teaching session? (Select all that apply.)
   a. Appropriate treatment is for 6 months' duration.
   b. It can be applied as a lotion to all body parts.
   c. Clobetasol is a super-high-potency corticosteroid.
   d. Maximum dose is 50 g/week.
   e. Occlusive dressing speeds healing.

49

Pituitary, Thyroid, Parathyroid, and Adrenal Disorders

http://evolve.elsevier.com/McCuistion/pharmacology

OBJECTIVES

- Differentiate the actions and uses of the hormones from the pituitary, thyroid, parathyroid, and adrenal glands: thyroxine (T_4), triiodothyronine (T_3), calcitonin, parathyroid hormone (PTH), mineralocorticoids, and glucocorticoids.
- Differentiate the side effects of thyroxine (T_4) and triiodothyronine (T_3).

- Apply the Clinical Judgment [Nursing Process], including patient teaching, for drug therapy related to hormonal replacement or hormonal inhibition for the pituitary, thyroid, parathyroid, and adrenal glands.

OUTLINE

This chapter describes drugs used for hormonal replacement and for inhibition of hormonal secretion from the pituitary, thyroid, parathyroid, and adrenal glands. Before reading this chapter, review the endocrine glands and their associated hormones. Knowledge of the various endocrine glands and their respective hormones and functions facilitates an understanding of the drugs that act on the endocrine glands.

PITUITARY GLAND

Anterior Lobe

The pituitary gland, or hypophysis, has an anterior lobe and a posterior lobe (Fig. 49.1). The anterior pituitary gland, called the adenohypophysis, secretes hormones that target glands and tissues, including:
- Growth hormone (GH), which stimulates growth in tissue and bone
- Thyroid-stimulating hormone (TSH), which acts on the thyroid gland
- Adrenocorticotropic hormone (ACTH), which stimulates the adrenal gland

- Gonadotropins (follicle-stimulating hormone [FSH] and luteinizing hormone [LH]), which affect the ovaries and testes
- Prolactin (PRL), which primarily affects the breast tissues

The amount of each hormone secreted from the anterior pituitary gland is regulated by a negative feedback system. If excess hormone is secreted from the target gland, hormonal release from the anterior pituitary gland is suppressed. If there is a lack of hormone secretion from the target gland, there will be an increase in that particular anterior pituitary hormone (Fig. 49.2). Drugs with adenohypophyseal properties used to stimulate or inhibit glandular activity for GH, TSH, ACTH, and PRL are discussed according to their therapeutic use.

Growth Hormone

Two hypothalamic hormones regulate GH: (1) GH-releasing hormone (GH-RH; somatropin) and (2) GH-inhibiting hormone (GH-IH; somatostatin). GH does not have a specific target gland. It affects body tissues and bone; GH replacement stimulates linear growth when there are GH deficiencies. GH drugs cannot be given orally because they are

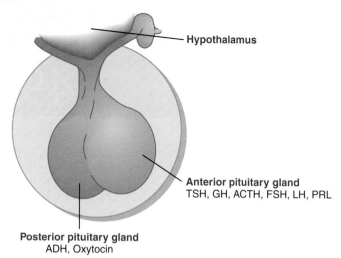

Fig. 49.1 The anterior and posterior pituitary glands. *ACTH,* Adrenocorticotropic hormone; *ADH,* antidiuretic hormone; *FSH,* follicle-stimulating hormone; *GH,* growth hormone; *LH,* luteinizing hormone; *PRL,* prolactin; *TSH,* thyroid-stimulating hormone.

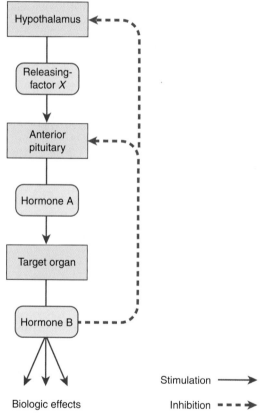

Fig. 49.2 Negative feedback loop of hypothalamus and pituitary. (From Burcham, J., & Rosenthal, L. [2016]. *Lehne's pharmacology for nursing care* [9th ed.]. St. Louis: Elsevier.)

inactivated by gastrointestinal (GI) enzymes. Subcutaneous (subcut) or intramuscular (IM) administration of GH is necessary.

If a child's height is well below the standard for a specified age, GH deficiency may be the cause, and dwarfism can result. Because of the cost, tests are performed to determine whether GH replacement therapy is essential. GH stimulation test (GHST) with insulin tolerance test (ITT) is labor intensive and can cause severe hypoglycemia. Macimorelin is a GH secretagogue and, after an oral dose, can measure the stimulated GH levels.

Because GH acts on newly forming bone, it must be administered before the epiphyses are fused. Administration of GH over several years can increase height by a foot. However, prolonged GH therapy can antagonize insulin secretion, eventually causing diabetes mellitus. Athletes should be advised not to take GH to build muscle and physique because of its effects on blood glucose along with other serious side effects. Table 49.1 lists the drugs used to replace or inhibit GH and gives their dosages, uses, and considerations.

Drug Therapy: Growth Hormone Deficiency. Somatropin is a GH used to treat growth failure in children because of GH deficiency. Somatropin is a product that has an identical amino acid sequence as human GH (hGH); it is contraindicated in pediatric patients who have growth deficiency due to Prader-Willi syndrome, in those who are severely obese, or in those who have severe respiratory impairment because fatalities associated with GH can occur. A second hGH, somapacitan, was recently approved by the FDA for adults with GH deficiency. GH products not approved by the FDA are being consumed among healthy adults to decrease signs of aging, such as lean muscle mass and increased body fat. Even though hGH increases muscle mass, it does not translate to improved strength. Furthermore, research indicates that these persons are at risk for complications, such as type 2 diabetes, fluid retention, gynecomastia, and certain cancers. Corticosteroids can inhibit the effects of somatropin; therefore they should not be taken concurrently. Somatropin can enhance the effects of antidiabetics and can cause hypoglycemia.

Side effects and adverse effects. Somatropin can cause paresthesia, arthralgia, myalgia, peripheral edema, weakness, and cephalgia. Metabolic complications include glucose fluctuations, hypothyroidism, and hematuria. Flulike symptoms and hyperpigmentation of the skin can also occur. Adverse reactions include seizures, intracranial hypertension, and secondary malignancy (e.g., leukemia).

Drug Therapy: Growth Hormone Excess. Gigantism, excessive growth during childhood, and acromegaly, excessive growth after puberty, can occur with GH hypersecretion; these are frequently caused by a pituitary tumor. If the tumor cannot be destroyed by radiation, GH receptor antagonists (e.g., pegvisomant), somatostatin analogues (e.g., lanreotide, octreotide), and dopamine agonists (e.g., bromocriptine) act by either blocking GH receptor sites or by inhibiting secretion of GH.

Pegvisomant blocks GH receptor sites, preventing abnormal growth by normalizing insulin-like growth factor 1 (IGF-1) level, and it is given by injection. Common side effects include hyperhidrosis, cephalgia, and fatigue. Adverse effects include chest pain, hypertension, and elevated hepatic transaminases.

Lanreotide is an analogue of somatostatin that has actions similar to those of endogenous somatostatin. The effects of reduced GH are dose related and have a duration of at least 28 days after a single injection; therefore injections are given every 4 weeks. Lanreotide is available in depot formulation and is administered deep in the subcutaneous layer. Common side effects include mild GI symptoms: diarrhea, abdominal pain, nausea, vomiting, constipation, weight loss, and flatulence.

Octreotide is a synthetic somatostatin-inhibiting secretion of GH. It is available in immediate-release and depot formulations. Immediate-release formulations are given by thrice-daily subcutaneous injection, and depot injection is administered once monthly. Common side effects include GI upsets such as nausea, bloating, and flatus. Adverse effects include cardiac toxicity, such as bradycardia and arrhythmia.

Bromocriptine, a dopamine agonist, inhibits the secretion of GH caused by pituitary adenomas. It is available in oral form and has fewer side effects than other treatments for hyperpituitarism, which include GI symptoms (e.g., nausea, anorexia, dyspepsia, and xerostomia). Adverse effects include cardiac toxicity (e.g., hypertension, myocardial infarction [MI], and angina) and cerebrovascular toxicity (e.g., stroke and seizure). Bromocriptine should be discontinued if hypertension occurs due to pregnancy (e.g., preeclampsia, eclampsia, or pregnancy-induced hypertension).

Thyroid-Stimulating Hormone

The adenohypophysis secretes thyroid-stimulating hormone (TSH) in response to thyroid-releasing hormone (TRH) from the hypothalamus. TSH stimulates the thyroid gland to release thyroxine (T_4) and triiodothyronine (T_3, or liothyronine). Excess TSH secretion can cause hyperthyroidism, and a TSH deficit can cause hypothyroidism. Hypothyroidism may be caused by a thyroid gland disorder (primary cause) or a decrease in TSH secretion (secondary cause). Thyrotropin, a purified extract of TSH for thyroid cancer, is used as a diagnostic agent to differentiate between primary and secondary hypothyroidism. Side effects caused by thyrotropin include symptoms of hyperthyroidism. Other side effects include urticaria, rash, pruritus, and flushing.

Table 49.1 lists the drug used to replace TSH and its dosages, uses, and considerations.

TABLE 49.1 Drug Therapies for Pituitary Disorders

Generic	Route and Dosage	Uses and Considerations
ANTERIOR LOBE		
Growth Hormone (GH-RH)		
Somapacitan	A: Subcut: Initial dose 1.5 mg; then increase q2–4 weeks by 0.5–1.5 mg until desired response; not to exceed 8 mg q week.	For GH deficiency in adults. Contraindicated in persons with active malignancy, diabetic eye disease, acute critical illness, including respiratory failure. PB: >99%; t½: 2–3 d
Somatropin	C: Subcut/IM: Dosing is based on brand names and is individualized for each patient; review the clinician's orders carefully.	For GH deficiency for adults and growth failure in children. Contraindicated in children with epiphyseal closure, patients with active neoplastic disease, and those with acute critical illness. Do not administer intravenously. Therapy is discontinued when final height is achieved if given for growth failure. Read clinician's orders carefully for the trade name; dosing is *not* interchangeable. PB: 20%; t½: 20–30 min
Growth Hormone Suppressant Drugs		
Bromocriptine mesylate	Acromegaly: A: PO: 1.25–2.5 mg/d at bedtime for 3 d; *maint:* 20–30 mg/d in divided doses; *max:* 100 mg/d Prolactinemia/pituitary adenoma: A/C ≥16 y: PO: 1.25–2.5 mg/d; titrate dose at 2–7 d intervals as needed; *max:* 30 mg/d C 11–15 y: PO: 1.25–2.5 mg/d, may titrate to 10 mg/d	For acromegaly, pituitary adenoma, and hyperprolactinemia. Also used with pituitary radiation or surgery to decrease GH levels. Decreases lactation and prolactinemia. Take with food. PB: >90%; t½: 3 h
Lanreotide acetate	Acromegaly: A: Subcut: Initially 90 mg q4wk for 3 mo, then adjust dose based on GH, IGF-1, and clinical symptoms q4wk NET: A: Subcut: 120 mg q4wk	For acromegaly and NET. PB: 79%–83%; t½: 23–30 d
Octreotide acetate	A: Subcut: 50–200 mcg tid A: IM: 20 mg q4wk for 3 mo, then adjust according to serum GH and IGF-1 levels	For acromegaly. Injectable depot suspension is for IM use only. PB: 65%; t½: 1.7 h
Pegvisomant	A: Subcut: Give a 40-mg loading dose, then 10 mg/d; adjust in increments of 5 mg; *max:* 30 mg/d	For acromegaly. IGF-1 concentrations should be measured q4–6wk. PB: UK; t½: 6 d
Thyroid-Stimulating Hormone (TSH)		
Thyrotropin	Thyroid cancer: A: IM: 0.9 mg into gluteus maximus, repeat in 24 h for 2 doses; *max:* 0.9 mg/d	For thyroid cancer. Radioiodine study follows last injection. PB: UK; t½: 15–35 h
Adrenocorticotropic Hormone (ACTH)		
Corticotropin	Immunosuppressant: A: IM/subcut: 40–80 units q24–72h Do *not* discontinue abruptly; dose must be tapered. ACTH deficiency diagnosis: A: IM/subcut: Up to 80 units MS exacerbations: A: IM/subcut: 80–120 units/d in divided doses for 2–3 wk	For ACTH deficiency diagnostic, MS, and infantile spasms. Administer only to patients with adrenal responsiveness. Repository gel must be room temperature before administration. Do not overpressurize vial during withdrawal. PB: UK: t½: 15 min
Cosyntropin	A: IM/IV: 0.25 mg over 2 min or slow infusion over 6 h	For diagnostic testing to differentiate between pituitary and adrenal cause of adrenal insufficiency. Obtain plasma cortisol level before and 30–60 min after administration. PB: UK; t½: 7 min

Continued

TABLE 49.1   Drug Therapies for Pituitary Disorders—cont'd

Generic	Route and Dosage	Uses and Considerations
POSTERIOR LOBE		

Antidiuretic Hormone (ADH)

Generic	Route and Dosage	Uses and Considerations
Desmopressin acetate	DI: A: PO: Initial dose 0.05 mg bid, then titrate to response. A: IN: Initial dose is 10 mcg in the evening, then titrate to response. A: IV/subcut: 2–4 mcg/d given in 2 divided doses daily Hemophilia A or von Willebrand disease: A: IN: One spray in 1–2 nostrils based on weight for 1–2 doses. A: IV/subcut: 0.3 mcg/kg/dose, then titrate to response.	For DI, hemophilia A, and von Willebrand disease. Desmopressin can have a long duration of action (5–21 h). PB: UK; t½: 1.5–2.5 h
Vasopressin	A: IM/subcut: 5–10 units q3–4h or 2–3 × daily PRN	For central DI. Can also be given intranasally. Aspirate IM injections; avoid injection into a blood vessel. PB: none; t½: 10–20 min
Demeclocycline	A: PO: 600–1200 mg/d in 3–4 divided doses	For off-label treatment of SIADH. PB: 65%–90%; t½: 10–17 h, increases to 42–68 h in patients with severe renal impairment
Conivaptan	A: IV: LD 20 mg over 30 min; *maint:* 20 mg continuous IV over 24 h; then 20 mg/d for 1–3 d; may titrate up to 40 mg/d; *max:* 4 d of therapy	For symptomatic euvolemic hyponatremia associated with SIADH. PB: 99%; t½: 5–8 h
Tolvaptan	A: PO: Initially 15 mg/d, then 15–30 mg/d; *max:* 60 mg/d for up to 30 d; adjust dose in 24-h increment.	For symptomatic hypervolemic or euvolemic hyponatremia. Avoid fluid restriction during the first 24 h of therapy. PB: 99%; t½: 12 h

A, Adult; *bid,* twice daily; *C,* child; *d,* day; *DI,* diabetes insipidus; *GH,* growth hormone; *h,* hour; *IGF,* insulin-like growth factor; *IN,* intranasal; *h,* hour; *IM,* intramuscular; *IN,* intranasal; *IV,* intravenous; *LD,* loading dose; *maint,* maintenance; *max,* maximum dosage; *min,* minute; *mo,* month; *MS,* multiple sclerosis; *NET,* neuroendocrine tumor; *q,* every; *PB,* protein binding; *PO,* by mouth; *PRN,* as needed; *SIADH,* syndrome of inappropriate diuretic hormone; *subcut,* subcutaneous; *t½,* half-life; *tid,* three times daily; *UK,* unknown; *wk,* week; *y,* year; *>,* greater than; *<,* less than; *≥,* greater than or equal to; *≤,* less than or equal to.

Adrenocorticotropic Hormone

The hypothalamus releases corticotropin-releasing factor (CRF), which stimulates the pituitary corticotrophs to secrete adreno-corticotropic hormone (ACTH), which stimulates the release of glucocorticoids (cortisol), mineralocorticoids (aldosterone), and androgen from the adrenal cortex and catecholamines (epinephrine and norepinephrine) from the adrenal medulla. Usually, ACTH and cortisol secretions follow a diurnal rhythm, in which the ACTH and cortisol secretion is higher in the early morning and then decreases throughout the day. Stresses such as surgery, sepsis, and trauma override the diurnal rhythm, causing an increase in secretions of ACTH and cortisol. Hypocortisolism, or adrenal insufficiency, can occur and may be due to inadequate secretion of ACTH or dysfunction of the adrenal glands. Cosyntropin (synthetic ACTH) or corticotropin (exogenous ACTH) is administered to establish the endocrine gland responsible for the inadequate serum cortisol. Table 49.1 lists the drugs used to replace ACTH and their dosages, uses, and considerations.

Cosyntropin, a synthetic ACTH, is only approved for diagnostic purposes and is less potent and less allergenic than corticotropin. Cosyntropin stimulates the production and release of cortisol, corticosterone, and androgens from the adrenal cortex. It is administered via IM or intravenous (IV) routes. Plasma cortisol concentrations should be measured just before (basal) and 30 to 60 minutes after administration; normal response is the doubling of the basal cortisol level. Caution is advised when administering cosyntropin in patients receiving diuretics; cosyntropin can increase electrolyte loss. Patients taking estrogens can have an abnormal decreased response to the ACTH stimulation test. Side

effects and adverse effects include bradycardia, hypertension, sinus tachycardia, and peripheral edema.

The ACTH drug corticotropin is primarily used to diagnose adrenal gland disorders, treat multiple sclerosis (MS), and treat infantile spasms; it is rarely used for corticosteroid-responsive disorders. Corticotropin is available as repository corticotropin injection (RCI), which is administered via IM or subcut routes. RCI controls the synthesis of ACTH from cholesterol, which stimulates adrenal glands in releasing its hormones. The effects of RCI are primarily due to the glucocorticoid from the adrenal cortex. RCI decreases the symptoms of MS during its exacerbation phase. ⚡ The drug should be tapered over a 2-week period for infantile spasms to avoid adrenal insufficiency. Corticotropin has numerous drug interactions. Diuretics and anti-*Pseudomonas* penicillins, such as piperacillin, can decrease the serum potassium level (hypokalemia). If the patient is taking a digitalis preparation and hypokalemia is present, digitalis toxicity can result. Phenytoin, rifampin, and barbiturates increase the metabolic rate, which can decrease the effect of the ACTH drug. Persons with diabetes may need increased insulin and oral antidiabetic (hypoglycemic) drugs because ACTH stimulates cortisol secretion, which increases the blood glucose level.

Side Effects and Adverse Effects. Side effects and adverse reactions are due to the activity of the adrenal glands and their hormones. See Table 49.2 for the physiologic data for hypoadrenalism and hyperadrenalism.

Prolactin

The primary function of prolactin (PRL) is stimulation of breast tissue for milk production. PRL deficiency (*hypoprolactinemia*) is generally without symptoms except during breastfeeding, when it

TABLE 49.2	Physiologic Effects: Adrenal Hyposecretion and Hypersecretion	
Body System	**Adrenal Hyposecretion (Addison Disease)**	**Adrenal Hypersecretion (Cushing Syndrome)**
Metabolism: Glucose Protein Fat	Hypoglycemia, muscle weakness, weight loss	Hyperglycemia, muscle wasting; thinning of skin; poor wound healing; osteoporosis; fat accumulation in face (moon face), back of neck (buffalo hump), and trunk (protruding abdomen); hyperlipidemia; high cholesterol; weight gain
Central nervous system	Apathy, depression, fatigue, irritability	Increased neural activity, mood elevation, irritability, seizures, weakness, fatigue
Integument	Hyperpigmentation	Easy bruising, striae, plethora, and excess hair growth to face (hirsutism), neck, chest, abdomen, and thighs
Eyes	None	Cataract formation
Cardiovascular	Tachycardia, hypotension, orthostatic hypotension, cardiovascular collapse, syncope, dizziness	Hypertension, edema, heart failure
Gastrointestinal	Nausea, vomiting, diarrhea, abdominal pain, anorexia	Peptic ulcers
Hematology	Anemia	Increased red blood cell count and neutrophils, impaired clotting
Reproductive	Irregular menses or amenorrhea	Amenorrhea, decreased fertility and libido
Fluids and electrolytes	Hypovolemia, hyponatremia, hyperkalemia	Hypervolemia, hypernatremia, hypokalemia

can cause lactation disruption. Excess PRL (*hyperprolactinemia*) produces symptoms in both males and females. Males may develop excess breast tissue (*gynecomastia*) and may lactate (*galactorrhea*), and excess PRL decreases sperm production. Females with excess PRL can experience lactation that is not pregnancy related, or they can develop amenorrhea. Excess PRL can be treated with dopamine agonists (e.g., bromocriptine, cabergoline). Cabergoline is better tolerated, has a longer half-life, and offers more convenient dosing than bromocriptine. Dopamine agonists are discussed in Chapter 20.

Posterior Lobe

The posterior pituitary gland, known as the neurohypophysis, secretes antidiuretic hormone (ADH) and oxytocin. ADH and oxytocin are produced by the hypothalamus and travel by way of the hypophysial portal system into the posterior pituitary gland for storage and secretion. (Oxytocin is discussed in Chapter 54.) Table 49.1 lists the drugs used to replace or inhibit ADH and their dosages, uses, and considerations.

ADH promotes water reabsorption from the renal tubules to maintain water balance in the body fluids. When there is a deficiency of ADH, large amounts of water are excreted by the kidneys. This condition, called diabetes insipidus (DI), can lead to severe fluid volume deficit and electrolyte imbalances. Head injury and brain tumors resulting in trauma to the hypothalamus and pituitary gland can cause DI. Fluid and electrolyte balances must be closely monitored in these patients, and ADH replacement may be needed. The ADH preparations vasopressin and desmopressin acetate can be administered intranasally or by injection. Desmopressin is also used in managing patients with bleeding disorders due to hemophilia A or von Willebrand disease type 1. Unlike vasopressin, desmopressin does not induce the release of ACTH, nor does it increase serum cortisol level. It is available as a nasal spray, as an oral tablet, and in parenteral formulations. ADH is contraindicated in patients with moderate to severe renal disease and in patients with hyponatremia or a history of such. Side effects and adverse reactions include hyponatremia, cephalgia, dyspepsia, diarrhea, nausea, and vomiting. Seizures may occur due to hyponatremia. Hypotension and tachycardia can occur due to hypovolemia.

When secretion of ADH from the posterior pituitary gland is excessive, the most common cause is small cell carcinoma of the lung. Medications, other malignancies, and stressors (e.g., pain, infection, anxiety, trauma) may also be causative factors. These conditions lead to an excessive amount of water retention expanding the intracellular and intravascular volume known as syndrome of inappropriate antidiuretic hormone (SIADH). This increased fluid volume causes enhanced glomerular filtration and decreased tubular sodium reabsorption. Natriuresis, excretion of urinary sodium, can occur and can cause hyponatremia. SIADH can be treated by fluid restrictions, by hypertonic saline, or by drugs such as demeclocycline, conivaptan, and tolvaptan.

Demeclocycline is a tetracycline antibiotic that can induce nephrogenic DI within 5 days of starting treatment that is reversed in 2 to 6 days after cessation of treatment. The most common complaint with demeclocycline is photosensitivity. As with other tetracyclines, dental discoloration and enamel hypoplasia can occur. Fluid and electrolytes must be monitored closely.

Vaptans (e.g., conivaptan and tolvaptan) are vasopressin receptor antagonists and are indicated for the treatment of euvolemic hyponatremia in SIADH. Their effects increase serum sodium and free water clearance. [!] Conivaptan is contraindicated in patients with corn allergy. Common complications with conivaptan therapy are injection site reactions such as phlebitis, pain, edema, and pruritus; therefore the drug must be administered only in large veins, and infusion sites should be rotated every 24 hours. Other common side effects and adverse reactions include orthostatic hypotension, syncope, hypertension, atrial fibrillation, and electrolyte imbalances.

Tolvaptan is given orally. It has black-box warnings for patients with alcoholism, hepatic disease, and malnutrition; tolvaptan should be avoided in these patients. Common side effects and adverse reactions are related to loss of fluids (e.g., thirst, dry mouth, constipation, hyperglycemia, dizziness, and weakness). Fluid and serum electrolytes must be closely monitored.

Vaptans are contraindicated in patients with hypovolemia. Fluid restrictions should be avoided during therapy to prevent sudden increase in serum sodium.

Table 49.1 lists the drugs used for pituitary disorders and their dosages, uses, and considerations.

◎ CLINICAL JUDGMENT [NURSING PROCESS]

Pituitary Hormones

Concept: Hormonal Regulation
- The ability of the body to maintain homeostasis by the regulation, secretion, and action of hormones associated with the endocrine system

Recognize Cues [Assessment]
- Obtain baseline vital signs for future comparison. Report abnormal results.
- Assess fluid, hydration, and electrolyte statuses. Report abnormal findings.
- Assess patient for an infectious process. Corticotropin can suppress signs and symptoms of infection.
- Note the patient's physical growth. If a child, compare growth with reported standards. Report findings.

Analyze Cues and Prioritize Hypothesis [Patient Problems]
- Hormonal imbalance related to the body's inability to regulate and secrete appropriate hormones
- Need for health teaching related to complex drug regimen

Generate Solutions [Planning]
- The patient will be free from any pituitary disorder with the appropriate drug regimen.
- The patient will understand the drug regimen.
- The patient will remain free of infection.

Take Action [Nursing Interventions]
Antidiuretic Hormone (ADH)
- Monitor vital signs. Increased heart rate and decreased systolic pressure can indicate fluid volume loss resulting from decreased ADH production. With less ADH secretion, more water is excreted, decreasing vascular fluid (hypovolemia).
- Record urinary output. Increased output can indicate fluid loss caused by a decrease in ADH.
- Obtain daily weight. A liter of fluid weighs approximately 2.2 pounds.

Growth Hormone (GH)
- Monitor blood glucose and electrolyte levels in patients receiving GH. Hyperglycemia can occur with high doses.

Repository Corticotropin
- Monitor the growth and development of a child receiving corticotropin.
- Observe the patient's weight. Check for edema if weight gain occurs. A side effect of repository corticotropin is sodium and water retention.

- Watch carefully for adverse effects when corticotropin is discontinued. Dose should be tapered and not stopped abruptly because adrenal hypofunction may result.
- Check laboratory findings, especially electrolyte levels and glucose. Electrolyte replacement may be necessary, and corticotropin can increase blood glucose.
- Observe for any signs of infection. Corticotropin is an antiinflammatory and can suppress the immune function, increasing the risk for infection.

Patient Teaching
General
Growth Hormone
- Suggest that the patient or family monitor the patient's growth rate.
- Individuals in some cultural groups may misunderstand the purpose and use of GH. The health care provider must emphasize that these are *not* drugs for building muscles and that they can cause many serious side effects, such as diabetes mellitus, when abused.

Corticotropin
- Advise patients to adhere to the drug regimen. Discontinuation of certain drugs, such as corticotropin, can cause hypofunction of the gland being stimulated.
- Direct patients to decrease salt intake to decrease or avoid edema. Potassium supplementation may be needed.

Side Effects
Growth Hormone
- Advise athletes not to take GH because of side effects. GH can be effective for children whose height is markedly below the expected norm for their age and for adults with confirmed diagnosis of GH deficiency. Because GH acts on newly forming bone, administer before the epiphyses are fused in children.
- Inform patients with diabetes to closely monitor blood glucose levels. Insulin regulation may be necessary.
- Instruct patients to monitor weight due to possible fluid retention.

Corticotropin
- Teach patients to report side effects such as muscle weakness, edema, petechiae, ecchymosis, decrease in growth, decreased wound healing, and menstrual irregularities.

Evaluate Outcomes [Evaluation]
- Evaluate effectiveness of drug therapy.

THYROID GLAND

The thyroid gland is an important regulator for many of the bodily functions. The three hormones produced and secreted by the thyroid gland are triiodothyronine (T_3); thyroxine (T_4), which helps with metabolism; and, to a lesser extent, calcitonin for regulating serum calcium. A majority of thyroid hormone is synthesized as T_4, which is then converted to T_3 to act on target cells. Iodide, an inorganic form of iodine, is needed for the synthesis of T_3 and T_4. These are carried in the blood by thyroxine-binding globulin (TBG) and albumin, which protect the hormones from being degraded. T_3 is more potent than T_4, and only unbound (free) T_3 and T_4 have biologic actions and produce a hormonal response.

Negative feedback mechanisms regulate hormone secretion from the thyroid gland. The hypothalamus releases thyrotropin-releasing hormone (TRH), which stimulates the release of TSH from the pituitary gland. TSH stimulates the synthesis and release of T_3 and T_4 from the thyroid gland. Excess free T_3 and T_4 inhibit the hypothalamus-pituitary-thyroid (HPT) axis, which results in decreased TRH and TSH secretion. Too low of an amount of T_3 and T_4 increases the function of the HPT axis.

For thyroid deficiency (hypothyroidism), synthetic thyroid hormones may be prescribed either alone or in combination. When the thyroid gland secretes an overabundance of thyroid hormone (hyperthyroidism), antithyroid drugs are usually indicated.

Hypothyroidism

Hypothyroidism, a decrease in thyroid hormone secretion, can have a primary cause (thyroid gland disorder), a secondary cause (lack of TSH secretion [pituitary disorder]), or a tertiary cause (lack of TRH [hypothalamus disorder]). Primary hypothyroidism occurs more frequently. Decreased T_4 and elevated TSH levels indicate primary hypothyroidism, the causes of which are acute or chronic inflammation of the thyroid gland, radioiodine therapy, excess intake of antithyroid drugs, or surgical removal of the thyroid gland. Myxedema is severe hypothyroidism in the adult; symptoms include lethargy; apathy; memory impairment; emotional changes; slow speech; a deep, coarse voice; edema of the eyelids and face; dry skin; cold intolerance; slow pulse; constipation; weight gain; and abnormal menses. In children, hypothyroidism can have a congenital onset that can cause delayed physical and mental growth (cretinism) or onset may be prepubertal (juvenile hypothyroidism). Drugs that contain T_3 and T_4, alone or in combination, are used to treat hypothyroidism. Exogenous thyroid hormones are contraindicated in patients with thyrotoxicosis, acute myocardial infarction (AMI), and adrenal insufficiency. Because thyroid hormones are catabolized by the hepatic system, drugs with hepatic enzyme–inducing properties (e.g., carbamazepine, hydantoins, rifabutin) should be used with caution. Elevated serum calcium levels could also be related to hypothyroidism; exogenous calcitonin may also be prescribed.

Thyroid Drugs

Levothyroxine sodium is the drug of choice for replacement therapy for the treatment of primary hypothyroidism. It increases the levels of T_4 and metabolically is deiodinated to T_3. Levothyroxine is also used to treat simple goiter and chronic lymphocytic (Hashimoto) thyroiditis. Prototype Drug Chart: Levothyroxine Sodium lists the pharmacologic data for levothyroxine sodium.

Liothyronine is a synthetic T_3 with a biologic half-life of 2.5 days with rapid onset of action (within a few hours). Liothyronine is indicated for use as replacement or supplemental treatment for hypothyroidism of any etiology. Unlike levothyroxine, liothyronine does not need to be deiodinated, which increases the availability

---

📋 PROTOTYPE DRUG CHART

Levothyroxine Sodium

Drug Class	Dosage
Thyroid hormone	Primary hypothyroidism, with/without goiter, in otherwise healthy persons: A: PO: Initially 1.6 mcg/kg/d; *maint:* 50–200 mcg/d; increase in increments of 12.5–25 mcg at 6- to 8-wk intervals. Other dosing is also available.

Contraindications	Drug-Lab-Food Interactions
Absolute contraindications: Thyrotoxicosis and myocardial infarction *Caution:* Adrenal insufficiency; cardiovascular disease, including cardiac arrhythmias, hypertension, and angina pectoris; diabetes mellitus; osteoporosis; hypopituitarism; dysphagia	Drug: Many drug-drug interactions exist and may alter the therapeutic effects of thyroid hormone replacement. Increased cardiac insufficiency occurs when levothyroxine is taken with sympathomimetics (e.g., epinephrine); levothyroxine increases the effects of anticoagulants, TCAs, vasopressors, decongestants, corticosteroids; decreases effects of antidiabetics (oral and insulin), digitalis products, beta blockers; decreased absorption of levothyroxine occurs with estrogens, antacids, cholestyramine, colestipol, sucralfate, and simethicone. Ketamines can worsen hypertension and tachycardia. Hepatic inducers (e.g., carbamazepine, barbiturates, hydantoins) increase the metabolism of thyroid hormones. Food: Drug should be taken on an empty stomach at least 30–60 min before breakfast and other medications. Tablets may be crushed and mixed in a small amount (5–10 mL) of water; use immediately after mixing. Do not mix with enteral or soy-based feedings. Certain food and beverages inhibit the absorption of thyroid hormones. Herb: Celery seed may reduce thyroid hormones.

Pharmacokinetics	Pharmacodynamics
Absorption: PO: 40%–80% Distribution: PB: 99% Metabolism: t½: 3–10 d depending on initial thyroid state Excretion: Urine (80%) and feces (20%)	PO: Onset: 3–5 d; IV: 6–8 h Peak: 24 h (IV) to several weeks (PO) Duration: Several weeks

Therapeutic Effects/Uses
To treat hypothyroidism, myxedema, goiter, and thyroid cancer Mechanism of Action: Increases metabolic rate, oxygen consumption, utilization and mobilization of glycogen stores; promotes gluconeogenesis and body growth; stimulates protein synthesis

Side Effects	Adverse Reactions
Nausea, vomiting, anorexia, diarrhea, cramps, tremors, nervousness, irritability, insomnia, headache, weight loss, diaphoresis, and amenorrhea; usually due to undermedication or overmedication	Tachycardia, hypertension, palpitations, osteoporosis, and seizures; usually due to overmedication. Other adverse reactions include urticaria, rash, and alopecia. *Life-threatening:* Thyroid crisis, angina pectoris, cardiac dysrhythmias (atrial fibrillation), cardiovascular collapse

A, Adult; *d,* day; *h,* hour; *IV,* intravenous; *maint,* maintenance; *min,* minutes; *PB,* protein binding; *PO,* by mouth; *t½,* half-life; *TCA,* tricyclic antidepressant; *wk,* week; *y,* year; >, greater than; ≤, less than or equal to.

for use by the body tissues. Liothyronine is better absorbed from the GI tract (over 95%) than levothyroxine, and because of its rapid onset of action and short half-life, it is frequently used as initial therapy for treating myxedema. Liothyronine is available for oral or IV administration.

Desiccated thyroid is a naturally occurring thyroid hormone from porcine thyroid glands. It contains both levothyroxine and liothyronine. Desiccated thyroid is used to treat hypothyroidism due to thyroid atrophy, thyroid hormone deficiency, and goiter.

Liotrix is a mixture of levothyroxine sodium and liothyronine sodium in a 4-to-1 ratio by weight, respectively. For treating hypothyroidism, there is no significant advantage to using liotrix over levothyroxine sodium alone, because levothyroxine converts T_4 to T_3 in the peripheral tissues.

Table 49.3 lists the natural and synthetic thyroid preparations and their dosages, uses, and considerations.

Hyperthyroidism

Hyperthyroidism is an increase in circulating T_3 and T_4 levels, which usually results from an overactive thyroid gland or excessive output of thyroid hormones from one or more thyroid nodules. Hyperthyroidism may be mild, with few symptoms, or it may be severe, as in thyroid storm, in which death may occur from vascular collapse. Graves disease, or thyrotoxicosis, is the most common type of hyperthyroidism caused by hyperfunction of the thyroid gland. It is characterized by a rapid pulse (*tachycardia*), palpitations, excessive perspiration (*hyperhidrosis*), heat intolerance, nervousness, irritability, bulging eyes (*exophthalmos*), and weight loss.

Hyperthyroidism can be treated by surgical removal of a portion of the thyroid gland (subtotal thyroidectomy), radioactive iodine therapy, or antithyroid drugs, which inhibit either synthesis or release of thyroid hormone. Any of these treatments can cause hypothyroidism. By blocking beta receptors, propranolol can control cardiac symptoms that result from hyperthyroidism, such as palpitations and tachycardia.

Antithyroid Drugs

The purpose of antithyroid drugs is to reduce the excessive secretion of thyroid hormones by inhibiting thyroid secretion. The use of surgery (subtotal thyroidectomy) and radioiodine therapy frequently leads to permanent hypothyroidism; these patients will need to be on thyroid replacement therapy. Thiourea derivatives (thioamides) are the drugs of choice used to decrease thyroid hormone production. This drug group interferes with synthesis of thyroid hormone. Thiourea derivatives do *not* destroy thyroid tissue; rather, they block thyroid action.

TABLE 49.3	Drug Therapies for Thyroid Disorders	
Generic	**Route and Dosage**	**Uses and Considerations**
Thyroid Replacements: Hypothyroidism		
Desiccated thyroid (porcine)	A: PO: Initially, 15–30 mg/d; *maint:* 60–120 mg/d; can increase 15 mg/d q2–3wk	For hypothyroidism and goiter. PB: >99%; t½: T_3, 2 d; T_4, 6–7 d
Levothyroxine sodium	See Prototype Drug Chart: Levothyroxine Sodium	
Liothyronine sodium	A: PO: Initially, 5–100 mcg/d; *maint:* 25–100 mcg/d Myxedema coma: A: IV: Initially, 25–50 mcg; subsequent doses based on clinical condition q4–12h to avoid hormone fluctuations	For hypothyroidism, myxedema, thyroiditis, hyperthyroidism diagnosis, cretinism, and goiter. Must be administered with glucocorticoid when treating myxedema coma with IV liothyronine. PB: 99%; t½: 2.5 d
Synthetic levothyroxine	A: PO: 25–100 mcg T_4/12.5–25 mcg T_3/d Dosages must be individualized based on clinical response and thyroid levels.	For hypothyroidism, goiter, and hyperthyroidism diagnosis. T_4T_3 drug. PB: 99%; t½: T_3, 2.5 d; T_4, 3–10 d
Antithyroid Drugs: Hyperthyroidism		
Thioamides Methimazole	A: PO: 15–60 mg/d in 1–3 divided doses	For hyperthyroidism, Graves disease, thyrotoxicosis. Inhibits thyroid hormone synthesis. Dosages greater than 40 mg/d may increase risk of agranulocytosis. PB: 0%; t½: 5–9 h
Propylthiouracil	A: PO: 300–900 mg/d divided q8h, then 100–150 mg/d divided q8h	For patients with hyperthyroidism or Graves disease who are intolerant of methimazole and are unable to receive surgery or radioiodine therapy; inhibits conversion of T_4 and T_3. PB: 60%–80%; t½: 1 h
Iodine Potassium iodide	A: PO: 0.27 mL three times daily for 10–14 d before surgery Dilute drug and administer after meals; sip through a straw to avoid discoloration of teeth.	For hyperthyroidism and thyrotoxicosis to suppress thyroid function before surgery. Maximum effect is achieved after 10–15 d. Drug is absorbed from the GI tract as iodinated amino acids and is excreted renally. PB: UK; t½: UK

A, Adult; *Adol*, adolescent; *d*, day; *GI*, gastrointestinal; *h*, hour; *IV*, intravenous; *maint*, maintenance; *PB*, protein binding; *PO*, by mouth; *q*, every; *t½*, half-life; *T₄*, thyroxine; *T₃*, triiodothyronine; *UK*, unknown; *wk*, week; *y*, year; >, greater than; <, less than; ≥, greater than or equal to.

Propylthiouracil (PTU) and methimazole are effective thioamide antithyroid drugs. They are used to control overactive thyroid due to Graves disease, toxic nodular goiter, or multinodular goiter; they are also used before radioiodine treatment or thyroid surgery. Methimazole does not inhibit peripheral conversion of T_4 to T_3 as does PTU; however, it is 10 times more potent, it has a longer half-life than PTU, and the euthyroid state is achieved in 2 to 4 months. It is the preferred antithyroid because of the less severe side effects. Methimazole is rapidly absorbed from the GI tract. Prolonged use of thioamides may cause goiter because of increased TSH secretion and inhibited T_4 and T_3 synthesis. Minimal doses of thioamides should be given when indicated to avoid goiter formation.

Strong iodide preparations such as potassium iodide have been used to suppress thyroid function for patients who are undergoing subtotal thyroidectomy because of Graves disease. Table 49.3 lists the antithyroid drugs used to treat hyperthyroidism along with their dosages, uses, and considerations.

Drug Interactions. Antithyroid drugs interact with many other drugs. When used with oral anticoagulants (e.g., warfarin), they can cause an increase in the anticoagulation effect. In addition, thyroid drugs decrease the effect of insulin and oral antidiabetics, digoxin and lithium increase the action of thyroid drugs, and phenytoin increases serum T_3 level.

⊚ CLINICAL JUDGMENT [NURSING PROCESS]

Thyroid Hormones: Replacement and Antithyroid Drugs

Concept: Hormonal Regulation
- The ability of the body to maintain homeostasis by the regulation, secretion, and action of hormones associated with the endocrine system

Recognize Cues [Assessment]
- Determine baseline vital signs, including weight changes, for future comparisons. Report abnormal results.
- Report any abnormal results of serum triiodothyronine (T_3), thyroxine (T_4), and thyroid-stimulating hormone (TSH) levels.
- Obtain a history of drugs and herbal products the patient is taking.
- ⚡ Assess for signs and symptoms of thyroid crisis (thyroid storm), including tachycardia, cardiac dysrhythmias, fever, heart failure, flushed skin, apathy, confusion, behavioral changes, and, later, hypotension and vascular collapse. Thyroid crisis can result from a thyroidectomy (excess thyroid hormones released), abrupt withdrawal of antithyroid drug, excess ingestion of thyroid hormone, or failure to give antithyroid medication before thyroid surgery.

Analyze Cues and Prioritize Hypothesis [Patient Problems]
- Altered functional ability related to imbalanced thyroid hormone
- Need for health teaching related to complex drug regimen
- General decreased tissue perfusion related to imbalanced thyroid hormone

Generate Solutions [Planning]
- The patient will report an improved activity level within 1 to 4 weeks of thyroid treatments.
- The patient will report decreased signs and symptoms of hypothyroidism within 2 to 4 weeks with prescribed thyroid drug replacement, and the patient will not experience side effects.
- The patient will report decreased signs and symptoms of hyperthyroidism in 1 to 3 weeks with prescribed antithyroid drug.

Take Action [Nursing Interventions]
- Record vital signs. With *hypothyroidism*, temperature, heart rate, and blood pressure usually decrease. With *hyperthyroidism*, tachycardia and palpitations usually occur.
- Monitor the patient's weight. Weight gain commonly occurs in patients with hypothyroidism.
- Obtain a pregnancy test, complete blood count (CBC), complete metabolic panel (CMP), liver function test (LFT), and electrocardiograph (ECG).
- Report periodic TSH, T_3, and T_4.

Patient Teaching
General
- Encourage patients to take drug at the same time each day in relation to meals. Levothyroxine is taken 30–60 minutes before any food or medications.
- Teach patients to check warnings on over-the-counter (OTC) drug labels. Avoid OTC drugs that caution against use by persons with heart or thyroid disease.
- Suggest that patients carry a MedicAlert identification card, tag, or bracelet that shows the health condition and the drug used to treat it.
- Instruct patients that certain foods can interfere with the absorption of thyroid hormones (e.g., soy products [estrogen], cruciferous vegetables [broccoli and cabbage], iodized salt, shellfish [iodine], and coffee).
- Instruct patients to take drugs as instructed; abrupt changes may lead to increased thyroid dysfunction.
- Recognize that family members may need guidance in understanding the disease processes of hypothyroidism or hyperthyroidism. Support patients and family members who may lack knowledge of prescribed drug therapy for management of thyroid conditions. Additional time in explanations and a written plan of care in the native language may be necessary for non-English-speaking persons.

Side Effects
- Direct patients to report symptoms of hyperthyroidism (tachycardia, chest pain, palpitations, excess sweating) caused by drug accumulation or overdosing.
- Demonstrate to patients how to take that pulse rate. Instruct patients to monitor pulse rate and to report increases or marked decreases in the rate.
- Teach patients the side effects of antithyroid drugs: skin rash, hives, nausea, alopecia, loss of hair pigment, petechiae or ecchymoses, and weakness.
- Advise patients to contact their health care provider if sore throat and fever occur while taking antithyroid drugs. A serious adverse reaction of antithyroid drugs is agranulocytosis (loss of white blood cells). CBC should be monitored for leukopenia.

Evaluate Outcomes [Evaluation]
- Evaluate both effectiveness of the treatment and drug compliance.
- Continue monitoring for side effects from drug accumulation or overdosing.
- Evaluate the patient's knowledge of the medication regimen.

TABLE 49.4 Drug Therapies for Parathyroid Disorders

Generic	Route and Dosage	Uses and Considerations
Hypoparathyroidism and Hypocalcemia: Vitamin D Analogues		
Calcitriol	See Prototype Drug Chart: Calcitriol	
Ergocalciferol	Hypoparathyroidism: C: PO: 1250–5000 mcg/d with calcium supplements	Prohormone for hypoparathyroidism. Enhances calcium and phosphorus absorption. Long duration of action. PB: UK; t½: UK
Hyperparathyroidism and Hypercalcemia		
Calcitonin-salmon	Hypercalcemia: A: IM/subcut: 4 IU/kg q12h, can increase to 8 IU/kg q12h; *max:* 8 IU/kg q6h Paget disease: A: IM/subcut: 50–100 IU/1–3 × wk	For hypercalcemia and Paget disease of bone (osteitis deformans). Calcitonin decreases serum calcium by binding at receptor sites on osteoclast. PB: UK; t½: 1 h
Cinacalcet	A: PO: Initially 30 mg bid; titrate in 30 mg increments q2–4wk; *max:* 360 mg/d	For hyperparathyroidism and hypercalcemia. Check serum calcium 1 wk after initiating treatment and 2 months thereafter. Administer with food. PB: 93%–97%; t½: 30–40 h

A, Adult; *bid*, twice daily; *C*, child; *d*, day; *h*, hour; *IM*, intramuscular; *IU*, international units; *max*, maximum; *PB*, protein binding; *PO*, by mouth; *q*, every; *subcut*, subcutaneous; *t½*, half-life; *UK*, unknown; *wk*, week.

PARATHYROID GLANDS

The parathyroid glands secrete parathyroid hormone (PTH), or parathormone, which regulates serum calcium levels in a number of ways:

- It enhances the release of calcium from the bones.
- It enhances calcium reabsorption in the renal tubules.
- It enhances calcium absorption in the intestines by increasing the production of activated vitamin D.

A decrease (negative feedback) in serum calcium stimulates the release of PTH. Calcitonin, one of three thyroid hormones, decreases serum calcium levels by promoting osteoclast activity in bones and calcium excretion by the kidneys and intestines.

For PTH deficiency, PTH analogues are used. Surgical removal (parathyroidectomy) is a common treatment for hyperparathyroidism. Calcimimetic drugs, which mimic calcium in the blood, prevent the parathyroid gland from releasing PTH.

Hypoparathyroidism

Damage to the parathyroid glands is a common cause of hypoparathyroidism. Hypomagnesemia (low serum magnesium) can also cause PTH deficiency. Other causes of hypocalcemia (serum calcium deficit) include vitamin D deficiency, renal impairment, or diuretic therapy; PTH replacement helps correct the calcium deficit. The action of PTH is to promote calcium absorption from the GI tract, promote reabsorption of calcium from the renal tubules, and activate vitamin D. Table 49.4 lists the drugs used to treat hypoparathyroidism and hyperparathyroidism and their dosages, uses, and considerations.

Calcitriol

Calcitriol is a vitamin D analogue that promotes calcium absorption from the GI tract and promotes secretion of calcium from bone to the bloodstream. Prototype Drug Chart: Calcitriol lists the pharmacologic data for calcitriol.

Hyperparathyroidism

Hyperparathyroidism can be caused by malignancies of the parathyroid glands or ectopic PTH hormone secretion from lung cancer, hyperthyroidism, or prolonged immobility, during which calcium is lost from bone. Partial or full parathyroidectomy is the most common treatment for primary hyperparathyroidism. Calcitonin-salmon, calcimimetics, and bisphosphonates are used to treat patients affected by hyperparathyroidism.

Calcitonin-salmon prevents bone loss and fractures, increases bone density, and alleviates pain due to fractures and bone metastasis. Calcitonin is not as effective as other drugs for hyperparathyroidism. Calcitonin is contraindicated in patients allergic to fish. Common side effects include allergic reactions, GI symptoms (e.g., nausea and vomiting), cephalgia, and hypocalcemia. Adverse reactions due to severe hypocalcemia (e.g., tetany and seizures) can also occur.

Calcimimetics, such as cinacalcet, are used in patients with hyperparathyroidism due to chronic renal disease and parathyroid cancer, and it is also used in those who are unable to undergo parathyroidectomy. Cinacalcet mimics calcium in circulation, increasing the sensitivity of the calcium-sensing receptors of the cells of the parathyroid gland, thereby reducing PTH secretion. This action causes a decrease in serum calcium and slows the progression of bone disease. Because of the hypocalcemic effect, cinacalcet is contraindicated in patients with hypocalcemia. Chapter 12 discusses calcium imbalances more in depth.

Bisphosphonates (e.g., alendronate, etidronate, ibandronate, and risedronate) block osteoclast activities, thereby inhibiting mineralization or resorption of the bone, which may lessen osteoporosis caused by hyperparathyroidism. Before treatment with bisphosphonates, bone mineral density measurements should be obtained at baseline and periodically thereafter. Serum calcium concentration should be obtained, and any hypocalcemia must be corrected before bisphosphonate therapy. Adequate intake of calcium and vitamin D is essential during therapy. Oral bisphosphonates are contraindicated in patients who are unable to sit or stand upright for at least 30 minutes after administration or who have esophageal strictures. During therapy, transient hypocalcemia and hypophosphatemia can occur. Other side effects include abdominal and musculoskeletal pain, GI upsets, hypotension, and fever. Individual bisphosphonates are discussed in Chapter 52.

📄 PROTOTYPE DRUG CHART

Calcitriol

Drug Class	Dosage
Vitamin D analogue	A: PO: 0.25–2 mcg/d

Contraindications	Drug-Lab-Food Interactions
Absolute contraindications: Hypersensitivity, hypercalcemia, hypervitaminosis D *Caution:* Cardiovascular disease, renal calculi, renal failure, hyperphosphatemia, dehydration, excess sunlight exposure, malabsorption syndrome, hypocalcemia	Drug: Increased cardiac dysrhythmias with digoxin, verapamil; decreased calcitriol absorption with cholestyramine; decreased calcitriol effects with ketoconazole, barbiturates; enhanced calcitriol effects with thiazide diuretics Calcitriol decreases the effects of estrogen. Lab: Increased serum calcium with thiazide diuretics, calcium supplements, calcium-rich foods; decreased serum calcium with low magnesium

Pharmacokinetics	Pharmacodynamics
Absorption: PO: Well absorbed Distribution: PB: 99% Metabolism: t½: 3–8 h adult; 27 h children Excretion: Feces (50%), urine (16%)	PO: Onset: 2–6 h Peak: 3–6 h Duration: 3–5 d

Therapeutic Effects/Uses
To treat parathyroid disorders (hyperparathyroidism and hypoparathyroidism) and to manage hypocalcemia in chronic renal failure Mechanism of Action: Calcitriol enhances calcium deposits into bones by the active form of vitamin D's metabolite, calcitriol. Calcitriol reabsorbs calcium by the kidneys, enhances intestinal absorption of dietary calcium, and decreases serum phosphate, bone resorption, and parathyroid hormone levels.

Side Effects	Adverse Reactions
Side effects are generally early signs of hypercalcemia: fatigue, weakness, somnolence, cephalgia, nausea, vomiting, diarrhea, cramps, drowsiness, dizziness, vertigo, metallic taste, lethargy, constipation, and xerostomia.	Adverse effects are late signs of hypercalcemia: anorexia, photophobia, dehydration, cardiac arrhythmias, decreased libido, hypertension, sensory disturbances, hypercalciuria, hypercalcemia, and hyperphosphatemia.

A, Adult; *d,* day; *h,* hour; *PB,* protein binding; *PO,* by mouth; *t½,* half-life; *y,* year; ≥, greater than or equal to.

◎ CLINICAL JUDGMENT [NURSING PROCESS]

Parathyroid Hormone Insufficiencies

Concept: Hormonal Regulation
- The ability of the body to maintain homeostasis by the regulation, secretion, and action of hormones associated with the endocrine system

Recognize Cues [Assessment]
- Note serum calcium level and report abnormal results.
- ⚠ Assess for symptoms of tetany in hypocalcemia: twitching of the mouth, tingling and numbness of fingers, carpopedal spasm, spasmodic contractions, and laryngeal spasm.

Analyze Cues and Prioritize Hypothesis [Patient Problems]
- Hyper- or hypocalcemia related to hormonal imbalance and therapeutic regimen
- Need for health teaching related to complex drug regimen
- Disrupted fluid and electrolytes related to side effects of drug regimen

Generate Solutions [Planning]
- The patient will maintain a serum calcium level within the normal range.
- The patient will report no or minimal side effects.

Take Action [Nursing Interventions]
- Monitor serum calcium level. The normal reference range is 8 to 10 mg/dL; serum calcium below 8 mg/dL indicates hypocalcemia. Total serum calcium greater than 10.5 mg/dL indicates hypercalcemia.

Patient Teaching
General
- Advise women to inform their health care provider about pregnancy status before taking calcitonin preparations.
- Encourage patients to check over-the-counter (OTC) drugs for possible calcium content, especially if the patient has an elevated serum calcium level. Some vitamins and antacids contain calcium. Tell patients to contact their health care provider before taking drugs with calcium.

Side Effects
- Direct patients to report symptoms of hypocalcemia (e.g., tetany).
- Teach patients to report signs and symptoms of hypercalcemia, which include bone pain, anorexia, nausea, vomiting, thirst, constipation, lethargy, bradycardia, and polyuria.

Evaluate Outcomes [Evaluation]
- Monitor effectiveness of drug therapy (e.g., serum calcium level, signs and symptoms of hypercalcemia or hypocalcemia).
- Continue monitoring for signs and symptoms of calcium imbalances.
- Evaluate the patient's knowledge of medication regimen.

ADRENAL GLANDS

The paired adrenal glands consist of the adrenal medulla and adrenal cortex. Hormones secreted from the adrenal medulla are epinephrine and norepinephrine (catecholamines); Chapters 15 and 55 further discuss these hormones. The adrenal cortex produces two types of steroid hormones, glucocorticoids (cortisol) and mineralocorticoids (aldosterone), and, to a lesser extent, the adrenal androgens and estrogens. Steroids are secreted by the adrenal cortex in response to signals from the hypothalamus-pituitary-adrenal (HPA) axis; the levels are regulated by the negative feedback mechanism. A decrease in serum steroid levels (hypocortisolism) increases CRF and ACTH secretions from the hypothalamus and anterior pituitary gland, respectively; these stimulate the adrenal glands to secrete and release steroids. An increased serum steroid level (hypercortisolism) inhibits the HPA axis, resulting in fewer steroids being released. A decrease in steroid secretion is called *adrenal hyposecretion* (adrenal insufficiency, or Addison disease), and an increase in steroid secretion is called *adrenal hypersecretion* (Cushing syndrome). Corticosteroids are also described in Chapter 24.

❗ Because of the influences of steroids on electrolytes and on carbohydrate, protein, and fat metabolism, hypocortisolism can result in serious illness or death.

⚡ PATIENT SAFETY

Do not Confuse…
- **Calcitonin** with **calcitriol** or **calcium**
- **Levothyroxine** with **liothyronine**
- **Somatropin** with **somatostatin** or **sandostatin**

Glucocorticoids

Glucocorticoids are the most potent natural cortisol produced by the body and are influenced by ACTH, which is released from the anterior pituitary gland. Its functions include having an effect on the inflammatory response (see Chapter 24), metabolism, growth, and biorhythms. Glucocorticoids also affect carbohydrate, protein, and fat metabolism and muscle and blood cell activities. Indications for glucocorticoid therapy include trauma, surgery, inflammation, emotional upsets, and anxiety. Table 49.2 lists the physiologic aspects of adrenal hyposecretion (Addison disease) and hypersecretion (Cushing syndrome).

Most of the glucocorticoid drugs, frequently called *cortisone drugs,* are synthetically produced. These drugs have several routes of administration: oral, parenteral (IM or IV), topical (creams, ointments, lotions), and aerosol (inhaler). Drugs administered via the (seldom used) IM route should be administered deep into the muscle; subcutaneous administration is not recommended.

Glucocorticoids are used to treat many diseases and health problems, including inflammatory, allergic, and debilitating conditions. Among the inflammatory conditions that may require glucocorticoids are autoimmune disorders (e.g., MS, rheumatoid arthritis, myasthenia gravis), ulcerative colitis, glomerulonephritis, shock, ocular and vascular inflammation, polyarteritis nodosa, and hepatitis. Allergic conditions include asthma, drug reactions, contact dermatitis, and anaphylaxis. Debilitating conditions are mainly caused by malignancies. Organ transplant recipients may require glucocorticoids to prevent organ rejection.

There are many glucocorticoids, some more potent than others. Dexamethasone has been used to treat severe inflammatory responses that result from head trauma or allergic reactions. An inexpensive glucocorticoid frequently prescribed is prednisone. Prototype Drug Chart: Prednisone lists the pharmacologic data for prednisone.

Commonly used glucocorticoid drugs and their dosages, uses, and considerations are listed in Table 49.5. Drugs used for adrenocortical insufficiency contain both glucocorticoids and mineralocorticoids, whereas drugs with antiinflammatory or immunosuppressive properties contain mostly glucocorticoids with minimal mineralocorticoid activity.

Side Effects and Adverse Effects. Side effects and adverse reactions of glucocorticoids that result from high doses or prolonged use include increased blood glucose, abnormal fat deposits in the face and trunk (so-called *moon face* and *buffalo hump*), decreased extremity size, muscle wasting, edema, sodium and water retention, hypertension, euphoria or psychosis, thinned skin with purpura, increased intraocular pressure (glaucoma), peptic ulcers, and growth retardation. Long-term use of glucocorticoid drugs can cause adrenal atrophy (loss of adrenal gland function). ❗ When drug therapy is discontinued, the dose should be tapered to allow the adrenal cortex to produce cortisol and other corticosteroids. Abrupt withdrawal of the drug can result in severe adrenocortical insufficiency.

Drug Interactions. Glucocorticoids increase the potency of drugs taken concurrently, including aspirin and nonsteroidal antiinflammatory drugs (NSAIDs), thus increasing the risk of GI bleeding and ulceration. Use of potassium-wasting diuretics (e.g., furosemide) with glucocorticoids increases potassium loss, resulting in hypokalemia.

Barbiturates, phenytoin, and rifampin decrease the effect of prednisone because they increase glucocorticoid metabolism. Larger doses of glucocorticoids may be required to achieve the desired effect. Prolonged use of glucocorticoids can cause severe muscle weakness.

Dexamethasone, a potent glucocorticoid, interacts with many drugs. Phenytoin, theophylline, rifampin, barbiturates, and antacids decrease the action of dexamethasone, whereas estrogen and NSAIDs such as aspirin increase its action. Dexamethasone decreases the effects of oral antidiabetics. Glucocorticoids can increase blood glucose levels, so insulin or oral antidiabetic drug dosage may need to be increased. When the drug is given with diuretics or anti-*Pseudomonas* penicillin preparations, the serum potassium level may decrease markedly.

Herbal products such as cascara sagrada, yellow dock, and licorice can potentiate the effects of corticosteroids, which can worsen potassium depletion.

Mineralocorticoids

Mineralocorticoids promote sodium retention and potassium and hydrogen excretion in the renal tubules. The primary mineralocorticoid is aldosterone, which is controlled by the renin-angiotensin-aldosterone system (RAAS). Mineralocorticoids maintain fluid balance by promoting the reabsorption of sodium from the renal tubules. Sodium attracts water, resulting in water retention. When *hypovolemia* (a decrease in circulating fluid) occurs, more aldosterone is secreted to increase sodium and water retention, thereby restoring fluid balance. With sodium reabsorption, potassium is lost and hypokalemia (potassium deficit) can occur. Some glucocorticoid drugs also contain mineralocorticoid properties; these include cortisone and hydrocortisone. A severe decrease in the mineralocorticoid can lead to hypotension and vascular collapse, as seen in Addison disease. Mineralocorticoid deficiency usually occurs with glucocorticoid deficiency, frequently called *corticosteroid deficiency.*

Fludrocortisone is an oral mineralocorticoid that can be given with a glucocorticoid. Even though fludrocortisone has significant glucocorticoid activity, it is not appreciable at usual therapeutic doses. Fludrocortisone mimics the actions of endogenous aldosterone, facilitating sodium resorption and promoting hydrogen ion and potassium excretion. In larger doses, it can inhibit endogenous hormone secretions of adrenal cortex and pituitary gland, causing a negative nitrogen balance;

TABLE 49.5 Drug Therapies for Adrenal Disorders

Generic	Route and Dosage	Uses and Considerations
GLUCOCORTICOIDS		
Short Acting		
Cortisone acetate	A: PO: 12–50 mg/d in divided doses to simulate normal diurnal adrenal rhythm	For adrenocortical insufficiency. Give with fludrocortisone (mineralocorticoid). Give oral dose with food to minimize GI irritation. PB: 90%; t½: 8–12 h
Hydrocortisone	Primary adrenocortical insufficiency: Hydrocortisone or hydrocortisone *cypionate*: A: PO 20–240 mg/d in 2–4 divided doses Hydrocortisone sodium *phosphate*: A: IM/IV/subcut: 15–240 mg/d twice daily (q12h). Hydrocortisone sodium *succinate*: A: IV/IM: 100–500 mg repeated in 2-, 4-, or 6-h intervals Hydrocortisone *acetate* suspension: A: IM: 15–240 mg once daily	For adrenocortical insufficiency. Given IV or IM (hydrocortisone sodium succinate) for crisis prophylaxis in ill patients or those undergoing surgery. Hydrocortisone sodium phosphate (subcut/IV/IM), hydrocortisone sodium succinate (IV/IM), and hydrocortisone acetate suspension (IM only) are for acute adrenal insufficiency. Oral hydrocortisone is also available for primary adrenocortical insufficiency. Oral dosages in this table are for primary adrenal insufficiency. Administer with meals to minimize GI irritation. Daily doses should be given in the morning to coincide with the body's normal cortisol secretion. Acetate formulations should never be given intravenously. PB: 90%; t½: 1–2 h
Intermediate Acting		
Methylprednisolone	A: PO: 4–48 mg/d in 4 divided doses Methylprednisolone *acetate*: A: IM: 10–120 mg; subsequent doses determined by clinical response Methylprednisolone sodium *succinate*: A: IV/IM: 10–40 mg over several minutes; subsequent dosages determined by clinical response	For adrenocortical insufficiency. Has little to no mineralocorticoid properties. Dosing is highly variable. Administer oral dosages with meals to minimize GI irritation. Acetate formulation should never be given intravenously. PB: UK; t½: 3–3.5 h
Prednisolone	A: PO: 5–60 mg/d in 1–2 doses	For parenteral use in primary or secondary adrenocortical insufficiency. Prednisolone is a potent steroid that can be injected into joints and soft tissue. Must be given concomitantly with a mineralocorticoid. PB: 70%–90%; t½: 2–4 h
Prednisone	See Prototype Drug Chart: Prednisone	
Long Acting		
Betamethasone (PO), betamethasone sodium phosphate/betamethasone acetate susp (IM)	A: PO: 0.6–7.2 mg/d in single or divided doses Injectable suspension: A: IM: 0.5–9 mg/d divided q12h Other regimen is available	Synthetic glucocorticoids with minimal mineralocorticoid properties are used as antiinflammatory or immunosuppressive agents; must be used in conjunction with a mineralocorticoid for primary or secondary adrenocortical insufficiency. Dosing is variable and depends on indications. Should be taken with food. PB: 64%; t½: 6.5 h
Dexamethasone	Adrenocortical insufficiency: A: PO: 0.75–9 mg/d in 2–4 divided doses or IV/IM: 0.5–9 mg/d q6–12h	Synthetic glucocorticoids with little or no mineralocorticoid activity. Longest acting corticosteroid. Must use a mineralocorticoid when treating adrenal insufficiency. Higher oral doses are used for dexamethasone suppression test for Cushing syndrome. Give oral dose with food. PB: UK; t½: 1.8–3.5 h
MINERALOCORTICOIDS		
Fludrocortisone	A: PO: 0.1–0.2 mg/d. If hypertension occurs due to therapy, decrease dose to 0.05 mg once daily	For adrenocortical insufficiency (Addison disease). To be used as a supplement to hydrocortisone or cortisone. Circulating drug is bound to protein and transcortin. Only the unbound drugs are active. May be administered without regard to food. PB: 42%; t½: 3.5 h

A, Adult; *d,* day; *GI,* gastrointestinal; *h,* hour; *IM,* intramuscular; *IV,* intravenous; *PB,* protein binding; *PO,* by mouth; *q,* every; *subcut,* subcutaneous; *susp,* suspension; *t½,* half-life; *UK,* unknown.

therefore a high-protein diet is usually indicated. Because potassium excretion occurs with the use of mineralocorticoids, serum potassium level should be monitored. Other adverse effects include fluid imbalance, fluid overload, and hypertension. These usually indicate overdosage, at which point fludrocortisone should be discontinued and then resumed at lower doses. Hypokalemia may cause metabolic alkalosis, which can cause GI symptoms (nausea and vomiting), orthostatic hypotension, cardiac rhythm changes, weakness, anorexia, and myalgia. Commonly used mineralocorticoid drugs and their dosages, uses, and considerations are listed in Table 49.5.

📄 **PROTOTYPE DRUG CHART**

Prednisone

Drug Class	Dosage
Glucocorticoid/corticosteroid	Dosage is individualized and highly variable depending on the severity of the disease and on patient response. A: PO: 5–60 mg/d in single or divided doses Delayed-release tablets release drug approximately 4 h after the first dose

Contraindications	Drug-Lab-Food Interactions
Contraindication: Untreated serious infections, hypersensitivity, varicella *Caution:* Psychosis, diabetes mellitus, renal disease, heart failure, myocardial infarction, hypertension, osteoporosis, cirrhosis, diverticulitis, hypothyroidism, myasthenia gravis, ulcerative colitis, seizures, visual disturbances, GI disorders, ocular herpes simplex	Drug: Additive effects occur with other immunosuppressive drugs when taken concurrently with corticosteroids. Increased corticosteroid levels are seen with estrogens, diltiazem, ketoconazole; decreased levels are seen with barbiturates, phenytoin, and rifampin. Concurrent use of aspirin and NSAIDs increase GI toxicity; concurrent use of diuretics and amphotericin B increases potassium depletion; concurrent use with cardiac glycosides increases risk of dysrhythmias and digitalis toxicity; concurrent use with bupropion lowers seizure threshold Herb: Level is decreased with ephedra (Ma-huang). Lab: Hyperglycemia, false-positive TB test

Pharmacokinetics	Pharmacodynamics
Absorption: PO: Well absorbed Distribution: PB: 65%–91% Metabolism: t½: 2–3 h Excretion: In urine	PO: Onset: UK Peak: 1–2 h Duration: 1 h (plasma); 18–36 h (biologic)

Therapeutic Effects/Uses	
Adrenocortical insufficiency, Addison disease Mechanism of Action: Suppresses inflammation, immune responses (humoral), and adrenal function; has mild mineralocorticoid activity	

Side Effects	Adverse Reactions
Fluid and sodium retention, nausea, diarrhea, abdominal distension, increased appetite, sweating, headache, depression, flushing, mood changes, cataracts, amenorrhea, anorexia, Cushing syndrome, psychosis, immunosuppression, HPA suppression, hypercholesterolemia, elevated hepatic transaminases	Angioedema, cardiac arrhythmia, avascular necrosis, osteoporosis, fractures, cardiac arrest, cardiomyopathy, GI ulceration, exfoliative dermatitis, GI bleeding and perforation, CHF, increased ICP, lupus-like symptoms, pancreatitis, pulmonary edema, ocular disease, CVA, tendon rupture, thromboembolism

A, Adult; *CHF*, congestive heart failure; *CVA*, cerebrovascular accident; *d*, day; *GI*, gastrointestinal; *h*, hour; *HPA*, hypothalamic-pituitary-adrenal axis; *ICP*, intracranial pressure; *NSAID*, nonsteroidal antiinflammatory drug; *PB*, protein binding; *PO*, by mouth; *t½*, half-life; *TB*, tuberculosis; *UK*, unknown.

◎ **CLINICAL JUDGMENT [NURSING PROCESS]**

Adrenal Hormones: Corticosteroids

Concept: Hormonal Regulation
- The ability of the body to maintain homeostasis by the regulation, secretion, and action of hormones associated with the endocrine system

Recognize Cues [Assessment]
- Note baseline vital signs for future comparisons.
- ⚡ Assess laboratory test results, especially serum electrolytes and blood glucose. The serum potassium level usually decreases and blood glucose level increases when a corticosteroid, such as prednisone, is taken over an extended period.
- Obtain the patient's weight and urine output for future comparisons. Corticosteroids can cause fluid retention and weight gain.
- Assess the patient's medical and herbal history. Report if the patient has glaucoma, cataracts, peptic ulcer, psychiatric problems, or diabetes mellitus. Glucocorticoids can intensify these health problems.

Analyze Cues and Prioritize Hypothesis [Patient Problems]
- Disrupted fluid and electrolyte balance related to treatment regimen
- Decreased immunity, risk for
- Decreased self-concept, risk for

Generate Solutions [Planning]
- The patient will report decreased signs and symptoms of inflammation.
- The patient will report minimal side effects from glucocorticoid therapy.
- The patient will not develop new or worsening infection.
- The patient will have increased knowledge of the medication regimen.

Take Action [Nursing Interventions]
- Determine vital signs. Corticosteroids such as prednisone can increase blood pressure and sodium and water retention.

CLINICAL JUDGMENT [NURSING PROCESS]—CONT'D

Adrenal Hormones: Corticosteroids

- Administer corticosteroids only as ordered. Routes of administration include oral, intramuscular (IM; not in deltoid muscle), intravenous (IV), aerosol, and topical. Apply topical corticosteroids in thin layers (see Chapter 45). Rashes, infection, and purpura should be noted and reported.
- Record weight. Report a weight gain of 5 lb in 2 days; this could indicate water retention due to sodium reabsorption from hyperaldosteronism.
- Monitor laboratory values, especially serum electrolytes and blood glucose. The serum potassium level could decrease to less than 3.5 mEq/L, and serum sodium and glucose could increase.
- Watch for signs and symptoms of hypokalemia: nausea, vomiting, muscular weakness, abdominal distension, paralytic ileus, and irregular heart rate.
- Assess for side effects from corticosteroid drugs when therapy has lasted more than 10 days and drug is taken in high dosages. Cortisone preparations should not be abruptly stopped because adrenal crisis can result.
- Monitor older adults for signs and symptoms of increased osteoporosis. Some corticosteroids promote calcium loss from bone.

Patient Teaching
General
- Advise patients to take drugs as prescribed, and caution patients not to abruptly stop drugs. When the drug is discontinued, the dose is tapered over 1 to 2 weeks.
- Direct patients not to take cortisone preparations (oral or topical) during pregnancy unless necessary and prescribed by the health care provider. Drugs may be harmful to the fetus.
- ⚡ Inform patients that certain herbal laxatives and diuretics may interact with corticosteroid drug therapy and may increase the severity of hypokalemia.

- Teach patients to avoid large crowds and persons with respiratory infections, because corticosteroids can suppress the immune system.
- Teach patients receiving corticosteroids to inform other health care providers of all drugs taken.
- Encourage patients to carry a medical alert identification card, tag, or bracelet stating that corticosteroids are taken.
- Teach patients proper use of the drug.
- Counsel patients to take cortisone preparations at mealtime or with food to prevent irritation of gastric mucosa.
- Advise patients to eat foods rich in potassium, such as fresh and dried fruits, vegetables, meats, and nuts. Some corticosteroid preparations promote potassium loss.
- Explain to the family that the patient is not "dumb" or "uninterested" but has an adrenal problem. Explain that symptoms do not go away and may be progressive if prescribed therapy is not followed.

Side Effects
- Teach patients to report signs and symptoms of Cushing syndrome: moon face, puffy eyelids, edema in the feet, increased bruising, dizziness, bleeding, and menstrual irregularity.

Evaluate Outcomes [Evaluation]
- Evaluate effectiveness of corticosteroid therapy. If clinical manifestations have not improved, a change in drug therapy may be necessary.
- Continue monitoring for side effects, especially when a patient is receiving high doses of corticosteroids.
- Evaluate the patient's knowledge of the therapy.

CRITICAL THINKING SINGLE EPISODE CASE STUDY

SLO: Apply the clinical judgment [nursing process] on a patient requiring hormonal therapy.

NGN Item Type: Cloze

Cognitive Skills: Analyze cues

A 68-year-old female presented to the clinic with complaints of fatigue and weight gain over a 6-month time frame. On further assessment, the nurse noted the following:

- Blood pressure 114/72 mm Hg
- Heart rate 54 beats per minute
- Respiratory rate 14 breaths per minute
- Oxygen saturation 97% on room air
- Dry skin
- Voice hoarseness
- Muscle weakness
- Mildly enlarged thyroid gland
- Hemoglobin 13 g/L
- Hematocrit 40%
- Serum sodium 138 mEq/L
- Serum potassium 4.1 mEq/L
- Serum calcium 9.8 mg/dL
- Serum albumin 3.8 g/dL
- Serum total protein 6.9 g/dL
- Thyroid-stimulating hormone 10 mIU/L

Choose the *most likely* options for the information missing from the statements below by selecting from the list of options provided.

The nurse suspects _____1_____, and when reviewing T_3 and T_4 levels, the nurse would expect the levels to be _____2_____. The nurse reports the assessment findings to the patient's medical provider, anticipating an order of _____3_____.

Option 1	Option 2	Option 3
Secondary hypoadrenalism	Decreased	Cinacalcet
Primary hypoparathyroidism	Increased	Prednisone
Primary hyperpituitarism	Normal	Alendronate
Primary hypothyroidism		Somatropin
Secondary hyperadrenalism		Propylthiouracil
		Levothyroxine

Answers:

The nurse suspects **primary hypothyroidism**, and when reviewing T_3 and T_4 levels, the nurse would expect the levels to be **decreased**. The nurse reports the assessment findings to the patient's medical provider, anticipating an order of **levothyroxine**.

Rationale:

The patient is exhibiting clinical manifestations of *primary hypothyroidism*, indicated by a TSH level of 10 mIU/L, which is elevated (normal TSH levels 0.5 to 5 mIU/L). TSH levels would be increased if there is not enough circulating thyroid hormone (T_3 and T_4). With primary hypothyroidism, total T_3 and T_4 levels would be decreased. The patient would be prescribed levothyroxine to replace the deficiency.

Secondary hypoadrenalism is a deficiency of the adrenal glands due to other causes, such as hypopituitarism. The adrenal glands do not produce their hormones because the pituitary gland does not release adrenocorticotropic hormone (ACTH). Hypoadrenalism can result in decreased serum sodium and increased serum potassium; the serum sodium and potassium levels are normal. Primary hypoparathyroidism is a deficiency of the parathyroid gland, which regulates

Continued

CRITICAL THINKING SINGLE EPISODE CASE STUDY—CONT'D

serum calcium. The serum calcium levels were normal. Hyperpituitarism could cause an elevated TSH level; but its other hormones, such as ACTH, would cause an increased activity to its respective endocrine gland, such as the adrenals. However, serum electrolytes (sodium and potassium) are normal. If the adrenal glands were hyperactive, serum sodium would be elevated, and serum potassium would most likely be decreased. Fatigue decreases metabolism, which can cause weight gain. Secondary hyperadrenalism can result in increased serum sodium and decreased serum potassium; these were normal. Fatigue could be due to anemia; however, the patient's hemoglobin and hematocrit were normal.

References

Endocrine Society. (2019). Hypothyroidism. Retrieved from https://www.hormone.org/diseases-and-conditions/hypothyroidism

Endocrine Society. (2019). The endocrine system. https://www.hormone.org/what-is-endocrinology/the-endocrine-system

Endocrine Society. (2020). Hypoparathyroidism. Retrieved from https://www.hormone.org/diseases-and-conditions/hypoparathyroidism

Lab tests online. Retrieved from https://labtestsonline.org/

▌ REVIEW QUESTIONS

1. A patient is receiving the drug somatropin. Which drug action would the nurse anticipate?
   a. Act as an antiinflammatory agent
   b. Increase metabolic rate and oxygen consumption
   c. Stimulate growth in long bones at epiphyseal plates
   d. Promote water reabsorption from the renal tubules

2. A patient is given desmopressin acetate. The nurse knows that this drug is used to treat which condition?
   a. Gigantism
   b. Diabetes mellitus
   c. Diabetes insipidus
   d. Adrenal insufficiency

3. A patient is taking levothyroxine. For which adverse effect would the nurse monitor?
   a. Tachycardia
   b. Drowsiness
   c. Constipation
   d. Weight gain

4. A patient has just begun taking calcitriol. Which nursing action would the nurse do?
   a. Monitor the patient's weight.
   b. Monitor serum calcium levels.
   c. Teach side effects of alopecia and petechiae.
   d. Instruct the patient to avoid persons with respiratory infections.

5. A patient is given corticotropin. The nurse knows to monitor the patient for which condition?
   a. Weight gain
   b. Hyperkalemia
   c. Hypoglycemia
   d. Dehydration

6. The nurse is administering prednisone to a newly admitted patient who is taking multiple other drugs. The nurse would consider which drug interaction with prednisone? (Select all that apply.)
   a. Cardiac and central nervous system actions are increased when drug is taken with an adrenergic agent.
   b. Potassium-wasting diuretics increase potassium loss, resulting in hypokalemia.
   c. Risk for gastrointestinal bleeding and ulceration increases when drug is taken with aspirin or other nonsteroidal antiinflammatory drugs (NSAIDs).
   d. The action of prednisone is decreased when taken with phenytoin because phenytoin increases glucocorticoid metabolism.
   e. Risk for dysrhythmias and digitalis toxicity increase when drug is taken with cardiac glycosides.
   f. Dosage of antidiabetic agents may need to be decreased when taken concurrently with glucocorticoids.

7. The nurse is administering vasopressin to a patient. Which nursing intervention is indicated when administering vasopressin? (Select all that apply.)
   a. Record urinary output.
   b. Observe the patient's weight and note edema.
   c. Monitor the patient for decreased blood pressure.
   d. Closely monitor the patient's blood glucose levels.
   e. Monitor the patient's pulse for increased heart rate.
   f. Record the patient's daily calcium levels.

50

Antidiabetics

http://evolve.elsevier.com/McCuistion/pharmacology

OBJECTIVES

- Compare type 1 and type 2 diabetes mellitus.
- Describe the symptoms of diabetes mellitus.
- Differentiate symptoms of hypoglycemic reaction and hyperglycemia.
- Compare onset, peak, and duration of rapid-acting, short-acting, intermediate-acting, and long-acting insulins.
- Compare the action of oral antidiabetic drugs and their side effects.
- Differentiate between the actions of insulin, oral antidiabetic agents, and glucagon.
- Apply the Clinical Judgment [Nursing Process] to the patient taking insulin and oral antidiabetic agents.

OUTLINE

INTRODUCTION

The pancreas, located to the left of and behind the stomach, is both an exocrine and an endocrine gland. The exocrine section of the pancreas secretes digestive enzymes into the duodenum. The endocrine section has cell clusters called *islets of Langerhans*. The alpha islet cells produce glucagon, which breaks glycogen down to glucose in the liver, and the beta cells secrete insulin, which regulates glucose metabolism. Insulin is an antidiabetic agent used to control diabetes mellitus. Antidiabetic drugs are discussed in this chapter.

Antidiabetic drugs are used primarily to control diabetes mellitus, a chronic disease that affects carbohydrate metabolism. The two groups of antidiabetic agents are insulin and oral hypoglycemic (antidiabetic) drugs. Insulin, a protein secreted from the beta cells of the pancreas, is necessary for carbohydrate metabolism and plays an important role in protein and fat metabolism. The beta cells make up 75% of the pancreas, and the alpha cells that secrete glucagons—a hyperglycemic substance—occupy approximately 20% of the pancreas. Oral hypoglycemic drugs, also known as oral antidiabetic drugs (to avoid confusion with the term *hypoglycemic reaction*), are synthetic preparations that stimulate insulin release or otherwise alter the metabolic response to hyperglycemia.

DIABETES MELLITUS

Diabetes mellitus, a chronic disease that results from deficient glucose metabolism, is caused by insufficient insulin secretion from the beta cells. This results in high blood glucose (*hyperglycemia*). Diabetes mellitus is characterized by the three *p*'s: polyuria (increased urine output), polydipsia (increased thirst), and polyphagia (increased hunger). Diabetes *mellitus* is a disorder of the pancreas, whereas diabetes *insipidus* is a disorder of the posterior pituitary gland, discussed in detail in Chapter 46.

The four types of diabetes are presented in Table 50.1. Viral infections, environmental conditions, and genetic factors contribute to the onset of type 1 diabetes mellitus. Type 2 diabetes mellitus is the most common type of diabetes. Some sources suggest that heredity and obesity are the major factors that cause type 2 diabetes. With type 2 diabetes, there is some beta-cell function with varying amounts of insulin secretion. Hyperglycemia may be controlled for some type 2 diabetes patients with oral antidiabetic *(hypoglycemic)* drugs and a diet prescribed by the American Diabetes Association (ADA); however, about one-third of patients with type 2 diabetes need insulin. Patients with type 2 diabetes who use one or two oral antidiabetic drugs may become insulin dependent years later.

TABLE 50.1 Types and Occurrences of Diabetes Mellitus

Types of Diabetes Mellitus	Percentage of Occurrences
Type 1	10%–12%
Type 2	85%–90%
Secondary diabetes (medications, hormonal changes)	2%–3%
Gestational diabetes mellitus	1% (2%–5% of all pregnancies)

Certain drugs increase blood glucose and can cause hyperglycemia, called *secondary diabetes mellitus* in prediabetic persons. These include glucocorticoids (cortisone, prednisone), thiazide diuretics (hydrochlorothiazide), and epinephrine. Usually the blood glucose level returns to normal after the drug is discontinued.

During the second and third trimesters of pregnancy, the levels of the hormones progesterone, cortisol, and human placental lactogen (hPL) increase. These increased hormone levels can inhibit insulin usage. This is a contributing factor for the occurrence of gestational diabetes mellitus (GDM). Glucose is then mobilized from the tissue and from lipid storage sites. After pregnancy, the blood glucose level may decrease; however, some patients may develop diabetes mellitus, whereas others may develop type 2 diabetes in later years.

Insulin

Insulin is released from the beta cells of the islets of Langerhans in response to an increase in blood glucose. Oral glucose load is more effective in raising the serum insulin level than an intravenous (IV) glucose load. Insulin promotes the uptake of glucose, amino acids, and fatty acids and converts them to substances that are stored in body cells. Glucose is converted to glycogen in the liver and muscle for future glucose needs, thereby lowering the blood glucose level. The normal range for fasting blood glucose is 70 to 99 mg/dL for a person without diabetes. When the blood glucose level is greater than 180 mg/dL, *glycosuria*—glucose in the urine—can occur. Increased blood glucose acts as an osmotic diuretic, causing polyuria. When blood glucose remains elevated (>200 mg/dL), diabetes mellitus occurs.

Hemoglobin A1c (HbA1c), a derivative of the interaction of glucose with hemoglobin in red blood cells (RBCs), is used for the diagnosis of diabetes as recommended by the ADA. Because RBCs have a life span of approximately 120 days, the HbA1c level reflects the average glucose level for up to 3 months. In monitoring treatment, the goal is to keep the diabetic patient's HbA1c below 7%. For diagnostic purposes, an HbA1c level of 5% or less indicates that the patient does *not* have diabetes, 5.7% to 6.4% indicates prediabetes, and 6.5% or greater indicates a diagnosis of diabetes mellitus.

Beta-Cell Secretion of Insulin

The beta cells in the pancreas secrete approximately 0.2 to 0.5 units/kg/day of insulin. A patient who weighs 70 kg (154 pounds) secretes 14 to 35 units of insulin per day, although more insulin secretion may occur if the person consumes more calories. A patient with diabetes mellitus may require 0.2 to 1 units/kg/day. The higher range may be because of obesity, stress, or tissue insulin resistance.

⚠ Commercially Prepared Insulin

Early insulin preparations utilized pancreas tissue extracted from animals—either pigs or cattle. Pork insulin is structurally closer to human insulin than beef insulin. Today, insulins are currently manufactured biosynthetically using recombinant DNA technology. *Human insulin* duplicates insulin produced by the pancreas of the human body; examples of human insulin include Humulin R and Novolin N. The use of human insulin has a low incidence of both allergic effects and insulin resistance. *Human insulin analogues* are modifications of human insulin with alterations in onset and duration of action. Insulin lispro and insulin aspart are examples of human insulin analogues.

Insulins are usually administered subcutaneously. Abdominal injections of insulin are absorbed faster than those at other body sites and have been found to be more consistent.

The concentration of insulin is 100 units/mL or 500 units/mL (U100/mL or U500/mL, respectively), and the insulin is packaged in a 10-mL vial. Insulin in 500 units/mL is only available in short-acting

regular insulin. Insulin in 500 units/mL is seldom used except in emergencies and for patients with serious insulin resistance (>200 U/day). Insulin in 40 units/mL is no longer used in the United States, although it is still used in other countries. Insulin syringes are typically marked in units of 100 U/mL or 50 U/0.5 mL for insulin U100. Insulin syringes must be used for accurate dosing. To prevent dosage errors, the nurse must be certain that there is a match of the insulin concentration with the calibration of units on the insulin syringe. Before use, the patient or nurse must roll—not shake—cloudy insulin bottles to ensure that the insulin and its ingredients are well mixed. Shaking a bottle of insulin can cause bubbles, which can lead to an inaccurate dose. Insulin requirements vary; usually less insulin is needed with increased exercise, and more insulin is needed with infections and high fever.

Administration of Insulin

Insulin is a protein and cannot be administered orally because gastrointestinal (GI) secretions destroy the insulin structure. It is administered subcutaneously at a 45- to 90-degree angle. The 90-degree angle is made by raising the skin and fatty tissue, and the insulin is injected into the pocket between the fat and the muscle. In a thin person with little fatty tissue, the 45- to 60-degree angle is used. Regular insulin is the *only* type that can be administered intravenously.

The site and depth of insulin injection affect absorption. Insulin absorption is greater when given in the abdomen than when given in the thigh or buttocks. Heat and massage could increase subcutaneous absorption, and cooling the subcutaneous area can decrease absorption.

Insulin is usually given in the morning before breakfast, and it can be given several times a day. Insulin injection sites should be rotated to prevent lipodystrophy, tissue atrophy or hypertrophy, which can interfere with insulin absorption. *Lipoatrophy,* tissue atrophy, is a depression under the skin surface that primarily occurs in women and children; *lipohypertrophy,* tissue hypertrophy, is a raised lump or knot on the skin surface and is more common in men. It is frequently caused by repeated injections into the same site. The patient needs to develop a "site rotation pattern" to avoid lipodystrophy and to promote insulin absorption. There are various insulin rotation programs, such as an 8-day rotation schedule in which insulin is given at a different site each day. The ADA suggests that insulin be injected daily at a chosen site for 1 week. Injections should be 1.5 inches (a knuckle length) apart each day. When a patient requires two insulin injections a day, morning and evening, one site should be chosen on the right side (morning) and one on the left side (evening). Fig. 50.1 illustrates the sites for insulin injections. A record of injection area sites and dates administered should be kept.

Illness and stress increase the need for insulin, so doses should *not* be withheld during illness, including infections and stress. Hyperglycemia and ketoacidosis may result from insufficient insulin.

Types of Insulin

Several standard types of insulin are available that include rapid-, short-, intermediate-, or long-acting types and combinations of these. *Rapid- and short-acting insulins* are in a clear solution without any added substance to prolong insulin action. *Intermediate-acting insulins* are cloudy and may contain protamine, a protein that prolongs the action of insulin, or zinc, which also slows the onset of action and prolongs the duration of activity.

Rapid-acting insulins include insulin lispro (human analogue), human insulin aspart (recombinant DNA [rDNA] origin), insulin glulisine, and human oral inhalation insulin. Insulin lispro is formed by reversing two amino acids in human regular insulin. Insulin aspart

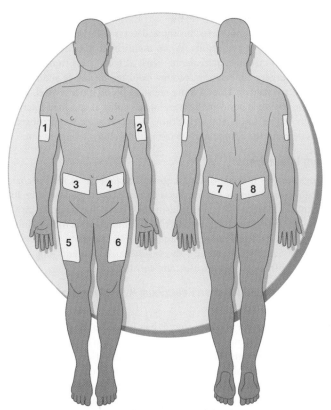

Fig. 50.1 Sites for insulin injection.

(rDNA origin) is another human insulin analogue in which a single amino acid (proline) has been substituted with aspartic acid to help prevent the molecules from clumping together to allow quicker entry into blood circulation. Insulin lispro, insulin aspart, insulin glulisine, and human oral inhalation insulin act faster than regular insulin, so they must be administered within 10 to 15 minutes before mealtime (food should be present before administering these insulins). Patients who are insulin dependent and take rapid-acting insulin usually require intermediate-acting insulin as well.

Short-acting insulin has an onset of action of 30 minutes. The peak action occurs in 1.5 to 3.5 hours, and the duration of action is 4 to 12 hours. Regular (unmodified, crystalline) insulin is short-acting insulin that can be administered intravenously or subcutaneously. Regular insulin is generally given 30 to 60 minutes before meals.

Intermediate-acting insulins include neutral protamine Hagedorn (NPH). Isophane insulins like NPH contain protamine, a protein that prolongs the action of insulin. The onset of intermediate-acting insulin is 1 to 2 hours, peak action occurs in 4 to 12 hours, and the duration of action is 14 to 24 hours.

Insulin glargine is long-acting insulin with an onset of 1 to 1.5 hours. It is evenly distributed over a 24-hour duration of action; therefore it is administered once a day, usually at bedtime. The incidence of nocturnal hypoglycemia is not as common as with other insulins because of its continuous sustained release. Insulin detemir is another long-acting insulin that peaks in 6 to 8 hours and lasts for 24 hours, and insulin degludec, a *long-acting insulin,* has an onset of 1 hour, peaks at 12 hours, and lasts for 42 hours; these insulins are analogues of human insulin. Glargine was the first long-acting rDNA-origin human insulin for patients with types 1 and 2 diabetes. Glargine, detemir, and degludec are available in a prefilled cartridge for the OptiPen insulin pen device. Some patients complain of more pain at the injection site with the administration of glargine than with NPH insulin.

Combination insulins are commercially premixed. These include NPH 70/regular 30 and NPH 50/regular 50. These combinations are widely used. The NPH 70/regular 30 is available in vials or as prefilled disposable pens. The exterior of an insulin pen resembles a fountain pen. It can be stored at room temperature for up to 10 days. With these combinations of insulin, the patient does not have to mix regular and NPH insulins as long as one of these combinations is effective. However, some patients need less than 25% or 30% regular insulin and more intermediate-acting insulin. These patients need to mix the two insulins in the prescribed proportions.

Regular insulin can be mixed with other insulin in the same syringe. However, mixing insulin can alter the absorption rate.

Insulin Resistance

Antibodies develop over time in persons taking animal insulin. This can slow the onset of insulin action and extend its duration of action. Antibody development can cause insulin resistance and insulin allergy, and obesity can also be a causative factor for insulin resistance. Skin tests with different insulin preparations may be performed to determine whether an allergic effect is present. Human and regular insulins produce fewer allergens.

Storage of Insulin

Unopened insulin vials are refrigerated until needed. Once an insulin vial has been opened, it may be kept at room temperature for 1 month or in the refrigerator for 3 months; insulin is less irritating to the tissues when injected at room temperature. Insulin vials should not be put in the freezer, nor should they be placed in direct sunlight or in a high-temperature area. Prefilled syringes should be stored in the refrigerator and should be used within 1 to 2 weeks. Opened insulin vials lose their strength after approximately 3 months.

Prototype Drug Chart: Insulins lists the pharmacologic data for the different types of insulin.

Pharmacokinetics. All insulins can be administered subcutaneously, but only regular insulin can be given intravenously. The half-life varies. Insulin is metabolized by the liver and muscle and is excreted in the urine.

Pharmacodynamics. Insulin lowers blood glucose by promoting the use of glucose by the body's cells. Insulin is also active in the storage of glucose as glycogen in muscles. The onset of action of rapid-acting insulin given subcutaneously is approximately 10 to 30 minutes. The onset of action of regular insulin is 30 minutes given subcutaneously and 15 minutes given intravenously. The onset of action of intermediate-acting insulin is 1.5 hours. The peak action of insulins is important because of the possibility of a hypoglycemic reaction (insulin shock) occurring during that time. The peak action for rapid-acting insulin is approximately 30 to 90 minutes. The peak time for regular insulin is 1.5 to 3.5 hours; for intermediate-acting insulin, the peak time is 4 to 12 hours. The nurse needs to assess for signs and symptoms of hypoglycemic reaction, such as nervousness, tremors, confusion, sweating, and increased pulse rate. Orange juice, sugar-sweetened beverages, or hard candy should be kept available to be given if a reaction occurs. If the patient is unable to ingest fast-acting carbohydrates, glucagon may be given. Glucagon promotes the breakdown of glycogen in the liver and raises blood glucose within 10 minutes.

Regular insulin can be given several times a day, especially during the regulation of insulin dosage. Intermediate- and long-acting insulins are usually administered once a day. Regular insulin can be mixed with intermediate-acting NPH insulin, especially if rapid onset of action is needed. When switching from one type of insulin to another, the patient may require a dose adjustment because human insulin has a shorter duration of action.

📄 PROTOTYPE DRUG CHART

⚠️ *Insulins*

Drug Class	Dosage

Antidiabetic: Insulin
Lispro, rapid acting
Regular, short acting
NPH, intermediate acting
Glargine, long acting
	Must be individualized and varies
	    according to patient's blood glucose
	    and health status

Contraindications	Drug-Lab-Food Interactions

Hypersensitivity, hypoglycemia,
    rosiglitazone use
Caution: Hypokalemia, fever,
    surgery or trauma, vomiting,
    infection, diarrhea, ketoacidosis,
    renal or hepatic impairment,
    breastfeeding, and older adults
	Drug: Increased hypoglycemic effect
	    with aspirin, oral anticoagulants,
	    alcohol, oral hypoglycemics, beta
	    blockers, ACE inhibitors, ARBs,
	    TCAs, MAOIs, and tetracycline;
	    decreased hypoglycemic effect
	    with thiazides, glucocorticoids,
	    oral contraceptives, thyroid drugs,
	    furosemide, bumetanide, phenytoin,
	    fluoroquinolones, smoking, and
	    green tea

Pharmacokinetics	Pharmacodynamics

Absorption: Lispro and regular,
    rapidly absorbed from subcut
    injection site; NPH is absorbed
    at a slower rate; glargine is
    absorbed at a slow, evenly
    distributed rate.
Distribution: PB: UK
Metabolism: t½: Varies with type
    of insulin
Excretion: Mostly in urine
	Lispro:
	Subcut: Onset: 15–30 min
	Peak: 30–90 min
	Duration: 3–5 h
	Regular:
	Subcut: Onset: 30 min
	Peak: 1.5–3.5 h
	Duration: 4–12 h
	NPH:
	Subcut: Onset: 1.5 h
	Peak: 4–12 h
	Duration: 14–24 h
	Glargine:
	Subcut: Onset: 1–1.5 h
	Peak: None
	Duration: 24 h

Therapeutic Effects/Uses

To control type 1 diabetes mellitus, to lower blood glucose
Mechanism of Action: Promotes use of glucose by body cells

Side Effects	Adverse Reactions

Headache, diarrhea, abdominal
    pain, infection, influenza,
    sinusitis, nasopharyngitis,
    weight gain, back pain,
    injection site reaction,
    lipodystrophy, peripheral
    neuropathy/edema
	Tachycardia, hypoglycemia, Somogyi
	    effect, hypokalemia
	Life-threatening: Insulin shock,
	    anaphylaxis, angioedema,
	    bronchospasm

ACE, Angiotensin-converting enzyme; *ARB,* angiotensin II–receptor blocker; *h,* hour; *MAOI,* monoamine oxidase inhibitor; *min,* minute; *NPH,* neutral protamine Hagedorn; *PB,* protein binding; *subcut,* subcutaneous; *t½,* half-life; *TCA,* tricyclic antidepressant; *UK,* unknown; *UTI,* urinary tract infection.

Sliding-Scale Insulin Coverage

Insulin may be administered in adjusted doses that depend on individual blood glucose test results. When the diabetic patient has extreme variances in insulin requirements—such as with stress from hospitalization, surgery, illness, or infection—adjusted dosing or sliding-scale insulin coverage provides a more constant blood glucose level. Blood glucose testing is performed several times a day at specified intervals, usually before meals and at bedtime. A preset scale usually involves directions for the administration of rapid- or short-acting insulin.

Drug Interactions

Drugs such as thiazide diuretics, glucocorticoids (cortisone preparations), thyroid agents, and estrogen increase blood glucose; therefore the insulin dosage may need adjustment. Drugs that decrease insulin needs are tricyclic antidepressants (TCAs), monoamine oxidase inhibitors (MAOIs), aspirin products, and oral anticoagulants.

Table 50.2 lists the rapid-, short-, intermediate-, and long-acting insulins with their dosages, uses, and considerations.

Side Effects and Adverse Reactions: Hypoglycemic Reactions and Ketoacidosis

When more insulin is administered than is needed for glucose metabolism, a hypoglycemic reaction, or insulin shock, occurs. The person may exhibit nervousness, trembling, and lack of coordination; have cold and clammy skin; and complain of a headache. Some patients become combative and incoherent. Giving sugar orally or intravenously increases the use of insulin, and the symptoms disappear immediately.

In response to an excessive dose of insulin, diabetic patients may develop what is known as the *Somogyi effect,* a hypoglycemic condition that usually occurs in the predawn hours of 2:00 a.m. to 4:00 a.m. wherein a rapid decrease in blood glucose during the nighttime hours stimulates a release of hormones (cortisol, glucagon, and epinephrine) to increase blood glucose by lipolysis, gluconeogenesis, and glycogenolysis. Management of the Somogyi effect involves monitoring blood glucose between 2:00 a.m. and 4:00 a.m. and reducing the bedtime insulin dosage.

Hyperglycemia on awakening is known as the *dawn phenomenon.* The patient usually awakens with a headache and reports night sweats and nightmares. Management of the dawn phenomenon involves increasing the bedtime dose of insulin.

With an inadequate amount of insulin, sugar cannot be metabolized, and fat catabolism occurs. The use of fatty acids (ketones) for energy causes ketoacidosis (diabetic acidosis or diabetic coma). Table 50.3 lists the signs and symptoms of hypoglycemic reaction and ketoacidosis.

Insulin Pen Injectors

An insulin pen resembles a fountain pen but contains a disposable needle and a disposable insulin-filled cartridge. Insulin pens come in two types, prefilled and reusable, and are considered to deliver a more accurate dose than the traditional 100-unit syringe and vial.

To operate the insulin pen, the insulin dose is obtained by turning the dial to the number of insulin units needed. The capacity of these prefilled and reusable insulin pens is 150 to 300 units, or 1.5 to 3 mL; the 1.5-mL replaceable cartridges for insulin pens are being phased out. Insulin pens available on the market include the NovoLog FlexPen (Novo Nordisk), Humalog KwikPen (Lilly), Apidra SoloSTAR (Sanofi-Aventis), Lantus SoloSTAR (Sanofi), and Levemir FlexPen (Novo Nordisk). Insulin pens tend to be more expensive than other delivery systems, but their advantages may outweigh the extra cost.

The use of insulin pens increases the patient's compliance with the insulin regimen. The convenience of the pen is most appealing, and

! TABLE 50.2   Antidiabetics: Insulins

| Drug | Half-Life | ACTION | | |
		Onset	Peak	Duration
Rapid-Acting Insulins				
Insulin lispro	1 h	15–30 min	30–90 min	3–5 h
Insulin aspart	1.5 h	10–20 min	40–50 min	3–5 h
Insulin glulisine	5–6 min	20–30 min	55 min	1.5 h
Oral inhalation insulin	2–3.5 h	12–15 min	53 min	2.5 h
Short-Acting Insulins				
Insulin regular	1.5 h	Subcut: 30 min IV: 15 min	Subcut: 1.5–3.5 h IV: 15–30 min	Subcut: 4–12 h IV: 2–6 h
Intermediate-Acting Insulins				
Insulin isophane NPH	5–6 min	1.5 h	4–12 h	14–24 h
Long-Acting Insulins				
Insulin glargine	5–6 min	1–1.5 h	None	24 h
Insulin detemir	5–6 min	1–2 h	6–8 h	24 h
Insulin degludec	25 h	1 h	12 h	42 h

h, Hour; *IV*, intravenous; *min*, minute; *NPH*, neutral protamine Hagedorn; *subcut*, subcutaneous.

TABLE 50.3   Hypoglycemic Reaction and Diabetic Ketoacidosis

Reaction	Signs and Symptoms
Hypoglycemic reaction (insulin shock)	Headache, lightheadedness Nervousness, apprehension Tremor Excess perspiration; cold, clammy skin Tachycardia Slurred speech Memory lapse, confusion, seizures Blood glucose <60 mg/dL
Diabetic ketoacidosis (hyperglycemic reaction)	Extreme thirst Polyuria Fruity breath odor Kussmaul breathing (deep, rapid, labored, distressed, dyspneic) Rapid, thready pulse Dry mucous membranes, poor skin turgor Blood glucose >250 mg/dL

>, Greater than; <, less than.

patients may choose to use the insulin pen for its portability; it can be used at work or while traveling, whereas the traditional method for administering insulin may be used at other times. The cost of insulin in vials is somewhat less than the prefilled pens, but most patients state that less injection pain is associated with insulin pens than with the traditional insulin syringe.

Insulin Pumps

Insulin pumps are an alternative to daily insulin injections used in association with blood glucose monitoring and carbohydrate counting. These computerized devices have an insulin reservoir and programming capacity to deliver continuous rapid-acting insulin in varying amounts at different times throughout a 24-hour period. These pumps are smaller than most mobile phones, and the types of insulin pumps include implantable and portable. The *implantable insulin pump* is surgically implanted in the abdomen and delivers both basal infusion (continuous release of a small amount of insulin) and bolus (additional) doses with meals. It is administered intraperitoneally. With the use of implantable insulin pumps, fewer hypoglycemic reactions occur, and blood glucose levels are controlled. Long-term effectiveness of the pump is currently under study.

External or *portable insulin pumps*, also called *continuous subcutaneous insulin infusion* (CSII), may have a tube or infusion set placed under the skin. The needle is inserted into the abdomen, upper thigh, or upper arm. This type of pump is worn outside the body and is placed in a pocket or bra. The external tubeless pump lies directly on the skin and injects insulin through the skin without tubes. The external insulin pump keeps blood glucose levels as close to normal as possible. This insulin pump is a battery-operated device that uses rapid-acting insulin, which is stored in a reservoir syringe placed inside the device. It delivers both basal insulin infusion and bolus doses with meals. Infusions are programmed by the patient. About three basal rates are programmed per day; however, the patient can adjust the rate according to changes in activity. The patient pushes a button to deliver a bolus dose at meals. Only rapid-acting insulin is used; modified (NPH) insulins are not used because of unpredictable control of blood glucose. The pump delivers exactly as much insulin as the patient programs.

The ongoing insulin delivery therapy helps decrease the risk of severe hypoglycemic reaction and maintains tight glucose (glycemic) control. Glucose levels should be monitored at least four times daily with an insulin pump. The patient must count carbohydrates and bolus doses before meals.

Most insulin pumps have a (time and day) memory of the last 24 boluses. An alarm sounds so the patient can take appropriate action when insulin is not delivered or when there is an oncoming low or high. Newer pumps have an automatic shutoff for 1 to 2 hours during periods of low blood glucose. This feature is designed for patients who may not hear the alarm and for those in whom blood glucose is allowed to elevate. The pump can be disconnected from the insertion site for bathing, swimming, and other activities; however, it is recommended that it not be discontinued for longer than 1 to 2 hours.

Success of insulin pump therapy depends on the individual's knowledge and compliance related to insulin use and the diabetic state. The person with type 1 diabetes mellitus may benefit most from the use of insulin pump therapy. This insulin delivery method is considered more effective than the use of multiple injections of regular and modified types of insulins, and it lessens the long-term diabetic complications. Studies have shown that myocardial infarction, renal disease, nerve damage, eye damage, and death have all been greatly reduced by tight blood glucose control. Also, HbA1c levels, neuropathy pain, and sexual performance have improved with the use of insulin pump control.

Insulin Jet Injectors

Insulin jet injectors shoot insulin, without a needle, directly through the skin into the fatty tissue. Because the insulin is delivered under high pressure, stinging, pain, burning, and bruising may occur. This method of insulin insertion is not indicated for children or older adults. This type of device is also expensive, costing approximately 2 to 10 times as much as the subcutaneous dose.

⚠ Oral Antidiabetic (Hypoglycemic) Drugs

First- and Second-Generation Sulfonylureas

Oral antidiabetic drugs, also called *oral hypoglycemics,* should be used by those with type 2 diabetes; persons with type 1 diabetes should not use them. However, pramlintide is used to treat both type 1 and type 2 diabetes. Patients with type 2 diabetes have some degree of insulin secretion by the pancreas. The sulfonylureas, a group of antidiabetics

---

◎ CLINICAL JUDGMENT [NURSING PROCESS]

Antidiabetics: Insulin

Concept: Glucose Regulation
- The process of maintaining normal glucose levels

Recognize Cues [Assessment]
- Identify the drugs a patient currently takes. Certain drugs such as alcohol, aspirin, oral anticoagulants, oral antidiabetics, beta blockers, tricyclic antidepressants (TCAs), monoamine oxidase inhibitors (MAOIs), and tetracycline increase the hypoglycemic effect when taken with insulin. Note that thiazides, glucocorticoids, oral contraceptives, thyroid drugs, and smoking can increase blood glucose.
- Assess the type of insulin and dosage. Note whether it is given once or multiple times a day.
- Note blood pressure (BP), heart rate, and blood glucose levels. Tachycardia and heart palpitations may occur with hypoglycemia, and hypotension may occur with hyperglycemia. Report abnormal findings.
- Determine the patient's knowledge of diabetes mellitus and use of insulins.
- Check for signs and symptoms of hypoglycemic reaction (insulin shock), hyperglycemia, or ketoacidosis.

Analyze Cues and Prioritize Hypothesis [Patient Problems]
- Hypoglycemia
- Metabolic acidosis
- Hyperglycemia
- Reduced glucose regulation
- Hyponatremia
- Fatigue

Generate Solutions [Planning]
- The patient will maintain fasting blood glucose levels within normal values (80 to 130 mg/dL).
- The patient will self-administer insulin correctly.

Take Action [Nursing Interventions]
- Monitor vital signs. Tachycardia can occur during insulin reaction.
- Determine blood glucose levels and report changes.
- Monitor the patient's hemoglobin A1c (HbA1c) to provide feedback of diabetic control.
- Prepare a teaching plan based on the patient's knowledge of the health problem, diet, and drug therapy.

Patient Teaching
General
- ⚡ Teach patients to recognize and immediately report symptoms of *hypoglycemic* (insulin) reaction—such as headache, nervousness, sweating, tremors, rapid pulse—and those of *hyperglycemic* reaction (diabetic acidosis): thirst, increased urine output, and a sweet, fruity breath odor.
- Advise patients that hypoglycemic reactions are more likely to occur during peak action time. Most diabetic patients know whether they are having a hypoglycemic reaction, but some have a higher tolerance to low blood glucose and can have a severe reaction without realizing it.
- Explain that orange juice, sugar-containing drinks, and hard candy may be used when a hypoglycemic reaction begins.
- Teach family members to administer glucagon by injection if a patient has a hypoglycemic reaction and cannot drink sugar-containing fluid.
- Inform patients that certain herbs may interact with insulin and oral antidiabetic drugs. A hypoglycemic or hyperglycemic effect might occur.
- Teach patients about the necessity of compliance with prescribed insulin therapy and diet. HbA1c provides the most accurate picture of optimal diabetic control.
- ⚡ Advise patients to carry a MedicAlert card, tag, or bracelet that indicates the health problem and the insulin dosage.

Self-Administration
- Instruct patients on how to check blood glucose with a glucometer (OneTouch AccuSure, GlucoSure, Accu-Chek).
- Teach patients about the care of insulin containers and syringes. Inform patients taking neutral protamine Hagedorn (NPH) insulin with regular insulin that regular insulin is drawn up before NPH insulin.

Diet
- Advise patients taking insulin to eat the prescribed diet on a consistent schedule. Diet information may be obtained from the American Diabetes Association (ADA) or from a nutritionist.

Evaluate Outcomes [Evaluation]
- Evaluate the effectiveness of insulin therapy by noting whether the blood glucose level is within the accepted range.
- Establish the patient's ability to perform self-care.
- Determine the patient's knowledge of the signs and symptoms of hypoglycemic or hyperglycemic reaction.

COMPLEMENTARY AND ALTERNATIVE THERAPIES
Antidiabetic Agents

- Chromium may decrease insulin requirements.
- Black cohosh may potentiate the hypoglycemic effects of insulin and oral antidiabetic drugs.
- Garlic, bitter melon, aloe, and gymnema can increase insulin levels and therefore may cause hypoglycemia when used with insulin or oral antidiabetic drugs. They can have a direct hypoglycemic effect.
- Ginseng can cause hypoglycemia when taken with insulin or an oral antidiabetic (hypoglycemic) drug.
- Bilberry may increase hypoglycemia when taken with insulin or oral antidiabetics.
- Rosemary and stinging nettle decrease the therapeutic effect of insulin and oral antidiabetic drugs (have a hyperglycemic effect).
- Milk thistle may improve insulin sensitivity.
- Hawthorn may potentiate hypoglycemia when taken with insulin or oral antidiabetics.
- Ginkgo may cause hypoglycemia when taken with glipizide, may enhance effectiveness of metformin, may increase drug level of pioglitazone, and may decrease effectiveness of tolbutamide.
- St. John's wort may alter metabolism of repaglinide and affect blood glucose level when taken with tolbutamide.

chemically related to sulfonamides but lacking antibacterial activity, stimulate pancreatic beta cells to secrete more insulin. This increases the insulin cell receptors, which increases the ability of the cells to bind insulin for glucose metabolism.

The sulfonylureas are classified as first- and second-generation drugs. First-generation sulfonylureas are divided into short-, intermediate-, and long-acting antidiabetics. Tolbutamide is a first-generation, short-acting sulfonylurea; tolazamide is a first-generation, intermediate-acting sulfonylurea; and chlorpropamide is a first-generation, long-acting sulfonylurea.

Second-generation sulfonylureas increase the tissue response to insulin and decrease glucose production by the liver. They have greater hypoglycemic potency than the first-generation sulfonylureas. Effective doses for the second-generation drugs are lower than for the first-generation drugs; the second-generation drugs also have a longer duration of action and cause fewer side effects. The second-generation drugs also have less displacement potential from protein-binding sites by other highly protein-bound drugs, such as salicylates and warfarin, than do first-generation drugs. Second-generation sulfonylureas should *not* be used when liver or kidney dysfunction is present. A hypoglycemic reaction is more likely to occur in older adults.

Second-generation sulfonylureas include glimepiride and glipizide, which directly stimulate the beta cells to secrete insulin, thus decreasing the blood glucose level. Glimepiride improves postprandial glucose levels and may be used in combination with insulin in persons with type 2 diabetes. Side effects include blurred vision, diarrhea, weight gain, and hyponatremia.

Table 50.4 lists the sulfonylureas and their dosages, uses, and considerations. Prototype Drug Chart: Glipizide lists the pharmacologic data for the second-generation sulfonylurea glipizide.

Pharmacokinetics. Glipizide is well absorbed from the GI tract and is highly protein bound. Glipizide is metabolized by the liver. The primary metabolites are inactive and are excreted mainly in urine.

PROTOTYPE DRUG CHART
Glipizide

Drug Class
Glipizide: Sulfonylurea, second generation

Dosage
Regular release:
A: PO: Initially 2.5–5 mg/d 30 min before breakfast; *maint:* 10–15 mg/d; *max:* 40 mg/d
Extended release:
A: PO: Initially 2.5–5 mg/d with breakfast; *maint:* 5–10 mg/d; *max:* 20 mg/d

Contraindications
Diabetic ketoacidosis, glipizide and sulfonamide hypersensitivity
Caution: Hepatic or renal impairment, older adults, malnutrition, adrenal or pituitary insufficiency, type 1 diabetes, trauma, infection, fever, surgery, G6PD deficiency, diarrhea, GI obstruction, vomiting, thyroid disease, breastfeeding

Drug-Lab-Food Interactions
Drug: Alcohol may produce disulfiram-like reaction (flushing, headache, sweating, nausea, violent vomiting, weakness). Beta blockers, aspirin, systemic azole antifungals, clarithromycin, oral anticoagulants, MAOIs, atypical antipsychotics, salicylates, probenecid, sulfonamides, antacids, cimetidine, clofibrate, and phenylbutazone may potentiate hypoglycemia. Oral contraceptives, thiazide diuretics, glucocorticoids, phenothiazines, and anticonvulsants may enhance hyperglycemia.
Lab: Altered liver function tests
Food: Green tea may potentiate hypoglycemia.

Pharmacokinetics
Absorption: Rapidly absorbed from GI tract
Distribution: PB: 99%
Metabolism: t½: 2–5 h
Excretion: Primarily in urine

Pharmacodynamics
Regular release: PO: Onset: 90 min
Peak: 1–3 h
Duration: 12–24 h
Extended release: PO: Onset: UK
Peak: 6–12 h
Duration: UK

Therapeutic Effects/Uses
To control hyperglycemia in type 2 diabetes mellitus
Mechanism of Action: Directly stimulates beta cells in the pancreas to secrete insulin; indirectly alters sensitivity of peripheral insulin receptors, allowing increased insulin binding

Side Effects
Drowsiness, dizziness, headache, confusion, blurred vision, anxiety, hyperhidrosis, insomnia, dyspepsia, flatulence, nausea, vomiting, constipation, diarrhea, tremor, arthralgia, myalgia, weight gain, paresthesia

Adverse Reactions
Hypoglycemia, hyponatremia, angioedema, porphyria, GI bleeding
Life-threatening: Agranulocytosis, aplastic anemia, leukopenia, thrombocytopenia, pancytopenia, hepatic failure, SIADH

A, Adult; *d,* day; *GI,* gastrointestinal; *G6PD,* glucose-6-phosphate dehydrogenase deficiency; *h,* hour; *maint,* maintenance; *MAOI,* monoamine oxidase inhibitor; *max,* maximum; *min,* minute; *PB,* protein binding; *PO,* by mouth; *SIADH,* syndrome of inappropriate antidiuretic hormone; *t½,* half-life; *UK,* unknown.

! TABLE 50.4   Antidiabetics

Drug	Route and Dosage	Uses and Considerations
First-Generation Sulfonylureas: Short Acting		
Tolbutamide	A: PO: Initially 1–2 g/d in 1–3 divided doses; *maint:* 250–2000 g/d in 1–3 divided doses; *max:* 3 g/d	For managing type 2 diabetes mellitus. May cause headache, dysgeusia, nausea, pyrosis, weight gain, hypoglycemia, weakness, and fatigue. PB: 98%; t½: 4.5–6.5 h
First-Generation Sulfonylureas: Intermediate Acting		
Tolazamide	A: PO: Initially 100–250 mg/d with breakfast; *max:* 1 g/d	For managing type 2 diabetes mellitus. May cause headache, dizziness, fatigue, weight gain, hypoglycemia, and weakness. PB: 94%; t½: 7 h
First-Generation Sulfonylureas: Long Acting		
Chlorpropamide	A: PO: Initially 250 mg/d; *max:* 750 mg/d	For managing type 2 diabetes. Avoid administration to older adults. May cause anorexia, nausea, vomiting, diarrhea, hypoglycemia, weight gain, and pruritus. PB: 60%–90%; t½: 36 h
Second-Generation Sulfonylureas		
Glipizide	See Prototype Drug Chart: Glipizide	
Glyburide	A: PO: Initially 2.5–5 mg/d conventional form or 1.5–3 mg/d micronized form with breakfast; *max:* 20 mg/d conventional form, 12 mg/d micronized form	For managing type 2 diabetes. May cause blurred vision, hypoglycemia, hyponatremia, weight gain, erythema, rash, nausea, dyspepsia, pruritus, and pyrosis. PB: 99%; t½: 10 h
Glimepiride	A: PO: Initially 1–2 mg/d with breakfast; *maint:* 1–4 mg/d; *max:* 8 mg/d	For managing type 2 diabetes. May cause dizziness, weakness, headache, nausea, weight gain, and hypoglycemia. PB: 99.5%; t½: 5–9 h
Nonsulfonylureas		
Biguanides		
Metformin	See Prototype Drug Chart: Metformin	
Alpha-Glucosidase Inhibitors		
Acarbose	A: PO: Initially 25 mg tid with first bite of each meal; *maint:* 50–100 mg tid; *max:* 150 mg/d if <60 kg, 300 mg/d if >60 kg	For managing type 2 diabetes mellitus. May cause flatulence, diarrhea, anemia, weight loss, abdominal pain, and edema. PB: UK; t½: 2 h
Miglitol	A: PO: Initially 25 mg tid with first bite of each meal; *max:* 300 mg/d	For managing type 2 diabetes. May cause rash, elevated hepatic enzymes, nausea, flatulence, diarrhea, abdominal pain, and GI bleeding. PB: <4%; t½: 2 h
Thiazolidinediones (Insulin-Enhancing Agents)		
Pioglitazone hydrochloride	A: PO: 15–30 mg/d; *max:* 45 mg/d	For managing type 2 diabetes. May cause headache, dizziness, peripheral edema, hypertension, infection, myalgia, weight gain, sinusitis, edema, pharyngitis, back pain, hypoglycemia, flatulence, and diarrhea. PB: 99%; t½: 3–7 h
Rosiglitazone	A: PO: Initially 4 mg/d; *max:* 8 mg/d	For managing type 2 diabetes. May cause headache, weight gain, edema, abdominal pain, nausea, diarrhea, bone fractures, infection, arthralgia, and hypoglycemia. PB: 99.8%; t½: 3–4 h
Meglitinides		
Repaglinide	A: PO: Initially 0.5–2 mg 30 min ac bid/qid; *max:* 16 mg/d	For managing type 2 diabetes mellitus. May cause headache, hypoglycemia, infection, back pain, arthralgia, rhinitis, dyspepsia, nausea, and diarrhea. PB: 98%; t½: 1 h
Nateglinide	A: PO: 60–120 mg tid ac; *max:* 360 mg/d	For managing type 2 diabetes mellitus. May cause infection, back pain, cough, hypoglycemia, arthropathy, and diarrhea. PB: 98%; t½: 1.5 h
Dipeptidyl Peptidase 4 Inhibitors		
Sitagliptin phosphate	A: PO: 100 mg/d; *max:* 100 mg/d	For managing type 2 diabetes. May cause headache, nasopharyngitis, stomatitis, infection, peripheral edema, nausea, abdominal pain, diarrhea, and hypoglycemia. PB: 38%; t½: 12.4 h
Saxagliptin	A: PO: 2.5–5 mg/d; *max:* 5 mg/d	For managing type 2 diabetes mellitus. May cause headache, hypoglycemia, nasopharyngitis, sinusitis, infection, peripheral edema, vomiting, and abdominal pain. PB: 0%; t½: 2.5 h
Linagliptin	A: PO: 5 mg/d; *max:* 5 mg/d	For managing type 2 diabetes mellitus. May cause hypoglycemia, diarrhea, cough, and nasopharyngitis. PB: 70%–80%; t½: 12 h
Alogliptin	A: PO: 25 mg/d; *max:* 25 mg/d	For managing type 2 diabetes mellitus. May cause headache, hypoglycemia, nasopharyngitis, infection, and elevated hepatic enzymes. PB: 20%; t½: 21 h

⚠ TABLE 50.4   Antidiabetics—cont'd

Drug	Route and Dosage	Uses and Considerations
Selective Sodium-Glucose Co-Transporter 2 Inhibitor		
Canagliflozin	A: PO: Initially 100 mg/d before first meal; *max:* 300 mg/d	For managing type 2 diabetes mellitus. May cause infection, candidiasis, diuresis, cystitis, vaginitis, polyuria, increased urinary urgency/frequency, nocturia, and hypoglycemia. PB: 99%; t½: 10.6–13.1 h
Dapagliflozin	A: PO: Initially 5 mg/d in the morning; *max:* 10 mg/d	For managing type 2 diabetes mellitus. May cause nasopharyngitis, cystitis, candidiasis, hypercholesterolemia, hypoglycemia, hyperphosphatemia, infection, vaginitis, diuresis, and prostatitis. PB: 91%; t½: 12.9 h
Empagliflozin	A: PO: Initially 10 mg/d in the morning; *max:* 25 mg/d	For managing type 2 diabetes mellitus. May cause infection, candidiasis, cystitis, vaginitis, hypercholesterolemia, hypoglycemia, diuresis, pharyngitis, hyperlipidemia, polyuria, and increased urinary frequency. PB: 86.2%; t½: 12.4 h
Ertugliflozin	A: PO: 5 mg/d in morning; *max:* 15 mg/d	For type 2 diabetes mellitus. May cause candidiasis, diuresis, infection, cystitis, dysuria, headache, hypoglycemia, and hypovolemia. PB: 94%; t½: 17 h
Amylin Analogue		
Pramlintide	Type 1: A: Subcut: Initially 15 mcg ac, then 30–60 mcg; *max:* 120 mcg/dose Type 2: A: Subcut: Initially 60 mcg ac, then 60–120 mcg; *max:* 120 mcg/dose	For managing types 1 and 2 diabetes mellitus as an adjunct to insulin therapy. May cause headache, dizziness, cough, fatigue, arthralgia, pharyngitis, nausea, anorexia, vomiting, abdominal pain, and hypoglycemia. PB: 40%; t½: 48 min
Glucagon-Like Peptide 1 Agonists		
Exenatide	Regular release: A: Subcut: Initially 5 mcg bid within 60 min before morning and evening meals; *max:* 20 mcg/d Extended release: A: Subcut: 2 mg/wk; *max:* 2 mg/wk	For managing type 2 diabetes mellitus. May cause antibody formation, fatigue, headache, restlessness, dizziness, weakness, anorexia, nausea, dyspepsia, GERD, vomiting, diarrhea, constipation, hypoglycemia, and injection site reaction. PB: UK; t½: 2.4 h
Liraglutide	A: Subcut: Initially 0.6 mg/d for 1 wk; *max:* 1.8 mg/d	For managing type 2 diabetes mellitus and obesity. May cause injection site reaction, headache, dizziness, fatigue, anorexia, dyspepsia, nausea, vomiting, diarrhea, constipation, hypoglycemia, tachycardia, palpitations, and antibody formation. PB: 98%; t½: 12–13 h
Dulaglutide	A: Subcut: Initially 0.75 mg/wk; *max:* 4.5 mg/wk	For managing type 2 diabetes mellitus. May cause fatigue, anorexia, nausea, vomiting, diarrhea, abdominal pain, dyspepsia, constipation, tachycardia, and hypoglycemia. PB: UK; t½: 5 d
Lixisenatide	A: Subcut: Initially 10 mcg/d within 1 h before morning meal; *max:* 20 mcg/d	For type 2 diabetes mellitus. May cause headache, dizziness, dyspepsia, nausea, vomiting, diarrhea, constipation, hypoglycemia, and injection site reaction. PB: UK; t½: 3 h
Semaglutide	A: Subcut: 0.25 mg/wk; *max:* 1 mg/wkA: PO: 3 mg/d 30 min before breakfast for 30 d, then may increase to 7 mg/d for 30 d, then may increase to 14 mg/d; *max:* 14 mg/d	For type 2 diabetes mellitus. May cause nausea, abdominal pain, diarrhea, vomiting, constipation, dyspepsia, flatulence, GERD, fatigue, headache, hypoglycemia, and retinopathy. PB: 99%; t½: 1 wk
Fixed-Combination Oral Antidiabetic Drugs		
Glyburide-metformin	A: PO: Initially 1.25/250 mg/d (glyburide/metformin) or bid with meals; increase dose at 2-wk intervals; *max:* 20/2000 mg/d	For managing type 2 diabetes mellitus. May cause headache, weakness, dizziness, dyspepsia, flatulence, nausea, vomiting, diarrhea, abdominal pain, and hypoglycemia. PB: metformin 0%, glyburide 99%; t½: metformin 6.2–17.6 h, glyburide 10 h
Sitagliptin-metformin	Immediate release, extended release: A: PO: Initially give dose already being taken; *max:* sitagliptin 100 mg, metformin 2000 mg/d	For managing type 2 diabetes mellitus. May cause weakness, headache, anorexia, dysgeusia, dyspepsia, abdominal pain, diarrhea, flatulence, nasopharyngitis, infection, and peripheral edema. PB: metformin 0%, sitagliptin 38%; t½: metformin 6.2–17.6 h, sitagliptin 12.4 h
Linagliptin-metformin	Immediate release: A: PO: Initially linagliptin 2.5 mg/metformin 500 mg bid with meals; *max:* 5 mg linagliptin, 2000 mg metformin	For managing type 2 diabetes mellitus. May cause dyspepsia, nausea, vomiting, diarrhea, abdominal pain, weakness, nasopharyngitis, headache, flatulence, vitamin B_{12} deficiency, and hypoglycemia. PB: metformin 0%, linagliptin 70%–80%; t½: metformin 6.2–17.2 h, linagliptin 12 h
Dapagliflozin-metformin	A: PO: Initially 5 mg dapagliflozin, 500 mg metformin/d; *max:* 10 mg dapagliflozin, 2000 mg metformin	For managing type 2 diabetes mellitus. May cause headache, diuresis, metallic taste, vomiting, dyspepsia, diarrhea, flatulence, abdominal pain, infection, pharyngitis, cystitis, candidiasis, vaginitis, and vitamin B_{12} deficiency. PB: metformin 0%, dapagliflozin 91%; t½: metformin 6.2–17.6 h, dapagliflozin 12.9

Continued

⚠ TABLE 50.4 **Antidiabetics—cont'd**

Drug	Route and Dosage	Uses and Considerations
Empagliflozin-metformin	Immediate release, Extended release: A: PO: Individualize doses bid with meals; *max:* 25 mg empagliflozin, 2000 mg metformin	For managing type 2 diabetes mellitus. May cause weakness, nausea, diarrhea, pharyngitis, headache, abdominal pain, dysgeusia, vaginitis, candidiasis, cystitis, hypercholesterolemia, vitamin B_{12} deficiency, infection, and diuresis. PB: metformin 0%, empagliflozin 86.2%; t½: metformin 6.2–17.6 h, empagliflozin 12.4 h
Dapagliflozin-saxagliptin	A: PO: Initially dapagliflozin 5 mg/d, saxagliptin 5 mg/d in morning; *max:* dapagliflozin 10 mg/d and saxagliptin 5 mg/d	For type 2 diabetes mellitus. May cause diuresis, candidiasis, cystitis, infection, pharyngitis, prostatitis, vaginitis, and headache. PB: saxagliptin 0%, dapagliflozin 91%; t½: saxagliptin 2.5 h, dapagliflozin 12.9 h
Lixisenatide-insulin glargine	A: Subcut: 15–30 units glargine, 5–10 mcg lixisenatide/d; *max:* 60 units glargine, 20 mcg lixisenatide/d	For type 2 diabetes mellitus. May cause hypoglycemia, antibody formation, infection, nausea, diarrhea, nasopharyngitis, headache, and injection site reaction. PB: UK; t½: insulin glargine 5–6 min, lixisenatide 3 h
Liraglutide-insulin degludec	A: Subcut: degludec 16–50 units, liraglutide 0.58–1.8 mg; *max:* insulin gludec 50 units, 1.8 mg liraglutide/d	For type 2 diabetes mellitus. May cause antibody formation, headache, nausea, diarrhea, nasopharyngitis, and hypoglycemia. PB: degludec 99%, liraglutide 98%; t½: degludec 25 h, liraglutide 12–13 h
Hypoglycemic Drugs		
Glucagon	A: Subcut/IM/IV: 1 mg, may repeat in 15 min as needed	For hypoglycemia. May cause nausea, vomiting, abdominal pain, hypo/hypertension, tachycardia, headache, and hypo/hyperglycemia, PB: UK; t½: IM 26–45 min, IV 8–18 min
Diazoxide	A: PO: Initially 3 mg/kg/d in 3 divided doses q8h; *maint:* 3–8 mg/kg/d in divided doses q8–12h	For hypoglycemia. May cause dizziness, nausea, vomiting, weakness, hypotension, hyperuricemia, hyperglycemia, and diabetic ketoacidosis. PB: 90%; t½: 21–36 h
Dasiglucagon	A: Subcut: 0.6 mg, may repeat in 15 min if no response	For severe hypoglycemia in patients with diabetes mellitus. May cause headache, dizziness, injection site reaction, nausea, vomiting, diarrhea, antibody formation, bradycardia, palpitations, and hypo/hypertension. PB: UK; t{1/2}: 30 min

A, Adult; *ac*, before meals; *bid*, twice a day; *d*, day; *GI*, gastrointestinal; *h*, hour; *HF*, heart failure; *maint*, maintenance; *max*, maximum; *min*, minute; *PB*, protein binding; *PO*, by mouth; *qid*, four times a day; *subcut*, subcutaneous; *t½*, half-life; *tid*, three times a day; *UK*, unknown; *URI*, upper respiratory infection; *UTI*, urinary tract infection; *wk*, week; *>*, greater than; *<*, less than.

Pharmacodynamics. Glipizide is the most common sulfonylurea drug prescribed for type 2 diabetes mellitus. It lowers blood glucose by stimulating pancreatic beta cells to secrete insulin. The onset of action usually occurs within 90 minutes, and the peak action time is 1 to 3 hours. Glipizide is normally given once a day in the morning because of its long duration of action of 24 hours.

Side Effects, Adverse Reactions, and Contraindications. The side effects of most oral antidiabetic drugs are similar to those of insulin. The major side effect of sulfonylureas is hypoglycemia. Taking antidiabetic drugs without adequate food can lead to an insulin reaction with signs and symptoms such as irritability, sweating, tremors, dizziness, confusion, extreme hunger, and anxiety. Adverse reactions include hematologic disorders such as aplastic anemia, leukopenia, and thrombocytopenia. Hyperhidrosis, nausea, vomiting, and hepatic failure may also occur. Sulfonylureas are contraindicated in type 1 diabetes (no functioning beta cells), diabetic ketoacidosis, and sulfonamide hypersensitivity. Caution is used when giving to patients during stress, surgery, fever, or severe infection.

Drug Interactions. Aspirin, oral anticoagulants, MAOIs, sulfonamides, and cimetidine can increase the action of sulfonylureas, especially first-generation ones, by binding to plasma proteins and displacing sulfonylureas. Because this causes increased free sulfonylurea, hypoglycemia can result. The action of sulfonylureas is decreased by concurrent administration of thiazide diuretics, phenothiazines, phenytoin, and corticosteroids. Patients should

be alerted not to drink alcohol while taking sulfonylureas because alcohol increases the half-life, and a disulfiram-like reaction can result (flushing, headache, sweating, nausea, vomiting, and weakness).

Nonsulfonylureas

Expanding knowledge of glucose metabolism has revealed new mechanisms for the management of type 2 diabetes. The drugs metformin and acarbose use different methods to control serum glucose levels after a meal. Unlike the sulfonylureas, which enhance insulin release and receptor interaction, these drugs affect the hepatic and GI production of glucose.

Biguanides: Metformin

Metformin is a biguanide compound that acts by decreasing hepatic production of glucose from stored glycogen. This diminishes the increase in serum glucose after a meal and blunts the degree of postprandial hyperglycemia. Metformin also decreases the absorption of glucose from the small intestine, and there is evidence that it increases insulin receptor sensitivity as well as peripheral glucose uptake at the cellular level. Unlike sulfonylureas, metformin does *not* produce hypoglycemia or hyperglycemia, although it can cause GI disturbances.

Metformin is 51% to 60% bioavailable and is absorbed primarily from the small intestine. It does not undergo hepatic metabolism and is eliminated unchanged in the urine. It is not recommended for patients with renal impairment. Monotherapy with metformin is effective; however, when combined with a sulfonylurea, the drug is useful in cases that are resistant to oral antidiabetics (hypoglycemics). Metformin therapy should be withheld for 48 hours before and after administration of IV contrast because lactic acidosis or acute renal failure may develop.

Alpha-Glucosidase Inhibitors: Acarbose and Miglitol

Acarbose acts by inhibiting the digestive enzyme in the small intestine that is responsible for the release of glucose from complex carbohydrates in the diet. By inhibiting alpha glucosidase, absorption of complex carbohydrates is delayed. Acarbose has no demonstrated systemic effects and is not absorbed into the body in significant amounts. Acarbose is intended for use in patients who do not achieve results with diet alone. Miglitol, like acarbose, inhibits alpha glucosides. Miglitol is absorbed from the GI tract. Acarbose and miglitol do not cause hypoglycemia, but if taken with a sulfonylurea or insulin, hypoglycemia could occur.

Thiazolidinediones

Pioglitazone and rosiglitazone are examples of thiazolidinedione drugs. Both drugs are contraindicated in class III and IV heart failure due to dose-related fluid retention. These two drugs can be prescribed as monotherapy or combined with other oral antidiabetic drugs. Pioglitazone can be taken in combination with sulfonylurea or insulin, and rosiglitazone may be combined with metformin (Prototype Drug Chart: Metformin). These drugs decrease insulin resistance and improve blood glucose control.

Meglitinides

Repaglinide and nateglinide are classified as meglitinide oral antidiabetic agents. They stimulate the beta cells to release insulin. The action of repaglinide and nateglinide is similar to that of sulfonylureas. These agents can be used alone or in combination with metformin for patients with type 2 diabetes mellitus; they are short-acting antidiabetic drugs. Repaglinide and nateglinide should be avoided or given with caution to patients with liver dysfunction because of a possible decreased liver metabolism rate; more of the drug could remain in the body, which could cause a hypoglycemic reaction.

Incretin Modifier

The oral antidiabetics sitagliptin phosphate and saxagliptin are classified as *incretin modifiers*, also called *dipeptidyl peptidase 4 (DPP-4) inhibitors* and *gliptins*, for treatment of type 2 diabetes mellitus. The action of DPP-4 inhibitors is to increase the level of incretin hormones, increase insulin secretion, and decrease glucagon secretion to reduce glucose production. This incretin modifier is used as an adjunct treatment with exercise and diet to reduce both fasting and postprandial plasma glucose levels. Pramlintide is given subcutaneously in abdomen and thigh immediately before each major meal. Never administer in the arm; absorption is unpredictable.

Guidelines for Oral Antidiabetic (Hypoglycemic) Therapy for Type 2 Diabetes

The following are criteria for the use of oral antidiabetic drugs:
- Onset of diabetes mellitus at 40 years of age or older
- Diagnosis of diabetes within the past 5 years
- Normal weight or overweight
- Fasting blood glucose of 200 mg/dL or less
- Fewer than 40 units of insulin required per day
- Normal renal and hepatic function

PROTOTYPE DRUG CHART

⚠ *Metformin*

Drug Class	Dosage
Metformin: Biguanide	Immediate release: A: PO: Initially 500 mg bid or 850 mg/d with meals; increase dose gradually; *max:* 2550 mg/d Extended release: A: PO: 500 mg/d with evening meal; *max:* 2500 mg/d

Contraindications	Drug-Lab-Food Interactions
Hypersensitivity, diabetic ketoacidosis, renal failure *Caution:* Pregnancy, children, infection, fever, trauma, surgery, hepatic dysfunction, adrenal insufficiency, alcohol abuse, cardiac disease, dehydration, diarrhea, breastfeeding, heart failure, older adults	Drug: ACE inhibitors, ARBs, calcium channel blockers, beta blockers, procainamide, quinidine, digoxin, MAOIs, furosemide, alcohol, cimetidine, ranitidine, oral contraceptives, sulfonamides, azole antifungals, trimethoprim, vancomycin, and quinine may potentiate hypoglycemia. Nicotine, triamterene, thiazide diuretics, niacin, phenytoin, phenothiazines, and atypical antipsychotics may cause hyperglycemia. Lab: Altered liver function tests Food: Green tea may lead to hypoglycemia.

Pharmacokinetics	Pharmacodynamics
Absorption: 51%–60% absorbed Distribution: PB: 0% Metabolism: t½: 6.2–17.6 h Excretion: Primarily in urine	PO: Onset: UK Peak: Regular release 2.5 h; extended release 4–8 h Duration: UK

Therapeutic Effects/Uses

To control hyperglycemia in type 2 diabetes mellitus

Mechanism of Action: Increases binding of insulin to receptors, improves tissue sensitivity to insulin, increases glucose transport to skeletal muscles and fatty tissues, decreases glucose production in the liver by reducing gluconeogenesis, and reduces glucose absorption from intestines

Side Effects	Adverse Reactions
Dizziness, headache, weakness, flushing, chills, dysgeusia, hyperhidrosis, metallic taste, anorexia, dyspepsia, nausea, vomiting, flatulence, diarrhea, abdominal pain, weight loss, infection, vitamin B_{12} deficiency, myalgia	Palpitations, chest pain, hypoglycemia, metabolic acidosis *Life-threatening:* Lactic acidosis, megaloblastic anemia, hepatic impairment

A, Adult; *ACE,* angiotensin-converting enzyme; *ARB,* angiotensin II–receptor blocker; *bid,* twice daily; *d,* day; *h,* hour; *MAOI,* monoamine oxidase inhibitor; *max,* maximum; *PB,* protein binding; *PO,* by mouth; *t½,* half-life; *UK,* unknown.

CLINICAL JUDGMENT [NURSING PROCESS]

Oral Antidiabetics

Concept: Glucose Regulation
- The process of sustaining normal glucose levels

Recognize Cues [Assessment]
- Identify drugs the patient currently takes. Aspirin, alcohol, sulfonamides, oral contraceptives, and monoamine oxidase inhibitors (MAOIs) increase the hypoglycemic effect; a decrease in oral antidiabetic drug may be needed. Glucocorticoids (cortisone), thiazide diuretics, and estrogen increase blood glucose.
- Note vital signs and blood glucose levels and report abnormal findings.
- Determine the patient's knowledge of diabetes mellitus and use of oral antidiabetics.

Analyze Cues and Prioritize Hypothesis [Patient Problems]
- Hypoglycemia
- Metabolic acidosis
- Hyperglycemia
- Reduced glucose regulation
- Hyponatremia
- Fatigue

Generate Solutions [Planning]
- The patient will maintain fasting blood glucose within normal serum levels (80 to 130 mg/dL).
- The patient will adhere to a prescribed diet, blood testing, and drug regimen.
- The patient will demonstrate knowledge of oral hypoglycemics and their importance.

Take Action [Nursing Interventions]
- Determine vital signs. Oral antidiabetics increase cardiac function and oxygen consumption, which can lead to cardiac dysrhythmias.
- Administer oral antidiabetics with food to minimize gastric upset.
- Monitor blood glucose levels, and report changes.
- Prepare a teaching plan based on the patient's knowledge of health problems, diet, and drug therapy.

Patient Teaching
General

- Advise patients that a hypoglycemic (insulin) reaction can occur when taking an oral hypoglycemic drug, especially sulfonylureas. Such drugs stimulate the release of insulin from beta cells of the pancreas. Oral antidiabetics are not insulin. Normally, patients with diabetes mellitus type 1 do not have functioning beta cells and should not take oral antidiabetics, only insulin. Sulfonylureas are prescribed for patients with diabetes mellitus type 2.
- ⚡ Teach patients to recognize symptoms of a hypoglycemic reaction—headache, nervousness, sweating, tremors, and rapid pulse—and hyperglycemic reaction, which include thirst, increased urine output, and a sweet, fruity breath odor.
- Explain that insulin might be needed instead of an oral antidiabetic drug during stress, surgery, or serious infection. Blood glucose levels are usually elevated during stressful times.
- Tell patients about the necessity for compliance with a diet and drug regimen.
- ⚡ Advise patients to carry a MedicAlert card, tag, or bracelet that indicates their health problem and the antidiabetic dosage.

Self-Administration
- Teach patients how to check blood glucose levels with a glucometer. Patients should record and report abnormal results.

Side Effects
- Advise patients to report side effects such as vomiting, diarrhea, and rash.

Diet
- ⚡ Caution patients not to ingest alcohol with antidiabetic drugs to avoid a hypoglycemic reaction.
- Advise patients taking oral antidiabetics to eat the prescribed diet on schedule. Delaying or missing a meal can cause hypoglycemia.
- Explain the use of orange juice, sugar-containing drinks, or hard candy when a hypoglycemic reaction begins. Explain the importance of reporting such problems to a health care provider.
- Direct patients to take oral antidiabetics with food to decrease gastric irritation.

Evaluate Outcomes [Evaluation]
- Evaluate the effectiveness of drug therapy by noting whether blood glucose levels are within the accepted range.
- Determine the patient's knowledge of the diabetic regimen.

Other Antidiabetic Agents

Exenatide and liraglutide are in a classification of antidiabetic drugs known as *incretin mimetics,* also called *glucagon-like peptide 1 (GLP-1) agonists.* These drugs improve beta-cell responsiveness, which improves glucose control in people with type 2 diabetes mellitus. The actions of exenatide and liraglutide are to enhance insulin secretion, increase beta-cell responsiveness, suppress glucagon secretion, slow gastric emptying, and reduce food intake. Exenatide and liraglutide are not a substitute for insulin and should not be administered to patients with type 1 diabetes mellitus, diabetic ketoacidosis, severe renal dysfunction, or severe GI disease. Common adverse effects that occur with exenatide include headache, dizziness, jitteriness, nausea, vomiting, and diarrhea. Exenatide is administered by injectable prefilled pens in twice-a-day dosing and has significantly improved HbA1c levels and weight loss in many patients. Liraglutide is given subcutaneously once a day in the arm, abdomen, or thigh.

Pramlintide acetate is another antidiabetic agent in a classification called *amylin analogues,* approved by the US Food and Drug Association (FDA) for adults with type 1 and type 2 diabetes mellitus. The primary purpose of pramlintide is to improve postprandial glucose control in diabetic patients who are using insulin but are unable to achieve and maintain glucose control. The actions of pramlintide are to suppress glucagon secretion, slow gastric emptying, and modulate appetite by inducing satiety. Suppression of glucagon secretion reduces postprandial hepatic glucose for approximately 3 hours. By slowing gastric emptying, the absorption rate of glucose is reduced; satiety promotes reduced food intake. Common adverse effects include dizziness, anorexia, nausea, vomiting, and fatigue. Pramlintide is administered by subcutaneous injection before meals in the abdomen or thigh; it is never given in the arm.

Hyperglycemic Drugs

Glucagon

Glucagon is a hyperglycemic hormone secreted by alpha cells of the islets of Langerhans in the pancreas. Glucagon increases blood glucose by stimulating glycogenolysis (glycogen breakdown) in the liver. It protects the body cells, especially those in the brain and retina, by providing the nutrients and energy needed to maintain body function.

Glucagon is available for parenteral use (subcutaneous, intramuscular [IM], and IV). It is used to treat insulin-induced hypoglycemia when other methods of providing glucose are not available. For example, the patient may be semiconscious or unconscious and unable to ingest sugar-containing products. Patients with diabetes who are prone to severe hypoglycemic reactions (insulin shock) should keep glucagon in the home, and family members should be taught how to administer subcutaneous or IM injections during an emergency hypoglycemic reaction. The blood glucose level begins to increase within 10 minutes after administration.

Diazoxide

Oral diazoxide, which is chemically related to thiazide diuretics, increases blood glucose by inhibiting insulin release from the beta cells and stimulating release of epinephrine from the adrenal medulla. This drug is *not* indicated for hypoglycemic reaction; rather, it is used to treat hypoglycemia caused by hyperinsulinism.

Diazoxide has a long half-life and is highly protein bound. Its onset of action is 1 hour, and the duration of action is 8 hours. Most of the drug is excreted unchanged in urine.

CRITICAL THINKING SINGLE EPISODE CASE STUDY

Cognitive Skill: Generate solutions [Matrix]
Objective: Care of a patient with type 2 diabetes mellitus prescribed an antidiabetic drug.

A 62-year-old female with type 2 diabetes mellitus presented to the emergency department and was admitted to the hospital with a diagnosis of hypoglycemic reaction and a blood sugar of 50 mg/dL. The patient's prescribed diabetic medication is repaglinide 2 mg/three times a day 30 minutes before meals. After reviewing the patient's admit orders, the nurse notes that the patient forgot the morning dose of repaglinide and took the dose at bedtime. The next morning, the patient self-administered the ordered dose of repaglinide and did not eat breakfast, causing the patient to become hypoglycemic.

The patient will be discharged today. The nurse is preparing the discharge teaching for this patient.
Use an X for the nursing instruction that is indicated (appropriate or necessary) or contraindicated (could be harmful) for this patient's care.

Nursing Instruction	Indicated	Contraindicated
Take the 2 mg dose of repaglinide, as ordered, three times a day followed by a full meal.		
You may increase the dose of repaglinide if your blood glucose increases without notifying your health care provider.		
Adverse reactions associated with repaglinide are anxiety, diarrhea, infection, headache, drowsiness, and hypoglycemic reaction. If experienced, notify your provider.		
Repaglinide is classified as an alpha-glucosidase inhibitor.		
Take your blood sugar prior to self-administering repaglinide. If it is < 70 mg/dL (3.9 mmol/L), notify your health care provider before taking the drug.		
A diabetic patient does not have to follow a special diet and may eat whatever they want.		
Instruct the patient in signs of hypoglycemic reaction: headache, nervousness, sweating, trembling, and rapid pulse. If experienced, the patient should immediately drink a glass of orange juice, take their blood sugar, and notify their health care provider.		

Answers

Nursing Instruction	Indicated	Contraindicated
Take the 2 mg dose of repaglinide, as ordered, three times a day followed by a full meal.	X	
You may increase the dose of repaglinide if your blood glucose increases without notifying your health care provider.		X
Adverse reactions associated with repaglinide are anxiety, diarrhea, infection, headache, drowsiness, and hypoglycemic reaction. If experienced, notify your provider.	X	
Repaglinide is classified as an alpha-glucosidase inhibitor.		X
Take your blood sugar prior to self-administering repaglinide. If it is < 70 mg/dL (3.9 mmol/L), notify your health care provider before taking the drug.	X	
A diabetic patient does not have to follow a special diet and may eat whatever they want.		X
Instruct the patient in signs of hypoglycemic reaction: headache, nervousness, sweating, trembling, and rapid pulse. If experienced, the patient should immediately drink a glass of orange juice, take their blood sugar, and notify their health care provider.	X	

Rationale

Repaglinide is an antidiabetic drug. It is classified as a meglitinide drug whose purpose is to treat type 2 diabetes by working in the pancreas to sequentially block certain potassium channels, create an influx of calcium, and induce insulin secretion. It is usually taken in tablet form and should be taken as ordered by the patient's provider, with food, to avoid hypoglycemic reactions. Adverse reactions are correctly listed as anxiety, diarrhea, infection, headache, drowsiness, and hypoglycemic reaction. In following correct diabetes care, the patient should perform a glucometer check prior to administration and, if it is less than 70 mg/dL, hold the drug and notify their health care provider to avoid a hypoglycemic reaction. It is important for the nurse to review symptoms of a hypoglycemic reaction, correctly stated as headache, nervousness, sweating, trembling, and rapid pulse. It is also important to tell the patient to drink a glass of orange juice, which will increase the patient's blood sugar, and to repeat the glucometer check and notify their health care provider. The patient should never increase or decrease the ordered dose of repaglinide without health care provider knowledge and new orders. Repaglinide is not classified as an alpha-glucosidase inhibitor. It is very important for a diabetic to follow a diabetic diet as ordered by their health care provider.

References

McCuistion, L., et al, *Pharmacology: A Patient-Centered Nursing Process Approach* (10th ed), 1922, Chapter 47, pp. 623–635; Burchum R., & Rosenthal L. D., *Lehne's Pharmacology for Nursing Care* (10th ed), 2019, Chapter 57, pp. 674–710.

REVIEW QUESTIONS

1. A patient is diagnosed with type 2 diabetes mellitus. The nurse is aware that which statement is true about this patient?
   a. The patient is most likely a teenager.
   b. The patient is most likely a child younger than 10 years.
   c. Heredity and obesity are major causative factors.
   d. Viral infections contribute most to disease development.

2. Antidiabetic drugs are designed to control signs and symptoms of diabetes mellitus. The nurse primarily expects a decrease in which?
   a. Blood glucose
   b. Fat metabolism
   c. Glycogen storage
   d. Protein mobilization

3. A patient is to receive insulin before breakfast, and the time of breakfast tray delivery is variable. The nurse knows that which insulin should not be administered until the breakfast tray has arrived and the patient is ready to eat?
   a. NPH
   b. Lispro
   c. Glargine
   d. Regular

4. A patient is receiving a daily dose of NPH insulin at 7:30 a.m. The nurse expects the peak effect of this drug to occur at what time?
   a. 8:15 a.m.
   b. 10:30 a.m.
   c. 5:00 p.m.
   d. 11:00 p.m.

5. A patient is prescribed glipizide. The nurse knows that which side effects and adverse effects may be expected? (Select all that apply.)
   a. Tachypnea
   b. Tachycardia
   c. Increased alertness
   d. Increased weight gain
   e. Visual disturbances
   f. Hyperhidrosis

6. A nurse is teaching a patient how to recognize symptoms of hypoglycemia. Which symptoms should be included in the teaching? (Select all that apply.)
   a. Headache
   b. Nervousness
   c. Bradycardia
   d. Sweating
   e. Thirst
   f. Sweet breath odor

7. A patient is newly diagnosed with type 1 diabetes mellitus and requires daily insulin injections. Which instructions should the nurse include in the teaching of insulin administration? (Select all that apply.)
   a. Teach family members how to administer glucagon by injection when the patient has a hyperglycemic reaction.
   b. Instruct the patient about the necessity for compliance with prescribed insulin therapy.
   c. Teach the patient that hypoglycemic reactions are more likely to occur at the onset of action time.
   d. Instruct the patient in the care and handling of the insulin container and syringe.

51

Urinary Disorders

http://evolve.elsevier.com/McCuistion/pharmacology

OBJECTIVES

- Compare the groups of drugs that are urinary antiseptics and antiinfectives.
- Describe the side effects and adverse reactions to urinary antiseptics and antiinfectives.

- Differentiate the uses for a urinary analgesic, a urinary stimulant, and a urinary antispasmodic/antimuscarinic/anticholinergic.
- Apply the Clinical Judgment [Nursing Process], including teaching, to nursing care of the patient receiving urinary antiseptic/antiinfective drugs.

OUTLINE

INTRODUCTION

This chapter discusses agents prescribed to combat disease-producing microorganisms. Included in this unit are antiseptics, antibacterials, analgesics, stimulants, antispasmodics, antimuscarinics, anticholinergics, and other drugs for urinary tract disorders. Common disorders of the urinary tract are presented in this unit. Urinary tract infections (UTIs), acute cystitis, and pyelonephritis are focused on.

Disease-producing organisms may be gram-positive or gram-negative bacteria, viruses, or fungi. The degree to which they are pathogenic depends on the microorganism and its virulence. This chapter addresses drugs for urinary tract disorders.

Fig. 51.1 illustrates the various sites of infection in the upper and lower urinary tracts. Fig. 51.2 illustrates the female and male urethra, showing the female urethra being the shortest.

The largest number of urinary tract disorders are caused by urinary tract infections (UTIs), microbial infections of any part of the urinary tract. The infection may be referred to as an *upper UTI*, such as pyelonephritis, or a *lower UTI*, such as cystitis, urethritis, or prostatitis. A group of drugs called urinary antiseptics/ antiinfectives prevents bacterial growth in the kidneys and bladder, but these drugs are not effective for systemic infections. When given in lower dosages, urinary antiseptics/antiinfectives have a bacteriostatic effect—that is, they inhibit bacterial growth. When given in higher dosages, they also have a bactericidal (bacteria killing) effect. Urinary antiseptics/antiinfectives are presented in this chapter, along with urinary analgesics, which relieve pain and burning in the urinary tract; urinary stimulants, agents that increase the tone of urinary muscles; and urinary antispasmodics/antimuscarinics. Chapter 26 presents further discussions of antibiotics used to treat UTIs, such as fluoroquinolones and sulfonamides. Diuretics are discussed in Chapter 38.

Acute cystitis, a lower UTI, frequently occurs in female patients because of the short urethra. It is more common in women of childbearing age, older women, and young girls. Acute cystitis is commonly caused by *Escherichia coli* (also called *E. coli*). Other bacterial causes include the gram-positive *Staphylococcus saprophyticus* and gram-negative *Klebsiella, Proteus,* and *Pseudomonas* species. Symptoms of cystitis include pain and burning on urination and urinary frequency and urgency. A urine culture is usually obtained before the start of any antiinfective/antibiotic drug therapy. In male patients, a lower UTI is most likely prostatitis with symptoms similar to cystitis.

Acute pyelonephritis, an upper UTI, is commonly seen in women of childbearing age, older women, and young girls. *E. coli* is the most common organism to cause pyelonephritis. Symptoms include chills, high fever, flank pain, pain during urination, urinary frequency and urgency, and pyuria. The bacterial count in the urine is greater than 100,000 bacteria/mL. In severe cases, the patient may be hospitalized and may receive intravenous (IV) antibiotics (e.g., an aminoglycoside or piperacillin-tazobactam).

Commonly used agents for treating UTIs are nitrofurantoin and trimethoprim-sulfamethoxazole (TMP-SMZ). Treatment may consist of a single double-strength dose of the chosen drug, a 3-day course, or the traditional method of 7 to 14 days of drug dosing. Fosfomycin tromethamine, a nitrofurantoin prototype drug, is effective for UTIs as a single-dose treatment. Other agents used to treat UTIs include third-generation cephalosporins (cefixime, cefpodoxime

proxetil, or ceftibuten), fourth-generation cephalosporins (cefepime), fifth-generation cephalosporins (ceftolozane-tazobactam), and fluoroquinolones, such as ofloxacin, ciprofloxacin, and levofloxacin. For uncomplicated UTIs, fluoroquinolones, especially levofloxacin, may be used only when other options are not available as the risk generally outweighs the benefits. With severe UTIs, IV drug therapy followed by oral drug therapy is usually recommended.

URINARY ANTISEPTICS/ANTIINFECTIVES AND ANTIBIOTICS

Urinary antiseptics/antiinfectives are limited to the treatment of UTIs. Drug action occurs in the renal tubule and bladder, where it is effective in reducing bacterial growth. A urinalysis, as well as a culture and sensitivity test, is usually performed before the initiation of drug therapy. As bactericidal agents, these drugs have the potential to cause superinfections. The urinary antiseptics/antiinfectives are fosfomycin tromethamine, nitrofurantoin, methenamine hippurate, trimethoprim, ertapenem, sulfonamides, fluoroquinolones, beta-lactams, polypeptides, aminoglycosides, and cephalosporins.

Trimethoprim and Trimethoprim-Sulfamethoxazole

Trimethoprim can be used alone for the treatment of UTIs, but it is usually used in combination with a sulfonamide, sulfamethoxazole (the combined generic preparation is called *TMP-SMZ*), to prevent the occurrence of trimethoprim-resistant organisms. TMP-SMZ is discussed further in Chapter 26, and it is used in the treatment and prevention of acute and chronic UTIs. The amount of TMP-SMZ in the prostatic fluid is about two to three times greater than the amount in the vascular fluid.

Pharmacokinetics. TMP-SMZ is well absorbed from the gastrointestinal (GI) tract. The drug may be taken with food, water, or milk to decrease GI distress, which includes anorexia, nausea, vomiting, abdominal pain, and diarrhea. TMP-SMZ is moderately protein bound at 44% for TMP and 70% for SMZ. The half-life is 8 to 10 hours for TMP and 6 to 12 hours for SMZ.

Pharmacodynamics. The combination of trimethoprim and sulfamethoxazole in a 1:5 ratio increases its bactericidal activity. This drug combination produces slow-acting bactericidal effects against most gram-positive and gram-negative organisms, especially strains of *S. aureus*, including methicillin-resistant *S. aureus* (MRSA), and also *Shigella* and *Proteus* species. The peak action of TMP-SMZ is 1 to 4 hours.

The nursing process for TMP-SMZ is applicable to the other urinary antiseptics/antiinfectives.

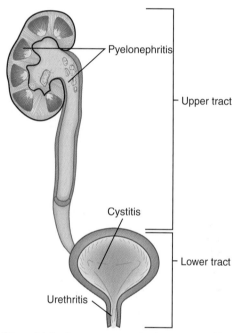

Fig. 51.1 Sites of infectious processes in the upper and lower urinary tracts.

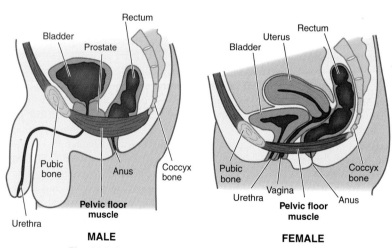

Fig. 51.2 Shorter urethra in the female than in the male.

CLINICAL JUDGMENT [NURSING PROCESS]

Urinary Antiinfectives

Concept: Infection
- A condition in which infective microorganisms have invaded a part of the body

Recognize Cues [Assessment]
- Obtain a history from the patient of clinical problems with urinary tract infection (UTI), incontinence, or other urinary tract disorders.
- Assess the patient for signs and symptoms of UTI: pain or burning sensation on urination and frequency and urgency of urination.
- Monitor complete blood count (CBC) regularly in patients on long-term therapy.
- Monitor urine culture and sensitivity results.
- Assess renal and hepatic function.
- Determine urine pH. A pH of 5.5 is desired, but alkalization of the urine is not recommended.

Analyze Cues and Prioritize Hypothesis [Patient Problems]
- Acute pain
- Discomfort
- Decreased sensation
- Changes in elimination

Generate Solutions [Planning]
- The patient will state within 10 days that she does not have pain or burning upon urination.

Take Action [Nursing Interventions]
- Monitor urinary output and urine specific gravity. Careful attention to output is required when administering urinary antiseptics to patients with anuria and oliguria. Report promptly any decrease in urine output.
- Obtain urine culture to identify infecting organism before initiation of drug therapy to treat UTI.
- Observe the patient for side effects and adverse reactions to urinary antiseptic drugs. Peripheral neuropathy (tingling, numbness of extremities) may result from renal insufficiency (inability to excrete drug) or long-term use of nitrofurantoin. Peripheral neuropathy may be irreversible.

Patient Teaching
General
- Teach patients not to crush tablets or open capsules.
- Advise patients to rinse the mouth thoroughly after taking oral nitrofurantoin. The drug can stain teeth.
- Encourage patients to avoid antacids because they interfere with drug absorption.

- Teach patients to shake suspensions well before administration and to protect them from freezing.
- ⚡ Warn patients not to drive a motor vehicle or operate dangerous machinery; the drug may cause drowsiness.
- Advise female patients to immediately report pregnancy to their health care provider.

Diet
- Inform patients to increase fluids and take the drug with food to minimize GI upset.

Side Effects
- Advise the patient to drink an adequate amount of fluids.
- Encourage the patient to report any signs of secondary fungal or bacterial infection (superinfection) such as stomatitis or anogenital discharge or itching.

Nitrofurantoin
- Alert the patient that urine may turn a harmless brown color.
- Direct the patient to report a sudden onset of dyspnea, chest pain, cough, fever, and chills to health care provider.

Methenamine
- Educate patients to drink cranberry juice, eat plums, or take vitamin C (with approval of the health care provider) to keep urine acidic. Foods that are alkaline, such as milk and some vegetables, may increase urine pH. Urine pH should be less than 5.5 for the antiseptic to be effective.

Fluoroquinolones
- ⚡ Warn patients to avoid operating hazardous machinery or driving a car while taking the drug, especially if dizziness is present.
- Encourage patients to take the drug with food and to avoid antacids because they interfere with drug absorption.
- Direct patients to report any signs of superinfection or secondary fungal or bacterial infection.

Trimethoprim and Trimethoprim-Sulfamethoxazole
- Tell patients to avoid excessive exposure to sunlight when taking nitrofurantoin.

Evaluate Outcomes [Evaluation]
- Evaluate the effectiveness of the urinary antiinfectives in alleviating UTI. The patient should be free of side effects and adverse reactions to the drug.

Methenamine

Methenamine produces a bactericidal effect when the urine pH is less than 5.5. It is effective against gram-positive and gram-negative organisms, especially *E. coli*, *Enterococcus* and *Proteus* species, and *Pseudomonas aeruginosa*. It is used for chronic UTIs. Methenamine should not be taken with sulfonamides because crystalluria is likely to occur. Methenamine is absorbed readily from the GI tract, and approximately 90% of the drug is excreted in the urine unchanged. Methenamine forms ammonia and formaldehyde in acid urine; therefore the urine needs to be acidified to exert a bactericidal action. Cranberry juice (several 8-ounce glasses per day), ascorbic acid, and ammonium chloride can be taken to decrease the urine pH.

Nitrofurantoin

Nitrofurantoin was first prescribed to treat UTIs in 1953. It is bacteriostatic or bactericidal, depending on the drug dosage, and it is effective against many gram-positive and gram-negative organisms, especially *E. coli*. It is used to treat cystitis and UTIs. Nitrofurantoin is usually taken with food to decrease GI distress, which includes anorexia, nausea, vomiting, abdominal pain, and diarrhea. Decreased absorption occurs when the drug is taken with antacids. With normal renal function, nitrofurantoin is rapidly eliminated because of its short half-life; however, it accumulates in the serum with urinary dysfunction.

When nitrofurantoin is given in low doses for prophylactic use, the drug has a bacteriostatic effect. However, higher concentrations of nitrofurantoin cause a bactericidal effect, and it is effective against many gram-positive and gram-negative organisms such as *E. coli*, *Staphylococcus aureus*, streptococci, and *Neisseria* and *Klebsiella* species. If sudden onset of dyspnea, chest pain, cough, fever, and chills develops, the patient should contact the health care provider. Symptoms resolve after discontinuing the drug.

Fluoroquinolones (Quinolones)

Fluoroquinolones are one of the groups of urinary antibacterials that are effective against strains of *Acinetobacter, Chlamydia, Clostridium, Klebsiella, Staphylococcus,* and *Streptococcus* species that cause lower UTIs; they include ciprofloxacin, ofloxacin, and levofloxacin. Fluoroquinolones should be reserved for patients who have no alternative treatment options due to their harsh adverse reactions of tendon rupture, peripheral neuropathy, central nervous system effects, and exacerbation of myasthenia gravis. The drug dosage must be decreased when renal dysfunction is present. The half-lives of these drugs are ordinarily 2 to 8 hours, but half-lives are prolonged in patients with renal dysfunction. Table 51.1 lists the urinary antiseptics/antiinfectives and their dosages, uses, and considerations. Due to the serious adverse reactions of fluoroquinolones, they are used with caution for complicated UTIs and acute pyelonephritis and levofloxacin is only used for uncomplicated UTIs when no other options are available. Levofloxacin is illustrated in Prototype Drug Chart: Levofloxacin in Chapter 26.

Side Effects and Adverse Reactions

Nitrofurantoin. Side effects of nitrofurantoin include GI disturbances such as anorexia, nausea, vomiting, diarrhea, and abdominal pain and pulmonary reactions such as dyspnea, chest pain, and cough.

Methenamine. Methenamine has side effects that include nausea, dysuria, hematuria, and crystalluria.

Trimethoprim-Sulfamethoxazole. GI symptoms such as anorexia, nausea, and vomiting and skin problems such as rash and pruritus can accompany TMP-SMZ use.

Fluoroquinolones. Side effects of ciprofloxacin and ofloxacin include headaches, dizziness, nausea, vomiting, diarrhea, visual impairment, rash, and pruritus. Serious adverse reactions include peripheral neuropathy, tendinitis, and tendon rupture. Fluoroquinolones may exacerbate muscle weakness in patients with myasthenia gravis. Direct patients to stop taking fluoroquinolones immediately if experiencing serious adverse reactions and notify health care provider.

TABLE 51.1	**Antiseptics and Urinary Antiinfectives**	
Generic Name	**Route and Dosage**	**Uses and Considerations**
Fosfomycin tromethamine	Cystitis: A/Females: PO: 3-g packet dissolved in 4 oz water as a single dose	For cystitis and UTIs in females. May cause headache, rhinitis, vaginitis, dysuria, hematuria, superinfection, CDAD, nausea, and diarrhea. PB: 0%; t½: 3–9 h
Methenamine hippurate	A: PO: 1 g bid pc and at bedtime; *max:* 2 g/d	For cystitis and UTIs. May cause crystalluria, rash, nausea, hematuria, dysuria, elevated hepatic enzymes, and urinary frequency. PB: UK; t½: 4 h
Nitrofurantoin	A: PO: 50–100 mg q6h with meals and at bedtime for 3–7 d	For cystitis and UTIs. May cause headache, dizziness, drowsiness, peripheral neruopathy, anorexia, abdominal pain, nausea, vomiting, diarrhea, elevated hepatic enzymes, brown urine discoloration, blood dyscrasias, and CDAD. PB: 20%–60%; t½: 20 min
Trimethoprim	UTIs: A: PO: 100 mg q12h or 200 mg/d for 10–14 d; *max:* 200 mg/d	For cystitis and UTIs. May cause rash, pruritus, diarrhea, nausea, vomiting, superinfection, and CDAD. PB: 45%; t½: 8–10 h
Ertapenem	UTI: A: IM/IV: 1 g/d for 10–14 d; *max:* 1 g/d	For UTIs, community-acquired pneumonia, and intraabdominal, skin, and diabetic foot infections. May cause headache, drowsiness, confusion, cough, agitation, nausea, vomiting, diarrhea, abdominal pain, dysuria, and CDAD. PB: 95%; t½: 4.5 h
Sulfonamides		
Trimethoprim sulfamethoxazole (TMP-SMZ)	UTIs: A: PO: TMP 160 mg, SMZ 800 mg q12h for 3–14 d A: IV: 8–10 mg/kg/d in 2–4 divided doses for 7–14 d	For cystitis, UTIs, bronchitis, otitis media, pneumonia, traveler's diarrhea, and shigellosis. May cause rash, pruritus, headache, anorexia, nausea, vomiting, abdominal pain, diarrhea, crystalluria, arthralgia, myalgia, and CDAD. PB: TMP, 44%; SMZ, 70%; t½: TMP, 8–10 h; SMZ, 6–12 h
Quinolones (Fluoroquinolones)		
Ciprofloxacin	UTIs: Regular release: A/Females: PO: 250 mg q12h for 3 d; *max:* 1.5 g/d Extended release: A females: PO: 500 mg/d for 3 d; *max:* 1 g/d A: IV: 200–400 mg q12h for 7–14 d; *max:* 1.2 g/d	For respiratory, urinary, skin, bone, joint, eye, ear, intradominal, and anthrax infections. May cause irritability, conjunctival hyperemia, ocular pruritus, visual impairment, pharyngitis, tendon rupture, dysgeusia, nausea, vomiting, abdominal pain, diarrhea, CDAD, superinfection, and corneal deposits. PB: 20%–40%; t½: 4 h
Ofloxacin	UTIs: A: PO: 200 mg q12h for 3–10 d; *max:* 800 mg/d	For respiratory, urinary, eye, ear, bacterial prostatitis, STI, and skin infections. May cause headaches, dizziness, insomnia, dysgeusia, nausea, vomiting, diarrhea, CDAD, pruritus, rash, visual impairment, peripheral neuropathy, polyuria, candidiasis, superinfection, tendinitis, and tendon rupture. PB: 20%–32%; t½: 4–8 h
Beta-Lactam		
Aztreonam	UTIs: A: IM/IV: 500 mg to 1 g q8–12h; *max:* 8 g/d	For bacteremia and intraabdominal, respiratory, skin, gynecologic, and UTIs. May cause injection site reaction, CDAD, neutropenia, rash, abdominal pain, fever, cough, wheezing, elevated hepatic enzymes, and nasal congestion. PB: 56%–65%; t½: 1.7 h

TABLE 51.1   Antiseptics and Urinary Antiinfectives—cont'd

Generic Name	Route and Dosage	Uses and Considerations
Polypeptide		
Polymyxin B sulfate	UTIs: A: IV: 15,000–25,000 units/kg/d in divided doses q12h or as a continuous infusion; *max:* 25,000 units/kg/d A: IM: 25,000–30,000 units/kg/d in divided doses q4–6h; *max:* 30,000 units/kg/d	For meningitis, bacteremia, and ophthalmic and urinary tract infections. May cause dizziness, drowsiness, confusion, blurred vision, headache, paresthesias, hematuria, superinfection, neurotoxicity, and nephrotoxicity. PB: UK; t½: 4–6 h
Aminoglycoside		
Plazomicin	A: IV: 15 mg/kg q24h for 4–7 d Trough: Less than 3 mcg/mL	For complicated UTIs including pyelonephritis. May cause headache, diarrhea, hypertension, vomiting, nausea, and renal failure. PB: 20%; t½: 3–4 h
Cephalosporin		
Cefiderocol	A: IV: 2 g q8h for 7-14 d; *max:* 6 g/d	For UTIs. May cause dry mouth, nausea, vomiting, diarrhea, constipation, rash, elevated hepatic enzymes, hypo/hyperkalemia, hypocalcemia, hypomagnesemia, and injection site reaction. PB: 40%–60%; t½: 2–3 h
Combinations		
Imipenem and cilastatin sodium	UTIs: A: IV: 500–1g mg q6h or 1 g q8h; *max:* 4 g/d	For respiratory, bone, intraabdominal, urinary, gynecologic, skin, and joint infections; septicemia; and endocarditis. May cause anuria, seizures, nausea, diarrhea, oliguria, candidiasis, injection site reaction, and CDAD. PB: imipenem, 20%; cilastatin, 40%; t½: 1 h
Imipenem, cilastatin, and relebactam	UTIs: A: IV: imipenem 500 mg, cilastatin 500 mg, relebactam 250 mg q6h for 4–14 d	For UTIs and complicated intra-abdominal infections. May cause headache, hypertension, fever, erythema, nausea, diarrhea, phlebitis, injection site reaction, anemia, hypokalemia, hyponatremia, and elevated hepatic enzymes. PB: imipenem 20%, cilastatin 40%, relebactam 22%; t½: imipenem 1 h, cilastatin 3.9–6.3 h, relebactam 1.2 h
Ceftazidime and avibactam	UTIs: A: IV: 2.5 g (ceftazidime 2 g and avibactam 500 mg) q8h over 2 h for 7–14 d; *max:* 7.5 g/d (6 g ceftazidime and 1.5 g avibactam)	For intraabdominal, respiratory, and UTIs. May cause anxiety, headache, dizziness, nausea, constipation, abdominal pain, diarrhea, vomiting, pruritis, CDAD, hypokalemia, and superinfection. PB: ceftazidime 10%, avibactam 5%–8%; t½: ceftazidime 1.5–2 h, avibactam 2 h
Ceftolozane and tazobactam	UTIs: A: IV: 1.5 g (1 g ceftolozane and 0.5 g tazobactam) q8h for 7 d; *max:* 9 g/d (6 g ceftolozane and 3 g tazobactam)	For respiratory and intraabdominal infections, and UTIs. May cause headache, insomnia, dyspnea, nausea, vomiting, diarrhea, constipation, intracranial bleeding, renal failure, elevated hepatic enzymes, CDAD, hypokalemia, and fever. PB: ceftolozane 16%–21%, tazobactam 30%; t½: ceftolozane 3–4 h, tazobactam 2–3 h
Meropenem and vaborbactam	A: IV: 2 g meropenem, 2 g vaborbactam q8h up to 14 d; *max:* 6 g meropenem, 6 g vaborbactam/d	For UTIs. May cause headache, fever, injection site reaction, phlebitis, hypokalemia, nausea, elevated hepatic enzymes, diarrhea, superinfection, and CDAD. PB: meropenem, 2%; vaborbactam, 33%; t½: meropenem, 1.22 h; vaborbactam, 1.68 h

A, Adult; *bid,* twice a day; *BUN,* blood urea nitrogen; *CDAD, Clostridium difficile*–associated diarrhea; *d,* day; *GI,* gastrointestinal; *h,* hour; *IM,* intramuscular; *IV,* intravenous; *max,* maximum dosage; *min,* minute; *mo,* month; *PB,* protein binding; *pc,* after meals; *PO,* by mouth; *q,* every; *qid,* four times a day; *t½,* half-life; *UK,* unknown; *UTI,* urinary tract infection; *y,* year; *>,* greater than.

Drug-Drug Interactions

The following drug-drug interactions can occur with the use of urinary antiseptics/antiinfectives:

- Antacids decrease nitrofurantoin absorption.
- Sodium bicarbonate inhibits the action of methenamine.
- Methenamine taken with sulfonamides increases the risk of crystalluria.
- Most urinary antiseptics cause false-positive Clinitest (glucose urine test) results.

URINARY ANALGESICS

Phenazopyridine

Phenazopyridine hydrochloride, an azo dye, and dimethyl sulfoxide (also called DMSO) are urinary analgesics that are used to relieve the urinary pain, burning sensation, frequency, and urgency of urination that are symptomatic of cystitis. Phenazopyridine can cause methemoglobinemia, hemolytic anemia, and renal and hepatic dysfunction. The urine becomes a harmless reddish-orange because of the phenazopyridine dye. Phenazopyridine can alter the glucose urine test (Clinitest); therefore a blood test should be used to monitor glucose levels. Dimethyl sulfoxide may cause a garlic-like taste and skin hyperpigmentation.

URINARY STIMULANTS

When bladder function is decreased or lost as a result of (1) a neurogenic bladder (a dysfunction caused by a lesion of the nervous system), (2) a spinal cord injury (paraplegia, hemiplegia), or (3) a severe head injury, a parasympathomimetic may be used to stimulate micturition (urination). The drug of choice, bethanechol chloride, is a urinary stimulant also known as a *direct-acting parasympathomimetic.* The drug action is to increase bladder tone by increasing tone of the detrusor urinal muscle, which produces a contraction strong enough to stimulate urination. This drug is contraindicated in patients with a peptic ulcer. Bethanechol is discussed in detail in Chapter 16.

URINARY ANTISPASMODICS/ANTIMUSCARINICS/ANTICHOLINERGICS

Urinary tract spasms resulting from infection or injury can be relieved with antispasmodics that have a direct action on the smooth muscles of the urinary tract. This group of drugs—mirabegron, oxybutynin, and flavoxate—is contraindicated for use if urinary or GI obstruction is present or if the patient has glaucoma. Caution should be used when given to older adults, tobacco smokers, or contact lens wearers, as well as the patient who has a bladder flow obstruction, prostatic hypertrophy, GERD, or hepatic disorder. Antispasmodics have the same effects as antimuscarinics, agents that block parasympathetic nerve impulses; parasympatholytics; and

anticholinergics (see Chapter 16). Tolterodine tartrate, trospium chloride, and solifenacin succinate are antimuscarinic/anticholinergic drugs used to control an overactive bladder, which causes frequency in urination. These drugs also decrease urgency and urinary incontinence. Antispasmodics/antimuscarinics/anticholinergics frequently have side effects including blurred vision, headache, dizziness, dry mouth, constipation, and tachycardia. The patient taking these drugs should be taught to report urinary retention, severe dizziness, blurred vision, palpitations, and confusion. Table 51.2 lists drugs that are urinary analgesics, stimulants, and antispasmodics/antimuscarinics/anticholinergics. Solifenacin is the most frequently prescribed drug for overactive bladder and urinary incontinence. See Prototype Drug Chart: Solifenacin Succinate.

TABLE 51.2　Urinary Analgesics, Stimulants, and Antispasmodics

Generic	Route and Dosage	Uses and Considerations
Urinary Analgesics		
Phenazopyridine hydrochloride	A: PO: 200 mg tid pc for 2 days; *max:* 600 mg/d	For cystitis, dysuria, and urgency. May cause headache, contact lens discoloration, urine discoloration, elevated hepatic enzymes, and rash. Do not use long term for undiagnosed urinary tract pain. PB: UK; t½: UK
Dimethyl sulfoxide	Bladder instillation: 50 mL of 50% sol retained for 15 min; repeat q2wk until relief	For cystitis. May cause infection, bladder discomfort and spasm, cystitis, dysgeusia, and anaphylaxis. PB: UK; t½: UK
Urinary Stimulants		
Bethanechol chloride	A: PO: 5–10 mg q1h until effective response or 50 mg given; *maint:* 10–50 mg tid/qid 1 h ac or 2 h pc; *max:* 200 mg/d A: Subcut: 5 mg tid/qid PRN; *max:* 40 mg/d	For urinary retention and neurogenic bladder. May cause headache, dizziness, flushing, nausea, vomiting, diarrhea, abdominal cramps, urinary urgency and frequency. PB: UK; t½: UK
Urinary Antispasmodics		
Flavoxate hydrochloride	A: PO: 100–200 mg tid/qid	For urinary urgency and incontinence, dysuria, and overactive bladder. May cause headache, drowsiness, confusion, dry mouth, nausea, vomiting, blurred vision, palpitations, dysuria, and tachycardia. PB: UK; t½: UK
Oxybutynin chloride	Immediate release: A: PO: 5 mg bid/qid; *max:* 20 mg/d Older A: PO: 2.5 mg bid/tid; *max:* 20 mg/d Extended release: A: PO: 5–10 mg/d; *max:* 30 mg/d	For neurogenic and overactive bladder. May cause drowsiness, dizziness, headache, insomnia, blurred vision, dry mouth, nausea, diarrhea, constipation, urinary retention, erythema, and skin irritation. PB: 99%; t½: IR 2–5 h, ER 13 h
Mirabegron	A: PO: 25 mg/d; *max:* 50 mg/d	For urinary incontinence and overactive bladder. May cause headache, dizziness, dry mouth, nasopharyngitis, infection, constipation, urinary retention, back pain, and hypertension. PB: 71%; t½: 50 h
Antimuscarinics/Anticholinergics		
Tolterodine tartrate	Immediate release: A: PO: 1–2 mg bid; *max:* 4 mg/d Extended release: A: PO: 2–4 mg/d; *max:* 4 mg/d	For overactive bladder. May cause headache, dizziness, drowsiness, fatigue, arthralgia, blurred vision, dry mouth, dyspepsia, diarrhea, constipation, and abdominal pain. Contraindicated in narrow-angle glaucoma and urinary retention. PB: 96%; t½: regular release, 2–4 h; extended release, 7–18 h
Trospium chloride	A: PO: 20 mg bid; *max:* 60 mg/d Extended release: A: PO: 60 mg/d in the morning	For overactive bladder. May cause headache, fatigue, dry conjunctiva/cornea of eye, dyspepsia, flatulence, nausea, abdominal pain, urinary retention, dry mouth, and constipation. PB: 48%–85%; t½: regular release, 20 h; extended release, 35 h
Solifenacin succinate	See Prototype Drug Chart: Solifenacin Succinate	
Desmopressin	Nocturia: A: 50–64 y: Intranasal: 1 spray (0.83–1.66 mcg) in 1 nostril 30 min before bedtime Female A: SL: 27.7 mcg/d 1 h before bedtime without water Male A: SL: 55.3 mcg/d 1 h before bedtime without water	For controlling nocturia, polydipsia, and polyuria. Fluid should be restricted to a minimum 1 h before administration and for at least 8 h after. May cause dizziness, hyponatremia, xerostomia, headache, pharyngitis, rhinitis, sneezing, nasal congestion, and hypertension. PB: UK; t½: 2.8 h
Fesoterodine	A: PO: Initially 4 mg/d; *max:* 8 mg/d	For overactive bladder. May cause dry conjunctiva/cornea of eye, weight gain, abdominal pain, diarrhea, nausea, headache, dry mouth, constipation, and infection. PB: 50%; t½: 7 h

TABLE 51.2   Urinary Analgesics, Stimulants, and Antispasmodics—cont'd

Generic	Route and Dosage	Uses and Considerations
Darifenacin hydrobromide	Extended release: A: PO: Initially 7.5 mg/d, then in 2 wk 15 mg/d; *max:* 15 mg/d	For overactive bladder and urinary incontinence. May cause headache, dizziness, dry conjunctiva/cornea of eye, weakness, dry mouth, dyspepsia, abdominal pain, nausea, vomiting, and constipation. PB: 98%; t½: 13–19 h
Vibegron	A: PO: 75 mg/d; *max:* 75 mg/d	For overactive bladder. May cause headache, infection, pharyngitis, dry mouth, nausea, diarrhea, constipation, hot flashes, and urinary retention. PB: 50%; t½: 30.8 h

A, Adult; *ac,* before meals; *bid,* twice a day; *d,* day; *GERD,* gastroesophageal reflux disease; *GI,* gastrointestinal; *h,* hour; *max,* maximum; *min,* minute; *PB,* protein binding; *pc,* after meals; *PO,* by mouth; *PRN,* as needed; *q,* every; *qid,* four times a day; *sol,* solution; *subcut,* subcutaneous; *t½,* half-life; *tid,* three times a day; *UK,* unknown; *wk,* week; *y,* year; *>,* greater than.

📄 PROTOTYPE DRUG CHART

Solifenacin Succinate

Drug Class	**Dosage**
Urinary antimuscarinic, anticholinergic, bladder antispasmodic	A: PO: Initially 5 mg/d, then up to 10 mg/d; *max:* 10 mg/d

Contraindications	**Drug-Lab-Food Interactions**
Hypersensitivity, glaucoma, gastroparesis, GI obstruction, urinary retention *Caution:* Rheumatoid arthritis, hypomagnesemia, hypokalemia, hypocalcemia, renal/hepatic impairment, angioedema, older A, bradycardia, dysrhythmias, CAD, heart failure, breastfeeding, contact lenses wearers	Drug: Antagonizes action of cisapride and metoclopramide; potentiates dysrhythmias and torsades de pointes with fluconazole, chlorpromazine, citalopram, droperidol, haloperidol, risperidone, azithromycin, and fluoroquinolones

Pharmacokinetics	**Pharmacodynamics**
Absorption: Well absorbed Distribution: PB: 98% Metabolism: t½: 45–68 h Excretion: Urine, feces	PO: Onset: UK Peak: 3–8 h Duration: UK

Therapeutic Effects/Uses

To treat overactive bladder and urinary incontinence
Mechanism of Action: Exerts selective muscarinic receptor antagonist effect on all muscarinic receptors; depresses voluntary and involuntary bladder contractions, salivary gland secretion, gastric ciliary muscle, and CNS.

Side Effects	**Adverse Reactions**
Blurred vision, dizziness, fatigue, cough, pharyngitis, dry mouth, nausea, vomiting, abdominal pain, constipation, dyspepsia, cystitis, urinary retention, peripheral edema	Palpitations, hypertension, tachycardia, GI obstruction, angioedema *Life-threatening:* Dysrhythmias, hyperkalemia, torsades de pointes

A, Adult; *CAD,* coronary artery disease; *CNS,* central nervous system; *d,* day; *GERD,* gastroesophageal reflux disease; *GI,* gastrointestinal; *h,* hours; *max,* maximum dosage; *PB,* protein binding; *PO,* by mouth; *t½,* half-life; *UK,* unknown.

▮ CRITICAL THINKING CASE STUDY

A 29-year-old woman has complained to her health care provider of painful urinary frequency and urgency. The patient has an elevated temperature. A urine specimen indicates that the patient has a urinary tract infection (UTI). The health care provider prescribes trimethoprim-sulfamethoxazole (TMP-SMZ) double-strength tablets (trimethoprim 160 mg, sulfamethoxazole 800 mg) twice a day for 14 days.

1. What other information should the health care provider obtain from the patient?

2. Why was TMP-SMZ prescribed? Explain your answer.

3. What should the health care provider discuss with the patient in regard to taking the drug and its possible side effects? What other information should F.L. receive?

4. What is the recommended follow-up care for the patient?

5. What other drugs might be used instead of TMP-SMZ? Would one urinary antiinfective drug be more effective than another? Explain your answer.

REVIEW QUESTIONS

1. A patient is taking nitrofurantoin. What will the nurse teach the patient?
   a. Expect the urine to turn brown.
   b. Keep the urine acidic by drinking milk.
   c. Rinse the mouth after taking oral nitrofurantoin to avoid staining teeth.
   d. Take an antacid with oral nitrofurantoin to avoid gastrointestinal distress.

2. A patient complains about a burning sensation and pain when urinating. Which urinary analgesic does the nurse suspect will be ordered?
   a. Tolterodine
   b. Oxybutynin
   c. Bethanechol
   d. Phenazopyridine

3. A patient is taking the urinary antiseptic methenamine for a urinary tract infection (UTI). The nurse understands that this drug should *not* be given concurrently with which other drug to avoid crystalluria?
   a. Ertapenem
   b. Ciprofloxacin
   c. Fosfomycin
   d. Trimethoprim-sulfamethoxazole

4. A patient is receiving solifenacin succinate. The nurse knows that this drug is used to treat which condition?
   a. Chronic cystitis
   b. Urinary tract stones
   c. Urinary tract infection
   d. Overactive bladder
   e. Urinary retention
   f. Neurogenic bladder

5. The patient is taking tolterodine. The nurse plans to teach the patient to report which condition?
   a. Alkaline urine
   b. Urinary retention
   c. Excessive tearing
   d. Reddish-orange urine

Pregnancy and Preterm Labor

Christina DiMaggio Boudreaux, RN, BSN, IBCLC

http://evolve.elsevier.com/McCuistion/pharmacology

OBJECTIVES

- Explain potential health-promoting and detrimental effects of substances ingested during pregnancy.
- Describe the drugs that alter uterine muscle contractility.
- Discuss drug therapy used during preterm labor to decrease the incidence or severity of neonatal respiratory dysfunction.
- Compare systemic and regional treatments for pain control during labor.
- Describe the drugs used in gestational hypertension.
- Using the Clinical Judgment [Nursing Process] model, describe patient teaching associated with drugs used for pregnancy and preterm labor.

OUTLINE

PHYSIOLOGY OF PREGNANCY

Pregnancy elicits many changes in the normal physiology of the body, which means that the expected pharmacokinetics of drugs is also changed during pregnancy.

Changes in drug action during pregnancy include the (1) effect of circulating steroid hormones on the liver's metabolism of drugs; (2) reduced gastrointestinal (GI) motility and increased gastric pH; (3) increased glomerular filtration rate and increased renal perfusion, resulting in more rapid renal excretion of drugs; (4) expanded maternal circulating blood volume, resulting in dilution of drugs; and (5) alteration in the clearance of drugs in later pregnancy, resulting in a decrease in serum and tissue concentrations of drugs. Because of alterations in the normal physiology of the body, drugs should not be ordered in lower doses with longer intervals between doses because of the possibility of subtherapeutic serum concentrations.

Other factors, such as late pregnancy and labor, can alter the half-lives of some drugs. Labor can actually increase the half-life of some drugs. It is also believed that drug clearance can decrease as a result of reduced blood flow associated with uterine contractions when a patient is in supine position.

There is also concern about the effects of certain disease states on medication usage during pregnancy. Disorders such as diabetes mellitus and gestational hypertension may result in decreased renal perfusion and subsequent drug accumulation.

The placenta plays an important role in drug use and metabolism. It was once thought that the placenta played a barrier role, but it is now known that the placenta has an important function as the organ of exchange for numerous substances, including drugs. It allows some substances to transfer quickly or slowly between mother and fetus, depending on variables such as (1) maternal and fetal blood flow; (2) molecular weight of the substance (low-molecular-weight substances cross more readily than do high-molecular-weight substances; most drugs have a low molecular weight, so they readily cross the placenta); (3) degree of ionization of the drug molecule (the more ionized the molecule, the less readily it crosses the placenta); (4) degree of protein binding (highly bound drugs do not cross readily); (5) metabolic activity of the placenta (the metabolic activity can bio-transform molecules into active metabolites that can affect the fetus); and (6) maternal dose.

Guidelines for drug administration during pregnancy must include determination that the benefits of prescribing a drug outweigh potential short- or long-term risks to the maternal-fetal system. Careful selection and monitoring for the minimum effective dose for the shortest interval in the therapeutic range are required. Consideration must be given to alterations related to the physiologic changes of pregnancy.

Liver metabolism of drugs is much slower in the fetus because of immaturity of the liver, which can cause more evident or longer drug effects on the fetus than on the mother. The degree of fetal exposure to a drug and its breakdown products are more important to fetal outcome than the rate at which the drug is transported to the fetus.

The mechanisms by which drugs cross the placenta are analogous to the way in which drugs infiltrate breast tissue. Lactation results in increased blood flow to the breasts, and drugs accumulate in adipose breast tissue through simple diffusion. Long-term effects on infants from drugs in breast milk are unknown, but drugs that accumulate in breast milk are known, and the breastfeeding patient should be alerted to the potential accumulation.

Despite prenatal education, public service announcements, and information conveyed through the media, use of legal and illicit drugs by pregnant patients continues. Additionally, health care providers may prescribe drugs for maternal disorders that indirectly affect the fetus. It is estimated that half the drugs taken by pregnant patients are over-the-counter (OTC) drugs. The drugs most commonly ingested during pregnancy are iron supplements, vitamins, antiemetics, antacids, stool softeners, nasal decongestants, mild analgesics, and antibiotics. Although many drugs required by pregnant patients can be used safely, pregnant patients should be discouraged from using OTC drugs until they consult with their health care provider.

Drugs conclusively determined to be safe for the embryo are limited in number. Clinical trials can be resources for reliable drug information; however, it is unethical to test for the safety and efficacy of drugs in pregnant patients. Animal studies are required during drug testing, but the information obtained from such studies is difficult to extrapolate to humans.

There are many known teratogens, substances that cause developmental abnormalities. Timing, dose, and duration of exposure are crucial in determining the teratogenicity of a given drug. In humans, the teratogenic period begins 2 weeks after conception, before which the embryo is not susceptible to teratogenesis. After this 2-week point in fetal development, however, exposure to teratogens may result in either death of the embryo or minor cellular damage without congenital birth defects. Gestational week 2 through week 12 (first trimester) is the period of organogenesis, in which major structures and organs develop.

THERAPEUTIC DRUGS AND USE OF HERBS IN PREGNANCY

The most common indications for use of drugs during pregnancy are to supplement nutrition with iron, vitamins, and minerals and to treat nausea and vomiting, gastric acidity, and mild discomforts; however, caution must be exercised.

 COMPLEMENTARY AND ALTERNATIVE THERAPIES

Pregnancy

Herbal preparations are not generally recommended during pregnancy. In particular, the following herbs should be avoided:

- Feverfew, rosemary, and sage are emmenagogues that stimulate blood flow in the uterus.
- Kava decreases platelets.
- Dong-quai, garlic, and ginkgo biloba increase bleeding when used with anticoagulants.
- Ginseng may decrease the action of anticoagulants.
- St. John's wort has mutagenic effects on the cells of the developing embryo and fetus.
- Pennyroyal, rue, tansy, and blue cohosh taken orally or topically can be abortifacient.

Iron

During pregnancy, approximately twice the normal amount of iron is needed to meet fetal and maternal daily requirements: 27 mg/day during pregnancy compared with 18 mg/day for nonpregnant women 19 to 30 years of age.

The Centers for Disease Control and Prevention (CDC) now recommends starting a low-dose iron supplement, such as 30 mg/day with the first prenatal appointment. In most cases, this will be found in a prenatal vitamin. The goal is to prevent maternal iron deficiency anemia, not supply the fetus. The fetus is adequately supplied through the placenta. The greatest iron demand occurs in the third trimester: 22.4 mg/day, compared with 6.4 mg/day in the first trimester and 18.8 mg/day in the second trimester.

Although a normal diet generally provides the 18-mg recommended daily allowance (RDA) of iron for nonpregnant patients, pregnant patients at risk for anemia are usually instructed to supplement with 60 to 120 mg of elemental iron per day. The elemental iron content of the most common iron salts includes ferrous sulfate 20% (325 mg of ferrous sulfate is equivalent to 65 mg elemental iron), exsiccated ferrous sulfate 30%, ferrous gluconate 12%, and ferrous fumarate 33%. The estimated net iron cost of pregnancy is approximately 600 to 800 mg. This iron cost is due to the iron use by the fetus, placenta, and increased red blood cell (RBC) volume. Patients are advised to continue supplements for 6 weeks postpartum.

Pregnant patients generally have decreased hematocrit early in the third trimester. Those with levels below 30% will have their supplemental iron dosages increased, and a complete blood count (CBC) with platelet and ferritin will be measured. In those with true iron-deficiency anemia, response to iron supplementation is usually noted in 5 to 7 days with a modest reticulocytosis and an increase in hemoglobin in 3 weeks. No teratogenic effects have been reported with physiologic doses. In contrast, increasing evidence has associated prenatal iron supplementation with glucose impairment and hypertension in midpregnancy. Many OTC and prescription iron products (Table 52.1) are available in varying dosages, which differ in the amount of elemental iron contained in the form of iron salts.

Adverse Reactions

Common side effects of iron supplements include nausea, constipation, black tarry stools, GI irritation, epigastric pain, vomiting, discoloration of urine, and diarrhea.

Nursing Implications

Liquid forms can cause temporary tooth discoloration and therefore should be diluted and administered through a straw. Iron supplements

TABLE 52.1   Iron Products

Generic	Route and Dosage	Uses and Considerations
Iron salts (ferrous sulfate, ferrous gluconate, ferrous fumarate) *Caution:* Read the label carefully. The amount of elemental iron differs according to the formulation.	PO: 15 mg PO once/d in the first trimester; 27 mg PO once/d during the last 2 trimesters.	Prevention and treatment of iron-deficiency anemia and prophylaxis for iron deficiency in pregnancy. Replaces iron stores needed for RBC development. Absorption PO is 5%–30% in intestines; therefore GI side effects may occur. Toxic reactions include pallor, hematemesis, shock, cardiovascular collapse, and metabolic acidosis. Contraindicated in patients with hypersensitivity or peptic ulcer. Decreased absorption of zinc, tetracycline, and penicillamine and increased absorption with ascorbic acid, such as orange juice; decreased absorption with antacids, eggs, milk, coffee, and tea. Take at bedtime to avoid GI upset. Use straw for elixir to prevent staining of teeth, swallow tab/cap whole with full glass of water or juice, preferably on an empty stomach. Sit upright 30 min after dose to decrease reflux. Increase fluids, activity, and dietary bulk. Keep out of reach of children. Peak reticulocytosis: 5–10 d; hemoglobin values increase in 2–4 wk PB: To transferrin; t½: UK; onset: 3–10 d; duration: 3–4 mo Pregnancy Considerations: Iron crosses the placenta and fetal stores are obtained from the mother. Untreated iron-deficiency anemia during pregnancy may be associated with an increased risk of low birth weight, preterm delivery, and perinatal mortality, as well as postpartum depression in mother and decreased mental functioning in the offspring. Treatment improves maternal hematologic status and neonatal birth weight.

cap, Capsule; *d,* day; *GI,* gastrointestinal; *min,* minutes; *mo,* months; *PB,* protein binding; *PO,* by mouth; *RBC,* red blood cell; *t½,* half-life; *tab,* tablet; *UK,* unknown; *wk,* weeks.

are best absorbed when administered with water or juice on an empty stomach. Vitamin C increases the absorption of iron. If gastric irritation does occur, administer the iron with food. Iron supplementation may inhibit the absorption of several drugs, and appropriate separation of doses should be followed (e.g., iron supplementation should be administered 2 hours before or 4 hours after antacids). Additional examples of drugs that may require separation in dose include levodopa, levothyroxine, methyldopa, penicillins, quinolones, and tetracyclines. For the same reasons, do not administer iron with milk, cereal, tea, coffee, or eggs.

Folic Acid

Folic acid supplementation as part of preconception planning improves the outcome of pregnancy. During pregnancy, folic acid (vitamin B$_9$, folate) is needed in increased amounts. Folic acid deficiency early in pregnancy can result in spontaneous abortion or birth defects, especially neural tube defects (NTDs); a failure of the embryonic neural tube to close properly can lead to spina bifida or skull and brain malformations. Deficiency of folic acid may also contribute to premature birth, low birth weight, and premature separation of the placenta (abruptio placentae). In the United States approximately 4000 pregnancies a year are affected by NTDs. Controlled clinical trials have demonstrated that folic acid supplementation can reduce this incidence by as much as 50%.

Normally, the RDA for folic acid is 180 mcg, but the US Preventive Services Task Force recommends that women who are planning pregnancy take a supplement containing 400 mcg to 800 mcg of folic acid 1 month before and for the first 2 to 3 months after conception. The American Congress of Obstetricians and Gynecologists (ACOG) recommends that all women of childbearing age ingest 400 mcg of folic acid daily for birth defect prevention and 600 mcg during pregnancy. The reasoning behind the ACOG recommendation is the high incidence of unplanned and unrecognized pregnancies.

The neural tube closes within the first 4 weeks of pregnancy (18 to 26 days after conception); therefore it is important that women consume the recommended amounts of folic acid every day. For patients who have had a pregnancy affected by an NTD, higher doses of folic acid are recommended: 4000 mcg starting 1 to 3 months before conception.

The recommended amount should be ingested from folate-rich foods, such as dark green leafy vegetables, asparagus, papaya, strawberries, and oranges; from folate-enriched foods, such as bread, rice, cornmeal, pasta, and cereal; and from supplementation because the amount of naturally occurring folic acid ingested in foods varies from day to day and the folic acid from these sources is not well absorbed.

Adverse Reactions

Side effects include flushing, malaise, erythema, pruritus, skin rash, and, in rare cases, allergic bronchospasm. Patients should be aware that folic acid supplementation may cause urine to turn more intensely yellow in color.

Multiple Vitamins

Prenatal vitamin preparations are routinely recommended for pregnant women. These preparations generally supply vitamins A, B-complex, B$_{12}$, C, calcium, D, E, iron, and other minerals.

Inadequate nutrition cannot be rectified through supplements alone; vitamins are used most effectively by the body when taken with meals, and calories and protein are not supplied by supplements.

Large doses of vitamins and minerals above the recommended amounts do not improve health and may cause harm to the pregnant patient and fetus. Some vitamins and minerals can be teratogenic or toxic when taken in large amounts.

Drugs for Minor Discomforts of Pregnancy

Many complaints associated with pregnancy are related to the GI tract and include nausea and vomiting, heartburn, and constipation. The etiology of nausea and vomiting is unclear, although research suggests that it is probably related to an increase in human chorionic gonadotropin (hCG) levels during pregnancy. Increased progesterone during pregnancy, which relaxes smooth muscle, contributes to heartburn and constipation. The elevation in female sex hormones during pregnancy changes the motility of the GI tract, and the enlarging uterus displaces the bowel.

Nausea and Vomiting

Nausea and vomiting ("morning sickness") during early pregnancy are major complaints for about 88% of pregnant patients, but hyperemesis gravidarum—severe nausea and vomiting that may require hospitalization for hydration and nutrition—occurs with a much lower incidence (1% to 3%). Nonpharmacologic measures to decrease nausea and vomiting include (1) eating crackers, dry toast, or other carbohydrates before rising; (2) avoiding high-fat or highly seasoned foods; (3) eating small, frequent meals; (4) drinking fluids between, rather than with, meals; (5) drinking apple juice or flat soda between meals; (6) eating a high-protein bedtime snack; (7) stopping smoking; and (8) taking an iron supplement at bedtime. These measures work well for most patients, but if vomiting is severe, fluid replacement and pharmacologic measures may be necessary.

The US Food and Drug Administration (FDA) has approved pyridoxine hydrochloride and doxylamine succinate for treatment of morning sickness. Table 52.2 lists drugs used for management of nausea and vomiting during pregnancy with their dosages, uses, and considerations.

Iron supplementation during pregnancy may add to the problems of nausea and vomiting. Taking these supplements with food or at bedtime may help decrease gastric distress. Prenatal vitamins should be taken at the time of day the patient is least likely to experience emesis because a high incidence of nausea and vomiting is associated with prenatal vitamins. For patients with continued iron-induced gastric distress, many health care providers recommend taking two children's chewable multivitamins with iron. Salting food to taste may help replace vomited chloride; foods rich in potassium and magnesium may also help replace lost nutrients.

Patients whose symptoms persist and who experience weight loss and dehydration may require intravenous (IV) rehydration, including replacement of electrolytes and vitamins, as well as antiemetic therapy. (See Table 52.2 for drugs used for management of nausea and vomiting during pregnancy.)

TABLE 52.2	Drugs for Management of Nausea and Vomiting During Pregnancy[a]	
Generic	**Route and Dosage**	**Uses and Considerations**
Vitamin		
Pyridoxine (B$_6$) (Also available as combination drug with doxylamine)	PO: 10–25 mg 3–4 times a day. May be given alone or in combination with doxylamine. Adjust dose based on severity of symptoms	In the United States, B$_6$ is the drug of choice for nausea and vomiting in pregnancy; it is a coenzyme for various metabolic functions, including metabolism of proteins, carbohydrates, and fats. Side effects include fatigue, headache, nausea, somnolence, and sensory neuropathy. Absorbed in the jejunum, metabolized in the liver, excreted in urine. Peak plasma time: 5–6 h (pyridoxine); t½: 15–20 d Pregnancy Considerations: Used to treat nausea and vomiting of pregnancy. Crosses the placenta. No problems reported.
Antihistamine Plus Vitamin B$_6$ Analogue		
Doxylamine succinate 10 mg/pyridoxine 10 mg	PO: 2 tabs at bedtime	Mechanism of Action: Competes with histamine for H$_1$ receptor sites on effector cells. Side effects include CNS depression, which may impair physical or mental ability. Patients must be cautioned about performing tasks that require mental alertness, like driving or operating machinery. Effects may be potentiated when used with other sedative drugs. Contraindicated in women with known hypersensitivity to doxylamine succinate or any other component of the drug. MAOIs intensify and prolong the adverse CNS effects. Has anticholinergic properties and should be used with caution in women with asthma, increased intraocular pressure, narrow-angle glaucoma, stenosing peptic ulcer, pyloroduodenal obstruction, and urinary bladder neck obstruction. Not for use by nursing mothers. Administer on an empty stomach with a glass of water. Swallow tablets whole; do not chew, crush, or split. Pregnancy Considerations: Doxylamine succinate and pyridoxine hydrochloride are recommended individually and in combination for use in pregnant women to manage nausea and vomiting of pregnancy. Crosses the placenta. No problems reported. ⚡ Not recommended for use during lactation. Primarily metabolized in the liver; excreted in the kidney; peak: 2–4 h; t½: 10–12 h, PB: UK
Phenothiazines		
Promethazine	PO/IV/IM/PR: 12.5–25 mg q4–6h PRN ❗ Black Box Warning: Promethazine injections can cause severe tissue injury, including gangrene, necrosis, abscess, erythema, edema, severe spasms of distal vessels, phlebitis, sensory loss, and paralysis.	Blocks postsynaptic mesolimbic dopaminergic receptors in the brain; exhibits a strong α-adrenergic blocking effect and depresses release of hypothalamic and hypophyseal hormones; competes with histamine for H$_1$ receptor. Side effects include dizziness, agitation, drowsiness, excitation, fatigue, insomnia, photosensitivity reactions, nausea, vomiting, and constipation. Contraindicated in patients with CNS depression or hypersensitivity to the drug or any component. Use caution in patients with cardiovascular disease; not recommended for subcut or intraarterial administration; injection may contain sulfites, which may cause allergic reaction. Pregnancy Considerations: Approved for use as an antiemetic for pregnancy; however, other drugs are recommended as initial therapy for the treatment of nausea and vomiting of pregnancy. t½: 9–16 h; onset: PO/IM, 20 min; IV, 3–5 min; duration: 4–6 h but may have effects up to 12 h; PB: 93%; excretion: urine, feces as inactive metabolites.

TABLE 52.2	**Drugs for Management of Nausea and Vomiting During Pregnancy[a]—cont'd**

Generic	Route and Dosage	Uses and Considerations
Prokinetic Agents		
Metoclopramide	PO/IM/IV: 5–10 mg q 8 hours	Blocks dopamine receptors in the CTZ; causes enhanced motility and accelerated gastric emptying without stimulating secretions Side effects include restlessness, drowsiness, diarrhea, weakness, insomnia, depression, and tardive dyskinesia. ⚠ *Black Box Warning:* Contraindicated in patients with hypersensitivity to the drug or any component; GI obstruction, perforation, or hemorrhage; pheochromocytoma; history of seizure disorder, history of hypertension, or history of tardive dyskinesia Onset of Action: PO: 30–60 min, IM: 10–15 min, IV: 1–3 min Duration: 1–2 h; t½: 4–7 h PB: 30% Pregnancy Considerations: Crosses the placenta and can be detected in cord blood and amniotic fluid. Metoclopramide is one of the agents that may be considered for adjunctive treatment of nausea and vomiting of pregnancy when symptoms persist after initial pharmacologic therapy. PO/IM therapy may be given in patients who are not dehydrated; IV therapy should be used when dehydration is present.
Other		
Ondansetron	PO/IV: 4–8 mg 2–3 times/d It is recommended that ondansetron is only reserved for severe hyperemesis gravidarum or when conventional treatments are not effective.	Antiemetic; selective 5-HT₃ receptor antagonist that blocks serotonin both peripherally on vagal nerve terminals and centrally in the CTZ. Side effects include headache, constipation, diarrhea, and malaise/fatigue. Contraindicated in patients with hypersensitivity to the drug or other selective 5-HT₃ antagonists *Caution:* Use as scheduled, not PRN. Use with caution in patients who have congenital/medical conditions that cause prolonged QT interval or who take medications that prolong QT interval. Drug interactions: Drugs that alter the activity of liver enzymes. Pregnancy Considerations: Crosses the placenta. Although ondansetron has been evaluated for the treatment of nausea and vomiting of pregnancy, current guidelines note data related to fetal safety are conflicting, so it is generally reserved for use when other agents have failed. Onset: 30 min; duration: 4–8 h; t½: 3–6 h

CNS, Central nervous system; *CTZ*, chemoreceptor trigger zone; *d*, day; *GI*, gastrointestinal; *GU*, genitourinary; *H₁*, histamine₁; *h*, hour; *IM*, intramuscular; *IV*, intravenous; *MAOI*, monoamine oxidase inhibitor; *min*, minute; *PO*, by mouth; *PR*, by rectum; *PRN*, as needed; *qid*, four times a day; *subcut*, subcutaneously; *t½*, half-life; *tabs*, tablets; *tid*, three times a day.
[a]Recommendation not implied.

Heartburn

Heartburn, or *pyrosis*, is a burning sensation in the epigastric and sternal regions related to reflux of acidic stomach contents. Approximately 80% of pregnant patients are affected with pyrosis. *The normal increase in the hormone progesterone causes decreased motility of the GI tract during pregnancy.* Progesterone also relaxes the cardiac sphincter—the sphincter that leads into the stomach from the esophagus, also called the *lower esophageal sphincter*—making reflux activity, or *reverse peristalsis*, more likely. During pregnancy, digestion and gastric emptying are slower than in the nonpregnant state. Heartburn is common when a pregnant patient sits or lies down soon after eating a normal meal, only to have her gravid uterus exert upward pressure on her stomach, causing increased reflux activity and the perception of hyperacidity. Heartburn is a disorder of the second and third trimesters of pregnancy.

Nonpharmacologic measures are preferred in the management of heartburn. These include (1) limiting the size of meals; (2) avoiding highly seasoned or greasy foods; (3) avoiding gas-forming foods (e.g., cabbage, onions); (4) eating slowly and chewing thoroughly; (5) avoiding citrus juices; (6) drinking adequate fluids, but not with meals; and (7) avoiding reclining immediately after eating.

Antacids should be considered first-line therapy if the patient does not respond to nonpharmacologic therapy. The antacids of choice for the pregnant patient include nonsystemic low-sodium products (those considered dietetically sodium free) that contain aluminum and magnesium (in the form of hydroxide) in combination. Discourage long-term use or large doses of magnesium antacids because fetal renal, respiratory, cardiovascular, and muscle problems may result. Chewable calcium carbonate tablets are frequently taken by pregnant patients for heartburn, but because they are calcium based, excessive use may contribute to constipation.

Most patients do not realize that remedies commonly used by nonpregnant patients (e.g., baking soda, sodium bicarbonate) can be harmful during pregnancy. Selection of the wrong antacid can result in diarrhea, constipation, or electrolyte imbalance. A combination of nonpharmacologic measures and minimal use of safe antacids should effectively meet the pregnant patient's needs.

Liquid antacids are the preparations most commonly used in pregnancy because of their uniform dissolution, rapid action, and greater activity. Tablets are also acceptable, particularly for convenience, provided they are thoroughly chewed and the patient maintains adequate fluid intake.

Histamine₂ (H₂)-receptor antagonists can be used during pregnancy, but only if their use is recommended by a health care provider and initial treatment with antacids has failed. The teratogenicity of these medications is unknown. H₂-receptor antagonists work by competitively and reversibly binding to the histamine receptors of the parietal cells, causing a reduction in gastric acid secretion. The onset of action is generally in 1 hour and can persist for 6 to 12 hours.

There is even less experience with the use of proton pump inhibitors. These medications work to suppress gastric acid secretion by inhibiting the proton pump on the surface of the parietal cells. Omeprazole, which is now OTC, is not recommended for use in pregnancy except when the benefits outweigh the risks and after other medications and initial treatments have failed. Encourage patients to discuss all options with their health care provider before taking any medication during pregnancy.

Table 52.3 presents medications for heartburn commonly used during pregnancy.

Constipation

Constipation is a frequent occurrence during pregnancy. Its cause may be related to hormonal changes—specifically progesterone, which decreases GI motility. As with heartburn, nonpharmacologic treatments for constipation should be tried first. These include (1) increased fluid intake, (2) increased dietary fiber intake, and (3) moderate physical exercise. If these methods do not work, pharmacological interventions may be indicated, and the safest drugs are bulk-forming preparations that contain fiber because they are not systemically absorbed. Also, docusate sodium, a stool softener, would be appropriate as first-line treatment during pregnancy. Drugs that should be reserved for occasional use include magnesium hydroxide, magnesium citrate, lactulose, sorbitol, bisacodyl, and senna.

Castor oil should be avoided during pregnancy because it can stimulate uterine contractions. Mineral oil should also be avoided because it can reduce the absorption of fat-soluble vitamins such as vitamin K. Low levels of vitamin K in the neonate can result in hemorrhage.

Pain

Through week 26 of pregnancy, headaches that result from hormonally induced body changes, sinus congestion, or eye strain are quite common. It is not unusual for the pregnant patient to experience backaches, joint pains, round ligament pain (resulting in mild abdominal aches and twinges), and pain from minor injuries. Nonpharmacologic pain relief measures should be tried initially, including rest; a calming environment; relaxation exercises; alteration in routine; mental imagery; ice packs; warm, moist heat; postural changes; correct body mechanics; and changes in footwear.

Acetaminophen. Acetaminophen, a para-aminophenol analgesic, is the most commonly ingested nonprescription drug during pregnancy. Acetaminophen may be used during all trimesters of pregnancy in therapeutic doses on a short-term basis for its analgesic and antipyretic effects. The drug is a weak prostaglandin inhibitor and does not have significant antiinflammatory effects. See Prototype Drug Chart: Acetaminophen in Chapter 25 for the pharmacologic data.

TABLE 52.3	Over-the-Counter Antacids Commonly Used in Pregnancy	
Generic	**Route and Dosage**	**Uses and Considerations**
Aluminum hydroxide	A: PO: Oral Susp 40-60 mL per dose every 3-6 hours OTC: A: PO 10 mL 5-6 times/d	Used to counteract hyperacidity in pregnancy Contains 320 mg of aluminum hydroxide gel per 300-mg tab or per 5 mL; ANC 8 contains saccharin and sorbitol. OTC preparation for heartburn secondary to reflux; it neutralizes gastric acidity. Side effects include constipation, fecal discoloration, fecal impaction, nausea, vomiting, stomach cramps. Adverse reactions include dehydration, hypophosphatemia (long-term use), GI obstruction. Pregnancy Considerations: Nonpharmacological treatments, such as dietary and lifestyle modifications, are preferred. If antacids are warranted, most aluminum-containing antacids that are considered acceptable when used in recommended doses for dyspepsia during pregnancy and prevention of adverse events should aspiration occur during labor. PB: UK; onset: 15–30 min; peak: 0.5 h; duration: 1–3 h; t½: UK *max:* not to exceed recommended dose in 24/h
Magnesium hydroxide and aluminum hydroxide with simethicone	PO: Multiple formulations available OTC—take as directed[a]	Antiflatulent and neutralizes gastric acid. Provides relief of acid indigestion, heartburn, sour stomach or upset stomach and flatus associated with these symptoms. Liquid: Each 5 mL contains 400 mg aluminum hydroxide; 400 mg magnesium hydroxide; 40 mg simethicone, parabens, saccharin, and sorbitol; and 2 mg sodium. Tablets: Each contains 200 mg aluminum hydroxide, 200 mg magnesium hydroxide, and 20 mg simethicone. Tabs must be chewed thoroughly. Administer 1 hour after meals or between meals. Shake suspension well before administering. Adverse effects include acid rebound. Aluminum-based antacids may cause constipation, whereas magnesium-based antacids have a laxative effect. Aluminum and magnesium–based combination antacids are given to balance the constipation and laxative effects. Do not administer magnesium-based antacids to patients with renal disease. *Drug interactions:* Concurrent administration with digoxin, indomethacin, or iron salts may decrease absorption of these drugs. Decreased pharmacologic effect with antacids and benzodiazepines, captopril, corticosteroids, fluoroquinolones, H₂ antagonists, hydantoins, ketoconazole, penicillamine, phenothiazines, salicylates, and ticlopidine. Increased pharmacologic effect with levodopa, sulfonylureas, and valproic acid. Pregnancy Considerations: Crosses the placenta but is considered acceptable during pregnancy and labor. PB: UK; t½: UK

ANC, Acid-neutralizing capacity (per tablet or 5 mL); *d,* day; *GI,* gastrointestinal; *h,* hour; *H₂,* histamine 2; *min,* minute; *OTC,* over-the-counter; *PB,* protein binding; *PO,* by mouth; *susp,* suspension; *t½,* half-life; *tab,* tablet; *tsp,* teaspoon; *UK,* unknown.

Pharmacokinetics. The rate of absorption of acetaminophen is dependent on the rate of gastric emptying. Acetaminophen is 10% to 25% protein bound and crosses the placenta during pregnancy; it is also found in low concentrations in breast milk. Acetaminophen is partially hepatically metabolized into inactive metabolites; however, a highly active metabolite (*N*-acetyl-*p*-benzoquinone) produced when the drug is taken in large doses can have potential liver and kidney toxicity. The half-life is 2 to 3 hours. There is no concrete evidence of fetal anomalies associated with the use of acetaminophen, and no adverse effects have been noted in breastfed infants of patients who used the drug while pregnant or breastfeeding.

Pharmacodynamics. The maximum daily dose of acetaminophen is 3000 mg per day and use during pregnancy should not exceed this because of potential for kidney and liver toxicity. The drug should be taken at 4- to 6-hour intervals. Onset of effects after oral ingestion is within 10 to 30 minutes, peak action occurs at 1 to 2 hours, and duration is from 3 to 5 hours.

Manufacturers of OTC products that contain acetaminophen have lowered the maximum daily dose recommendation to 3000 mg due to the frequency of overdose with acetaminophen. One reason for the high frequency of overdose is that patients may take multiple OTC products that contain acetaminophen.

Most patients without preexisting renal or hepatic disease tolerate acetaminophen without adverse drug effects. Patients with hypersensitivity to the compound should not use it. Acetaminophen should be used cautiously in patients who are at risk for infection because of the possibility of masking signs and symptoms. The most frequent adverse reactions are skin eruptions, urticaria, unusual bruising, erythema, hypoglycemia, jaundice, hemolytic anemia, neutropenia, leukopenia, pancytopenia, and thrombocytopenia.

Aspirin and Ibuprofen. Aspirin, a salicylate, is classified as a mild analgesic. It is a nonsteroidal antiinflammatory drug (NSAID), more specifically a prostaglandin synthetase inhibitor with antipyretic, analgesic, and antiinflammatory properties.

Aspirin can inhibit the initiation of labor and may prolong labor through its effects on uterine contractility; therefore its use is not recommended during pregnancy. Aspirin use late in pregnancy is also associated with greater maternal blood loss at delivery, and there may be increased risk for anemia in pregnancy and of antepartum hemorrhage. Hemostasis is affected in the newborn whose mother ingested aspirin during the last 2 months of pregnancy even without use during the week of delivery. Platelets are unable to aggregate to form clots, and it appears that this is *not* a reversible effect after delivery; the infant must wait for its own bone marrow to produce new platelets. Ibuprofen is also an NSAID and a prostaglandin synthetase inhibitor with antipyretic, analgesic, and antiinflammatory properties. Bleeding risks are similar to those reported with aspirin, although ibuprofen causes less inhibition of platelet aggregation than aspirin formulations. If taken late in pregnancy, ibuprofen may cause premature closure of the ductus arteriosus; therefore ibuprofen use is contraindicated during the third trimester and during labor and delivery.

Antidepressant Drugs

Depressive disorders and exposure to antidepressant drugs have been associated with adverse birth outcomes. Adverse outcomes have included low birth weight (LBW), infants born small for gestational age (SGA), preterm delivery, and increased neonatal irritability and decreased attentiveness. Use of selective serotonin reuptake inhibitors (SSRIs) in pregnancy is associated with LBW and SGA infants. Preterm delivery (before 37 weeks) is significantly higher in patients taking SSRIs and tricyclic antidepressants (TCAs). Although TCA use in pregnancy has not been associated with structural malformations, in utero exposure has been linked to neonatal jitteriness and irritability. *Poor neonatal adaptation*—a term for transient symptoms such as tachypnea, irritability, hypoglycemia, and weak cry—has been reported in neonates exposed to SSRIs in late pregnancy. Options for treatment for pregnant patients include psychotherapy alone or in conjunction with pharmacologic therapy as determined by the health care provider.

◎ CLINICAL JUDGMENT [NURSING PROCESS]

Antepartum Drugs

Concept: Reproduction
- Reproduction is the process by which offspring is produced. Nurses perform assessments on their antepartum patients to determine their course of drugs and care.

Recognize Cues [Assessment]
- Gather comprehensive medical and drug history to include illicit, herbal, and pharmacologic formulations and nonpharmacologic interventions, such as acupuncture.
- Obtain baseline vital signs.
- Identify patients at risk for substance abuse and collaborate with other professionals to plan strategies to minimize risks.
- Assess drug history to determine whether antacid use will interfere with absorption of the drug.
- Review history of aspirin use when admitting a patient in labor. If aspirin has been used, alert staff and monitor for increased bleeding.
- Ascertain any medical history of alcoholism, liver disease, viral infection, or renal deficiencies. Acetaminophen should be used cautiously in these patients.
- Assess group B *Streptococcus* colonization in pregnancy for treatment and neonatal prevention.

Analyze Cues and Prioritize Hypotheses [Patient Problems]
- Anxiety
- Potential for decreased adherence
- Need for patient teaching

Generate Solutions [Planning]
- The patient will verbalize the name and side effects of at least one pharmacologic and nonpharmacologic treatment used during pregnancy.
- The patient will discuss drugs and herbal supplements with a health care provider or pharmacist before use.

Take Action [Nursing Interventions]
General
- Discuss the importance of prenatal care and discuss the patient's fears.
- Instruct on nonpharmacologic and pharmacologic measures to relieve common pregnancy discomforts.
- Instruct the patient on tobacco, alcohol, or drug treatment programs if appropriate.
- Counsel the patient on nutritional and therapeutic supplements needed during pregnancy.
- Monitor hemoglobin/hematocrit of the prenatal patient per agency protocol.

Continued

◎ CLINICAL JUDGMENT [NURSING PROCESS]—CONT'D

Antepartum Drugs

Iron
- Instruct the patient about nausea, constipation, and bowel habit changes if they are taking iron preparations.
- Instruct the patient to dilute liquid iron preparations and take through a plastic straw to prevent discoloration of teeth. Giving iron with orange juice, which is high in ascorbic acid, enhances absorption.
- Store iron in a light-resistant container.
- Assess for a false-positive result of occult blood in the stool that may occur in patients taking iron.

Patient Teaching
General
- Advise the patient that tobacco, alcohol, and heavy caffeine use may have adverse effects on the fetus.
- Encourage the patient to speak with their health care provider before taking drugs—illicit, over-the-counter (OTC), or prescribed drugs—because of their teratogenic potential.
- Instruct the patient planning to breastfeed to discuss drugs—illicit, OTC, and prescribed—with their health care provider.

Aspirin, Acetaminophen, and Ibuprofen
- Advise the patient to take acetaminophen, rather than aspirin, during pregnancy; aspirin and ibuprofen are particularly contraindicated during the third trimester.
- Instruct the patient against ingesting multiple OTC pain or cough/cold preparations because many OTC products contain acetaminophen.

Antepartum Drugs
- Advise the patient not to refrain from taking nonsteroidal antiinflammatory drugs (NSAIDs) with acetaminophen.
- Advise the patient not to take NSAIDS after the second trimester.

Caffeine, Alcohol, and Nicotine
- Advise the patient to limit coffee ingestion to 1 cup per day and to limit other sources of caffeine (tea, soda, chocolate, certain drugs).
- Encourage the patient to limit and space caffeine intake evenly throughout the day because caffeine passes readily to the fetus, which cannot metabolize it. Caffeine can decrease intervillous placental blood flow.
- Advise the patient to discuss use of caffeine products with their health care provider.
- Advise the patient to use decaffeinated products or to dilute caffeinated products.
- Advise the patient to discuss use of herbal products with their health care provider (see Complementary and Alternative Therapies box).
- Instruct the patient who plans to breastfeed that 1% of caffeine consumed will appear in breast milk within 15 minutes. Therefore although one cup of coffee is fine, it is not wise to drink several cups of coffee in succession; excess caffeine will accumulate in the infant's tissues because it lacks the enzymes to adequately clear the caffeine for 7 to 9 months after birth.
- Advise the pregnant patient not to drink alcohol because no safe level has been determined; emphasize that even *minimal* exposure can result in fetal alcohol effect (FAE), and moderate/excessive exposure may result in fetal alcohol syndrome (FAS).
- Advise the patient that smoking can cause loss of nutrients such as vitamins A and C, folic acid, cobalamin, and calcium. Tobacco use may contribute to shortened gestation and low-birth-weight infants.

Antacids
- Advise the patient that antacids should not be taken within 1 hour of taking an enteric-coated tablet because the acid-resistant coating may dissolve in the increased alkaline condition of the stomach and the medication will not be released in the intestine as intended. Stomach upset may result.
- Instruct the patient to store antacid liquid suspensions at room temperature or to place them under refrigeration to improve palatability; advise that suspensions should not be frozen and that the bottle must be shaken well before ingesting.

Iron
- Advise the patient about dietary sources of iron, including red meat, nuts and seeds, wheat germ, spinach, broccoli, prunes, and iron-fortified cereal.
- Instruct the patient that, if supplemental iron is taken between meals, increased absorption—and increased side effects—may result. Taking iron 1 hour before meals is suggested. Give with orange juice or water but not with milk or antacids.

Self-Administration of Iron and Antacids
- Advise the patient to swallow iron tablets whole, not crush them. Liquid iron preparations are taken with a plastic straw to avoid staining teeth.
- Instruct the patient not to take antacids with iron; antacids impair absorption and are generally discouraged during pregnancy. Iron and antacids should be taken 2 hours apart if both are prescribed.

Side Effects of Iron and Antacids
- Advise the patient to keep iron tablets away from children. Iron tablets look like candy, and death has been reported in small children. Iron is a leading cause of fatal poisoning in children.
- Advise the patient there may be a change in bowel habits when taking antacids. Aluminum and calcium carbonate products can cause constipation, whereas magnesium products can cause diarrhea. Many antacids contain a combination of ingredients to reduce adverse effects.

Evaluate Outcomes [Evaluation]
- Evaluate effectiveness of prescribed drug therapy. Report side effects.
- Evaluate the patient's understanding of possible effects on the fetus from maternal use of drugs (prescribed, OTC, and illicit) and tobacco or alcohol.

DRUGS THAT DECREASE UTERINE MUSCLE CONTRACTILITY

Preterm Labor

Preterm labor (PTL) is defined as cervical changes and uterine contractions that occur between 20 and 37 weeks of pregnancy. *Preterm birth* is any birth that occurs before the completion of 37 weeks of pregnancy, regardless of birth weight. Complications related to preterm birth account for more newborn and infant deaths than any other cause. PTL occurs in 12% of pregnancies.

Although PTL has no single known cause, certain risk factors have been identified: maternal age younger than 18 years or older than 40 years, low socioeconomic status, previous history of preterm delivery (17% to 37% chance of recurrence), intrauterine infections (e.g., bacterial vaginosis), polyhydramnios, multiple gestation, uterine anomalies, antepartum hemorrhage, smoking, drug use, urinary tract infections, and incompetent cervix. Attempts to arrest PTL are contraindicated in (1) pregnancy of less than 20 weeks' gestation (confirmed by ultrasound), (2) bulging or premature rupture of membranes (PROM), (3) confirmed fetal death or anomalies incompatible with life, (4)

TABLE 52.4 Drugs Used to Decrease Uterine Contractility

Generic	Route and Dosage	Uses and Considerations
Beta-Adrenergic Agents		
Terbutaline	Subcut: 0.25 mg q20min–3h; hold for pulse >120 beats/min. Continuous Subcut infusion 50 to 100 mcg/h; *max:* 100 mcg/h Follow agency protocol for specific directives plus individual health care provider's orders. See Black Box Warning.[a]	Relaxes bronchial and uterine smooth muscle by acting on β_2-receptors. Used for acute, short-term, less than 72 hours tocolysis "off-label" use. Partially metabolized in liver, excreted in urine and feces. Drug rapidly crosses the placenta, increases maternal pulse and FHR; monitor MHR. Breastfeeding is *not* contraindicated because of short half-life. Additive effect with CNS depressants (narcotics, sedative-hypnotics) and neuromuscular blocking agents *Contraindication:* Hypersensitivity to terbutaline, sympathomimetic amines, or any component of the formulation. Pregnancy Considerations: Crosses the placenta. US **!** *Black Box Warning:* Not FDA approved for prolonged tocolysis. May be used for 48 hours, short-term prolongation of pregnancy to allow for administration of antenatal steroids. Should not be used before fetal viability or when the risks of use to the fetus or mother are greater than the risk of preterm birth. Onset: 6–15 min; PB: 25%; peak: 30–60 min; duration: 1.5–4 h; t½: 2.9–14 h
Calcium Antagonists		
Magnesium sulfate	See Table 52.6	

CNS, Central nervous system; *cont,* continuous; *FHR,* fetal heart rate; *h,* hour; *max,* maximum; *MHR,* maternal heart rate; *min,* minutes; *PB,* protein binding; *q,* every; *subcut,* subcutaneously; *t½,* half-life; *>,* greater than.
[a]*Black-Box Warning:* The United States Food and Drug Administration has concluded that the risk of serious adverse events outweighs any potential benefit to pregnant women receiving prolonged tocolytic treatment beyond 48 to 72 hours.

maternal hemorrhage and evidence of severe fetal compromise, and (5) chorioamnionitis.

Nonpharmacologic treatment measures for PTL include bed rest, hydration (ingestion of 6 to 8 glasses of fluids daily or more, IV fluid bolus), pelvic rest (no sexual intercourse or douching), and screening for intrauterine and urinary tract infections. Patient assessment includes uterine activity (frequency, duration, and intensity), vaginal bleeding or discharge, and fetal monitoring.

Tocolytic Therapy

When patients in true PTL (with cervical change) have no contraindications, they become candidates for tocolytic therapy—drug therapy to decrease uterine muscle contractions. No medication has been approved by the FDA as a tocolytic, so medications used for this reason are considered "off-label" use. The goals in tocolytic therapy are to (1) interrupt or inhibit uterine contractions to create additional time for fetal maturation in utero, (2) delay delivery so antenatal corticosteroids can be delivered to facilitate fetal lung maturation, and (3) allow safe transport of the patient to an appropriate facility if required. Table 52.4 lists the drugs used to decrease preterm uterine contractions and their dosages, uses, and considerations.

Beta-Sympathomimetic Drugs

Beta-sympathomimetic drugs act by stimulating β_2-receptors on uterine smooth muscle. The frequency and intensity of uterine contractions decrease as the muscle relaxes. Terbutaline is used in the late second and early third trimesters, more commonly limited to a single-dose therapy as an acute tocolytic. Terbutaline can effectively decrease uterine contractions; however, use of terbutaline in the United States has decreased with increased awareness of its effects on maternal and fetal cardiovascular systems and free placental passage. The FDA recommends that *injectable* terbutaline should not be used in pregnant women for prevention of PTL or prolonged treatment (beyond 48 to 72 hours) secondary to the risk of maternal cardiac problems and death (see http://www.fda.gov/drugs/drugsafety/ucm243539.htm).

⚡ ***Pregnancy Considerations.*** Black Box Warning: Not FDA approved and should not be used for prolonged tocolysis (more than 48 to 72 hours). Adverse events observed in pregnant women include arrhythmias, increased heart rate, hyperglycemia, hypokalemia, myocardial ischemia, pulmonary edema. Heart rate may be increased in the fetus and hypoglycemia in neonates has been observed.

⚡ PATIENT SAFETY

Do not Confuse...
- **Methylergonovine**, used to *stimulate* uterine contractions in the prevention and treatment of postpartum hemorrhage, with **terbutaline sulfate**, used to *decrease* uterine contractions in PTL. These drugs have the same packaging but opposite actions. Both are amber ampules with amber plastic packaging and colored neckbands wrapped in foil. Do not store together. Manufacturers of terbutaline are now packaging this drug in vials, but some ampules may still be in circulation.

Pharmacokinetics. Patients with contractions may be initially given subcutaneous terbutaline 0.25 mg every 20 minutes to 3 hours if the maternal pulse is less than 120 beats/min. Patients are monitored to determine whether and when contractions diminish or cease. Terbutaline is minimally protein bound (25%) and is metabolized via the liver to inactive metabolites. Its half-life is 11 to 16 hours.

Pharmacodynamics. Subcutaneous terbutaline has an onset of action of 6 to 15 minutes, a peak serum concentration level in 30 to 60 minutes, and a duration of action of 1.5 to 4 hours subcutaneously.

Adverse Reactions. Maternal side effects include tremors, dizziness, nervousness, tachycardia, hypotension, chest pain, palpitations, nausea, vomiting, hyperglycemia, and hypokalemia. Many of these effects are associated with terbutaline's cross-reactivity with β_1-adrenergic receptors. More serious adverse reactions include pulmonary edema, dysrhythmias, ketoacidosis, and anaphylactic shock. Fetal side effects include tachycardia and potential hypoglycemia resulting from fetal hyperinsulinemia caused by maternal hyperglycemia. Terbutaline is contraindicated in patients with cardiac disease and in those with poorly controlled hyperthyroidism or diabetes mellitus.

Drug Interactions. The increased effects of general anesthetics can produce additive hypotension. Pulmonary edema can occur with concurrent use of corticosteroids. Cardiovascular effects may be additive with other sympathomimetic drugs.

Magnesium Sulfate

Parenteral magnesium sulfate, a calcium antagonist and central nervous system (CNS) depressant, relaxes the smooth muscle of the uterus through calcium displacement and can be given as an "off-label" use for PTL. Administered intravenously, the drug has a direct depressant effect on uterine muscle contractility. This drug is excreted by the kidneys and crosses the placenta. Magnesium sulfate is administered as a 4 to 6 g IV loading dose over 20 to 30 minutes followed by a 1 to 2 g/h for at least 24 hours. Magnesium sulfate can be used up to 48 hours in women at risk of delivery within 7 days; however, it is not the preferred tocolytic. Magnesium sulfate therapy is contraindicated in patients who have myasthenia gravis, neuromuscular disease, impaired kidney function, or recent myocardial infarction (MI). Patients with renal impairment may require adjusted dosages.

Adverse Reactions. Dosage-related side effects in the patient include flushing, feelings of increased warmth, perspiration, dizziness, nausea, headache, lethargy, slurred speech, sluggishness, nasal congestion, heavy eyelids, blurred vision, decreased GI action, increased pulse rate, and hypotension. Increased severity is evidenced by depressed reflexes, confusion, and magnesium toxicity (respiratory depression and arrest, circulatory collapse, cardiac arrest). Decreased fetal heart rate (FHR) variability is one side effect, and side effects in the neonate are respiratory depression, slight hypotonia with diminished reflexes, and lethargy for 24 to 48 hours. If maternal neurologic, respiratory, or cardiac depression is evidenced, the antidote is calcium gluconate (1 g IV push over 3 minutes).

Nursing Interventions During Tocolytic Therapy

- Monitor vital signs, FHR, fetal activity, and uterine activity as ordered. Report respirations of fewer than 12 per minute, which may indicate magnesium sulfate toxicity.
- Monitor intake and output (I&O). Report urinary output below 30 mL/h.
- Assess breath and bowel sounds as ordered or at least every 4 hours.
- Assess deep tendon reflexes (DTRs) and clonus before initiation of therapy and as ordered. Notify the health care provider of changes in DTRs (areflexia or hyporeflexia) and clonus.
- Assess pain and uterine contractions.

◎ CLINICAL JUDGMENT [NURSING PROCESS]

Beta₂-Adrenergic Agonists: Terbutaline

Concept: Reproduction
- Reproduction is the process by which offspring is produced. Nurses perform assessments on their antepartum patients to determine course of drugs and care.

Recognize Cues [Assessment]
- Identify risks for preterm labor (PTL) early in pregnancy.
- When a patient has preterm uterine contractions, obtain a history, complete physical assessment, vital signs, fetal heart rate (FHR), and urine specimen for screening for intrauterine infection and urinary tract infection.

Analyze Cues and Prioritize Hypothesis [Patient Problems]
- Anxiety
- Potential for decreased adherence
- Need for patient teaching

Generate Solutions [Planning]
- The patient will remain free of uterine contractions.
- The patient will verbalize the need to maintain fluid intake to decrease contractions.
- The patient will maintain a left-side lying position.
- The patient will remain free of progressive cervical change.

Take Action [Nursing Interventions]
- Monitor vital signs, FHR, and fetal and uterine activity as ordered.
- Maintain the patient in a left lateral position as much as possible to facilitate uteroplacental perfusion.
- Monitor vital signs per facility's protocol, specifically maternal pulse. Report maternal heart rate (MHR) greater than 130 beats/min.
- Report auscultated cardiac dysrhythmias. An electrocardiogram (ECG) may be ordered.
- Auscultate breath sounds every 4 hours. Notify the health care provider if respirations are more than 30 per minute, or <12 per minute, or if the breath quality changes (e.g., wheezes, rales, coughing).

- Monitor daily weight at the same time every day to assess fluid overload; implement strict intake and output (I&O) measurement.
- Report baseline FHR over 180 beats/min or any significant increase in uterine contractions from pretreatment baseline.
- Report persistence of uterine contractions despite tocolytic therapy.
- Report leakage of amniotic fluid, vaginal bleeding or discharge, and complaints of rectal pressure.
- Assess for the presence of maternal hyperglycemia and hypokalemia and hypoglycemia in the newborn delivered within 5 hours of discontinued β-sympathomimetic drugs.

Patient Teaching
General
- Advise the patient of signs and symptoms of PTL: menstrual-type cramps, sensations of pelvic pressure, low backache, increased vaginal discharge, and abdominal discomfort.
- Instruct the patient who experiences PTL contractions that her initial action should be to void, recline on her left side to increase uterine blood flow, and drink extra fluids. Emphasize that she should notify her health care provider if uterine contractions do not cease or if they increase in frequency.
- Explain side effects of β-sympathomimetic drugs. Report heart palpitations or dizziness to the health care provider.
- Advise the patient to contact her health care provider before taking any other drugs while on tocolytic drug therapy.

Evaluate Outcomes [Evaluation]
- Evaluate effectiveness of the tocolytic drug by noting six or fewer uterine contractions in 1 hour or per the health care provider's order.
- Evaluate the patient's understanding of nonpharmacologic measures for decreasing preterm contractions: bed rest, increasing oral fluid intake, pelvic rest, and lying on the left side.
- Continue monitoring the patient's vital signs, FHR, and uterine activity. Report any change immediately.

- Weigh daily at the same time.
- Monitor serum magnesium levels as ordered (therapeutic level is 4 to 7 mg/dL).
- Have available calcium gluconate (1 g given IV over 3 minutes) as an antidote.
- Assess the newborn for 24 to 48 hours for magnesium effects if drug was given to the mother before delivery.

CORTICOSTEROID THERAPY IN PRETERM LABOR

The desired outcome of tocolytic therapy is to delay birth long enough to allow time for corticosteroids to reach maximum benefit. Patients at risk for preterm delivery (24 to 34 weeks' gestation) should receive antenatal corticosteroid therapy with betamethasone or dexamethasone. An off-label use, administration of antenatal corticosteroids accelerates lung maturation and lung surfactant development in the fetus in utero, decreasing the incidence and severity of respiratory distress syndrome (RDS) and increasing survival of preterm infants. Antenatal therapy decreases infant mortality, RDS, and intraventricular bleeds in neonates born between 24 and 34 gestational weeks. The effects and benefits of corticosteroid administration are believed to begin 24 hours after administration, and they last for up to 1 week. The goal is to delay delivery by 48 hours to maximize the effect of the glucocorticoids.

Surfactant is made up of two major phospholipids: sphingomyelin and lecithin. Sphingomyelin initially develops in greater quantity than lecithin from about the 24th week. However, by the 33rd to 35th weeks of gestation, lecithin production peaks, making the ratio of the two substances about 2:1 in favor of lecithin. This lecithin/sphingomyelin (L/S) ratio is measured in the amniotic fluid and is a predictor of fetal lung maturity and risk for neonatal RDS.

Patients with gestational hypertension, PROM, placental insufficiency, or some types of diabetes and those who abuse narcotics may have amniotic fluid with higher than expected L/S ratios for the gestational date because of a stress-induced increase in endogenous corticosteroid production.

Betamethasone

Betamethasone is recommended for women between 24 to 34 weeks of gestation, including those with ruptured membranes or multiple gestations, who are at risk of delivering within 7 days. A single course of 12 mg IM every 24 hours for a total of 2 doses may be appropriate in some women beginning at 23 weeks' gestation or late preterm between 34 to 36 weeks and 6 days. A single repeat course may be considered in some women with pregnancies less than 34 weeks' gestation at risk for delivering within 7 days and who had their last dose of corticosteroids more than 14 days prior.

Adverse Reactions. Side effects of betamethasone include headache, vertigo, edema, bradycardia, arrhythmias, malaise, hypertension, increased sweating, petechiae, ecchymoses, facial erythema, and seizures.

Dexamethasone

In clinical controlled trials, evidence is insufficient to recommend betamethasone over dexamethasone, because the two have not been directly compared. Investigations have noted a trend of decreased risk of neonatal cystic periventricular leukomalacia and intraventricular hemorrhage with exposure to betamethasone over dexamethasone. Dexamethasone has a rapid onset of action and a shorter duration; therefore it must be prescribed in a shorter frequency compared with betamethasone. The recommended antepartum regimen for dexamethasone is 6 mg IM every 12 hours for 4 doses.

⚡ PATIENT SAFETY

Do not Confuse...
- **Dexamethasone**, a corticosteroid used to accelerate fetal lung maturity during weeks 24 to 34 of gestation, with **desoximetasone**, which is used to treat inflammation from corticosteroid-responsive dermatoses.

Adverse Reactions. The potential adverse reactions associated with dexamethasone therapy include insomnia, nervousness, increased appetite, headache, hypersensitivity reactions, and arthralgias. Table 52.5 lists the prenatal drugs used for surfactant development and their dosages, uses, and considerations.

DRUGS FOR GESTATIONAL HYPERTENSION

Gestational hypertension, elevated blood pressure (BP) after 20 gestational weeks in patients normotensive before pregnancy, is the most common serious complication of pregnancy and can have devastating maternal and fetal effects. Gestational hypertension has replaced the term *pregnancy-induced hypertension,* still commonly used in clinical

---

◎ CLINICAL JUDGMENT [NURSING PROCESS]

Betamethasone

Concept: Reproduction
- Reproduction is the process by which offspring is produced. Nurses perform assessments on their antepartum patients to determine course of drugs and care.

Recognize Cues [Assessment]
- Assess for history of hypersensitivity.
- Assess vital signs; report abnormal findings.
- Assess fetal heart rate (FHR).

Analyze Cues and Prioritize Hypotheses [Patient Problems]
- Anxiety
- Potential for decreased adherence
- Need for patient teaching

Generate Solutions [Planning]
- The patient will remain free of preterm uterine contractions for 24 hours allowing betamethasone to be delivered to improve fetal lung function

Take Action [Nursing Interventions]
- Shake the suspension well.
- Avoid exposing the suspension to excessive heat or light.
- Avoid local muscle atrophy; inject drug into a large muscle, not the deltoid.
- Monitor maternal vital signs.
- Maintain accurate input and output (I&O) measurements.
- Assess blood glucose in patients with diabetes mellitus.

Evaluate Outcomes [Evaluation]
- Continue monitoring patient vital signs. Report changes.
- Continue monitoring FHR. Report any changes.
- Monitor the neonate for hypoglycemia and presence of neonatal sepsis.

TABLE 52.5 Prenatal Therapy for Surfactant Development

Generic	Route and Dosage	Uses and Considerations
Betamethasone	A: Pregnant females IM: 12 mg q 24 h × 2 dose	Corticosteroid. Given to prevent RDS in preterm infants by injecting the mother before delivery to stimulate surfactant production in fetal lung. Not effective in treating preterm infant after delivery. Most effective if given at least 24 h (preferably 48–72 h) but less than 7 d before delivery in week 33 or before. Contraindicated in severe gestational hypertension and in systemic fungal infection. Simultaneous use with terbutaline may enhance risk for pulmonary edema. Not usually given with ruptured membranes; may mask signs of chorioamnionitis. Metabolized in liver and excreted by kidneys; crosses placenta; enters breast milk. Therapy less effective with multifetal birth and with male infants. Pregnancy Considerations: Crosses the placenta. Recommended for women between 24 and 34 weeks' gestation who are at risk of delivering within 7 days. A single course may be considered for women beginning at 23 weeks' gestation who are at risk for delivering within 7 days. Multiple repeat courses are not recommended; however, in women with pregnancies less than 34 weeks at risk for delivery within 7 days who had a course greater than 14 days prior, a repeat course may be considered. PB: 64%; onset: 1–3 h; peak: 10–36 min; duration: 7–14 d; t½: 6.5 h
Dexamethasone	IM: 6 mg q12h × 4 doses	Same as betamethasone but shorter half-life and more significant variation in circulating serum levels. Pregnancy Considerations: Same as betamethasone.

d, Days; *h*, hours; *IM*, intramuscular; *IV*, intravenous; *min*, minutes; *PB*, protein binding; *q*, every; *RDS*, respiratory distress syndrome; *t½*, half-life.

discussions but no longer correct. With proper management of gestational hypertension, the prognosis for both patient and infant is good. Hypertensive disorders are reported in 10% to 20% of all pregnant patients, with 5% to 8% of all pregnancies reflecting the incidence of preeclampsia (gestational hypertension with proteinuria). Historically, preeclampsia was the presence of hypertension (systolic BP >140 or diastolic BP >90) and proteinuria (>300 mg in a 24-hour urine collection) in a normotensive patient after 20 weeks' gestation. However, "The Task Force Report – Hypertension in Pregnancy" issued by ACOG in November 2013 concluded that preeclampsia can be diagnosed without high levels of protein in the urine.

The cause of preeclampsia remains unknown, although numerous hypotheses exist. The pathophysiology is believed to be related to decreased levels of vasodilating prostaglandins with resulting vasospasm. Preeclampsia stresses all organs of the body, resulting in severe hypertension, often increased protein in the urine, headaches, visual problems, and edema of the hands and feet. About 5% of preeclampsia patients progress to eclampsia, in which seizure activity occurs. Early diagnosis of preeclampsia with appropriate treatment keeps most patients from progressing to this stage.

One severe sequela of preeclampsia is defined by its symptoms—*he*molysis, *e*levated *l*iver enzymes, and *l*ow *p*latelet count—and is therefore known as HELLP syndrome, which occurs in about 2% to 12% of patients with gestational hypertension. Patients who manifest severe preeclampsia are most likely to also have HELLP syndrome.

In addition to delivery of an uncompromised fetus and psychological support for the patient and family, two primary treatment goals in preeclampsia are reduction of vasospasm and prevention of seizures.

Delivery of the infant and placenta (products of conception) is the only known cure for preeclampsia. Vaginal delivery is preferred so that anesthesia and surgical risks will not be added. Labor induction via cervical ripening may be initiated to facilitate labor. For a vaginal delivery, epidural anesthesia or combined epidural and spinal anesthesia is frequently performed for pain management while promoting uteroplacental circulation. Maternal hypotension is a significant concern for hypertensive patients who have epidurals. In contrast, patients with worsening preeclampsia or fetal distress may be delivered via cesarean section. Patients with HELLP syndrome may have their labor induced for a vaginal delivery at 32 or more weeks' gestation. For patients with HELLP syndrome who are at less than 32 weeks' gestation, cesarean delivery may be considered.

If HELLP syndrome progresses to the point of eclampsia (maternal seizure), delivery is generally postponed for 1 to 3 hours if fetal status allows. The labor induction or cesarean delivery is an additional stressor for the patient who exhibits acidosis and hypoxia resulting from seizure. Ideally, once vital signs are stabilized with improved urinary output and decreased acidosis/hypoxia, delivery is pursued.

Nonpharmacologic treatments for preeclampsia include activity reduction; lying on the left side; eating a nutritious, balanced diet; and drinking six to eight 8-ounce glasses of water a day. Studies have shown that nonpharmacologic treatments have not had clinically beneficial effects; therefore drug therapy is commonly used for treatment.

Drugs Used to Treat Preeclampsia

Methyldopa is considered the first-line therapy for mild preeclampsia because it's been widely used in pregnant patients and its safety and efficacy has been established.

Hydralazine is recommended for use in the management of acute-onset, severe hypertension (systolic BP ≥160 mm Hg or diastolic BP ≥110 mm Hg. Oral: immediate release 10 mg given, may repeat with 20 mg dose in 20 min if needed). If treatment for chronic hypertension of pregnancy is needed, other oral agents are preferred as initial therapy.

Magnesium sulfate is used for severe preeclampsia for prevention of eclampsia. Table 52.6 lists the commonly used drugs for treating preeclampsia along with their dosages, uses, and considerations.

Adverse Reactions of Methyldopa

Observe the patient for peripheral edema, anxiety, nightmares, drowsiness, headache, dry mouth, drug-induced fever, and mental depression. These are the most common potential adverse reactions.

TABLE 52.6   Drugs Used in Severe Preeclampsia

Generic	Route and Dosage	Uses and Considerations
Magnesium sulfate	IV: 4–6 g loading dose in 100 mL over 20 min; followed by 2–4 g/h continuous infusion for at least 24 h postpartum IM: Same dose but is not the preferred route	Prevention and treatment of seizures related to preeclampsia. Calcium antagonist and CNS depressant. Decreases acetylcholine from motor nerves, which blocks neuromuscular transmission and decreases incidence of seizures. Secondary effect is reduction in BP as magnesium sulfate relaxes smooth muscle. Secondarily affects peripheral vascular system with increased uterine blood flow caused by vasodilation and some transient BP decrease during the first hour; also inhibits uterine contractions. Depresses DTRs and respiration; maintenance dose depends on reflexes, respiratory rate, urinary output, and magnesium level. Main risk is production of abnormally high serum magnesium levels. Therapeutic levels range from 4 to 7 mEq/L; effective in preventing seizures. Patient at risk if respiratory rate <12/min, urinary output <30 mL/h, DTR absent or hyporeflexic. Patellar reflexes disappear with serum magnesium levels of 8–10 mEq/L. Maternal respiratory depression may occur with levels >10–15 mEq/L; cardiac arrest occurs with levels >20–25 mEq/L. Notify health care provider if any of the previously discussed issues occur. Absorbed magnesium is excreted by kidneys; excreted in breast milk, but breastfeeding is not contraindicated. Use with caution in patients with renal impairment. Contraindicated in patients with myasthenia gravis. Relative contraindications: myocardial damage or heart block Pregnancy Considerations: Although not recommended during 2 h before delivery, stopping magnesium before cesarean delivery is not recommended and can increase risk of seizures. PB: 30%; onset: IV, immediate; IM, 1 h; duration: IV, 30 min; IM, 3–4 h; t½: UK Antidote: Calcium gluconate 1 g slow IV push over 3 min
Hydralazine hydrochloride	IV: 5–10 mg q20min; *max cumulative total:* 20 mg or until BP is controlled	Antihypertensive agent. Causes arteriolar vasodilation. Usually lowers diastolic BP more than systolic BP. Objective is to maintain diastolic BP of 90–110 mm Hg. Usually well tolerated; maternal tachycardia and increased cardiac output and oxygen consumption may occur. Usually not given to pregnant preeclamptic patients with diastolic BP >105 mm Hg because of risk for reduced intervillous blood flow. Patients with impaired renal function may require lower doses. Pregnancy Considerations: Crosses the placenta. Recommended for use in the management of acute-onset, severe hypertension with preeclampsia or eclampsia in pregnant and postpartum women. Parenteral: Onset, 5–20 min; peak, 10–80 min; PB: 87%, duration, up to 12 hours; t½: 3–7 hours
Methyldopa	PO: 250 mg bid, *max:* 3 g/d IV: 250–500 mg infused over 30–60 min q 6 h	Stimulates central α-adrenergic receptors, resulting in decreased sympathetic outflow to heart, kidneys, and peripheral vasculature. *Contraindication:* Hypersensitivity to drug or any component, active hepatic disease, liver disorders previously associated with use of methyldopa, concurrent use of MAOIs *Caution:* Sedation is usually transient during initial treatment and during dosage increases. Pregnancy Considerations: Used to treat chronic maternal hypertension during pregnancy; however, other agents are preferred for control of acute hypertension. Onset: 3–6 h; peak: 2–4 h; duration: 10–16 h (multiple doses: 24–48 h)
Labetalol	IV: 20 mg over 2 min May increase dose q 10m by 20–40 mg to a max dose of 80 mg; *max cumulative dose:* 300 mg After the initial dose, may initiate a continuous infusion of 1–2 mg/min	Blocks α-, β₁-, and β₂-adrenergic receptor sites. Monitor BP frequently. Adverse effects: orthostatic hypotension; dizziness; ventricular arrhythmia. Pregnancy Considerations: Recommended for the use in management of acute-onset, severe hypertension with preeclampsia or eclampsia in pregnant or postpartum women. Onset: 2–5 min; peak: 5–15 min; duration: 2–18 h (dose dependent); t½: 5.5 h

bid, Twice daily; *BP*, blood pressure; *CNS*, central nervous system; *d*, day; *DTR*, deep tendon reflex; *h*, hour; *IM*, intramuscular; *IV*, intravenous; *MAOI*, monoamine oxidase inhibitor; *max*, maximum; *min*, minutes; *PB*, protein binding; *PO*, by mouth; *q*, every; *t½*, half-life; *UK*, unknown; *>*, greater than; *<*, less than.

Adverse Reactions of Hydralazine

Observe the patient for headache, nausea, vomiting, nasal congestion, dizziness, tachycardia, palpitations, and angina pectoris. Avoid a sudden decrease in maternal BP, which may cause fetal hypoxia.

Adverse Reactions of Magnesium Sulfate

Early signs of increased magnesium levels include lethargy, flushing, feelings of increased warmth, perspiration, thirst, sedation, heavy eyelids, slurred speech, hypotension, DTR, and decreased muscle tone. Therapeutic magnesium levels are 4 to 7 mEq/L. Loss of patellar reflexes is

◎ CLINICAL JUDGMENT [NURSING PROCESS]

Gestational Hypertension

Concept: Perfusion

- Perfusion is the passage of blood and blood products through the circulatory system to organs or tissues to deliver oxygen and nutrients to cells, such as to the uterus and fetus.

Recognize Cues [Assessment]

- Review baseline vital signs from early pregnancy and blood pressure (BP) readings during prenatal visits.
- Identify patient history that may predispose the patient to preeclampsia.

Analyze Cues and Prioritize Hypotheses [Patient Problems]

- Hypertension
- Decreased tissue perfusion to the uterus and fetus
- Anxiety

Generate Solutions [Planning]

- The patient will maintain BP within acceptable ranges.
- The patient will verbalize understanding of preeclampsia and its etiology, signs and symptoms, and nonpharmacologic and pharmacologic treatment measures.
- The patient will understand and comply with the planned preeclampsia treatment regimen.
- The patient will maintain adequate perfusion to the fetus.
- The patient will maintain a therapeutic magnesium level.
- The patient will verbalize the need for a magnesium sulfate infusion for at least 24 hours postpartum.

Take Action [Nursing Interventions]

Magnesium Sulfate

- Provide continuous electronic fetal monitoring.
- Monitor for maternal toxicity. Lethargy and weakness resulting from blocking of neuromuscular transmission. Diaphoresis, flushing, feelings of warmth, and nasal congestion are results of vasodilation from relaxation of smooth muscle.
- Have available airway suction, resuscitation equipment, and emergency drugs in the event it is needed.
- Have available the antidote for magnesium sulfate in the event it is needed: calcium gluconate 1 g IV given over 3 minutes.
- Maintain the patient in a left lateral recumbent position in a low-stimulation environment. Provide close observation and monitoring.
- Monitor BP, pulse, and respiratory rate per agency protocol; monitor deep tendon reflexes (DTRs), clonus, and intake and output (I&O) every hour. Some health care providers will request manual BP measurements.
- Monitor temperature, breath sounds, and bowel sounds every 4 hours.
- Assess the patient's urine for protein every hour.
- Assess for epigastric pain, headache, visual symptoms (blurred vision and scotoma), sensory changes, edema, level of consciousness, and seizure activity on an ongoing basis.
- Monitor serum magnesium levels according to agency protocol for a range between 4 and 7 mEq/ L.
- Immediately notify the health care provider if the patient experiences a decrease or change in their level of consciousness; fewer than 12 respirations per minute; absence of DTR; urinary output below 30 mL/h; systolic BP of 160 mm Hg or more, unless ordered otherwise; magnesium level greater than 7 mEq/L; absent bowel sounds or altered breath sounds; epigastric pain or right upper quadrant pain (associated with hepatic edema causing stretching of the liver capsule); headache; visual symptoms (blurred vision and scotoma); sensory changes; change in affect or level of consciousness; or seizure activity.

- Monitor laboratory reports for low platelet count, elevated liver enzymes (aspartate aminotransferase [AST], lactate dehydrogenase [LDH]), and bilirubin levels. Observe for evidence of excessive bleeding.
- Monitor fetal status. Fetal heart rate (FHR) baseline should remain at 110 to 160 beats/min.
- Monitor 24-hour urinary protein laboratory results if ordered (≥300 mg/day is abnormal).
- Monitor the patient for signs and symptoms of magnesium toxicity.
- Monitor the newborn patient for effects of placental exposure to excess magnesium sulfate. Although infrequent, newborn side effects include lethargy, neurologic or respiratory depression, and muscle hypotonia.

Hydralazine

- Monitor BP frequently with an electronic BP monitoring device during drug administration.
- Maintain maintenance of diastolic BP between 90 and 110 mm Hg or as ordered.
- Observe for changes in level of consciousness and headache.
- Monitor I&O to avoid deficiency (hypotensive episodes) or overload (hypertension).
- Monitor FHR.

Patient Teaching

General

- Explain preeclampsia and its implications for the patient, fetus, and newborn.
- Provide information about nonpharmacologic and pharmacologic treatment measures for preeclampsia.
- Advise avoiding exposure to the common cold, flu, and other infectious diseases.
- Instruct the patient with diabetes to have their glucose level taken as ordered.

Side Effects

- Advise the patient to report immediately any breathing difficulty, weakness, or dizziness.
- Advise the patient to report changes in stool, easy bruising, bleeding, blurred vision, unusual weight gain, and emotional changes.

Safety

- Advise the patient to lie in the left lateral recumbent position and explain the rationale.
- Instruct the patient in the signs and symptoms of progressive preeclampsia and when to seek medical assistance.
- Instruct the patient that fetal well-being will be assessed through biophysical profile (BPP), nonstress test (NST), or contraction stress test (CST) at frequent intervals, depending on the health care provider and preeclampsia severity (e.g., NST and/or BPP 1 to 2 times per week until delivery).
- Instruct the parents regarding the possibility of seizures and appropriate actions if a seizure occurs.

Diet

- Provide nutritional counseling regarding a nutritious, balanced diet.
- Discuss the importance of adequate fluid intake.

Magnesium Sulfate

- Instruct the patient in the necessity of having an indwelling catheter, infusion pump, continuous fetal monitoring, and assessment of DTRs and clonus. Explain that therapy will extend into the postpartum period 24 to 48 hours, depending on the agency and health care provider.

⊙ CLINICAL JUDGMENT [NURSING PROCESS]—CONT'D

Gestational Hypertension

- Instruct the patient about visitor restrictions and the need for a low-stimulation environment.
- Advise the patient that a flushing feeling or a warm sensation may occur.
- Advise the patient nausea and vomiting during the initial loading dose may occur.
- Advise the patient that evidence of magnesium levels within the therapeutic range includes decreased appetite, some speech slurring, double vision, and weakness.

Hydralazine

- Instruct the patient that after administration their BP and pulse will be constantly monitored until the patient remains stable, then every 15 minutes thereafter. Explain that an electronic BP monitor may be used to obtain constant readings. Some health care providers will request manual BP measurements.

- Instruct the patient in the need for careful monitoring of their I&O.
- Advise the patient it is possible they may experience a headache as a side effect of the drug.

Evaluate Outcomes [Evaluation]

- Evaluate effectiveness of therapy to reduce BP.
- Continue monitoring vital signs. Report any changes.
- Document the patient's response to the teaching and learning opportunities provided for instruction.
- Document any knowledge deficits concerning preeclampsia treatment modalities and outcomes.
- Assess and document the fetal well-being secondary to treatment with drugs as evidenced by fetal monitoring and fetal movement assessment.
- Monitor maternal physiologic changes in relation to magnesium sulfate levels.
- Continue monitoring FHR. Report any changes.

often the first sign of magnesium toxicity and may be seen at 8 to 10 mEq/L. Respiratory depression may manifest at levels greater than 10 to 15 mEq/L, and cardiac arrest may manifest at levels greater than 20 to 25 mEq/L.

Decreased variability is commonly seen on the FHR tracing. If the patient received magnesium sulfate close to the time of delivery, the neonate may exhibit low Apgar scores, hypotonia, lethargy, weakness, and potential respiratory distress. The fetal level of magnesium generally reaches more than 90% of maternal levels within 3 hours of administration, but the greater risk to the fetus is from maternal preeclampsia, with resulting decreased placental blood flow and intrauterine growth retardation.

▮ CRITICAL THINKING CASE STUDY

A 30-year-old female (gravida 3, para 0) has a history of spontaneous abortion at 10 weeks' gestation and a preterm delivery and demise of a neonate at 21 weeks' gestation. At her 28-week prenatal visit, she reports increased clear vaginal discharge and feelings of pelvic pressure. Examination of her cervix reveals 2-cm dilation and a presenting fetal part low in the pelvis. The patient is admitted to the hospital and uterine activity is documented. Magnesium sulfate therapy is ordered for treatment of preterm labor. The nurse prepares for IV magnesium sulfate administration.

1. How will magnesium sulfate therapy be initiated? What intervals and dosages should be anticipated?
2. What maternal and fetal side effects will the nurse expect to observe?

3. What would the patient be told about the drug effects she will experience?
4. How would the nurse respond to the patient's questions about the risks of preterm delivery?

After 24 hours of magnesium sulfate therapy, uterine contractions have been reduced to two to three per hour. The patient is to be discharged home, and the nurse is preparing her discharge teaching.

5. What instructions would the nurse give the patient about her activity and diet?
6. The patient asks whether the side effects of magnesium sulfate will continue. What is an appropriate nursing response?
7. What signs and symptoms would the patient be advised to report?

▮ REVIEW QUESTIONS

1. A patient in her first trimester of pregnancy calls the nurse to ask for suggestions on decreasing nausea in the morning when she awakens. Which nonpharmacologic measures would the nurse be aware of to decrease nausea and vomiting? (Select all that apply.)
   a. Eating dry toast before rising
   b. Eating small frequent meals
   c. Eating a high-protein bedtime snack
   d. Eating high-fat foods
2. When nonpharmacological treatment fails for constipation, which drug would be a first-line treatment for constipation during pregnancy?
   a. Docusate sodium
   b. Magnesium citrate
   c. Castor oil
   d. Mineral oil

3. The nurse is teaching a pregnant client how to decrease the gastrointestinal distress she experiences with prenatal vitamins. Which instruction would the nurse provide?
   a. Take her vitamins between meals
   b. Eat when she takes her vitamins
   c. Drink orange juice when she takes her vitamins
   d. Drink milk when she takes her vitamins
4. The nurse, working with a preconceptional couple at an infertility clinic, advises the woman to take which supplement for at least 3 months before becoming pregnant?
   a. Iron
   b. Ginger
   c. Folic acid
   d. Vitamin B_6

5. A patient with severe preeclampsia is on magnesium sulfate. Which initial action by the nurse would be most appropriate for a magnesium sulfate level of 7 mEq/L?
   a. Continue to monitor the patient because this level is therapeutic.
   b. Contact the health care provider and report the level.
   c. Prepare to administer 1 g of calcium gluconate.
   d. Turn the patient on her left side and administer 10 liters of oxygen by nasal cannula.

6. Which assessment finding is most concerning when examining a client in preterm labor who is receiving magnesium sulfate?
   a. Feelings of lethargy
   b. Feelings of warmth
   c. Loss of patellar reflexes
   d. Positive clonus +2 bilaterally

7. The patient has been receiving magnesium sulfate intravenously for 24 hours to treat severe preeclampsia. On assessment, the nurse finds a temperature of 37.3°C (99°F), pulse of 88, respirations at 14, blood pressure of 138/76, 2+ patellar reflexes, and negative ankle clonus. Which intervention would be most appropriate for the nurse to take?
   a. Obtain a stat magnesium sulfate level.
   b. Discontinue magnesium sulfate.
   c. Contact the health care provider.
   d. Continue to monitor the patient.

8. A primigravida patient, 8 gestational weeks, is at the prenatal clinic for her first examination with complaints of nausea and vomiting "every morning." Which comment made by the patient would indicate the need for further instruction?
   a. "My friend gave me ginger cookies to eat."
   b. "I have been eating dry crackers before I get up."
   c. "I have tried to avoid foods with strong smells."
   d. "I have been drinking chamomile tea every day."

9. The nurse working in labor and delivery is reviewing messages to be returned to patients. Which statement made by the patient would the nurse respond to first?
   a. "I'm 32 weeks pregnant and taking calcium carbonate for my heartburn. Is there anything else I can take?"
   b. "I'm 38 weeks pregnant and taking ibuprofen for my backache. Should I take aspirin too?"
   c. "I'm 8 weeks pregnant and taking folic acid. Will it hurt me or the baby if I stop?"
   d. "I checked my blood glucose with a friend's machine and it was 120 mg/dL. I'm not diabetic. Is that normal?"

10. A young adolescent—gravida 1, para 0—is admitted to labor and delivery with preterm labor at 29 weeks' gestation. Which nursing interventions would the nurse include? (Select all that apply.)
    a. Administration of antenatal glucocorticoid
    b. Order a complete liver function profile
    c. Bed rest in the left lateral position
    d. Administration of bolus intravenous fluids
    e. Administration of tocolytics
    f. Administration of an antihypertensive

11. A patient is planning to become pregnant. Which actions would the nurse counsel the patient to initiate before she stops taking her oral contraceptive? (Select all that apply.)
    a. Stop smoking immediately.
    b. Take omega-6 fatty acids every day.
    c. Take a multivitamin every day.
    d. Stop taking over-the-counter acetaminophen.
    e. See her health care provider.

53

Labor, Delivery, and Postpartum

Christina DiMaggio Boudreaux, RN, BSN, IBCLC

http://evolve.elsevier.com/McCuistion/pharmacology

OBJECTIVES

- Critique systemic and regional medications for their action, pain control during labor, side effects, and nursing implications.
- Describe the nursing process and patient teaching associated with the drugs used during labor and delivery.
- Compare drugs used to enhance uterine contractility during labor and after placental expulsion along with their action, side effects, and nursing implications.

- Discuss the purpose, action, side effects, and nursing implications of the drugs commonly administered during the postpartum period.
- Describe the Clinical Judgment [Nursing Process] and patient teaching related to drugs used during the postpartum period immediately after delivery.

OUTLINE

DRUGS FOR PAIN CONTROL DURING LABOR

Labor and delivery are divided into four stages. During the first stage, the *dilating stage,* cervical effacement and dilation occur; the cervix thins and becomes fully dilated at 10 cm. The first stage consists of three phases categorized by cervical dilation: the *latent phase* (0 to 4 cm), the *active phase* (4 to 7 cm), and the *transition phase* (8 to 10 cm). The second stage of labor, the *pelvic stage,* begins with complete cervical dilation and ends with delivery of the newborn. During the third stage of labor, *placental separation and expulsion,* the placenta separates from the uterine wall and is delivered. The fourth stage of labor, *early postpartum,* comprises the first 4 hours after the delivery of the placenta and is a period of physiologic stabilization for the mother and initiation of familial attachment.

During the first stage of labor, uterine contractions produce progressive cervical effacement and dilation. As the first stage of labor progresses, uterine contractions become stronger, longer, and more frequent, and discomfort increases. Pain and discomfort in labor are caused by uterine contraction, cervical dilation and effacement, hypoxia of the contracting myometrium, and perineal pressure from the presenting part. Pain perception is influenced by physiologic, psychological, social, and cultural factors—in particular, the woman's past experiences with pain, anticipation of pain, fear and anxiety, knowledge deficit of the labor and delivery process, and involvement of support persons.

Before administering pharmacologic treatment, nonpharmacologic measures should be initiated. Nonpharmacologic measures for pain relief during labor include (1) ambulation, (2) effleurage and counterpressure, (3) touch and massage, (4) changing positions and rocking, (5) engaging support persons, (6) breathing and relaxation techniques, (7) transcutaneous electrical nerve stimulation, (8) application of heat and cold, (9) aromatherapy, and (10) hydrotherapy (warm-water baths or showers).

Other nonpharmacologic measures include alternative and complementary drugs. Of particular concern is the use of herbal supplements, especially in late pregnancy, to stimulate labor. Patients may self-administer, or the practice may be part of their traditional beliefs and framework of health. Concerns with herbal supplements are related to the often numerous physiologically active components of the herbs, adulterants, inconsistent dosing, and lack of proven efficacy. Herbs taken in late pregnancy may contribute to preterm labor or increased bleeding during delivery. Nurses must be sensitive to the use of herbal supplements and health practices during pregnancy, specifically in the later gestational weeks.

When pharmacologic intervention is needed for pain relief, drugs are used as an adjunct to nonpharmacologic measures. Drugs should be selected not only to decrease the patient's pain but also to minimize side effects for the patient and the fetus or neonate. Pain relief during labor can be obtained with systemic analgesics and regional anesthesia; that is, injection of a drug near the nerves or spinal canal to numb a specific area of the body (Fig. 53.1). Analgesics alter the patient's perception and sensation of pain without producing unconsciousness.

Analgesia and Sedation

Systemic drugs used during labor include sedative-hypnotics, opioid agonists, and mixed opioid agonist-antagonists. These drugs should be administered at the onset of the uterine contraction because parenteral administration at the onset decreases neonatal drug exposure because blood flow is decreased to the uterus and fetus.

Table 53.1 lists the analgesics and sedatives commonly used during labor, delivery, and postpartum and their dosages, uses, and considerations.

The sedative-tranquilizer drugs are most commonly given for false or latent labor or with ruptured membranes without true labor. These drugs may also be administered to minimize maternal anxiety and fear, and although they promote rest and relaxation, they do not provide pain relief. The sedative drugs most commonly used are barbiturates or hypnotics (e.g., pentobarbital sodium). Other drugs, such as hydroxyzine, can be given alone during early labor or in combination

with opioid agonists when the patient is in active labor. In addition to decreasing anxiety and apprehension, hydroxyzine potentiates the analgesic action of the opioids and minimizes emesis. Promethazine, also a phenothiazine derivative, has been noted in studies to impair the analgesic efficacy of opioids and is now only labeled for nausea and vomiting.

> ⚡ **PATIENT SAFETY**
>
> Do not confuse...
> • **Pentobarbital with phenobarbital.**

The second group of drugs given for active labor is the opioid agonists. These drugs may be administered parenterally or via regional blocks. When administered with neuraxial anesthesia, a lower dose of anesthetic is required for effective pain relief, thereby minimizing side effects. These drugs interfere with pain impulses at the subcortical level of the brain. Opioids interact with the mu and kappa receptors.

Of the narcotic agonists, meperidine was the most commonly prescribed synthetic opioid for pain control during labor for many years; however, current guidelines do not recommend it to treat pain during labor. Opioids are further discussed in Chapter 25.

The third group of systemic drugs used for pain relief in labor is opioids with mixed opioid agonist-antagonist effects. These drugs exert their effects at more than one site and are often an agonist at one site and an antagonist at another. The two most commonly used opioid agonist-antagonist drugs are butorphanol tartrate and nalbuphine.

Side Effects and Adverse Reactions

Adverse effects of sedative-hypnotic drugs (pentobarbital) include paradoxically increased pain and excitability, lethargy, subdued mood, decreased sensory perception, and hypotension. Fetal and neonatal side effects include decreased fetal heart rate (FHR) variability; neonatal respiratory depression, sleepiness, hypotonia; and delayed breastfeeding with poor sucking response for up to 4 days.

Side effects of phenothiazine derivatives and antiemetic antihistamines (e.g., promethazine, hydroxyzine) include confusion, disorientation, excess sedation, dizziness, hypotension, tachycardia, blurred vision, headache, restlessness, weakness, and urinary retention with promethazine; drowsiness, dry mouth, dizziness, headache, blurred vision, dysuria, urinary retention, and constipation with hydroxyzine. Decreased FHR variability can occur, and the neonate can experience moderate central nervous system (CNS) depression, hypotonia, lethargy, poor feeding, and hypothermia.

The adverse effects of opioids depend on the responses activated by the mu and kappa receptors. Activation of mu receptors results in analgesia, sedation, euphoria, decreased gastrointestinal (GI) motility, respiratory depression, and physiologic dependence. Activation of kappa receptors results in analgesia, decreased GI motility, miosis, and sedation. When parenterally administered, the side effects of opioids include nausea, vomiting, sedation, orthostatic hypotension, pruritus, and maternal and neonatal respiratory depression. The associated nausea and vomiting result from stimulation of the chemoreceptor trigger zone in the medulla. Motor block is another concern; mothers may not walk after delivery until they are able to maintain a straight leg raise against downward pressure applied by the practitioner. Fetal and neonatal effects include decreased FHR variability, depression of neonatal respirations, and depression of neonatal neurobehavior. For example, neonatal respiratory depression occurs within 2 to 3 hours after administering meperidine and may require reversal by administration of naloxone. Through inhibition of both mu and kappa receptors, naloxone may reverse the

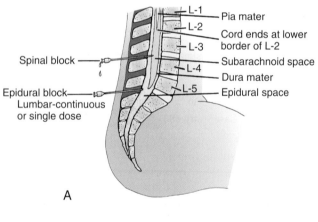

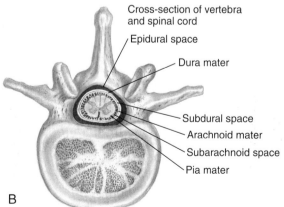

Fig. 53.1 (A) Membranes and spaces of spinal cord and levels of sacral, lumbar, and thoracic nerves. (B) Cross-section of vertebra and spinal cord. (From Lowdermilk, D., Perry, S., Cashion, C., & Alden, K. [2012]. *Maternity and women's health care* [10th ed.]. St. Louis: Mosby.)

TABLE 53.1 Analgesics Used During Labor, Delivery, and Postpartum

Drug	Route and Dosage	Uses and Considerations
Sedative-Hypnotics		
Pentobarbital	IV: 100 mg (common initial dose for 70 kg patient). IM: 150 to 200 mg use as a reduced dosage in debilitated patients.	Short-acting barbiturate and sedative for latent phase of labor Mechanism of action: Depresses the sensory cortex, decreases motor activity, alters cerebella function and produces sedation Side effects: Bradycardia, hypotension, syncope, anxiety, confusion, and hallucinations Onset: Immediate: 3–5 min. PB: 45–70%; t½: 15–50 h [!] An increased incidence of fetal abnormalities may occur after maternal use. Respiratory depression may occur in the newborn when administered to the mother during labor; resuscitation equipment should be readily available. Not contraindicated but should be used with caution
Promethazine	IM/IV: Early labor: 50 mg Established labor: 25–75 mg in combination with analgesic at reduced dosage; may repeat every 4 hours for up to 2 additional doses (*Max:* 100 mg/day while in labor)	A phenothiazine antihistamine and antiemetic often given with opioids as an adjunct to increase sedation and reduce nausea and vomiting in labor. Do not give subcutaneously [!] *Black Box Warning:* Severe tissue damage has been seen with injections and extravasation, which can result in necrosis and gangrene; use the Z-track method for IM injection to prevent or reduce complications, and dilute IV doses and give over 10–15 min. Instruct patients to report signs of pain and burning with administration Side effects: Blurred vision, CNS depression, orthostatic hypotension Pregnancy Considerations: Crosses the placenta and platelet aggregation may be inhibited in newborns after maternal use within 2 weeks of delivery. It is indicated for use during labor for obstetric sedation and may be used alone or as an adjunct to opioid analgesics. Also approved for use as an antiemetic in pregnancy; however, other agents are recommended as initial therapy for the treatment of nausea and vomiting of pregnancy. Onset: IM: 20 min; IV: 3–5 min; duration: 4–6h (up to 12 h). PB: 93%; t½: 9–16h. PB: 35%–55%; t½: 22 h
Hydroxyzine	Anxiety: PO: 25–100 mg qid PRN Preoperative sedation: IM: 50–100 mg as a single dose	Anxiolytic antiemetic antihistamine used as a preoperative and postoperative adjunct therapy to reduce opioid dosage, treat anxiety and control emesis in labor Side effects: CNS depression Onset: PO: 15–30 min; IM: rapid peak: 2 h; duration: 2–36 h. PB: UK; t½: 3–7 h [⚡] Acute High Alert: Crosses the placenta and possible withdrawal symptoms have been observed in neonates after chronic maternal use during pregnancy. Use of hydroxyzine early in pregnancy is contraindicated
Narcotic Agonists		
Fentanyl citrate	IV: 50–100 mcg Give IV over 1–2 min, may repeat q1–2h PRN; muscle rigidity may occur when IV administration is too rapid Regional anesthesia: Initial 50–100 mcg bolus, then 10–15 mL/h of bupivacaine and fentanyl continuous infusion	[!] A synthetic opiate that is 100 times as potent as morphine. Used as pain relief as adjunct to regional anesthesia Side effects: Constipation, nausea and vomiting, dyspnea, confusion, dizziness, fatigue, headache, CNS depression Contraindicated in patients with severe asthma Onset: IV, 1–2 min; peak: IV, 3–5 min; duration: IV, 30–60 min. PB: 79–87%; t½: 2–4 h [!] Blackbox Warning: Crosses the placenta and can cause respiratory depression in the newborn and life-threatening withdrawal symptoms, especially in prolonged maternal use. Make sure resuscitation equipment is readily available for the newborn. Fentanyl patches have not been studied and therefore are not recommended in pregnancy
Morphine sulfate	Only given as adjunct to regional anesthesia at 1/10 of the IV dose IV dose: 2–5 mg every 3–4 h PRN	An opioid that binds to CNS opiate receptors and inhibits ascending pain pathways; used for adjunct to regional anesthesia for pain in delivery Side effects: CNS depression, constipation, hypotension Monitor for CNS and respiratory depression. Have naloxone available as antidote Onset: IV, 3–10 min; peak: IV, 20 min; duration: IV, 3–5 h. PB: 30%–35%; t½: 2–4 h [!] *Black Box Warning:* Crosses the placenta. Watch for respiratory depression in the newborn and life-threatening withdrawal symptoms, especially with prolonged maternal use. Have resuscitation equipment for newborn readily available

Continued

TABLE 53.1 Analgesics Used During Labor, Delivery, and Postpartum—cont'd

Drug	Route and Dosage	Uses and Considerations
Mixed Opioid Agonist-Antagonists		
Butorphanol tartrate	IM/IV: 1–2 mg; may repeat in 4 hours	Mixed opioid agonist-antagonist used for relief of moderate to severe pain. Used in pregnancies >37 wk with no fetal distress. Use alternative analgesic if delivery is anticipated in 4 h or less Side effects: CNS depression, hypotension, constipation Onset: 5–10 min; peak: 4–5 min; duration: 3–4 h. PB: 80%; t½: 2.5–4 h ⚠ Blackbox Warning: Crosses the placenta. May temporarily affect the heart rate of the fetus, causing abnormal patterns. Prolonged use in pregnancy can cause neonatal opioid withdrawal syndrome. Have resuscitation equipment readily available
Nalbuphine hydrochloride	Surgical anesthesia supplement: IV: 0.3–3 mg/kg over 10–15 min; *maintenance:* 0.25–0.5 mg/kg as required	Mixed opioid agonist-antagonist narcotic used as adjunct to anesthesia Side effects: Respiratory depression; constipation, hypotension Onset: 2–3 min; peak: 2–3 min; duration: 3–6 h. PB: 50%; t½: 5 h ⚠ Blackbox Warning: Crosses Placenta; may cause respiratory depression in newborn; abnormal heart rate, and severe bradycardia. Have resuscitation equipment and naloxone on hand to reverse bradycardia
Postpartum Perineal Wounds and Hemorrhoids		
Benzocaine, aerosol 20%	Spray liberally tid/qid 6–12 inches from the perineum after perineal cleansing	A local anesthetic that inhibits impulses from sensory nerves by decreasing permeability of the cell membrane to sodium ions; it is hydrolyzed in plasma and liver (to a lesser extent) by cholinesterase and is eliminated as metabolites in urine. Drug is well absorbed from mucous membranes and traumatized skin and is contraindicated in patients with secondary bacterial infection of tissue and known hypersensitivity. Side effects: rash, hives, itching, redness Peak: 1 min; duration: 30–60 min. PB: UK; t½: UK Pregnancy Considerations: When used in moderation, not associated with significant risk of adverse pregnancy outcomes
Witch hazel or pramoxine premedicated pads	Apply premoistened pads up to 6 times daily, especially after bowel movements	Witch hazel is one of the safest and most natural postpartum vaginal care options for local irritation and discomfort of hemorrhoids and episiotomies Precipitates protein, causing tissue to contract. May be refrigerated in the original container for additional comfort. If liquid, pour over ice and dip absorbent pads into solution; change when diluted. Medical intervention should be sought if rectal bleeding is present. Side effect: local irritation (discontinue use) PB: UK; t½: UK Pregnancy Considerations: Not associated with significant risk of pregnancy outcomes
Hydrocortisone acetate 25 mg	Insert 1 suppository bid rectally for 2 wk Wear gloves to administer	Acts as an antiinflammatory agent to relieve pain and itching from irritated anorectal tissue. Contraindicated in patients with known hypersensitivity. Discontinue if tissue infection occurs. If anorectal symptoms do not improve in 7 days or if bleeding, protrusion, or seepage occurs, inform the health care provider. Do not use if fourth-degree perineal laceration is present. It is unknown whether drug is excreted in breast milk; use cautiously Onset, peak, and duration are unknown Pregnancy Considerations: Not associated with significant risk of adverse pregnancy outcomes when used in moderation; however, there may be an increased risk of low-birth-weight infants after maternal use of potent or very potent topical products
Dibucaine ointment, USP 1%	Apply to cleansed rectum 3–4 times daily, using no more than 30 g in 24 h	Topical anesthetic with the same action as benzocaine. Do not use near eyes or over denuded surfaces or blistered areas or if rectal bleeding is present. Do not use with known hypersensitivity to amide-type anesthetics. Side effects include burning, tenderness, irritation, inflammation, contact dermatitis, urticaria, cutaneous lesions, and edema Onset: Within 15 min; peak: UK; duration: 2–4 h.

bid, Twice daily; *CNS,* central nervous system; *cont.,* continuous; *FHR,* fetal heart rate; *h,* hour; *IM,* intramuscular; *IV,* intravenous; *max,* maximum; *min,* minute; *PB,* protein binding; *PO,* by mouth; *PRN,* as needed; *q,* every; *qid,* four times daily; *subcut,* subcutaneously; *t½,* half-life; *tid,* three times daily; *UK,* unknown; *USP,* US Pharmacopeia; *wk,* weeks; *>,* greater than.

effects of opioids. It is important to note that with maternal administration of naloxone, there will be a subsequent increase in pain.

Opioid agonist drugs can cause orthostatic hypotension, nausea, vomiting, headache, sedation, hypotension, confusion, decreased FHR variability, and neonatal CNS depression.

Mixed opioid agonist-antagonist drugs (e.g., butorphanol tartrate, nalbuphine) can cause nausea, clamminess, sweating, sedation, respiratory depression, vertigo, lethargy, headache, and flush. Side effects in the fetus and neonate include decreased FHR variability, moderate CNS depression, hypotonia at birth, and mild behavioral depression.

Anesthesia: Local, Regional, and General

Anesthesia in labor and delivery represents the loss of painful sensations with or without loss of consciousness. Two types of pain are experienced in childbirth, visceral and somatic. Visceral pain occurs during the first two stages of labor from uterine contractions and the pressure of the stretching cervix. *Somatic pain* is caused by pressure of the presenting part and by stretching of the perineum and vagina. This is the pain of the transition phase and the second stage of labor. Table 53.2 lists the anesthetics used during labor and delivery and their dosages, uses, and considerations.

Regional Anesthesia. Regional anesthesia achieves pain relief during labor and delivery without loss of consciousness. Injected local anesthetic agents temporarily block conduction of painful impulses along sensory nerve pathways to the brain. Regional anesthesia allows the patient to experience labor and childbirth with relief from discomfort in the blocked area while maintaining consciousness. The two primary types of anesthesia are *local anesthetics* for local infiltration (e.g., episiotomy) and *regional blocks* (e.g., epidural, spinal). The most common types of peridural anesthesia are spinal, epidural, and combined spinal-epidural blocks. Other, less commonly administered regional blocks include caudal, paracervical, and pudendal blocks. The anesthesiologist or nurse anesthetist is responsible for administering regional anesthesia. Nurses may assist and monitor the patient for drug effectiveness and side effects during and after administration.

◎ CLINICAL JUDGMENT [NURSING PROCESS]

Pain Control Drugs

Concept: Pain
- Pain is the discomfort caused by an injury or illness, such as in labor and delivery.

Recognize Cues [Assessment]
- Assess the patient's level of pain.
- Assess the patient's beliefs regarding labor and expectations related to pain experiences.
- Assess for use of complementary and alternative medicine (CAM), including supplements, at any point during the pregnancy.
- Assess for drug history to ascertain the potential for drug interactions.
- Obtain vital signs (blood pressure [BP], heart rate [HR]), respiratory status, quality of uterine contractions, degree of effacement and dilation, and fetal heart rate (FHR) before and after administration of an analgesic and monitor the effectiveness of pain management.
- Assess the laboring patient's behavior for relaxation and progress of labor in relation to expected norms.
- Assess the patient's verbal and nonverbal behavior for data supportive or nonsupportive of coping with labor.

Analyze Cues and Prioritize Hypotheses [Patient Problems]
- Pain
- Discomfort
- Communication
- Reduced functional ability
- Confusion
- Decreased ability to cope
- Need for health teaching

Generate Solutions [Planning]
- The patient will verbalize a decrease in pain on a scale of 1 to 10 or per the agency's pain scale.
- The patient will demonstrate minimal to no side effects from pain control drugs during labor.

Take Action [Nursing Interventions]
- Assess the patient's parity, obstetric delivery history, and anticipated time until delivery.

- Offer analgesia appropriate for the stage and phase of labor and anticipated method of delivery. Encourage the patient and their support person to participate in decision making about analgesia.
- Document the administration of drugs per agency protocol.
- Provide appropriate safety measures after administration of drugs.
- Monitor the patient's vital signs, heart rate, and breathing pattern.
- ⚡ Check a compatibility chart for mixing of drugs.
- Verify that correct antidote drugs are available.
- Administer drugs before pain and anxiety reach maximum intensity within agency protocol, safe obstetric practice, and patient preferences.
- Assess the patient's level of pain using an agency-appropriate pain scale 30 to 60 minutes after analgesic administration.
- Monitor FHR, assessing for fetal well-being before and during any drug administration.
- Instruct the patient to request assistance with ambulation and to keep the bed rails up when the patient is nonambulatory.
- Monitor the patient's urine output.

Patient Teaching
General
- Advise the patient concerning (1) drugs ordered, (2) route of administration and reason, (3) expected effects of the drug on labor, and (4) potential drug effects on the mother and the fetus or neonate.
- Advise the patient that most drugs used for pain relief in labor and delivery are not given by mouth because the GI tract functions more slowly during labor and drug absorption is decreased, making the oral route ineffective.
- Instruct the patient about safety precautions to be used while receiving the drug, including (1) positioning in bed, (2) use of side rails, and (3) assistance with ambulation.

Evaluate Outcomes [Evaluation]
- Evaluate effectiveness of the drug in alleviating pain.
- Evaluate fear and anxiety in regard to pain and the ability to cope with labor.
- Monitor maternal respirations, heart rate, BP, uterine contractions, dilation and effacement, and FHR for alterations from baseline. Report deviations beyond those expected with normally progressing labor.
- Document findings using agency protocol and obstetric nursing standards of care.

TABLE 53.2   Anesthetic Used in Obstetrics[a]

Drug	Route and Dosage	Uses and Considerations
Chloroprocaine	Lumbar epidural block: 2% or 3%, 2–2.5 mL per segment; usual start volume is 15–25 mL; *max:* single dose (with epinephrine 1:200,000), 14 mg/kg; total dose, 750 mg	An ester-type local anesthetic that stabilizes the neuronal membranes and prevents initiation and transmission of nerve impulses, affecting local anesthetic actions (local or pudendal block) Side effects: hypotension, bradycardia, restlessness, anxiety, dizziness, tremors Onset of action: 6–12 min; duration: Up to 60 min. PB: UK; t½: 21–25 sec ⚡ Pregnancy Considerations: Rapidly crosses placenta and may cause varying degrees of fetal and neonatal toxicity. Have resuscitation equipment near
Tetracaine 0.2%, 0.3%	Spinal anesthesia: Lower abdomen: 10 mg of 0.3% Perineum: 5mg of 0.3% Saddle block: 2–4 mg of 0.2%; *max:* 15 mg Other anesthesia dosages available	An ester-type local anesthetic that blocks both initiation and conduction of nerve impulses by decreasing neuronal membrane permeability to sodium ions; a low spinal block or spinal anesthesia for cesarean delivery Adverse reactions: hypotension, chills, dizziness, drowsiness, nausea, vomiting, tremors, seizures Duration of action: 1.5–3 h. PB: UK; t½: UK ⚡ Pregnancy Considerations: Crosses placenta, fetal monitoring is recommended
Lidocaine injectable	Doses vary per procedure, see packaging; *max:* 4 mg/kg/dose or 300 mg per procedure when used without epinephrine	Suppresses automaticity of conduction tissue by increasing the electrical stimulation threshold of the ventricle; blocks both initiation and conduction of nerve impulses by decreasing neuronal membrane permeability to sodium ions Side effects: headache, bradycardia, hypotension, anxiety, dizziness, n/v, tremors Onset: 45–90 s; duration: 10–20 min. PB 60%–80%; t½: 1.5–2 h ❗ Blackbox Warning: Crosses placenta. Approved for obstetric analgesia, however, adverse reactions have been noted in fetus/neonate, with affecting CNS, heart, or peripheral vascular tone. Fetal heart rate monitoring is recommended, as well as emergency equipment being on hand. Cumulative total from all routes of administration should be considered
Bupivacaine	Epidural block: 3–4 mL increments IV or intrathecal administration of 10–20 mL of 0.25% or 0.5%	Epidural or spinal for labor and cesarean delivery; blocks both initiation and conduction of nerve impulses by decreasing neuronal membrane permeability to sodium ions Adverse effects: Bradycardia, hypotension, arrhythmias, anxiety, nausea, vomiting Onset: Up to 17 min; duration: epidural, 2–7.7 h; spinal, 1.5–2.5 h. PB: 84%–95%; t½: 2.7 h ❗ *Black Box Warning:* The 75% concentration is not recommended for obstetric anesthesia; reports of cardiac arrest with difficult resuscitation and death have been reported
Ropivacaine	Lumbar epidural block for cesarean section: 20–30 mL dose of 0.5% solution or 15–20 mL of 0.75% solution in incremental doses Doses available for vaginal obstetric anesthesia as incremental administration or continuous infusion	Epidural for cesarean delivery; blocks both initiation and conduction of nerve impulses by decreasing neuronal membrane permeability to sodium ions Adverse effects: hypotension, bradycardia, nausea, vomiting, back pain, hypertension and tachycardia Position pregnant woman in left lateral position to prevent compression of the uterus Onset: 3–15 min; duration: 3–15 h. PB: UK; t½: 5–7 h ⚡ Pregnancy Considerations: Crosses placenta, which can result in fetal/neonatal effects of CNS and cardiovascular depression. Fetal monitoring and resuscitation equipment required

abd, Abdomen; *h,* hour; *IV,* intravenous; *max,* maximum dosage; *min,* minute; *n/v,* ; *PB,* protein binding; *t½,* half-life; *UK,* unknown.

[a]The following nursing considerations apply to all types of epidurals: Use a test dose (3 mL of lidocaine 1.5% with 1:200,000 epinephrine) to confirm correct catheter placement. If a local anesthetic is injected into a vein, the patient may experience dizziness, ringing in the ears, numbness, a metallic taste in the mouth, or a toxic response. Maternal lateral positioning is done to prevent aortocaval compression. Maternal diastolic blood pressure (BP) should be less than 110 mm Hg before initiating the epidural. When maternal hypotension occurs, place the patient on her left side, infuse IV fluids rapidly, and administer ephedrine 5 to 10 mg IV or 100 mcg phenylephrine IV. Repeat as necessary. Monitor BP every 1 to 2 min for the first 10 min, then every 10 to 30 min until the block wears off. Assess the level of analgesia. After administration of the anesthetic, assess motor strength before ambulation.

Local Anesthesia. Women receiving parenteral analgesic for labor and delivery may require more focused anesthesia for episiotomies and repair of perineal lacerations. Local anesthetic drugs such as lidocaine may be administered. Burning at the site of injection is the most common side effect.

Regional Anesthesia. Spinal anesthesia, also known as a *saddle block*, is injected in the subarachnoid space at the T10 to S5 dermatome. This anesthesia may be administered as a single dose or as a combined spinal-epidural block. Spinal anesthesia is administered immediately before delivery or late in the second stage, when the fetal head is on the perineal floor. Drugs frequently administered either alone or in combination with the local anesthetic for a vaginal delivery include bupivacaine with fentanyl. Dosages vary depending on whether administration of the anesthetic agent is plain or with epinephrine. Bupivacaine 0.75% concentration is *not* recommended for obstetric anesthesia due to reports of cardiac arrest with difficult resuscitation or death. Spinal anesthesia has a rapid onset, requires less local anesthetic, and may be used with high-risk patients. Postdural puncture headache is a primary concern and occurs 6 to 48 hours after dural puncture; it may also occur after accidental dural puncture with epidural anesthesia. Treatment for postdural headache includes analgesics, increased fluids, and bed rest. An epidural blood patch is the most effective means to treat postdural headache.

Lumbar epidurals may be administered as a single injection, by intermittent injection, as continuous patient-controlled epidural anesthesia (PCEA), or as a combined spinal-epidural block. Epidurals may be administered as a single anesthetic drug or with opioids or epinephrine. Most frequently, patients now receive a continuous epidural infusion, which provides more consistent drug levels and more effective pain relief. Rescue doses are given as necessary to achieve pain relief. Opioids are administered with a local anesthetic to more effectively control the somatic pain of transition and second-stage labor (see Tables 53.1 and 53.2).

Another additive to the local anesthetic is epinephrine, which increases the duration of the local anesthetic, decreases its uptake and clearance from the cerebrospinal fluid (CSF), and enhances the intensity of the neural blockade. Single and intermittent injections have wide variations in drug levels and provide less effective control of pain. A continuous lumbar epidural allows a more evenly spaced drug level; less anesthetic is required to provide more effective pain control. Continuous-infusion PCEA gives the patient better control of her anesthesia. Often, single and intermittent injections and PCEA will require rescue doses to improve analgesia.

Lastly, combined spinal-epidural analgesia couples the rapid analgesia and specificity of catheter placement of spinal anesthesia with the continuous infusion via catheter of epidural anesthesia, providing pain relief for later labor.

Controversy exists regarding the effect of regional analgesia, specifically epidurals, on the progress of labor. Some studies indicate no significant effect on labor, whereas other research has demonstrated a decreased maternal urge to push and increased length of labor.

General Anesthesia. General anesthesia, although rarely used, may be necessary for emergency deliveries, when spinal or epidural anesthesia is contraindicated. It allows for rapid anesthesia induction and control of the airway. Before the administration of general anesthesia, antacids or other drugs that reduce gastric secretions are given to decrease gastric acidity. See Unit XIII: Gastrointestinal Drugs for more information on acid reducers. More commonly, spinal or epidural anesthesia is administered for cesarean births. Spinal anesthesia is the more common choice for cesarean delivery because of rapid onset,

◉ CLINICAL JUDGMENT [NURSING PROCESS]

Regional Anesthetics

Concept: Pain
- Pain is the discomfort caused by an injury or illness, such as in labor and delivery.

Recognize Cues [Assessment]
- Check the patient's history for drug sensitivity to local anesthetic agents.
- Assess the patient's labor plan with expectations for coping with labor and beliefs about use of analgesia and anesthesia.
- Assess the patient's knowledge about regional anesthesia.
- Assess cervical dilation and effacement and labor progress.
- Monitor fetal status.
- Review the patient's history for contraindications to regional anesthesia; notify the anesthesia provider.

Analyze Cues and Prioritize Hypothesis [Patient Problems]
- Discomfort
- Communication
- Reduced functional ability
- Pain
- Coping
- Anxiety

Generate Solutions [Planning]
- The patient will verbalize the desired amount of pain relief during labor.
- The patient will remain normotensive and will maintain a normal pulse rate; fetal heart rate (FHR) will remain within normal parameters. The patient will maintain minimal to no side effects from anesthesia.
- The patient will maintain urine output.
- The patient will be able to discuss use of regional anesthesia for labor and delivery pain control.

Take Action [Nursing Interventions]
General
- Assess hydration status before regional anesthesia is given; monitor for anesthetic hypotensive effects. Provide bolus intravenous (IV) fluids as ordered, usually 500 to 1000 mL before regional anesthesia administration.

- Insert an indwelling urinary catheter before administration to monitor maternal fluid status.
- Position and support the patient on the left side or as instructed by the anesthesia provider.
- Monitor labor progress for any decrease in frequency or intensity of uterine contractions.
- Monitor maternal vital signs and FHR.
- Supply oxygen and emergency drugs, including ephedrine and antihistamines, along with resuscitation equipment in the event it may be needed.
- Monitor for postdural puncture headache; notify the anesthesia provider.

Spinal
- Assess uterine contractions; anesthetic drugs must be given immediately after a contraction.
- Monitor blood pressure (BP) for hypotensive effects per agency protocol; this is generally a decrease in systolic BP greater than 20% to 30% of baseline or below 100 mm Hg.
- Have a supply of oxygen with positive-pressure ventilation equipment readily available.
- Assess level of analgesia after administration and sensory and motor status after delivery.
- Document procedures per agency protocol.

Epidural
- Ensure that the patient has 500 to 1000 mL IV bolus of an isotonic solution before the procedure to increase circulatory volume and prevent maternal hypotension.
- Monitor FHR and progress of labor, and keep in mind that anesthetic can inhibit fetal descent.
- Monitor BP for hypotensive effects per agency protocol.
- Assess the level of analgesia after administration.
- Maintain the patient on the left side and increase the rate of IV fluids per agency protocol if maternal hypotension occurs, notify the health care provider immediately.

Continued

CLINICAL JUDGMENT [NURSING PROCESS]—CONT'D

Regional Anesthetic

- Assess for bladder distension. If voiding cues are unsuccessful (e.g., placement in semi-Fowler position, privacy, running water over the perineum, running water over the hand), catheterize the patient.
- Assess the patient's sensory and motor status before ambulation after delivery.
- Manage the patient's pain by ongoing pain assessments. If the nature of the patient's pain changes, contact the anesthesia provider to evaluate anesthesia needs.
- Document procedures per agency protocol.

Caudal

- Place the patient in the position requested by the anesthesia provider for administration.

Paracervical Block

- Maintain continuous FHR monitoring for fetal bradycardia after administration.
- Monitor maternal BP.

Patient Teaching
General

- Discuss technique, potential benefits, and side effects of the patient's particular method of anesthesia.

Side Effects

- Instruct the patient that regional anesthetics may slow labor and there may be a need for a drug to enhance uterine contractions.

- Assess the patient for postdural puncture headache after spinal anesthesia or after accidental dural puncture with epidural anesthesia.
- Advise the patient that bed rest, oral analgesics, caffeine, or an autologous blood patch may be used for relief of headache pain.

Skill

- Instruct the patient how to curl into position for epidural administration.
- Instruct the patient that forceps or vacuum extraction may be needed for delivery because of reduction of the "urge to push" sensation.
- Instruct the patient how to assume the left lateral or other position as requested by the anesthesia provider for caudal anesthesia.
- Advise the patient receiving epidural anesthesia they will have an IV and close monitoring of FHR and uterine contractions secondary to anesthesia.

Evaluate Outcomes [Evaluation]

- Evaluate BP compared with preprocedure baseline; evaluate FHR for alterations in variability and for decelerations.
- Evaluate effectiveness of anesthetic in relieving discomfort.
- Evaluate for uniformity of anesthesia; if there is lateralization or if it is "patchy," notify the anesthesia provider.
- Assess for bladder distension. If voiding cues are unsuccessful, catheterize the patient.
- Assess the patient's sensory and motor status before ambulation after delivery.
- Evaluate the uterine fundus for firmness.

---

increased reliability, and improvement in spinal needle design (smaller gauge and shape [Sprotte needle]) with subsequent reduction in postdural headaches. With spinal anesthesia, the local anesthetic most commonly administered is bupivacaine with fentanyl; pain relief begins in 5 minutes and lasts for approximately 2 hours. With the additives, spinal anesthesia provides 18 to 24 hours of pain relief. For epidural inductions, the test dose of lidocaine with epinephrine—followed by administration of local anesthetics—is given. This is followed by a bolus or maintenance infusion with anesthetics with or without opioids and/or epinephrine to maintain maternal comfort. The nurse should assess the level of analgesia and motor block at least hourly. Monitor for complications, such as cardiovascular or CNS toxicity, postdural puncture headache, fetal bradycardia, or respiratory depression.

Absolute Contraindications to Regional Anesthesia

- Severe gestational hypertension (increased risk of profound hypotension associated with the underlying disease state)
- Coagulation disorders and risk of bleeding secondary to decreased platelets (the patient should have a normal partial thromboplastin time and platelet count)
- Generalized sepsis or local infection at the needle insertion site

DRUGS THAT ENHANCE UTERINE MUSCLE CONTRACTILITY

Uterotropic drugs enhance uterine contractility by stimulating the smooth muscle of the uterus. Oxytocin, the ergot alkaloids, and some prostaglandins constitute the uterotropics.

Oxytocin is synthesized in the hypothalamus and is transported to nerve endings in the posterior pituitary gland. The hormone is released by the nerve endings under appropriate stimulation; capillaries absorb the substance and carry it into the general circulation, where

it facilitates uterine smooth muscle contraction. Table 53.3 lists drugs commonly used for cervical ripening and uterine contraction.

In the presence of adequate estrogen levels, those normally achieved by the third trimester, IV oxytocin stimulates uterine contraction. Oxytocin prepared in a synthetic form is approved by the US Food and Drug Administration (FDA) for labor induction, the process of causing or initiating labor, and also for labor augmentation.

Before labor induction begins, risks and benefits and the status of the mother and fetus must be assessed, and informed consent for induction must be obtained. The gestational age of the fetus must be considered, together with the position of the fetus (head down and deep in the pelvis) and the size of the fetus in relation to the mother's pelvis. Cervical ripening, or softening of the cervix, is also assessed; the cervix is ripe and thus ready for induction when it is soft and progressing in effacement and partial dilation. An objective measurement called the Bishop score assists in predicting whether labor induction may be successful, and it is used to assess readiness for induction. Elements assessed in the modified Bishop scoring system are (1) dilation, (2) effacement, (3) station, (4) cervical consistency, and (5) cervical position. Modified Bishop scores of 8 or greater are associated with a successful labor induction.

In pregnant women at or near term with a medical or obstetric indication for labor induction, cervical ripening and effacement for cervical dilation are obtained with the administration of dinoprostone, a naturally occurring form of PGE$_2$. It is thought that intracervically or intravaginally administered PGE$_2$ acts to create cervical effacement and softening through a combination of contraction-inducing and cervical-ripening properties, possibly secondary to an increased submucosal water content and collagen degradation resulting from collagenase secretion in response to PGE$_2$. One approach uses prefilled syringes of commercially prepared dinoprostone cervical gel, 0.5 mg, which is introduced just inside the cervical os. A second approach

TABLE 53.3 Cervical Ripening and Uterine Contractions

Drug	Route and Dosage	Uses and Considerations
Cervical Ripening		
Dinoprostone cervical gel, 0.5 mg	Contains 0.5 mg of dinoprostone in 2.5 mL of gel for intracervical use Before beginning oxytocin after dinoprostone cervical gel administration, there should be a 6- to 12-h delay	Naturally occurring form of prostaglandin E_2 (PGE_2). Used to ripen an unfavorable cervix at or near term in women needing labor induction. Must be at room temperature before administration and is administered by sterile technique, using catheter supplied and inserted into the cervical canal. Patient is to remain recumbent 15–30 min after administration of gel and 2 h after insert Adverse effects: hypersensitivity reactions including anaphylaxis, GI distress, uterine contractions, back pain PB: UK; t½: 2.5–5 min; onset: 10 min; peak: 30–45 min; duration: 12 h ⚡ Pregnancy Considerations: Fetal distress without corresponding maternal uterine hyperstimulation. Abnormal fetal heart rate and distress. Fetal monitoring and resuscitation equipment required ❗ Blackbox Warning: Requires specialized care setting that can provide immediate intensive care facility and an experienced clinical to over see use and monitoring.
Dinoprostone vaginal inserts, 10 mg	Contains 10 mg of dinoprostone in a timed-release insert that supplies 0.3 mg/h. Insert is left in place for 12 h. Oxytocin may be started 30–60 min after removal of an insert. In contrast to gel, inserts may be removed with FHR decelerations or uterine hyperstimulation Ripening an unfavorable cervix: 10 mg over 12 h; remove 12 h after insertion or at onset of active labor	Assess cervical dilation and effacement at time of insertion. After administration, patient remains in a lying position for 30 min to 2 h. Monitor FHR and uterine stimulation. Have medication available for frequent GI side effects of abdominal cramping, diarrhea, nausea, and vomiting. If uterine hyperstimulation occurs, remove the insert and have oxygen or beta-adrenergic drugs to treat. Onset: 10 min; peak: UK; duration: up to 2–3 h. PB: UK; t½: 2.5–5 min ⚡ Pregnancy Considerations: Crosses placenta. Fetal distress and abnormal heart rate can occur. Fetal monitoring and resuscitation equipment required ❗ Blackbox Warning: Requires specialized care setting that can provide immediate intensive care facility and an experienced clinical to oversee use and monitoring.
Uterine Contraction		
Oxytocin	See Prototype Drug Chart: Oxytocin	
Carboprost tromethamine	IM: Initially, 0.25 mg; repeat every 15–90 min as needed *Max total dose:* 2 mg (8 doses)	Naturally occurring prostaglandin F_2-alpha. Direct stimulation of uterine smooth muscle. Treatment of postpartum hemorrhage secondary to uterine atony. Give deep IM rotating sites if repeat injections are required. Contraindicated before delivery of placenta. Use with caution in patients with acute renal disease, cardiac disease, hypertension, PID, and asthma. *Adverse reactions:* Diarrhea, nausea, vomiting, fever, and abdominal pain with cramps. PB: UK; t½: 8 min; peak: 30 min Pregnancy Considerations: Intended for use after delivery of the infant and placenta
Methylergonovine maleate	PO: 0.2 mg 3–4 times daily in the puerperium for up to 7 d IM: 0.2 mg after delivery of anterior shoulder (if full obstetric supervision), after delivery of placenta, or postpartum; repeat q2–4h. Oral doses may follow parenteral administration IV: Same as for IM but slowly over 1 min with careful monitoring of BP (IV route for acute emergencies only [e.g., bleeding])	Prevention and treatment of postpartum hemorrhage, subinvolution, and postabortion hemorrhage. Exhibits similar smooth muscle action to ergotamine but primarily affects smooth muscle, producing sustained contractions and shortening the third stage of labor. Not routinely administered IV because of possible sudden hypertensive and cerebrovascular accidents; limit use in patients with hypertension (especially IV). Contraindicated with maternal sepsis, labor induction, threatened spontaneous abortion Do *not* use with vasodepressors, other ergot alkaloids, or vasoconstrictors. Appears in breast milk, but interference with breastfeeding is less than with ergonovine. *Adverse reactions:* Transient hypertension, diaphoresis, palpitations, dizziness, headache, nausea, vomiting, tinnitus, transient chest pain, dyspnea, bradycardia, angina, hallucinations, seizures Onset of Action: Oral 5–10 min; IM: 2–5 min; IV: immediate; duration: Oral/IM: 3 h; IV: 45 min. PB: UK; t½: 3 h Pregnancy Considerations: Intended for use after delivery of the infant and is contraindicated during pregnancy

BP, Blood pressure; *d*, day; *FHR*, fetal heart rate; *GI*, gastrointestinal; *h*, hour; *IM*, intramuscular; *IV*, intravenous; *max*, maximum; *min*, minute; *PB*, protein binding; *PID*, pelvic inflammatory disease; *PO*, by mouth; *q*, every; *t½*, half-life; *UK*, unknown.

is the placement in the posterior vaginal fornix of a vaginal insert of dinoprostone containing 10 mg of controlled release dinoprostone at 0.3 mg/h.

Side effects associated with the use of prostaglandins include uterine hyperstimulation, which can be treated with terbutaline sulfate. Uncommonly, some patients experience chills, fever, vomiting, and diarrhea. Contraindications to the use of prostaglandins include active vaginal bleeding and known allergies to prostaglandins. With hepatic or renal disease, cautious use of PGE_2 is recommended; use of PGE_2 is contraindicated in patients with glaucoma.

Table 53.3 lists the dosages, uses, and considerations for administration of dinoprostone for cervical ripening.

📋 **PROTOTYPE DRUG CHART**

Oxytocin

Drug Class	Dosage
Oxytocic agent Used to induce labor during pregnancy, to control postpartum hemorrhage, and to prevent uterine atony postdelivery Pregnancy Considerations: To be used for medical rather than elective induction of labor. Small amounts of exogenous oxytocin are expected to reach the fetal circulation. Nonteratogenic adverse reaction is reported in the neonate as well the mother	For induction or augmentation of labor: Dilute 10 units (1 amp) of oxytocin in 1000 mL lactated Ringer's solution for 10 milliunits/mL Connect to primary IV line close to needle site as a piggyback line. IV: Low-dose regimen: Start with 0.5–1 milliunits/min; gradually increase dose in increments of 1–2 milliunits/min q30–60 until desired contraction pattern is established. Dose may be decreased by similar increments after desired frequency of contractions is reached and cervix is 5–6 cm dilated. Infuse up to 6 milliunits/min. Provides oxytocin levels similar to those of spontaneous labor; rates >9 milliunits/min are rarely required. High-dose regimen: Start with 6 milliunits/min; may increase 3–6 milliunits/min q15–60 min until desired contraction pattern is established. If uterine hyperstimulation, decrease dose to 3 milliunits/min; may be further decreased to 1 milliunits/min. For reduction and control of postpartum hemorrhage and postdelivery uterine contractions: IV: 10–40 units added to 1000 mL compatible IV solution; infuse at a rate to prevent uterine atony. IM: 3–10 units after delivery of the placenta

Contraindications	Drug-Lab-Food Interactions
Proven cephalopelvic disproportion, fetal intolerance of labor, hypersensitivity, anticipated nonvaginal delivery; intranasal spray is contraindicated in pregnancy. ⚠ *Black Box Warning:* To be used for medical, rather than elective, induction of labor	Drug: Hypertension can occur with vasopressors, and hypotension and/or bradycardia can occur with cyclopropane anesthetics. Herbals: Black cohosh, cottonroot, squaw vine, and cinnamon can have a synergistic effect to oxytocin.

Pharmacokinetics	Pharmacodynamics
Absorption: Not well absorbed PO; intranasal and IM absorption is very rapid. Distribution: Low PB; widely distributed in extracellular fluid; minute amounts in fetal circulation Metabolism: t½: 1–9 min; rapidly metabolized in liver Excretion: In urine	IM: Onset: 3–5 min Peak: 40 min Duration: 2–3 h IV: Onset: Within 1 min Peak: UK Duration: 1 h Intranasal: Onset: Minutes Peak: UK Duration: UK

Therapeutic Effects/Uses

To induce or augment labor contractions; to treat uterine atony (intranasal spray)
Mechanism of Action: Oxytocin promotes uterine contractions by increasing intracellular concentrations of calcium in uterine myometrial tissue, thereby increasing the activity of the calcium-dependent phosphorylating enzyme myosin light-chain kinase.

Side Effects	Adverse Reactions
Maternal effects with undiluted IV use include hypertension, dysrhythmias, uterine hyperstimulation (contractions lasting at least 2 min or 5 or more contractions in a 10-min window), and tachysystole (6 or more uterine contractions in a 20-min window).	Seizures; water intoxication can occur if given in electrolyte-free solution or at a rate greater than 20 milliunits/min. (Water intoxication is manifested by nausea, vomiting, hypotension, tachycardia, and cardiac arrhythmias.) *Life-threatening:* Maternal intracranial hemorrhage, cardiac dysrhythmias, asphyxia; fetal jaundice, hypoxia

amp, Ampule; *h,* hour; *IM,* intramuscular; *IV,* intravenous; *min,* minute; *PB,* protein binding; *PO,* by mouth; *q,* every; *t½,* half-life; *UK,* unknown; *>,* greater than.

Oxytocin

In addition to labor induction, IV oxytocin can also be used for labor augmentation, stimulation of effective uterine contractions once labor has begun. It facilitates smooth muscle contraction in the uterus of a patient already in labor but experiencing inadequate uterine contractility, tightening and shortening of uterine muscles. The patient with uterine inertia, uterine inactivity or hypotonic contractions, may be more responsive to oxytocin than the patient who has not begun labor; therefore a lower starting dose will be needed.

In both labor induction and labor augmentation, oxytocin is infused at a prescribed individualized dosage rate, and this rate is increased, decreased, or maintained at fixed intervals based on uterine and fetal response. The objective is to establish an

⊚ CLINICAL JUDGMENT [NURSING PROCESS]

Enhancement of Uterine Contractility: Oxytocin

Concept: Comfort
- Comfort is the easing or alleviating a person's pain, grief, or distress.

Recognize Cues [Assessment]
- Confirm term gestation before inducing or augmenting labor and obtain the patient's informed consent.
- Collect accurate baseline data before beginning infusion, including maternal pulse and blood pressure (BP), uterine history, uterine activity, and fetal heart rate (FHR) pattern.
- Interview the patient and review the history to ascertain that no contraindications exist.

Analyze Cues and Prioritize Hypothesis [Patient Problems]
- Pain
- Discomfort
- Reduced functional ability

Generate Solutions [Planning]
- The patient will have enhanced uterine contractions without adverse maternal or fetal effects.
- The patient will maintain vital signs within acceptable ranges throughout labor, delivery, and the postpartum period.
- The patient will demonstrate FHR that is normal in rate, pattern, and variability throughout labor and delivery.

Take Action [Nursing Interventions]
- Have a supply of tocolytic drugs, such as terbutaline, and oxygen readily available.
- Monitor the patient's intake and output.
- Monitor maternal pulse and BP, uterine activity, and FHR during oxytocin infusion.
- Maintain the patient in a sitting or lateral recumbent position to promote placental infusion.
- Monitor for signs of uterine rupture, which include FHR decelerations, sudden increased pain, loss of uterine contractions, hemorrhage, and rapidly developing hypovolemic shock.
- Use an intravenous (IV) pump to administer all intravenous drugs.

Patient Teaching
- Inform the patient the drug is given intravenously and the dosage is adjusted in response to the uterine contraction pattern.

Evaluate Outcomes [Evaluation]
- Evaluate for effective labor progress.
- Monitor maternal vital signs every 30 to 60 minutes and with every increment in dose and monitor FHR every 15 minutes and with every increment in dose during the first stage of labor and every 5 minutes in the second stage of labor. Report changes in vital signs and FHR, specifically late decelerations, and report any vaginal bleeding.

---

adequate contraction pattern that promotes labor progress, generally represented by contractions every 2 to 3 minutes that last for 50 to 60 seconds with moderate intensity. It is important that the patient receiving oxytocin *not* experience uterine hyperstimulation, which causes markedly increased pain and compromised FHR patterns secondary to impaired placental perfusion. Continuous nursing observation during labor induction or augmentation is critical. The need for an accurate infusion rate requires the use of an infusion pump with oxytocin as an IV piggyback line. Once cervical dilation has reached 5 to 6 cm and an adequate contraction pattern is evident, the rate of oxytocin infusion can often be slowed or stopped.

After delivery, oxytocin 10 to 40 units is usually added to an existing IV solution to help the uterus stay contracted and close the uterine sinuses at the placental site. The maximum concentration should be 40 units per 1000 mL IV fluid. Prototype Drug Chart: Oxytocin lists the pharmacologic data for oxytocin.

The peak concentration time is unknown for all methods of administration, but the onset of action of IM oxytocin is 3 to 5 minutes, and the duration of action is 2 to 3 hours; the onset of action of IV oxytocin is immediate, and the duration of action is 1 hour.

The medication is diluted and administered by IV piggyback for induction or augmentation of labor. Oxytocin is diluted in a variety of ways and is administered via infusion pump in milliunits-per-minute dosing with the volume determined by the dilution. IV administration of undiluted oxytocin is not recommended because of the risk of a sudden acute hypotensive response.

Concurrent use of vasopressors can result in severe hypertension, whereas hypotension can occur with concurrent use of cyclopropane anesthesia and with undiluted IV push administration. The Institute for Safe Medication Practices (ISMP) includes oxytocin on its list of high-alert medications because of its heightened risk of causing significant harm when used in error.

Other Drugs That Enhance Uterine Contractions: Ergot Alkaloids

The ergot alkaloids, one of a large group of alkaloids derived from fungi, act by direct smooth muscle cell receptor stimulation. These drugs are *not* used during labor because they can cause sustained uterine contractions (tetanic contractions), which would result in fetal hypoxia and could rupture the uterus. In addition, the uterus becomes more sensitive to these drugs. After delivery, however, sustained contractions are effective to prevent or control postpartum hemorrhage and to promote uterine involution.

The most commonly used ergot derivative is methylergonovine maleate, which can be given by mouth but is most frequently administered intramuscularly. IV administration is not recommended and is used only in emergency situations. If IV methylergonovine maleate is given, administer 0.2 mg over 1 minute. Transient significant elevations in BP can occur, particularly after IV infusion. Patients with preexisting or gestational hypertension or peripheral vascular diseases should *not* receive ergot derivatives. Table 53.3 lists commonly used uterotonic drugs and their dosages, uses, and considerations.

Side Effects and Adverse Reactions

Side effects of ergot alkaloids include uterine cramping, nausea and vomiting, dizziness, hypertension with IV administration, sweating, tinnitus, chest pain, dyspnea, itching, and sudden severe headache. Signs of ergot toxicity, also called ergotism, include pain in the arms, legs, and lower back; numbness; cold hands and feet; muscular weakness; diarrhea; hallucinations; seizures; and blood hypercoagulability.

TABLE 53.4	Nonpharmacologic Measures for Common Postpartum Needs
Indication	**Intervention**
Uterine contractions	Patient is positioned on the abdomen with a pillow under the abdomen for 20–30 min for 3–4 d.
	Distraction, breathing techniques, therapeutic touch, relaxation, guided imagery, and ambulation may be used.
	No heat should be applied to the abdomen because of the risk of uterine relaxation and increased bleeding.
Perineal wound resulting from episiotomy or laceration	Ice packs made with a nonlatex glove filled with crushed ice and covered in a thin, absorbent material to protect tissue are applied for 6–8 h after delivery.
	The patient is positioned on her side as much as possible with a pillow between the legs; early and frequent ambulation and perineal exercises (Kegels) are encouraged.
	A cool sitz bath should be taken 2–3 h after delivery along with warm sitz baths 12–24 h after delivery two to three times daily.
	The perineum is cleansed front to back using a peri-spray squeeze bottle or cleansing shower.
	Keep area around the stitches clean and dry and change pads every 2–3 h
	Patient is advised to tighten the buttocks or squeeze them together before sitting and to sit tall and flat, not rolled back onto the coccyx.
	No tampons, douches, or feminine hygiene sprays should be used until advised by the health care provider.
	Advise no intercourse until after lochia has ceased or as advised by the health care provider.
Hemorrhoids	As previously mentioned but particularly:
	Apply ice packs to area several times a day
	Modified left lateral recumbent position position to help increase venous return
	Warm, moist heat or sitz bath
	Witch hazel pads (e.g., Tucks)
	Alternate cold and warm treatments as directed
Lactation suppression	Tight bra worn continuously for 10–14 d
	Normal fluid intake
	No manipulation or stimulation of breasts
	Pyridoxine (vitamin B$_6$) 200 mg for 5 d
Engorgement	Same as for lactation suppression as previously discussed plus ice to the axillary area of the breasts if bottle feeding or warm compresses if breastfeeding; cold cabbage leaves placed inside the bra may also be helpful.
	If breastfeeding, express a small amount of colostrum or milk by hand before putting the infant to the breast to facilitate latching on.
Sore or cracked nipples	Wear absorbent breast pads to keep moisture away from nipples.
	Do not use soap on nipples.
	Air-dry nipples after nursing.
	After nursing, express a small amount of breast milk on nipples to use as a protective lubricant.
	After nursing, apply hypoallergenic purified lanolin to nipples as a protective lubricant to promote healing.
	For cracked nipples, use comfort gel pads (hydrogel pads).
	Do not use nipple shields because they can promote chafing.
	Do not limit the infant's nursing time; if the milk ducts are not emptied, increased pressure can occur.
	Ensure proper positioning for feeding and initiate nursing on the less sore nipple.
	After feeding, the infant may instinctively suck during attempts to disengage: break the suction with your little finger to prevent pulling on the nipple.

d, Day; *h*, hour; *min*, minute.

DRUGS USED DURING THE POSTPARTUM PERIOD

During the puerperium, the period from delivery until 6 weeks postpartum, the mother's body physically recovers from antepartal and intrapartal stressors and returns to its prepregnant state.

Pharmacologic and nonpharmacologic measures commonly used during the postpartum period have five primary purposes: (1) to prevent uterine atony and postpartum hemorrhage; (2) to relieve pain from uterine contractions, perineal wounds, and hemorrhoids; (3) to enhance or suppress lactation, production and release of milk by the mammary glands; (4) to promote bowel function; and (5) to enhance immunity (Tables 53.4 and 53.5).

Whenever possible, nonpharmacologic measures are preferred to the use of drugs or are used in conjunction with drugs. Postpartum nursing care ideally occurs as a partnership between the nurse and the new family. To enhance health and wellness, the nurse collaborates with the mother and family to strengthen the new mother's self-confidence and ability to handle her own health challenges. The nurse's role in this system is threefold:

🌿 COMPLEMENTARY AND ALTERNATIVE THERAPIES

Herbal Supplements and Lactation

Because little is known about the safety of herbal supplements, they are not generally recommended during lactation. Breastfeeding patients should be advised to check with their health care provider before taking any herbal supplements; those contraindicated for breastfeeding patients include aloe, belladonna, black tea, bromelain, buckthorn bark, burdock, cat's claw, chondroitin, comfrey, echinacea, ephedra (Ma-huang), eucalyptus, flaxseed, kava, lavender, licorice, milk thistle, pennyroyal, and saw palmetto. This list is not exhaustive. Again, it is important to check with the health care provider on all complementary and alternative therapies used during lactation.

TABLE 53.5   Promote Postpartum Bowel Function

Generic	Route and Dosage	Uses and Considerations
Docusate sodium, docusate calcium (various dosages available)	50–360 mg/d PO in 1–4 divided doses; *max:* 360 mg/d for docusate sodium; 240 mg/d for docusate calcium	Reduces surface tension of the oil-water interface of the stool, resulting in enhanced incorporation of water and fat and subsequent stool softening. Docusate salts are interchangeable (Na, Ca, or K is clinically insignificant). Do not use concomitantly with mineral oil. Do not use for more than 1 wk. Prolonged, frequent, or excessive use may cause bowel dependence or electrolyte imbalance. Contraindicated in patients with intestinal obstruction, acute abdominal pain, nausea, or vomiting. Compatible with breastfeeding Side effect is rash Onset: 12–72 h. PB: NA; t½: NA Pregnancy Considerations: Hypomagnesemia was reported in a newborn after chronic maternal use throughout pregnancy. Nonpharmacologic treatment is preferred initially.
Sennosides 8.6 mg tab or 8.8 mg/5 mL	PO: 1–2 tabs bid; take with a full glass of water or 10–15 mL at bedtime	A stimulant laxative that acts on the colon as a local irritant to promote peristalsis and bowel evacuation; also increases moisture content of stool by accumulating fluids in the intestine. Metabolized in liver, eliminated in feces (viable) and urine. Drug interactions may occur with MAOIs, disulfiram, metronidazole, and procarbazine. May discolor urine or feces. May create laxative dependence and loss of bowel function with prolonged use Side effects: abdominal cramps, diarrhea, nausea/vomiting Contraindicated in patients with fluid and electrolyte disturbances, abdominal pain, and nausea and vomiting; excreted in breast milk Onset: 8–12 h but may require up to 24 h. PB: NA; t½: NA Pregnancy Considerations: Agents other than senna are preferred as initial treatment of constipation when pregnant. Not recommended for chronic use, but may be used intermittently
Bisacodyl (10 mg supp or 5 mg tab)	PO: 5–15 mg once daily PR: 1 supp as a single dose *Max:* PO: 15 mg/d; PR 10 mg/d	Stimulant laxative; irritates smooth muscle of the intestine and possibly the colon and intramural plexus; alters water and electrolyte secretion, increasing intestinal fluid and producing a laxative effect. After oral or rectal administration, 5% absorbed systemically; metabolized in the liver to conjugated metabolites; excreted in breast milk, bile, and urine. Do not crush tablets or give within 1 h of milk or antacid because enteric coating may dissolve, resulting in abdominal cramping and vomiting. Side effects include abdominal cramps, nausea, vomiting, rectal burning, electrolyte and fluid acidosis or alkalosis, and hypocalcemia. Onset: PO, 6–10 h; PR, 15 min–1 h Pregnancy Considerations: Not recommended for chronic use
Magnesium hydroxide Magnesium concentrate is three times as potent as regular-strength product.	PO: 15–60 mL reg susp or 15–30 mL conc susp per d, preferably at bedtime; may be taken in divided doses Tab: 2–4 caplets/d, preferably at bedtime; may be taken in divided doses	A laxative that acts by increasing and retaining water in the intestinal lumen, causing distension that stimulates peristalsis and bowel elimination. Absorbed drug is excreted in kidneys; unabsorbed drug is excreted in feces. Drug poses a risk to patients with renal failure because 15%–30% of the magnesium is systemically absorbed. Use with caution in patients with impaired renal function; hypermagnesemia and toxicity may occur as a result of decreased renal clearance of absorbed magnesium. Contraindicated in patients with colostomy, ileostomy, abdominal pain, nausea, vomiting, fecal impaction, and renal failure. Drug interactions may occur with tetracyclines, digoxin, indomethacin, iron salts, or isoniazid Side effects are abdominal cramps and nausea. Adverse reactions include hypotension, hypermagnesemia, muscle weakness, and respiratory depression. Onset: 4–8 h. Pregnancy Considerations: Magnesium crosses the placenta; however, serum concentrations in the fetus are similar to those in the mother and considered acceptable for treating heartburn of pregnancy
Simethicone	PO: 40–125 mg qid after meals and at bedtime; *max:* 500 mg/d	An antiflatulent that acts by dispersing and preventing formation of mucus-surrounded gas pockets in the GI tract; drug changes the surface tension of gas bubbles and allows them to coalesce, making them easier to eliminate as belching and rectal flatus. Tablets must be chewed thoroughly before swallowing; follow with a full glass of water. Drug is excreted unchanged in feces; may interfere with results of guaiac tests of gastric aspirates, but no other side effects are known. Do *not* take double doses to make up for missed doses. Store below 104°F (40°C) in a well-closed container. Onset: UK. t½: UK Pregnancy Considerations: Not absorbed systemically after oral administration; therefore does not cross the placenta

bid, Twice daily; *Ca,* calcium; *conc,* concentration; *d,* day; *GI,* gastrointestinal; *h,* hour; *K,* potassium; *MAOI,* monoamine oxidase inhibitor; *max,* maximum dosage; *min,* minute; *Na,* sodium; *NA,* not applicable; *PB,* protein binding; *PO,* by mouth; *PR,* per rectum; *qid,* four times a day; *reg,* regular; *supp,* suppository; *susp,* suspension; *t½,* half-life; *tab,* tablet; *UK,* unknown; *wk,* week.

- To assess and discuss postpartal physical changes and pain management with the patient and determine healing progress within a standard and effectiveness of medications
- To teach the patient and administer postpartal medications
- To teach the patient and administer opioid analgesics as prescribed when pain control by nonnarcotics is ineffective

Pain Relief for Uterine Contractions

Afterbirth pains may occur during the first few days postpartum, when uterine tissue experiences ischemia during contractions, particularly in multiparous patients and when breastfeeding. Nonsteroidal agents may be used to control postpartal discomfort and pain; opioid agents are reserved for more severe pain, such as that experienced by the patient after cesarean delivery, tubal ligation, or extensive perineal laceration. Table 53.1 lists systemic analgesics commonly used during the postpartum period.

Because some systemic analgesics can cause decreased alertness, it is important for the nurse to observe the patient as she cares for her newborn to ensure safety. Patients who receive opioids should be assessed for bowel function and respirations. With continued opioid use, patient assessment of bowel history is necessary because these drugs can exacerbate the constipation of pregnancy. During the intrapartum period, women are NPO (nothing by mouth) or ingest limited liquids and are not ambulatory, all factors that contribute to decreased bowel activity. In addition, respiratory assessment is important for patients receiving opioids because respiratory depression may occur. Frequently, nonsteroidal drugs like ibuprofen are used to control postpartum discomfort and pain. Nonsteroidal antiinflammatory drugs (NSAIDs) inhibit the enzyme cyclooxygenase (COX), of which there are two isoenzymes, COX-1 and COX-2; both decrease prostaglandin synthesis. These drugs are effective in relieving mild to moderate pain caused by postpartum uterine contractions, episiotomy, hemorrhoids, and perineal wounds. NSAIDs commonly cause GI irritation, and it is recommended that patients take them with a full glass of water or with food to minimize GI distress. With administration of NSAIDs, a lower narcotic dosage may control pain as a result of the additive analgesic effect. The use of NSAIDs requires ongoing assessment for GI bleeding. These drugs inhibit platelet synthesis and may prolong bleeding time. Patient teaching with this category of drugs is important because some NSAIDs may be purchased over the counter (OTC). Patient teaching includes avoidance of these drugs while pregnant if symptoms of GI bleeding occur (dark, tarry stools; blood in urine; coffee-ground emesis) and avoidance of the concurrent use of alcohol, aspirin, and corticosteroids, which may increase the risk for GI toxicity.

Pain Relief for Perineal Wounds and Hemorrhoids

Pregnancy and the delivery process increase pressure to the perineal soft tissue, causing it to become ecchymotic or edematous. Increased edema, ecchymosis, and pain may occur if an episiotomy, incision made to enlarge the vaginal opening to facilitate newborn delivery, or perineal laceration is present. The perineum is assessed for *r*edness, *e*cchymosis, *e*dema, *d*ischarge, and *a*pproximation (REEDA). In addition, hemorrhoids that developed during pregnancy may be exacerbated by the pushing during labor. Comfort measures—ice packs immediately after birth, tightening of the buttocks before sitting, use of peri-bottles, and cool or warm sitz baths—and selected topical agents such as witch hazel and dibucaine ointment may relieve pain and minimize discomfort (see Table 53.1). Note that rectal suppositories should *not* be used by women with fourth-degree perineal lacerations.

 CLINICAL JUDGMENT [NURSING PROCESS]

Pain Relief for Perineal Wounds and Hemorrhoids

Concept: Pain
- Pain is the discomfort caused by an injury or illness.

Recognize Cues [Assessment]
- Assess the patient's pain using an agency pain scale.
- Assess the perineal area for wounds and hemorrhoids (size, color, location, pain scale, REEDA [redness, ecchymosis, edema, discharge, and approximation]).
- Assess for presence of infection at the perineal site; avoid use of benzocaine on infected perineal tissue.

Analyze Cues and Prioritize Hypotheses [Patient Problems]
- Pain
- Infection

Generate Solutions [Planning]
- The patient will report decreased perineal discomfort with the use of topical sprays, compresses, sitz baths, and ointments.
- The patient will be free of signs and symptoms of infection.

Take Action [Nursing Interventions]
- Teach the patient about use of the peri-bottle. Use warm, direct water on the perineum from front to back (clean to dirty).
- Instruct the patient not to use benzocaine spray when perineal infection is present.
- Shake the spray can and administer benzocaine 6 to 12 inches from the perineum with the patient lying on their side, top leg up and forward, to provide maximum exposure. This can also be done with one foot on the toilet seat.
- Apply witch hazel compresses (glycerin and witch hazel or witch hazel solution) with an ice pack and a peri-pad cold to the affected area.
- Store pramoxine and hydrocortisone acetate suppositories below 86°F (30°C) but protect them from freezing. Use gloves for administration.

- Assess to determine whether the patient is ready to switch to a preparation without hydrocortisone (the goal is to discontinue use of suppositories as quickly as possible if the patient is breastfeeding).
- Instruct carefully the use of pramoxine hydrochloride (HCl). Instruct the patient to place the agent inside the anus, which is not generally done with an obstetric patient because they may have perineal wounds that extend into the anus. Rectal suppositories should not be used by patients with fourth-degree perineal laceration.

Patient Teaching
General
- Describe the process of perineal wound healing.
- Explain the expected action and side effects. With witch hazel, a cooling, soothing sensation will provide relief. Ointment and suppositories will soothe, lubricate, and coat mucous membranes. Pramoxine HCl is not chemically related to the "-caine" type of local anesthetics, and there is a decreased chance of cross-sensitivity reactions in patients who are allergic to other local anesthetics.
- Advise patients that the drug is not for prolonged use (no more than 7 days) or for application to a large area.
- Instruct that topical analgesia lasts for several hours after use.
- Advise the patient to store suppositories below 86°F (30°C) so they do not melt, and do not freeze. Counsel the patient with bleeding hemorrhoids to use the drug carefully and to keep their health care provider (HCP) informed if the condition exacerbates or does not improve within 7 days.

Self-Administration: Perineal Wounds—Topical Spray Containing Benzocaine
- Apply three to four times daily or as directed.
- Apply without touching sensitive areas.
- Instruct the patient to administer the spray by either lying on their side in bed while spraying from behind or by standing with one foot on a chair or toilet seat and to hold the can 6 to 12 inches from the affected area.

⊙ CLINICAL JUDGMENT [NURSING PROCESS]—CONT'D

Pain Relief for Perineal Wounds and Hemorrhoids

- Avoid contact of medication with eyes.
- Assess use of complementary and alternative medicine (CAM), including herbal supplements.
- Instruct the patient not to use a perineal heat lamp after application because this could cause tissue burns.
- Notify the health care provider if exacerbation of symptoms recurs within a few days.
- Keep all medications out of children's reach in the postpartum unit the home. If ingested, contact a poison control center immediately.
- Store below 120°F (49°C). Dispose of empty cans without puncturing or incinerating.

Self-Administration: Hemorrhoids and Perineal Wounds—Witch Hazel Compresses

- Apply by pouring liquid witch hazel over chipped ice; place soft, clean, absorbent squares in the solution; squeeze each square to eliminate excess moisture, and fold and place the moist square against the episiotomy site or hemorrhoids.
- Instruct the patient using commercial medicated pads that the entire container may be placed in the refrigerator.
- Avoid touching the surface of the pad placed next to the perineal wound.
- Instruct the patient when to change the compress and how to place the ice bag and peri-pad over the compress.
- Instruct the patient not to insert medicated pads into the rectum.
- Keep all products out of children's reach.
- Instruct the patient use is not recommended if rectal bleeding is present.
- Discontinue use if local irritation occurs.

Self-Administration: Hemorrhoids—Ointment and Suppositories

- Apply ointment externally in the postpartum period.
- Place the suppository in the lower portion of the anal canal. Caution must be used because products usually are not inserted rectally if fourth-degree lacerations are present.
- Apply a small quantity of ointment onto a 2-inch square gauze pad; place inside the peri-pad against the swollen anorectal tissue approximately five times per day.
- Instruct the patient if a suppository is ordered to keep it refrigerated but not frozen. Remove the wrapper before inserting the suppository in the rectum (hold the suppository upright and peel evenly down the sides). Do not hold the suppository for a prolonged period; it will melt. If a suppository softens before use, hold it in the foil wrapper under cold water for 2 to 3 minutes.
- Assess the patient for hypersensitivity to any components of the ointment.
- Avoid contact of medication with eyes.
- Instruct the patient that ointment may occasionally cause a burning sensation, especially if anal tissue is not intact.

- Discontinue use and consult the HCP if erythema, irritation, edema, or pain develops or increases.
- Notify the health care provider if bleeding occurs.

Self-Administration: Hydrocortisone and Pramoxine and Pramoxine Hydrochloride

- Instruct the patient that the product is for anal or perianal use only and is not to be inserted into the rectum.
- Shake the can vigorously before use and fully extend the applicator plunger; hold the can upright to fill the applicator. Express the contents of the applicator onto a 2-inch square gauze pad and place it inside the peri-pad and against the rectum.
- Instruct the patient to use two to three times daily and after bowel movements.
- Wash the applicator by taking it apart after each use and rinsing it with warm water.
- Keep the aerosol container out of children's reach in the postpartum unit and later in the home.
- Store below 120°F (49°C).
- Dispose of the aerosol container without puncturing or incinerating it.
- Avoid contact of medication with eyes.
- Instruct the patient that it is unknown whether topical administration of corticosteroids results in sufficient systemic absorption to produce detectable quantities in breast milk. Burning, itching, irritation, dryness, and folliculitis may occur, especially if occlusive dressings are used.

Self-Administration: Dibucaine Ointment, 1%

- Express ointment from the applicator on a tissue or 2-inch square gauze pad and place it against the anus. Do not insert the applicator into the rectum. Effects should occur within 15 minutes and should last for 2 to 4 hours. Ointment is poorly absorbed through intact skin but is well absorbed through mucous membranes and excoriated skin.
- Instruct the patient to not use near eyes, over denuded surfaces or blistered areas, or if there is rectal bleeding.
- Advise the patient to not use more than one tube (30-g size) in 24 hours.
- Keep all medication out of children's reach.
- Assess the patient for any known hypersensitivity to amide-type anesthetics; if so, dibucaine ointment is contraindicated.
- Instruct the patient that local side effects may include burning, tenderness, irritation, inflammation, and contact dermatitis; inform the health care provider if these occur. Other side effects may include edema, cutaneous lesions, and urticaria.

Evaluate Outcomes [Evaluation]

- Reevaluate the patient's perception of pain after use of nonpharmacologic and pharmacologic measures. Identify the need for additional patient teaching.
- Reassess perineal and anal tissues for integrity, healing, and side effects.

Side Effects and Adverse Reactions

The most commonly reported side effects of topical or local agents include burning, stinging, tenderness, edema, rash, tissue irritation, and sloughing, in addition to tissue necrosis, tissue death caused by disease or injury. The most commonly reported side effects of hydrocortisone local or topical drugs include burning, pruritus, irritation, dryness, folliculitis (skin inflammation resulting from contact with an irritating substance or allergen), allergic contact dermatitis, and secondary infection. These side effects are more likely to occur when occlusive (i.e., obstructive) dressings are used.

Lactation Suppression

Due to severe side effects such as thrombophlebitis and potential carcinogenic effects, medications that were once prescribed for lactation suppression are no longer used. Nonpharmacologic measures are currently recommended for lactation suppression, such as wearing a well-fitted support bra or breast binder continuously for 72 hours after giving birth and avoiding breast stimulation, including running warm water over the breast and expressing milk.

If breast engorgement occurs while trying to suppress lactation, ice packs to the breasts (15 minutes on and 45 minutes off each hour) can help decrease the discomfort and swelling. The use of cabbage leaves is often recommended to help decrease engorgement. It is recommended that the woman wear a cold cabbage leaf over each breast inside of her bra and replace the leaves each time they wilt. A mild analgesic can help decrease discomfort during this time (see Table 53.1).

Promotion of Bowel Function

Constipation is common during the postpartum period. The residual effects of progesterone on smooth muscle decrease peristalsis. This decrease in peristalsis—added to decreased liquid intake during labor,

 CLINICAL JUDGMENT [NURSING PROCESS]

Laxatives

Concept: Elimination
- Elimination is the act of discharging or excreting waste products from the body.

Recognize Cues [Assessment]
- Obtain a history of bowel problems by noting the time of delivery, predelivery food and fluid intake, ambulation and activity, and predelivery bowel habits. Obtain a history of bowel problems.
- Assess bowel sounds in all four quadrants, particularly after cesarean delivery, and note abdominal distension.
- Assess the perineal area for wounds, hemorrhoids, and episiotomy (REEDA).

Analyze Cues and Prioritize Hypotheses [Patient Problems]
- Pain
- Discomfort
- Constipation

Generate Solutions [Planning]
- The patient will have a bowel movement by 2 to 4 days postpartum.
- The patient will resume a normal bowel elimination pattern within 4 to 6 weeks.

Take Action [Nursing Interventions]
Docusate Sodium and Sennosides
- Store at room temperature.
- Instruct the patient if a liquid preparation is ordered, it may be taken with milk or fruit juice to mask the bitter taste.
- Instruct the patient to always consume with a full glass of water.
- Assess for a history of laxative dependence.
- Instruct the patient that drug interactions may occur with mineral oil, phenolphthalein, or aspirin.

Bisacodyl
- Store tablets and suppositories below 77°F (25°C) and avoid excess humidity.
- Instruct the patient to not crush tablets.
- Instruct the patient not to administer within 1 to 2 hours of milk or antacid because enteric coating may dissolve, resulting in abdominal cramping and vomiting.
- Consume with a full glass of water.

Magnesium Hydroxide
- Shake the container well.
- Instruct the patient not to take 1 to 2 hours before or after oral drugs because of the effects on absorption.
- Consume with a full glass of water.
- Advise the patient that milk of magnesia concentrate is three times as potent as the regular-strength product.
- Administer laxatives 1 hour before or 1 hour after any oral antibiotic.

Senna
- Protect senna from light and heat.

Simethicone
- Administer after meals and at bedtime.

- Instruct the patient if chewable tablets are ordered, the tablets must be chewed thoroughly before swallowing and followed with a full glass of water.

Patient Teaching
General
- Advise patients that stool softeners are given to enable bowel movement without straining.
- Advise patients that measures to prevent and treat constipation include drinking 6 to 8 glasses of fluid per day, ingesting foods high in fiber (bran, fruits, vegetables), and increasing daily ambulation and activity. Instruct patients to avoid or minimize ingestion of gas-forming foods (beans, cabbage, onions) and to increase ambulation and other activity.
- Advise patients regarding temperature and storage requirements for particular drugs.
- Instruct the patient prolonged, frequent, or excessive use may result in electrolyte imbalance or dependence on the drug.
- Advise the patient that many laxatives contain sodium. Instruct them to check with their health care provider or pharmacist before using any laxative if they are on a low-sodium diet.

Docusate Sodium and Sennosides With Docusate Sodium
- Advise patients to drink at least six 8-oz glasses of liquid daily and to drink one glass of fluid with each dose. Patients should not take the drug if they are already taking mineral oil or having acute abdominal pain, nausea, vomiting, or signs of intestinal obstruction. Patients should not use products for longer than 1 week, and they should report skin rash or stomach or intestinal cramping that does not diminish.

Senna
- Instruct the patient that senna may change urine and feces to a yellow-green color; advise discontinuation of senna if abdominal pain, nausea, or vomiting occurs.

Magnesium Hydroxide
- Advise the patient that laxative action generally occurs in 4 to 8 hours.
- Instruct the patient that magnesium hydroxide should be taken with a full glass of water.
- Instruct the patient to note whether the drug is in regular or concentrated form; the concentrate is three times more potent than the regular-strength product.
- Advise the patient that the drug may interact with tetracyclines, digoxin, indomethacin, iron salts, and isoniazid. Instruct the patient to notify their health care provider if any of these drugs are used.
- Instruct the patient to report any muscular weakness, diarrhea, or abdominal cramps.

Simethicone
- Advise the patient that simethicone will help relieve flatus and associated pain and that it should be taken after meals; if chewable tablets are ordered, instruct patients to chew tablets thoroughly and to drink a full glass of water afterward. If a dose is missed, the patient should take it as soon as possible but should not take double doses.

Evaluate Outcomes [Evaluation]
- Evaluate for the return of regular bowel function.

decreased activity, and relaxation of the abdominal muscles—amplifies the problem. Patients who deliver by cesarean are even more likely to experience constipation and flatus (intestinal gas). Nonpharmacologic measures such as high-fiber foods, early ambulation, drinking at least 64 ounces of fluids per day, and promptly responding to the defecation urge are generally instituted after delivery.

Pharmacologic measures include the use of stool softeners, laxative stimulants, and for the postcesarean patient, antiflatulents to treat excessive gas in the stomach and intestines (see Table 53.5).

IMMUNIZATIONS

Rh$_0$(D) Immune Globulin

The Rh factor is a protein found on the surface of red blood cells. If a patient's blood cells have this protein, they are considered Rh positive; if not, they are negative.

A patient who lacks the (Rh) factor in her own blood (an Rh-negative mother) may carry a fetus who is either Rh negative or Rh positive. During pregnancy, minimal amounts of fetal blood can cross the placenta. Also, abortion, either spontaneous, therapeutic, or induced; amniocentesis; ectopic pregnancy; and placenta previa or abruption can result in some mixing of maternal and fetal blood. Subsequently, anti-D antibodies develop in an Rh-negative mother with an Rh-positive fetus; with the development of these antibodies, the mother becomes sensitized against the Rh factor. If mother and fetus are both Rh negative, no incompatibility exists to trigger this maternal antibody response, but if the fetus is Rh positive, the Rh-negative mother is at risk for Rh sensitization (i.e., development of protective

antibodies against incompatible Rh-positive blood). Initially, immune globulin M (IgM) is formed and does not cross the placenta. Later, IgD antibodies develop, which may cross the placenta with isoimmunization to the D antigen with subsequent hemolysis of fetal red blood cells (RBCs). Prenatal IgD isoimmunization occurs in approximately 1% to 2% of Rh-negative women. In later exposure, as with subsequent pregnancies, there is a more rapid IgG (secondary) immune response and an increased potential for fetal hemolysis in an Rh-positive fetus. Once formed, the protective antibodies remain throughout life and may result in hemolytic difficulties for fetuses in subsequent pregnancies. Maternal blood is assessed for the anti-D antibody at the initial prenatal laboratory evaluation and at 26 to 28 gestational weeks. Rh0(D) immune globulin is routinely administered to women with maternal/fetal blood mixing, such as after abortion or with threatened abortion at any stage of gestation with continuation of the pregnancy, obstetric manipulation or trauma, or ectopic pregnancy. If abortion occurs up to and including 12 weeks' gestation, the microdose is administered if less than 2.5 mL of Rh-incompatible RBCs were administered. During the postpartum period, Rh$_0$(D) immune globulin should be administered within 72 hours; therefore one full dose (300 mcg) is given postpartum if the newborn is Rh positive, as antepartum prophylaxis at 26 to 28 weeks' gestation, and after amniocentesis, chorionic villus sampling, and percutaneous umbilical blood sampling. For women with abruption, previa, cesarean births, or manual placental removal, a Kleihauer-Betke analysis (serum test) should be done because more than 15 mL of fetal-maternal hemorrhage of Rh-positive RBCs may have occurred, necessitating an increased dose of Rh$_0$(D) immune globulin. When 15 mL or more of Rh-positive RBCs is suspected, a fetal RBC count

---

◎ CLINICAL JUDGMENT [NURSING PROCESS]

Rh$_0$(D) Immune Globulin

Concept: Perfusion
- Perfusion is the passage of blood and blood products through the circulatory system to organs or tissues to deliver oxygen and nutrients to cells, such as to the uterus and fetus.

Recognize Cues [Assessment]
- Determine blood type and Rh status of all prenatal patients.
- Assess the patient's understanding of their own and their partner's Rh status.
- Asses the patient by inquiring about previous pregnancies and outcomes; ask whether the patient has ever received Rh$_0$(D) immune globulin.
- Follow agency policy for Rh blood testing for the patient and infant at the time of delivery.
- Assess postpartum data concerning the neonate's Rh type. If the infant is Rh negative, drug is not needed. If the infant is Rh positive and the Rh-negative mother is not sensitized (negative indirect Coombs test) and the infant has a negative direct Coombs test, the mother is a candidate to receive the injection to prevent antibody production or "sensitization."
- Obtain the patient's written consent before administration. Some agencies require a refusal form if the drug is declined.
- Assess for a history of allergy to immune globulin products.

Analyze Cues and Prioritize Hypotheses [Patient Problems]
- Hypersensitivity reaction
- Reduced perfusion

Generate Solutions [Planning]
- The patient will receive Rh$_0$(D) immune globulin as indicated within 72 hours after delivery or abortion.

- The patient will be able to discuss Rh sensitization and actions indicated during subsequent pregnancies.

Take Action [Nursing Interventions]
- Assess and document Rh workup and eligibility of the patient to receive the drug. Convey information in a verbal report and in the patient's record according to agency policy.
- Assess the lot numbers on vials and laboratory slips for agreement before administration; check expiration dates. Check the identification band and laboratory slip for matching numbers. Return required slips to the laboratory or blood bank.
- Administer Rh$_0$(D) immune globulin and dose (microdose/standard dose) according to gestational weeks, exposure and route, provider orders, and agency protocol. Administer intramuscularly, normally in the deltoid, within 72 hours after delivery. If more than 72 hours have passed, administer as soon as possible up to 28 days, although a lesser degree of protection may result.
- Administration of IV Rh$_0$(D) immune globulin is possible but infrequent. Check provider orders and dosage. For IV administration, reconstitute with normal saline. Store at 36° to 46°F (2° to 8°C).
- Always have a supply of epinephrine available to treat anaphylaxis.

Patient Teaching
General
- Explain the action, purpose, and side effects of prescribed drugs.
- Advise patients to avoid live virus vaccines for 3 months after administration.
- Provide written documentation of the date of administration for the patient's personal health record.

Evaluate Outcomes [Evaluation]
- Evaluate the patient's understanding of the need for Rh$_0$(D) immune globulin.

should be performed to determine the appropriate dose of $Rh_0(D)$ immune globulin.

The Rh sensitization process can be prevented through the administration of $Rh_0(D)$ immune globulin to unsensitized Rh-negative women after each actual or potential exposure to Rh-positive blood.

Side Effects and Adverse Reactions

Adverse reactions to $Rh_0(D)$ immune globulin include hypotension, chills, dizziness, fever, headache, pruritus, rash, abdominal pain, diarrhea, and injection site reactions (discomfort, mild pain, redness, swelling).

Rubella Vaccine

Maternal rubella, also called *German measles,* is a potentially devastating infection for the fetus, depending on gestational age. If an unimmunized woman (rubella titer <1:10 or negative titer) contracts the virus during the first trimester, a high rate of abortion and neurologic and developmental sequelae associated with congenital rubella syndrome (transmission of the rubella virus to the fetus via the placenta) may result. Cataracts, glaucoma, deafness, heart defects, and mental retardation are seen with this syndrome. When infection occurs after the first trimester, there is less risk of fetal damage because of the developmental stage of the fetus. There is no treatment for maternal or congenital rubella infection. The goals are immunization and prevention of rubella in patients of childbearing age.

Side Effects and Adverse Reactions

Side effects of the rubella vaccine are generally mild and temporary. Burning or stinging at the injection site is caused by the acidic pH of

---

> ### ⚡ PATIENT SAFETY
>
> **Do not confuse...**
> 1. **Fentanyl citrate**, used as an adjunct to general or regional anesthesia or for persistent moderate to severe postoperative pain, with **sufentanil**, an agent used to induce anesthesia in combination with other drugs or as the sole anesthetic agent.

the vaccine. Regional lymphadenopathy, urticaria (skin rash caused by an allergic reaction), rash, malaise, sore throat, fever, headache, polyneuritis, arthralgia, and moderate fever are occasionally seen.

POSTPARTUM DEPRESSION

Postpartum depression is intense feelings of sadness, anxiety, or despair preventing patients from performing their daily tasks and occurring 1 to 3 weeks after childbirth, but may occur up to a year after giving birth, related to changes in hormone levels. Patients with a history of depression before or during pregnancy have an increased risk of developing postpartum depression. Postpartum depression may be treated with therapy in combination with antidepressants.

Brexanolone is a new medication approved in March 2019 indicated for treatment of postpartum depression. Guidelines list that it must be given in a monitored health care setting, where patients can be monitored for hypoxia and excessive sedation. See Chapter 23, Antidepressants and Mood Stabilizers, for more information on antidepressants.

▌ CRITICAL THINKING CASE STUDY

A patient, who is gravida 3, para 0, is at 42 weeks' gestation. At her prenatal visit, her health care provider notes signs and symptoms of pregnancy-induced hypertension and advises the patient about a plan to induce labor after administration of prostaglandin gel. The patient asks the nurse, "Can you help me understand all of this?"

1. What objective tool (scoring system) can be used to predict the extent to which the patient's cervix is "ripe" and therefore favorable for successful induction?

The patient's health care provider orders dinoprostone gel for use in the cervix.

2. What will be accomplished with use of the gel?
3. Who will administer the gel?
4. How often can the gel be administered?
5. How long after the last dose of gel can the IV oxytocic medication be started to induce labor?
6. Why is there a waiting period before starting the oxytocin?

Further questioning reveals that the patient has been ingesting a pregnancy tonic that includes herbal supplements since 36 weeks' gestation.

7. List three concerns specific to pregnancy.

It is 16 hours since she first had the gel applied. Responding to her call light, the nurse finds the patient in the bathroom, upset because she feels nauseated and is occasionally vomiting a little stomach fluid and complaining that her stool is watery. "Is something wrong?" she asks.

8. Analysis of the data about the patient's symptoms supports what conclusion?
9. What nursing actions might be taken to support the patient?
10. When the patient returns to bed and the external fetal monitor is reapplied, what data would the nurse collect, record, and report to the obstetric provider?

It is 24 hours since the patient had the first gel instillation and 6 hours since her last insertion. A vaginal examination reveals her cervix is soft, 50% effaced, and 3 cm dilated, and the presenting part is at 2 station. Contractions are 5 minutes apart and mild, and the health care provider elects to begin an oxytocin infusion.

11. The patient asks how "a medicine running into my arm is able to make my uterus contract." How would the nurse explain the mechanism of action of oxytocin?
12. Why is intravenous oxytocin infused through a secondary line attached as a piggyback to the primary line? At which port along the primary line is the piggyback inserted and why?
13. Why is oxytocin administered via infusion pump? What is the measurement for dosing?
14. In regard to the IV equipment setup, what actions would be taken as safety measures before starting the oxytocin?
15. The nurse would have which drugs readily available in the event of an emergency with the oxytocin?
16. What information should be recorded during the infusion?
17. While setting up the oxytocin infusion, a new nurse being precepted to labor and delivery asks what criteria are used to know when to slow the rate or stop the infusion. The nurse correctly responds that contractions should be _____ minutes apart with _____ intensity, and the cervix would be dilated at least _____ cm.
18. Address the following if uterine hyperstimulation occurs: Position the patient; rationale: _____IV fluids; rationale: _____Oxygen; rationale: _____
19. The patient asks what side effects can occur if she receives a continuous lumbar epidural. What is the appropriate response?

REVIEW QUESTIONS

1. A patient (gravida 3, para 2, at 40.6 weeks' gestation) asks, "Is there anything we can do to start labor besides medication? I'm so ready to have this baby." Which response is appropriate by the nurse?
   a. There is nothing we can do to increase labor and hasten the birth of the baby.
   b. Amniocentesis is ordered to ensure the lungs are mature before we start labor.
   c. Some women may begin a brisk walking program to precipitate labor.
   d. If the cervix is ripe, the health care provider will initiate medication to soften the cervix and initiate beginning of labor.

2. A patient is to receive 10 mg nalbuphine by slow intravenous push for pain relief during labor. During which phase of uterine contractions would the nurse plan to administer nalbuphine?
   a. During the uterine contraction
   b. At the end of the uterine contraction
   c. Between uterine contractions
   d. At any time during the contraction

3. A patient received butorphanol 2 mg intravenously 10 minutes before delivery. Which nursing action is appropriate?
   a. Administer butorphanol subcutaneously
   b. Have naloxone available
   c. Administer intravenous fluid bolus
   d. Place oxygen 10 L by nasal cannula

4. A patient is to have lumbar epidural anesthesia. Which nursing action is appropriate?
   a. Administer citric acid/sodium citrate
   b. Administer promethazine
   c. Infuse 500 to 1000 mL of a crystalloid intravenous solution
   d. Administer Rh0(D) immune globulin injection

5. A 33-year-old patient in active labor is experiencing "back labor" with intense pain in her lower back. Which nursing intervention would be most effective?
   a. Counterpressure against the sacrum
   b. Pant-blow breathing techniques
   c. Effleurage
   d. Conscious relaxation or guided imagery

6. A patient has an epidural for pain control during labor. During the assessment, the nurse notes a drop in the client's blood pressure. Which priority nursing intervention would the nurse do?
   a. Administer low-flow oxygen.
   b. Turn her on her left side.
   c. Assess her urinary output.
   d. Monitor her vaginal bleeding.

7. A patient is to have an emergency cesarean delivery due to late fetal decelerations. Before surgery, the nurse administers an antacid, citric acid/sodium citrate. Which patient response would indicate effective patient teaching regarding this drug?
   a. Citric acid/sodium citrate will prevent infection after the cesarean section.
   b. The drug will neutralize the contents in my stomach.
   c. The citric acid/sodium citrate will reduce the need to use pain drug after the cesarean delivery.
   d. This drug is administered to prevent vomiting after the cesarean section.

8. Spinal anesthesia with morphine is administered to a patient for pain relief during cesarean section. She complains of itching. The nurse prepares to administer which drug?
   a. Diphenhydramine
   b. Ephedrine sulfate
   c. Butorphanol tartrate
   d. Lidocaine

9. A patient (gravida 2, para 1) is admitted to labor and delivery at 39.6 weeks' gestation in active labor. The health care provider performs an amniotomy. Which nursing intervention would be a priority?
   a. Monitoring uterine contractions.
   b. Checking fetal heart rate
   c. Assessing cervical dilation and effacement
   d. Checking umbilical cord compression

10. A patient in labor is to have an epidural administered. Which nursing interventions would the nurse perform before the epidural is administered? (Select all that apply.)
    a. Infuse 500 to 1000 mL of the ordered IV fluids.
    b. Monitor maternal blood pressure and fetal heart rate.
    c. Insert indwelling urinary catheter and monitor output.
    d. Position and support patient on left side as ordered by the health care provider.
    e. Position the patient in a lithotomy position to assist with delivery.
    f. Administer 2 L/min of oxygen via nasal cannula.

54

Neonatal and Newborn

This chapter focuses on drugs commonly administered to the neonate, which includes late preterm newborns immediately after delivery.

As discussed in Chapter 49, a thorough medical history, such as acquired immunodeficiency syndrome (AIDS), Group B *streptococcal* infection, and viral hepatitis B or hepatitis C, should be conducted. Labor is determined to be preterm if it commences before 37 weeks of pregnancy. If there are no contraindications to halting preterm labor, tocolytic therapy is administered to delay birth (see Chapter 49 for more information on pregnancy and preterm labor drugs). However, when preterm labor is not arrested, premature delivery of the neonate occurs, which puts the newborn at risk for health problems. Premature neonates are at risk for respiratory distress, hypothermia, hypoglycemia, and hyperbilirubinemia, and they may have feeding difficulties.

DRUGS ADMINISTERED TO PRETERM NEONATES

Synthetic Surfactant

Respiratory distress syndrome (RDS) can occur because of immature lung development and breathing control and decreased airway muscle tone and surfactant level. Surfactant, a lipoprotein, is necessary to decrease the surface tension of the alveoli (air sacs) to allow the lungs to fill with air and prevent the alveoli from deflating. Immature lungs have lower than normal levels of surfactant; the more premature the neonate is, the higher the chance of RDS. One approach used to minimize respiratory difficulties in the preterm neonate is surfactant replacement. Supplementing the amount of endogenous surfactant available to maintain distension of the alveolar sacs is the focus of this therapy.

Beractant intratracheal (IT) suspension, a natural bovine lung extract, contains phospholipids, neutral lipids, fatty acids, and surfactant-associated proteins. It is administered intratracheal (IT) for prophylaxis and treatment of RDS in premature infants <1250 g birth weight or with evidence of surfactant deficiency within 15 minutes of birth, or in a neonate with confirmed RDS requiring endotracheal (ET) intubation given within 8 hours of birth.

Calfactant, recently approved by the US Food and Drug Administration for use in infants, is a bovine-derived lung surfactant similar to beractant. Calfactant contains phospholipids, neutral lipids, fatty acids, and two low-molecular-weight, hydrophobic, surfactant-associated proteins. It is indicated for prevention of RDS in premature infants at high risk and for rescue of neonates who develop RDS.

Poractant alfa is a porcine lung surfactant and is indicated for rescue treatment, whereas beractant and calfactant are approved for prophylaxis and rescue treatment. Poractant alfa replaces pulmonary surfactant, which is deficient in some premature neonates. Each of these products defines *prophylactic* and *rescue* use differently and has different dosing and administration requirements. Table 54.1 lists the surfactant drugs used for prevention and treatment of RDS along with their dosages, uses, and considerations.

Based on clinical response and outcomes in neonates, most clinicians feel there is little difference between the currently available natural and synthetic exogenous surfactant products.

All exogenous surfactants require a patent ET tube for administration and specified alterations in positioning the infant throughout the procedure to ensure even drug dispersion. These precise position changes allow gravity to assist in the distribution of the product in the lungs, particularly at the alveolar surface.

Crackles and moist breath sounds may be a transient finding after administration of these products, particularly with beractant. Exogenous surfactant can cause postadministration complications such as hyperoxia (excessive oxygenation) and hypocarbia (decreased carbon dioxide [CO_2]). Additionally, transient endotracheal reflux can obstruct the ET tube and lead to oxygen desaturation, cyanosis, bradycardia, and apnea. These issues do not usually lead to serious long-term complications when properly managed. Unless obvious signs of airway obstruction are noted, suctioning should not be performed immediately after administration of supplemental surfactant. Dosing is slowed or halted if the infant (1) becomes dusky-colored, (2) becomes agitated, (3) experiences transient bradycardia, (4) has oxygen saturation increases of more than 95%, (5)

TABLE 54.1 Exogenous Surfactant Therapy for Prevention and Treatment of Respiratory Distress Syndrome

Generic	Route and Dosage	Uses and Considerations
Beractant	PN: IT: 4 mL/kg per dose divided into four equal amounts; administer each quarter amount separately followed by repositioning and extra ventilation; repeat q6h; *max:* 100 mg/kg (birth weight) dose or 4 mL/kg (birth weight) dosed intratracheally	Indicated for prevention and treatment (rescue) of RDS in premature neonates. Drug must be given by health care personnel experienced with intubation and the use of ventilators for prevention or rescue in treatment of RDS. Administer through a 5-French end-hole catheter as a dosing catheter inserted into an ET tube; *do not shake;* do not reconstitute; warm 20 min at room temperature or in the hand for at least 8 min. Reposition infant to distribute drug, followed by ventilation for 20 s after each quarter dose.
Calfactant	PN: IT: 3 mL/kg (approx. 100 mg/kg of birth weight) IT; divided into 2 doses. Each dose administered gradually over a total of 20 to 30 breaths, with small bursts of drug administration occurring only during inspiration phase. Between doses the infant is repositioned. Wait at least 12 h before re-dosing; *max:* 100 mg/kg birth weight (3 mL/kg birth weight) dosed IT	Indicated for prevention and treatment (rescue) of RDS in premature neonates. Drug must be given by health care personnel experienced with intubation and the use of ventilators for prevention or rescue in treatment of RDS. Administer through a side port adaptor or a 5-French end-hole catheter inserted into the proximal end of the ET tube.
Poractant alfa	PN: IT: 2.5 mL/kg per dose divided in two equal amounts; administer each half amount to each main bronchus followed by repositioning and monitoring respiratory status; repeat q12h; *max:* 2.5 mL/kg (birth weight) dosed IT	Poractant alfa is indicated for the treatment ("rescue") of respiratory distress syndrome (RDS) in premature infants. Drug must be given by health care personnel experienced with intubation and the use of ventilators and RDS. Slowly warm to room temperature; do not reconstitute; do not shake; gently invert to obtain uniform suspension. Draw dose with a 20-gauge or larger needle; do *not* filter or dilute; administer via a 5-French end-hole catheter inserted into the proximal end of the ET tube.

approx., Approximately; *ET,* endotracheal; *h,* hour; *IT,* intratracheal; *min,* minute; *PN,* premature neonate; *q,* every; *RDS,* respiratory distress syndrome; *s,* second; *wk,* weeks; <, less than; ≤, less than or equal to.

experiences improved chest expansion, or (6) has arterial or transcutaneous CO_2 levels below 30 mm Hg. Suctioning before dosing decreases the chance for ET tube blockage during dosing. No long-term complications or sequelae of synthetic surfactant therapy have been reported. Surfactant replacement therapy has been found effective in reducing the severity of RDS; rapid improvements in lung compliance and oxygenation may require immediate decreases in ventilator settings to prevent lung overdistension and pulmonary air leak.

Surfactant drugs are administered by medical personnel experienced with ventilators and intubation of their patient population. Administration is a two-person procedure. It should be performed by at least one medical practitioner or a neonatal nurse practitioner (NNP) who administers the surfactant, and one registered nurse as the assistant.

DRUGS ADMINISTERED TO FULL-TERM, HEALTHY NEONATES

Newborns should receive eye care (e.g., erythromycin ophthalmic ointment), phytonadione, and immunizations for hepatitis B (www.who.int). Additionally, an antiinfective agent (e.g., chlorhexidine) may be applied to the cord stump during the first few hours after birth and for up to 1 week for at-risk newborns and newborns born in homes.

Erythromycin Ophthalmic Ointment

A common antiinfective administered to a newborn's eyes within the first hour of birth is erythromycin ophthalmic ointment. Erythromycin ointment serves as a simple, harmless, cost-effective means of preventing blindness. The blindness in question results from infection with sexually transmitted infections, chlamydia and gonorrhea. Both infections can progress rapidly in newborns' eyes, damaging the clear part over the pupils (corneas) and causing irreversible harm. Ocular irritation and redness can occur from the use of erythromycin ophthalmic ointment.

Phytonadione

Phytonadione, a synthetic vitamin K, is a fat-soluble vitamin given to newborns to prevent vitamin K–deficiency bleeding (VKDB). This can result in a life-threatening disease called hemorrhagic disease of the newborn. Vitamin K deficiency is one of the most common causes of bleeding in a healthy infant. Newborns are inherently vitamin K deficient at birth due to lower stores of vitamin K in their immature system, as well as a decreased ability to utilize vitamin K. The newborn lacks appropriate intestinal flora to synthesize vitamin K.

It is administered as a single-dose injection. Side effects include pain and edema at the injection site. Some allergic reactions, manifested by urticaria and rash, have been reported. Neonates who receive larger doses may exhibit hyperbilirubinemia and jaundice resulting from competition for binding sites.

Table 54.2 covers erythromycin and phytonadione and their dosages, uses, and considerations.

Immunizations

The American Academy of Pediatrics and the Centers for Disease Control and Prevention (CDC) have recommended that immunization against hepatitis B virus (HBV) begin in the newborn period. HBV infection may result in serious long-term liver disease, cancer, and

TABLE 54.2 Drugs Administered to Newborns

Generic	Route and Dosage	Uses and Considerations
Erythromycin ophthalmic ointment	Neonate ophthalmic 0.5%: within 1 h of delivery and without touching the tip of the tube to the eye, fingertips, or any other surface, place a 1-cm ribbon of ointment in the lower conjunctival sac of each eye, beginning at the inner canthus from the inner to outer eye	Prevention of ophthalmia neonatorum, an eye infection among newborns, and protection against gonococcal and chlamydial conjunctivitis. Most states mandate erythromycin ophthalmic ointment but consult your facility's policy. Do not flush eyes after installation. Use new tube for each infant.
Hepatitis B immune globulin (HBIG)	IM: 0.5 mL within 12 h after birth into the anterolateral thigh (vastus lateralis)	For newborns of mothers positive for HBsAg for passive immunity; obtain consents from parents. Initiate recombinant HB as a separate injection at different sites; aspiration is not required.
Phytonadione	0.5–1 mg into the anterolateral thigh (vastus lateralis) within 1 h after birth; check health care provider or agency standing orders for dosage	An anticoagulant antagonist for prevention of hemorrhagic disease of the newborn. Drug is readily absorbed after IM administration.
Hepatitis B vaccine, recombinant	IM/subcut: 0.5 mL (5 mcg) within 24 h after birth (first dose); subsequent doses at 1 and 6 mo of age into anterolateral thigh (vastus lateralis)	Stimulates the immune system to produce anti–HBsAg antibodies without the risk of developing active infection. Because hepatitis D occurs only in persons infected with hepatitis B, recombinant HB protects against hepatitis D. Protection usually occurs 1 mo after the third dose.

h, Hour; *HB,* hepatitis B; *HBsAg,* hepatitis B surface antigen; *IM,* intramuscularly; *mo,* month; *subcut,* subcutaneous.

◎ CLINICAL JUDGMENT [NURSING PROCESS]

Drug Administered to Preterm Neonate: Synthetic Surfactant

Concept: Oxygenation
- *Oxygenation* refers to the process of providing cells with oxygen. The act of breathing depends on a functioning respiratory system that provides oxygen to the cells. Nurses encounter alterations in patient's oxygenation. Those who care for the neonatal population must quickly detect problems in oxygenation and act to prevent respiratory distress and death in the infant.

Recognize Cues [Assessment]
- Obtain informed consent. Separate consents are needed for multifetal births.
- Assess the patient's vital signs, perform a physical examination, and monitor arterial blood gases (ABGs).

Analyze Cues and Prioritize Hypothesis [Patient Problems]
- Decreased gas exchange
- Decreased tissue perfusion
- Decreased ability to cope (parents)

Generate Solutions [Planning]
- The patient's oxygen requirement and respiratory effort will decrease.
- The patient will experience no respiratory distress after surfactant administration.
- The patient will breathe without the assistance of mechanical ventilation and experience adequate oxygenation.
- The patient will maintain a patent airway.

Take Action [Nursing Interventions]
- Continuously monitor the patient's vital signs before, during, and after surfactant therapy.
- Assess the patient to ensure adequate respiratory status is maintained.
- Assist the multidisciplinary team (physician or neonatal nurse) as needed.
- Monitor ABGs and obtain a chest radiography study.
- Maintain adequate respiratory status.
- Position and reposition the patient as needed for equal distribution of surfactant throughout the lungs.
- Support and educate the parents.
- Acknowledge the parents' concerns regarding the well-being of the newborn.
- Provide an interpreter if patient's parents have a language barrier.
- Provide health information written in the patient's primary language.

Patient Teaching
- Explain to parents what respiratory distress syndrome (RDS) is and how surfactant helps the neonate.
- Explain to parents the purpose of multiple monitoring devices to reduce unrealistic fears about the neonate's condition.
- Ensure informed consent for drug usage.
- Encourage parents to verbalize their understanding about risks associated with use of the drug.

Evaluate Outcomes [Evaluation]
- Evaluate preadministration breath sounds, ABGs, respiratory status, and ventilator pressure readings to compare with postadministration findings.
- Evaluate the effectiveness of teaching to parents.

death in adulthood. The goal of immunization is to reduce the number of chronic carriers of the virus in the population, thus decreasing the prevalence of HBV infection.

In pregnancy, HBV transmission occurs vertically—that is, by perinatal transmission—primarily at the time of delivery. Hepatitis B immune globulin (HBIG) is given to infants born to mothers who are positive for hepatitis B surface antigen (HBsAg). HBIG provides the newborn passive protection against HBV. Adverse effects of the injection include pain, tenderness, and erythema at the injection site. Hypotension, erythematous rash, and anaphylaxis after receiving HBIG can also occur.

A three-dose series vaccine for hepatitis B, recombinant hepatitis B, is indicated for HBV prophylaxis in infants; the first injection is given at birth. The second and third injections are administered at 1-month and 2-month intervals by the pediatrician. Newborns who for a medical reason do not get the vaccine at birth should receive

◎ CLINICAL JUDGMENT [NURSING PROCESS]

Drugs Administered to Full-Term, Healthy Neonates

Concept: Caring Interventions

- Caring interventions are performed by the nurse during medication administration. These interventions ensure safe practice outcomes. The interventions are the result of scientific research, best practice guidelines, composed by the professional body of nursing for quality care and safe practice.

Recognize Cues [Assessment]

- Assess the patient for signs of distress such as cyanosis, bleeding, ecchymosis, apnea, fever, and hypotension.
- Assess the mother's hepatitis B virus (HBV) status.
- Assess the parents' knowledge of treatments (e.g., medications and immunizations) given to their newborn.

Analyze Cues and Prioritize Hypothesis [Patient Problems]

- Potential injury
- Need for health teaching (parental)
- Anxiety (parental)

Generate Solutions [Planning]

- The patient will experience minimal or no side effects from drugs routinely administered after delivery.
- Parents will express understanding of medications and immunizations given to their newborn.

Take Action [Nursing Interventions]

- Obtain parental consents for immunizations.
- Provide immediate skin-to-skin contact between mother and infant while preparing medications and immunizations. Skin-to-skin contact in the first hour of birth prevents hypothermia and promotes breastfeeding.
- Wear gloves for administration of medications and immunizations.
- Prepare to administer hepatitis B immune globulin (HBIG) to the patient if the mother is hepatitis B surface antigen (HBsAg) positive.
- Prepare and administer drugs and immunizations according to the manufacturer's instructions while the patient maintains contact with the mother's skin.

- Administer erythromycin ophthalmic ointment *before* administration of phytonadione and hepatitis B injections. The patient may cry after injections, making administration of ophthalmic ointment more difficult.
- Monitor for any reactions, such as redness and swelling in and around the eye from the eye ointment or redness, swelling, or ecchymosis at injection sites. Monitor for any respiratory distress (e.g., grunting, apnea, nasal flaring).
- Acknowledge parent concerns about immunizations.
- Provide printed literature on hepatitis B and other immunizations.
- It is important for nurses to be sensitive to the family's traditions and beliefs.
- It is important for the nurse to establish rapport with the patient's parents.

Patient Teaching

- Instruct parents regarding the action, purpose, and side effects of medications and immunizations.
- Inform parents that any edema around the eyes usually disappears within 24 to 48 hours.
- Explain to parents the difference between HBIG and recombinant hepatitis B (HB) injections.
- Instruct parents regarding childhood immunizations as recommended by current immunization schedules and inform them when repeat doses should be given. Give parents written information regarding the patient's immunization record and vaccination schedule.
- Document administration of hepatitis B vaccine on the patient's immunization record.
- Instruct parents on the signs and symptoms of adverse effects and when to notify the nurse.

Evaluate Outcomes [Evaluation]

- Evaluate for newborn bleeding, particularly on days 2 and 3 after administration of phytonadione.
- Evaluate for drug hypersensitivity or side effects.
- Evaluate parents' understanding about medications administered to their newborn.

---

their first dose as soon as possible and complete all three doses at the recommended intervals. The dose is administered intramuscular in the anterolateral thigh area to the vastus lateralis muscle. Hepatitis B, recombinant (HB) can provide active immunity against HBV by stimulating the immune system to produce antibodies against hepatitis B (anti–hepatitis B antigen), and it can be given concurrently with HBIG if the infant is born to an HBsAg-positive mother. Recombinant HB is given as separate injection administered to separate sites. Adverse effects from recombinant HB are generally mild and include pain, tenderness, pruritus, erythema, swelling, and induration at the injection site. It is mandatory that a parent sign a consent form before the infant receives an HBV immunization.

Table 54.2 lists HBIG and recombinant HB and their dosages, uses, and considerations.

▮ CRITICAL THINKING CASE STUDY

The patient is an 18-year-old female, admitted to the hospital for labor induction/augmentation with signs and symptoms of gestational hypertension at 42 weeks' gestation (gravida 4, para 1). The delivery occurred at 6:00 a.m. by vacuum extraction. The baby, weighing 8 lb 7 oz, had Apgar scores of 7 and 9. The infant is alert and active. Immediately after the delivery, the nurse assesses and prioritizes nursing care needs.

1. What steps should the nurse follow to instill ointment into the patient's eyes?

2. What should the infant's mother be taught about the side effects of eye prophylaxis?
3. How should the nurse explain the reason for the vitamin K injection for the infant patient in terms the mother can understand?
4. Which newborn patients are eligible to receive the hepatitis B vaccine?
5. How many doses constitute the total series of the hepatitis B vaccine, and what is the duration for these?

REVIEW QUESTIONS

1. A patient asks the nurse why her baby is receiving a vitamin K injection. The nurse's best response is based on what knowledge?

   a. Vitamin K is important because it increases the newborn's platelets.

   b. A newborn baby's metabolism is too immature to produce vitamin K.

   c. A newborn lacks appropriate intestinal flora to synthesize vitamin K.

   d. Vitamin K isn't produced in bone marrow until an infant is 8 days old.

2. It is mandatory to have maternal signed consent before administering which newborn drug?

   a. Erythromycin eye ointment

   b. Phytonadione (Vitamin K^1)

   c. Hepatitis B vaccine series

   d. Betamethasone injection

3. The nurse is mentoring a new graduate who is preparing to administer the phytonadione injection to a newborn. Which muscle sites selected by the new graduate would indicate the need for further teaching? (Select all that apply.)

   a. Anterolateral thigh

   b. Gluteus maximus

   c. Rectus femoris

   d. Vastus lateralis

   e. Vastus medialis

4. The nurse is preparing to administer an ophthalmic drug to a newborn. Education for the parents includes which fact about the drug?

   a. All infants born preterm receive an ophthalmic drug to protect their eyes.

   b. Eye ointments are given in the lower bottom of the eye from the inner to the outer eye.

   c. This drug will prevent congenital ophthalmic diseases and must be given.

   d. Infants with a negative direct Coombs test receive this drug to protect vision.

5. A newborn is admitted to the nursery, and the nurse reviews the maternal history. It is important that the nurse assess the mother's status specific to which infectious process(es)? (Select all that apply.)

   a. Rubeola (Measles)

   b. Hepatitis A

   c. Hepatitis B

   d. HIV/AIDS

   e. Group B *Streptococcus*

6. A neonate whose mother is positive for the hepatitis B surface antigen (HBsAg) is admitted to the nursery. Which immunizations are appropriate for this neonate? (Select all that apply.)

   a. Hepatitis B immune globulin (HBIG)

   b. Recombinant hepatitis B (HB)

   c. *Haemophilus influenzae* type B

   d. Hepatitis A vaccine

   e. Cobalamin (Vitamin B$_{12}$)

Women's Reproductive Health

Christina DiMaggio Boudreaux, RN, BSN, IBCLC

http://evolve.elsevier.com/McCuistion/pharmacology

OBJECTIVES

- Recognize that successful contraception is essential to the health and well-being of women.
- Describe methods of contraception commonly prescribed, patient selection, mechanisms of action, and possible side effects.
- Identify specific nursing actions that will enhance successful contraception for women and their partners.
- Describe the Clinical Judgment [Nursing Process], including teaching and risk-benefit–alternative education associated with drugs used for contraception and family planning.
- Explain the pathophysiology of women's health conditions, pharmacologic therapies, and expected outcomes of pharmacologic therapies.
- Understand pharmacologic interventions used in the treatment of female infertility.

- Describe the mechanism of action for ovulatory stimulation therapy.
- Identify drug therapies used for common gynecologic conditions, such as dysfunctional uterine bleeding, endometriosis, dysmenorrhea, and premenstrual syndrome.
- Describe the Clinical Judgment [Nursing Process], including teaching, related to drugs used in women's health and infertility.
- Provide information for nonpharmacologic and pharmacologic interventions for women experiencing menopausal symptoms.
- Differentiate among types of drugs used for osteoporosis.
- Describe the Clinical Judgment [Nursing Process], including teaching and risk-benefit–alternative education associated with drugs used for menopausal symptoms.

OUTLINE

Women have specific health care needs throughout their reproductive and postreproductive life cycle. A woman's reproductive life cycle begins with menarche, the start of spontaneous menstruation, and continues through menopause, the permanent cessation of menstruation. Successful contraception is essential to the health and well-being of sexually active women of reproductive age. During the reproductive years, many disorders can occur in women's health. These gynecologic conditions interfere with a woman's overall health and well-being and may impede her ability to become pregnant.

Successful adaptation to menopause, control of menopausal symptoms, and continued sexual health are essential to the well-being of older women. This chapter reviews pharmacologic products that may be used throughout the reproductive and menopausal life cycle of women as well as typical drug regimens used for disorders in women's health. Drugs for female infertility are also addressed with an emphasis on drugs that stimulate ovulation.

DRUGS USED FOR CONTRACEPTION

Combined Hormonal Contraceptives

Combined hormonal contraceptives (CHCs) are one of the most commonly used methods of reversible contraception in the world because of their ease of use, high degree of effectiveness (92% to 99.3% effective), and relative safety. Research has shown that higher doses of estrogen increase the risk for venous thromboembolism (VTE), myocardial infarction (MI), and stroke. Subsequently, low-dose oral contraceptives (OCs) and, more recently, ultra-low-dose OCs have been introduced to reduce the risk of dangerous side effects. Research continues to focus on actual and potential short- and long-term benefits and risks associated with use of low-dose OCs, particularly in the areas of heart and circulatory risks as well as carcinogenesis. Clinical studies also continue to investigate the venous circulatory effects of new-generation progestins.

CHC formulations are differentiated based on the strength of the estrogen component, the type of progestin used, and whether estrogen or progesterone (and androgen) activity predominates. Increased estrogenic activity may include side effects such as cyclic breast changes, dysmenorrhea (painful periods), menorrhagia (heavy periods), chloasma (hyperpigmentation of the skin), and VTE, whereas decreased estrogenic activity can cause amenorrhea (absence of periods) or spotting at certain points in the cycle. Increased progestational activity can cause weight gain, depression, fatigue, and decreased libido, and a lack of progestational activity may cause breakthrough bleeding (BTB) and headaches. BTB is an episode of bleeding that occurs during the active pill cycle of CHCs. It is more common at the start of CHC use, when there is a change to the type of pill being taken, and with progestin-only preparations of contraception. There is no evidence that an episode of BTB is associated with a decrease in the CHC's effectiveness if the patient continues to take the pill daily as prescribed. Increased androgenic activity may cause acne, hirsutism, edema, and cholestatic jaundice. The estrogens and progestins in OC pills also effect the uterine endometrium, which may cause changes in the patient's periods that can include irregular bleeding, heavy or light periods, or spotting between periods. The undesirable side effects of hormonal contraception products are discussed later in this chapter.

Most women on CHC products experience shorter, lighter periods. Other advantages with CHCs are decreased blood loss and uterine cramps, elimination of mittelschmerz (midcycle pain usually associated with ovulation), reduction of symptoms in many forms of benign breast disorders, and prevention of physiologic ovarian cysts. CHC products also reduce the incidence of pelvic inflammatory disease (PID), ectopic pregnancy, endometrial and ovarian cancer risk, and deaths from colorectal cancer. CHC products do *not* reduce the incidence of sexually transmitted infections (STIs; see Chapter 57 for further discussion of STIs.)

The goal of therapy is to identify the product that offers the best contraceptive protection while producing the fewest unwanted side effects. It is important to note that the effectiveness of OCs can also be compromised by concurrent use of some drugs (e.g., antibiotics) or herbal products.

COMPLEMENTARY AND ALTERNATIVE THERAPIES

St. John's Wort

- St. John's wort may decrease the level of contraceptive hormones in the bloodstream, reducing the effectiveness of combined hormonal contraceptives (CHCs). This may result in breakthrough bleeding and/or spontaneous ovulation.
- Chasteberry extract should be used with caution with CHCs or hormone therapy because it may alter contraceptive hormone levels in the body and can make them less effective.
- Other herbal remedies that may alter the effectiveness of contraceptive hormones include dong quai, black cohosh, and red clover.

All combined hormonal contraceptives (CHCs) contain a synthetic version of *estrogen* and a compound known as *progestin*. Ethinyl estradiol (EE) is the most commonly used synthetic estrogen found in CHCs. Progestins are natural or synthetic hormones that have *progesterone-like* effects. *Progesterone* is the naturally occurring sex hormone produced in the ovaries of women; *progestogen* refers to any synthetically produced progesterone compound. Almost all progestins are derivatives of testosterone, a steroid hormone classified under the androgen group that binds to and activates the progesterone receptors. The term *progestin* will be used to describe the compound used in CHC products. Not only do progestins have contraceptive properties, they also serve to balance out the effects of estrogen.

One of eight different types of progestins is used in CHC products. Norethindrone, norethindrone acetate, and ethynodiol diacetate are first-generation progestin compounds (estrane family) and were the earliest progestin formulations to be used in OCs. Second-generation progestins (gonane family) include norgestrel and levonorgestrel (LNG). Third-generation progestins include desogestrel and norgestimate. The new-generation progestins have a higher efficacy rating and fewer effects on lipid and carbohydrate metabolism compared with their earlier counterparts. They also have fewer androgenic side effects, which are described later in this chapter.

Drospirenone (DRSP) is a fourth-generation progestin. It is an analogue of spironolactone. As with spironolactone, a potassium-sparing diuretic, DRSP can increase serum potassium levels in women taking DRSP-containing OCs, altering water and electrolyte balance.

The amount of estrogen and type of progestin determine bioactivity and possible side effects of CHC products. The combination of estrogen and the selected progestin have an effect on the uterine endometrium; therefore the lowest effective dose that successfully prevents conception should be used (Table 55.1).

Mechanism of Action

The estrogen component of CHC products inhibits ovulation by preventing the formation of a dominant follicle. When a dominant follicle does not mature, estrogen remains at a consistent level and is unable to reach the peak level needed to stimulate the luteinizing hormone (LH) surge. The progestin component also suppresses the LH surge. When the LH surge is suppressed, ovulation is prevented, and pregnancy does not occur. Any cycle in which ovulation does not occur, whether induced by drugs or naturally occurring, is called an anovulatory cycle. CHCs produce drug-induced anovulatory cycles. The estrogen component of CHC products also stabilizes the uterine endometrium, inhibiting proliferation and secretory changes, and decreasing the occurrence of irregular or heavy bleeding. The progestational effects of progestin change the endometrium to make it less favorable for implantation of a fertilized ovum. In addition, progestins affect the quantity and viscosity of the cervical mucus, making it thick and hostile to sperm penetration. Progestins alter the motility of both the muscles of the fallopian tube and the cilia within the tube, impeding the movement of the ovum through the tube.

Route of Delivery

There are several routes of administration for CHC products. Most women are familiar with oral contraception, in which a pill is ingested daily that is absorbed by the gastrointestinal (GI) tract and metabolized by the liver. However, CHC products can also be administered through transvaginal and transdermal routes. The advantage of these alternative sites is avoiding GI absorption and the initial metabolism by the liver, or the *first-pass effect*. Theoretically, side effects such as nausea and vomiting, heart and circulatory risks, and nonadherence with a daily dosage regimen can be avoided.

TABLE 55.1 Oral Combined Hormonal Contraceptives

Drug	Route and Dosage	Uses and Considerations
Combination products containing norethindrone and ethinyl estradiol	Oral: 1 tablet PO daily 21-tablet package: 1 tablet daily for 21 consecutive days followed by 7 days off. A new course begins on the 8th day after a tablet is taken. 28-tablet package: 1 tablet daily without interruption taken at the same time each day Schedule 1: Start the first Sunday after onset of menstruation (while using additional contraception for 7 days) Schedule 2: Start the first day of menstrual cycle.	Estrogen and progestin combination used for contraception and for treatment of moderate acne vulgaris in females 15 years and older who have achieved menarche, are unresponsive to topical treatments, have no contraindications to CHC use, and plan to stay on therapy for 6 months or longer. *Contraindications:* History of or current thrombophlebitis, DVT, PE, CVA, CAD, valve disease, hypertension, diabetes mellitus with vascular involvement, migraines in women >35 y, cancers, neoplasms, and tumors. Cardiovascular side effects are increased in women who smoke, especially those >35 y and in those who use CHCs. Absorption: Rapid; PB: >95%; t½: 19–24 h Pregnancy Considerations: Use in pregnancy is contraindicated. Treatment should be discontinued immediately if pregnancy occurs. ⚡ Blackbox warning: Cigarette smoking increases the risk of serious cardiovascular events while using combination oral contraceptives.
Combination products containing levonorgestrel (LNG) and ethinyl estradiol (EE)	Same	Estrogen and progestin combination used for contraception and postcoital emergency contraception. Contraindications and blackbox warnings are same as previously discussed; use with caution in patients with depression, and monitor patients on thyroid replacement therapy, who may require higher doses of thyroid hormone while receiving estrogens. PB: 95%–99%; t½: EE 12–23 h, LNG 22–49 h Pregnancy Considerations: Use is contraindicated in pregnant women; discontinue treatment if pregnancy occurs. Recommended waiting 4–6 weeks postpartum before starting this combination due to increased risk of venous thromboembolism. When used for emergency contraception, a barrier contraceptive method is recommended after use or abstinence for 7 days.
Combination products containing norgestrel and EE, ethynodiol diacetate and EE, and desogestrel and EE	Same	Combination progesterone and estrogen used for contraception. Contraindications include most of the same as previously discussed, current thrombophlebitis, DVT, PE, CVA, CAD, valve disease, hypertension, diabetes mellitus with vascular involvement, migraines in women over 35 y, cancers, neoplasm, tumors; cardiovascular side effects are increased in women who smoke, especially those over 35 y. Some evidence has suggested there is an increased risk for VTE in obese women (BMI greater than or equal to 30 kg/m²) using CHCs. Caution in patients with history of depression. Absorption: Rapid; PB: 95%–99%; t½: EE 12–23 h; t½: Norgestrel 22–49 h Pregnancy Considerations: Contraindicated in pregnancy
Combination products containing drospirenone (DRSP) and EE	Same	Estrogen and progestin combination used for contraception, for acne treatment in adults, and for PMDD. Same contraindications and blackbox warnings as previously discussed PB: 97%–98%; t½: 24–30 h Pregnancy Considerations: Contraindicated in pregnancy
Combination products containing norgestimate and EE	Same	Estrogen and progestin combination used for contraception and for acne treatment in adults. Same contraindications and blackbox warnings as previously discussed PB: 97%–99%; t½: 16–38 h Contraindicated in pregnancy
Combination with folate in the form of EE–DRSP–levomefolate calcium	Same	Estrogen and progestin combination used for contraception, acne, and PMDD. Same contraindications and blackbox warnings as previously discussed PB: 97%–99%; t½: DRSP 31 h, EE 24 h (approx.), levomefolate calcium 4–5 h (approx.) Contraindicated in pregnancy

CAD, Coronary artery disease; *CHC*, combined hormonal contraceptive; *CVA*, cerebrovascular accident; *DRSP*, drospirenone; *DVT*, deep venous thrombosis; *EE*, ethinyl estradiol; *h*, hours; *LNG*, levonorgestrel; *PB*, protein binding; *PE*, pulmonary embolus; *PMDD*, premenstrual dysphoric disorder; *PO*, by mouth; *t½*, half-life; *y*, year; *>*, greater than.

Types of Combined Hormonal Contraceptives

Combination pills are classified as either monophasic or multiphasic (biphasic, triphasic, or four-phasic). The *monophasics* provide a fixed ratio of estrogen to progestin throughout the menstrual cycle. In *biphasics,* the amount of estrogen is fixed throughout the cycle, but the amount of progestin varies; it is reduced in the first half to provide for some proliferation of the endometrium and is increased in the second half to promote secretory development of the endometrium. This simulates the normal physiologic process of menstruation while still inhibiting ovulation. The *triphasics* deliver low doses of both hormones with minimal side effects because the amounts of estrogen and progesterone both vary throughout the cycle in different ratios during the phases. The *four-phasics* deliver varying doses of estradiol valerate (1, 2, or 3 mg) and dienogest (0, 2, or 3 mg) throughout the cycle.

Withdrawal Bleeding

Most of the monophasic, biphasic, and triphasic CHC products are packaged in both 21- and 28-day tablet packs. In the 21-day tablet packs, 21 days of active pills that contain estrogen and progestin are followed by a 7-day "pill-free" period. A new pack of pills is started after the 7-day pill-free period. In the 28-day tablet pack, 21 days of active pills are followed by 7 days of inert pills, called *counters.* The patient takes one pill daily and begins a new pack the day after the last counter is taken. During the hormone-free period (counters) or the 7-day pill-free period, the level of estrogen and progestin decreases to allow for a breakdown of the endometrial lining. This causes a pseudomenstruation known as withdrawal bleeding or *withdrawal menses.* The withdrawal bleeding is not a true menstrual period, and the bleeding experienced by a woman can vary in amount and duration.

There are CHCs that provide ferrous fumarate, an iron compound, or folic acid, a B vitamin, during the hormone-free period. Ferrous fumarate provides supplementation during the phase of withdrawal bleeding, promoting healthy iron stores in women and protecting against menstrual-associated iron-deficiency anemia. Folic acid reduces the risk of neural tube defect should the woman become pregnant on OCs or shortly after discontinuation.

Withdrawal bleeding periods are scheduled monthly to mimic a normal 28-day menstrual cycle; however, researchers have established that a monthly episode of withdrawal bleeding is not necessary to maintain a healthy uterus. CHCs are available that (1) decrease the number of withdrawal menses per year by having 81 to 84 continuous days of active pills and 7 days of less-active pills, resulting in four withdrawal menses per year, or (2) eliminate withdrawal bleeding altogether by continuous oral administration of active pills.

Extended-Use and Continuous-Use Combined Hormonal Contraception

Extended-use CHC delays menstruation, whereas continuous-use eliminates menstruation. Extended-use contraceptives contain continuing dosing pills with EE and LNG in a 91-day pill regimen. This includes 84 days of active pills and 7 days of inert pills. This drug causes withdrawal bleeding four times a year. Patients may experience uterine bleeding in an irregular pattern.

With continuous-dose CHCs, menses is completely eliminated, making these products beneficial for women with menses disorders such as menorrhagia (heavy periods), metrorrhagia (irregular bleeding between periods, usually heavy), endometriosis, dysmenorrhea, premenstrual syndrome (PMS), and physiologic ovarian cyst formation.

Ethinyl Estradiol and Norelgestromin Transdermal Patch

This is a weekly form of CHC patch that delivers 35 mcg EE and 150 mcg norelgestromin every 24 hours through a transdermal system. The system is a thin plastic patch placed on the skin of the buttocks, stomach, upper outer arm, or upper torso. The patch is placed once a week for 3 weeks in a row. The fourth week is patch-free to allow for withdrawal bleeding. The patch should be placed on clean, dry skin; placement on or near the breasts should be avoided because of the estrogen component, and the site of the patch placement should be rotated to avoid skin irritation. If the patch partially or completely detaches from the skin, a new patch should be placed. When used correctly, the patch is 92% to 99.3% effective at preventing pregnancy on a monthly basis.

The patch works in a similar manner to CHC pills by inhibiting ovulation, thickening cervical mucus to prevent sperm penetration, and preventing a fertilized egg from implanting in the uterus. Advantages include not having to remember to take a pill daily, as well as a decrease of menstrual flow, cramping, acne, iron-deficiency anemia, excess body hair, premenstrual symptoms, and vaginal dryness. As with CHC pills, the patch reduces the risk for ovarian and endometrial cancers, PID, breast and ovarian cysts, and osteoporosis (loss of bone mass) that predisposes women to fractures. With the patch, occurrences of ectopic pregnancy are also reduced. As with all CHC products, the ability to become pregnant quickly returns when discontinued.

Disadvantages of the patch include skin reaction at the site of application, menstrual cramps, and a change in vision or the inability to wear contact lenses; it is not as effective for women who weigh more than 198 lb. Due to the peak levels of estrogen remaining constant during the week the patch is in place, women are exposed to 60% more estrogen than with oral contraception. Therefore EE and norelgestromin transdermal patch carry a boxed warning stating that it exposes women to higher risk for VTE. Women being prescribed the transdermal route of CHCs should be notified of potential risks, and the patch should be used with extreme caution in any patient with increased risk for VTE. Women who are older than 35 years and smoke should not use the transdermal patch. Other side effects include temporary irregular bleeding, weight gain or loss, breast tenderness, and nausea.

Ethinyl Estradiol and Etonogestrel Transvaginal Contraception

The EE and etonogestrel transvaginal ring is a 2-inch flexible indwelling ring inserted vaginally and left in place continuously for 3 consecutive weeks, then removed for 1 week. It releases 15 mcg of EE and 120 mcg of progestin etonogestrel daily, similar to the quantities of estrogen and progestin found in lower-dose CHC products. As with the transdermal patch, patients may be exposed to higher level of estrogen; however, studies have been inconclusive, and the US Food and Drug Administration (FDA) has placed no additional warnings on the ring at this time. Theoretic effectiveness and typical effectiveness rates are 98% and 92%, similar to those of other leading CHCs. The patient inserts the ring during the first 5 days of the menstrual cycle and removes the ring after 3 weeks, remains "ring-free" for 1 week (for withdrawal menses), and then inserts a new ring. Backup contraception is recommended during the first 7 days after the first ring is placed. During this time, the hormones reach an appropriate protective level. After this, contraceptive effects are expected to be continuous provided the ring is correctly inserted. Correct insertion involves placing the ring into the middle or upper third of the vagina. Unlike the diaphragm, it does not need to be placed near or over the cervix. It is the close proximity of the ring to the vaginal mucosa that causes absorption of steroid hormones to occur. The ring remains in place during intercourse, tampon use, or administration of intravaginal drugs. If the ring slips out, it can be rinsed with lukewarm water and reinserted into the vagina. It should be reinserted within 3 hours after becoming dislodged; if the ring remains out for more than 3 hours, additional contraception is required until the ring has been in place for 7 days. Possible side effects include vaginal discharge, irritation, or infection. Other associated risks are the same as for low-dose CHCs and are increased in patients who smoke.

Segesterone acetate and EE transvaginal ring is another combination hormonal contraceptive vaginal ring. Ethinyl estradiol is a potent synthetic estrogen, and segesterone is a synthetic progestin. Contraindications are listed as the same as EE transvaginal ring at this time.

Pharmacokinetics. EE is rapidly absorbed orally and reaches peak serum concentration in 1 to 2 hours. It undergoes significant first-pass metabolism resulting in 40% bioavailability. EE is 98.5% protein bound. It is excreted as metabolites via feces and urine. It undergoes some enterohepatic circulation.

The steroid hormones in the transvaginal ring are rapidly absorbed through the vaginal mucosa. Etonogestrel in the transvaginal ring has a bioavailability of 100%; bioavailability of EE is 55%. The transdermal patch also bypasses the hepatic portal system. Avoiding first-pass metabolism through the liver has the potential to decrease adverse drug interactions. The norelgestromin in the patch binds to albumin. Levels of serum steroid hormones in the patch reach constant levels of contraceptive efficacy within 48 hours. Serum hormone levels are rapidly reached, and blood levels do not fluctuate as much as is seen with OC products.

Progestin Contraceptives

Progestin contraceptives do not contain estrogen. The estrogen component of contraceptives increases the risk of circulatory disorders; therefore progestin-only contraceptives allow contraception to be available for women who cannot take CHCs. Advantages of progestin contraceptive include relative safety, ease of use, spontaneity of sexual intercourse, and reversibility. However, because the estrogen component is missing, these products have a higher incidence of irregular bleeding and spotting as well as the possibility of depression, mood changes, decreased libido, fatigue, and weight gain. Progestin contraceptives do not protect women against STIs. Women who cannot take estrogen but may be candidates for progestin contraceptives include patients with a personal or strong family history of VTE or heart disease, breast-feeding patients, smokers older than 35 years of age, and women with uncontrolled hypertension.

Progestin-Only Oral Contraceptive Pills

The progestin-only oral contraceptive pill (POP), called the *minipill*, has four mechanisms of action: (1) it alters cervical mucus, making it thick and viscous, which blocks sperm penetration; (2) it interferes with the endometrial lining, which makes implantation difficult; (3) it decreases peristalsis in the fallopian tubes, slowing the transport of ovum; and (4) in approximately 50% of cycles, it interferes with the LH surge and thereby inhibits ovulation.

POPs contain 0.35 mg of norethindrone. The minipill is taken continuously, without a break for withdrawal bleeding. Patients should be instructed to take the minipill daily within a 3-hour window. Risk for pregnancy will increase if a patient misses a dose of POP because they do not suppress the release of follicle stimulating hormone (FSH) and LH to the same degree as the combination hormone pills.

Depot Medroxyprogesterone Acetate

Depot medroxyprogesterone acetate (DMPA) is a highly effective, long-acting injectable progestin with theoretic and typical use efficacy rates of 99% and 97%, respectively. This makes DMPA one of the most effective hormonal methods of contraception. It appeals to women because it is discreet and has a convenient dosing schedule; DMPA is popular with adolescents for these same reasons. Injectable progestin is administered in a flexible dosing schedule every 11 to 13 weeks. The

mechanism of action of DMPA relies on the progestational activities: thickening of the cervical mucus, thinning of the uterine endometrium, and a decrease in fallopian tube motility. Because the progestin in DMPA reaches a higher circulating level than with POPs, DMPA inhibits both FSH and LH secretion from the anterior pituitary gland. This results in both anovulation (lack of ovulation) and amenorrhea. Because FSH and LH secretion is inhibited, formation of a dominant follicle is inhibited, and the production of estrogen in the body is greatly decreased. However, the patient experiences a hypo-estrogen state, which can affect bone mineral density (BMD).

The DMPA vial or prefilled syringe should be vigorously shaken just before administration to ensure a uniform drug suspension. DMPA 150 mg/1 mL is given by deep intramuscular (IM) injection into the ventral gluteus or deltoid muscle. The site should *not* be massaged after injection, and the injection site must be documented so that sites can be rotated. The patient is given a personalized calendar for subsequent doses and should return for another injection within 13 weeks. If the patient is late for her injection by even 1 day, pregnancy should be ruled out before resuming treatment.

As with OCs, DMPA does not protect against STIs. Due to the hypo-estrogenic state produced by DMPA, bone reabsorption exceeds bone formation. This results in a reduction of BMD, greatest during the first 1 to 2 years of DMPA use. After discontinuation of DMPA, BMD substantially improves (more so at the spine than hips) but may not be completely reversible. Based on these data, the FDA issued a boxed warning recommending DMPA be discontinued after 2 years of continuous use, unless other methods of contraception are inadequate. Many professional provider organizations agree that the concerns of the 2-consecutive-year limit given by the FDA and the BMD effects of DMPA should not prevent the practitioner from considering the benefit-risk ratio for each individual patient. The American Congress of Obstetricians and Gynecologists (ACOG) stated in a committee opinion that "the possible adverse effects of DMPA must be carefully balanced against the significant personal and public health impact of unintended pregnancy." The benefits, risks, and alternatives and the prevention of BMD loss while taking DMPA must be discussed with the patient before administration of the product.

Women taking DMPA should be instructed to increase calcium and vitamin D intake to the daily recommended allowance for their age and to participate in regular weight-bearing exercises. DMPA is safe to receive immediately postpartum, and women can breastfeed while using this contraceptive without affecting milk supply. The most common side effects include initially irregular uterine bleeding or spotting. Menstruation may cease about 1 year after starting. In addition, DMPA has been shown to cause progressive weight gain in some women. Other side effects include breast tenderness and an increase in depression. The drug is contraindicated in cases of undiagnosed vaginal bleeding and known or suspected pregnancy. Caution should be used in giving DMPA postpartum in women who are at risk for or have a history of postpartum depression.

DMPA formulated for subcutaneous injection is available as an injectable suspension of 104 mg/0.65 mL. It is administered to women every 12 to 14 weeks. This drug has the same mechanism of action, benefits, and risks as DMPA for intramuscular injection, and women should be counseled about the potential loss of BMD. Women taking DMPA have a slower return to fertility than those using other hormonal methods of contraception.

Progestin Implant

A progestin implant is a single-rod device that contains 68 mg of etonogestrel; it is implanted in the inner side of the upper nondominant arm. It needs to be removed no later than 3 years after the date of insertion; it may be replaced with a new implant at the time of removal. The progestin implant contains barium, a radiopaque substance that can help locate the device on two-dimensional radiography, ultrasound, magnetic resonance imaging (MRI), and computed tomography (CT) scanning if necessary. Also, the device comes in a preloaded application system that reduces insertion errors. The progestin implant may not be as effective in women who have a body mass index (BMI) greater than 30 (obese) or who are on drugs that induce liver enzymes. Theoretic and typical effectiveness rates for implantable progestins are the same, at 99.6%.

Pharmacokinetics. Progestin contraceptives are well absorbed from the GI tract. Peak plasma levels occur 1 to 2 hours after ingestion, depending on the particular compound. Norethynodrel and ethynodiol diacetate are converted to norethindrone. Norgestrel and LNG are 100% bioavailable and do not undergo first-pass liver metabolism; norethindrone undergoes first-pass metabolism and is 65% available. The progestins are bound to plasma proteins and sex hormone–binding globulin. The half-life of norethindrone varies from 5 to 14 hours; the half-life of LNG is 11 to 45 hours.

DMPA provides higher peak levels of progestin than POPs and implantable progestins. Once injected, the levels of DMPA increase for 3 weeks, remain stable for a few days, then begin to decline. DMPA is undetectable in the blood between 120 and 200 days after injection. The formulation for subcutaneous administration of DMPA provides a slower and more sustained absorption than IM, permitting a lower dose. DMPA is 90% protein bound, metabolized in the liver, and excreted primarily in the urine.

A progestin implant is a sustained-release system that releases progestin at a level of 60 to 70 mcg/day during the first 6 weeks after insertion, declining to 35 to 45 mcg/day during the first year. This decreases to 30 to 40 mcg/day after 2 years of implantation and 25 to 30 mcg/day by the end of the third year. Bioavailability remains constant at 95%. Once the rod is inserted, effective contraceptive levels are reached within 8 hours.

Start Date and Dosing Schedule for Starting Hormonal Contraception Products

There are three ways to implement the start of hormonal contraception products unless otherwise indicated by the manufacturer. With the *first-day start method,* the contraception product is initiated on the first day a women experiences bleeding; the first day of bleeding is day 1 of the menstrual cycle. Days are then counted 2, 3, 4, 5, 6, and so on until the first-day bleeding begins again, usually around day 28. Most methods of contraception can be safely started on day 1 through day 5 of the menstrual cycle, when it is less likely that the patient has an early undiagnosed pregnancy. No back-up method of contraception is needed when the product is started on the first through fifth day of menstruation. Many products require a *Sunday start,* meaning the patient starts the tablets or patch on the Sunday after the first days of menstruation. If menstruation actually starts on Sunday, the patient starts her tablet or patch on that day. The Sunday start aids a woman in remembering the first day of her contraception cycle. If a patient starts the contraception later than day 5 of her menstrual cycle, a back-up form of contraception should be used for 7 days.

Special Considerations

DMPA and the transvaginal ring must be started within the first 5 days of the menstrual cycle. The continuous-dosing CHC products use a Sunday start only. If the patient is on a 21-day CHC regimen, the next pack should be started after the 7-day break whether bleeding

---

BOX 55.1 Guidelines for Missed Doses of Oral Contraceptives

Combined Hormonal Contraceptives
One Tablet
Take the tablet as soon as the missed dose is realized.
Take the next tablet as scheduled.

Two Tablets
Take two tablets as soon as the missed dose is realized and two tablets the next day.
Use a back-up method of contraception for the rest of the cycle.

Three Tablets
Discontinue the present pack and allow for withdrawal bleeding. Start a new package of tablets 7 days after the last tablet is taken. Use another form of contraception until tablets have been taken for 7 consecutive days.

Progestin-Only Pills
One or More Tablets
Take the tablet as soon as the missed dose is realized and follow with the next tablet at the regular time *plus* use a back-up method of contraception for 48 hours.

---

has stopped or not. With 28-day packs, a pill is taken daily without stopping regardless of the bleeding pattern. Usually, withdrawal menses occur in a cyclic fashion. In multiphasic preparations, the day 1 pill is clearly marked, and the tablets are taken in the order noted. A difference in the color of the tablets delineates the change in the dose of estrogen or progestin through the phases. With the POP, a pill is taken daily without a break. To increase effectiveness, all OCs should be taken at the same time daily. With the POP, women should strictly adhere to this instruction.

Missed Doses

Box 55.1 provides guidelines for patients on how to handle missing a dose of their OC.

Contraindications

Not every patient is a candidate for use of CHCs. Box 55.2 lists contraindications to CHC use.

Drug Interactions

The effectiveness of some drugs is impaired by CHC products; other drugs impair the effectiveness of CHCs and progestin contraceptives. Box 55.3 shows drugs that may have interactive effects with CHCs. Patients receiving low-dose formulations of OCs need to be particularly cautious about potential interactions. If a patient is taking a drug that affects estrogen absorption or metabolism, a CHC with a higher dose of EE may be prescribed.

Potential Side Effects and Adverse Reactions

Most of the untoward side effects are related to differences in the estrogen-progestin ratio of the products and the patient's response to these differences. Side effects primarily caused by an excess of estrogen include nausea, vomiting, dizziness, fluid retention, edema, bloating, breast enlargement, breast tenderness, chloasma (slightly more in dark-skinned patients on higher-dose tablets who are exposed to sunlight), leg cramps, decreased tearing, corneal curvature alteration,

BOX 55.2 Contraindications for Combined Hormonal Contraceptives

Absolute Contraindications

- Pregnancy (known or suspected)
- Venous thrombosis history or risk factors
- Vascular disease, including coronary artery disease and cerebrovascular accident (CVA) and past or current history of deep venous thrombosis (DVT) or pulmonary embolism
- Liver disease, including cirrhosis, viral hepatitis, and benign or malignant liver tumors
- Undiagnosed vaginal bleeding or known or suspected endometrial cancer
- Breast cancer
- Tobacco use of more than 15 cigarettes per day in a patient older than 35 years of age

Cautious Use

- Hypertension with associated vascular disease
- Hypertension with blood pressure greater than 160/100 mm Hg
- Hyperlipidemia
- Diabetes mellitus complicated by neuropathy, retinopathy, nephropathy, or vascular disease
- Diabetes mellitus for more than 20 years' duration
- Postpartum fewer than 3 weeks
- Lactation fewer than 6 weeks
- Age greater than 35 years and smoking fewer than 15 cigarettes per day
- Hypercoagulation disorders
- Prolonged immobility
- Use of drugs that affect liver enzymes (e.g., anticonvulsants, rifampin)

visual changes, vascular headache, and hypertension (in about 1% to 5% of previously normotensive patients within the first few months).

Side effects primarily caused by estrogen deficiency include vaginal bleeding (BTB, especially in the first few cycles after starting therapy) that lasts several days, usually during days 1 to 14; *oligomenorrhea* (very scant periods), especially after long-term use; nervousness; and *dyspareunia* (painful sexual intercourse) secondary to atrophic vaginitis.

Side effects primarily caused by an excess of progestin include increased appetite, weight gain, oily skin and scalp, acne, depression, vulvovaginal candidiasis (vaginitis from the yeast microbe *Candida*), excess hair growth, decreased breast size, and amenorrhea after cessation of use (1% to 2% of patients).

Side effects primarily caused by progestin deficiency include dysmenorrhea, bleeding late in the cycle (days 15 to 21), heavy menstrual flow with clots, or amenorrhea. There may also be changes in laboratory values, including thyroid and liver function, blood glucose, and triglycerides.

CHCs may increase the vascularity of the cervical epithelium, extend the area of cervical ectopy, and alter certain immune parameters. Advise pill users to use male or female latex or polyurethane condoms unless they are confident that both partners are free of human immunodeficiency virus (HIV) and other STIs.

Adverse reactions of a more severe nature include cardiovascular and carcinogenetic risks.

Cardiovascular

There is an increased risk for hypertension (usually seen within 3 months after initiating CHCs in women with preexisting risk) and

BOX 55.3 Drugs That Interact With Combined Hormonal Contraceptives

Drugs That Decrease the Effectiveness of Combined Hormonal Contraceptives

Use a higher-dose pill or an alternative form of contraception (if the drug is continuous).

Use a back-up method for the duration of treatment plus 7 days (if drug is short term).

Anticonvulsant Drugs

Carbamazepine
Hydantoins (ethotoin, mephenytoin, phenytoin)
Succinimide anticonvulsants (ethosuximide)

Antituberculin Drugs

Rifampin

Antifungal Drugs

Griseofulvin

Antibiotics

Amoxicillin
Ampicillin
Doxycycline
Metronidazole
Minocycline
Neomycin

Nitrofurantoin
Penicillin
Tetracycline

Barbiturates

Phenobarbital
Primidone

Hypnotics and Sedatives

Benzodiazepines

Migraine Drugs

Topiramate

Drugs That May Increase Combined Hormonal Contraceptive Activity

Acetaminophen
Ascorbic acid
Fluconazole

Other Drug Interactions

An alternative method of contraception is necessary.
Anticoagulants: CHCs increase clotting factors and decrease the effectiveness of anticoagulants.
Anticonvulsants: CHCs may increase the risk for seizure.

CHC, Combined hormonal contraceptive.

arterial blood clot complications such as MI, pulmonary embolus, and cerebrovascular accident (CVA) in women using CHCs compared with women who are not using CHCs. However, in terms of absolute risk for adolescents and women, the rate of dangerous complications from hormonal methods of contraception is extremely low because women younger than 50 years rarely experience heart attack or stroke. The risk for hypertension in women younger than 35 years is also low. Hormonal methods of contraception that contain DRSP or etonogestrel may double a woman's risk for venous thromboembolic events. Cardiovascular risks are increased in women older than 35 years who smoke, women older than 45 years, and women with hypertension that is undiagnosed or uncontrolled by drugs.

Carcinogenesis

Long-term use of CHCs may increase the risk for breast cancer in younger women, but the risk is minimal. Breast cancer risk returns to normal 10 years or more after discontinuing CHCs. There is also an increased risk for benign liver tumors. Risk for cervical cancer is slightly increased, which is thought to be because CHCs change cervical epithelium, making it more susceptible to the high-risk pathogenic strains of human papillomavirus (HPV) and because condoms may be used less frequently in prevention of STIs. Women who use hormonal methods of contraception have a greatly reduced risk for ovarian and endometrial cancers, and the protective effect is directly related to the duration of time the method is used.

CLINICAL JUDGMENT [NURSING PROCESS]

Combined Hormonal Contraceptives

Concept: Hormonal Regulation
- Hormonal regulation involves substances working together to promote healthy development of female sex characteristics during puberty and adulthood to ensure or delay fertility.

Recognize Cues [Assessment]
- Obtain a record of the patient's drug, supplement, and complementary and alternative medicine (CAM) use.
- Obtain baseline vital signs that include temperature, pulse, and respirations; blood pressure (BP); weight; and height. Calculate body mass index (BMI) and report any abnormal findings.
- Obtain a complete menstrual history that includes age at menarche, menstrual pattern, cycle length, duration, and amount of bleeding and the first day of the last menstrual period (LMP).
- Determine the patient's pregnancy status.
- Obtain a family medical history specific to contraindications for combined hormonal contraceptives (CHCs) and progestin contraceptives.
- Obtain a family history of premenopausal breast cancer.
- Assess for domestic violence, intimate partner violence, and past or recent sexual abuse/assault.
- Obtain a medical history, assessing for history of allergies to drugs, smoking, hypertension, and the contraindications to CHCs listed in Box 55.2.
- Obtain a complete obstetric and gynecologic history that includes gravida, parity, abortion (spontaneous, therapeutic, or elective); age at first and last pregnancy; time frame between pregnancies; complications during pregnancy, delivery, and postpartum; genetic anomalies and health of children; time since the last Papanicolaou (Pap) test; history of abnormal Pap testing; history of gynecologic and/or sexual infections; gynecologic problems and/or surgeries; and gynecologic anomalies.
- Obtain a complete sexual history that includes sexual expression and sexual risk practices, history of sexually transmitted infections (STIs) and treatment, and past or present sexual abuse and/or assault.
- Recognize the need for periodic reassessment of baseline data and side effects. Most patients should be seen 1 to 3 months after beginning a contraceptive regimen.

Analyze Cues and Prioritize Hypothesis [Patient Problems]
- Discomfort
- Potential for nonadherence
- Confusion
- Coping
- Anxiety
- Need for patient teaching

Generate Solutions [Planning]
- The patient with contraindications to hormonal contraception will be determined by evaluation of risk-benefit method.
- The patient will verbalize the difference between CHCs and progestin contraceptives and their various routes of administration.
- The patient will verbalize understanding of the bleeding patterns associated with both types of contraceptives by reporting menstrual changes that occur.
- The patient will choose a contraceptive method suitable to their lifestyle and health status.
- The patient will understand and verbalize the pros and cons of contraception through use of the BRAIDED method. This method is recommended by the Department of Health and Human Services to provide regulations concerning guidance for informed consent of contraceptive methods. BRAIDED method: discuss **benefits** (advantages, positive aspects, and both theoretic and actual effective rates of the method), **risks** (dangers, complications, disadvantages, and failure rates), **alternatives** (other contraception options available), **inquiries** (opportunity for the patient to ask questions about options proposed), **decision** (deciding on a method with opportunity to change the decision as needed), **explanation** (health care teaching specific to the method chosen), and **documentation**.
- The patient will verbalize the dosing schedule and use of contraceptive method chosen.
- The patient will receive instruction on how to report dangerous cardiovascular side effects to the health care provider (HCP) by using the ACHES acronym. (ACHES acronym: *abdominal pain* [severe]; *chest pain* or shortness of breath; *headaches* [severe], dizziness, weakness, numbness, or speech difficulties; *eye disorders*, which includes blurring or loss of vision; and *severe* leg pain or swelling in the calf or thigh).
- The patient will verbalize understanding of the ACHES acronym.
- The patient will take oral contraceptives (OCs) as prescribed and report adverse side effects to the HCP.
- The patient will demonstrate and report comfort with placement of the transvaginal ring and will report adverse side effects that occur.
- The patient will verbalize the specific scheduling needs for progestin-only pills.
- The patient will verbalize the initiation and scheduling of depot medroxyprogesterone acetate (DMPA) injections and the need for weight-bearing exercises and calcium supplementation.
- The patient will be instructed to schedule follow-up appointments as needed.

Take Action [Nursing Interventions]
- Assist the patient with obtaining informed consent for the initiation of contraceptives through the BRAIDED method.

⊚ CLINICAL JUDGMENT [NURSING PROCESS]—CONT'D

Combined Hormonal Contraceptives

- Instruct and have the patient verbalize the complications and side effects of their particular contraceptive method.
- Instruct the patient about alternatives to the method (including abstinence and no method).
- Instruct the patient about their patient's right and responsibility.
- Instruct the patient in a format that is understandable to the patient and have the patient verbalize their understanding.
- Assess the patient for misconceptions and provide factual, evidence-based information when instructing the patient.
- Encourage the patient's effective use of the chosen contraceptive method.
- Ensure the patient understands the start date, continuation of drug, and appropriate follow-up.
- Provide the patient with alternative forms of contraceptive therapy because a percentage of patients on hormonal contraceptives will abandon the method within 1 year; and encourage the patient to seek care with a qualified health care provider before discontinuing any method of contraception.
- Discuss with the nonnursing mother that it's suggested they begin CHCs 4 to 6 weeks postpartum, regardless of whether menstruation has spontaneously occurred. Some sources indicate that a CHC method can be initiated as early as 3 weeks postpartum.
- Instruct nonnursing and nursing mothers they may begin DMPA immediately postpartum if there is no increased risk for postpartum depression. Progestin-only oral contraceptive pills (POPs) can be started at 4 to 6 weeks postpartum.
- Instruct the patient that CHCs may decrease milk production in patients who are breastfeeding. CHCs can be used by breastfeeding mothers, but these methods should be initiated after breastfeeding is well established. This is usually 2 to 3 months after the birth, although some sources state that 6 weeks is sufficient. Always check with the HCP.

Patient Teaching
General
- Instruct the patient that contraceptive drugs should be used only under the direction of a qualified HCP.
- Advise the patient that concurrent use of certain drugs and herbal products decreases the effectiveness of hormonal contraceptives. The patient should use a second form of contraception during use of these drugs and herbal supplements for 7 days after discontinuing counteracting drugs.
- Instruct the patient that hormonal methods of contraception do *not* prevent transmission of STIs or the pathogen that causes human immunodeficiency virus (HIV) infection. If a patient is at risk for STI or HIV infection, condoms should be used concurrently with the CHC method, and safe-sex practices should be discussed. Inform patients regarding proper condom use.

Safety
- ⚡ Instruct the patient not to smoke tobacco because of increased cardiovascular risks.
- Advise the patient to use a barrier method of contraception as needed during the first 7 days of contraception use if the method is started 5 days or more after the first day of the menstrual period. Instruct the patient on how to use barrier methods properly.
- Instruct the patient about how to manage missed pills. Provide instruction for missed POPs and on patch, ring, and injection methods. Review instructions for emergency contraception.
- Advise the patient to report any effects from hormonal contraception to the HCP so therapy can be adjusted to suit their needs. Encourage the patient not to discontinue use of the method until an adequate trial time frame has been completed, which should be at least 3 to 6 months.

- ⚡ Instruct the patient that HCPs should be advised of CHC use before surgery in which immobilization for an extended period may be needed.
- Encourage the patient to report any irregular bleeding to the HCP; this may require a change in dose or another type of hormonal contraceptive method.
- Advise the patient to always report use of hormonal contraceptives when seeing a HCP because of possible synergistic or antagonistic responses to other drugs and therapies.
- Advise the nursing mother that the use of CHCs may decrease the quantity and quality of breast milk.

Side Effects
- ⚡ Advise the patient that rare but serious side effects can occur, including venous thromboembolism (VTE), myocardial infarction (MI), cerebral vascular accident (CVA), and retinal vein thrombosis.
- ⚡ Instruct the patient in the ACHES acronym for reporting symptoms of dangerous cardiovascular side effects to their health care provider (abdominal pain, chest pain, headaches, eye problems, swelling and /or aching in the legs and thighs).
- Instruct the patient to notify their HCP immediately if any of these symptoms occur.
- Advise the patient that menstrual flow may be less in amount and duration because of thinning of the endometrial lining with CHCs and progestin contraceptives.
- Advise the patient of menstrual changes that can occur at the start of combined estrogen-progestin contraception use, when changing types of hormonal contraception products, and with progestin contraceptives.
- Determine whether the patient wears contact lenses and discuss alterations in the shape of the cornea and dry eyes that may occur due to decreased tearing. If this occurs, the patient should consult their optometrist.
- Instruct the patient who experiences post-CHC amenorrhea that 95% of women have regular periods within 12 to 18 months. Advise the patient that those who participate in endurance fitness activities may have increased post-CHC amenorrhea.
- Advise the patient of a possible decrease in libido caused by an alteration in vaginal secretions and decreased levels of testosterone.
- Ensure the patient understands the ability to return to fertility after discontinuing a hormonal contraception product and the time frame in which pregnancy can be expected.
- Ensure a safe transition between contraceptive methods if a change in method is desired.

Skill
- Instruct the patient in breast health awareness and self-examination.
- Instruct the patient how to inspect genitalia for abnormalities and note changes in vaginal secretions.
- Show the patient the packet of pills and discuss how to recognize start dates and follow the sequential pill dosing. Demonstrate how to remove the pill from the pill packet.
- Instruct the patient how to place and remove transdermal contraception patches.
- Instruct the patient how to place and remove transvaginal contraception rings.
- Instruct the patient how to use a calendar to record placement and removal of transvaginal rings or transdermal patches.
- Advise the patient to return for a DMPA injection within the 13-week time frame.

Continued

CLINICAL JUDGMENT [NURSING PROCESS]—CONT'D

Combined Hormonal Contraceptives

Diet
- Counsel the patient to moderate caffeine intake, because elimination of caffeine may be decreased as a result of prescribed CHC products.
- Instruct the patient to take OCs with a snack or after meals to help eliminate nausea.
- Advise the patient using DMPA to increase calcium and vitamin D intake and to do 15 to 30 minutes of weight-bearing exercises 3 to 4 times per week.
- Discuss foods that increase iron and iron absorption.

Evaluate Outcomes [Evaluation]
- Encourage the patient in planning follow-up evaluations.
- Evaluate the patient's adherence with the hormonal contraceptive regimen; assess for changes in sexual partners and/or health status that may compromise the method.

Preventing Fertilization

CHCs can be used to prevent fertilization after an incidence of unprotected vaginal intercourse or failure of a contraceptive method. The method involves taking 2 to 5 OC pills at one time. This raises both estrogen and progestin levels to delay or prevent ovulation; it interferes with tubal transport of the embryo, egg, or sperm; and it changes the hormones necessary for the preparation of the uterine lining. Using this method decreases the risk for pregnancy by 75% for each act of sexual intercourse. The major side effect is nausea; to prevent this, an OTC antinausea medicine should be taken 1 hour before CHC administration. Antihistamines are the most commonly used OTC drug for nausea, and some are marketed specifically for this purpose. Antihistamines include diphenhydramine, dimenhydrinate, and meclizine. Irregular menstrual bleeding is another side effect. If a woman does not begin menstruation within a few days of the expected time, a pregnancy test should be performed. Patients who are unable to take estrogen should *not* take CHCs as emergency contraception (EC).

Family planning agencies and women's health organizations provide a full list of CHC pills along with the dosage and administration regimen for these products when used for EC. Treatment should be initiated within 72 hours of intercourse. The sooner a plan is initiated, the more effective it will be at preventing pregnancy.

The first EC pill available in the United States was approved in 1999; it was known as Plan B (LNG, a progestin-only pill). In 2006 the FDA approved this drug without a prescription for women 18 years of age or older. In 2009 the FDA stated that both men and women can obtain this drug without a prescription if they are older than 17 years. Those younger than 17 years need a prescription.

The EC pill should be taken within 72 hours after intercourse, but it is still effective 120 hours afterward. If taken within 24 hours of intercourse, EC reduces the risk of pregnancy by 95%. Just 12 hours after the initial 24-hour postcoital period, the effectiveness rate of EC decreases to approximately 60%. In Plan B One-Step, one 1.5 mg LNG tablet is taken. If Next Choice is used, one 0.75 mg tablet is taken, followed by another 12 hours later. If vomiting occurs within 3 hours, the dose should be repeated. Less nausea is associated with this drug than with estrogen-containing EC methods.

DRUGS USED TO TREAT DISORDERS IN WOMEN'S HEALTH

Common reasons women seek gynecologic health care include alterations in menstrual cycle, menstrual or pelvic pain, and changes in vaginal secretions. Included within these broad categories are irregular uterine bleeding, dysmenorrhea, and PMS. This section describes common disorders in women's health and presents current pharmacologic approaches to management.

Irregular or Abnormal Uterine Bleeding

Irregular uterine bleeding is a term that describes many different medical conditions or pathologies related to the menstrual cycle. Irregular uterine bleeding, also known as *abnormal uterine bleeding* (AUB), is a common reason women seek gynecologic care. AUB encompasses a wide range of variable bleeding patterns in women, such as amenorrhea, menorrhagia, metrorrhagia, menometrorrhagia, intramenstrual bleeding, and dysfunctional uterine bleeding (DUB).

Amenorrhea

Amenorrhea is the absence of menses. *Primary amenorrhea* is defined as an absence of menses by 14 years of age *without* secondary sex characteristics or an absence of menses by 16 years of age *with* secondary sex characteristics. Primary amenorrhea may be caused by abnormalities in the structures of the female reproductive tract, chromosomal alterations, or endocrine disorders. Many times, the cause is just a physiologic delay in the onset of menstruation. *Secondary amenorrhea* is the absence of a spontaneous menstrual period for 6 consecutive months in women who have experienced menstrual cycles in the past. Pregnancy is the most common reason a patient may experience amenorrhea, as well as breastfeeding and menopause; therefore secondary amenorrhea is a *symptom* of these normal physiologic processes. Other causes of secondary amenorrhea include anovulatory cycles (cycles without ovulation), hypothyroidism or hyperthyroidism, and hyperprolactinemia (high levels of the hormone prolactin, which stimulates lactation). Extreme weight loss and anorexia can also cause amenorrhea.

After assessment of the patient's health history and a physical examination; after laboratory testing to include FSH, serum prolactin (PRL), thyroid-stimulating hormone (TSH), and serum estradiol (ES); and after pregnancy has been ruled out, a *progestin withdrawal test* may be administered to determine the underlying cause of amenorrhea. This test uses an oral progestin administered for a limited time to confirm that the hypothalamic-pituitary-ovarian (HPO) responses—that is, the hormonal system that mediates the menstrual cycle—are intact.

With the progestin withdrawal test, a patient is given medroxyprogesterone 10 mg for 10 days. The progestational activity thickens the endometrial lining and increases secretory activity. When the drug is discontinued, progesterone levels decrease, resulting in a breakdown of the endometrial lining and withdrawal bleeding. Withdrawal bleeding should occur within 7 to 10 days after completing the drug, which indicates that the HPO axis (the menstrual cycle) is functioning in providing the hormones necessary to regulate the menstrual cycle. Even the smallest amount of bleeding, such as one incidence of scant spotting, is considered a positive test. However, if no withdrawal bleeding occurs, other pathophysiologic problems may exist, and further evaluation and diagnostic testing by the health care provider are needed.

Polycystic Ovarian Syndrome

Another common cause of secondary amenorrhea is polycystic ovarian syndrome (PCOS), a disorder in the metabolism of androgens and estrogen. PCOS may be caused by dysfunction of the HPO axis. Women with PCOS experience menstrual dysfunction, anovulation, hyperandrogenism, hirsutism, infertility, obesity, metabolic syndrome, diabetes, and obstructive sleep apnea.

Diet and exercise are first-line treatment for PCOS. Weight loss of 5% to 10% has been shown to improve overall metabolic status and reduce serum androgen concentrations. Pharmacologic treatment of PCOS is used to treat anovulation, hirsutism, and menstrual irregularities. To manage menstrual irregularities, low-dose CHCs are prescribed. With the addition of the progestin in the CHC product and a cycling of a monthly withdrawal menses (or four times per year, depending on the product), the risks of unopposed estrogen on the endometrium are significantly reduced.

For women who are attempting to conceive and in whom weight loss has not restored ovulation, new studies have shown that letrozole, an aromatase inhibitor, is now the first-line ovulation induction agent over clomiphene citrate for women with PCOS, although it is an off-label use. Clomiphene citrate can still be used, but studies have shown that it is less effective for live birth rates than letrozole. Metformin has been used with clomiphene citrate, although current guidelines recommend against the use of metformin in obese women with PCOS, except in women with glucose intolerance not corrected with lifestyle changes.

Abnormal Uterine Bleeding Patterns

The normal menstrual cycle occurs every 25 to 35 days and lasts 2 to 7 days, with an estimated blood loss of no more than 80 mL. Menorrhagia is *regular* uterine bleeding greater than 80 mL or lasting more than 7 days. Women with menorrhagia may describe their periods as very heavy or state the need to change a tampon or sanitary pad frequently. Metrorrhagia is *irregular* uterine bleeding greater than 80 mL or lasting more than 7 days. Women with metrorrhagia describe their periods as irregular and heavy. They may state that they have no idea when bleeding will occur and that, when it does happen, it will soak through sanitary products or clothing. Menometrorrhagia is a combination of these two. *Intramenstrual bleeding* is an episode of bleeding, usually light, that occurs between menstrual periods.

A common complaint that brings a woman into the gynecologic health care setting is that she is having menstrual cycles that are suddenly different from the pattern she usually experiences. In women of reproductive age, pregnancy should always be considered first as the possible cause of AUB. However, AUB can result from physiologic processes such as stress, severe dieting and weight loss, eating disorders, or excessive exercise. Irregular bleeding patterns are a sign of decreasing ovarian function or approach of menopause in older women. AUB can also be caused by pathologic processes such as endocrine disorders, thyroid disease, leiomyomata (benign tumors in the uterus), ovarian cysts, infections of the genital tract, or cancer. If a woman is pregnant, uterine bleeding may indicate ectopic pregnancy or impending miscarriage. Some pharmacologic drugs, substances, and herbal preparations can also cause irregular bleeding, including anticoagulants, antipsychotics, benzodiazepines, hormone therapy (HT), ginkgo, ginseng, and soy products. Once physiologic, pathologic, and pharmaceutic causes have been ruled out, the patient may be diagnosed with DUB.

Dysfunctional Uterine Bleeding

DUB is the most common classification of irregular bleeding. Diagnosis of DUB is made when no organic pathology can be determined to cause the irregular bleeding. Pharmacologic treatment of DUB primarily involves normalizing the bleeding pattern and correcting anemia

that may have resulted from chronic or acute blood loss. In the normal physiologic menstrual cycle, estrogen and progesterone levels are low during menstruation. Once estrogen levels start to rise with the formation of a dominant follicle, uterine bleeding is effectively stopped, ending menstruation. Increasing levels of estrogen by administration of an estrogen drug product is usually effective in stopping prolonged DUB.

Because estrogen is *never* used alone in treatment, and because of the detrimental effects of unopposed estrogen on the uterine endometrium and the risk for endometrial cancer, estrogen-progestin combination products are used. Progestins alone are not as effective as estrogen in reducing an episode of acute bleeding; however, because *prolonged* progestin administration causes atrophy of the endometrial lining, progestins can be very effective if long-term control is needed. DMPA by IM injection and a levonorgestrel-intrauterine system (LNG-IUS) inserted into the uterus are among the products used for extended progestin therapy.

Pharmacologic Management of Irregular Bleeding

Nonsteroidal antiinflammatory drugs (NSAIDs) can be used for the treatment of menorrhagia, reducing bleeding by 25% to 35%. NSAIDs block the production of prostaglandin, which decreases both excessive bleeding and uterine cramps. Common NSAIDs used for menorrhagia are mefenamic acid, ibuprofen, and naproxen sodium. Only mefenamic acid has FDA approval for menorrhagia. Although approved for the treatment of dysmenorrhea, ibuprofen and naproxen sodium are used by providers as off-label options in the treatment of menorrhagia. The correct dosage of mefenamic acid is 500 mg by mouth (PO) once, followed by 250 mg PO every 6 hours as needed for 2 to 3 days. Mefenamic acid should be taken with food to avoid gastric upset. Tranexamic acid may also be given at 1300 mg three times a day for a maximum of 5 days. Tranexamic acid inhibits plasminogen binding sites, thus decreasing plasmin formation and fibrinolysis, reducing blood loss by 40% to 60%.

CHCs can be used to decrease and regulate DUB. The increase in estrogen suppresses endometrial development, restores predictable bleeding, and reduces menstrual flow. Reduction in flow should be seen within 24 hours. If a heavy flow continues for more than 48 hours, the patient should be reevaluated. Benefits, risks, and patient instructions are the same as if the product were being used for contraception. Women who are not candidates for estrogen therapy (ET) or CHCs should be excluded. Women using a CHC product for DUB should see their periods normalize within the first 3 months of use. Patients can continue the method for contraception, or they can discontinue use in 6 to 9 months, depending on the effectiveness in controlling bleeding.

Progestins are not as effective as estrogens at reducing episodes of irregular bleeding. However, progestins are effective in the long-term treatment of AUB and may be the method of choice in women who have contraindications to estrogen use. Progestins are given cyclically (e.g., norethindrone acetate 2.5 to 5 mg PO daily for 21 days or medroxyprogesterone 10 mg/day for 21 days) to produce a monthly withdrawal bleeding. DMPA and the LNG-IUS are also used for treatment of DUB. Long-term use of progesterone has an atrophic effect on the uterine endometrium, consequently decreasing incidences of irregular bleeding. Women using DMPA or the LNG-IUS for DUB should see heavy bleeding patterns decrease within 3 to 6 months.

Dysmenorrhea

Dysmenorrhea, also called *cyclic pelvic pain* (CPP), is pelvic pain associated with the menstrual cycle. Other symptoms that may occur with the menstrual cycle are uterine cramping, lower back pain, abdominal cramps, changes in bowel patterns, increased bowel movements, and nausea and vomiting. Dysmenorrhea is experienced by approximately 80% of women in their late teens and early 20s, when it is more prevalent. It is the most common reason young women miss school or work. Dysmenorrhea is classified as either primary dysmenorrhea or secondary dysmenorrhea, depending on whether there is a known etiology for the menstrual pain. *Primary dysmenorrhea* is diagnosed when there is no apparent underlying pathology. It is caused by larger-than-normal amounts of prostaglandins at the start of the menstrual period. Prostaglandins cause arterioles in the uterus to contract, decreasing blood flow to the endometrium. All of these mechanisms are necessary for breakdown of the endometrial lining and for menstruation to occur. However, this process causes increased pain in some women.

In *secondary dysmenorrhea,* there is an underlying cause for the pelvic pain. Conditions that may cause secondary dysmenorrhea are urinary tract infections (UTIs), PID, irritable bowel syndrome (IBS), uterine leiomyomata (fibroids), and endometriosis.

Pharmacologic Management of Dysmenorrhea

Nonsteroidal Antiinflammatory Drugs. NSAIDs block pain by preventing synthesis of prostaglandins. The mechanism of drug action is the inhibition of cyclooxygenase (COX). The COX enzyme converts arachidonic acid into prostaglandins, which cause constriction of the uterine arterioles, necrosis of the endometrial lining, uterine contractions, and menstrual pain. Usually nonselective and COX-2 inhibitors are used. The most commonly used NSAIDs for relief of pain associated with dysmenorrhea include naproxen sodium, diclofenac potassium, ibuprofen, naproxen, celecoxib, and mefenamic acid. Many NSAIDs can be purchased over the counter, so the nurse should include health information about the benefits, risks, and alternatives as well as specific dosage amounts, drug interactions, and administration instructions. Some drugs (diclofenac potassium, celecoxib, and mefenamic acid) are by prescription only. Patients must understand the differences in these drugs and avoid them if they have allergies to, or side effects from, any of the ingredients. Patients should avoid taking two different NSAID drugs at the same time. GI upset is a common side effect of NSAIDs, so most drugs in this category should be taken with food and water. NSAIDs can also be taken with an antacid or calcium supplement to prevent GI upset. NSAIDS carry a US blackbox warning that they can cause an increased risk of serious and potentially fatal cardiovascular events such as myocardial infarction and stroke. Always use the lowest effective dose for the shortest time.

Combined Hormonal Contraceptives. CHCs are effective in the treatment of dysmenorrhea. CHCs reduce the thickness of the uterine endometrium. The 24/4 day CHCs shorten withdrawal bleeding periods, and the extended-use CHCs decrease the number of withdrawal menses per year or eliminate them altogether. DMPA, progestin implants, and LNG-IUS decrease dysmenorrhea in patients who are candidates for these methods. Long-term progestin-only products cause atrophy of the uterine lining, limiting the occurrence of dysmenorrhea and the amount of bleeding during menstruation.

Endometriosis

Endometriosis is the abnormal location of endometrial tissue outside the uterus. The tissue is known as *ectopic endometrial implants.* It is a common cause of dysmenorrhea, chronic pelvic pain, and infertility. The ectopic endometrial implants can be found affixed to the ovaries, the posterior surface of the uterus, the uterosacral ligaments, the broad ligaments, or the bowel. They also can be found on other organs within the pelvic or thoracic cavity. The ectopic endometrial implants respond to hormonal control, particularly estrogen, in the same way as the normal endometrial tissue located inside the uterus. Thus when menstruation occurs, the ectopic endometrial implants proliferate and then bleed. As the number of menstrual cycles increases, inflammation of

surrounding organ tissue, scar tissue formation, and adhesions result, causing pelvic pain.

Diagnosis of endometriosis is based on laparoscopic evidence of endometrial tissue, or implants, outside the uterus. The most common symptoms of endometriosis are dysmenorrhea and pelvic pain, sometimes including chronic pelvic pain, which lasts more than 6 months and is not associated specifically with menstruation. The patient may experience back pain; painful, sometimes bloody bowel movements; and dyspareunia (painful sexual intercourse). An increased number of women with endometriosis experience primary or secondary infertility; although a specific cause linking the two has not been established, it is theorized that the ectopic endometrial implants or the resultant scar tissue and adhesions obstruct or affect the motility of the fallopian tubes or other reproductive organs. Affected women have an increased risk for ectopic pregnancy.

Pharmacologic Management of Endometriosis

Pharmaceutic treatment strategies for endometriosis include drugs that decrease the amounts of circulating estrogen and limit or eliminate menstruation. This interrupts internal bleeding and irritation associated with the ectopic endometrial implants and may even cause them to recede.

Combined Hormonal Contraceptives. These drugs suppress gonadotropin-releasing hormone (GnRH) release, prevent ovulation, and cause atrophy of the uterine lining, actions thought to relieve pelvic pain by causing a regression of the endometrial implants. CHCs relieve the pain of endometriosis in approximately 75% of women. Extended-use CHCs can also manage endometriosis by causing fewer cycles per year or eliminating withdrawal menses altogether.

Progestin Therapy. These drugs suppress ovulation and cause long-term endometrial atrophy. They also inhibit GnRH release, similar to CHCs. Over time, progestins can shrink or eliminate endometrial implants. The most commonly used progestin is DMPA, with which 70% to 90% of patients experience relief of symptoms associated with endometriosis. This effect may last months after discontinuing the drug. Benefits and risks are the same as if using DMPA for contraception, so concerns for BMD loss and prevention, irregular bleeding or amenorrhea, possible weight gain, and mood changes should be discussed with the patient. The injection is given every 11 to 13 weeks.

Alternatively, norethindrone acetate may be taken at 5 mg PO daily for 2 weeks, then increasing the dose by 2.5 mg every 2 weeks until a dose of 15 mg per day is reached and continued for 6 to 9 months.

Gonadotropin-Releasing Hormone Agonists. For women who experience severe symptoms of infitility (endometriosis) and who NSAIDs, CHCs, or progestins do not help, GnRH agonists may be used. GnRH agonists are potent drugs that inhibit GnRH release and create a hypoestrogenic environment. The side effects are menopause-like and include hot flashes, atrophic vaginitis, vaginal dryness, decreased sex drive, and potential for bone loss. Leuprolide is administered either 3.75 mg IM monthly or 11.25 mg IM every 3 months. Leuprolide should be initiated in the first 3 days of the menstrual cycle because its use is contraindicated in pregnancy. Women may be able to become pregnant on leuprolide, so a barrier method of contraception should be used. The total duration of therapy should not exceed 6 months. Leuprolide can be used alone or in combination with norethindrone acetate.

Alternatively, nafarelin nasal spray is administered in a divided 400 mcg daily dose, with 1 spray (200 mcg) into one nostril in the morning and 1 spray (200 mcg) into the other nostril in the evening, starting between days 2 to 4 of menstrual cycle, for up to 6 months. Side effects of GnRH agonists include decreased bone density, ovarian cysts, and depression. Use cautiously in patients who experience these symptoms before treatment.

Elagolix is a new GnRH antagonist that was approved by the FDA in July 2018. The recommended dose is 150 mg once daily for max of 24 months used for the management of moderate to severe pain associated with endometriosis. Elagolix is contraindicated in pregnancy, known osteoporosis, and severe hepatic impairment. Adverse effects include irregular bleeding, decreased bone density, hepatic impairment, and depression.

Premenstrual Syndrome

Premenstrual syndrome (PMS) comprises a collection of cyclic physical symptoms and perimenopausal mood alterations. Symptoms increase in the 2 weeks before menstruation and subside after menses begins. These physical, emotional, and behavioral symptoms interfere to varying degrees with a woman's ability to function.

PMS can result in decreased work effectiveness and mood variations. PMS affects as many as 90% of all adult women, with less than 5% experiencing a more severe form of PMS, called premenstrual dysphoric disorder (PMDD) (http://www.women's health.gov). The hallmark of PMS and PMDD is that symptoms occur in a repetitive pattern during the luteal phase (days 15 to 28) of the menstrual cycle and decrease significantly in the early follicular phase (days 1 to 14).

There is no universal agreement about the definition, etiology, symptoms, or treatment of PMS. Researchers theorize that the etiology of PMS could be hormonal excess or deficits, fluid or sodium retention, or nutritional deficiencies. It is also proposed that an imbalance exists in the HPO axis function. Other hypotheses center on the neuroregulatory effects of estrogen and progesterone on the release or uptake of serotonin.

A patient can help with the diagnosis of PMS by recording three variables on a perimenstrual assessment calendar: (1) group of symptoms, (2) severity of symptoms, and (3) effect on function (degree of distress). Diagnosis of PMS can be made when the patient's symptoms consistently occur in a cyclic pattern at least 1 week before the menstruation cycle and decrease significantly after menses begins. Symptoms usually have a negative effect on the ability to function effectively. Other endocrine abnormalities must be ruled out. Also, it should be noted that not every symptom associated with the menstrual cycle is indicative of PMS.

Symptoms of Premenstrual Syndrome

Physical symptoms of PMS include breast soreness, constipation or diarrhea, bloating in lower abdomen, headache, backache, fatigue, acne flare-ups, and alterations in sleep patterns.

Emotional or mental symptoms of PMS include irritability or hostile behavior, appetite changes, trouble with concentration, anxiety, depression, mood swings, and decreased sexual desire.

Nonpharmacologic Treatment of Premenstrual Syndrome

Nonpharmacologic treatment modalities are very important in treating women with PMS. Therapies include expression of empathy, support from family and friends, exercise, and dietary changes. Aerobic exercise improves general health, increases endorphin levels, and may facilitate an overall sense of well-being. Dietary changes include limiting salty foods, alcohol, caffeine, and concentrated sweets. Eating four to six small, high-carbohydrate, low-fat meals may also help relieve some symptoms. Stress-reduction exercises are also helpful. These measures may help the patient feel proactive regarding her diagnosis of PMS.

Pharmacologic Treatment of Premenstrual Syndrome

Antidepressant Drugs. PMS is improved with selective serotonin reuptake inhibitors (SSRIs). Symptom relief includes a decrease in irritability, mood swings, fatigue, tension, and breast tenderness. SSRIs block the reuptake of serotonin into nerve terminals in the central nervous system (CNS), regulating serotonin use by the brain. The most commonly used SSRIs are fluoxetine and sertraline, paroxetine, citalopram, and escitalopram. Venlafaxine, a serotonin norepinephrine reuptake inhibitor (SNRI), has also demonstrated relief in patients with severe PMS symptoms but is not considered a first-line agent (see Chapter 23 for further information on antidepressants). SSRIs may be taken continuously, during the luteal phase only (drug is started on day 14 of the cycle and discontinued with menses), or as intermittent therapy beginning with symptom onset and discontinuing after the first few days of menses. Determining a treatment regimen depends on history and physical, patient preference, and predictability of symptoms.

Hormonal Therapy. Long-term suppression of ovulation has been shown to decrease cyclic physical discomforts and to normalize mood variations in some women. Combined hormonal contraception such as those containing the progestin DRSP along with a shorter (4-day) pill-free interval or transdermal and transvaginal HT can be used in this manner. Caution should be used with progestin-only products because they may exacerbate symptoms of depression.

DRUGS USED TO PROMOTE FERTILITY

Infertility is defined as the inability to conceive a child after 12 months of unprotected sexual intercourse. Women older than 35 years may be considered infertile after 6 months of attempting pregnancy. Infertility is considered *primary infertility* if a couple has never conceived or has never carried a pregnancy to term. *Secondary infertility* describes a couple who has conceived and brought a pregnancy to term but is unable to conceive afterward. Approximately 15% to 20% of couples in the United States experience infertility. Fertility rates decrease in both men and women as they get older; however, the risk for infertility increases more abruptly in women than in men as women reach the end of the reproductive life cycle. The monthly chance of achieving pregnancy decreases to 5% after 40 years of age.

Assessing the Infertile Couple

Causes of infertility are numerous. Infertility can be attributed to a female factor, a male factor, and, many times, a combination of both. (Male infertility is discussed in depth in Chapter 56.) In the female partner, the most common causes for infertility are alterations in ovarian function and anatomic disorders. Alterations in ovarian function are categorized as *ovulatory dysfunction disorders*. Any process, whether a disease state or the normal biologic process of aging, that causes anovulation or a decrease in ovulation cycles will affect the process of conception. Many of these women present with irregular menstrual periods. Causes of ovulatory dysfunction include alterations in the HPO axis, such as metabolic disorders (most commonly PCOS), and age approaching the end of the reproductive spectrum. Fertility declines sharply in women after 35 years of age, and infertility becomes a factor from 38 to 40 years of age. Endocrine disorders such as hyperprolactinemia (increase in circulating prolactin, the hormone that promotes breastfeeding) or thyroid disorders (hypothyroidism or hyperthyroidism) can also cause anovulatory cycles. Ovulation can be disrupted by eating disorders (anorexia and bulimia) and by stress.

The most common anatomic disorder is blocked fallopian tubes. Blocked tubes can be the result of a history of STI or PID. STIs, treated or undiagnosed, and PID can lead to scarring within the tubes, impeding sperm or ovum transport. A previous ectopic pregnancy or other tubal surgery can also result in infertility. Other causes include endometriosis, uterine leiomyomata (fibroids), or scarring within the uterine endometrium. (See Chapter 56 for male infertility discussion.)

Treatment of infertility depends on the cause. A general health assessment of the infertile couple includes (1) complete health history, including nutritional, reproductive, and social histories; drugs; herbal and illicit drug use; and gynecologic, menstrual, obstetric, and sexual histories as they pertain to each partner; (2) complete physical examinations with breast and pelvic examinations of the female partner and examination of male genitalia and function; (3) Pap testing, HPV testing, collections of cultures for STI testing; and (4) laboratory tests and other diagnostic tests. Semen evaluation is also necessary.

The leading cause of infertility in women is ovulatory dysfunction (most often, PCOS). The first line of pharmacologic treatment for ovulatory dysfunction is usually induction of ovulation by oral drug therapy.

Induction of Ovulation

Clomiphene citrate (CC) is a selective estrogen receptor modulator (SERM) that competes for estrogen receptors within the hypothalamus. With the binding of CC to the estrogen receptors, the hypothalamus receives a signal that circulating estrogen levels are low. This sets the hypothalamus in motion to secrete more GnRH, thus stimulating the HPO axis. The GnRH instructs the anterior pituitary gland to release FSH and LH to initiate a response from the ovarian follicles. Estrogen levels increase in response to FSH and LH, and a follicle becomes dominant, producing the level of estrogen needed for the LH surge. The

TABLE 55.2 Ovulatory Stimulants and Ovulation Control

Drug	Route and Dosage	Use and Considerations
Clomiphene citrate	See Prototype Drug Chart: Clomiphene Citrate	
Letrozole	Oral: 2.5 mg once daily for 5 days, starting on day 3, 4, or 5 following menses or progestin-induced bleed; may increase by 5 mg/day for max of 7.5 mg/day, studied in up to 5 cycles	Inhibits aromatase and may increase the release of FSH by blocking estradiol production. Androgens that would normally be converted to estrogens may accumulate in the ovaries, thereby increasing the sensitivity of ovarian follicles to FSH. Unlike clomiphene, it does not deplete estrogen receptors, which may be important for inducing mono-ovulation and also for preventing negative changes in the endometrium and cervical mucus. Contraindications: Hypersensitivity to letrozole or any component; pregnancy PB, plasma: Weak; t½: About 2 days
GnRH analogues Agonists: nafarelin Antagonists: cetrorelix, ganirelix	**Nafarelin:** Spray up to 400 mcg/d (200 mcg per nostril bid) **Cetrorelix:** 0.25 mg in a single dose subcut daily on stimulation day 5 or day 7 or 3 mg subcut in a single dose on stimulation day 7 (to control day of LH surge) **Ganirelix:** 250 mcg subcut once daily after initiating FSH, during mid to late follicular stage	Enhances ovulation stimulation for IVF cycles by suppression of a spontaneous LH surge and controls the fertility cycle, improving pregnancy outcomes. Contraindications: Hypersensitivity or previous severe reaction; latex allergies; rule out pregnancy before initiating treatment. Teach patient proper injection procedures and syringe disposal; ultrasound before initiating treatment to assess follicle size. Should only be prescribed by a fertility specialist. PB: 81.9%; Duration: less than 48 h; Absorption: rapid; t½: 12.8–16.2h Pregnancy Considerations: Contraindicated in pregnancy
Menotropins	Subcut: 250 units once daily beginning on cycle day 2 or 3; menotropins may be administered together with urofollitropin, and the total initial dose of both products combined should not exceed 225 units (menotropins 150 units and urofollitropin 75 units). Adjustments should not be made more frequently than once every 2 days and should not exceed 75–100 units per adjustment based on ultrasound monitoring of ovarian response and/or measurement of serum estradiol.	Possesses the same activities as FSH and LH; will induce ovulation in women with hypothalamic amenorrhea. Risks include ovarian hyperstimulation and multiple gestation Contraindications: hypersensitivity, tumors, abnormal uterine bleeding, history of ovarian cysts, pregnancy t½: 11–13 h following multiple doses; peak 18 h; excreted in urine Pregnancy Considerations: Contraindicated in women who are already pregnant
Recombinant FSH, follitropin alpha, recombinant LH, hCG, or recombinant hCG	Recombinant FSH: Subcut or IM injection; dosage individualized for each patient, usually 75–150 units/d, early follicular phase continuing for 10–14 d Recombinant LH: Subcut 75 units given along with an FSH or recombinant FSH Recombinant hCG: 250 mcg prefilled syringe; subcut injection given 1 d after last dose of gonadotropin (FSH and/or LH) 5000–10,000 units IM 1 d after last dose of gonadotropin (FSH and/or LH)	Recombinant FSH possesses the same hormonal activities as FSH. Ovarian hyperstimulation remains a risk, although minimal, with recombinant products. Multiple gestation is a risk, which is reduced by careful monitoring. Avoid use with herbal supplements that contain black or blue cohosh. PB: UK; t½: IM 23–77 h, subcut 13–35 h Pregnancy Considerations: Contraindicated in pregnancy

bid, Twice daily; *d*, day; *FSH*, follicle-stimulating hormone; *GnRH*, gonadotropin-releasing hormone; *h*, hour; *hCG*, human chorionic gonadotropin; *hMG*, human menopausal gonadotropin; *IM*, intramuscular; *IVF*, in vitro fertilization; *LH*, luteinizing hormone; *max*, maximum dosage; *PB*, protein binding; *subcut*, subcutaneously; *t½*, half-life; *UK*, unknown.

PROTOTYPE DRUG CHART

Clomiphene Citrate

Drug Class	Route and Dosage
Ovulation stimulant	A: PO: 50–100 mg/d; start with 50 mg for days 5–9 of the cycle
	If ovulation does not occur with 50 mg/d, increase the next course to 100 mg/d; *max:* 100 mg/d; maximum sequential cycles is three
	Under strict supervision by physicians specializing in infertility, as much as 200 mg/d may be used, but these high amounts greatly increase the risk for side effects

Contraindications	Drug-Lab-Food Interactions
Pregnancy, undiagnosed vaginal bleeding, depression, fibroids, hepatic dysfunction, thrombophlebitis, primary pituitary or ovarian failure	Drug: None are significant; danazol may inhibit response; drug decreases effects of ethinyl estradiol. Lab: Increases serum thyroxine

Pharmacokinetics	Pharmacodynamics
Absorption: Readily absorbed from GI tract	PO: Onset: 5–10 d
Distribution: PB: UK	Peak: 6 h
Metabolism: t½: 5–8 d	Duration: UK
Excretion: In feces	Pregnancy Considerations: Use is contraindicated in females who are already pregnant.

Therapeutic Effects/Uses
To stimulate ovarian follicle growth
Mechanism of Action: Stimulates release of follicle-stimulating hormone and luteinizing hormone.

Side Effects	Adverse Reactions
Breast discomfort, fatigue, dizziness, depression, anxiety, nausea, vomiting, constipation, increased appetite, headache, flatulence, multiple gestation, hot flashes, fluid retention	Visual disturbances, abdominal pain, weight gain, hair loss, ovarian hyperstimulation, anxiety, ovarian cysts, ectopic pregnancy

A, Adult; *d,* day; *GI,* gastrointestinal; *max,* maximum dosage; *PB,* protein binding; *PO,* by mouth; *t½,* half-life; *UK,* unknown.

LH surge causes release of an ovum from the dominant follicle. It is important for LH to reach a level high enough to produce an ovulatory cycle and that the timing of the LH surge be at the height of follicle formation, which is midcycle.

CC is the most commonly used ovulation stimulant. Women with PCOS may need concurrent treatment for hyperinsulinemia with metformin. Although metformin is known to help regulate the menstrual cycle and promote ovulation, it should not be used specifically for ovulation induction.

New studies have shown that letrozole has higher results in live birth rates when used to promote ovulation, but it is not approved by the FDA for this use; however, it has been recommended in several studies as a first-line therapy over clomiphene. Letrozole 2.5 mg once daily for 5 days, starting on day 3, 4, or 5 following menses or progestin-induced bleed; may increase to 5 mg/day for 5 days in subsequent cycles if ovulation does not occur. Dosing of up to 5 cycles is used.

In women with PCOS who have not responded to CC or other therapies, gonadotropin therapy may be an option. Menotropins may be used under the direction of an infertility prescriber to help stimulate follicle maturation and promote ovulation. Monitor for ovarian hyperstimulation syndrome (OHSS), a medical emergency presenting with acute abdominal pain and distension, nausea, vomiting, diarrhea, and weight gain, along with gross ovarian enlargement, ascites, dyspnea, oliguria, and pleural effusion. OHSS may result in death.

These therapies supply women with exogenous hormones to enhance the normal physiologic process of the menstrual cycle, promoting ovulation and increasing the probability of conception; the use of another gonadotropin, human chorionic gonadotropin (hCG), triggers ovulation when ovarian follicles are mature (as determined by ultrasonography). The corpus luteum provides for adequate levels of both estrogen and, more importantly, progesterone to maintain the uterine endometrium and a pregnancy, should one occur. These drugs are more potent than CC and have an increased risk for multiple births (up to 36%). Further details are listed in Table 55.2.

Pharmacokinetics. CC is readily absorbed from the GI tract. It is partially metabolized in the liver and is primarily excreted in the feces via biliary elimination. CC has a half-life of about 5 days.

Pharmacodynamics. The mechanism of action of CC is unknown, but it is hypothesized that it competes with estrogen at receptor sites. The perception of decreased circulating estrogen by the hypothalamus and pituitary gland triggers the negative feedback response that increases secretion of FSH and LH. The results are ovarian stimulation, maturation of the ovarian follicle, ovulation, and development of the corpus luteum.

Side Effects

Side effects of CC include breast discomfort, fatigue, dizziness, depression, nausea, increased appetite, dermatitis, urticaria, anxiety, weakness, heavier menses, vasomotor flushing, and abdominal bloating or pain. Antiestrogenic effects include interference with endometrial maturation and cervical mucus production. Paradoxically, this may interfere with fertilization or implantation.

◎ CLINICAL JUDGMENT [NURSING PROCESS]

Infertility

Concept: Hormonal Regulation

- Hormonal regulation involves substances working together to promote healthy development of female sex characteristics during puberty and adulthood to ensure or delay fertility.

Recognize Cues [Assessment]

- Assess the patient's general health history, including drug and herbal product use.
- Assess the patient's reproductive and sexual histories, include the following: history of abnormal Papanicolaou (Pap) testing and treatment; history of sexually transmitted infections (STIs) and treatment; past use of contraception methods; pelvic surgery; and pregnancy and birth history and complications.
- Assess the complete menstrual history, including menarche; last menstrual period (LMP); length, duration, and flow of bleeding; and any signs or symptoms related to the menstrual cycle.
- Assess sexual practices of the couple to include use of lubricants, timing, and technique of intercourse.
- Assess the couple's mental health status and refer to a support group or counseling as needed. Infertility can be isolating because many couples may have several peers who are pregnant or already have children.
- Instruct the couple about the diagnostic tests to evaluate the cause of infertility. Once this is determined, conditions that contraindicate the treatment of choice are ruled out.
- Discuss with the couple's their interpretation of infertility. Ascertain the effect on their relationship. The nurse should help the couple discuss their feelings in a safe, supportive environment.

Analyze Cues and Prioritize Hypothesis [Patient Problems]

- Discomfort
- Potential for nonadherence
- Decreased self-esteem
- Anxiety
- Need for patient teaching
- Reduced sexual expression
- Grieving
- Need for patient teaching

Generate Solutions [Planning]

- The patient will understand the normal physiologic process of conception.
- The patient will identify basic concepts that increase fertility.
- The patient will adhere to the medical regimen with minimal adverse effects physically, psychologically, emotionally, and spiritually.
- The patient will report adverse effects of treatment or pharmacologic therapy.
- The patient will recognize that the long-term goal is a successful pregnancy. If pregnancy cannot be achieved, the patient will be able to consider alternatives and make the transition with confidence, with the relationship and sense of self-worth intact.
- The patient will recognize that many treatment regimens for infertility must be repeated before successful conception is attained.

Take Action [Nursing Interventions]

General

- Initiate teaching to assist the patient and their partner in understanding the menstrual cycle; patterns and symptoms of ovulation; temperature changes with ovulation; specific physiologic signs of ovulation; use of ovulation predictor kits; and timing of sexual intercourse.
- Instruct the patient in the interrelationships among the menstrual cycle, ovulation, and coitus as they relate to conception.
- Advise the patient and their partner on the sexual techniques that enhance fertilization: placement of a pillow under the female's hips during coitus, and placement of the female in a supine position with the hips elevated for about 30 minutes after her partner ejaculates.
- Instruct the patient and their partner in the drug treatment regimens as prescribed by the provider. The patient and partner(s) will verbalize the treatment regimen and the expected outcomes of the treatment regimen.
- Facilitate the patient and their partner's psychological counseling and support.

Specific

- ⚡ Instruct the patient to report adverse effects such as abdominal pain or visual disturbances to the infertility specialist at once and to be cautious with tasks that require alertness. If a dose of the drug is missed, the patient should call the infertility specialist.
- Advise the patient that treatment increases the chance of multiple births.
- ⚡ Ensure that the patient understands the risks, benefits, and alternatives to pharmacologic therapy.

Patient Teaching

- Instruct the couple how to evaluate and record on a chart the female's basal body temperature and changes in the cervical mucus. The first day of menses is day 1 of the cycle. Ovulation is predicted by a 0.5°F drop in basal body temperature, followed by a 1°F rise. Over-the-counter (OTC) diagnostic kits for assessing ovulatory status can also be used to time coitus. The couple is advised to engage in coitus frequently from 4 days before to 3 days after ovulation.
- Advise the female partner to take the drug at the same time each day to maintain steady blood levels.
- Encourage the patient to verbalize concerns and express feelings about treatment successes and failures.

Evaluate Outcomes [Evaluation]

- Successful outcomes of fertility treatment include avoidance of ovarian hyperstimulation and other untoward effects. Pregnancy that results in the birth of a live infant fulfills the objectives of treatment. If pregnancy is not achieved, intervention is aimed at helping the couple consider alternatives to childbearing without any adverse effect on their self-esteem or harm to their relationship.

Adverse Reactions

Adverse reactions include bloating and stomach or pelvic pain, photophobia, diplopia, and decreased visual acuity. Patients may also experience hot flashes, breast discomfort, dizziness, headache, heavy menstrual periods, depression, nausea or vomiting, and fatigue. OHSS may occur.

Postmarket surveillance of CC has revealed the following fetal/neonatal abnormalities: delayed development, mental retardation, abnormal bone development, tissue malformation, abnormal organ development (including anencephaly), dwarfism, chromosomal disorders, and neural tube defects.

Contraindications

Contraindications for treatment with CC include undiagnosed vaginal bleeding, pregnancy, uterine fibroids, clinical depression, history of hepatic dysfunction or thromboembolic disease, and primary pituitary or ovarian failure. CC may cause existing ovarian cysts to enlarge. Contraindications to the use of other ovulatory stimulants are listed in Table 55.2.

Drug Interactions

There are no known significant drug interactions with CC. Danazol may inhibit patient response to CC, and CC may suppress response to EE. There are no known drug interactions with menotropins and HCG.

Other Drug Treatments

Endocrine disorders include hyperprolactinemia and thyroid disorders. In women with hyperprolactinemia, an elevated level of prolactin is the causative factor of infertility. Prolactin is a hormone secreted by the anterior pituitary gland and is elevated during pregnancy and postpartum to support milk production. Breastfeeding causes a natural rise in prolactin, and hyperprolactinemia can be seen in women who are or have recently discontinued breastfeeding.

Drug therapies such as haloperidol, metoclopramide, methyldopa, reserpine, and long-term CHC use have been known to cause hyperprolactinemia. The most common cause of pathologic hyperprolactinemia is a small, benign pituitary tumor called a *pituitary adenoma*. Regardless of the cause of hyperprolactinemia, most women can be treated with the ergot derivative bromocriptine, which binds to dopamine receptors in the pituitary gland and inhibits prolactin secretion. Treatment continues until pregnancy is confirmed. Clomiphene can be introduced if needed after 2 months.

MENOPAUSE

The transitional process experienced by women as they move from the reproductive years into the nonreproductive stage of life is called *menopause,* a naturally occurring event and part of the normal life cycle of women. It occurs for most women between their mid-40s and mid-50s but may start as early as the late 30s. Menopause has three stages: perimenopause or premenopause, menopause, and postmenopause, during which certain physiologic events occur. As women go through menopause, providers do not treat the cessation of menses but rather address the symptoms that may occur with the menopausal passage.

Perimenopause

The perimenopausal period includes the years before the natural cessation of spontaneous menstruation. During this period, menstrual variations become evident. Women may experience short cycles (<25 days), long cycles (>35 days), heavy bleeding, light bleeding, or periods of longer or shorter duration. Women may start to skip periods or abruptly stop menstruating altogether. Oligomenorrhea, very scant periods, and menorrhagia are common. Symptoms experienced during perimenopause are similar to those during menopause, with the exception that women in perimenopause continue to have some type of cyclic bleeding. The most common symptoms are hot flashes caused by a surge in LH levels and vaginal dryness caused by estrogen withdrawal. Other symptoms include insomnia, headaches, irritability or anxiety or other variations in mood, cognitive difficulties, memory lapses, joint aches, and decreased libido. These unpredictable changes may last a short period of time or they may last for several years.

There are a set number of follicles in the ovaries at birth. They are dormant throughout childhood and become active with puberty. Ovarian follicles are high in number during puberty and until 35 years of age, but the number of follicles steadily declines after 35 years of

age, and the decline is more rapid after 40 years of age. During the menstrual cycle, these follicles provide high levels of estrogen in the form of estradiol. The highest level of estradiol production in women occurs from puberty until the early 30s. Follicular growth, and therefore the secretion of estradiol, is under the influence of FSH and, to a lesser degree, LH, both of which are released by the anterior pituitary gland.

During the perimenopausal period, ovarian follicles become depleted, causing estrogen levels to diminish. The decrease in estrogen is gradual and allows for fluctuating levels of FSH and LH. Subsequently, menstrual cycles become anovulatory and therefore irregular. The onset of menstrual irregularity is one of the early indications of perimenopause. Symptoms are thought to be related to hormone fluctuations, particularly estrogen withdrawal, and increased levels of LH and FSH. Serum FSH testing is used as a marker of follicular activity, and an elevated level of FSH can be an indication of decreased ovarian function.

Menopause

Menopause is the permanent end of spontaneous menstruation caused by cessation of ovarian function. This natural event is documented as having occurred once a woman has stopped menstruating for 1 year. The triggering event is not known. Women who experience menopause before 40 years of age are said to have premature ovarian failure. Menopause can also occur abruptly as a secondary effect of oophorectomy (surgical removal of the ovaries), radiologic procedures in which ovarian function is destroyed, severe infection, or ovarian tumors or as a temporarily induced state for treatment of conditions such as endometriosis. During this transitional period, and with any episodes of menstrual changes or irregularities caused by perimenopause, women should use contraception until menstruation has ceased for 1 year if they do not want to become pregnant.

Postmenopause

Postmenopause is the stage when the body adapts to a new hormonal environment. The production of estrogen and progesterone from the ovaries decreases during the late premenopausal and early postmenopausal periods. The ovaries continue to secrete androgens (testosterone) in varying amounts as a result of the influence of increased LH levels. This surge in LH causes hot flashes: transient sensations of intense heat with or without sweating, tachycardia, and sleep disruption. During postmenopause, androstenedione—the main androgen secreted by the ovaries and adrenal cortex, which is present in reduced amounts after menopause—is converted into estrone, a naturally occurring estrogen formed in extraglandular tissues of the brain, liver, kidney, and adipose tissue. This represents the main source of available estrogen once the ovaries lose the ability to produce estradiol.

Hormone therapy (HT) significantly improves vasomotor symptoms and vaginal dryness, two frequently encountered symptoms of menopause. Vasomotor symptoms have the potential to disrupt sleep quality and to exacerbate irritability, mood swings, depression, and problems with concentration. The decrease in systemic estrogen seen in menopause can cause vaginal dryness, atrophic vaginitis, decreased libido, and negative effects on urinary health. Current guidelines do not support the use of HT for the prevention of cardiovascular disease, osteoporosis, or dementia.

The FDA has issued a boxed warning that states that HT should be used only for the treatment of menopausal symptoms, at the lowest dose possible, for the shortest duration possible, usually fewer than 5 years (Box 55.4). Most health care providers adhere to this practice when prescribing HT. Health teaching must be done with women in

⚡ PATIENT SAFETY

Do not confuse...

- **Combined hormonal contraceptive (CHC) products** with **HT products.** Oral, transdermal, and vaginal ring preparations for contraception and HT are dispensed in packages and boxes that are very similar. Once opened, CHC products and HT products may have the same disc-dispensing systems and splintered packaging and may have similar-appearing skin patches and vaginal rings.

BOX 55.4   FDA Boxed Warnings for Combined Hormonal Contraceptives (CHCs) and Hormone Therapy Products

CHCs: "Cigarette smoking increases the risk of serious cardiovascular side effects from oral contraceptive use. This risk increases with age and with heavy smoking (15 or more cigarettes per day) and is quite marked in women over 35 years of age. Women who use oral contraceptives should be strongly advised not to smoke."

Ethinyl estradiol and norelgestromin transdermal patch: "Do not use this transdermal patch if you smoke cigarettes and are over 35 years old. Smoking increases your risk of serious cardiovascular side effects (heart and blood vessel problems) from hormonal contraceptives, including death from heart attack, blood clots, or stroke. The risk increases with age and the number of cigarettes you smoke."

Ethinyl estradiol and etonogestrel transvaginal ring: "Cigarette smoking increases the risk of serious cardiovascular side effects from combination oral contraceptive use. This risk increases with age and with heavy smoking (15 or more cigarettes per day) and is quite marked in women over 35 years of age. Women who use combination hormonal contraceptives, including the transvaginal ring, should be strongly advised not to smoke."

Hormone replacement therapies with estrogen and estrogen plus progesterone: "Warning: Cardiovascular disorders, breast cancer, endometrial cancer and probable dementia [can occur]. … Estrogens, with or without progestins, should be prescribed at the lowest effective doses and for the shortest duration consistent with treatment goals and risks for the individual woman."

menopause to ensure that they are aware of the risks and benefits of hormone replacement therapy.

Pharmacologic Therapy for Perimenopausal and Menopausal Symptoms

Hormone Therapy

HT is used only for the relief of symptoms related to menopause, most commonly hot flashes, vaginal dryness, and associated sleep disorders. HT includes estrogen-progestin therapy (EPT) for use with women who have an intact uterus and ET for use with women who have had a hysterectomy, surgical removal of the uterus. It is the estrogen component in HT that relieves the symptoms of menopause. The progestin is added to protect the uterine endometrium from hyperplasia, an abnormal proliferation or overgrowth of tissue. When the uterus is exposed to unopposed estrogen—that is, estrogen without concurrent progestins—the

📄 PROTOTYPE DRUG CHART

Conjugated Estrogens

Drug	Route and Dosage
Estrogen replacement in menopause.	A: PO: 0.3 mg/d; give continuously, with no interruption in therapy, or cyclically Always use lowest effective dose; few patients require 1.25 mg/d PO or more Reevaluate the need for treatment q3–6mo

Contraindications	Drug-Lab-Food Interactions
Undiagnosed vaginal bleeding, pregnancy, lactation, severe liver disease, venous thrombosis, personal history of breast cancer *Caution:* Cardiovascular disease, severe renal disease, diabetes mellitus *Black Box Warning:* Absolute contraindications in myocardial infarction, new primary malignancy, stroke, thromboembolism, and dementia	Drug: Increased effects with corticosteroids; decreases effects of anticoagulants and oral hypoglycemics; decreased effects with rifampin, anticonvulsants, and barbiturates; toxicity with tricyclic antidepressants

Pharmacokinetics	Pharmacodynamics
Absorption: PO: Well absorbed Distribution: PB: Largely bound to sex hormone–binding globulin (SHBG) and albumin. Widely distributed; crosses placenta and enters breast milk Metabolism: t½: UK Excretion: In urine and bile	PO/IV: Onset: Rapid Peak: UK Duration: UK IM: Onset: Delayed

Therapeutic Effects/Uses	
For moderate to severe vasomotor symptoms of menopause and vaginal dryness/atrophy Mechanism of Action: Develops and maintains female genital system, breast, and secondary sex characteristics; increases synthesis of protein.	

Side Effects	Adverse Reactions
Nausea, vomiting, fluid retention, breast tenderness, leg cramps, breakthrough bleeding, chloasma	Jaundice, thromboembolic disorders, depression, hypercalcemia, gallbladder disease *Life-threatening:* Thromboembolism, CVA, PE, MI, endometrial cancer

A, Adult; *CVA,* cerebrovascular accident; *d,* day; *IM,* intramuscular; *IV,* intravenous; *MI,* myocardial infarction; *mo,* month; *PB,* protein binding; *PE,* pulmonary embolism; *PO,* by mouth; *t½,* half-life; *UK,* unknown.

endometrium becomes hyperplastic, potentiating the development of endometrial cancer. Estrogen alone can be used with women who have had a hysterectomy. With patients who still have their uterus, estrogen is taken together with the synthetic progestin. The progestin, however, has the potential to cause unpredictable uterine bleeding.

⚡ PATIENT SAFETY

Do not confuse...

- **Premarin** with **Prempro** or **Premphase:** Premarin is estrogen only for hormone replacement therapy. Both *Prempro* and *Premphase* have combined estrogen and progesterone for use by women with an intact uterus to prevent uterine hyperplasia when estrogen is used.

HT is available in oral preparations, transdermal applications, and vaginal preparations. Vaginal preparations are creams, suppositories, or rings. All vaginal preparations contain estrogen only and are very effective in treating vaginal dryness. FDA-approved estrogens used in HT are derived from natural sources and synthetic sources.

Conjugated equine estrogens (CEEs) are mixtures of natural estrogens isolated from the urine of pregnant mares (see Prototype Drug Chart: Conjugated Estrogens). Although CEEs are derived from nonhuman sources, they are naturally occurring estrogens. Synthetic estrogens include EE, which is the same estrogen found in CHC products.

Dosage Forms. The oral route is most commonly used because it is well tolerated by most patients and relatively easy to administer. It requires daily dosing. Some patients experience GI upsets, particularly nausea and vomiting. A patient with GI disorders such as colitis, IBS, peptic ulcer, or a malabsorption disorder may receive inconsistent doses with oral administration, necessitating the use of another route. Oral estrogens have a particularly beneficial effect on lipids by increasing high-density lipoproteins. Although the oral route does result in complete absorption from the GI tract, there is greater effect on liver proteins. In women with an intact uterus, oral estrogen is combined with a progesterone or progestin, completing the combined therapy. This can be given in a separate estrogen tablet combined with a separate progestin tablet (two oral pills taken daily) or in a combined estrogen-progestin tablet (one oral pill taken daily). Oral estrogens are typically used continuously. Common HT products include CEE, estradiol, synthetic conjugated estrogen, and esterified estrogen.

The transdermal skin patch is a convenient method to deliver HT because it does not require daily dosing. The patch is applied to intact skin in the prescribed dosage. Generally, the lower abdomen is used, but other sites may also be used. As with the transdermal patch used for contraception, the HT patch should not be placed on or near the breasts. The patch allows for absorption of the estrogen directly into the bloodstream through a membrane that limits the absorption rate. All types of transdermal patches, both estrogen-only and estrogen-progestin combination patches, contain plant-derived 17-β estradiol; many women prefer to take an estrogen derived from a plant source. The advantage is the same as the first-pass avoidance in CHC products using the transdermal route: the GI tract and liver are bypassed initially, which results in less nausea and vomiting and less effect on the hepatic system. Transdermal patches are changed twice a week or weekly, depending on the product, and they are used continuously. A progestin should be taken concurrently with the estrogen patch in women with an intact uterus.

HT is also available in topical gels, emulsions, and sprays; synthetic plant-based transdermal estradiol gels are applied once daily for the treatment of moderate to severe vasomotor symptoms. A thin film is applied to one arm from the shoulder to the wrist; the gel dries in 2 to 5 minutes. The dosage regimen is designed to deliver a specific amount of estradiol with each application.

With the topical HT products listed previously, a progestin should be taken concurrently in women who have an intact uterus. Medroxyprogesterone acetate (MPA) is the oral progestin most often administered in combination with estrogen. Other available products are norethindrone acetate and micronized progesterone. Combination products contain both estrogen and a progestin, which offers the added convenience of not having to take two pills daily. Combination products have the same adverse effects as estrogen-only and progestin-only HT.

Two combination transdermal products contain estrogen and progestin combinations to treat menopausal symptoms such as hot flashes. The transdermal patch allows for continuous delivery of hormones at much lower doses than in oral HT. This route avoids first-pass metabolism by the liver and may be better tolerated. Patients should be treated with the lowest effective dose and for the shortest duration consistent with treatment goals.

Vaginal cream preparations are used in the treatment of vaginal atrophy, which causes painful intercourse and urinary difficulties. There is estradiol cream and conjugated equine topical cream, which is an estrogen derivative. Both preparations are rapidly absorbed into the bloodstream via the mucous membranes that line the vagina. Vaginal creams may be used in conjunction with another method, such as tablets or the transdermal patch. However, vaginal creams do *not* need a progestin counter because they do not affect the uterine endometrium to the extent that oral and transdermal products will. Conjugated estrogen vaginal cream is usually delivered in a dose of 0.5 to 2 g/day intravaginally for 2 weeks; then the dosing is decreased to twice weekly for 3 weeks out of each month.

One estradiol vaginal ring is a low-dose estradiol-releasing ring containing 2 mg of estradiol per 90-day ring (7.5 mcg/24 hours). This ring is inserted into the upper portion of the vagina, where it releases the estradiol, providing a consistent low dose of estrogen for 3 months. It may be left in place during intercourse and during treatment for vaginal infections. It is used to treat local symptoms of urogenital atrophy.

Another estradiol vaginal ring consists of a low-dose estradiol-acetate releasing ring, made from silicone elastomer. This vaginal ring is available in two dosage strengths: 0.05 mg/day or 0.1 mg/day. This ring is inserted into the upper portion of the vagina, where it releases the estradiol, providing a consistent low dose of estrogen for 3 months. The lowest effective dose should be used. In women with an intact uterus, consideration should be given to adding progestin 10 to 14 days out of a 4-week menstrual cycle.

Vaginal estrogen tablets that contain estradiol can be inserted intravaginally once daily for 2 weeks. The dose is one 10-mcg tablet to be inserted once daily, and then the dose is decreased to one 10-mcg tablet twice weekly. Consideration should be given to adding progestin for 10 to 14 days out of a 4-week menstrual cycle if the woman's uterus is intact.

Contraindications. Contraindications to HT include pregnancy, history of endometrial cancer (when treatment for early endometrial cancer has been completed, it is no longer a contraindication to HT), personal history of breast cancer, history of thromboembolic disorders, acute liver disease or chronic impaired liver function, active gallbladder or pancreatic disease, coronary artery disease (CAD), undiagnosed vaginal bleeding, and endometriosis. Lifestyle factors such as smoking, known to enhance the risk of thromboembolism, should be considered in the treatment decision. The patient with a history of fibroid tumors is not started on HT for a full year after the last menstruation, because estrogen would likely result in tumor growth. The hypoestrogenic state associated with natural menopause usually causes existing fibroids to shrink. The presence of fibrocystic breast disease or diabetes may require extra caution.

Pharmacokinetics. CEEs are water soluble and well absorbed from the GI tract after tablet disintegration. Tablets are designed to release conjugated estrogens slowly over several hours. The estrogens are widely distributed in the body and circulate in the blood largely bound to sex hormone–binding globulin (SHBG) and albumin. Exogenous estrogens are metabolized in the liver, converted to metabolites, and excreted in the urine. Estrogens undergo enterohepatic recirculation.

Other Drugs for Perimenopausal/Menopausal Symptoms

Women who are not candidates for HT—more specifically, women with contraindications and breast cancer survivors—can be prescribed other drugs.

Selective Serotonin Reuptake Inhibitors and Serotonin Norepinephrine Reuptake Inhibitors. SSRIs and SNRIs reduce the number and severity of vasomotor symptoms in women. SSRIs also have the added benefit of reducing depression, which may relieve the irritability and mood changes associated with menopause. SSRIs and SNRIs can be gradually tapered in most postmenopausal women after 1 to 2 years of therapy.

Gabapentin. Gabapentin is an antiseizure drug that reduces the number and severity of nocturnal vasomotor symptoms in menopausal women. It should be administered in a single dose at bedtime. Gabapentin should be limited to those women who cannot take HT drugs and who have vasomotor symptoms that are affecting their quality of life. Gabapentin can cause drowsiness and should not be used concurrently with other drugs with similar precautions or if the patient's activities of daily living include those that would be affected or even dangerous if sleepiness, dizziness, or syncope should occur.

Clonidine. Clonidine, a drug used for hypertension, also reduces the number and severity of vasomotor symptoms in women. It is used for this purpose, though infrequently, due to its side effect profile, for women in whom HT is contraindicated. Blood pressure must be monitored at regular intervals, and the drug is discontinued if hypotension occurs.

Bremelanotide. Bremelanotide is an FDA-approved drug used for generalized hypoactive sexual disorders, or low sexual desire, experienced by perimenopausal women. Not recommended for use in postmenopause. It is an injectable melanocortin receptor agonist, and 1.75 mg is injected SC 45 minutes before sexual activity. It has a unique mechanism of action that helps activate the brain pathways involved in normal sexual responses. Bremelanotide transiently increases blood pressure and reduces heart rate after each dose; bremelanotide is contraindicated in patients with uncontrolled hypertension.

Osteoporosis

Osteoporosis is a progressive, debilitating skeletal disease that affects older men and women, with women older than 50 years being at greatest risk because the loss of estrogen during menopause is directly related to loss in BMD. Bone mass is at its highest density at 30 years of age and then steadily declines. Osteoporosis occurs through an imbalance of osteoblasts (bone-building cells) and osteoclasts (cells that break down bone), which causes bone reabsorption to accelerate. This imbalance causes both deterioration of the microstructure within the bone and a decrease in bone density. The loss of bone structure and "porous bone" fragility lead to an increased risk for fractures. Osteoporosis has significant morbidity and mortality in the United States. The most serious fracture site is the hip, and hip fracture is the second most common reason for older women to be placed in nursing homes, exceeded only by Alzheimer disease. Women who experience hip or vertebral fracture may have long-term, progressive, and debilitating health problems that can eventually lead to death. More than half of American women older than 50 years have some degree of osteopenia (low BMD) or osteoporosis (a severe decline in BMD).

Diagnosis of osteopenia and osteoporosis is made by axial skeletal measurements of bone density in the lumbar spine and hip through a dual-energy x-ray absorptiometry (DXA) scan. The World Health Organization (WHO) defines osteopenia and osteoporosis by translating the results of the DXA scan into a T score. Normal BMD is a T score of −1 or greater. Osteopenia is defined by a T score of −1 to −2.5, and osteoporosis is defined by a T score of −2.5 or less.

HT is no longer recommended for the *treatment* of osteoporosis; however, it may be considered as a *preventive* measure in postmenopausal women who are at risk, although not as first-line therapy. Women who have used HT for 5 years or more have been shown to have a 35% reduction in hip and vertebral fractures. Other drugs can manage osteoporosis and prevent fractures without the concerns raised by HT. These include bisphosphonates, which can reduce the breakdown of bone microstructure, and SERMs. SERMs are a new class of synthetic estrogens that act like estrogens in certain parts of the body, such as the bones, while leaving other parts unaffected. Contraindications to SERM therapy include past history of or risk for VTE and pregnancy. Caution is used in women with heart disease, risk of MI or stroke, and hepatic or renal insufficiency.

The side effects of oral bisphosphonates include nausea, abdominal or stomach pain, difficulty swallowing, esophageal inflammation, reflux, and ulcers. Injectable bisphosphonates do not have the GI side effects, and it can be easier for the patient to schedule a quarterly or yearly injection than to remember to take a daily or weekly pill. A rare complication of bisphosphonates is full or partial spontaneous femur fractures. Oral bisphosphonates should not be taken with aspirin, NSAIDs, or antacids. Contraindications to bisphosphonates include esophageal abnormalities or delayed emptying of the esophagus, inability to sit or stand for 30 minutes after oral ingestion, and hypocalcemia.

Nursing Interventions

Prevention of osteoporosis includes sufficient intake of calcium and vitamin D throughout the life span by either dietary intake or supplementation. The recommended daily requirement of calcium for women 19 to 50 years of age is 1000 mg/day, whereas women older than 50 years need 1200 mg/day. Calcium should be taken in divided doses and with adequate vitamin D to enhance absorption. The recommended daily allowance of vitamin D is 600 IU/day for women 19 to 70 years of age and 800 IU/day for women older than 70 years. All calcium preparations, with the exception of calcium citrate, should be taken with food. Smoking cessation should be encouraged because smoking interferes with vitamin D absorption. Alcohol consumption should be limited to one drink per day because alcohol reduces GI absorption of calcium. Weight-bearing exercise includes walking, jogging, low-impact aerobics, weight training, and yoga; these strengthen the bones, increase muscle strength, and enhance balance. Caution should be used in patients who are prescribed drugs that cause hypotension or dizziness. The patient should be assessed for fall risk, and the prevention of falls should be part of the nurse's health care teaching.

Drugs

Alendronate is a bisphosphonate used to treat osteopenia and osteoporosis. It is available in a daily or weekly dose. For prevention of osteoporosis, the oral weekly dose is 35 mg. For treatment, the oral weekly dose is 70 mg. Alendronate must be taken with 8 ounces of water 30 minutes before ingesting any food, liquids, or drug, and the patient must remain upright for 30 minutes. Once-a-week dosing has made this a first-line therapy. Common side effects include abdominal pain and acid reflux. Alendronate is also available with added vitamin D for enhanced absorption of calcium.

Ibandronate is a once-a-month bisphosphonate indicated for the treatment and prevention of osteoporosis in postmenopausal women. It comes in both oral and intravenous (IV) formulations. The oral dose has the same directions for use and side effects as the other bisphosphonates. Ibandronate can be administered as 150-mg once-monthly tablets or 3 mg every 3 months administered IV over 15 to 30 seconds.

Risedronate is also available in a daily or weekly dose. It has similar directions for use and side effects similar to the bisphosphonates. The dosing schedule is a 5-mg tablet once daily or a 35-mg tablet once weekly and should be taken immediately after breakfast with at least 4 ounces of water.

Zoledronic acid is a bisphosphonate that is administered IV in a 5-mg dose yearly for the treatment of osteoporosis; the dose should be administered over 15 minutes. Zoledronic acid can be given in a 5-mg dose every 2 years for prevention of osteoporosis.

Kidney failure is a rare but serious condition that may be associated with the use of bisphosphonates in patients with underlying renal disease or renal impairment. These drugs should not be used in patients with chronic kidney disease (CKD) and a glomerular filtration rate (GFR) lower than 30 to 35 mL/min.

Nurses should teach patients to advise their health care provider of any increased thigh or groin pain, which can be symptoms of rare, atypical femur fractures.

Studies suggest that some patients may be able to discontinue the use of these drugs after 3 to 5 years and still benefit from using bisphonates. It is recommended that the bone density test of the hip and spine be repeated after 2 years. Health care providers should reassess patients on an individual basis every 5 years to determine whether continued therapy is beneficial. It has been determined that bisphosphonates do work to improve osteoporosis; however, the time frame for safe use of these drugs needs to be investigated. Research is ongoing to determine whether the use of bisphosphonates increases the risk for esophageal cancer, which is extremely rare in women.

Raloxifene is an SERM that increases BMD, decreases bone turnover, and reduces vertebral fractures. A secondary analysis of osteoporotic women treated with raloxifene showed a decrease in the risk for breast cancer. Side effects include hot flashes and increased risk for deep venous thrombosis (DVT). Raloxifene is taken orally once a day in a 60-mg tablet. Patients need to take calcium and vitamin D to prevent or treat hypocalcemia while taking this drug.

Teriparatide is a parathyroid hormone used for treatment of postmenopausal osteoporosis, and it is administered 20 mcg subcutaneously on a daily basis for 2 years. It can be used by both men and women who have had a fracture related to osteoporosis or who have multiple risk factors for fracture and cannot use other osteoporosis treatments. The patient can be taught self-administration.

Calcitonin-salmon is composed of calcitonin, a naturally occurring hormone that regulates calcium in the body and promotes bone metabolism. It is administered 100 units subcutaneously or IM every day to every other day. Another delivery option is via intranasal spray in a 200-IU dose administered daily.

Denosumab is a monoclonal antibody and bone-modifying agent used in women who are at a high risk for osteoporotic fracture, who have had a fracture, or who have not had improvement in T score after using the bisphosphonates for osteoporosis. A 60-mg dose is given subcutaneously every 6 months. Patients need to take calcium and vitamin D to prevent or treat hypocalcemia while taking this drug.

Romosozumab is a parenteral humanized IgG2 monoclonal antibody and sclerostin inhibitor for the treatment of osteoporosis in postmenopausal women at high risk for fracture and for those who have failed or could not tolerate other osteoporosis therapy. It is administered in 2 subcutaneous consecutive injections (105 mg each) for a total dose of 210 mg once monthly for 12 months. It is recommended to initiate bisphosphonate or denosumab therapy to maintain bone mineral density gains following the 12 months. It is contraindicated in patients with myocardial infarction or stroke.

◎ CLINICAL JUDGMENT [NURSING PROCESS]

Management of Symptomatic Menopausal Women

Concept: Hormonal Regulation

- Hormonal regulation involves substances normally present in the body to promote fertility in adulthood that decrease during the aging process and can cause many symptoms and complications if not regulated.

Recognize Cues [Assessment]

- Obtain a history of patient's drug and supplement intake.
- Obtain baseline vital signs that include temperature, pulse, respirations, blood pressure (BP), and weight and height. Report abnormal findings.
- Obtain a family history to assess for risk factors regarding osteoporosis and osteoporotic fractures; cardiovascular risks, including coronary artery disease, ischemic and hemorrhagic stroke, and venous thromboembolism (VTE); cognitive disorders; and cancers that affect women.
- Obtain a history of allergies to drugs, foods, and supplements.
- Obtain a medical-surgical history, asking about present or past hypertension; falls and fractures; cardiovascular disease; cerebral vascular disorders; hepatic, renal, and urinary tract disorders and infections; gastrointestinal (GI) problems; neurologic disorders; and past systemic infections. Assess for past and present history of cancer. Ask about previous surgeries, in particular gynecologic or pelvic surgery.
- Assess for smoking, alcohol, and illicit drug use. Assess risk for falls and fractures, self-care concerns, and ability to take drugs.

- Obtain a complete menstrual history including age at menarche and age at menopause. If the patient is perimenopausal, assess menstrual pattern; cycle length, duration, and amount of bleeding; first day of last menstrual period (LMP); and method used for contraception. If the patient is in menopause, assess past and present menopausal symptoms along with their effects on quality of life. Assess for any incidence of postmenopausal bleeding.
- Obtain a full gynecologic history, including the last Papanicolaou (Pap) testing results, history of abnormal Pap testing and colposcopy, and gynecologic problems, disorders, and surgeries.
- Obtain a complete sexual history, including sexual expression and sexual risk practices, menopausal symptoms and effects on sexual expression, and past or present sexual abuse and/or assault.
- Assess the patient's perception of menopause and knowledge of nonpharmacologic and pharmacologic hormone therapies.

Analyze Cues and Prioritize Hypothesis [Patient Problems]

- Discomfort
- Confusion
- Potential for injury
- Anxiety
- Need for patient teaching

Continued

⊚ CLINICAL JUDGMENT [NURSING PROCESS]—CONT'D

Management of Symptomatic Menopausal Women

Generate Solutions [Planning]

- The patient's risks and benefits associated with hormone therapy (HT) will be evaluated on an individual basis.
- The patient will verbalize menopausal symptoms and will understand nonpharmacologic and pharmacologic measures that may aid in alleviating symptoms.
- The patient will choose the route of administration that is best suited for their lifestyle and will increase safety and effective use of the product.
- The patient will report side effects that occur to the health care provider (HCP).
- The patient will self-administer their prescribed medication: oral, transdermal, topical, or vaginal drugs.
- The patient will place the patch as directed and will report any adverse side effects that occur.
- The patient will be comfortable with vaginal placement of drugs.
- The patient will report abnormal uterine bleeding (AUB) and other side effects associated with HT.
- The patient will verbalize the dosing schedule, risks, benefits, and alternatives of their treatment.
- The patient will schedule follow-up appointments as needed.

Take Action [Nursing Interventions]

- ⚡ Instruct the patient about the nature of menopause, its potential effects, and the benefits, risks, and alternatives of both nonpharmacologic and pharmacologic treatment modalities.
- Determine the patient's misconceptions about HT and provide factual, research-based information.
- Assist the patient in using the BRAIDED method for HT therapy.
- Instruct the patient in the effective use of HT.
- Supply various health community sites with educational materials concerning HT.

Patient Teaching

General

- ⚡ Review with the patient the risks, benefits, and alternatives for use of HT.
- Review with the patient contraindications to HT.
- Advise the patient to have breast and pelvic examinations and a Pap test before starting HT.
- Instruct the patient that warm weather and stress exacerbate hot flashes.
- Advise the patient to use a fan, drink cool liquids, and decrease intake of caffeine and spicy foods.
- ⚡ Instruct the patient on HT therapy to have a medical follow-up every 6 to 12 months, including a BP check, a clinical breast examination, and a pelvic examination.
- Instruct the patient in the need to use a method of contraception until 1 year after cessation of spontaneous menstruation.

- Suggest to patient the use of a water-soluble vaginal lubricant to reduce painful intercourse (dyspareunia) and prevent trauma.
- Advise the patient to decrease use of antihistamines and decongestants if experiencing vaginal dryness.
- Advise the patient to wear cotton underwear and pantyhose with a cotton liner, and to avoid douches and feminine hygiene products.
- Suggest the patient take HT oral drugs after meals to avoid nausea and vomiting.
- Advise the patient that some vaginal bleeding may be expected and that it should stop 3 to 6 months after starting HT.
- Instruct the patient to carry sanitary pads or tampons for breakthrough bleeding (BTB) or irregular menstruation.
- Advise the patient to report any heavy bleeding or irregular bleeding patterns and to have their hematocrit and hemoglobin levels evaluated.
- Advise the patient that after HT is discontinued, there may be a recurrence of menopausal signs and symptoms such as hot flashes.
- Instruct the patient wanting to stop HT that it should be done with guidance by the health care provider.

Self-Administration

- Instruct the patient about breast health and regular breast self-examination.
- Advise the patient to list on their calendar regular Pap screening due dates.
- Instruct the patient in the application of vaginal cream and suggest the use of minipads.
- Instruct the patient in the application of the transdermal patch, such as checking the edges to ensure adequate contact to the skin; always placing the patch on the abdomen (except the waistline); rotating sites with at least 1 week before reuse of a site; never to use the breast area as a site; never to put the patch on an irritated or oily skin; and never to reapply the patch if it loosens.
- Advise the patient about appropriate use of gels, sprays, and mists.

Balanced Diet and Exercise

- Instruct the patient about osteoporosis prevention and encourage (1) with the HCP's clearance both a walking and weight-bearing exercise program; (2) a well-balanced diet high in fiber, vegetables, fruits, whole grains, and plant proteins and low in animal proteins and sugar; (3) supplementation with 1000 mg/day of calcium (if <50 years of age) or 1200 mg/day (if >50 years of age) and vitamin D 600 IU/day if <70 years of age; (4) smoking cessation and reduced alcohol consumption.

Evaluate Outcomes [Evaluation]

- Evaluate the effectiveness of nonpharmacologic or pharmacologic measures for premenopausal symptoms.
- Determine whether side effects occur. Plan alternative measures to control menopausal symptoms with the patient.
- Plan follow-up appointments and health care screenings.

CRITICAL THINKING UNFOLDING CASE STUDY

Objective: Apply knowledge of women's reproductive health as it relates to menopause.

A 52-year-old woman presents to the health clinic for an early morning appointment to see the healthcare provider for a check-up. She is complaining of fatigue and decreased libido. The provider obtains baseline vital signs, including temperature, pulse, respirations, blood pressure, weight, and height. Her history includes three live births and no miscarriages. Patient has no known allergies. The only reported medication is a multivitamin taken by mouth every morning.

Question 1

Cognitive Skill: Recognize cues [enhanced hot spot]

The nurse documents the following assessment findings:

- Blood pressure 118/78 mm Hg, heart rate 72 bpm
- Complains of intense feelings of heat
- Temperature of 98.6°F, respirations 20 breaths per minute
- Complains of nighttime sweating
- No history of abnormal Pap smears
- Reports no menstrual cycle in a year

CRITICAL THINKING UNFOLDING CASE STUDY—CONT'D

- Reports vaginal dryness and painful intercourse
- Routine postmenopausal pregnancy test negative
- Patient is 5.0 ft in height and weighs 240 lb.

Highlight or place a checkmark next to the assessment findings that require follow up by the nurse.

Answers:
- Blood pressure 118/78 mm Hg, heart rate 72 bpm
- Complains of intense feelings of heat
- Temperature of 98.6°F, respirations 20 breaths per minute
- Complains of nighttime sweating
- No history of abnormal Pap smears
- Reports no menstrual cycle in a year
- Reports vaginal dryness and painful intercourse
- Routine postmenopausal pregnancy test negative
- Patient is 5.0 ft in height and weighs 240 lb.

Rationale
Symptoms of menopause are the same as those of perimenopause. The only difference is that with menopause there is no menstrual period. Menopause is caused by a change in the balance of the sex hormones, which occurs with age. The most common symptoms are hot flashes, feelings of heat, nighttime sweating resulting from a surge in luteinizing hormone (LH) levels, and vaginal dryness caused by estrogen withdrawal. Other symptoms include insomnia; headaches; irritability, anxiety, or other variations in mood; cognitive difficulties; memory lapses; joint aches; and decreased libido. Patient's blood pressure, temperature, and respirations are within normal ranges. The patient does not have a history of abnormal Pap smears, which indicates no pre-diagnostic problems. The postmenopausal pregnancy test is negative, which rules out pregnancy as she has not had a menstrual cycle in a year.

Reference
Chapter 55 Women's Reproductive Health, pages 703–708 (Menopause/Perimenopause). Lewis, et al, *Medical Surgical Nursing*, 10th ed, Ch 53 pgs. 1242–1267.

Question 2
Cognitive Skill: Analyze cues [cloze]

The nurse documents the following assessment findings:
- Blood pressure 118/78 mm Hg, heart rate 72 bpm
- Complains of intense feelings of heat
- Temperature of 98.6°F, respirations 20 breaths per minute
- Complains of nighttime sweating
- No history of abnormal Pap smears
- Reports no menstrual cycle in a year
- Reports vaginal dryness and painful intercourse
- Routine postmenopausal pregnancy test negative
- Patient is 5.0 ft in height and weighs 240 lb.

Choose the most likely options for the information missing from the statements below by selecting from the lists of options provided.

Based on the patient's assessment data, the provider determines that the patient's diagnosis _____(1)_____. The provider explains that possible hormonal irregularity can cause _____(2)_____, _____(2)_____, and _____(2)_____. Due to the patient's height and weight, which indicate a BMI of obesity, the provider instructs the patient to _____(3)_____ and _____(3)_____.

OPTION 1	OPTION 2	OPTION 3
Pregnancy	Vaginal dryness	Make sensible diet choices
Menopause	Increased libido	Incorporate a diet high in fat

OPTION 1	OPTION 2	OPTION 3
Infertility	Decreased libido	Decrease fluid intake
Endometriosis	Feelings of cold hands and feet	Institute a walking program
Amenorrhea	Feelings of heat with nighttime sweating	Drink 3 carbonated sodas a day
Urinary tract infection	Hypotension and dizziness	Decrease daily activity

Answers
Based on the patient's assessment data, the provider determines that the patient's diagnosis is menopause. The provider explains that possible hormonal irregularity can cause vaginal dryness, decreased libido, and feelings of heat with nighttime sweating. Due to the patient's height and weight, which indicate a BMI of obesity, the provider instructs the patient to make sensible diet choices and institute a daily walking program.

Rationale
Menopause happens when the ovaries stop producing the hormone estrogen and no longer release an egg each month. Amenorrhea and infertility are symptoms of menopause. During menopause, pregnancy is rare. Endometriosis affects the menstrual cycle, and a small percentage of women do experience endometriosis in the postmenopausal phase, but not this patient. Urinary tract infections are a symptom of menopause; as vaginal tissue thins, women are more prone to infection. Due to the lack of estrogen, common symptoms are nighttime sweating, vaginal dryness, and decreased libido, which are caused by a surge in lutenizing hormone (LH) levels.

Increased libido and feelings of cold hands and feet are not associated with menopause. In menopause, a patient usually will not experience hypotension and dizziness. There is usually weight gain and a sensitivity to salt intake, which may cause hypertension. Due to the patient's height of 5.0 ft and weight of 240 lb., the patient has a BMI of 46.9. A BMI >30 suggests obesity, which is why the provider encourages sensible diet choices and instituting a walking program. A high-fat diet, decreased fluid intake, and decreased daily activity are not helpful advice for this overweight patient.

Reference
Chapter 55 Women's Reproductive Health, pages 703–708 (Menopause/Perimenopause). Lewis, et al, *Medical Surgical Nursing*, 10th ed, CH 53 pgs. 1242–1267.

Question 3
Cognitive Skill: Prioritize hypotheses [extended multiple response]

Due to the patient's symptoms, the provider prescribes medications to help with the symptoms of menopause. Also, the provider plans to order additional testing for this patient.

Choose which medications and priority testing are most important for this patient. Select all that apply.

_____ a. Levothyroxine therapy
_____ b. Magnetic resonance imaging of chest (MRI)
_____ c. Oral estrogen 0.3 mg/day
_____ d. Oral progesterone 200 mg/day
_____ e. Combined hormonal contraceptive
_____ f. Mammogram testing
_____ g. DEXA bone density scan

Answers
_____ a. Levothyroxine therapy
_____ b. Magnetic resonance imaging of chest (MRI)
__X__ c. Oral estrogen 0.3 mg/day
__X__ d. Oral progesterone 200 mg/day

Continued

CRITICAL THINKING UNFOLDING CASE STUDY—CONT'D

_____ e. Combined hormonal contraceptive

__X__ f. Mammogram testing

__X__ g. DEXA bone density scan

Rationale

Estrogen is used for the relief of symptoms related to menopause, most commonly hot flashes, vaginal dryness, and associated sleep disorders. Progesterone is used for the prevention of endometrial hyperplasia associated with estrogen replacement therapy in postmenopausal women who have an intact uterus. Progesterone 200 mg PO is given as a single dose in the evening for 12 sequential days of every 28-day cycle of daily estrogen therapy. Women older than 50 years are at greatest risk for bone loss due to the loss of estrogen during menopause and should receive a DEXA scan/bone density test. Women over 50 years should have a mammogram and a bone density test every 1 to 2 years. Levothyroxine therapy is used to treat hypothyroidism. Patient's workup and complaints do not indicate the need for an MRI of chest. Patient is in menopause and does not require combined hormonal contraceptive.

Reference

Chapter 55 Women's Reproductive Health, pages 703–708, pg. 707, pg. 705 Osteoporosis. Lewis, et al, _Medical Surgical Nursing_, 10th ed, CH 53 pgs. 1242–1267.

Question 4

Cognitive Skill: Generate solutions [matrix]

The provider instructs the patient about hormonal therapy (HT).

Use an X for the health teachings listed below that are Indicated (appropriate or necessary) or Contraindicated (could be harmful) for the client's care at this time.

Health Teaching	Indicated	Contraindicated
Take HT after meals to avoid nausea and vomiting.		
You can stay on HT therapy forever.		
Decrease use of antihistamines if experiencing vaginal dryness.		
Must have medical follow-up every 6–12 months while on HT therapy.		
If you experience any vaginal bleeding, notify your provider.		
To help decrease hot flashes, use a fan, drink cool liquids, and decrease intake of caffeine and spicy foods.		

Answers

Health Teaching	Indicated	Contraindicated
Take HT after meals to avoid nausea and vomiting.	X	
You can stay on HT forever.		X
Decrease use of antihistamines if experiencing vaginal dryness.	X	
Must have medical follow-up every 6–12 months while on HT therapy.	X	
If you experience any vaginal bleeding, notify your provider.	X	

Health Teaching	Indicated	Contraindicated
To help decrease hot flashes, use a fan, drink cool liquids, and decrease intake of caffeine and spicy foods.	X	

Rationale

The following are indications for a patient taking hormonal therapy: Since conjugated estrogen may cause nausea and vomiting, it is suggested to take HT after meals. The FDA has issued a boxed warning that HT should only be used in the treatment of menopausal symptoms, at the lowest dose possible, for the shortest duration possible. It is contraindicated for a patient to remain on HT and it is recommended for use for less than a 5-year period of time. Patients must have follow up appointments every 6 to 12 months, including blood pressure checks with their provider. The use of antihistamines can have a drying effect inside the body, especially during menopause. This can result in vaginal dryness. Vaginal bleeding can be a serious sign of inflammation caused by low estrogen levels. Notify the provider at the first sign of vaginal bleeding. Spicy foods and caffeine narrow blood vessels, which precipitates in a hot flash. A common remedy is to use a fan or drink a cool (nonalcoholic, caffeine-free) drink, which will cause the hot feeling to subside.

Reference

Chapter 55 Women's Reproductive Health, pgs 703–705; Clinical Judgment [Nursing Process} care plan, pg 707 for Management of Symptomatic Menopausal Women. Lewis, et al, _Medical Surgical Nursing_, 10th ed, Ch 53 pgs 1242–1267.

Question 5

Cognitive Skill: Take action [Extended drag and drop]

Due to the patient's symptoms, the provider prescribes medications to help with the symptoms of menopause. Also, the provider plans to order additional testing for this patient.

After a month, the patient returns to the health clinic to receive the results of her DEXA scan/bone density and mammogram. The provider tells the patient that the mammogram is clear from cancer but the bone density test indicates osteopenia.

Indicate which provider response listed in the far-left column is appropriate for each question. Note that all responses will be used.

Provider's Response	Patient Questions	Appropriate Provider's Response to Patient Questions
1. You must increase your calcium intake.	What do I need to do to increase my calcium intake?	
2. You must increase your daily intake of vitamin D.	Can you explain how much vitamin D I should take daily?	
3. Do you understand why you must take vitamin D?	Explain to me why vitamin D is necessary.	
4. It is important to incorporate walking and weight-bearing exercises into your exercise routine.	What is weight-bearing exercise?	
5. The provider states, "I will order a new medicine called alendronate 35 mg per day."	Can you tell me more about this medication?	

CRITICAL THINKING UNFOLDING CASE STUDY—CONT'D

Provider's Response	Patient Questions	Appropriate Provider's Response to Patient Questions
6. It prevents osteoporosis. You must take it with 8 oz of water 30 min before ingesting any food, liquid, or drugs. Also, you must remain upright for 30 min after taking this drug.		
7. Walking, weight training, swimming, and yoga are weight-bearing and help to strengthen bones.		
8. Vitamin D helps with the absorption of calcium.		
9. The recommended intake of calcium for women over 50 years of age is 1200 mg/day.		
10. The recommended daily allowance of vitamin D is 600 IU/day for women your age.		

Answers

Provider's Response	Patient Questions	Appropriate Provider's Response to Patient Questions
1. You must increase your calcium intake.	What do I need to do to increase my calcium intake?	9. The recommended intake of calcium for women over 50 years of age is 1200 mg/day.
2. You must increase your daily intake of vitamin D.	Can you explain how much vitamin D I should take daily?	10. The recommended daily allowance of vitamin D is 600 IU/day for women your age.
3. Do you understand why you must take vitamin D?	Explain to me why vitamin D is necessary.	8. Vitamin D helps with the absorption of calcium.
4. It is important to incorporate walking and weight-bearing exercises into your exercise routine.	What is weight-bearing exercise?	7. Walking, weight training, swimming, and yoga are weight-bearing and help to strengthen bones.
5. The provider states, "I will order a new medicine called alendronate 35 mg per day."	Can you tell me more about this medication?	6. It prevents osteoporosis. You must take it with 8 oz of water 30 min before ingesting any food, liquid, or drugs. Also, you must remain upright for 30 min after taking this drug.

Rationale

Prevention and treatment of osteoporosis/osteopenia include sufficient intake of calcium and vitamin D. The recommended requirement of calcium for women 50 years or older is 1200 mg/d. The recommended daily allowance for vitamin D is 600 IU/d for women ages 19 to 70 years. Weight-bearing exercises include walking, jogging, low-impact aerobics, weight training, and yoga. These strengthen the bones, increase muscle strength, and enhance balance. Alendronate is a bisphosphonate used to treat osteopenia and osteoporosis. It must be taken with 8 oz of water 30 min before ingesting any food, liquids, or drugs, and the patient must remain upright for 30 min.

Reference

Chapter 55 Women's Reproductive Health, pages 703–708, Management of Symptomatic Menopausal Women, pg. 707, pg. 705, Osteoporosis. Lewis, et al, *Medical Surgical Nursing*, 10th ed, Ch 53 pgs 1242–1267.

Question 6

Cognitive Skill: Evaluate outcomes [matrix]

After a month, the patient returns to the health clinic to receive the results of her DEXA scan/bone density and mammogram. The provider tells the patient that the mammogram is clear from cancer, but the bone density test indicates osteopenia.

The provider assesses the patient for understanding and compliance. For each assessment finding, use an X to indicate whether teaching was effective (helped to meet expected outcomes) or ineffective (did not meet expected outcomes).

Assessment Findings	Effective	Ineffective
Patient reports feeling an increase in energy.		
Patient shows a 20-lb weight loss since initial visit.		
Patient indicates satisfactory libido.		
Patient reports still experiencing some vaginal dryness.		
Patient indicates improvements of hot flashes.		

Answers

Assessment Findings	Effective	Ineffective
Patient reports feeling an increase in energy.	X	
Patient shows a 20-lb weight loss since initial visit.	X	
Patient reports still experiencing some vaginal dryness.		X
Patient reports satisfactory libido.	X	
Patient indicates improvements of hot flashes.	X	

Rationale

HT significantly improves vasomotor symptoms including hot flashes, decreased libido, and vaginal dryness. The patient has achieved success except for vaginal dryness. The provider will order an over-the-counter topical to help with the vaginal dryness. Menopausal symptoms disrupt sleep, exacerbate irritability, and increase mood swings. The patient reports feeling more energy since these symptoms have improved and has added exercise to her daily routine, which has benefited her with a weight loss of 20 lb.

Reference

Chapter 55 Women's Reproductive Health; Menopause pgs. 702–709 and Clinical Judgment [Nursing Process] Care plan on pg 707. Lewis, et al, *Medical Surgical Nursing*, 10th ed, Ch 53, pgs 1242–1267.

REVIEW QUESTIONS

1. The nurse is preparing a teaching plan for combined hormonal contraceptive use. Which information should the nurse include in the teaching plan? (Select all that apply.)
   a. The patient should report abdominal pain, chest pain, headaches, blurred vision and visual disturbances, and severe leg pain.
   b. Combined hormonal contraceptives are safe for smokers older than 35 years who smoke fewer than 20 cigarettes per day.
   c. Combined hormonal contraceptive use will not protect patients from sexually transmitted infections.
   d. The pills can be missed but not for more than 12 hours.
   e. Vaginal spotting after starting combined hormonal contraceptives is a sign that the method is not effective in preventing pregnancy.

2. A 54-year-old menopausal patient comes into the gynecology office and is interested in hormone therapy. Which are indications for prescribing hormone therapy? (Select all that apply.)
   a. Assists in relief of hot flashes
   b. Prevention of breast cancer
   c. Prevention of cardiovascular disease
   d. Prevention of osteoporosis in at-risk patients
   e. Assists in relief of vaginal dryness

3. A 24-year-old patient tells the nurse that she would like to use the progestin-only pill for contraception. Nursing evaluation of this patient as a candidate for the progestin-only pill includes what?
   a. Ask the patient if she has given birth in the past
   b. Assess whether or not the patient has regular periods
   c. Assessing patient reliability in taking an oral pill daily
   d. Interviewing the patient about past smoking habits

4. A 39-year-old patient who smokes one pack of cigarettes (20) per day asks about a contraception method that is best for her. She is normotensive and has used combined hormonal contraceptives in the past. She is in a monogamous relationship and has had two children with no complications during pregnancy. She is not planning any more pregnancies. The nurse determines that which method would be best for this patient?
   a. Combined hormonal contraceptives
   b. A levonorgestrel intrauterine system
   c. Contraceptive that contain progestin only
   d. Levonorgestrel (systemic) progestin

5. The nurse is instructing a patient on the use of depot medroxyprogesterone acetate. Which statements are correct? (Select all that apply.)
   a. Patients usually do not have any changes in their periods.
   b. Patients should increase their intake of calcium.
   c. Patients can expect some irregular bleeding at first.
   d. Patients may use this contraceptive when breastfeeding.
   e. Patients will experience a decrease with postpartum depression.

6. The nurse is counseling a 62-year-old patient with a T score of −2.0 after her dual-energy x-ray absorptiometry scan. What is the best advice for this patient?
   a. The patient should take a daily calcium supplement, 1200 to 1500 mg orally in the morning.
   b. The patient's exercise program will include weight-bearing exercises like swimming and cycling.
   c. The patient most likely will be prescribed a drug of the bisphosphonate classification by the health care provider.
   d. The patient should supplement her diet with 1200 mg of calcium with vitamin D 600 IU orally once daily.

7. A 48-year-old patient arrives at the clinic to discuss her perimenopausal symptoms. She states that her last menstrual period was 8 months ago, and before that, her periods had been irregular. What is the most important nursing advice to give this patient?
   a. Hormone therapy is only used for hot flashes and vaginal dryness.
   b. The patient should be using some form of contraception to avoid pregnancy.
   c. The patient should have a dual-energy x-ray absorptiometry scan to test for osteopenia.
   d. At this time, herbal supplementation is probably best to relieve her perimenopausal symptoms.

8. A patient has been prescribed clomiphene citrate therapy by her doctor. The patient asks the nurse, "How does my new medicine work?" What can the nurse say to convey the mechanism of action of clomiphene citrate therapy to this patient? (Select all that apply.)
   a. This drug stimulates the ovaries, increasing the chance of ovulation.
   b. This drug increases circulating progesterone levels.
   c. This drug usually does not work on the first cycle.
   d. This drug helps the ovaries form multiple follicles.

56

Men's Reproductive Health

Jared Robertson III, RN, MN

http://evolve.elsevier.com/McCuistion/pharmacology

OBJECTIVES

- Describe the effects of gonadal hormone supplementation on the hypothalamic anterior pituitary feedback loop.
- Describe the role of testosterone therapy in managing developmental problems related to primary and secondary male sex characteristics and spermatogenesis.
- Differentiate common conditions for which androgen therapy and antiandrogen therapy are indicated.

- Describe those for whom androgen therapy is particularly risky.
- Assess patients for therapeutic and adverse effects of androgen therapy.
- Categorize commonly prescribed drugs that can impair male sexual function.
- Explain the Clinical Judgment [Nursing Process], including patient teaching, related to drugs used to treat male reproductive disorders.

OUTLINE

Reproductive health requires the production of adequate quantities of various hypothalamic, pituitary, and gonadal hormones as well as the appropriate hormone receptors. It requires normal development and patency of the reproductive tract. In addition, reproductive health implies that men and women at developmentally appropriate life stages are fertile (i.e., able to produce gametes [sperm or eggs]). Finally, reproductive health entails the ability to engage in sexual intercourse with ejaculation by the male.

Alterations in male reproductive health reflect a wide range of developmental, endocrine, infectious, inflammatory, hypertrophic, malignant, and psychoemotional processes. Review the introduction to this unit to gain a better understanding of ways in which reproductive health is affected, including anatomy and physiology, sperm production, regulation of male sexual functioning, and sexual intercourse.

The drug family most clearly associated with male reproductive processes is the androgens. Because synthetic anabolic steroids and antiandrogens affect male reproduction, they are also discussed.

DRUGS RELATED TO MALE REPRODUCTIVE DISORDERS

Androgens

Androgens, or male sex hormones, control the development and maintenance of sexual processes, accessory sexual organs, cellular metabolism, and bone and muscle growth. Testosterone, an anabolic

steroid, is the principal male sex hormone. It is the prototype of the androgen hormones, synthesized primarily in the testes and, to a lesser extent, in the adrenal cortex. In women, the ovaries synthesize small amounts of testosterone. In adult males, normal plasma concentrations of testosterone are 270 to 1070 ng/dL, with a slow decline of 1% per year after 30 years of age (Table 56.1). The Prototype Drug Chart: Testosterone Cypionate discusses the dosage, uses, and considerations for

TABLE 56.1 Testosterone Levels by Age

Age	T Level (ng/dL)
0–5 mo	75–400
6 mo–9 y	<7–20
10–11 y	<7–130
12–13 y	<7–800
14 y	<7–1200
15–16 y	100–1200
17–18 y	300–1200
19+ y	240–950
Avg. adult male	270–1070
30+ y	–1% per year

From Mayo Clinic Laboratories. (n.d.). Test ID: TTFB. Retrieved October 12, 2019, from https://www.mayocliniclabs.com/test-catalog/Clinical+and+Interpretive/83686.

PROTOTYPE DRUG CHART

Testosterone Cypionate

Drug Class	Dosage
Androgen CSS III	Male primary hypogonadism and hypogonadotropic hypogonadism: IM: 50–400 mg q2–4wk

Contraindications	Drug-Food Interactions
Hypersensitivity to drug or drug components, cottonseed oil, pregnancy, breastfeeding, male breast cancer, and prostate cancer *Caution:* Prostate cancer risk, benign prostatic hyperplasia, older adults, renal and/or hepatic impairment, risk of hypercalcemia, cardiovascular disease, heart failure, hyperlipidemia, diabetes, pulmonary disease, obesity, sleep apnea, polycythemia, and male patients trying to conceive	Drug: May decrease serum glucose, requiring insulin adjustment Herbal: St. John's wort may decrease concentration/effects Food: None known Lab: May increase Hgb, Hct, LDL, serum alkaline phosphatase, bilirubin, calcium, potassium, sodium, AST. May decrease HDL

Pharmacokinetics	Pharmacodynamics
Absorption: IM: Well absorbed Distribution: PB: 98% Metabolism: Liver; t½: 8 days Excretion: Urine 90%, feces 6%	IM: Onset: UK Peak: UK Duration: Cypionate/enanthate: 2–4 wk

Therapeutic Effects/Uses

Androgen replacement therapy in treatment of delayed male puberty, male hypogonadism (congenital or acquired)
Mechanism of Action: Binds to androgen receptors, producing multiple anabolic and androgenic effects.

Side Effects	Adverse Reactions
Abdominal pain, nausea, diarrhea, constipation, hives, irritation at injection site, increased salivation, mouth soreness, increased or decreased libido, insomnia, aggressive behavior, weakness, dizziness, pruritus, acne, masculinization, irregular menses, urinary urgency, gynecomastia, priapism, red skin, jaundice, sodium and water retention, allergic reaction, depression, habituation	*Life-threatening:* Hepatic necrosis, hepatitis, hepatic tumors, respiratory distress

CSS, Controlled Substances Schedule; *IM,* intramuscular; *min,* minute; *PB,* protein binding; *q,* every; *t½,* half-life; *UK,* unknown; *wk,* week.

this formulation of the drug. Table 56.2 presents additional formulations of testosterone available for use.

Pharmacokinetics. Testosterone secretion is greater in men than in women in most stages of life. About 98% of circulating testosterone is bound to both sex hormone–binding globulin (SHBG) and albumin protein, leaving about 2% unbound, or circulating free in the plasma; this unbound portion is biologically active. Estrogen elevates the production of SHBG, resulting in more protein-bound testosterone in women than in men. The half-life of endogenous, or naturally occurring, free testosterone in the blood is 10 to 20 minutes.

Because as much as 50% of testosterone is metabolized on its first pass through the hepatic circulation when taken orally, oral testosterone is not available for prescription in the United States. Testosterone can be combined with esters to form esterified testosterone in an oil base for intramuscular (IM) injection.

Ninety percent of testosterone is excreted in the urine as glucuronic and sulfuric acid conjugates and its metabolites. About 6% of the hormone is excreted unconjugated in the feces. Synthetic androgens may be excreted as unaltered hormone or as metabolites. In some tissues the action of testosterone depends on its reduction to 5-alpha-dihydrotestosterone (DHT), whereas in other tissues testosterone itself is the active hormone. In the central nervous system, the metabolite estradiol affects hormonal action.

Pharmacodynamics. Testosterone is responsible for the development of male sex characteristics. The biologic effects of testosterone may be mediated directly by testosterone or by its metabolites. Testosterone and dihydrotestosterone act as androgens

by way of a single androgen receptor officially designated NR3A. The hormones bind to sites on certain responsive genes, causing a change to take place in the target cell. The effects of the testosterone depend on which receptor it activates and the tissues in which these effects occur. The manufacture of protein within the target cells results in the buildup of cellular tissue (anabolism), especially in muscles. This leads to development of secondary sex characteristics such as pubic hair growth, beard and body hair growth, baldness, deepening of the male voice, thickening of the skin, sebaceous gland activity, increased musculature, bone development, and red blood cell formation.

Fetal testes begin to produce testosterone during the first 3 months in utero. After birth until just before puberty, production is negligible. During puberty, production increases rapidly and continues until later adulthood. As men age, the number of Leydig cells decreases, sperm production declines, and luteinizing hormone (LH) and follicle-stimulating hormone (FSH) levels rise. Levels of unbound testosterone are reduced in older men to one-third to one-fifth the peak value. If men experience osteoporosis and anemia, and if their testosterone levels are 300 ng/dL or less, testosterone replacement therapy should be considered.

Indications for Androgen Therapy

Table 56.2 lists the natural and synthetic androgens with their dosages, uses, and considerations. Androgen therapy is approved for use in androgen deficiency in males, specifically hypogonadism; replacement therapy for testicular failure in adult males; and delayed puberty in adolescents.

TABLE 56.2 Androgens (Controlled Substance, Schedule III)

Drug	Route and Dosage	Uses and Considerations
Natural Androgens		
Testosterone		
Testosterone nasal	Nasal: 5.5 mg per gel pump actuation; 1 pump actuation in each nostril 3 times/d	For primary male hypogonadism and male hypogonadotropic hypogonadism.
Transdermal testosterone patch	Transdermal patch: 2 mg/24 h or 4 mg/24 h patch; apply to nongenital skin; avoid bony areas	Drug is started at the full dose and adjusted according to tolerance and therapeutic response.
Testosterone topical gel	1% Gel: 50–100 mg once daily 2% Gel: 40–70 mg once daily	Less skin irritation occurs with the gel than with the patch. PB: 98%; t½: 10–100 min
Buccal testosterone	Buccal: 30 mg twice daily	
Testosterone pellet	Subcut implantable 75-mg pellets: implant two 75-mg pellets for each 25 mg testosterone propionate required weekly. Replace every 4–6 mo	For replacement therapy in conditions associated with a deficiency or absence of endogenous testosterone. PB: 98%; t½: 10–100 min
Testosterone cypionate	IM: 50–400 mg q3–4wk	For androgen replacement and delayed puberty; therapy generally lasts 3–4 y. PB: 98%; t½: 8 d
Synthetic Androgens		
Fluoxymesterone	PO: 5 mg 1–4 times/d	For androgen deficiency and palliative treatment of carcinoma of the breast. PB: 98%; t½: 29.2 h
Methyltestosterone	PO: 10–50 mg/d in divided doses initially; reduced for maintenance	For androgen deficiency and palliative treatment of carcinoma of the breast. PB: UK; t½: 2.5–3.5 h

d, Day; *h,* hour; *IM,* intramuscular; *min,* minute; *mo,* month; *PB,* protein binding; *PO,* by mouth; *q,* every; *subcut,* subcutaneous; *t½,* half-life; *UK,* unknown; *wk,* week; *y,* year.

Hypogonadism. The clearest indication for exogenous androgen therapy is hypogonadism. Male hypogonadism is a defect of the reproductive system that results in failure of the testes to produce testosterone, sperm, or both. Deficiency of sex hormones can result in defective primary or secondary sexual development, and defective sperm development can result in infertility. Hypogonadism is either *primary,* reflecting testicular abnormality, or *secondary,* reflecting hypothalamic or pituitary failure. A combination of disorders can also occur. Inadequate pituitary function will severely affect young boys and results in infertility and a lack of secondary sex characteristics. Adult men may experience testicular atrophy, impotence, decreased libido, decreased bone density, loss of muscle mass, hair loss, gynecomastia, fatigue, difficulty concentrating, or vasomotor flushing.

The timing and extent of treatment depend on the clinical manifestations. Because accelerated bone maturation can lead to premature closure of bone epiphyses and short stature, androgen therapy should be used cautiously in children and only by specialists aware of the adverse effects on bone maturation. Skeletal maturation must be monitored every 6 months by radiography of the hand and wrist. Artificial induction of puberty is undertaken only after boys reach 15 to 17 years of age and after hypothalamic and pituitary function has been assessed. A 4- to 6-month trial of androgen therapy is implemented, followed by a similar period of rest for reevaluation. If prolonged therapy is required, testosterone cypionate is used, 50 to 400 mg IM every 2 to 4 weeks. It should be given deep in the IM. Inspect vials visually for particulate matter and discoloration before administration, and warm and shake the vial to dissolve any crystals that may have formed during storage. It takes 3 or 4 years for sexual development to occur; plasma testosterone levels should be monitored and dosages adjusted as needed to maintain normal levels. If the serum testosterone level is below the normal range, the provider will adjust the dose upward. Therapy may be lifelong.

Testosterone may be administered buccally, nasally, transdermally, or parenterally. Drug selection depends on the balance of growth and sexual maturation desired and on the preferred route of administration. A buccal mucoadhesive system is available that provides a 30-mg dose every 12 hours. Advise the patient to place the rounded surface of the system against the gum above an incisor tooth and hold it firmly in place with finger over the lip and against the product for 30 seconds. To remove, slide gently downward toward the tooth to avoid scratching the gums. Sites must be rotated with each application. If the product falls off within the 12-hour dosing interval or if it falls out of position within 4 hours before next dose, remove it and apply a new system. The patient should not chew or swallow the system. Advise the patient to regularly inspect gums where the system has been applied. Testosterones are considered Schedule III controlled substances.

Transdermal testosterone (TT) patches achieve adequate serum concentrations when applied to the arm, back, or upper buttocks. TT patches can be applied to any healthy skin site other than the scrotum or bony areas. Daily application of one to two TT 2 mg/24 h or 4 mg/24 h skin patches at 10 p.m. results in serum testosterone concentrations approaching those of healthy young men. The first day of dosing results in morning serum testosterone concentrations within the normal range. There is no testosterone accumulation with continued use. After removal of TT patches, hypogonadal status returns within 24 hours. Keep testosterone gel out of reach of children.

Testosterone gel is applied to clean dry skin of shoulders or upper arms. It should not be applied to the genitals. Hands should be thoroughly washed with soap and water after application. Testosterone gel carries a boxed warning because it can be transferred to others through personal contact with skin or clothing. Children should avoid contact with unwashed application sites or application sites not covered by clothing. Children can experience virilization from secondary exposure. Caution is advised.

Side Effects

Hypogonadal men on androgen therapy may experience frequent erections or priapism (painful, continuous erection), gynecomastia (mammary gland enlargement in men), or urinary urgency. Continued use of androgens by normal men can halt spermatogenesis (formation of spermatozoa). The sperm count may be low (oligospermia) for 3 or more months after therapy is stopped.

Other side effects of androgen therapy include abdominal pain, nausea, insomnia, diarrhea or constipation, hives or redness at the injection site, increased salivation, mouth soreness, and increased or decreased sexual desire. Advise the patient to notify the health care provider if side effects persist, worsen, or are bothersome.

Adverse Reactions

Androgen therapy may cause hypercalcemia by stimulating bone resorption in immobilized patients and those with breast cancer. The drug should be discontinued and appropriate measures instituted if signs of hypercalcemia occur; signs include nausea and vomiting, lethargy, decreased muscle tone, polyuria, and increased urine and serum calcium.

Virilization refers to the development of male secondary sex characteristics in women or hypogonadal males. Such characteristics include growth of facial hair, acne and skin oiliness, and vocal huskiness. Menstrual irregularities or amenorrhea, suppressed ovulation or lactation, baldness or increased hair growth (hirsutism), and hypertrophy of the clitoris may develop in women undergoing androgen therapy. Although most adverse effects slowly reverse themselves after short-term therapy is completed, vocal changes may be permanent. With long-term therapy, as in the treatment of breast cancer, adverse effects may be irreversible.

Children may experience profound virilization as well as impaired bone growth. During pregnancy, androgens can cross the placenta and cause masculinization of the fetus. Virilization can occur in those secondarily exposed to testosterone gel and may cause teratogenic effects in fetuses. Women and children should not handle the gel and should avoid contact with application sites in men using testosterone gel.

Less frequent adverse effects include dizziness, weakness, changes in skin color, frequent headaches, confusion, respiratory distress, depression, pruritus, allergic skin rash, edema of the lower extremities, jaundice, bleeding, paresthesias, chills, polycythemia, muscle cramps, and sodium and water retention. Hepatocellular carcinoma can occur in patients who have received selected androgens for long-term therapy and in cases of abuse of androgenic hormones by athletes.

Serum cholesterol may become elevated during androgen therapy. Other alterations in laboratory tests include increased hematocrit, altered thyroid and liver function tests, and elevated urine 17-ketosteroids (a by-product of the breakdown of androgens). Rare complications of long-term therapy include hepatic necrosis, hepatic peliosis (blood-filled cysts), hepatic tumors, and leukopenia.

Contraindications

Androgen therapy is contraindicated during pregnancy and in individuals with nephrosis or those in the nephrotic phase of nephritis; it is also contraindicated in patients with hypercalcemia, pituitary insufficiency, hepatic dysfunction, benign prostatic hyperplasia (BPH), prostate cancer, or history of myocardial infarction. Men with breast cancer are not treated with androgens, nor are women whose breast cancer is not estrogen dependent.

Caution must be exercised when using androgen therapy in individuals with hypertension, hypercholesterolemia, coronary artery disease, renal disease, or seizure disorder. It is used with caution in infants and prepubertal children because of the potential for growth disturbances and in older men because of their increased risk for BPH and prostate cancer.

Drug Interactions

Androgens potentiate the effects of oral anticoagulants, necessitating a decrease in anticoagulant dosage. Androgens antagonize calcitonin and parathyroid hormones. Because androgens can decrease blood glucose in patients with diabetes, dosages of insulin or other antidiabetic agents may need to be reduced. Concurrent use of corticosteroids exacerbates the edema that can occur with androgen therapy. Barbiturates, phenytoin, and phenylbutazone decrease the effects of androgens.

Anabolic Steroids

Anabolic steroids, or anabolic-androgenic steroids (AASs), are a class of steroid hormones related to the hormone testosterone. They increase protein synthesis within cells, which results in the buildup of cellular tissue (anabolism), especially in muscles. Anabolic steroids also have androgenic and virilizing properties, including the development and maintenance of masculine characteristics such as the growth of the vocal cords and body hair. Although the American College of Sports Medicine notes that AASs, combined with sufficient diet and exercise, can contribute to increased lean body mass in some individuals, they also note it is in the best interest of all sports to eradicate the use of AASs by athletes due to the risk of serious harm or death in those who use AASs. ⚡ See Chapter 8 for further information.

Testosterone precursors available as nutritional supplements include androstenediol, androstenedione, and dehydroepiandrosterone (DHEA). Older teens are the heaviest users, but more than 500,000 junior high school students also use them. Marketed as "sport supplements" or "teen formulas," they can be purchased without a prescription in stores and on the Internet. A sudden dramatic increase in weight and body size, increased acne, and changes in mood and behavior can be signs of exogenous anabolic steroid use. Individuals using anabolic steroids may become more aggressive and physical, and health risks can result from long-term use or excessive intake of anabolic steroids; these effects include increased low-density lipoprotein (bad) cholesterol and decreased high-density lipoprotein (good) cholesterol, acne, high blood pressure, liver damage, and dangerous changes in the structure of the left ventricle of the heart. Adverse effects may not be recognized until years later. ⚡ See Chapter 8 for further information.

Two other steroids that have gained popularity, especially with athletes, are human chorionic gonadotropin (hCG) and tetrahydrogestrinone (THG); hCG is a hormone used to treat infertility and stimulate testosterone production, and THG is a potent androgen developed to escape detection on urine drug screens, although tests have since been developed for rapid screening. It is not approved by the US Food and Drug Administration (FDA) and is not legally marketed. All major athletic organizations prohibit the use of anabolic steroids, but their continued use despite bans has led to "antidoping" investigations and punitive action.

Antiandrogens

Antiandrogens, or androgen antagonists, block the synthesis or action of androgens (Table 56.3). These drugs are used in the treatment of BPH and advanced prostatic cancer and as hormonal therapy in the treatment of endometriosis. They may also be used to treat male-pattern baldness (MPB), acne, hirsutism, virilization syndrome in women, and precocious puberty in boys, although their effectiveness is not well established.

Gonadotropin-releasing hormone (GnRH), or a synthetic analogue such as leuprolide, is the most effective inhibitor of testosterone synthesis. When such agents are given over time, LH and testosterone

◎ CLINICAL JUDGMENT [NURSING PROCESS]

Androgens

Concept: Hormonal Regulation
- Physiologic mechanisms that regulate the secretion and action of hormones associated with the endocrine system

Recognize Cues [Assessment]
- Assess the reason for androgen therapy and the patient's perception of it. If delayed puberty is the indication, assess patient and family attitudes about the condition.
- Monitor weight, blood pressure, liver and thyroid function, hemoglobin and hematocrit, creatinine, clotting factors, glucose tolerance, serum lipids and electrolytes, and blood count before and throughout treatment. Note the presence of liver or endocrine dysfunction and any elevation in blood pressure.
- Note concomitant anticoagulant therapy.
- When a prepubertal child is treated, obtain hand and wrist radiographs before, every 6 months during, and after treatment to monitor growth.
- Appraise the patient's expressive affect during therapy, particularly aggressiveness in patients taking large doses. Self-concept is an important consideration in the patient on androgen therapy, particularly in children with delayed puberty and in women.

Analyze Cues and Prioritize Hypothesis [Patient Problems]
- Sexual expression
- Self-concept
- Weight gain
- Decreased self-esteem

Generate Solutions [Planning]
- Through collaboration, the patient agrees to (1) adhere to the prescribed regimen for taking drug and for monitoring, (2) use drug appropriately, (3) report adverse effects immediately, and (4) maintain a positive self-concept during long-term treatment.

Take Action [Nursing Interventions]
- Collaborate with the patient and family on proper administration of drugs, their reasons for use, and potential undesired effects. Review which effects warrant prompt medical attention (e.g., urinary problems, priapism, respiratory distress).

- Advise patients that an intermittent approach to treatment allows for monitoring of endocrine status between courses of androgen therapy. Explain the need to return to the health care facility for monitoring and confirm the patient's ability to do so. Arrange social service referrals if necessary.
- Counsel the family pursuing treatment for a child with delayed puberty about the range of normal development.
- Encourage patients to monitor muscle strength during treatment.
- Instruct patients to administer androgens as directed.
- Coach patients about good skin hygiene to decrease the severity of acne.
- Urge men undergoing androgen therapy to report priapism promptly so the drug dosage can be reduced to avoid subsequent erectile dysfunction (ED).
- Instruct men to report decreased urinary stream promptly so they can be evaluated for prostatic hypertrophy.
- Assess and review the nutritional intake to ensure adequate intake of essential nutrients.
- Counsel patients to record body weight several times per week. Restrict sodium if edema develops.
- Advise patients with elevated serum calcium of the need to drink 2 L per day or more of fluid to prevent kidney stones. Individuals on bed rest need range-of-motion exercises, whereas ambulatory patients need to engage in active weight-bearing. Hypercalcemia requires prompt medical attention because it can lead to cardiac arrest.

Evaluate Outcomes [Evaluation]
- Monitor the patient's ability to adhere to a treatment regimen and response to prescribed drugs. The ability to adhere to a treatment plan and discuss treatment and effects knowledgeably suggests that teaching has been effective and that the patient accepts the treatment.
- Ask the patient about therapeutic and adverse drug effects on follow-up visits. Monitoring of weight, blood pressure, and laboratory tests will continue throughout therapy with alterations in the plan of care as needed.
- Periodically assess children and women who experience virilizing effects or acne for the ability to cope with these changes and to maintain a positive self-concept.
- Assess sexual function when appropriate.

TABLE 56.3 Antiandrogens

Mechanism	Drugs
Inhibits gonadotropin release, suppressing levels of testosterone	Goserelin acetate Leuprolide acetate
Inhibits testosterone synthesis	Ketoconazole[a]
Blocks conversion of testosterone to dihydrotestosterone	Finasteride
Androgen receptor inhibitors	Flutamide Bicalutamide

[a]Off-label use for castration-resistant prostate cancer.

levels fall. Normally, GnRH is released in a pulsatile fashion, but the sustained activity of leuprolide leads to decreased production of FSH and LH. In the male, this activity stops testosterone production in the testes. In the female, it stops estrogen production in the ovaries. This drug should not be used in combination with herbal or dietary supplements such as black cohosh, chasteberry, or DHEA.

Ketoconazole, an antifungal drug, has testosterone-suppressing effects similar to those of GnRH analogues when given at doses higher than those required for antifungal activity (400 mg orally every 8 hours as opposed to 200 to 400 mg daily for the treatment of fungal infections). The mechanism of action of this non-GnRH drug is unclear. GnRH analogues act directly through their effect on testosterone production for the treatment of prostate cancer. Ketoconazole as treatment of prostate cancer is an off-label use.

Flutamide is an oral nonsteroidal antiandrogen drug used as an antihormonal agent in the treatment of metastatic prostate cancer. It is most effective when used simultaneously with luteinizing hormone–releasing hormone (LHRH) analogues such as leuprolide acetate. When used alone, the best response is seen in untreated patients. Flutamide is not effective in treating other hormonally dependent diseases such as breast cancer or BPH. Flutamide competes with androgens at androgen receptor sites in the prostate gland, blocking the conversion of testosterone to dihydrotestosterone; by doing so, it prevents the androgens from stimulating the prostate cancer cells to grow. Men receiving flutamide show elevations in plasma LH and testosterone levels. Bicalutamide is structurally related to flutamide but has a long plasma half-life that allows once-daily dosing, compared with thrice-daily dosing for flutamide. In addition, bicalutamide is more selective for the peripheral androgen receptor and has less activity at the central androgen receptor on the hypothalamic-pituitary axis.

Finasteride, a synthetic compound, inhibits conversion of testosterone to DHT. This orally active agent decreases the concentration of dihydrotestosterone in plasma and the prostate without elevated plasma concentrations of LH or testosterone. Finasteride is used to treat BPH and MPB. The recommended 5-mg daily dose of finasteride for BPH needs to be reevaluated at 6 months and periodically thereafter. The 1-mg dose of finasteride for MPB is taken once a day for 12 months, and continued treatment is recommended for sustained results. After discontinuation of therapy, reversal of effect is typically seen within 1 year. Adverse reactions include impotence, decreased libido, and decreased ejaculate. Women of childbearing age must not use finasteride and should not handle crushed or broken tablets because the active ingredient may cause abnormalities of a male fetus's sex organs.

Drugs Used in Other Male Reproductive Disorders

Delayed Puberty

Puberty is considered to be delayed when testicle enlargement, followed by penile growth and pubic hair development, has not begun by 14 years of age. Delay in growth may be a normal part of the maturation process, but the cause could also be androgen deficiency or a deficiency of growth hormone. Secretion of GnRH, LH, or FSH is insufficient in up to 5% of cases of delayed puberty. Treatment is only begun after 14 years of age, after a full evaluation, including serum LH, FSH, thyroid-stimulating hormone (TSH), and testosterone levels. Therapy with testosterone cypionate 50 mg IM every month, for 3 to 6 months or less before epiphyseal closure, may result in linear growth without adverse permanent effects on hypothalamic, pituitary, or gonadal maturation.

Pituitary, Thyroid, and Adrenal Disorders

Inadequate pituitary function can be another cause of hypogonadism. Menotropins are purified combination preparations of the human pituitary gonadotropins FSH and LH. These drugs are indicated when both LH and FSH levels are low. When given in combination with hCG, the drug stimulates testosterone production in men to encourage spermatogenesis when injected three times a week for 4 to 9 months to ensure adequate spermatozoa production. One ampule of a menotropin contains 75 international units each of LH and FSH. The initial dose is 75 to 150 international units subcutaneously (subcut) or 3 times per week. Subsequent doses are adjusted according to individual response but not exceeding 75 to 150 international units per adjustment; the maximum dose is 300 units 3 times per week. Use the lower abdomen (alternating sides) for subcut administration. Menotropin must be used immediately after reconstitution and must be protected from light. Advise patients to discard unused drug. Adverse effects include nausea, vomiting, diarrhea, gynecomastia, and fever.

Inadequate thyroid and adrenal gland function can also affect sexuality. Hypothyroidism, a deficiency in thyroid hormone, can be the result of insufficient thyroid hormone production or resistance to its effects at the target organs. The problem can be congenital or acquired. It can cause inhibited sexual desire, a lack of or decreased interest in sexual activity, and erectile dysfunction (ED). In Addison disease, there is a deficit of both cortisol and the mineralocorticoid aldosterone. Men with Addison disease may experience inhibited sexual desire, ED, or diminished fertility. Both hypothyroidism and Addison disease are highly responsive to replacement therapy with the appropriate hormones.

TABLE 56.4 Drugs That Cause Sexual Dysfunction in Males

Drug Category	Drugs or Drug Families
Anticholinergics	Atropine Scopolamine Benztropine Trihexyphenidyl
Antidepressants	Tricyclic antidepressants Monoamine oxidase inhibitors Selective serotonin reuptake inhibitors
Antihistamines	Diphenhydramine Hydroxyzine
Antihypertensives	Centrally acting alpha$_2$ agonists Alpha- and beta-receptor blockers Diuretics Angiotensin-converting enzyme inhibitors
Antipsychotics	Phenothiazines Thioxanthenes Butyrophenone
Antiulcer drugs	Cimetidine Ranitidine Famotidine
Sedatives and illicit drugs	Alcohol Barbiturates Diazepam Chlordiazepoxide Cannabis Cocaine Opiates Methadone
Others	Aminocaproic acid Baclofen Steroids Ethionamide Digoxin Chemotherapeutic agents Lithium

Sexual Dysfunction

Sexual dysfunction is the inability to experience sexual desire, erection, ejaculation, and/or detumescence—the four phases of the sexual response cycle in men. Inhibited sexual desire can result from androgen deficiency, an affective disorder, or discord in the sexual relationship. Many drugs can also cause sexual dysfunction (Table 56.4).

Ejaculatory dysfunction, impaired ejection of seminal fluid from the male urethra, can be psychogenic or a result of drug therapy, androgen deficiency, or sympathetic degeneration. Failure of detumescence (reduction of penile engorgement) is most commonly caused by penile disease, systemic disease, trauma, or adverse effects of drugs. Individuals who experience premature ejaculation related to excessive anxiety about sexual intercourse may be helped by treatment with one of the many antidepressants alone or in conjunction with psychotherapy.

Erectile dysfunction (ED) is the inability to achieve or maintain an erection satisfactory for sexual performance. ED happens when not enough blood flows to the penis during sexual stimulation. This may be caused by psychoemotional problems, diabetes, hypertension, lower urinary tract symptoms, pelvic surgery, vascular insufficiency, neurologic disorders, androgen deficiency or resistance, or diseases of the

TABLE 56.5 Phosphodiesterase-5 Inhibitors for Erectile Dysfunction

Generic	Onset/Duration	Side Effects	Drug Interactions
Avanafil 50–200 mg; not affected by food	Onset: 15–30 min Duration: 4–6 h Use once in 24 h	Abdominal symptoms such as diarrhea, heartburn, and upset stomach Abnormal vision such as blurring and sensitivity to light and blue-green color tint Dizziness Flushing Headache Nasal congestion Hearing loss/tinnitus	Nitrates: Isosorbide, nitroglycerin, amyl nitrate, butyl nitrate Alpha blockers: Alfuzosin, doxazosin, prazosin, tamsulosin, terazosin, amiodarone Antiinfective agents: Fluconazole, itraconazole, ketoconazole, clarithromycin, moxifloxacin, erythromycin Cardiac drugs: Disopyramide, procainamide, quinidine, sotalol, thioridazine, verapamil HIV protease inhibitors: Atazanavir, indinavir, ritonavir, saquinavir Other drugs: Methadone, pimozide, haloperidol
Sildenafil 25–100 mg; works best on an empty stomach	Onset: 30–60 min Duration: 4 h		
Tadalafil 5–20 mg; not affected by food	Onset: 15–60 min Duration: 24–36 h Max: 20 mg/dose once daily		
Vardenafil 5–20 mg; less effective with a high-fat meal	Onset: 25–30 min Duration: 4–5 h Max: 20 mg/dose once daily		

h, Hour; *HIV*, human immunodeficiency virus; *min*, minute.

penis. ED caused by vascular insufficiency is occasionally treated on a short-term basis by local vasoactive drugs, including papaverine, phentolamine, prostaglandin E, and nitroglycerin. Other drug options for the treatment of ED include oral drugs, drugs injected into the penis, intraurethral alprostadil, or testosterone.

A class of drugs called *phosphodiesterase inhibitors* facilitate erection by enhancing blood flow to the penis. Phosphodiesterase-5 (PDE-5) inhibitors are currently the most commonly used medical treatment for ED. These drugs have a high success rate, are easy to use, and often result in erection during sexual stimulation. The PDE-5 inhibitors currently approved by the FDA are sildenafil, tadalafil, vardenafil, and avanafil. PDE-5 inhibitors are taken before sexual activity with variations in effective start time and duration of benefit (Table 56.5).

Nitroglycerin and other nitrate drugs used to treat heart disease can cause a significant decrease in blood pressure when taken with PDE-5 inhibitors; therefore this class of drugs is contraindicated for use by any patient using organic nitrates in *any* form. Patients with a prescription for as-needed (PRN) sublingual nitroglycerin can take PDE-5 inhibitors but should still be cautioned about taking them concomitantly. Organic nitrates include nitroglycerin, isosorbide mononitrate, isosorbide nitrate, isosorbide dinitrate/phenobarbital, pentaerythritol tetranitrate, erythritol tetranitrate, and illicit substances (amyl nitrate/nitrite, butyl nitrate). Sildenafil is contraindicated in patients with significant cardiovascular disease and in individuals who have anatomic deformities or conditions that predispose them to priapism.

Studies have shown that vardenafil and tadalafil are safer for patients with heart failure or a history of myocardial infarctions. Like sildenafil, they are contraindicated if the patient is taking nitrate-containing drugs. Common side effects of these drugs are headache (most common), dyspepsia, nasal congestion, and nasopharyngitis. Other rare side effects can also occur, and the patient should be taught about them; these effects include blurred vision, photosensitivity, changes in color perception (especially blue and green), hearing loss, tinnitus, seizures, priapism, and urinary tract symptoms such as frequent or painful urination and cloudy or bloody urine. Patients are instructed to notify their health care provider of any side effects they experience.

The PDE-5 inhibitors interact with grapefruit juice and grapefruit products by increasing the amount of the PDE-5 inhibitor absorbed, thereby increasing the risk of side effects. Many drugs interact with PDE-5 inhibitors, so be sure to obtain a complete list of drugs taken by the patient.

Certain drugs are often abused by individuals seeking a heightened sexual experience. Amyl nitrate is commonly believed to be an aphrodisiac. Sudden death, myocardial infarction, and methemoglobinemia have been reported with its use. Cantharides (Spanish fly) causes bladder and urethral irritation, accounting for its use as a sexual stimulant. Permanent penile damage has been reported with its use.

⚡ PATIENT SAFETY

Do not confuse...
- **Lupron Depot-3 Month** with **Lupron Depot-Ped**
- **Anabolic steroids** with **corticosteroids**

Complementary and Alternative Medicine. To self-treat sexual problems or to enhance sexual performance, consumers use a wide variety of herbs and plant-derived compounds (phytochemicals). Despite new science-based therapies, men are attracted to phytochemicals because they are easy to obtain and may be cheaper than prescription drugs and therapies, procedures, or surgeries not covered by insurance. Consumers may mistakenly perceive natural products as providing health benefits beyond sexual performance because they can be purchased at nutrition centers or health food stores. Common herbs used for sexual health and performance include *Pausinystalia yohimbe*, *Panax quinquefolius*, ginkgo biloba, saw palmetto, muira puama, *Lepidium meyenii*, *Mondia whitei*, and *Tribulus terrestris*. Limited studies have been conducted on these products; all studies have yielded mixed results. As such, there is insufficient evidence to recommend any complementary or alternative medicine (CAM). Its benefits appear to reflect popular or cultural beliefs. Reports in health magazines and advertising are anecdotal and based on a small number of users. However, it is important for the nurse to be aware of CAM, because ED affects 50% of men between 50 and 70 years of age, but only 10% seek medical attention. These statistics indicate men may be choosing to use CAM to avoid the discomfort of discussing this sensitive topic with their health care provider.

Non–Sexually Transmitted Infections

Drugs used to treat acute or chronic prostatitis, orchitis, or epididymitis are the same as those used to treat urinary tract infections (see Chapter 51).

Benign Prostatic Hyperplasia. As a man ages, the glandular units in the prostate gland begin to undergo tissue hyperplasia, an abnormal increase in the number of cells, which results in prostatic hypertrophy, or enlargement of the gland. The exact cause of BPH is unknown, but its development is almost universal in older men. The enlarged prostate gland contributes to overall lower urinary tract symptoms either through direct bladder outlet obstruction or from resistance within the enlarged gland itself. The man experiences storage and/or voiding disturbances, such as a sensation of bladder fullness, frequency, nocturia, hesitation when trying to begin urinating, dribbling of urine, and ED. Although BPH is not a life-threatening condition, the effect of symptoms on quality of life can be significant. Because these are the same symptoms that prostate cancer may cause, the patient should have a prostate-specific antigen (PSA) blood test and may undergo a prostate biopsy to make sure no cancer is present. Traditionally, the primary goal of treatment has been to alleviate bothersome symptoms. More recently, treatment has also been focused on the alteration of disease progression and prevention of complications. Drugs from several pharmacologic classes are used; they include alpha-adrenergic antagonists (alpha blockers), 5-alpha-reductase inhibitors (5-ARIs), anticholinergics (only used in men without large postvoid residuals), and the PDE-5 inhibitor tadalafil. Choosing the correct medical treatment for BPH is complex (Table 56.6). The American Urological Association 2010 Guidelines are a useful reference on the effective evidence-based management of lower urinary tract symptoms caused by BPH. The guidelines advise a discussion of benefits and risks of each recommended treatment alternative (e.g., watchful waiting; medical, surgical, or minimally invasive surgical treatments). The choice of treatment is reached in a shared decision-making process between provider and patient.

With initiation of drug therapy, the patient should be followed every 1 to 3 months, depending on the class of drug chosen, to assess success and inquire about side effects. The patient with an enlarged prostate should avoid drugs that can cause urinary retention, such as anticholinergics, antihistamines, and decongestants.

Malignant Tumors. Prostatic cancer accounts for about 10% of all cancer deaths among American men. Most prostatic cancers are adenocarcinomas. Metastasis to lymph nodes, bone, lungs, liver, and adrenal glands is common. Prostatic cancer is often asymptomatic, but urinary obstruction is commonly the first sign. Treatment may include a combination of surgical resection, cryotherapy, antiandrogen administration, radiation therapy, chemotherapy, and pain management.

Testicular tumors peak in early adulthood. They include malignant germinal cell tumors and benign Leydig or Sertoli cell tumors. Treatment depends on the type and stage of the tumor. Surgical excision, radiation therapy, and chemotherapy are used alone or in combination.

Approximately 1% of breast cancer cases occur in men, most commonly after the 60 years of age. Treatment is similar for men and women and entails surgery, radiation therapy, chemotherapy, and endocrine therapy. Carcinoma of the penis represents less than 1% of all malignancies among men. In situ, treatment entails local excision, radiation therapy, and local application of 5-fluorouracil cream or solution. Invasive carcinoma is treated by surgical resection of the penis and the involved nodes. Radiation and chemotherapy follow as needed.

TABLE 56.6 Drugs Used for Treatment of Benign Prostatic Hyperplasia

Drug	Route and Dosage	Side Effects
5-Alpha-Reductase Inhibitors		
Finasteride	PO: 5 mg daily	Decreased libido, erectile dysfunction, orthostatic hypotension, gynecomastia
Dutasteride	PO: 0.5 mg daily	

Safety in Administration

Women of childbearing age must not handle crushed or broken tablets due to possible absorption and potential risk to male fetuses; immediately wash contact area with soap and water if contact occurs. Inform patients of an increase in high-grade prostate cancer in men treated with 5-alpha-reductase inhibitors indicated for BPH treatment. Inform patients that the volume of ejaculate may be decreased, and that impotence or decreased libido may occur. Instruct patients to promptly report to their physician any changes in breasts (lumps, pain, or nipple discharge).

Drug	Route and Dosage	Side Effects
Alpha-Adrenergic Blocking Agents		
Tamsulosin	PO: 0.4 mg/d 30 min after a meal; titrate up to 0.8 mg/d	Dizziness, headache, orthostatic hypotension, decreased libido, upper respiratory infection symptoms, priapism
Doxazosin	PO: Start 1 mg/d at bedtime; titrate up to 8 mg/d	
Terazosin	A: PO: Start 1 mg/d at bedtime; titrate up to 10 mg/d *max:* 20 mg/d	
Alfuzosin	PO: 10 mg/d after a meal	
Silodosin	PO: 8 mg/d with a meal	

Safety In Administration

Alpha-adrenergic blocking agents are also used to control blood pressure. To avoid hypotensive episodes, advise using at bedtime, and reconcile all drugs taken before adding another antihypertensive drug.
Instruct patients to take these drugs with food. Counsel about possible symptoms of postural hypotension (dizziness); caution patients about driving, operating machinery, or performing hazardous tasks while using these drugs. Inform patients that orgasm with reduced or no semen does not pose a safety concern and is reversible when the drug is stopped. Advise patients to notify their ophthalmologist about use before cataract surgery or other eye procedures.

Drug	Route and Dosage	Side Effects
Phosphodiesterase-5 Inhibitors		
Tadalafil	PO: 5 mg daily	See Table 56.5

Safety in Administration

Tadalafil should not be used by patients taking nitrates such as nitroglycerin because the combination may trigger an unsafe drop in blood pressure. Tadalafil should not be used with alpha blockers for the treatment of BPH because the combo therapy has not been adequately studied and may increase the risk of lowering blood pressure.

A, Adult; *BPH,* benign prostatic hyperplasia; *d,* day; *max,* maximum; *min,* minute; *PO,* by mouth.

CRITICAL THINKING CASE STUDY

The patient, 16 years of age, is a high school junior who is 59.3 inches tall and weighs 126 pounds. He is having increased feelings of discomfort about not fitting in with the other students at school because he has not yet begun sexual maturation. He is a good student and an accomplished violinist in the school orchestra. His father states that he also was a "late bloomer," but both parents are concerned about the patient's increasing social withdrawal and seem determined to seek medical intervention for him. The nurse at the clinic assesses the needs and status of the patient and his parents.

1. What is the patient's primary complaint?
2. What is concerning the patient's parents?
3. What information must be included in the history and physical examination?
4. What education should the nurse prepare before the parents decide whether to start their son on androgen therapy?

The decision is made to prescribe testosterone 30 mg every 12 hours by buccal tablet (held inside the cheek until it dissolves). The patient will be on this regimen for 4 months, during which time he is to come to the clinic at monthly intervals.

5. The patient asks why he will be treated for 4 months. What will the nurse reply?
6. About what adverse effects do the patient and his parents need to be educated?
7. What physical and psychosocial parameters will be assessed at the patient's monthly visits?
8. What special hygiene needs does the patient have while on this regimen?
9. When should the patient have x-rays taken? Explain your answer.

REVIEW QUESTIONS

1. A young male patient is referred to the nurse for initiation of intramuscular androgen therapy for hypogonadism. What information should the nurse give this patient? (Select all that apply.)
   a. A 4- to 6-month trial of androgen therapy will be followed by a period of rest for reevaluation.
   b. Sexual development will begin to occur immediately.
   c. Dosages may be adjusted based on periodic plasma testosterone levels.
   d. Growth will be monitored periodically by radiography.
   e. The patient should not consume alcohol.

2. A married man with two daughters is taking finasteride to treat benign prostatic hyperplasia. Which nursing assessment data are most critical in developing a care plan? (Select all that apply.)
   a. His spouse and children should not handle the drug.
   b. The drug may cause decreased libido and urinary retention.
   c. The dose needs to be reevaluated periodically.
   d. This drug may also cause his hair to grow.
   e. Using finasteride will not increase his risk for developing prostate cancer.

3. The nurse is discussing androgen therapy with a patient. Which statements will the nurse include in the patient education? (Select all that apply.)
   a. Lower extremity edema associated with androgen therapy can be increased by corticosteroids.
   b. Only men are prescribed androgen replacement therapy.
   c. Androgen therapy is safe in pregnancy.
   d. Androgen therapy can affect glucose levels, cholesterol, and thyroid and liver functioning.
   e. Androgen therapy may cause seizures.

4. During his annual physical examination, a patient tells the nurse he is in a new relationship and having some problems with erectile dysfunction. He is interested in nutrition and natural therapies. Which are the most appropriate responses by the nurse? (Select all that apply.)
   a. Herbal therapies are commonly used by men to enhance sexual performance.
   b. Side effects from using some herbal therapies include increased anxiety, frequent headaches, and trouble sleeping.
   c. Phytochemicals have been widely researched and are safe to use.
   d. Men who have cardiovascular, neurologic, or psychological problems should not use some of the herbal products.
   e. It is a good idea to increase intake of dietary vitamins.

5. The nurse is interviewing a man with erectile dysfunction who is interested in one of the phosphodiesterase inhibitors. Which response by the nurse is best for this patient?
   a. The onset of action varies among the different drugs in this class.
   b. These drugs should not be used if you take nitroglycerine for angina.
   c. Common side effects include headache, blurred vision, photosensitivity, changes in color perception, and urinary tract symptoms.
   d. There are many causes of sexual dysfunction in men, so a complete history and physical is the first step in treatment.

6. A 17-year-old is brought to the health care provider by his father because he has been taking nutritional supplements sold at the gym. Which assessment data are most critical in developing a care plan for this patient? (Select all that apply.)
   a. His blood pressure is low.
   b. His acne is worsening.
   c. He has been in several fistfights with other teenagers.
   d. He has gained 60 pounds.
   e. His liver function tests are abnormal.

7. A male patient presents with complaints of lower urinary tract symptoms, getting up three times at night to urinate, dribbling after urination, and feeling pressure throughout the day. Recent screening laboratory tests are normal. The health care provider starts him on doxazosin 1 mg at bedtime. What advice can the nurse give this patient? (Select all that apply.)
   a. Advise the patient about signs and symptoms of low blood pressure.
   b. Tell the patient to notify his ophthalmologist about the doxazosin use before cataract surgery.
   c. Caution the patient that he should not allow his wife to handle the medicine.
   d. Advise the patient to immediately report problematic prolonged erection.
   e. Instruct the patient to take the drug on an empty stomach.

57

Sexually Transmitted Infections

OBJECTIVES

- Describe the pharmacologic intervention for sexually transmitted infections (STIs) caused by bacterial and viral agents, parasites, and other pathogens.

- Relate Clinical Judgment [Nursing Process], including teaching, to the prevention of STIs.

OUTLINE

Each day, more than 1 million new cases of sexually transmitted infection (STI) occur worldwide. The incidence of STIs has been increasing since 2013. Young adults are at risk, particularly young women, but infections among men are also rising. More than 30 bacteria, viruses, and parasites can cause STIs. The most common bacterial pathogens are *Chlamydia, Neisseria gonorrhoeae,* and *Treponema pallidum* (syphilis); *Trichomonas* is a common parasite; and the most common viral pathogens are hepatitis B virus (HBV), herpes simplex virus (HSV), human immunodeficiency virus (HIV), and human papillomavirus (HPV). The majority of persons with STIs experience few or no symptoms, making it difficult to diagnose and treat to stop the spread of infections. STIs are spread through sexual contact, via blood or blood products, and through mother-to-child transmission during pregnancy and childbirth.

SEXUALLY TRANSMITTED INFECTIONS

Sexual transmission of pathogens can occur through breaks in the vaginal or cervical mucosa or in the skin covering the shaft or glans of the penis. Each act of coitus results in tiny, friction-induced fissures on these surfaces. Seminal fluid, spermatozoa, vaginal secretions, blood, and other body fluids can carry pathogens. Skin and mucosal lesions can be penetrated by microorganisms, and skin and mucosa can shed microorganisms.

Sexual contact can involve transmission of pathogens through the skin or mouth and via oral-genital, oral-anal, or hand-anal transmission of pathogens through breaks in the skin or mucosal surfaces or from inoculation by infectious body fluids. Anal penetration is particularly risky because of the likelihood of tissue trauma that results in the partner's exposure to enteric microorganisms. The risk for contracting an STI increases with substance abuse, imprisonment, sexual activity with a partner who has been imprisoned, sexual activity with individuals being paid for sex acts, and rape or sexual assault.

Patients who engage in sexual activity with multiple partners are at high risk for transmission of STIs, particularly HIV. The Centers for Disease Control and Prevention (CDC) reports the risk for getting STIs is markedly increased among individuals who have more than one sexual partner per year versus those who have fewer partners. It should be noted that 5.2% of men between the ages of 15 and 44 report having five or more partners in a 12-month period, and 2% of women report the same. Additionally, 21.8% of men between the ages of 15 and 44 report having had 15 or more sexual partners, and 10.6% of women report the same.

Other high-risk practices are anal or vaginal intercourse without a condom, hand-anal contact, contact with menstrual blood during sexual activity, use of an enema before anal intercourse, and urination on broken skin or inside the body. Refer to Fig. 57.1 for guidelines provided by the CDC on the prevention of STIs.

STIs are often manifested as multiple infections. Individuals undergoing treatment for one STI should be assessed for others, including HIV. This is especially true if genital or perianal ulcerations are present.

Vertical transmission is the passage of infecting organisms from mother to neonate. Microbes can travel up the reproductive tract from the vagina or cervix and enter the intrauterine environment. Organisms that are of little consequence to healthy adults can be devastating to a fetus. Transmission can also occur through contact with the mother's blood at birth or through breast milk, as in the case of HIV and HBV. Many STIs, such as syphilis, are transmitted through the placenta and membranes. Others, such as the herpes simplex virus type 2 (HSV-2), require actual contact by the infant with microorganisms in the birth canal. Because of the risk for blindness caused by *Chlamydia trachomatis* and *N. gonorrhoeae,* erythromycin ointment is routinely administered in the eyes of neonates as prophylaxis. This is usually done within the first hour after birth.

CDC guidelines for the primary treatment of some STI pathogens are listed in Table 57.1; the most common pathogens are discussed

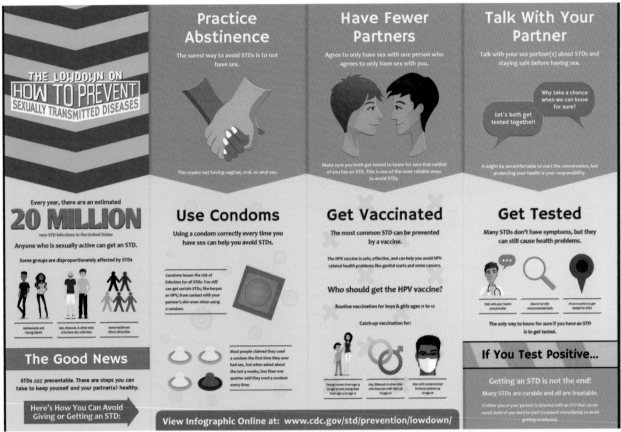

Fig. 57.1 How to prevent sexually transmitted infections. (From Centers for Disease Control and Prevention. [2016]. *How you can prevent sexually transmitted diseases.* Retrieved from www.cdc.gov/std/prevention.)

in the following section. All sexual contacts of an infected individual should be informed of the exposure so they can be treated. Partners should refrain from sexual activity until each is clear of infection on follow-up evaluation or, at the very least, condoms should be used until each is clear of infection.

SEXUALLY TRANSMITTED PATHOGENS

The information in this chapter comes directly from the 2015 treatment guidelines for STIs, available at www.cdc.gov/std/tg2015/default.htm.

Bacterial Pathogens

Sexually transmitted bacterial pathogens can be effectively treated with antibiotic therapy. When present, common symptoms include vaginal discharge, urethral discharge or burning (in men), genital ulcers, and abdominal pain.

Bacterial Vaginosis

Bacterial vaginosis (BV) causes a large amount of homogenous, thin, white vaginal discharge with a strong fishy odor. In BV, normal, healthy bacteria in the vagina—lactobacilli—are replaced with anaerobic bacteria, most commonly *Gardnerella vaginalis, Mycoplasma hominis, Ureaplasma urealyticum,* or *Prevotella, Porphyromonas, Bacteroides, Peptostreptococcus,* and *Mobiluncus* species. BV can be transmitted via sexual contact but is not considered an STI; however, having BV can increase a woman's risk for getting an STI due to the imbalance in vaginal bacteria.

BV is treated with metronidazole 500 mg by mouth (PO) twice a day for 7 days. Because metronidazole can cause stomach upset, it should be taken with food or a full glass of water or milk. Alcohol causes severe nausea and vomiting when ingested with metronidazole, so patients should be instructed not to drink alcoholic beverages or use products that contain alcohol, such as mouthwash, for the duration of drug therapy and for 48 hours after treatment.

Vaginal preparations are also effective in treating BV, such as metronidazole gel 0.75%, one 5-g applicator intravaginally at bedtime for 5 nights; clindamycin cream 2%, one 5-g applicator intravaginally at bedtime for 5 days; or clindamycin ovules, 100 mg intravaginally at bedtime for 3 days.

Oral drugs that are alternatives to metronidazole include tinidazole, either 2 g orally once a day for 2 days or 1 g orally once a day for 5 days, or clindamycin 300 mg orally twice a day for 7 days. Tinidazole has the same precautions with alcohol as metronidazole and should be taken with food. Tinidazole causes slightly less gastrointestinal (GI) upset than metronidazole. Patients taking clindamycin should be instructed to notify their health care provider if diarrhea develops because it may be an indication of *Clostridium difficile*–associated diarrhea (CDAD). Treating BV is especially important for pregnant women because of the risk of spontaneous abortion, delivery of premature or low-birth-weight babies, or pelvic infection developing after delivery. Metronidazole (oral or intravaginal) and clindamycin (oral) are the drugs of choice in pregnancy, and tinidazole should *not* be used during the first trimester of pregnancy. *None* of the drugs should be used by nursing mothers because these drugs are excreted in breast milk.

TABLE 57.1   Current Guidelines for Other Sexually Transmitted Infections

Pathogen	Primary Therapy	Notes
Chancroid *(Haemophilus ducreyi)*	Azithromycin PO: 1 g, single dose *or* ceftriaxone IM: 250 mg, single dose *or* ciprofloxacin PO: 500 mg bid for 3 d *or* erythromycin base PO: 500 mg tid for 7 d Data suggest ciprofloxacin presents a low risk to the fetus during pregnancy with a potential for toxicity during breastfeeding; therefore alternate drugs should be used during pregnancy and lactation.	Regardless of whether symptoms of the disease are present, sex partners of patients who have chancroid should be examined and treated if they had sexual contact with the patient during the 10 days preceding the patient's onset of symptoms. Men who are uncircumcised and patients with HIV infection do not respond as well to treatment as persons who are circumcised or HIV-negative. Patients should be tested for HIV infection at the time chancroid is diagnosed.
Klebsiella granulomatis (granuloma inguinale)	Recommended regimen: Azithromycin PO: 1 g/wk or 500 mg/d for at least 3 wk and until all lesions have completely healed Alternative regimens: Doxycycline PO: 100 mg bid for at least 3 wk and until all lesions have completely healed *or* ciprofloxacin PO: 750 mg bid for at least 3 wk and until all lesions have completely healed *or* erythromycin base PO: 500 mg four times a day for at least 3 wk and until all lesions have completely healed *or* trimethoprim-sulfamethoxazole PO: One double-strength (160 mg/800 mg) tablet bid for at least 3 wk and until all lesions have completely healed	All persons who receive a diagnosis of granuloma inguinale should be tested for HIV. Persons who have had sexual contact with a patient who has granuloma inguinale within the 60 days before onset of the patient's symptoms should be examined and offered therapy. Doxycycline should be avoided in the second and third trimesters of pregnancy because of the risk for discoloration of teeth and bones, but it is compatible with breastfeeding. Data suggest that ciprofloxacin presents a low risk to the fetus during pregnancy. Alternate drugs should be used during pregnancy and lactation.
Hepatitis A virus (HAV)	Patients with acute HAV usually require only supportive care, with no restrictions in diet or activity. Hospitalization might be necessary for patients who become dehydrated because of nausea and vomiting and is critical for patients with signs or symptoms of acute liver failure.	Vaccination is the most effective means of preventing HAV transmission among persons at risk for infection (see Chapter 31 for a discussion on vaccines).
Hepatitis B virus (HBV)	No specific therapy is available for persons with acute hepatitis B; treatment is supportive.	Two products have been approved for hepatitis B prevention: hepatitis B immune globulin (HBIG; recommended dose is 0.06 mL/kg IM × 1) for postexposure prophylaxis and hepatitis B vaccine (see Chapter 31 for a discussion on vaccines).
Hepatitis C virus (HCV)	The treatment of HCV is constantly changing; please see www.hcvguidelines.org for the latest recommendations.	No vaccine for hepatitis C is available, and prophylaxis with immune globulin is not effective in preventing HCV infection after exposure.
Lymphogranuloma venereum (LGV; *C. trachomatis* serovars)	Recommended regimen: Doxycycline PO: 100 mg bid for 21 d Alternative regimen: Erythromycin base PO: 500 mg four times a day for 21 d Pregnant and lactating women should be treated with erythromycin. Doxycycline should be avoided in the second and third trimesters of pregnancy because of risk for discoloration of teeth and bones, but it is compatible with breastfeeding.	Persons who have had sexual contact with a patient who has LGV within the 60 days before onset of the patient's symptoms should be examined and tested for urethral, cervical, or rectal chlamydial infection depending on anatomic site of exposure. They should be presumptively treated with an antichlamydial regimen (azithromycin 1 g PO single dose or doxycycline 100 mg PO bid for 7 d).
Mycoplasma genitalium	Uncomplicated infection: Doxycycline 100 mg 2 × daily for 7 days followed by azithromycin 1 g × 1, then 500 daily × 2 Complicated infection or macrolide-resistant *M. genitalium*: Moxifloxacin 400 mg daily × 14 days	*M. genitalium* lacks a cell wall; thus antibiotics targeting cell-wall biosynthesis (e.g., beta-lactams, including penicillins and cephalosporins) are ineffective against this organism. Sex partners should be managed according to guidelines for patients with nongonococcal urethritis (NGU), cervicitis, and PID.

bid, Twice daily; *d,* day; *HIV,* human immunodeficiency virus; *IM,* intramuscularly; *NSAID,* nonsteroidal antiinflammatory drug; *PO,* by mouth; *tid,* three times daily; *wk,* weeks.

From Centers for Disease Control and Prevention. (2015). *2015 Sexually transmitted diseases treatment guidelines.* Retrieved from https://www.cdc.gov/std/tg2015/default.htm.

Chlamydia

Chlamydia trachomatis is the most common STI in the United States in young adults. This infection is most often asymptomatic. Women who contract the infection are at risk for developing pelvic inflammatory disease (PID), ectopic pregnancies, and infertility. Because of this, it is recommended that all sexually active women under the age of 25 be screened annually for *C. trachomatis* and that all women over 25 be screened based on risk factors.

The CDC recommends azithromycin 1 g orally in a single dose as treatment for *C. trachomatis* infections or doxycycline 100 mg orally twice a day for 7 days. Alternatively, erythromycin base 500 mg orally four times a day for 7 days, erythromycin ethylsuccinate 800 mg orally four times a day for 7 days, levofloxacin 500 mg orally once daily for 7 days, or ofloxacin 300 mg orally twice a day for 7 days may be given.

Doxycycline is contraindicated in the second and third trimesters of pregnancy. In the case of a chlamydial infection during pregnancy, azithromycin 1 g orally in a single dose is the treatment of choice. Alternatively, amoxicillin 500 mg orally three times a day for 7 days may be given. If neither azithromycin nor amoxicillin is an option, erythromycin may be used.

Neonates may contract *C. trachomatis* from exposure to the mother's infected cervix during delivery. It most frequently presents as conjunctivitis that develops 5 to 12 days after delivery; however, *C. trachomatis* can also cause pneumonia in infants between 1 and 3 months old. Prenatal screening and treatment is the best means of prevention. Erythromycin ophthalmic ointment, administered to prevent gonococcal ophthalmia, may also prevent conjunctivitis caused by *C. trachomatis*.

Persons treated for *Chlamydia* infection should be instructed to abstain from sexual intercourse for 7 days after single-dose therapy or until a 7-day regimen is completed. Partners should be treated if they had sexual contact during the 60 days preceding the onset of symptoms or diagnosis.

Gonorrhea

In the United States gonorrhea is the second most common communicable disease. In men, infection by *N. gonorrhoeae* causes a greenish-yellow or whitish discharge from the penis, accompanied by burning with urination. These symptoms usually prompt them to seek evaluation and treatment but often not until they have spread the infection to others. In women, *N. gonorrhoeae* is frequently asymptomatic. Left untreated, women with *N. gonorrhoeae* infections develop PID, which can cause tubal scarring that leads to ectopic pregnancies and infertility. Oral infections caused by *N. gonorrhoeae* cause sore throat and trouble swallowing; on examination, the pharynx resembles strep throat.

Due to developing resistance to azithromycin, in uncomplicated *N. gonorrhoeae* infection in adolescents and adults, two-drug therapy is no longer recommended. Treatment of uncomplicated *N. gonorrhoeae* should be with ceftriaxone 500 mg IM as a single dose. Treatment of co-infection with *Chlamydia trachomatis*, or when chlamydia is not excluded, should be with oral doxycycline 100 mg twice a day for 7 days.

Neonates may contract *N. gonorrhoeae* from exposure to the mother's infected cervix during delivery. The infection most frequently presents as an acute illness that develops 2 to 5 days after delivery. Prenatal screening and treatment are the best means of prevention, and most states require neonates to be administered erythromycin (0.5%) ophthalmic ointment in each eye in a single application at birth to prevent conjunctivitis caused by *N. gonorrhoeae*.

Persons receiving treatment for gonorrhea should be instructed to abstain from sexual activity for 7 days after treatment. Persons diagnosed with gonorrhea should also be tested for *Chlamydia*, syphilis, and HIV. Partners should be treated if they had sexual contact during the 60 days preceding the onset of symptoms or diagnosis.

Syphilis

Syphilis is caused by the bacteria *Treponema pallidum;* if not treated early in the infectious process, it produces systemic disease that can be fatal. The disease is divided into three stages: primary, secondary, and tertiary.

Primary syphilis infections present with a sore, or chancre, at the site where the infection entered the body—typically, the penis in men and outer genitals or inner vagina in women. It is usually painless. The chancre develops about 3 weeks after exposure and resolves in 3 to 6 weeks without treatment. During this stage, the person is very contagious, even after the chancre has resolved.

Secondary syphilis is characterized by a skin rash that appears 2 to 8 weeks after the chancre. It may occur anywhere on the body, commonly on the hands and soles of the feet; the rash usually does not itch. Mucocutaneous lesions, fever, fatigue, sore throat, and lymphadenopathy may occur as well. The rash usually resolves in about 2 months. During this stage, the person remains very contagious, even after the rash has resolved. After the rash has resolved, a period that lasts anywhere from 1 year to 20 years goes by without any symptoms. This is called the latent stage, and it occurs in persons who have gone untreated. A person may remain contagious during the latent period, and diagnosis can only be made through blood testing.

Tertiary syphilis may occur as early as 1 year after infection or at any time during an untreated person's lifetime. Large sores inside the body or on the skin occur in the tertiary stage, along with cardiovascular and ocular syphilis and neurosyphilis. Examination of the cerebral spinal fluid (CSF) should be done in persons in the tertiary stage to determine neurologic involvement, even in the absence of clinical neurologic findings.

To diagnose syphilis, two types of serologic testing are necessary to avoid false positives. One test should be a nontreponemal antibody test (e.g., rapid plasma reagin [RPR] or Venereal Disease Research Laboratory [VDRL]) that tests for antibodies produced when a person has syphilis, although it may be produced in other diseases as well (e.g., Lyme disease or malaria). The other test should be a treponemal antibody test (e.g., fluorescent treponemal antibody absorption [FTA-ABS] or *T. pallidum* particle agglutination assay [TP-PA]), a test for antibodies that specifically target *T. pallidum*.

Treatment for primary and secondary syphilis is benzathine penicillin G, 2.4 million units given IM in one dose. Infants and children should be treated with benzathine penicillin G 50,000 units/kg IM up to the adult dose of 2.4 million units in a single dose, and these patients should be followed up with by a pediatric infectious disease specialist.

Adults with early latent syphilis should be treated with benzathine penicillin G 2.4 million units IM in a single dose; those with late latent syphilis or latent syphilis of unknown duration should receive benzathine penicillin G 7.2 million units total, administered as three doses of 2.4 million units IM each at 1-week intervals. Infants and children with early latent syphilis should be treated with benzathine penicillin G 50,000 units/kg IM, up to the adult dose of 2.4 million units in a single dose; those with late latent syphilis should receive benzathine penicillin G 50,000 units/kg IM, up to the adult dose of 2.4 million units, administered as three doses at 1-week intervals (total 150,000 units/kg up to the adult total dose of 7.2 million units). Infants and children should be managed by a pediatric infectious disease specialist.

Persons with tertiary syphilis should receive CSF analysis before initiating treatment. Those with normal CSF should receive benzathine penicillin G 7.2 million units total, administered as three doses of 2.4 million units IM each at 1-week intervals. Those with neurosyphilis or ocular syphilis should receive aqueous crystalline penicillin G 18 to 24 million units per day, administered as 3 to 4 million units IV every 4 hours or as a continuous infusion for 10 to 14 days. Alternatively, persons with neurosyphilis or ocular syphilis may be treated with procaine penicillin G 2.4 million units IM once daily plus probenecid 500 mg orally four times a day, both for 10 to 14 days. This alternative treatment should only be given to persons whose adherence can be ensured.

Pregnant women can pass syphilis to their fetus, with potentially fatal consequences. According to the CDC, cases of congenital syphilis have doubled since 2013. Benzathine penicillin G is the only treatment for syphilis during pregnancy. Pregnant women with syphilis in any stage who report they are allergic to penicillin should undergo penicillin allergy skin testing and desensitization and then should be treated with penicillin.

Partners should be treated if they had sexual contact during the 90 days preceding the diagnosis of primary, secondary, or early latent syphilis even if serologic testing is negative. If greater than 90 days, treatment should be initiated if serologic testing is positive or if testing is not available. All persons with syphilis at any stage should be tested for HIV.

Viral Pathogens

Infection caused by viral pathogens is not curable, although medication therapy is palliative. These include herpes simplex virus 1 (HSV-1; cross-contaminated from oral to genital) and HSV-2, HPV, and HIV.

Herpes Simplex Virus

Genital herpes is a lifelong viral infection. Two types of HSV can cause genital herpes: HSV-1 and HSV-2. Most cases of recurrent genital herpes are caused by HSV-2. Approximately 50 million people in the United States are infected with genital herpes. However, an increasing number of herpes infections are caused by HSV-1. Both types of the virus cause lesions that look like blisters, which crust over and scab. They may last for 2 to 4 weeks. The lesions may be accompanied by fever, lymphadenopathy, headache, and painful urination. Most HSV-2 cases go undiagnosed and are transmitted by people unaware that they have the infection or who are asymptomatic when transmission occurs.

Antiviral drugs are beneficial to most symptomatic patients and are the mainstay of management. It is imperative that nurses counsel patients with herpes regarding sexual and perinatal transmission and methods to reduce transmission.

Systemic antiviral drugs can control some of the signs and symptoms of genital herpes during initial and recurrent episodes or when used for daily suppressive therapy. However, these do not cure herpes or reduce the frequency and severity of recurrent episodes after drug discontinuation. Three antiviral drugs are used in the management of genital herpes: (1) acyclovir, (2) valacyclovir, and (3) famciclovir.

Recommendations for drug therapy of initial genital herpes infections is recommended using acyclovir 400 mg orally three times a day for 7 to 10 days, acyclovir 200 mg orally five times a day for 7 to 10 days, valacyclovir 1 g orally twice a day for 7 to 10 days, or famciclovir 250 mg orally three times a day for 7 to 10 days. Treatment can be extended if healing is incomplete after 10 days of therapy.

Suppressive therapy reduces the frequency of genital herpes recurrences by 70% to 80% in patients who have frequent recurrences. Recommended regimens are acyclovir 400 mg orally twice a day, valacyclovir 500 mg orally once a day, valacyclovir 1 g orally once a day, or famciclovir 250 mg orally twice a day. Valacyclovir 500 mg once a day might be less effective than other valacyclovir or acyclovir dosing regimens in persons who have 10 episodes or more per year.

For episodic treatment to be effective, treatment should begin within 1 day of lesion onset or during the prodrome (e.g., burning, itching, or tingling) that occurs anywhere from 30 minutes to a couple of days before some outbreaks. Patients should be provided with a prescription for the drug with instructions to initiate treatment immediately when symptoms begin. The recommended regimens for episodic therapy are acyclovir 400 mg orally three times a day for 5 days, acyclovir 800 mg orally twice a day for 5 days, acyclovir 800 mg orally three times a day for 2 days, valacyclovir 500 mg orally twice a day for 3 days, valacyclovir 1 g orally once a day for 5 days, famciclovir 125 mg orally twice daily for 5 days, famciclovir 1 g orally twice daily for 1 day, or famciclovir 500 mg once, followed by 250 mg twice daily for 2 days.

Sexual partners should be evaluated, treated if symptomatic, and counseled. Asymptomatic sex partners should be questioned about a history of genital lesions and offered serologic testing for HSV infection.

The risk of vertical transmission is high (30% to 50%) among women who become infected near the time of delivery and low (<1%) among women with a prenatal history of herpes or those who become infected early in the pregnancy. Prevention of vertical transmission depends on both preventing infection during late pregnancy and avoiding exposure to viral shedding during delivery. The recommended drug regimen for suppressive therapy of pregnant women with recurrent genital herpes is acyclovir 400 mg orally three times a day or valacyclovir 500 mg orally twice a day with treatment recommended starting at 36 weeks of gestation.

Human Immunodeficiency Virus

Two to 4 weeks after exposure, HIV infection typically presents with an acute flulike syndrome that includes fever, fatigue, rash, pharyngitis, and lymphadenopathy. HIV is a chronic illness that progressively depletes CD4 T lymphocytes and ends with symptomatic acquired immunodeficiency syndrome (AIDS). Early diagnosis and treatment is essential to reduce the risk of transmitting HIV to others and to maintain quality of life.

Persons with acute HIV infection are at high risk for transmitting HIV to their partner because the concentration of virus in blood and genital secretions is extremely elevated. Antiretroviral therapy (ART) during acute HIV infection is recommended because it substantially reduces transmission to others. See Chapter 32 for drugs used to treat HIV.

Partners (sexual partners and those with whom needles and syringes are shared) should be notified concerning possible exposure to HIV. Early diagnosis and treatment reduces the risk for further HIV transmission. Partner notification for HIV infection should be confidential.

All pregnant women should be tested for HIV infection during the first prenatal visit. A second test during the third trimester, preferably at less than 36 weeks' gestation, is recommended for those known to be at high risk for HIV.

Human Papillomavirus

Of the roughly 100 types of HPV infection that have been identified, nearly 40 infect the genital area. Most HPV infections are self-limited and asymptomatic, and most sexually active persons will become infected with HPV at some point in their lifetime. High-risk HPV infections (e.g., HPV types 16 and 18) cause most cervical, penile, vulvar, vaginal, anal, and oropharyngeal cancers. Low-risk HPV infection (e.g., HPV types 6 and 11) causes genital warts and recurrent respiratory papillomatosis. Screening with the Papanicolaou ("Pap") test can detect cervical dysplasia, which can be a precursor to cervical cancer if left untreated. Whereas the Pap test can determine whether the cervical cells are abnormal, an HPV test specifically looks for high-risk HPV in cervical cells.

There are several HPV vaccines approved for use in the United States: a bivalent vaccine that prevents infection with HPV types 16 and 18, which cause 66% of all cervical cancers; a quadrivalent vaccine that prevents infection with HPV types 6, 11, 16, and 18, which cause 90% of all genital warts; and a 9-valent vaccine that prevents infection with HPV types 6, 11, 16, 18, 31, 33, 45, 52, and 58. See Chapter 31 for a discussion on vaccines.

Because most HPV infections do no harm, they do not require treatment and tend to resolve on their own. Because of this, antiviral therapy is not recommended. Treatment is aimed at removal of genital warts and precancerous lesions and treatment of cervical cancer and includes cryotherapy (freezing) or a loop electrosurgical excision procedure (LEEP) to cut away abnormal tissue.

Condom use can lower the risk of transmitting and developing HPV infections. Limiting the number of sex partners can also reduce the risk for HPV. However, abstaining from sexual activity is the most reliable method for preventing HPV infection.

Other Pathogens

Pediculosis Pubis

Persons with pediculosis pubis, a parasitic infection caused by *Phthirus pubis,* usually seek treatment because of extreme pruritus of the body part or area where the lice are moving and laying egg cases. Infected persons may also notice lice or nits on their pubic hair. Pediculosis pubis is usually transmitted by sexual contact.

Recommended treatment is with a permethrin 1% cream rinse applied to affected areas and washed off after 10 minutes or pyrethrins with piperonyl butoxide applied to the affected area and washed off after 10 minutes. Alternatively, malathion 0.5% lotion can be applied to affected areas and washed off after 8 to 12 hours, or ivermectin 250 mcg/kg can be given orally and repeated in 2 weeks.

Sexual partners within the previous month should be treated, and bedding and clothing must be decontaminated. Sexual contact should be avoided until treatment is complete. Pregnant and lactating women should be treated with either permethrin or pyrethrins with piperonyl butoxide.

Scabies

Infection with *Sarcoptes scabiei* causes pruritus, which takes up to several weeks to develop. Scabies in adults frequently is sexually acquired, although scabies in children usually is not.

Treatment consists of permethrin 5% cream applied to all areas of the body from the neck down and washed off after 8 to 14 hours or ivermectin 200 mcg/kg orally, repeated in 2 weeks. Permethrin is the treatment of choice for infants and young children. Alternatively, lindane 1%—either 1 oz of lotion or 30 g of cream—applied in a thin layer to all areas of the body from the neck down and thoroughly washed off after 8 hours may be used; however, pregnant women, infants, and children under 10 years of age should *not* be treated with lindane.

Bedding and clothing should be decontaminated by either machine washing, machine drying using the hottest cycle, or dry cleaning; alternatively, bedding and clothing should be removed from body contact for at least 72 hours. Persons who have had sexual, close personal, or household contact with the patient within the month preceding scabies infestation should be examined and treated if infected.

Ivermectin likely poses a low risk to pregnant women and is likely compatible with breastfeeding; however, because of limited data regarding ivermectin use in pregnant and lactating women, permethrin is the preferred treatment

Trichomoniasis

The protozoan parasite *Trichomonas vaginalis* is the most common curable STI in the United States. Nearly 7.5 million cases occur annually. Most people with *T. vaginalis* (70% to 85%) have minimal or no symptoms. Men may develop urethritis, epididymitis, or prostatitis. Some infected women may develop a diffuse vaginal discharge that is malodorous and yellow green, with or without vulvar irritation.

The nitroimidazoles are the only class of antimicrobials effective against *T. vaginalis.* Metronidazole and tinidazole are approved for oral or parenteral treatment of trichomoniasis. The recommended regimen is metronidazole 2 g orally in a single dose or tinidazole 2 g orally in a single dose. Alternatively, metronidazole 500 mg orally twice a day for 7 days may be used.

Alcohol should be avoided during treatment with nitroimidazoles to prevent the likelihood of a disulfiram-like reaction. Abstinence from alcohol use should continue for 24 hours after completion of metronidazole or 72 hours after completion of tinidazole. Concurrent treatment of all sex partners is critical to prevent transmission and reinfection.

T. vaginalis is readily passed between sex partners. The best way to prevent infection is through consistent and correct use of condoms. Partners of men who have been circumcised might have a somewhat reduced risk of *T. vaginalis* infection.

T. vaginalis infection in pregnant women is associated with premature rupture of membranes, preterm delivery, and delivery of a low-birth-weight infant. The recommended treatment regimen in pregnant women is metronidazole 2 g orally in a single dose.

Vulvovaginal Candidiasis

Vulvovaginal candidiasis (VVC) is usually caused by *Candida albicans* but may also be caused by other *Candida* species. Typical symptoms of VVC include pruritus, vaginal soreness, dyspareunia, external dysuria, and abnormal vaginal discharge. Signs include vulvar edema, fissures, excoriations, and a thick, curdy vaginal discharge.

Treatment with topically applied azole drugs results in symptomatic relief and negative cultures in 80% to 90% of patients who complete therapy. A variety of over-the-counter (OTC) and prescription drugs may be used to treat VVC. Treatment regimens include OTC and prescription intravaginal agents.

Over-the-Counter Intravaginal Agents. Clotrimazole 1% cream 5 g intravaginally daily for 7 to 14 days, clotrimazole 2% cream 5 g intravaginally daily for 3 days, miconazole 2% cream 5 g intravaginally daily for 7 days, miconazole 4% cream 5 g intravaginally daily for 3 days, one miconazole 100-mg vaginal suppository daily for 7 days, one miconazole 200-mg vaginal suppository daily for 3 days, one miconazole 1200 mg vaginal suppository, or tioconazole 6.5% ointment 5 g intravaginally in a single application.

Prescription Intravaginal Agents. Butoconazole 2% cream (single-dose bioadhesive product) 5 g intravaginally in a single application, terconazole 0.4% cream 5 g intravaginally daily for 7 days, terconazole 0.8% cream 5 g intravaginally daily for 3 days, or one terconazole 80 mg vaginal suppository daily for 3 days. Alternatively, an oral drug—fluconazole 150 mg orally in a single dose—may be used.

Topical agents usually cause no systemic side effects, although local burning or irritation might occur. Oral azoles occasionally cause nausea, abdominal pain, and headache.

VVC occurs frequently during pregnancy. Only topical azole therapies, applied for 7 days, are recommended for use among pregnant women. Uncomplicated VVC is not usually acquired through sexual intercourse, thus treatment of sexual partners is not necessary.

PREVENTION OF SEXUALLY TRANSMITTED INFECTIONS

Because STIs can threaten reproductive health, neonatal health, fertility, and even life, early diagnosis and treatment are crucial but are less effective than prevention. Please review the information in Box 57.1 and in the Nursing Process box that discusses STI prevention.

◎ CLINICAL JUDGMENT [NURSING PROCESS]

Sexually Transmitted Infections

Concept: Safety

- Protection of the patient from potential or actual harm; is a basic human need

Concept: Sexuality

- A person's sexual expression and function

Recognize Cues [Assessment]

- Assess use of barrier methods and the patient's ability to obtain them.
- Assess patient history before gathering physical data. Address less sensitive issues before more personal ones so trust can first be established. Use the term *partner* when discussing sexual activity, rather than judgment-laden terms such as *wife* or *boyfriend*. Include the following questions for all patients, regardless of gender or sexual orientation: "Do you have sex with women?" and "Do you have sex with men?" Include information regarding the number of sexual partners.
- Assess history of drug use.
- Assess history of sexually transmitted infections (STIs).
- Assess support systems.
- Complete a review of body systems and obtain a general health history and a gynecologic history that includes reproductive history; also review lifestyle and social habits and identify known allergies.
- Physical examination includes inspection and palpation of the mouth, oropharynx, throat and lymph nodes, abdomen, and inguinal lymph systems. Also perform a physical examination of the genitalia and other points of potential inoculation.

Analyze Cues and Prioritize Hypothesis [Patient Problems]

- Need for health teaching
- Sexual expression
- Potential decreased adherence
- Decreased self-esteem

Generate Solutions [Planning]

- The patient will abstain from sexual contact until infection is treated and adopt risk-reducing sexual behaviors.
- The patient will identify signs and symptoms of STIs.
- The patient will verbalize when to seek medical attention.
- The patient will remain free from STIs.

Take Action [Nursing Interventions]

- Observe and report signs of infections (e.g., redness, discharge, fever).
- Note laboratory findings as appropriate.
- Ensure understanding of appropriate transmission-based precautions.
- Ensure an understanding of appropriate personal hygiene.
- Ensure responsible use of antibiotics.
- Discuss the risks for developing STIs with all patients, even older adults.
- Discuss condom use negotiation; counsel patients on effective use of condoms.
- See Fig. 57.2 for the right way to use a male condom.
- Review modes of transmission of STIs, the relationship of all STIs to human immunodeficiency virus (HIV) infection, and how HIV risk is avoided.
- Use a medical interpreter of the same sex and culture, especially for sensitive topics.

Evaluate Outcomes [Evaluation]

- The intervention has been successful if patients and their partners are successfully treated and remain free of infection.
- The patient is able to avoid sexual practices that carry risk for acquiring STIs, including intercourse without the use of a condom.

BOX 57.1   Special Topic: Sexually Transmitted Infections in the Older Adult

The rates of *Chlamydia*, gonorrhea, and syphilis have more than doubled in adults over 50 years of age in recent years. Over 15% of newly diagnosed cases of HIV occur in adults over 50 years of age. This spike in sexually transmitted infections (STIs) is felt to be related to a combination of factors:

- Patients are reluctant to bring up the issue with their health care providers and their health care providers are reluctant to bring up the issue with the patient.
- Older adults may not consider oral or anal sex as a way to transmit STIs.
- We are living longer and have higher divorce rates than past generations, leading to increased numbers of older adults entering the dating scene.
- Postmenopausal changes in women (e.g., decreased vaginal lubrication) put them at increased risk for infection.

- The availability of drugs for erectile dysfunction makes sex possible for an increased number of older men.
- Rates of condom use are low because condoms were used to prevent pregnancy in previous generations, not to prevent STIs.

Nurses must discuss the risks for developing STIs with their older adult patients and should provide information on prevention. Nurses should not make the faulty assumption that older adults do not engage in sexual activity. Among men, 85% report that sex is important in their relationships; 61% of women report that sex is important in their relationships. Among older adults, 28% have sex at least once a week. However, only 12% of men and 32% of women use condoms.

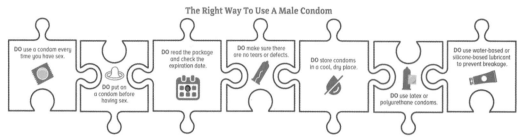

Fig. 57.2 How to use a male condom. (From Centers for Disease Control and Prevention. [2016]. *The right way to use a male condom.* Retrieved from www.cdc.gov/condomeffectiveness/male-condom-use.html.)

CRITICAL THINKING SINGLE EPISODE CASE STUDY

Cognitive Skill: Take action

Item Type: Extended multiple response

A 16-year-old female comes to the clinic, reporting her partner has noted a whitish penile discharge and has burning with urination. She states she has been sexually active, both orally and vaginally, for 2 years and has had four partners during this time. She denies using any barrier methods to avoid infection and is not on any other form of birth control. The patient also reports a sore throat. She denies any cough or congestion, headache, nausea, vomiting, or diarrhea. She denies any burning, urgency, or frequency of urination or vaginal discharge. The patient is living with her 62-year-old grandmother, along with her older brother. Her mother and father lost their parenteral rights due to abuse. She admits to vaping cannabis for the past few years and drinks hard liquor when out with her boyfriends. She is a year behind in school and has frequent tardiness and absences. Her blood pressure is 105/60 mm Hg, heart rate is 66 beats per minute, respirations 12 breaths per minute, and temperature 98.9°F. She is 5'8" tall and weighs 110 pounds (BMI 16.72 kg/m²) The nurse spends time talking with the patient before she is discharged from the clinic and providing necessary teaching and support.

What nursing actions are appropriate for the patient at this time? Select all that apply.

_____a. Administer ceftriaxone 250 mg intramuscular as a single dose, as ordered.

_____b. Teach the patient appropriate use of condoms.

_____c. Review the modes of sexually transmitted infection transmission with the patient.

_____d. Assess the patient's support systems and make referrals as necessary.

_____e. Administer azithromycin 1 g orally as a single dose, as ordered.

_____f. Discuss with patient the necessity of her partner coming to the clinic for treatment.

_____g. Administer ceftriaxone 500 mg intramuscular as a single dose, as ordered.

_____h. Instruct the patient to abstain from sexual activity for seven days after treatment.

Answer

__X__a. Administer ceftriaxone 250 mg intramuscular as a single dose, as ordered.

__X__b. Teach the patient appropriate use of condoms.

_____c. Review the modes of sexually transmitted infection transmission with the patient.

_____d. Assess the patient's support systems and make referrals, as necessary.

__X__e. Administer azithromycin 1 g orally as a single dose, as ordered.

__X__f. Discuss with patient the necessity of her partner coming to the clinic for treatment.

__X__g. Administer ceftriaxone 500 mg intramuscular as a single dose, as ordered.

__X__h. Instruct the patient to abstain from sexual activity for seven days after treatment.

Rationale

Due to developing resistance to azithromycin, in uncomplicated *N. gonorrhea* in adolescents and adults two-drug therapy is no longer recommended. Treatment of uncomplicated *N. gonorrhea* should be with ceftriaxone 500 mg intramuscular as a single dose. Appropriate nursing actions include assessing support systems and counseling patients on effective condom use, and the modes of sexually transmitted infection transmission should be reviewed with the patient. Partners should be treated if they had sexual contract during the 60 days preceding onset of symptoms or diagnosis. In this scenario, the partner is symptomatic as well and should be treated. Persons receiving treatment for gonorrhea should be instructed to abstain from sexual activity for 7 days after treatment.

▮ REVIEW QUESTIONS

1. A patient at the sexually transmitted infection clinic asks why he was not prescribed antibiotics. He has been diagnosed with herpes simplex virus type 2. The nurse's best response is based on what knowledge? (Select all that apply.)
   a. Antibiotics will not lessen the symptoms of herpes simplex virus.
   b. Herpes simplex virus can be cured with antiviral medications only.
   c. Antibiotics are used to successfully treat viral infections.
   d. Herpes simplex virus symptoms may be relieved with palliative antiviral medications.
   e. Antibiotics combined with antiviral medications are the best treatment for herpes simplex virus type 2 infections.

2. The nurse is teaching a group of junior high school students about preventing sexually transmitted infections if they are sexually active. Which of the following are the best methods of prevention? (Select all that apply).
   a. Douching after intercourse
   b. Monogamy
   c. Vaccination
   d. Consistent condom use
   e. Use of spermicidal creams

3. Which one of the following regimens is an appropriate treatment for episodic genital herpes infection?
   a. Acyclovir 400 mg orally three times a day for 5 days
   b. Famciclovir 2 g orally twice daily for 1 day
   c. Acyclovir 1 g orally once a day for 5 days
   d. Valacyclovir 500 mg orally twice a day for 7 days

4. The nurse is reviewing a patient's medications; she knows treatment of vulvovaginal candidiasis includes which drug?
   a. Metronidazole
   b. Fluconazole
   c. Metformin
   d. Ibuprofen

5. Your patient with primary syphilis has an order for penicillin G benzathine 2.4 million units IM × 1. You have available penicillin G benzathine 600,000 units per mL; how many mL will be administered?

6. When teaching a group of students about *Chlamydia*, which of the following should the health care provider emphasize? (Select all that apply).
   a. Most people who have *Chlamydia* have no symptoms.
   b. Good handwashing technique is the best way to prevent chlamydial infections.
   c. *Chlamydia* is the least common of all the major sexually transmitted infections.
   d. Burning and pain with urination may be a symptom of chlamydial infections.
   e. *Chlamydia* has no effect on future pregnancies.

7. A patient diagnosed with trichomoniasis is being treated with a nitroimidazole. When teaching the patient about this medication, which of the following is the most important for the nurse to include?
   a. Call our office if you experience any tendon pain or tenderness.
   b. You should avoid milk or dairy products during therapy.
   c. Do not drink alcohol while you are taking this medication.
   d. Report the occurrence of pain in your upper abdomen immediately.

8. Your patient calls stating she stopped taking the oral metronidazole that was prescribed because her symptoms resolved, and she wanted to drink at her best friend's bridal shower. As her nurse, what is your best response?
   a. No serious complications can happen from untreated *T. vaginalis*, so don't worry.
   b. Without treatment, the organism remains in your body, and you remain contagious.
   c. Because your symptoms are gone, there is no need to complete the course of metronidazole.
   d. If symptoms return, come back.

Adult and Pediatric Emergency Drugs

Linda Laskowski-Jones, MS, APRN, ACNS-BC, CEN, NEA-BC, FAWM, FAAN

http://evolve.elsevier.com/McCuistion/pharmacology

OBJECTIVES

- Describe indications for the emergency drugs listed in this chapter.
- Define the basic mechanism of action for each emergency drug.
- Discuss pertinent nursing considerations and actions specific for each drug.

- Explain how to properly administer emergency drugs.
- Describe significant adverse effects of each drug.

OUTLINE

INTRODUCTION

This final unit focuses on adult and pediatric first-line emergency drugs. This chapter considers oxygen as an emergency drug and discusses pharmacologic treatment for five categories of emergency situations: (1) cardiac disorders, (2) intracranial hypertension, (3) poisoning, (4) shock, and (5) hypertensive crises and pulmonary edema. Specific drug protocols and dosages for the pediatric patient are included when appropriate.

The drugs described in this chapter are first-line agents used to treat selected common emergency situations. Nurses must have knowledge of the indications and actions of these drugs because medical and surgical emergencies can occur in virtually any area of nursing practice. Learning key nursing implications *before* a crisis situation enables the nurse to function at the highest possible level when the patient requires life-saving intervention.

At the end of the discussion of each group of emergency drugs is a summary prototype drug chart that contains dosages and indications. Common adult dosages are listed in the drug charts; pediatric dosages may vary widely depending on the child's age and weight. For the purpose of drug dosing, advanced life support (ALS) guidelines consider adults to be older than 8 years and children to be 8 years or younger; infants are younger than 1 year. The drug charts list only the most common indications and dosages for the emergency drugs discussed; they do *not* describe all possible uses and dosing regimens for each drug.

OXYGEN AS AN EMERGENCY DRUG

Oxygen can be classified as a drug because it can have both beneficial and adverse effects on the body based on the amount and manner in which it is administered. Oxygen is essential to life—without it, brain death begins within 6 minutes. Inadequate oxygenation produces hypoxemia, inadequate oxygen in the blood, and leads to significant physiologic sequelae to all body systems; therefore oxygen is a first-line drug for all emergency situations in which hypoxemia poses a physiologic threat. Oxygen is a pulmonary vasodilator and a cerebral vasoconstrictor. Depending on the circumstances, adequate oxygenation may be all that is necessary to effectively treat physiologic disturbances that arise from hypoxemia, such as chest pain, bradycardia, and cardiac dysrhythmias. However, current evidence suggests that more liberal oxygen administration may be associated with increased mortality in patients who are not hypoxemic.

Before the other pharmacologic drugs discussed in this chapter are administered, ensure that the patient's airway and breathing are addressed to promote normoxemia, typically defined as an oxygen saturation between 94% and 99% depending on the patient's diagnosis and physiologic state. Giving a drug to treat a disorder brought on by hypoxemia without effectively correcting the cause of the hypoxemia is ineffective and ultimately does not produce the desired outcome. Pulse oximetry, which provides a digital display of oxygen saturation, is an essential monitoring tool that should be used in emergency situations to assess the adequacy of oxygenation and guide further interventions. Ideally oxygen saturation should be titrated based upon defined clinical parameters. For example, a patient who was successfully resuscitated from cardiac arrest should have oxygen delivered to achieve pulse oximetry readings in a range of 92% to 98%, while a patient who had a stroke should achieve oxygen saturation of greater than 94%. Increasing the saturation beyond the goal saturation range with supplemental oxygen may produce detrimental effects. It is also important to recognize that certain pathophysiologic states can make pulse oximetry readings inaccurate. These conditions include vasoconstriction, severe anemia, hypothermia, carbon monoxide poisoning, and shock.

The ambient room air contains approximately 21% oxygen. When patients breathe room air, the oxygen they inspire constitutes 21% of the total volume of gas they take in with each breath. This measure is termed the fraction of inspired oxygen (FiO_2). Patients with hypoxemia due to severe physiologic stress from shock states, major trauma with hemodynamic instability, and cardiac arrest initially require supplemental oxygen in high concentrations (i.e., an FiO_2 approaching 100%). The initial emergency oxygen delivery devices of choice for these conditions include a nonrebreather mask with an oxygen reservoir (oxygen flow rate set at 10 to 15 L/min) for spontaneously breathing patients and a bag valve mask device attached to an oxygen source at a flow rate of 15 L/min for patients who require assisted ventilation until definitive airway management and a mechanical ventilator are available.

Although caution must be exercised for patients with chronic obstructive pulmonary disease (COPD), who may lose their hypoxic respiratory drive when given oxygen in high concentration, oxygen should never be denied to a patient who needs it. In the case of COPD, the nurse should be prepared to ventilate the patient manually with a bag valve mask if respiratory depression or arrest occurs. Some patients in respiratory distress as a result of obstructive pulmonary disease or acute cardiogenic pulmonary edema may also benefit from oxygen therapy delivered through noninvasive mask ventilation via a continuous positive airway pressure (CPAP) or bilevel positive airway pressure (BiPAP) circuit; these devices deliver oxygen via a positive-pressure mechanism.

Whatever the underlying injury or disease process, as the patient's condition stabilizes, the oxygen concentration should be decreased to achieve the goal range, typically an arterial oxygen saturation between 94% and 96%. An FiO_2 above 50% for a prolonged period can lead to oxygen toxicity and other detrimental effects in both adults and children.

For situations that do not involve severe physiologic stress, supplemental oxygen delivered by nasal cannula at 1 to 6 L/min or by simple face mask at 6 to 10 L/min may be considered. Young children may better tolerate a face tent with a high oxygen flow of 10 to 15 L than a face mask. Current evidence suggests that oxygen administration to hemodynamically stable patients without heart failure who are normoxemic may offer no therapeutic benefit, may be detrimental, and should be avoided.

EMERGENCY DRUGS FOR CARDIAC DISORDERS

Drugs described in this section are indicated for cardiac emergencies such as angina, myocardial infarction ([MI] heart attack), disturbances of cardiac rate or rhythm, and cardiac arrest. In a resuscitation situation, the foundation of patient therapy is based upon proper oxygenation and ventilation, performance of optimal cardiopulmonary resuscitation (CPR), and application of electrical therapy (cardioversion and defibrillation) according to established treatment algorithms and standards. Drugs are used as adjuncts in synchrony with these efforts when indicated to enhance the likelihood of a successful outcome. These drugs often must be prepared and administered rapidly. A sound knowledge base and easy access to the drugs and necessary equipment are essential for the best patient response in a cardiac emergency. In many emergency situations, detailed personal, medical, drug, and herbal histories are unavailable. Treatment is based on patient presentation.

Aspirin

The nonenteric form of aspirin is a first-line emergency drug used to decrease platelet aggregation in the management of acute coronary syndromes and MI. It is best administered immediately upon the onset of chest pain in doses of 162 to 325 mg orally. The patient should be asked to chew the tablet to speed absorption of the drug instead of swallowing the tablet whole. For patients experiencing nausea and vomiting, an aspirin rectal suppository in a dose of 300 mg can be given as an alternative. Contraindications to aspirin administration include a true drug allergy, presence of cerebral hemorrhage on computed tomography (CT) scan, and recent gastrointestinal (GI) bleeding.

Nitroglycerin

Nitroglycerin dilates coronary arteries and improves blood flow to an ischemic myocardium. It is therefore the treatment of choice for angina pectoris (chest pain) and MI. Nitroglycerin is also considered a first-line drug in the management of patients with acute cardiogenic pulmonary edema due to its ability to decrease both preload and afterload. A focused prescription drug history is essential before administration, even in emergency situations, because nitroglycerin in combination with drugs for erectile dysfunction (i.e., sildenafil, vardenafil, tadalafil) causes profound hypotension that may be refractory to treatment when taken within a 24- to 48-hour period. This combination is contraindicated. Nitroglycerin is available in sublingual, translingual aerosol spray, oral, topical, and intravenous (IV) forms. Only the sublingual, translingual aerosol spray, and IV preparations are discussed.

Sublingual nitroglycerin (0.3- to 0.6-mg tablets) and the translingual aerosol spray (0.4 mg metered dose) preparations are indicated for patients experiencing an acute anginal attack who have a systolic blood pressure above 90 mm Hg. The patient is taught to sit or lie down and moisten 1 sublingual nitroglycerin tablet with saliva and then place it under the tongue to allow it to dissolve slowly. If the chest pain is not relieved, sublingual nitroglycerin may be repeated at 5-minute intervals—as long as the patient's systolic blood pressure remains above 90 mm Hg—until a total of 3 tablets have been taken. Patients prescribed the translingual aerosol preparation should be reminded that the spray should not be inhaled. Instead, it should be sprayed onto or under the tongue. The patient should be instructed not to swallow for approximately 10 seconds to allow absorption of the drug. As with sublingual nitroglycerin, up to 3 doses may be taken within 15 minutes. If pain persists despite 3 doses of the sublingual tablet or aerosol forms, further interventions are necessary in an emergency or critical care setting. An ambulance should be called if the patient is outside the hospital, and blood pressure and heart rate must be monitored closely. Hypotension is a common adverse effect, especially the first time a patient takes nitroglycerin. Tachycardia, an abnormally high heart rate in adults (>100 beats/min), or, uncommonly, bradycardia, a slow heart rate, also may occur. Patients who take sublingual tablets or translingual aerosol spray nitroglycerin while wearing a nitroglycerin patch may be at higher risk for hypotension. This situation warrants caution. However, individuals who take daily nitroglycerin can develop tolerance to the drug, which can provide some protection against hypotension. If hypotension persists or worsens, the nitroglycerin patch may need to be removed. To prevent arcing and the potential for skin burns, the nitroglycerin patch, like other medication patches in the area of the pads or paddles, must be removed before cardioversion or defibrillation.

Intravenous nitroglycerin is reserved for patients with unstable angina or AMI. A continuous infusion is usually initiated at a rate of 5 mcg/min and titrated by 5 mcg/min every 3 to 5 minutes based on chest pain and blood pressure response. Maximum rate of titration is 20 mcg/min every 3 to 5 minutes. Continuous blood pressure and heart monitoring are required because hypotension is a common adverse effect. Hypotension usually is treated by reducing or discontinuing the nitroglycerin infusion (see Chapter 37) and by placing the patient in a supine position with legs elevated if tolerated.

Morphine Sulfate

Morphine sulfate, an opiate analgesic, is used to treat the chest pain associated with ST-segment elevation myocardial infarction (STEMI) if unrelieved by nitroglycerin administration. It also is indicated for acute cardiogenic pulmonary edema. Morphine relieves pain, dilates venous vessels, and reduces the workload on the heart. The standard dosage of morphine sulfate is 1 to 4 mg IV over 1 to 5 minutes, repeated every 5 to 30 minutes until chest pain is relieved. Because respiratory depression and hypotension are common adverse effects, the drug must be administered slowly and must be carefully titrated to achieve the desired therapeutic effects. Close patient monitoring is essential. It is important to realize that although morphine can produce respiratory depression, this drug can also relieve the dyspnea caused by pulmonary edema. In this situation, respiratory distress is not a contraindication to morphine administration. The opioid antagonist naloxone may be ordered to reverse the action of morphine if adverse effects pose a significant risk to the patient. The dose is 0.4 to 2 mg every 2 minutes as indicated (see Chapter 25).

Atropine Sulfate

Atropine sulfate is the primary drug indicated for the treatment of hemodynamically significant bradycardia and some types of heart block (e.g., atrioventricular [AV] block at the nodal level). Atropine acts to increase heart rate by inhibiting the action of the vagus nerve (parasympatholytic effect). Atropine sulfate is also used as an emergency drug to reverse the toxic effects of organophosphate pesticide and nerve agent exposure, which include bradycardia and excessive secretions.

In symptomatic bradycardia with hemodynamic compromise, atropine is administered IV in 1 mg doses at 3- to 5-minute intervals until the desired heart rate is achieved or until 3 mg is given. Dosing in this manner may be repeated every 3 to 5 minutes up to a maximum of 3 mg IV.

The adult IV atropine dose should never be less than 0.5 mg. Doses below 0.5 mg may produce a paradoxical bradycardia; at doses of 3 mg or greater, vagal activity is considered completely blocked, and further atropine administration may have no benefit. However, in the case of organophosphate insecticide or nerve agent poisoning, *very high* doses of atropine may be necessary to counteract the pathophysiologic effects of these toxins. Therefore, the typical dosing range and limits do not apply under these circumstances.

If venous access is not available in an emergency situation, atropine sulfate should be administered through the intraosseous (IO) route.

Continuous cardiac and blood pressure monitoring is essential for the patient who receives atropine sulfate. Significant adverse effects include cardiac dysrhythmias, tachycardia, myocardial ischemia, restlessness, anxiety, mydriasis, thirst, and urinary retention. See Chapter 16 for more information on atropine and other anticholinergics.

Pediatric Implications

The definition of bradycardia is variable and age specific for the pediatric population. Knowledge of normal ranges is essential. Because cardiac output is dependent on heart rate in infants younger than 6 months, bradycardia (heart rate <100 beats/min for infants) must be treated. In fact, a heart rate less than 60 beats/min in an infant requires performance of CPR. Before administration of drugs, efforts always should be targeted first toward restoring adequate ventilation and oxygenation. For the neonate with a spontaneous heart rate of less than 80 beats/min, epinephrine 0.01 mg/kg IV or IO every 3 to 5 minutes as indicated should be given before atropine to elevate the heart rate because stressed neonates quickly deplete their own stores of catecholamines. If these interventions do not produce the desired clinical response, atropine is indicated in the presence of increased vagal tone or AV block. Other pediatric indications for atropine include management of organophosphate toxicity and as pretreatment to prevent bradycardia after succinylcholine administration during rapid-sequence intubation, although this specific indication is currently controversial.

The pediatric dose of atropine is 0.02 mg/kg IV or IO. It is important to be cognizant that in the pediatric population, the minimum single dose is 0.1 mg, and the maximum single dose is 0.5 mg IV. The maximum total pediatric dose is 1 mg in a child and 3 mg in an adolescent (defined as an individual who has reached puberty). Note that when referring to general age groupings of patients, *infants* are considered to be younger than 1 year; a *child* is considered to be 1 year of age to adolescence (puberty), and an *adult* is considered to be an adolescent or older. See Chapters 6, 10, and 11 for more information on pediatric medication dosing and monitoring.

Adenosine

Adenosine is the first-line drug of choice to treat paroxysmal supraventricular tachycardia (PSVT), a sudden, uncontrolled, rapid rhythm that exceeds 150 ventricular beats/min in adults and originates above the ventricles. The goal is to convert PSVT to sinus rhythm. Adenosine, a natural substance found in all body cells, slows impulse conduction through the heart's AV node, interrupts dysrhythmia-producing reentry pathways, and restores a normal rhythm in patients with PSVT.

Because the half-life is less than 5 seconds, adenosine is best administered rapidly via a peripheral IV site in the port most proximal to the patient as a 6 mg IV bolus over 1 second followed by a saline flush and immediate elevation of the arm. A 12 mg bolus may be given 1 to 2 minutes after the initial dose using the same procedure if PSVT persists. The 12-mg dose may be repeated once if indicated for persistent PSVT. Higher doses are not recommended.

Nursing considerations include continuous cardiac monitoring and frequent assessment of vital signs. Adenosine is inhibited by methylxanthines such as caffeine and theophylline, so higher doses may be needed. Although usually transient, ventricular ectopy, bradycardia, flushing, chest pain, and dyspnea may occur. In addition, a short period of asystole may follow injection of adenosine (up to 15 seconds). Spontaneous cardiac activity typically resumes. Adenosine is contraindicated in patients with poison- or drug-related tachycardia, second- and third-degree heart block, and sick sinus syndrome except those with functioning pacemakers. If the tachycardia originated in the ventricles, the patient could deteriorate and become hypotensive after adenosine administration. Adenosine is contraindicated in patients with bronchospastic disease because it may induce bronchospasm. See Chapter 37 for more information on antidysrhythmic drugs.

Pediatric Implications

Adenosine is used to treat narrow complex PSVT in pediatric patients who do not have evidence of cardiopulmonary compromise such as an altered mental status, shock, or hypotension. The dose is 0.1 mg/kg as a rapid IV/IO bolus to a maximum first dose of 6 mg. If the PSVT does not resolve after the first dose, a second dose of 0.2 mg/kg as a rapid IV/IO bolus to a maximum second dose of 12 mg can be given. The same nursing considerations and precautions apply as described for adults.

Diltiazem

Diltiazem is a calcium channel blocker, and it is administered as an IV bolus to treat PSVT and to slow the ventricular response rate in atrial fibrillation or flutter. It is considered a second-line agent after adenosine. Diltiazem has less of a negative inotropic effect than other, similar calcium channel blockers, but it has strong negative chronotropic actions. Therefore IV diltiazem is less likely to cause cardiac depression but is very effective in controlling heart rate.

The usual initial bolus dose of IV diltiazem is 0.25 mg/kg given over 2 minutes. If the supraventricular tachycardia does not convert to a normal sinus rhythm in 15 minutes, a second IV bolus of 0.35 mg/kg over 2 minutes may be necessary. For ongoing control of the ventricular rate in patients with atrial fibrillation or flutter, a continuous infusion of diltiazem is indicated at a dose range of 5 to 15 mg/hour, titrated according to the desired heart rate.

The nurse must carefully monitor blood pressure and heart rate and rhythm after administering IV diltiazem. Arrhythmias, bradycardia, heart block, and hypotension may develop. Diltiazem can elevate serum digoxin levels, predisposing the patient to digitalis toxicity. Simultaneous use of calcium channel blockers and beta blockers is contraindicated because their negative inotropic and negative chronotropic effects are synergistic, causing myocardial depression and bradycardia. Other contraindications include preexisting heart failure, Wolff-Parkinson-White syndrome, heart block, or sick sinus syndrome in the patient without a pacemaker, and in advanced aortic stenosis.

Amiodarone

The IV form of amiodarone is considered a first-line drug in the ALS algorithms for the treatment of life-threatening ventricular dysrhythmias and cardiac arrest. It has alpha- and beta-adrenergic blocking effects and acts on sodium, potassium, and calcium channels. Indications for use include pulseless ventricular tachycardia and ventricular fibrillation (after defibrillation and epinephrine), hemodynamically stable ventricular tachycardia, PSVT refractory to adenosine, ventricular rate control in atrial fibrillation, and pharmacologic treatment of atrial fibrillation.

Amiodarone is especially good for patients with impaired heart function who have atrial and ventricular dysrhythmias. It has been found to be more effective and to have fewer proarrhythmic properties than other drugs with similar actions.

For patients who have a pulse (i.e., those *not* in cardiac arrest), amiodarone 150 mg IV is given over 10 minutes, followed by a continuous infusion of 1 mg/min for 6 hours. For patients in cardiac arrest with pulseless ventricular tachycardia or ventricular fibrillation, a dose of 300 mg diluted in 20 to 30 mL D_5W is given as a rapid infusion followed by a continuous infusion as described earlier. Additional doses of 150 mg may be given by rapid infusion if ventricular fibrillation or ventricular tachycardia recurs.

Significant adverse effects include hypotension and bradycardia; therefore the nurse would slow the infusion rate to prevent or treat these effects and be prepared to administer IV fluids, vasopressors, and agents to increase heart rate. A temporary pacemaker may be needed. Amiodarone has a very long half-life. It should not be given concurrently with other drugs that prolong QT interval on electrocardiography (ECG), such as procainamide.

Pediatric Implications

Amiodarone has an off-label use among pediatric patients. It is given for pulseless ventricular tachycardia and ventricular fibrillation as a 5 mg/kg rapid IV/IO bolus, which can be repeated up to a maximum dose of 15 mg/kg per 24 hours. For responsive children who have supraventricular (junctional and atrial) tachycardia and ventricular dysrhythmias with pulses present, amiodarone is given as a 5 mg/kg IV/IO loading dose (300 mg maximum) over 20 to 60 minutes and repeated to a maximum daily IV dose of 15 mg/kg per 24 hours in pediatric patients or 2.2 g per 24 hours in adolescents.

Lidocaine

As an alternative to amiodarone, lidocaine may be used to treat significant ventricular dysrhythmias, or irregular heartbeats, such as frequent premature ventricular contractions (PVCs), ventricular tachycardia, and ventricular fibrillation. Lidocaine exerts a local anesthetic effect on the heart, thus decreasing myocardial irritability. Typically, a patient with ventricular dysrhythmias is given a 1 to 1.5 mg/kg bolus of lidocaine, followed by 0.5 mg/kg to 0.75 mg/kg every 5 to 10 minutes until the dysrhythmia is controlled or a total dose of 3 mg/kg has been administered via the IV or IO route.

Important nursing considerations for the patient receiving lidocaine include continuous cardiac monitoring and assessment for signs and symptoms of lidocaine toxicity (e.g., confusion, drowsiness, hearing impairment, cardiac conduction defects, myocardial depression, muscle twitching, and seizures). Because lidocaine is metabolized by the liver, patients with hepatic impairment are at a higher risk for toxicity; other risks include heart failure, shock, and advanced age (>70 years). In these patients, the lidocaine dose may need to be reduced by as much as 50% (see Chapter 40). Lidocaine is contraindicated as a *prophylactic* agent to prevent ventricular dysrhythmias after AMI.

Pediatric Implications

Ventricular ectopy is uncommon in children; therefore metabolic causes should be suspected if ventricular dysrhythmias occur. The pediatric dose of lidocaine is 1 mg/kg IV or via the IO route, and the endotracheal tube (ETT) dose is 2 to 3 mg/kg. Prototype Drug Chart: Lidocaine Hydrochloride lists the pharmacologic data for lidocaine.

PROTOTYPE DRUG CHART

Lidocaine Hydrochloride

Drug Class	Dosage
Antidysrhythmic, class IB	A: IV/IO: 1–1.5 mg/kg; may repeat 0.5 mg/kg q5–10min; *max:* 3 mg/kg A: ETT: 2–4 mg/kg C: IV/IO: Initially: 1 mg/kg C: ETT: 2–3 mg/kg Therapeutic range: 2–6 mcg/mL
Contraindications	**Drug-Lab-Food Interactions**
Hypersensitivity, advanced atrioventricular block *Caution:* Liver disease, heart failure, older adults	Drug: Increased effects with phenytoin, quinidine, procainamide, propranolol; increased risk for toxicity with cimetidine, beta-adrenergic blockers
Pharmacokinetics	**Pharmacodynamics**
Absorption: IV Distribution: PB: 60%–80%; concentrates in adipose tissue Metabolism: t½: Initial: 7–30 min; terminal: 9–120 min Excretion: Through the liver	PO: Onset: 45–60 s Peak: 45–60 s Duration: 10–20 min
Therapeutic Effects/Uses	
Antiarrhythmic drug to treat ventricular dysrhythmias such as premature ventricular contractions (PVCs), ventricular tachycardia, and ventricular fibrillation Mechanism of Action: Decreases automaticity; increases electrical threshold of ventricle.	
Side Effects	**Adverse Reactions**
Drowsiness, confusion, dyspnea, lethargy, hypotension, nausea, vomiting	*Life-threatening:* Seizures, cardiac arrest

A, Adult; *C,* child; *ETT,* endotracheal tube; *IO,* intraosseous; *IV,* intravenous; *max,* maximum; *min,* minute; *PB,* protein binding; *PO,* by mouth; *q,* every; *s,* seconds; *t½,* half-life.

Procainamide

Procainamide is an antidysrhythmic drug prescribed for ventricular tachycardia, PVCs, and rapid supraventricular dysrhythmias unresponsive to adenosine. The typical IV loading dose of procainamide is 20 to 50 mg/min until the dysrhythmia is successfully treated. Other end points to procainamide administration include a total administration of 17 mg/kg of the drug, development of hypotension, and specific changes on the ECG (e.g., widening of the QRS complex by 50% or more). A continuous maintenance infusion of 1 to 4 mg/min may be ordered after the loading dose. A procainamide infusion should be avoided in patients with congestive heart failure and in those with a prolonged QT interval.

The nurse must monitor vital signs and the ECG with particular attention to heart rate and rhythm, blood pressure, and the width of the QRS complex. Procainamide administration can cause severe hypotension. Heart block, rhythm disturbances, and cardiac arrest can also occur. Procainamide is contraindicated in patients with torsades de pointes, an unusual polymorphic ventricular tachycardia often associated with a prolonged QT interval. Procainamide is eliminated via the kidneys; therefore patients with renal failure are at higher risk of adverse effects and often require a lower dosage.

Magnesium Sulfate

Magnesium is an essential element in multiple enzymatic reactions in the body, including function of the sodium-potassium adenosine triphosphatase (ATPase) pump. Its physiologic effects can be likened to a calcium channel blocker with neuromuscular blocking properties. Hypomagnesemia is associated with the development of atrial and ventricular dysrhythmias.

Magnesium sulfate is the drug of choice for torsades de pointes. It is administered by diluting 1 to 2 g (2 to 4 mL of a 50% solution) in 10 mL of D5W or normal saline. For cardiac arrest caused by torsades de pointes, magnesium is given by direct IV push or via the IO route over 5 to 20 minutes. For patients experiencing torsades de pointes who are not in cardiac arrest, a magnesium infusion of 1 to 2 g diluted in 50 to 100 mL of D5W or normal saline can be given IV/IO over 5 to 60 minutes.

Although magnesium toxicity is rare, the nurse should monitor the patient's response to magnesium administration. Hypotension is the most common adverse effect when magnesium is given by rapid IV push. Other effects include mild bradycardia, flush, and sweating. True hypermagnesemia can cause diarrhea, respiratory depression, deep tendon reflex impairment, flaccid paralysis, and circulatory collapse. Because magnesium is eliminated via the kidneys, it should be administered with caution in patients with renal impairment.

Pediatric Implications

Indications for magnesium sulfate in pediatric patients include torsades de pointes, hypomagnesemia, and status asthmaticus that is unresponsive to beta-adrenergic drugs. The magnesium sulfate dose is 25 to 50 mg/kg IV/IO (maximum dose of 2 g) given as a bolus for pulseless ventricular tachycardia, slowly over 10 to 20 minutes for ventricular tachycardia with pulses and over 15 to 30 minutes for status asthmaticus.

Epinephrine

Epinephrine is a catecholamine with alpha- and beta-adrenergic effects. It has multiple uses. Emergency cardiac indications for administration of IV/IO epinephrine include profound bradycardia and hypotension, asystole, pulseless ventricular tachycardia, and ventricular fibrillation. Epinephrine is thought to improve perfusion of the heart and brain in cardiac arrest states by constricting peripheral blood vessels. In addition, epinephrine increases the chances for successful electrical countershock (defibrillation) in ventricular fibrillation. ⚡ It is important to be aware that epinephrine is available in two primary concentrations: 1:1000 and 1:10,000. The 1:10,000 concentration is used when administering a single IV/IO dose of epinephrine. The 1:1000 form is used when preparing a continuous epinephrine infusion or when giving epinephrine via the intramuscular (IM) route. The subcutaneous (subcut) route should not be used for emergency epinephrine administration because absorption is unpredictable.

For profound bradycardia or hypotension, an epinephrine infusion may be ordered at 0.1 to 0.5 mcg/kg/min. For asystole, pulseless ventricular tachycardia, and ventricular fibrillation, epinephrine is administered in 1 mg doses (1:10,000 solution) IV/IO every 3 to 5 minutes until the desired clinical response—usually return of effective cardiac activity—is achieved. In pulseless ventricular tachycardia and ventricular fibrillation, epinephrine is administered after the second defibrillation is delivered during CPR.

Nursing implications for patients receiving epinephrine include constant cardiac and hemodynamic monitoring. Epinephrine can cause myocardial ischemia and cardiac dysrhythmias. It should never be administered in the same site as an alkaline solution, such as with sodium bicarbonate, because alkaline solutions inactivate epinephrine. In addition, the presence of metabolic or respiratory acidosis decreases the effectiveness of epinephrine. All efforts should be made to correct acid-base imbalances in the patient. More drug information about epinephrine and other adrenergic drugs can be found in Chapter 15.

⚡ **PATIENT SAFETY**

- Ensure that the correct concentration (1:1000 vs. 1:10,000) is administered. The 1:10,000 preparation is meant to be given intravenously.

Pediatric Implications

The pediatric dose of epinephrine is 0.01 mg/kg (1:10,000 solution) given every 3 to 5 minutes IV/IO for cardiac arrest. For profound bradycardia or hypotension in pediatric patients, a continuous infusion of epinephrine can be given at a dose of 0.1 mcg/kg/min via IV/IO. Higher doses may be considered.

Sodium Bicarbonate

Sodium bicarbonate is prescribed to treat severe metabolic acidosis as well as hyperkalemia and acidotic states related to specific drug overdose situations. Sodium bicarbonate is not considered a first-line drug for the treatment of cardiac arrest; it is preferentially given based on results of arterial blood gas analysis when acidosis is severe. The current standard is to give sodium bicarbonate only after adequate resuscitative efforts, including effective ventilation, IV fluids, and drug therapy, fail to correct the acidotic state in cardiopulmonary arrest. The standard initial IV dose of sodium bicarbonate is 1 mEq/kg. Subsequent dosing depends on arterial blood gas analysis and achievement of therapeutic targets.

Important nursing considerations relevant to sodium bicarbonate include careful monitoring of arterial blood gas analysis results. Sodium bicarbonate administration can lead to metabolic alkalosis, which may be very difficult to reverse and can have deleterious physiologic effects. Catecholamines such as epinephrine, norepinephrine,

and dopamine should not be infused in the same site as sodium bicarbonate because they are inactivated by solutions that contain sodium bicarbonate.

Table 58.1 lists emergency cardiac drugs and their dosages, uses, and considerations.

Pediatric Implications

If severe metabolic acidosis persists after attention has been directed at maintaining optimal ventilation and oxygenation, sodium bicarbonate may be given to the pediatric patient in a 1 mEq/kg dose via the IV or IO route. It may also be given as treatment for a tricyclic antidepressant (TCA) overdose. Sodium bicarbonate is hyperosmolar and should be diluted from an 8.4% solution (1 mEq/mL) to a 4.2% solution (0.5 mEq/mL) for infants.

EMERGENCY DRUG FOR INTRACRANIAL HYPERTENSION

Mannitol

Mannitol is an osmotic diuretic used in emergency, trauma, critical care, and neurosurgical settings to treat cerebral edema and to reduce increased intracranial pressure (intracranial hypertension), which may occur after head trauma, neurosurgery, malignancy, and with other types of intracranial pathology (see Chapter 41). Mannitol may be given as an IV bolus or via a continuous drip. The usual initial bolus dose of mannitol ranges from 0.25 g/kg to 1 g/kg IV of a 20% to 25% solution. Subsequent dosing is highly variable and is influenced by serum osmolality and the patient's blood pressure. In general, mannitol is held when serum osmolality exceeds 320 mOsm/kg or when hypotension is present. Mannitol is highly irritating to veins, and the nurse must use a filter needle when administering the drug because crystals may form in the solution and syringe and can be inadvertently injected. When a filter needle is used to draw up the mannitol, a *new* filter needle *must* be used to administer the mannitol IV. In addition, the nurse should carefully assess the patient's neurologic status; monitor blood pressure and laboratory studies, including electrolytes and serum osmolality; and keep accurate intake and output records to assess fluid volume status because diuresis may be substantial. Prototype Drug Chart: Mannitol lists the pharmacologic data for mannitol.

EMERGENCY DRUGS FOR DRUG OVERDOSE

Although numerous antidotes exist for specific types of drug overdose, the drugs presented in this section are most commonly prescribed in cases of drug overdose and ingestion of toxic substances, and pertinent exceptions are noted. Particular attention must be given to administration guidelines to achieve the best possible clinical outcome for the patient. These drugs are cross-referenced to their specialty chapters.

Naloxone

Naloxone is classified as an opioid antagonist. It reverses the effects of all opioid drugs (e.g., morphine, hydromorphone, fentanyl, codeine, oxycodone, heroin) by competitively binding to opioid receptor sites in the body. Naloxone is indicated for individuals who have taken an overdose of opioid drugs, those experiencing respiratory or cardiovascular depression or arrest from therapeutic doses of opioids given in a health care setting, and those brought to the emergency department in a coma or cardiac arrest of unknown etiology (which may be drug induced). Given the epidemic of opioid overdoses in the general community, there is a widespread effort in many states to make naloxone available to medical first responders and even to members of the lay public who frequently encounter drug misuse and abuse.

TABLE 58.1 Emergency Cardiac Drugs

Generic	Route and Dosage[a]	Uses and Considerations
Adenosine	A/C/Adol >50 kg: IV/IO: Initially 6 mg, then 12 mg in 1–2 min if needed C/Adol <50 kg: IV/IO: 0.1 mg/kg/dose. May repeat 0.2 mg/kg/dose	For paroxysmal supraventricular tachycardia PB: UK; t½: <10 s
Amiodarone	A: IV: With pulse: 150 mg over 10 min, then continuous infusion 1 mg/min for 6 h Cardiac arrest: 300 mg diluted in 20–30 mL D₅W rapidly; second dose 150 mg, followed by continuous infusion as previously discussed; *max:* 2.2 g/d	Part of ALS algorithm for treatment of both atrial and ventricular dysrhythmias PB: UK; t½: 26–107 d
Atropine sulfate	A: IV/IO: 1 mg; can repeat up to 0.04 mg/kg or 3 mg (max) C/Adol: IV: 0.02 mg/kg/dose, repeat up to 1 mg max in C; 3 mg max in Adol	For symptomatic bradycardia and asystole PB: 60%–80%; t½: 2–3 h
Diltiazem	A: IV: 0.25 mg/kg; repeat in 15 min at 0.35 mg/kg IV drip: 5–10 mg/h	For supraventricular tachycardia and atrial fibrillation and flutter PB: 80%; t½: 2–5h
Epinephrine	A: IV: 1 mg; may be repeated q3–5 min C/Adol: IV: 0.01 mg/kg/dose, may repeat q3–5 min C/Adol: ETT: 0.1 mg/kg/dose, may repeat q3–5 min	For cardiac arrest PB: UK; t½: UK
Lidocaine	See Prototype Drug Chart: Lidocaine	
Magnesium sulfate	A: Dilute 1–2 g (2–4 mL of 50% solution) in 10 mL of D₅W. Give IV/IO in cardiac arrest due to torsades de pointes over 5–20 min Torsades de pointes with a pulse: 1–2 g diluted in 50–100 mL of D₅W given IV over 5–60 min followed by continuous infusion of 0.5–1 g/h	Drug of choice for torsades de pointes after defibrillation in patients with a prolonged QT interval; rapid infusion can cause hypotension PB: 25%–35%; t½: 30 min
Morphine sulfate	A: IV: 1–5 mg q5–30 min	For chest pain, unstable angina, pulmonary edema PB: 35%; t½: 2–2.5 h
Nitroglycerin	A: SL: 0.3–0.6 mg; translingual aerosol spray: 0.4 mg metered dose, up to 3 tab/sprays within 15 min onto or under the tongue A: IV drip: Initially 5 mcg/min; titrate by 5 mcg/min q3–5 min; *max rate of titration:* 20 mcg/min q3–5 min	For chest pain, angina, unstable angina, MI; hypotension can occur *Contraindication:* With drugs for erectile dysfunction (e.g., sildenafil). PB: 60%; t½: 1–4 min
Procainamide hydrochloride	A: IV: 20–50 mg/min; *max:* 17 mg/kg; followed by 1–4 mg/min IV drip Recognized end points: Hypotension, QRS widens >50%, or total of 500 mg administered	For PVCs, ventricular tachycardia, ventricular fibrillation, atrial dysrhythmias PB: 20%; t½: 3–4 h
Sodium bicarbonate	A/C >2 y: IV: Initially 1 mEq/kg, then dose based on ABG results	For severe metabolic acidosis unresponsive to resuscitation, hyperkalemia, and certain types of drug overdoses. Not for routine use in cardiac arrest PB: UK; t½: UK

A, Adult; *ABG,* arterial blood gas; *ALS,* advanced life support; *Adol,* adolescent; *C,* child; *d,* day; *h,* hour; *IO,* intraosseous; *IV,* intravenous; *max,* maximum; *MI,* myocardial infarction; *min,* minute; *PB,* protein binding; *PVC,* premature ventricular contraction; *q,* every; *resp,* respiratory; *s,* second; *SL,* sublingual; *t½,* half-life; *tab,* tablet; *UK,* unknown; *y,* year; >, greater than; <, less than.
[a]Other dosing regimens for neonates, infants, and children are available.

The typical dose of naloxone for actual or suspected opioid overdose in adults is 0.4 to 2 mg IV administered every 2 minutes until the patient's condition improves to an acceptable level. If there is no improvement within 10 minutes after 10 mg of the drug has been injected, nonopioid drugs or disease must be suspected. Although ideally naloxone should be administered intravenously in emergency situations, it also may be given via IO, IM, subcut, and intranasal (IN) routes if IV access is not readily obtainable. The adult dose for the IN route is 1 mg per nostril. IN naloxone offers the advantages of a reduced risk of needlestick injuries as well as a readily accessible route of administration for rescuers and laypersons. Naloxone autoinjectors are also available to facilitate rapid IM administration by rescue personnel and members of the general public.

Because most opioid drugs have a longer duration of action than naloxone, the nurse must monitor the patient closely for signs and symptoms of recurrent opioid effects such as respiratory depression and hypotension. In this situation, naloxone administration may need to be repeated several times, or a continuous IV infusion may be

prescribed. Naloxone has no major opioid effects, but it can precipitate withdrawal symptoms in patients addicted to opioid drugs and, rarely, it can cause anaphylaxis. In addition, pulmonary edema has been reported after naloxone administration in patients who have had an overdose of morphine (see Chapter 25). Nurses also must be on guard for combative or violent behavior after naloxone administration, especially in patients who have overdosed on an illicit drug; having security personnel available to stand by is prudent. Prototype Drug Chart: Naloxone Hydrochloride lists the pharmacologic data for naloxone.

Pediatric Implications

For opioid reversal in children, give 0.1 mg/kg, repeating the drug as necessary by bolus every 2 minutes as needed up to 2 mg based upon desired therapeutic effects. Naloxone can be administered as an IV bolus, continuous infusion or via IO, IM, or subcut routes in children. If needed to maintain opioid reversal, a continuous IV or IO infusion of naloxone can be administered in a range of 0.002 to 0.16 mg/kg per hour.

📄 **PROTOTYPE DRUG CHART**

Mannitol

Drug Class	Dosage
Osmotic diuretic	A: IV: 0.25–1 g/kg q4h Dosing is highly individualized. Hold for serum osmolality >320 mOsm/kg

Contraindications	Drug-Lab-Food Interactions
Hypersensitivity, severe dehydration *Caution:* Pregnancy, breastfeeding, current intracranial bleeding	Drug: May decrease effectiveness with lithium

Pharmacokinetics	Pharmacodynamics
Absorption: IV Distribution: PB: Confined to extracellular space Metabolism: t½: 100 min Excretion: In urine	Decrease in intracranial pressure: IV: Onset: 30–60 min Peak: 1 h Duration: 6–8 h Diuresis: IV: Onset: 1–3 h Peak: 1 h Duration: 6–8 h

Therapeutic Effects/Uses	
To treat increased intracranial pressure, cerebral edema Mechanism of Action: Inhibits reabsorption of electrolytes and water by affecting pressure of glomerular filtrate.	

Side Effects	Adverse Reactions
Temporary volume expansion, hyponatremia/hypernatremia, hypokalemia/ hyperkalemia, dehydration, blurred vision, dry mouth	Pulmonary congestion, fluid/electrolyte imbalances *Life-threatening:* Convulsions

A, Adult; *h,* hour; *IV,* intravenous; *min,* minute; *PB,* protein binding; *q,* every; *t½,* half-life; *>,* greater than.

Flumazenil

Flumazenil is the reversal agent for the respiratory depressant and sedative effects of benzodiazepine drugs (e.g., diazepam, midazolam, chlordiazepoxide). It is administered to counteract the effects of benzodiazepines given as sedative or anesthetic drugs as well as to treat accidental or intentional benzodiazepine overdose. Flumazenil does not reverse the central nervous system (CNS) depressant effects of nonbenzodiazepine agents such as alcohol, opiates, and barbiturates, and may not reverse amnesia induced by benzodiazepines.

For suspected benzodiazepine overdose, flumazenil is given IV in an initial dose of 0.2 mg over 30 seconds. A second dose of 0.3 mg may be given over 30 seconds. A third dose and subsequent doses of 0.5 mg IV may be given every minute until the desired clinical response is achieved or until a total dose of 3 mg is given within an hour. If sedation occurs again, doses of flumazenil may be repeated at 20-minute intervals (not to exceed 1 mg at a time) to a total hourly dose of no more than 3 mg IV. If patients have only a partial response to 3 mg of flumazenil, additional doses may be administered slowly up to a 5 mg total dose. At that point, if the patient still has not responded to flumazenil, the cause of the depressed level of consciousness is a problem other than an adverse benzodiazepine effect.

Nursing considerations include careful assessment of respiratory rate and effort, blood pressure, and mental status. If the benzodiazepine is reversed too rapidly, patients may have emergence reactions in which they become agitated and confused and experience perceptual distortions. Because seizures are precipitated by benzodiazepine withdrawal, seizure precautions must be implemented for patients at risk (those with long-standing benzodiazepine use or abuse) and for those who have a known seizure disorder.

Activated Charcoal

Activated charcoal may be prescribed for poisoning as a means to prevent absorption of toxins into the body if the ingested substance is known to be affected by charcoal in the GI tract. A poison control center should be contacted as soon as possible to help guide medical therapy. In cases of known or suspected poisoning, activated charcoal is prepared as a slurry and is given to the patient orally or via a gastric tube, ideally within 30 minutes to 1 hour of ingestion, sometimes after gastric lavage. The dose is highly variable and is dependent on the amount of poison ingested, the age of the patient, and the type of activated charcoal formulation used. Activated charcoal dosing may need to be repeated for certain types of poisoning, particularly from drugs such as salicylates, slow-release drug preparations, and *Amanita phalloides* (death cap mushrooms), to name a few.

Because vomiting is a common adverse reaction, patients with an impaired gag reflex and/or an impaired mental status are at high risk for aspiration after ingesting activated charcoal. Aspiration pneumonia and death can occur. To promote safety, these patients may need intubation for airway protection followed by administration of the activated charcoal via a gastric tube. Activated charcoal should not be administered with milk products, because they decrease its adsorptive properties. Activated charcoal is ineffective and should not be given to patients who have ingested some forms of pesticides, hydrocarbons, alcohol, acids or alkalis, lithium, solvents, and iron supplements. A cathartic, a purgative that results in bowel movements, may be ordered after administration of activated charcoal to speed elimination of the charcoal-toxin complex from the body. The patient should be told that charcoal produces black stools.

Table 58.2 lists the emergency drugs for poisoning and their dosages, uses, and considerations.

EMERGENCY DRUGS FOR SHOCK

Drugs may be required to elevate blood pressure and to improve cardiac performance in various types of shock states. Therapeutic agents described in this section are primarily indicated in conditions such as cardiogenic, neurogenic, septic, anaphylactic, and insulin shock. A noteworthy exception to the list is hypovolemic shock, that resulting from loss of blood or fluid volume; drugs should never be used as the primary therapy to correct the hypotension associated with this condition. Administration of fluids or blood products or both is the only acceptable initial means to treat hypovolemic shock. However, if hypotension persists after appropriate volume resuscitation, vasoactive drugs may be necessary to elevate and sustain blood pressure. The drugs that follow are cross-referenced to their specialty chapters.

TABLE 58.2 Emergency Drugs for Drug Overdose

Generic	Route and Dosage	Uses and Considerations
Flumazenil	A: IV: Initially 0.2 mg over 30 s; additional doses of 0.3–0.5 mg are given over 30 s q1min as indicated. For resedation, may repeat at 20-min intervals to a total dose of no more than 3 mg per hour C/Adol: IV: Initially 0.01 mg/kg over 15 s, up to a max dose of 0.2 mg; may repeat at 1-min interval; *max:* 0.05 mg/kg or 1 mg, whichever is lower	Reversal agent for benzodiazepine overdose; may precipitate seizures in patients with long-term use or abuse of benzodiazepines and those with seizure disorders; may precipitate emergent reactions PB: 50%; t½: variable (40–80 min)
Naloxone	See Prototype Drug Chart: Naloxone	
Activated charcoal	A/C: PO: dose based on age, toxin, and formulation	For poisoning Onset: <1 min; PB: NA; t½: NA

A, Adult; *Adol,* adolescent; *C,* child; *IV,* intravenous; *max,* maximum; *min,* minute; *NA,* not applicable; *PB,* protein binding; *PO,* by mouth; *q,* every; *s,* second; *t½,* half-life; <, less than.

📄 PROTOTYPE DRUG CHART

Naloxone Hydrochloride

Drug Class	**Dosage**[a]
Opioid antagonist	A: IV/IM/IO/subcut/IN: 0.4–2 mg, repeating every 2–3 min PRN C: IV/IM/subcut/IO: age and weight based: 0.1–2 mg; may repeat q2–3 min PRN

Contraindications	**Drug-Lab-Food Interactions**
Hypersensitivity, respiratory depression *Caution:* Opioid-dependent patients, cardiac disease, breastfeeding neonates of opioid-dependent mothers	Drug: Naloxone can precipitate withdrawal in patients dependent on opioid analgesics. Lab: Urine vanillylmandelic acid (VMA), 5-hydroxyheptadecatrienoic acid (5-HIAA), urine glucose

Pharmacokinetics	**Pharmacodynamics**
Absorption: IM/subcut: Well absorbed Distribution: PB: UK Metabolism: t½: Adults: 1–4 h; neonates: 1–3 h Excretion: In urine metabolites	IM/IN/subcut: Onset: 2–5 min Peak: UK Duration: 1–4 h IV/IO: Onset: 1–2 min Peak: UK Duration: 1–4 h

Therapeutic Effects/Uses

To treat respiratory depression caused by opioids; to treat opioid-induced depressant effects and opioid overdose
Mechanism of Action: Blocks effects of opioids by competing for receptor sites.

Side Effects	**Adverse Reactions**
Negligible pharmacologic effect without opioids in the body	Nausea, vomiting, tremulousness, sweating, tachycardia, elevated blood pressure *Life-threatening:* Atrioventricular fibrillation, pulmonary edema (with overdose of morphine)

A, Adult; *C,* child; *h,* hour; *IM,* intramuscular; *IN,* intranasal; *IO,* intraosseous; *IV,* intravenous; *min,* minute; *PB,* protein-binding; *PRN,* as needed; *q,* every; *subcut,* subcutaneous; *t½,* half-life; *UK,* unknown.
[a]Other dosing regimens for neonates, infants, and children are available.

PROTOTYPE DRUG CHART

Dopamine Hydrochloride

Drug Class	Dosage
Adrenergic agonist	A: IV drip: 5–20 mcg/kg/min; >10 mcg/kg/min may be ordered if lower doses are ineffective. C/Adol: IV: 1–20 mcg/kg/min; titrate in increments of 2.5–5 mcg/kg/min.

Contraindications	Drug-Lab-Food Interactions
Hypersensitivity, tachydysrhythmias, ventricular fibrillation, pheochromocytomas *Caution:* Whether this drug is safe in children is unknown.	Drug: May result in hypertensive crisis when used within 2 wk of MAOIs; concurrent IV administration of phenytoin may result in hypotension and bradycardia; sodium bicarbonate solutions inactivate dopamine—do not administer these through the same IV line.

Pharmacokinetics	Pharmacodynamics
Absorption: IV Distribution: PB: UK Metabolism: t½: 2 min Excretion: In urine	IV: Onset: 1–2 min Peak: <5 min Duration: <10 min

Therapeutic Effects/Uses
To treat hypotension in shock states after adequate fluid and/or blood product resuscitation; to increase heart rate in atropine-refractory bradycardia Mechanism of Action: Stimulates receptors to cause cardiac stimulation; increases systemic vascular resistance.

Side Effects	Adverse Reactions
Palpitations, tachycardia, hypertension, ectopic beats, angina, IV line site irritation, piloerection, nausea, vomiting	Cardiac dysrhythmias, azotemia, tissue sloughing (from extravasation) *Life-threatening:* MI, gangrene in extremities (from vasoconstriction)

A, Adult; *Adol,* adolescent; *C,* child; *IV,* intravenous; *MAOI,* monoamine oxidase inhibitor; *MI,* myocardial infarction; *min,* minute; *PB,* protein binding; *t½,* half-life; *UK,* unknown; *wk,* week; >, greater than; <, less than.

Dopamine

Dopamine is a sympathomimetic agent often used to treat hypotension in shock states (see Chapter 15). Dopamine may also be used to increase heart rate (beta$_1$ effect) in bradycardic rhythms when atropine has not been effective. The typical dose range is 5 to 20 mcg/kg/min. Dopamine enhances cardiac output by increasing myocardial contractility and increasing heart rate (beta$_1$ effect), and it elevates blood pressure through vasoconstriction (alpha-adrenergic effect). Alpha effects predominate at higher doses—vasoconstriction of renal, mesenteric, and peripheral blood vessels occurs. Although sometimes necessary to maintain adequate blood pressure in severe shock, such vasoconstriction can lead to poor organ and tissue perfusion, decreased cardiac performance, and reduction of urine output. The lowest effective dose of dopamine should be used. Patients must be weaned gradually from dopamine; abrupt discontinuation of the infusion can cause severe hypotension.

Dopamine is typically mixed as a concentration of 200 to 800 mg in 250 mL D$_5$W or normal saline solution and is administered intravenously by an electronic infusion device for precision, preferably in a central vein. Sodium bicarbonate will inactivate dopamine; therefore it should not be infused in the same IV line. Continuous heart and blood pressure monitoring is essential. The nurse must carefully document vital signs, cardiac rhythm, and intake and output as prescribed. Significant adverse effects include tachycardia, dysrhythmias, myocardial ischemia, nausea, and vomiting. The IV site must be assessed hourly for signs of drug infiltration; extravasation (escape into tissues) of dopamine can produce tissue necrosis that may necessitate surgical debridement and skin grafting. If extravasation occurs, the site should be injected in multiple areas with phentolamine, 5 to 10 mg diluted in 10 to 15 mL of normal saline, to reduce or prevent tissue damage. Prototype Drug Chart: Dopamine Hydrochloride lists the pharmacologic data for dopamine.

⚡ PATIENT SAFETY

Do not confuse...
- **Dopamine** with **dobutamine**

Dobutamine

Dobutamine is a sympathomimetic drug with beta-adrenergic activities (see Chapter 15). The beta$_1$ effects include enhancing the force of myocardial contraction (positive inotropic effect) and increasing heart rate (positive chronotropic effect). The beta$_2$ effects produce mild vasodilation. Dobutamine is indicated in shock states when improvement in cardiac output and overall cardiac performance is desired. Blood pressure is elevated only through the increase in cardiac output. The usual IV dose range of dobutamine is 2 to 20 mcg/kg/min (titrated) administered via an electronic infusion device for precision. A typical concentration of dobutamine is 250 to 1000 mg mixed in 250 mL of D$_5$W or normal saline. Like dopamine, dobutamine administration should be tapered gradually as the patient's condition warrants; abrupt discontinuation can precipitate clinical deterioration.

Continuous cardiac and blood pressure monitoring is required for patients receiving dobutamine infusions. Adverse effects are dose related and include myocardial ischemia, tachycardia, dysrhythmias, headache, nausea, and tremors. The nurse must carefully monitor intake and output and assess for any signs or symptoms of myocardial ischemia such as chest pain or development of dysrhythmias.

Norepinephrine

Norepinephrine is a catecholamine with extremely potent vasoconstrictor actions (alpha-adrenergic effect) (see Chapter 15). It is used in shock states, often when drugs such as dopamine and dobutamine have failed to produce adequate blood pressure or as first-line alternative to dopamine. Like high-dose dopamine, the peripheral vasoconstriction that results has the potential to impair cardiac performance and decrease organ and tissue perfusion. In general, 4 mg of norepinephrine are added to 250 mL D$_5$W or normal saline solution for a concentration of 16 mcg/mL and are infused at 8 to 12 mcg/min initially, titrated down to a maintenance dose of 2–4 mcg/min as a continuous infusion. For adults with sepsis, a dosing range of 0.01 to 3 mcg/kg/min may be prescribed. Maximum titrated dose is 3.3 mcg/kg/min. Continuous cardiac monitoring and precise blood pressure monitoring are required. The drug must be tapered slowly; abrupt discontinuation can result in severe hypotension.

Nursing actions and considerations are the same as those for dopamine. Norepinephrine should not be used as an initial therapy to treat hypotension in hypovolemic patients; fluid, blood, or both must be administered to restore adequate volume first. Adverse effects of norepinephrine include myocardial ischemia, dysrhythmias, and impaired organ perfusion. Extravasation of norepinephrine causes tissue necrosis, so attention to the IV site is essential. If extravasation occurs, the area should be infiltrated with phentolamine, as was described for dopamine.

Pediatric Considerations

Norepinephrine is given to pediatric patients to treat hypotensive shock after adequate fluid administration via the IV/IO route in a dose range of 0.03 to 0.5 mcg/kg/min (titrated).

Epinephrine

Epinephrine is the drug of choice in the treatment of anaphylactic shock, an allergic response of the most serious type, brought about by an antibody-antigen reaction (see Chapter 15). Anaphylactic shock can be fatal if prompt treatment is not initiated. Severe bronchoconstriction and hypotension resulting from cardiovascular collapse are its hallmarks. Epinephrine is also indicated for an acute, severe asthmatic attack.

Administration of epinephrine causes bronchodilation, enhanced cardiac performance, and vasoconstriction to increase blood pressure. In severe asthma and anaphylactic shock, epinephrine is given in a dose range of 0.3 to 0.5 mg IM for adults (1:1000 solution). The IM route is used because it has a more predictable pattern of absorption than the subcutaneous route. Given the prevalence of severe allergic reactions to foods, drugs, and insect stings, epinephrine autoinjectors in both adult and pediatric formulations are available to facilitate rapid emergency IM administration of the drug by health care personnel in some settings as well as for self-administration by patients. As an alternative, epinephrine can be given in a dose of 0.05 to 0.1 mg IV over 5 to 10 minutes (1:10,000 solution) by healthcare personnel with cardiac monitoring capability. Epinephrine administration can be repeated every 5 to 15 minutes if necessary. For patients who do not respond to repeated doses of epinephrine, a continuous epinephrine infusion may be indicated at a starting rate of 0.1 mcg/kg/min, titrated to clinical response. The upper dosing limit is highly variable.

The patient who receives epinephrine must be closely monitored for tachycardia, cardiac dysrhythmias, hypertension, and angina. Patients who are given IV epinephrine must be on a cardiac monitor with resuscitation equipment immediately available. Other adverse effects include excitability, fear, anxiety, and restlessness. In addition, the nurse should be alert to the possibility that the anaphylactic response may recur and necessitate repeated treatment. For this reason, antihistamines and steroids are ordered as a standard component of treatment for an allergic reaction along with epinephrine. Diphenhydramine is a commonly prescribed antihistamine and is discussed later. Examples of steroids are hydrocortisone sodium succinate, prednisone, and methylprednisolone. After the initial dose, the steroids are slowly tapered over days to weeks to prevent recurrence.

Patient education should include strict avoidance of the agents responsible for the anaphylactic reaction and follow-up care with a health care provider. For some patients, such as those with severe allergic responses to insect stings or certain foods, the health care provider may prescribe an epinephrine kit, pen, or other type of autoinjector to be carried with the patient for self-medication in the event of contact with the antigen. Proper patient education regarding the use of the kit or pen is essential. See Chapter 1 for more information on patient teaching.

Albuterol

Albuterol is a beta-adrenergic bronchodilator (see Chapter 15) used to reverse bronchoconstriction in anaphylactic shock; asthma, inflammation and narrowing of the airways caused by enhanced responsiveness of the tracheobronchial system to a variety of stimuli; and COPD. In emergency situations, albuterol is typically administered via nebulizer (adults: 2.5–5 mg albuterol in the manufacturer's recommended volume and type of diluent). Albuterol is also supplied as a metered-dose inhaler (MDI), which the patient can carry to self-administer a "rescue" dose of the drug during an acute episode of bronchospasm. The nurse should assess breath sounds before and after administration; effectiveness is evidenced by relief of bronchospasm. In severe bronchospasm, wheezing may not be audible. As the bronchospasm is relieved, wheezing may become more pronounced, indicating that the drug is producing the desired therapeutic effect. Assessment of the patient's subjective feelings of respiratory distress before and after administration is especially important. Adverse effects of albuterol include tachycardia, tremor, nervousness, cardiac dysrhythmias, and hypertension. The patient who is prescribed an albuterol MDI should be taught how to properly use the device and to keep track of the remaining doses. Running out of the drug when a rescue dose is needed can produce life-threatening consequences in a severe asthma attack.

Diphenhydramine Hydrochloride

Diphenhydramine, an antihistamine, is administered with epinephrine to treat anaphylactic shock. This agent is effective for treating the histamine-induced tissue swelling and pruritus common to severe allergic reactions. The standard adult dose is 25 to 50 mg administered via IV or deep IM routes. Oral pill and liquid forms of the drug exist, but the parenteral form is preferred in emergencies. However, the patient may be instructed to keep an oral formulation on hand in the home setting for emergency self-administration during an allergic reaction before receiving medical assistance. An important tip for patient teaching is that liquid diphenhydramine is easier to swallow than a pill, especially in the presence of tissue edema in the mouth or throat. Adverse effects include drowsiness, sedation, confusion, vertigo, excitability, hypotension, tachycardia, GI disturbances, and dry mouth (see Chapter 35).

Dextrose 50%

Dextrose 50% is a concentrated, high-carbohydrate solution given to treat severe hypoglycemia, such as insulin-induced hypoglycemia or insulin shock (see Chapter 12). When hypoglycemia is known or suspected, and the patient's state of consciousness is impaired such that oral administration of sugar solutions is contraindicated, 50 mL of dextrose 50% is commonly ordered and is given as an IV bolus. Dextrose 50% is highly irritating to veins and should be administered in a large peripheral or central vein whenever possible; phlebitis can occur, and extravasation of the solution can cause tissue sloughing and necrosis. The nurse must monitor the patient's blood glucose carefully because hyperglycemia is common, especially after bolus injection. Urine output should be accurately recorded, because osmotic diuresis can occur when blood glucose is elevated, and a hyperosmolar state can result. Patient education must be centered on teaching about diabetes, nutrition, physical activity, and properly self-managing insulin or oral hypoglycemic agent administration.

Pediatric Implications

Glycogen stores in infants and children may be quickly depleted in stress states produced by severe illness. Because adequate amounts of glucose are essential to strong myocardial function as well as brain function, hypoglycemia must be corrected to provide the greatest chance for successful resuscitation. After determining that hypoglycemia is present by the fingerstick or heelstick method of rapid blood glucose testing, dextrose 25% or less may be administered per health care provider order. Because glucose is supplied in a 50% concentration, it must be diluted at least 1:1 in sterile water before administration to reduce its osmolarity and prevent sclerosis of peripheral veins. The standard dose is 0.5 to 1 g/kg IV or IO.

Glucagon

Glucagon is a pancreas-produced hormone that elevates blood glucose by stimulating glycogen breakdown (glycogenolysis). Glucagon, like dextrose 50%, is indicated in the treatment of severe hypoglycemia, such as that which results from insulin shock. In an emergency, when dextrose 50% is unavailable or cannot be administered intravenously, glucagon is an effective agent. Glucagon may be given via subcut, IM, or IV routes and produces the desired clinical effect within 10 to 15 minutes of administration due to the time necessary for glycogen to be converted to glucose. The standard dose for adults and children is 1 mg, which can be repeated in 15 minutes for persistent coma. If the coma has not resolved after two doses, dextrose 50% must be administered. Adverse effects from glucagon are uncommon but can include nausea, vomiting, and a hypersensitivity reaction that may produce bronchospasm and respiratory distress. Glucagon can also be used as a drug to reverse the effects of calcium channel blocker and beta blocker overdose; in this situation, 3.5 to 5 mg IV of glucagon is administered initially, followed by an IV infusion of 1 to 5 mg/h (see Chapter 50). In addition, glucagon dilates esophageal smooth muscle as well as the lower esophageal sphincter. It can be administered IV in the emergency department as a first-line agent to dilate the esophagus in an effort to relieve an esophageal food bolus or impaction.

Table 58.3 lists the emergency drugs for shock and their dosages, uses, and considerations.

EMERGENCY DRUGS FOR HYPERTENSIVE CRISES

A variety of pharmacologic agents may be prescribed to treat hypertensive crisis, generally defined as a systolic blood pressure that exceeds 180 to 200 mm Hg and a diastolic blood pressure that exceeds 120 mm Hg. Three of the most commonly prescribed drugs are discussed in this section. The drugs are cross-referenced to their specialty chapter.

Table 58.4 lists the emergency drugs for hypertensive crises and their dosages, uses, and considerations.

Labetalol

Labetalol is an alpha- and beta-adrenergic blocker that acts by inhibiting the effects of the sympathetic nervous system (see Chapter 15). Its pharmacologic actions include lowering heart rate, blood pressure, myocardial contractility, and myocardial oxygen consumption and reducing the vasoconstriction that results from sympathetic nervous system stimulation. This drug is indicated for the acute management of clinically significant hypertension in the presence of ischemic and hemorrhagic stroke as well as for hypertensive crisis.

Initially 10–20 mg of labetalol is administered IV push over 2 minutes. This starting dose can be repeated or doubled every 10 minutes until the desired clinical response is achieved up to a maximum dose of 300 mg. As an alternative approach, a continuous infusion of labetalol mixed with D_5W can be prepared to deliver 2–8 mg/min until the target therapeutic response is attained; the maximum dose with this approach is also 300 mg.

Important nursing considerations during the administration of labetalol include the use of an electronic infusion device for accurate continuous-infusion medication delivery, cardiac monitoring, and frequent blood

TABLE 58.3 Agents for Emergency Treatment of Shock

Generic	Route and Dosage[a]	Uses and Considerations
Albuterol	A: Nebulizer: 2.5–5 mg q20 min × 3 doses, then 2.5–10 mg q1–4h PRN C/Adol: 1.25–5 mg q20 min × 3 doses, then 2.5–10 mg q1–4h PRN	For bronchoconstriction secondary to anaphylactic shock, asthma, and COPD. Adverse effects include tachycardia, tremor, nervousness, cardiac dysrhythmias, and hypertension PB: UK; t½: 3.7–5 h
Dextrose 50%	A: IV: 10–25 g C: 0.5–1.0 g/kg IV of dextrose 25% sol	For insulin shock, severe hypoglycemia PB: UK; t½: UK
Diphenhydramine	A: IM/IV: 25–50 mg	For anaphylactic shock, acute allergic reaction PB: 98%–99%; t½: 3–8 h
Dobutamine	A: IV drip: 2–20 mcg/kg/min	For low cardiac output. Effects antagonized by beta blockers PB: UK; t½: 2 min
Dopamine hydrochloride	See Prototype Drug Chart: Dopamine Hydrochloride	
Epinephrine	A: IM: 0.3–0.5 mg (1:1000 sol); may repeat q5–15 min A: IV/IO: 0.05–0.1 mg (1:10,000 sol); may repeat q5–15 min A: ETT: 2–2.5 mg; may repeat q3–5 min C/Adol: IV: 0.03–0.2 mcg/kg/min; may repeat q3–5 min C ≥15 kg/Adol: IM: weight based: 0.15–0.3 mg/dose; may repeat q5–20 min	For anaphylactic shock, severe acute asthmatic attack. May cause hypertensive crisis with MAOIs, and increased dysrhythmias may occur with cardiac glycosides PB: UK; t½: UK
Glucagon	A: Subcut/IM/IV: 1 mg; may repeat once C/Adol: Subcut/IM/IV: weight based: 0.5–1 mg; may repeat once	Insulin shock, severe hypoglycemia, beta-blocker overdose (reverses effects of beta blockers) PB: UK; t½: 3–10 min
Norepinephrine	A: IV: Initially, up to 8–12 mcg/min, titrated in increments of 0.02 mcg/kg/min; max: 3.3 mcg/kg/min C: 0.03–0.5 mcg/kg/min IV/IO via continuous infusion; upper dosing limit highly variable	Hypotension not responsive to other therapies PB: UK; t½: UK

A, Adult; *Adol*, adolescent; *C*, child; *COPD*, chronic obstructive pulmonary disease; *ETT*, endotracheal tube; *h*, hour; *IM*, intramuscular; *IO*, intraosseous; *IV*, intravenous; *MAOIs*, monoamine oxidase inhibitors; *max*, maximum; *min*, minute; *PB*, protein binding; *PRN*, as needed; *q*, every; *sol*, solution; *subcut*, subcutaneous; *t½*, half-life; *UK*, unknown; ≥, greater than or equal to.
[a]Other dosing regimens for neonates, infants, and children are available.

TABLE 58.4 Emergency Drugs for Hypertensive Crises

Generic	Route and Dosage[a]	Uses and Considerations
Nitroprusside sodium	See Prototype Drug Chart: Nitroprusside Sodium	
Furosemide	A: IM/IV: Initially, 20–40 mg, titrate by 20 mg q2h PRN C: IM/IV: 1–2 mg/kg q6–12h; *max:* 6 mg/kg/dose	For acute pulmonary edema. Adverse effects include hypovolemia, dehydration, and electrolyte disturbances
Labetalol hydrochloride	A: IV: Initially, 20 mg over 2 min; additional doses of 20–80 mg q10min until desired response A: IV drip: 0.5–2 mg/min; titrate to response; *max:* 300 mg; continuous infusion 2 mg/min	For hypertension in CVA and for hypertensive crisis. Adverse effects include ventricular dysrhythmias, hypotension, and bronchospasm *Contraindications:* Bronchial asthma, COPD, severe bradycardia, heart failure

A, Adult; *C*, child; *COPD*, chronic obstructive pulmonary disease; *CVA*, cerebrovascular accident; *h*, hour; *IM*, intramuscular; *IV*, intravenous; *max*, maximum; *MI*, myocardial infarction; *min*, minute; *PRN*, as needed; *q*, every.
[a]Other dosing regimens for neonates, infants, and children are available.

pressure measurement. Documentation of blood pressure may need to be at least every 5 minutes during IV push dosing or at the initiation of the continuous infusion. Serious adverse effects include hypotension, bradycardia, ventricular dysrhythmias, and bronchospasm. Dizziness is also a frequently reported adverse reaction. Labetalol is contraindicated in patients with bronchial asthma or COPD because of the risk of bronchospasm and in patients with severe bradycardia or apparent heart failure.

Nitroprusside Sodium

Nitroprusside sodium is an IV drug used to reduce arterial blood pressure in hypertensive emergencies (see Chapter 39). The mechanism of action is immediate, direct arterial and venous vasodilation. Antihypertensive effects end when nitroprusside sodium is discontinued; blood pressure increases as soon as drug administration is stopped. Continuous and accurate blood pressure measurement is required. In general, 50 mg of nitroprusside sodium is mixed in 250 mL D_5W. The typical dose range for adults is 0.3 mcg/kg/min, titrated to the desired clinical response. The maximum dose is 10 mcg/kg/min.

There are several important nursing considerations:

- Nitroprusside sodium is rapidly inactivated by light; the IV bottle or bag must be wrapped with aluminum foil or another opaque material to protect the solution from degradation.
- Although a faint brown tint is typical, blue or brown discoloration of the solution indicates degradation and necessitates that the solution be discarded.
- When nitroprusside sodium therapy is prolonged, or when it is infused at the maximum dose of 10 mcg/kg/min for more than 10 minutes, patients are at risk for toxicity resulting from elevated serum thiocyanate or cyanide levels (by-products of drug metabolism). Signs and symptoms include metabolic acidosis, profound hypotension, dyspnea, dizziness, and vomiting. Serum thiocyanate levels should be monitored every 24 to 72 hours for patients receiving prolonged infusions of more than 2 mcg/kg/min. Patients with renal insufficiency or failure are at a higher risk because the metabolites are excreted in the urine.
- Patients should be placed on an oral antihypertensive agent as soon as possible so that nitroprusside sodium can be tapered slowly. Drug data for nitroprusside sodium are presented in Prototype Drug Chart: Nitroprusside Sodium.

📄 PROTOTYPE DRUG CHART

Nitroprusside Sodium

Drug Class	**Dosage**
Vasodilator	A/C: IV drip: Initially 0.3 mcg/kg/min, then titrate to desired response. Usual range is 0.2–10 mcg/kg/min

Contraindications	**Drug-Lab-Food Interactions**
Hypersensitivity, hypertension (compensatory), decreased cerebral perfusion, coarctation of the aorta *Caution:* Increased intracranial pressure	Drug: Antihypertensives, general anesthetics Note: Do not mix with any other drug in syringe or solution Lab: Decrease in Paco$_2$, pH

Pharmacokinetics	**Pharmacodynamics**
Absorption: IV only Distribution: PB: UK Metabolism: t½: <10 min Excretion: In urine	IV: Onset: 1–2 min Peak: Rapid Duration: 1–10 min

Therapeutic Effects/Uses

To treat hypertensive crisis and to decrease systemic vascular resistance to improve cardiac performance
Mechanism of Action: Stimulates smooth muscle of veins and arteries; produces peripheral vasodilation.

Side Effects	**Adverse Reactions**
Dizziness, headache, nausea, abdominal pain, sweating, palpitations, weakness, vomiting	Thiocyanate toxicity: hypotension, tinnitus, dyspnea, blurred vision, metabolic acidosis *Life-threatening:* Severe hypotension, loss of consciousness, profound cardiovascular depression

A, Adult; *C*, child; *IV*, intravenous; *min*, minute; *PB*, protein binding; *Paco$_2$*, partial pressure of carbon dioxide; *t½*, half-life; *UK*, unknown; *<*, less than.

Furosemide

Furosemide is classified as a *loop diuretic* that acts by inhibiting sodium and chloride reabsorption from the ascending loop of Henle and the proximal and distal tubules. It promotes the renal excretion of water, sodium, chloride, magnesium, hydrogen, and calcium, and it depletes potassium (see Chapter 41). Furosemide also has peripheral and renal vasodilating effects that can lower blood pressure. The main indications for use of furosemide as an emergency drug are acute pulmonary edema from left ventricular dysfunction and hypertensive crisis.

Furosemide is given as an initial bolus of 20 to 40 mg IV over 1 to 2 minutes. For patients who take furosemide on a regular basis, the effective dose may be much higher (up to 2 mg/kg). The vasodilatory effects occur *before* diuresis begins and act to lower blood pressure. Central venous pressure is reduced through a decrease in venous return to the heart once vasodilation is achieved. Diuresis should start within 5–10 minutes of drug administration and may continue for approximately 6 hours.

The most significant adverse effects are severe hypovolemia, dehydration, and electrolyte disturbances (hypokalemia, hypomagnesemia,

 COMPLEMENTARY AND ALTERNATIVE THERAPIES

Furosemide

Ginseng can inhibit the efficacy of furosemide. Licorice can promote potassium loss, which enhances the potential for severe hypokalemia. These products should not be taken concurrently with furosemide.

hyponatremia, and hypochloremia). Patients taking digitalis preparations are at an increased risk of digitalis toxicity from hypokalemia. The patient's fluid and electrolyte status, blood urea nitrogen (BUN), and creatinine must be carefully assessed before and after furosemide administration, including auscultation of breath sounds for rales, strict surveillance of intake and output, and review of laboratory data when available. Electrolyte and careful fluid replacement may be required during furosemide therapy to prevent physiologic consequences. The nurse must also exercise caution when giving nephrotoxic agents when furosemide is prescribed and in administering the drug to patients with sulfonamide sensitivity because furosemide is a sulfonamide derivative that can produce an allergic reaction.

CRITICAL THINKING SINGLE EPISODE CASE STUDY

SLO: Apply knowledge of pharmacodynamics of drugs to determine which medication effects require a follow-up by the nurse.

NGN Item Type: Extended drag and drop

Cognitive Skills: Take action

A 42-year-old male was brought to the emergency room by ground ambulance. The emergency medical technician (EMT) reported the patient has been having intermittent "indigestion" for 5 days and has been ingesting "Tums" with minimal relief. 911 was called when a friend noticed the patient grabbing his chest and was not able to "catch his breath." EMT administered oxygen 2 liters per nasal cannula, aspirin 325 mg orally, nitroglycerin (NTG) 0.4 mg sublingual × 3 tablets, and morphine 4 mg intravenously (IV). The electrocardiogram (ECG) en route did not reveal any acute coronary events. The nurse assists in transferring the patient onto a stretcher. The nurse follows the hospital protocol and places oxygen 2 liters per nasal cannula, attaches cardiac monitor, and inserts a second IV site while continuing to conduct a focused history and assessment.

Indicate which nursing action listed in the first column is appropriate for the clinical manifestation the nurse assessed in the second column. Note that not all nursing actions will be used while some of the nursing actions will be used more than once.

Nursing Action	Potential Clinical Manifestation	Appropriate Nursing Action for the Clinical Manifestation
No action other than monitor	Blood pressure of 98/68 mm Hg	
Administer morphine 2 mg intravenously	Heart rate of 73 beats per minute	
Administer diltiazem	Respiratory rate of 18 breaths per minute	
Obtain a 12-lead electrocardiogram	Pale, clammy skin	
Administer atropine sulfate	Bedside cardiac monitor with	
Notify the attending medical provider	Continued chest pain	
	Report of headaches	

Answers

Nursing Action	Potential Clinical Manifestation	Appropriate Nursing Action for the Clinical Manifestation
No action other than monitor	Blood pressure of 98/68 mm Hg	No action other than monitor
Administer morphine 2 mg intravenously	Heart rate of 73 beats per minute	No action other than monitor
Administer diltiazem	Respiratory rate of 18 breaths per minute	No action other than monitor
Obtain a 12-lead electrocardiogram	Pale, clammy skin	Obtain a 12-lead electrocardiogram
Administer atropine sulfate	Bedside cardiac monitor with	Obtain a 12-lead electrocardiogram
Administer nitroglycerin sublingual	Continued chest pain	Administer morphine 2 mg intravenously
	Reports of headaches	No action other than monitor

Rationale

The patient is most likely exhibiting angina pectoris with possible myocardial infarction with ST elevation. The initial goal for any cardiac event is to restore perfusion and prevent further damage to the myocardium. The patient's vital signs, which include blood pressure, heart rate, and respiratory rate, are within normal parameters and should be monitored. A decrease in blood pressure can occur as a side effect of nitroglycerin and morphine. The nurse would continue to monitor the vital signs and if continuing lowering of blood pressure occurs, the medical provider would be notified. However, a bedside cardiac monitor shows widened QRS complexes with ST-elevation; a 12-lead electrocardiogram would be obtained to determine if the patient is experiencing ST-elevated myocardial infarction (STEMI) or other cardiac abnormalities causing ST-elevation. Also, the nurse would continue to treat the chest pain with either nitroglycerin or morphine while monitoring blood pressure and heart rate. Because the patient continues to have chest pain after three doses of sublingual nitroglycerin, the nurse would administer morphine for the refractory chest pain. Headache is a common side effect after nitroglycerin due to

CRITICAL THINKING SINGLE EPISODE CASE STUDY—CONT'D

its vasodilatory effects and should be monitored. Atropine and diltiazem would not be administered. Atropine would be administered if the patient suddenly became bradycardic; diltiazem would be administered if the patient developed premature supraventricular tachycardia (PSVT) if his blood pressure is stable; otherwise, adenosine would be appropriate.

References:
Zafari, A.M., & Abdou, M.H. (May 7, 2019). Myocardial infarction treatment & management. Retrieved from https://emedicine.medscape.com/article/155919-treatment

▌CRITICAL THINKING CASE STUDY

A patient who is 19 years of age suffered a gunshot wound to the head and a spinal cord injury from a stab wound over the thoracic spine 1 hour ago. The patient was transported immediately from the injury scene to the trauma center by paramedics. Upon hospital arrival, the patient was awake and following simple commands, but the neurologic status has subsequently deteriorated. At this point, the patient has undergone initial resuscitation and a rapid diagnostic workup. The patient is now orally intubated, has two functional intravenous (IV) catheters—one peripheral line in the right forearm and one triple-lumen central line in the left subclavian vein—an oral gastric tube, and an indwelling urinary catheter. The patient's current vital signs are blood pressure (BP) 88/56, heart rate (HR) 56, temperature 96.8°F (36°C), and respiratory rate (RR) 16 on a mechanical ventilator. The patient's mother reported that DW is addicted to opioids, including heroin, and also abused oral diazepam and other street drugs.

The patient's diagnoses include a penetrating head injury with intracerebral hemorrhage diagnosed by computed tomography (CT) scan, a penetrating spinal cord injury at the T4 level, and drug abuse. The patient opens his eyes spontaneously and does not follow commands, and only the upper extremities withdraw; the lower extremities do not move.

1. On arrival at the trauma center, should the patient have received supplemental oxygen based on the pulse oximetry reading of 90%? What type of oxygen delivery device would be appropriate for the patient on initial presentation, with spontaneous breathing?

2. The physician orders 50 g of mannitol to be given now, IV push. On hand are several 50-mL vials of "mannitol, 25%" solution. How many milliliters of mannitol from this vial need to be drawn up into the syringe to administer 50 g?

3. Describe the type of needle that must be used when administering mannitol. Explain your answer. What size syringe would

be used? Which IV line would be used to administer the mannitol?

4. What are the indications for mannitol administration? List at least three nursing considerations when giving mannitol.

5. The patient has a history of heroin and diazepam abuse. List the reversal drugs that could be used if the trauma team believes recent illicit drug use may be a contributing factor to the altered mental state.

6. Because of the spinal cord injury, the patient is exhibiting signs of neurogenic shock: bradycardia, warm skin, and hypotension. What is the drug of choice that the nurse would keep at the bedside in case the patient requires emergency treatment for symptomatic bradycardia? Name the drug, its mechanism of action, and dosing considerations.

7. The physician orders dopamine 800 mg/250 mL D_5W, to be titrated to maintain systolic BP above 110 mm Hg. Which IV site would be the best choice for a continuous dopamine infusion in D.W.?

8. What is the consequence of dopamine extravasation?

9. Describe the treatment for dopamine extravasation.

10. What vital sign parameters must be monitored while the patient receives dopamine? Name at least four adverse effects of dopamine.

Antibiotics are initiated as prophylaxis for infection due to the nature of the patient's penetrating injuries. Upon infusion of the antibiotic, a full-body rash, swelling of the lips and tongue, and hypotension develop.

11. After antibiotic administration, what condition has developed in the patient?

12. What are the drugs of choice to treat the patient's condition now?

13. How can the nurse evaluate the effectiveness of these drugs?

▌REVIEW QUESTIONS

1. The nurse noted a patient's heart rate decreasing from 45 to 38 while administering atropine 0.3 mg IV. What is the most likely explanation?
   a. Atropine exerts its effects by stimulating the vagus nerve.
   b. The ordered dose was too low.
   c. Adenosine was indicated, not atropine.
   d. Atropine typically slows heart rate first and then increases it.

2. An older adult patient with a hip fracture became unresponsive 20 minutes after receiving morphine 3 mg intravenously. Which actions would the nurse take?
   a. Assess the patient, call for additional assistance, support breathing with a bag valve mask device as indicated, and prepare to administer flumazenil.
   b. Call the physician and report that the patient most likely suffered a stroke and now has elevated intracranial pressure; prepare to administer mannitol.

c. Assess the patient, call for additional assistance, support breathing with a bag valve mask device as indicated, and prepare to administer naloxone.
   d. Explain to the patient's family that the morphine is taking effect and that unresponsiveness is the desired outcome to best manage the pain.

3. The nurse is caring for a young patient with a closed head injury who has an intracranial pressure of 35 (normal <20) and serum osmolality of 330 mOsm/kg. The nurse would anticipate which action?
   a. Administration of mannitol
   b. Withholding mannitol at this time, but taking other measures to reduce intracranial pressure
   c. Administration of sodium nitroprusside
   d. Taking no action at this time because the patient has a serum osmolality of 330, which will offset the effects of the elevated intracranial pressure

4. A dopamine infusion was started in a patient's antecubital vein during resuscitation for profound hypotension, but the electronic infusion device is now sounding an alert for an occlusion. Which immediate concern would be most important for the nurse?
   a. Infiltration with phentolamine will be necessary if there is extravasation.
   b. An interruption in the infusion can produce hypotension in the patient.
   c. The device will need to be reported to the hospital's clinical engineering department for service.
   d. The patient could develop hypertension as a result of the alarm.

5. The nurse observes a short period of asystole on the cardiac monitor that resolves spontaneously immediately after administering adenosine IV to a patient who was experiencing paroxysmal supraventricular tachycardia. Which initial action is the most appropriate for the nurse?
   a. Call a code to report a cardiac arrest.
   b. Prepare epinephrine and atropine for intravenous administration.
   c. Initiate cardiopulmonary resuscitation (CPR).
   d. Closely observe the patient and the cardiac monitor.

6. The nurse practitioner has written a number of stat orders for drugs to treat a patient on the medical-surgical unit who has suffered an acute anaphylactic reaction with hives and bronchospasm during infusion of an IV antibiotic. Which priority drug would the nurse administer first?
   a. Steroid dose pack
   b. Dopamine
   c. Epinephrine
   d. Diphenhydramine

7. The nurse receives a stat order to administer 50% dextrose solution intravenously to a 1-year-old child with hypoglycemia. How should this drug best be prepared for safe administration to the child?
   a. Use a filter needle.
   b. Draw the drug into a tuberculin syringe.
   c. Dilute 1:1 with sterile water to produce dextrose 25%.
   d. Shake the solution vigorously before injection.

8. An unresponsive patient who was brought to the emergency department has been reportedly taking alprazolam for a severe anxiety disorder after the mother's death. Knowing this history, which drug would the nurse anticipate administering?
   a. Mannitol
   b. Naloxone
   c. Activated charcoal
   d. Flumazenil

9. A patient was admitted to the emergency department with a pulse oximeter reading of 85% after a successful prehospital resuscitation from cardiac arrest due to an asthma attack. Which initial drug would be most important to administer?
   a. Epinephrine
   b. Sodium bicarbonate
   c. Albuterol
   d. Oxygen

10. Which drug concentration is appropriate to administer in an order for epinephrine 0.3 mg IM to treat a severe allergic reaction in an adult patient?
    a. 1:10,000
    b. 1:1000
    c. 1:100
    d. 1:10

11. Upon preparing to administer activated charcoal by mouth to treat a patient who took an overdose of aspirin and several unknown drugs, the nurse notes that the patient has become very somnolent and eyes open only to a noxious stimulus. Which action by the nurse is most appropriate at this point?
    a. Immediately discuss the change in the patient's mental status with the nurse practitioner who wrote the activated charcoal orders so that the plan of care can be reevaluated.
    b. Immediately insert a nasogastric tube and administer the activated charcoal.
    c. Immediately elevate the head of the patient's stretcher, and coax the patient to drink the activated charcoal while applying noxious stimuli as necessary to maintain wakefulness.
    d. Give only half the dose now, and wait until the patient's mental status improves before giving the remainder of the dose.

12. A surgeon orders aspirin 325 mg by mouth to a patient who developed chest pain while undergoing a minor outpatient surgery for a mole removal from the leg. Which action is most appropriate by the nurse?
    a. Question the aspirin order because the patient just had a surgical procedure and might have bleeding complications.
    b. After checking for drug allergies, first instruct the patient to chew the aspirin tablet and then administer the aspirin.
    c. After checking for drug allergies, instruct the patient to swallow the aspirin tablet whole.
    d. Suggest to the surgeon that the enteric-coated form of aspirin might be better tolerated by the patient to avoid gastrointestinal distress.

Answers to Review Questions

Chapter 1
Answers: **1.** b; **2.** c; **3.** b; **4.** a, b, c, e; **5.** c; **6.** c; **7.** (1) c, (2) b, (3) d, (4) a, (5) f; (6) e.

Chapter 2
Answers: **1.** b; **2.** d; **3.** c; **4.** a; **5.** a, b, c, d; **6.** a, b, d, e; **7.** c; **8.** a; **9.** a, b, d; **10.** a, b, c; **11.** a; **12.** a.

Chapter 3
Answers: **1.** c, e; **2.** a; **3.** b; **4** a; **5.** a, b, d; **6.** a, b, c; **7.** a; **8.** d; **9.** c; **10.** b.

Chapter 4
Answers: **1.** d; **2.** a; **3.** a, b, c, d, e; **4.** d; **5.** a, b, c.

Chapter 5
Answers: **1.** a, b, c; **2.** b; **3.** b; **4.** b, e; **5.** a, c.

Chapter 6
Answers: **1.** d; **2.** c; **3.** c; **4.** a, c, e; **5.** a, b, e; **6.** a, d.

Chapter 7
Answers: **1.** a, b, c; **2.** c; **3.** a; **4.** c; **5.** a, c, e; **6.** b, c, e; **7.** a, b; **8.** b.

Chapter 8
Answers: **1.** c; **2.** a; **3.** b, c, e; **4.** a; **5.** a, b, c, e, f.

Chapter 9
Answers: **1.** a, c; **2.** b, c, d, e; **3.** a; **4.** d; **5.** b, c, d, e; **6.** a, d; **7.** d.

Chapter 10
Answers: **1.** a, b, d; **2.** d; **3.** d; **4.** b; **5.** b; **6.** b; **7.** a; **8.** a, c, d.

Chapter 11
See Answers to Practice Problems at the end of Chapter 11.

Chapter 12
Answers: **1.** a; **2.** b; **3.** c; **4.** d; **5.** a, b, c, e; **6.** b; **7.** a, b, d, e; **8.** a, b, e.

Chapter 13
Answers: **1.** d; **2.** a; **3.** b; **4.** a; **5.** c; **6.** c; **7.** b; **8.** b; **9.** d; **10.** b; **11.** c.

Chapter 14
Answers: **1.** c; **2.** b, c, d, e; **3.** c; **4.** a, b, d; **5.** d; **6.** a; **7.** a, b, d; **8.** b.

Chapter 15
Answers: **1.** a, b, d; **2.** c; **3.** c; **4.** d; **5.** b, c, d, e; **6.** a, b; **7.** b, c.

Chapter 16
Answers: **1.** b; **2.** c; **3.** a; **4.** d; **5.** b; **6.** d; **7.** a.

Chapter 17
Answers: **1.** d; **2.** d; **3.** c; **4.** a; **5.** c.

Chapter 18
Answers: **1.** a; **2.** c; **3.** d; **4.** c; **5.** b; **6.** d; **7.** a, b, c.

Chapter 19
Answers: **1.** c; **2.** b; **3.** c; **4.** c, d, e; **5.** a, b; **6.** b; **7.** d.

Chapter 20
Answers: **1.** b, c, d; **2.** d; **3.** d; **4.** c; **5.** b; **6.** a, b, c, e; **7.** a, b, c.

Chapter 21
Answers: **1.** b; **2.** b; **3.** c; **4.** d; **5.** a; **6.** a, c, d; **7.** b, c, d, e; **8.** c; **9.** a, b, d, e.

Chapter 22
Answers: **1.** b; **2.** a; **3.** d; **4.** a, b, c, d, e; **5.** a; **6.** b, c, d, e; **7.** a, b, c, f.

Chapter 23
Answers: **1.** d; **2.** a, c; **3.** a; **4.** b; **5.** d; **6.** a, b, c, d; **7.** a, b, e, f.

Chapter 24
Answers: **1.** c; **2.** c; **3.** a; **4.** a; **5.** a, c, d; **6.** a, b, c, e.

Chapter 25
Answers: **1.** c; **2.** b; **3.** c; **4.** b; **5.** a; **6.** a, b, c; **7.** a, c, e; **8.** a.

Chapter 26
Answers: **1.** a; **2.** a, b, c, d; **3.** a, b, d; **4.** c; **5.** b; **6.** d

Chapter 27
Answers: **1.** a, b, c, e; **2.** a, c, d, e, f; **3.** d; **4.** a.

Chapter 28
Answers: **1.** a; **2.** d; **3.** a, b, d, f; **4.** a, b, c, d, e.

Chapter 29
Answers: **1.** a; **2.** c; **3.** d; **4.** a, b, c, d; **5.** b.

Chapter 30
Answers: **1.** a; **2.** b; **3.** c; **4.** a, d, e, f; **5.** d; **6.** a, d, e; **7.** a.

Chapter 31
Answers: **1.** a; **2.** b; **3.** b; **4.** d; **5.** d; **6.** c.

Chapter 32
Answers: **1.** d; **2.** d; **3.** a; **4.** a, b, c, e; **5.** a, b, d.

Chapter 33
Answers: **1.** d; **2.** c; **3.** a, b, c, d; **4.** b; **5.** b.

Chapter 34
Answers: **1.** c; **2.** d; **3.** a; **4.** a; **5.** d; **6.** d; **7.** a, b; **8.** c.

Chapter 35
Answers: **1.** b; **2.** a; **3.** c; **4.** a; **5.** c; **6.** b; **7.** c; **8.** c; **9.** a, c, e; **10.** a, b, e.

Chapter 36
Answers: **1.** d; **2.** a; **3.** b; **4.** c; **5.** d; **6.** c; **7.** d; **8.** b; **9.** c.

Chapter 37
Answers: **1.** a; **2.** c; **3.** a; **4.** b; **5.** d; **6.** b.

Chapter 38
Answers: **1.** b; **2.** c; **3.** d; **4.** b; **5.** d; **6.** b, c, d, e.

Chapter 39
Answers: **1.** b, d, e; **2.** b; **3.** c; **4.** c; **5.** a.

Chapter 40
Answers: **1.** b; **2.** a; **3.** d; **4.** a; **5.** b; **6.** c; **7.** b; **8.** c; **9.** a, b, e.

Chapter 41
Answers: **1.** b; **2.** b, c, d, e; **3.** b; **4.** a; **5.** b; **6.** b; **7.** b.

Chapter 42
Answers: **1.** a, b, c, d; **2.** a; **3.** c; **4.** b; **5.** b; **6.** d; **7.** b; **8.** a, b, d, e.

Chapter 43
Answers: **1.** a, b, c, d, e; **2.** a; **3.** a; **4.** d; **5.** b; **6.** b; **7.** d.

Chapter 44
Answers: **1.** c; **2.** a; **3.** a; **4.** b; **5.** d; **6.** b; **7.** a; **8.** b, c, d.

Chapter 45
Answers: **1.** b; **2.** b; **3.** a; **4.** d; **5.** c; **6.** a, b, c, d, e.

Chapter 46
Answers: **1.** a; **2.** d; **3.** a, c, e, f; **4.** d; **5.** a, b, f; **6.** c.

Chapter 47
Answers: **1.** d; **2.** a; **3.** b; **4.** g, b, d, e, a, f, h, c; **5.** c; **6.** b, c.

Chapter 48
Answers: **1.** b; **2.** a, c, d; **3.** d; **4.** d; **5.** b, d; **6.** b, c; **7.** a, b, d; **8.** b, c, e; **9.** c, d.

Chapter 49
Answers: **1.** c; **2.** c; **3.** a; **4.** b; **5.** a; **6.** b, c, d, e; **7.** a, b, c, e.

Chapter 50
Answers: **1.** c; **2.** a; **3.** b; **4.** c; **5.** d, e; **6.** a, b, d; **7.** b, d.

Chapter 51
Answers: **1.** a; **2.** d; **3.** d; **4.** d; **5.** b.

Chapter 52
Answers: **1.** a, b, c; **2.** a; **3.** b; **4.** c; **5.** a; **6.** c; **7.** d; **8.** d; **9.** b; **10.** a, c, d, e; **11.** a, c, e.

Chapter 53
Answers: **1.** d; **2.** a; **3.** b; **4.** c; **5.** a; **6.** b; **7.** b; **8.** a; **9.** b; **10.** a, b, c, d.

Chapter 54
Answers: **1.** c; **2.** c; **3.** b, c, e; **4.** b; **5.** c, d, e; **6.** a, b, e.

Chapter 55
Answers: **1.** a, c; **2.** a, d, e; **3.** c; **4.** b; **5.** b, c, d; **6.** d; **7.** b; **8.** a, b, d.

Chapter 56
Answers: **1.** a, c, d; **2.** a, b, c, d; **3.** a, d; **4.** a, b, d; **5.** d; **6.** b, c, d, e; **7.** a, b, d.

Chapter 57
Answers: **1.** a, d; **2.** b, c, d; **3.** a; **4.** b; **5.** 4 mL IM × 1; **6.** a, d; **7.** c; **8.** b.

Chapter 58
Answers: **1.** b; **2.** c; **3.** b; **4.** b; **5.** d; **6.** c; **7.** c; **8.** d; **9.** d; **10.** b; **11.** a; **12.** b.

Solution Compatibility Chart

Intravenous Medication	D2½W	D5W	D10W	D5/¼NS	D5/½NS	D5NS	NS	½NS	R	LR	D5R	D5LR	Dextran 6%/D5W/NS	Fruc 10%/W/NS	Invert sug 10%/W/NS	Na Lactate ⅙ M
Acetazolamide	C	C	C	C	C	C	C	C	C	C	C	C	C	C	C	C
Acyclovir		C		C	C	C	C			C						
Aminophylline	C	C	C	C	C	C	C	C	C	C	C	C	C			C
Antithymocyte Globulin	C	C	C	C	C	C	C	C								
Ascorbic Acid	C	C	C	C	C	C	C	C	C	C	C	C	C	C	C	C
Aztreonam		C	C	C	C	C	C		C	C		C				C
Calcium Chloride		C	C	C	C	C	C		C	C	C	C				
Calcium Gluconate		C	C			C	C			C		C		W		C
Cefazolin Na		C	C	C	C	C	C		C	C		C			W	
Cefoperazone Na		C	C	C		C	C			C		C				
Cefotaxime Na		C	C	C	C	C	C			C					W	C
Cefotetan		C					C									
Cefoxitin Na		C	C	C	C	C	C		C	C		C			C	C
Ceftazidime		C	C	C	C	C	C		C	C					W	C
Ceftriaxone Na		C	C		C		C								W	C
Cefuroxime Na		C	C	C	C	C	C		C	C					W	C
Clindamycin		C	C		C	C	C			C	C					
Dexamethasone		C					C									
Dobutamine HCl		C	C		C	C	C	C		C		C				C
Dopamine HCl		C	C		C	C	C			C		C				C
Doxycycline		C				C	C		C						W	
Epinephrine	C	C	C	C	C	C	C		C	C	C	C	C	C	C	C
Famotidine		C	C				C			C						
Fentanyl		C					C									
Folic Acid		C					C									
Furosemide		C	C			C	C			C		C				C
Gentamicin		C	C				C		C	C						
Heparin Na	C	C*		C	C	C	C*	C	C		C	C	C	C	C	
Hydrocortisone Phosphate		C	C				C	C								
Hydrocortisone Na Succinate	C	C	C	C	C	C	C	C	C	C	C	C	C	C	C	C
Hydromorphone HCl		C	C		C	C	C	C	C	C	C	C		W		C
Imipenem-Cilastatin		C⁴	C⁴	C⁴	C⁴	C⁴	C¹⁰									
Insulin (Regular)		Cᴾ	C		C		Cᴾ			C	C					
Isoproterenol	C	Cᴾ	C	C	C	C	Cᴾ	C	C	C	C	C	C	C	C	C
Kanamycin		C	C			C	C				C					
Labetalol		C	C			C	C		C	C	C	C				
Lidocaine		Cᴾ			C	C	C	C		C		C				
Magnesium Sulfate		C					C			C						
Meperidine HCl	C	C	C	C	C	C	C	C	C	C	C	C	C	C	C	C
Meropenem		C¹	C¹	C¹		C¹	C⁴		C⁴	C⁴		C¹				C²

Intravenous Medication	D2½W	D5W	D10W	D5/¼NS	D5/½NS	D5NS	NS	½NS	R	LR	D5R	D5LR	Dextran 6%/D5W/NS	Fruc 10%/W/NS	Invert sug 10%/W/NS	Na Lactate ⅙ M
Metoclopramide HCl		C			C		C		C	C						
Morphine	C	C	C	C	C	C	C	C	C	C	C	C	C	C	C	C
Multivitamin		C	C			C	C			C				C	W	C
Nafcillin Na		C	C	C	C	C	C			C	C	C	C			C
Nitroglycerin		C*			C	C	C*	C		C		C				C
Norepinephrine		C^P				C^P				C						
Ondansetron HCl		C			C	C	C		C	C						
Oxacillin Na		C	C			C	C			C	C					
Pancuronium		C			C	C	C			C						
Papaverine	C	C	C	C	C	C	C	C	C	C			C	C	C	C
Penicillin G, K	C	C	C	C	C	C	C	C	C	C	C	C	C	C	C	
Pentobarbital Na	C	C*	C	C	C	C	C	C	C	C	C	C	C	C	C	C
Piperacillin/ Tazobactam		C					C			C*		NS				
Potassium Acetate		C	C				C			C		C				
Potassium Chloride	C	C	C	C	C	C	C	C	C	C	C	C	C	C	C	C
Potassium Phosphate	C	C	C	C	C	C	C	C					C	C	C	C
Prochlorperazine	C	C	C	C	C	C	C	C	C	C	C	C	C	C	C	C
Propranolol		C^P		C	C	C	C			C						
Pyridoxine HCl		C	C	C	C	C	C		C	C					C	C
Ranitidine		C	C	C		C				C						
Sodium Acetate		C	C			C	C	C	C			C				
Sodium Bicarbonate	C	C	C	C	C	C	C	C	C			C		C	C	C
Sodium Chloride	C	C	C	C	C	C	C	C	C	C	C	C	C	C	C	C
Succinylcholine	C	C	C	C	C	C	C	C	C	C	C	C	C	C	C	C
Thiamine	C	C	C	C	C	C	C	C	C	C	C	C	C	C	C	
Thiopental	C	C		C	C	C^6	C	C				C				C
Trace Metals		C	C			C	C			C						
Tranexamic Acid	C	C	C	C	C	C	C		C			C				
Warfarin		C	C		C	C	C*					C				
Zidovudine		C^P					C									

This chart is not all inclusive. It is based on manufacturer's recommendations and Trissel's.

KEY

C	= Compatible*	D5R	= 5% Dextrose in Ringer's solution
W	= Compatible in water not NS	D5LR	= 5% Dextrose in Lactated Ringer's solution
D2½W	= 2½% Dextrose in water	Dextran 6%/D5W/NS	= Dextran 6% in D5W or normal saline
D5W	= 5% Dextrose in water	Fruc 10%/W/NS	= Fructose 10% in water or normal saline
D10W	= 10% Dextrose in water	Invert sug 10%/W/NS	= Invert sugar 10% in water or normal saline
D5/¼NS	= 5% Dextrose in ¼ normal saline	Na Lactate ⅙ M	= Sodium lactate ⅙ M
D5/½NS	= 5% Dextrose in ½ normal saline	1	= Stable for 1 hour
D5NS	= 5% Dextrose in normal saline	2	= Stable for 2 hours
NS	= Normal saline	4	= Stable for 4 hours
½NS	= ½ Normal saline	6	= Stable for 6 hours
R	= Ringer's solution	10	= Stable for 10 hours
LR	= Lactated Ringer's solution	P	= Preferred diluent

Compatibility in various concentrations may vary; consult pharmacist.

Immunizations

Table 1   Recommended adult immunization schedule by age group, United States, 2021

Vaccine	19–26 years	27–49 years	50–64 years	≥65 years
Influenza inactivated (IIV) or Influenza recombinant (RIV4)	1 dose annually			
Influenza live, attenuated (LAIV4)	1 dose annually			
Tetanus, diphtheria, pertussis (Tdap or Td)	1 dose Tdap each pregnancy; 1 dose Td/Tdap for wound management (see notes); 1 dose Tdap, then Td or Tdap booster every 10 years			
Measles, mumps, rubella (MMR)	1 or 2 doses depending on indication (if born in 1957 or later)			
Varicella (VAR)	2 doses (if born in 1980 or later)		2 doses	
Zoster recombinant (RZV)			2 doses	
Human papillomavirus (HPV)	2 or 3 doses depending on age at initial vaccination or condition	27 through 45 years		
Pneumococcal conjugate (PCV13)	1 dose			1 dose
Pneumococcal polysaccharide (PPSV23)	1 or 2 doses depending on indication			1 dose
Hepatitis A (HepA)	2 or 3 doses depending on vaccine			
Hepatitis B (HepB)	2 or 3 doses depending on vaccine			
Meningococcal A, C, W, Y (MenACWY)	1 or 2 doses depending on indication, see notes for booster recommendations			
Meningococcal B (MenB)	19 through 23 years	2 or 3 doses depending on vaccine and indication, see notes for booster recommendations		
Haemophilus influenzae type b (Hib)	1 or 3 doses depending on indication			

Recommended vaccination for adults who meet age requirement, lack documentation of vaccination, or lack evidence of past infection

Recommended vaccination for adults with an additional risk factor or another indication

Recommended vaccination based on shared clinical decision-making

No recommendation/ not applicable

Table 2   Recommended adult immunization schedule by medical condition and other indications, United States, 2021

Vaccine	Pregnancy	Immuno-compromised (excluding HIV infection)	HIV infection CD4 count <200 mm³	HIV infection CD4 count ≥200 mm³	Asplenia, complement deficiencies	End-stage renal disease; or on hemodialysis	Heart or lung disease, alcoholism[1]	Chronic liver disease	Diabetes	Health care personnel[2]	Men who have sex with men
IIV or RIV4	1 dose annually										
LAIV4	Not recommended							Precaution		1 dose annually	
Tdap or Td	1 dose Tdap each pregnancy	1 dose Tdap, then Td or Tdap booster every 10 years									
MMR	Not recommended*	Not recommended	Not recommended	1 or 2 doses depending on indication							
VAR	Not recommended*	Not recommended	Not recommended	2 doses							
RZV				2 doses at age ≥50 years							
HPV	Not recommended*	3 doses through age 26 years	3 doses through age 26 years	2 or 3 doses through age 26 years depending on age at initial vaccination or condition							
PCV13				1 dose							
PPSV23				1, 2, or 3 doses depending on age and indication							
HepA				2 or 3 doses depending on vaccine							
HepB				2, 3, or 4 doses depending on vaccine or condition					<60 years / ≥60 years		
MenACWY				1 or 2 doses depending on indication, see notes for booster recommendations							
MenB	Precaution			2 or 3 doses depending on vaccine and indication, see notes for booster recommendations							
Hib		3 doses HSCT[3] recipients only			1 dose						

Legend:

- Recommended vaccination for adults who meet age requirement, lack documentation of vaccination, or lack evidence of past infection
- Recommended vaccination for adults with an additional risk factor or another indication
- Recommended vaccination based on shared clinical decision-making
- Precaution—vaccination might be indicated if benefit of protection outweighs risk of adverse reaction
- Not recommended/contraindicated—vaccine should not be administered.
- No recommendation/not applicable

*Vaccinate after pregnancy.

1. Precaution for LAIV4 does not apply to alcoholism. 2. See notes for influenza; hepatitis B; measles, mumps, and rubella; and varicella vaccinations. 3. Hematopoietic stem cell transplant.

Administration for Community Living: *2018 Profile of older Americans.* Retrieved from https://acl.gov/sites/default/files/Aging%20and%20Disability%20in%20America/2018OlderAmericansProfile.pdf, 2018.

Allen P: Will pharmacogenetics help your health?. Retrieved from https://health.usnews.com/health-news/patient-advice/articles/2015/10/23/will-pharmacogenetics-help-your-health, 2015.

American Academy of Dermatology at https://www.aad.org

American Academy of Ophthalmology: *What is macular degeneration?.* Retrieved from https://www.aao.org/eye-health/diseases/amd-macular-degeneration, 2020.

American Botanical Council: *Terminology.* Retrieved from http://abc.herbalgram.org/site/PageServer?pagename=Terminology, 2013.

American College of Cardiology/American Heart Association: *Guideline for the prevention, detection, evaluation and management of high blood pressure in adults*, 2019.

American College of Obstetricians and Gynecologists: *Antenatal corticosteroid therapy for fetal maturation.* Retrieved from https://m.acog.org, 2016.

American College of Obstetricians and Gynecologists. *ACOG Practice bulletin 194, Polycystic Ovary Syndrome.* 2018. Retrieved from https://m.acog.org.

American College of Obstetricians and Gynecologists. *ACOG Practice Bulletin No. 194: Polycystic Ovary Syndrome.* 2020. Retrieved from https://m.acog.org.

American College of Obstetricians and Gynecologists: *Preeclampsia and hypertension in pregnancy.* Retrieved from https://m.acog.org, 2018.

American College of Obstetricians and Gynecologists: *Morning sickness: nausea and vomiting of pregnancy.* Retrieved from https://www.m.acog.org, 2015.

American College of Obstetricians and Gynecologists: *Medications for pain relief during labor and delivery.* Retrieved from https://www.m.acog.org, 2018.

The American College of Obstetricians and Gynecologists: The Rh Factor: How it can affect your pregnancy. Retrieved from https://m.acog.org/Patients/FAQs/The Rh factor how it can affect your pregnancy.

The American Congress of Obstetricians and Gynecologists (ACOG): *Maternal safety bundle for severe hypertension in pregnancy. Safe motherhood initiative.* Retrieved from http://www.ACOG.com, 2017.

American Heart Association: *Guidelines for cardiopulmonary resuscitation and emergency cardiovascular care*, . https://eccguidelines.heart.org/index.php/circulation/cpr-ecc-guidelines-2/part-7-adult-advanced-cardiovascular-life-support/, 2015. Retrieved June 17, 2018.

American Nurses Association: *CDC: opioid use disorder prevalence up 333% among pregnant women*, Association Smart Brief, 2018. Retrieved from http://www:American Nurse's. . Association Smart Brief, 2018.

American Nurses Association: *Code of ethics for nurses with interpretive statements.* Retrieved July 23, 2019 from https://www.nursingworld.org/practice-policy/nursing-excellence/ethics/code-of-ethics-for-nurses/coe-view-only/, 2015.

American Society of Clinical Pharmacology: CAR T-Cell immunotherapy named advance of the year in annual ASCO report. , https://www.asco.org, 2018.

Association of Reproductive Health Professionals: *Extended or continuous use of combined hormonal contraceptive pills.* Retrieved from https://www.arhp.org/publications and resources.oc, 2014.

Bakall B, Hariprasad SM, Klein KA: Emerging gene therapy treatments for inherited retinal diseases, *Ophthalmic Surg Lasers Imaging Retina* 49(7):472–478, 2018, https://doi.org/10.3928/23258160-20180628-02.

Belluz J: *This new bill would add $9 billion for medical research. Here are 5 reasons critics are terrified*, VOX Science & Health, 2015. Retrieved from http://www.vox.com/2015/7/14/8961923/21st-century-cures-act.

Blaise K, Hayes Jr : *Professional nursing practice concept and perspective*, 7 ed, Upper Saddle River, NJ, 2016, Pearson.

Bodenheimer T. Teach-back: *A simple way to enhance patients' understanding.* Retrieved from https://aafp.org/fpm/2018/0700/p20.html, 2018.

Bonin M, Mewton N, Roubille F, et al.: Effect and safety of morphine use in acute anterior ST-segment elevation myocardial infarction, *JAHA* 7(4), 2018https://doi.org/10.1161/JAHA.117.006833. Retrieved September 20, 2018 https://www.ahajournals.org/doi/pdf/10.1161/JAHA.117.006833.

Bradley HC: *Renal transplantation.* Retrieved July 25, 2019 from https://emedicine.medscape.com/article/430128-overview, 2019.

Burchum J, Rosenthal L: *Lehne's pharmacology for nursing care*, ed 9, St. Louis, 2016, Elsevier.

Burchum JR, Rosenthal LD: *Lehne's pharmacology for nursing care*, ed 10, St Louis, 2019, Elsevier.

CancerQuest.org. *Biological Response Modifiers (BRM).* Retrieved from https://www.cancerquest.org/patients/treatments/biological-therapies, 2021.

CancerQuest.org. *Cancer Immunotherapy.* Retrieved from https://www.cancerquest.org/patients/treatments/immunotherapy, 2021.

Carlson NR: *Foundations of behavioral neuroscience*, ed 8, Upper Saddle River, NJ, 2010, Pearson.

Centers for Disease Control and Prevention. HIV in the United States and Dependent Areas. Retrieved from https://www.cdc.gov/hiv/statistics/overview/ataglance.html, 2021.

Centers for Disease Control and Prevention. Parasites - Malaria. Retrieved from https://www.cdc.gov/parasites/malaria/index.html, 2021.

Centers for Disease Control and Prevention: *The right way to use a male condom.* Retrieved from www.cdc.gov/condomeffectiveness/male-condom-use.html, 2016.

Centers for Disease Control and Prevention: *Medication safety program.* Retrieved July 24, 2019 from https://www.cdc.gov/medicationsafety/adult_adversedrugevents.html, 2017.

Centers for Disease Control and Prevention: Recommendations for women. Retrieved from https://www.cdc.gov/ncbddd/folicacid/recommendations.html.

Centers for Disease Control and Prevention: *2015 Sexually transmitted diseases treatment guidelines.* Retrieved from https://www.cdc.gov/std/tg2015/default.htm, 2015.

Centers for Disease Control and Prevention: Tuberculosis (TB). Retrieved from www.cdc.gov/tb/default.htm.

Centers for Disease Control and Prevention: *Vaccines & immunizations.* Retrieved July 25, 2019 from https://www.cdc.gov/vaccines/index.html?CDC_AA_refVal=https%3A%2F%2Fwww.cdc.gov%2Fvaccines%2Fdefault.htm, 2016.

Centers for Disease Control and Prevention. *V-safe After Vaccination Health Checker.* Retrieved from https://www.cdc.gov/coronavirus/2019-ncov/vaccines/safety/vsafe.html.

Chang KL, Weitzel K, Shmidt S: Pharmacogenetics: Using genetic information to guide drug therapy, *Am Fam Physician* 92(7):588–594, 2015. www.aafp.org/afp.

Cheek DJ: Pharmacogenomics: Strategies for individualized care, *Nursing2017CriticalCare* 12(1):23–27, 2017. www.nursingcriticalcare.com.

Cheek DJ: *Why nurses need to be informed about pharmacogenomics. Reflections on nursing leadership.* Retrieved from https://www.reflectionsonnursingleadership.org/features/more-features/Vol41_2_why-nurses-need-to-be-informed-about-pharmacogenomics, 2015.

Cheek DJ, Howington L: Patient care in the dawn of the genomic age, *Am Nurse Today* 12(3):16–22, 2017.

Chooniedass R, Temple B, Becker A: Epinephrine use for anaphylaxis: too seldom, too late: current practices and guidelines in healthcare, *Ann Allergy Asthma Immunol* 119:108–110, 2017.

Chu DK, Kim LH-Y, Young PJ, et al.: Mortality and morbidity in acutely ill adults treated with liberal versus conservative oxygen therapy (IOTA): a systematic review and meta-analysis, *The Lancet* 391(10131):1693–1705, 2018.

Clayton BD, Willihnganz MJ: *Basic pharmacology for nurses*, ed 17, St. Louis, 2017, Elsevier.

Clinic M: Labor & delivery, postpartum care. Retrieved from https://www.mayoclinic.org.

Clinical Info. Guidelines for the Use of Antiretroviral Agents in Adults and Adolescents Living with HIV. Retrieved from https://clinicalinfo.hiv.

gov/en/guidelines/adult-and-adolescent-arv/what-start-initial-combination-regimens-antiretroviral-naive?view=full, 2021.

Consumer Healthcare Products Association. (n.d.): Statistics on OTC use. Retrieved July 23, 2019 from https://www.chpa.org/MarketStats.aspx.

Council for Responsible Nutrition (CRN). *The science behind the supplements.* Retrieved from https://crnusa.org.

Department of Health: Human Services/Office on Women's Health. Premenstrual syndrome (PMS). Retrieved from https://www.womenshealth.gov.

Department of Health & Human Services/Office on Women's Health. Menopause. Retrieved from https://www.womenshealth.gov.

Divakaran S, Loscalzo J: The role of nitroglycerin and other nitrogen oxides in cardiovascular therapeutics, *J Am Coll Cardiol* 70(19):2393–2410, 2017.

DrugAbuse.com. (n.d.). http://drugabuse.com/library/drugs-a-z/; www.drugs.com

Drugs.com for Healthcare professionals. (n.d.). Retrieved from www.drugs.com/professionals.html

Drugs A-Z. Retrieved May 15, 2016, from www.drugs.com

Edmunds MW: *Introduction to clinical pharmacology*, ed 8, St. Louis, 2016, Mosby.

Epocrates. http://www.epocrates.com

Evans P: *8 incredible facts about the booming US marijuana industry.* Retrieved August 26, 2019 from https://markets.businessinsider.com/news/stocks/weed-us-marijuana-industry-facts-2019-5-1028177375#the-marijuana-industry-could-soon-be-worth-more-than-the-gdp-of-9-us-states1, 2019.

Farrukh: *The difference between active and passive transport.* Retrieved January 2, 2019 from https://hourstv.com/difference-between-active-and-passive-transport/, 2018.

Gahart B, Nazareno AR, Ortega MQ: *Intravenous medications*, ed 35, St Louis, 2019, Elsevier.

Gentili A, Adler RA: *Growth hormone replacement in older men?* Medscape. Retrieved from https://emedicine.medscape.com/article/126999-medication#2, 2020.

Giddens JF: *Concepts for nursing practice*, ed 2, St Louis, 2017, Elsevier.

GlobalRxPh: *Creatinine clearance adult.* Retrieved July 24, 2019 from https://globalrph.com/medcalcs/creatinine-clearance-adult/, 2017.

Gold Standard. http://www.clinicalpharmacology.com

Governing: *State marijuana Laws in 2019 Map.* Retrieved August 26, 2019 from https://www.governing.com/gov-data/safety-justice/state-marijuana-laws-map-medical-recreational.html, 2019.

Gummin DD, Mowry JB, Spyker DA, Brooks DE, Fraser MO, Banner W: 2016 Annual Report of the American Association of Poison Control Centers' National Poison Data System (NPDS): 34th annual report, *Clin Toxicol* 55(10):1072–1254, 2017, https://doi.org/10.1080/15563650.2017.1388087. Retrieved on September 20, 2018.

Government of Canada: *Controlled drugs and substances act.* Retrieved July 23, 2019 from https://laws-lois.justice.gc.ca/eng/acts/C-38.8/20180621/P1TT3xt3.html, 2018.

Guzman F (nd): Pharmacology corner. Retrieved on January 1, 2016, from http://pharmacologycorner.com/therapeutic-index/.

Haga SB, Mills R: Nurses' communication of pharmacogenetic tests results as part of discharge care, *Pharmacogenomics* 16(3):251–256, 2015, https://doi.org/10.2217/PGS.14.173.

Harvard Health Letter. *Sexually transmitted disease? At my age?* Retrieved from: https://www.health.harvard.edu/diseases-and-conditions/sexually-transmitted-disease-at-my-age, 2018.

Hastert JD: *H.R.1 - Medicare prescription drug, improvement, and modernization act of 2003.* Retrieved July 24, 2019 from https://www.congress.gov/bill/108th-congress/house-bill/1, 2003.

Hewitt J, Tower M, Latimer S: An education intervention to improve nursing students understanding of medication safety, *Nurses education in practice* 15(1):17–21, 2015.

Horvath AT, Misra K, Epner AK, Cooper GM, (n.d.): The diagnostic criteria for substance use disorders (addiction). Retrieved from www.amhc.org/1408-addictions/article/48502-the-diagnostic-criteria-for-substance-use-disorders-addiction.

Huether SE, McCance KL: *Understanding Pathophysiology*, ed 6, St Louis, 2017, Elsevier.

Human Research Protections (OHRP). (2014). U.S. Department of Health & Human Services. Retrieved from http://www.hhs.gov/ohrp/policy/consentckls.html

Ignatavicius D: Developing clinical judgment for professional nursing and the next generation NCLEX-RN examination, Missouri, 2021, Elsevier.

Ignatavicium D: *White paper: Using case studies to develop clinical judgment & ensure next generation NCLEX (NGN) success*, Missouri, 2021, Elsevier.

Ignatavicius DD, Workman ML, Rebar CR: *Medical-Surgical nursing: Concepts for interprofessional collaborative care*, ed 9, St Louis, 2018, Elsevier.

International Council for Harmonization of Technical Requirements for Pharmaceuticals for Human Use: *Integrated addendum to ICH E6(R1): Guideline for good clinical practice (E6(R2).* Retrieved from https://www.ich.org/fileadmin/Public_Web_Site/ICH_Products/Guidelines/Efficacy/E6/E6_R2__Step_4_2016_1109.pdf, 2016.

IQVIA Institute for human data science. Retrieved from. http://www.iqvia.com, 2018.

Lab Tests Online: *Pharmacogenetic tests.* Retrieved January 6, 2019 from https://labtestsonline.org/tests/pharmacogenetic-tests, 2018.

Lea DH: The role of pharmacogenomics in cancer, *Am Nurse Today* 5(10), 2010. Retrieved from https://www.americannursetoday.com/the-role-of-pharmacogenomics-in-cancer/.

Lewis SL, Bucher L, Heitkemper MM, Harding MM: *Medical-surgical nursing: assessment and management of clinical problems*, ed 10, St Louis, 2017, Elsevier.

Lexicomp Clinical Drug Information: http://www.wolterskluwercdi.com/lexicomp-online/.

Lilley LL, Collins SR, Snyder JS: *Pharmacology and the nursing process*, ed 8, St Louis, 2017, Elsevier.

Maddox TM, Januzzi JL, Allen LA, et al.; 2021 Update to the 2017 ACC Expert Consensus Decision Pathway for Optimization of Heart Failure Treatment: answers to 10 pivotal issues about heart failure with reduced ejection fraction: a Report of the American College of Cardiology Solution Set Oversight Committee, *J Am Coll Cardiol* 77(6):772–810.

Martin-Hijano L, Sainz B: The interactions between cancer stem cells and the innate-interferon signaling pathway, *Frontiers in Immunology* 11, 2020.

Maternal & Family Health Services: *Family planning protocols section 1 -Required family planning services: informed consent, .* https://www.maternal and family health services.org, 2013.

Mayo Clinic: Labor & delivery, postpartum care. Retrieved from https://www.mayoclinic.org.

McClary LM: *Essentials of medical genetics for nursing and health professionals: an interprofessional approach*, Burlington, MA, 2020, Jones & Bartlett Learning.

McCormick KA: Pharmacogenomics and documentation: new partnerships target optimal care quality and outcomes, *Nurs Manag* 48(5):32–40, 2017, https://doi.org/10.1097/01.NUMA.0000515793.26355.7f.

McKenry LM, Tessier E, Hogan MA: *Mosby's pharmacology in nursing*, ed 22, St. Louis, 2006, Elsevier.

Medscape.com. (n.d.). Drugs, OTCs & Herbals. Retrieved from http://reference.medscape.com/drugs

Mehta M., & Tudor, G.J. *Parkland formula.* StatPearls [Internet]. Retrieved from https://www.ncbi.nlm.nih.gov/books/NBK537190/#:~:text=The%20formula%20recommends%204%20milliliters,first%2024%20hours%20of%20care, 2020.

Meyer, D., Damm, T., & Jensen, K. Drug dosage adjustments in chronic kidney disease: the pharmacist's role. *Saskatchewan Drug Information Services College of Pharmacy and Nutrition, U of S*, 29(3): 4, 2012. Retrieved from https://www.rxfiles.ca/rxfiles/uploads/documents/ltc/HCPs/CKD/SDIS.Renal_newsletter.pdf

Montgomery S, Brouwer WA, Everett PC, et al.: Genetics in the clinical setting: what nurses need to know to provide the best patient care, *Am Nurse Today* 12(10):10–16, 2017.

Moreno JD, Schmidt U, Joffe S: The Nuremberg Code 70 years later, *Journal of the American Medical Association* 318(9):795–796, 2017, https://doi.org/10.1001/jama.2017.10265.

National Cancer Institute. *Cancer statistics.* Retrieved from cancer.gov/about-cancer/understanding/statistics, 2020.

National Council of State Boards of Nursing: *Next-generation-NCLEX.* Retrieved from: https://www.ncsbn.org.htm, 2021.

National Council of State Boards of Nursing. (n.d.): Substance use disorder in nursing. Retrieved July 24, 2019 from https://www.ncsbn.org/substance-use-in-nursing.htm.

National Center of State Boards of Nursing. *The NCSBN Clinical Judgment Measurement Model.* 2018. Retrieved from https://www.ncsbn.org/14798. htm.

National Institute on Drug Abuse: *Commonly abused drugs.* Retrieved May 15, 2016, from www.drugabuse.gov/drugs-abuse/, 2016.

National Institute on Drug Abuse (NIDA): *Media Guide.* Retrieved November 23, 2021, from https://archives.drugabuse.gov/publications/media-guide, 2018.

National Institute on Drug Abuse: *The science of drug abuse and addiction: the basics.* Retrieved May 16, 2016, from www.drugabuse.gov/publications/media-guide/science-drug-abuse-addiction-basics, 2014.

National Institute of General Medical Sciences: Pharmacogenomics: what is pharmacogenomics? [Fact Sheet]. Retrieved January 6, 2019 from https://www.nigms.nih.gov/education/pages/factsheet-pharmacogenomics.aspx, 2017.

National Kidney Foundation. (n.d.): Kidney transplant. Retrieved July 25, 2019 from https://www.kidney.org/atoz/content/kidney-transplant.

Neutropenic precautions. Retrieved 12/23/16 from https://www.cdc.gov/cancer/preventinfections/pdf/neutropenia.pdf

New FDA Pregnancy Categories (June 20, 2015). Retrieved from https://www.Drugus.com/pregnancy-categories.html

New Health Advisor: *How to use a female condom: Pictures and instructions.* Retrieved from www.newhealthadvisor.com/How-to-Use-Female-Condom-Picture.html, 2016.

North American Menopause Society (NAMS) T: *Menopause Hormone Therapy Benefits & Risks.* Menopause Relief/ Retrieved from https://www.menopause.org, 2019.

Office for Human Research Protections. https://www.hhs.gov/ohrp/

Parekh R: What is addiction?. Retrieved July 24, 2019 from https://www.psychiatry.org/patients-families/addiction/what-is-addiction, 2017.

Pelligrino B: *Immunosuppression.* Retrieved July 25, 2019 from https://emedicine.medscape.com/article/432316-overview#a3, 2016.

Pharmacogenomics Laboratory: Guideline-based decision support. Retrieved January 6, 2019 from https://ignite-genomics.org/wp-content/uploads/2016/03/26_PGx-lab-Marketing-Brochure.pdf.

PharmGKB*: What is pharmacogenomics?. Retrieved January 6, 2019 from https://www.pharmgkb.org/whatIsPharmacogenomics.

Piscitelli SC: *Space out drug discontinuations prior to "drug holiday"?.* Retrieved January 2, 2019 from https://www.medscape.com/viewarticle/413306, 2000.

Pinto JC, n.d.: Pediatric dosage development: where are we? [PowerPoint slides]. Retrieved from http://www.fda.gov/downloads/NewsEvents/MeetingsConferencesWorkshops/UCM415217.pdf.

Silvestri L: White paper: Higher-cognitive level questions a starting point for creating next generation NCLEX (NGN) test items, Missouri, 2021, Elsevier.

South Atlantic Association of Obstetricians & Gynecologists: Pentobarbital anesthesia in labor. Retrieved from https://www.sciencedirect.com/science/article/piv/0002937867902505

Substance Abuse and Mental Health Services Administration: *Substance use disorders.* Retrieved May 17, 2016, from www.samhsa.gov/disorders/substance-use/Preterm-Premature Labor and birth, 2015.

Substance Abuse and Mental Health Services Administration: Treatments for substance use disorders. Retrieved June 3, 2016, from www.samhsa.gov/treatment/substance-use-disorders, 2015.

Talwar A, Tsang CA, Price SE, Pratt RH, Walker WL, Schmit KM, Lunger AJ. Morbidity and mortality weekly report, March 22, 2019. Centers for Disease Control and Prevention: MMWR, 68:11. 257–262, 2019. Retrieved from https://www.cdc.gov/mmwr/volumes/68/wr/pdfs/mm6811a2-H.pdf

Umberger R, Holston EC, Hutson SP, Pierce M: Nursing genomics: Practice implications every nurse should know, *Nurs Clin N Am* 48:499–522, 2013, https://doi.org/10.1016/j.cnur.2013.08.006.

United States Drug Enforcement Administration: *Drug scheduling.* Retrieved January 2, 2019 from https://www.dea.gov/drug-scheduling, 2018.

U.S. Federal Drug Administration: *FDA approves new vaginal ring for one year of birth control.* Retrieved from https://www.fda.gov/ucm616541.htm, 2018.

U.S. Federal Drug Administration: *Drug trials snapshots: Orilissa.* Retrieved from https://www.fda.gov/ucm616534.htm, 2018.

U.S. Federal Drug Administration: *Milestones in U.S. Food and Drug law history.* Retrieved July 23, 2019 from https://www.fda.gov/about-fda/fdas-evolving-regulatory-powers/milestones-us-food-and-drug-law-history, 2018.

US Food and Drug Administration: *FDA approves weekly therapy for adult growth hormone deficiency.* Retrieved from https://www.fda.gov/drugs/drug-safety-and-availability/fda-approves-weekly-therapy-adult-growth-hormone-deficiency, 2020.

US Food & Drug Administration: *Critical path initiative.* Retrieved July 23, 2019 from https://www.fda.gov/science-research/science-and-research-special-topics/critical-path-initiative, 2018.

U.S. Federal Drug Administration. (n.d.): Requirements for all OTC products. Retrieved July 23, 2019 from https://www.accessdata.fda.gov/scripts/cder/training/OTC/topic4/topic4/da_01_04_0005.htm.

U.S. Federal Drug Administration: *The best way to take your over-the-counter pain reliever? Seriously.* Retrieved July 23, 2019 from https://www.fda.gov/drugs/safe-use-over-counter-pain-relievers-and-fever-reducers/best-way-take-your-over-counter-pain-reliever-seriously-four-panel-brochure, 2018.

U.S. Food and Drug Administration: Pediatric exclusivity study age group (C-DRG-00909). Retrieved from http://www.fda.gov/Drugs/DevelopmentApprovalProcess/FormsSubmissionRequirements/ElectronicSubmissions/DataStandardsManualmonographs/ucm071754.htm, 2014.

U.S. Pharmacopeia National Formulary. https://www.uspnf.com.

Vallerand AH, Sanoski CA: *Davis drug guide for nurses,* ed 15, Pennsylvania, 2017, F. A. Davis.

Vogel WH: Infusion reactions: Diagnosis, assessment and management, *Clin J Oncol Nurs* 14(2):E10–E21, 2010. Retrieved from http://chemotherapy.vc.ons.org/file_depot/0-10000000/0-10000/3365/folder/87592/Infusion+-Reactions+(Vogel+2010).pdf.

Wilson BA, Shannon M, Shields K: *Pearson nurse's drug guide,* ed 1, New York, 2017, Pearson.

World Health Organization. (n.d.): Lexicon of alcohol and drug terms published by the World Health Organization. Retrieved May 18, 2016, from http://www.who.int/substance_abuse/terminology/who_lexicon/en/.

World Health Organization. The International Pharmacopoeia (Ph. Int.). https://www.who.int/medicines/publications/pharmacopoeia/en/

World Health Organization Reproductive Health Library. WHO recommendation on daily oral iron and folic acid supplement (November 2016). The WHO Reproductive Health Library; Geneva: World Health Organization.

World Medical Association: *WMA declaration of Helsinki – ethical principles for medical research involving human subjects.* Retrieved July 23, 2019 from https://www.wma.net/policies-post/wma-declaration-of-helsinki-ethical-principles-for-medical-research-involving-human-subjects/, 2018.

A

absence seizure Formerly known as petit mal seizure

absorption Movement of a drug into the bloodstream after administration

acetylcholine (ACh) The neurotransmitter located at the ganglions and the parasympathetic terminal nerve endings

acetylcholinesterase (AChE) inhibitor An enzyme responsible for breaking down acetylcholine; also known as *cholinesterase*

acne vulgaris The formation of papules, nodules, and cysts on the face, neck, shoulders, and back that results from keratin plugs at the base of the pilosebaceous (oil) glands near the hair follicles

acquired immunodeficiency syndrome (AIDS) The most advanced stage of human immunodeficiency virus (HIV) infection

acquired resistance Resistance caused by prior exposure to an antibacterial

acromegaly Excessive growth after puberty

activated partial thromboplastin time (aPTT) A medical test that characterizes blood coagulation

active acquired artificial immunity Immunity that occurs when a weakened antigen or immunoglobulin (Ig) is injected into an individual as a vaccination, which then stimulates an immune response

active immunity Immunity that occurs when the body's immune response is stimulated by an antigen or when a pathogen enters the body

active transport A process that requires a carrier, such as an enzyme or protein, to move a drug against a concentration gradient

acute cystitis A lower urinary tract infection (UTI)

acute dystonia Characteristics of this reaction include muscle spasms of the face, tongue, neck, and back; facial grimacing; abnormal or involuntary upward eye movement; and laryngeal spasms that can impair respiration

acute myocardial infarction (AMI) Acute heart attack

acute pharyngitis Inflammation of the throat or "sore throat" caused by a virus, beta-hemolytic streptococci, or other bacteria

acute pyelonephritis An upper UTI

acute rhinitis Acute inflammation of the mucous membranes of the nose that usually accompanies the common cold

adequate intake (AI) The consumption and absorption of sufficient food, vitamins, and essential minerals necessary to maintain health

addiction A psychological and physical dependence upon a substance beyond normal voluntary control, usually after prolonged use

Addison disease An endocrine disorder of the adrenal glands causing adrenal hyposecretion of its hormones

additive effect When two drugs are administered in combination and the response is increased beyond what either could produce alone

adenohypophysis The anterior pituitary gland

adherence The extent to which a patient continues an agreed-on mode of treatment without close supervision

adjuvant A substance added to a vaccine to increase the body's immune response to the vaccine

adjuvant analgesic A generic term for a medication not designed to manage pain

adjuvant therapy A additional therapy added to the primary therapy

adrenal glands Consist of the adrenal medulla and adrenal cortex

adrenergic agonists A class of G-protein–coupled receptors that are targets of the catecholamines

adrenergic antagonists (adrenergic blockers) Drugs that block either the alpha or the beta receptor

adrenergic neuron antagonists (adrenergic neuron blockers) Drugs that block the release of norepinephrine from the sympathetic terminal neurons

adrenergic receptor Target of the catecholamines

adrenocorticotropic hormone (ACTH) An endocrine hormone secreted by the anterior pituitary gland that stimulates the release of glucocorticoids, mineralocorticoids, and androgen from the adrenal cortex and epinephrine and norepinephrine from the adrenal medulla

adsorbents Act by coating the wall of the gastrointestinal tract and adsorbing bacteria or toxins that cause diarrhea

adverse drug event (ADE) Any injury that occurs at the time a drug is used, regardless of whether it is identified as a cause of the injury

adverse drug reaction (ADR) Unintentional, unexpected reactions to drug therapy that occur at normal drug dosages

afterload Peripheral vascular resistance

age-related macular degeneration (AMD) Deterioration of the macula

aggregation Clumping together of platelets to form a clot

agonists Drugs that activate receptors and produce a desired response

akathisia A reaction in which the patient has trouble standing still, is restless, paces the floor, and is in constant motion

alcohol toxicity A life-threatening condition that can occur by drinking large amounts of alcohol over a short period of time

alkylating drugs Drugs that damage cellular DNA by cross-linkage of DNA strands, abnormal base pairing, or DNA strand breaks, thus preventing the reproduction of cancer cells

allergic rhinitis Caused by pollen or a foreign substance such as animal dander

alpha antagonists (alpha blockers) Drugs that promote vasodilation, causing a decrease in blood pressure

alternative health therapies The phenomenon of the dominant cultural group borrowing traditional health practices from less dominant groups

alveoli Air sacs

Alzheimer disease A chronic, progressive, neurodegenerative condition with marked cognitive dysfunction

amenorrhea Absence of menstrual periods

American Nurses Association Code of Ethics Developed as a guide for carrying out nursing responsibilities in a manner consistent with quality in nursing care and the ethical obligations of the profession

amphetamines Drugs that stimulate the cerebral cortex of the brain

ampule Glass container with a tapered neck

anabolism Buildup of cellular tissue

analeptic Acts on the brainstem and medulla to stimulate respiration

analgesic A drug prescribed for the relief of pain

anaphylactic shock An allergic response resulting in severe bronchoconstriction and hypotension resulting in cardiac collapse

anaphylaxis A serious, life-threatening allergic reaction to a specific vaccine or vaccine component

androgen A male sex hormone

anesthetic A drug that causes anesthesia

angina pectoris Chest pain

angle-closure glaucoma A condition in which the iris is situated close to the drainage angle, thus blocking the trabecular network; also known as closed-angle or narrow-angle glaucoma

anion A negative charge in ions

anorexiants Drugs thought to suppress appetite by stimulating the satiety center in the hypothalamic and limbic areas of the brain

anovulation Lack of ovulation

anovulatory The absence of ovulation

anoxia Absence of oxygen

antacids Promote ulcer healing by neutralizing hydrochloric acid and reducing pepsin activity

antagonistic effects The negative effect that one chemical or family of chemicals has on other chemicals

antagonists Drugs that prevent receptor activation and block a response

anthelmintics Agents that destroy worms

anthracycline A class of chemotherapeutic agents

antiandrogens Androgen antagonists that block the synthesis or action of androgens

antianginal drugs Medicines that relieve the symptoms of angina pectoris

antibacterials Substances that inhibit bacterial growth or kill bacteria and other microorganisms

antibiotic resistance Biologically occurring short chains of amino acid monomers linked by peptide (amide) bonds

antibodies Defend the body against pathogens

anticoagulants Prevent the formation of clots that inhibit circulation

antidepressants Drugs that treat depression and/or relieve the symptoms

antidiarrheals Agents used for treating diarrhea and decreasing hypermotility

antidiuretic hormone (ADH) A hormone made by the hypothalamus in the brain and stored in the posterior pituitary gland

antidysrhythmics (antiarrhythmics) Drugs that restore the cardiac rhythm to normal

antiemetics Antivomiting agents

antiflatulents Drugs that treat excessive gas in the stomach and intestines

antifungals Drugs used to treat fungal infections

antigen A toxin or other foreign substance that induces an immune response in the body, especially the production of antibodies

antihistamines Compete with histamine for receptor sites and prevent a histamine response

antihyperlipidemics Drugs used to lower lipoproteins

antihypertensives Drugs used to treat hypertension

antimalarials Drugs that provide treatment and prophylaxis for malaria

antimetabolite A chemical that interferes with various substances needed for normal cell function

antimicrobials Substances that inhibit bacterial growth or kill bacteria and other microorganisms

antimuscarinics Agents that block parasympathetic nerve impulses

antimycotic drugs Drugs used to treat fungal infections

antineoplastic drug An agent that destroys cancer cells

antioncogenes Genes that protect other genes

antiplatelets Used to prevent thrombosis in the arteries by suppressing platelet aggregation

antipsychotics Also known as *neuroleptics* or *psychotropics,* but the preferred name for this group is either *antipsychotics* or *neuroleptics*

antiretroviral therapy (ART) The combination of several antiretroviral medicines used to slow the rate at which human immunodeficiency virus (HIV) makes copies of itself in the body

antiseizure drugs Drugs used for epileptic seizures

antispasmodics Agents that block parasympathetic nerve impulses

antitumor antibiotics Agents that interfere with DNA replication and RNA transcription of cancer cells

antitussives Agents that act on the cough-control center in the medulla to suppress the cough reflex

antiviral drugs Agents used to prevent or delay the spread of viral infections

anxiolytics Also called *antianxiety drugs* or *sedative-hypnotics*

apolipoprotein A protein that combines with a lipid, such as cholesterol or triglyceride, to form a lipoprotein

apoptosis Programmed cell death

aqueous humor A clear fluid that flows continuously in and out of the chamber of the eye

assessment The phase during which a nurse gathers information from the patient about the patient's health and lifestyle

assimilation Occurs within and among cultural groups, such as when a minority group changes its ways to blend in with the dominant cultural group

asthma Hyperresponsiveness of the tracheobronchial system resulting in inflammation and narrowing of the airways

asystole The cessation of electrical activity within the heart

atonic seizure Loss of normal muscle tension; a seizure in which muscles suddenly lose strength

atrial fibrillation Cardiac dysrhythmia with rapid uncoordinated contractions of atrial myocardium

atrial flutter Cardiac dysrhythmia with rapid contractions of 200 to 300 beats/min

attention-deficit/hyperactivity disorder (ADHD) A disorder that might be caused by a dysregulation of the transmitter's serotonin, norepinephrine, and dopamine

attenuated viruses Viruses composed of live, attenuated microorganisms

atypical antidepressants Drugs used for major depression, reactive depression, and anxiety that affect one or two of the three neurotransmitters: serotonin, norepinephrine, and dopamine

atypical antipsychotics The second category of antipsychotics

autonomy The right to self-determination

B

bactericidal Bacteria killing

bacteriostatic Inhibits bacterial growth; may also be bactericidal (bacteria killing), depending on the drug dose, serum level, and pathogen

balanced anesthesia A combination of drugs frequently used in general anesthesia

barbiturates Long-, intermediate-, short-, and ultrashort-acting sedatives

basic formula The equation $D/H \times V = A$ to calculate the amount A to be administered, where D is the Desired dose; H is the drug on Hand; V is the Vehicle or Volume

Beers Criteria for Potentially Inappropriate Medication Use in Older Adults A document developed by a consensus panel of 12 experts in geriatric care to aid health care providers in the safe prescription and administration of drugs to older adults

beneficence The duty to protect research subjects from harm and to assess potential risks and possible benefits to ensure the benefits are greater than the risk

beta antagonists (beta blockers) May inhibit the action of albuterol

bioavailability The percentage of administered drug available for activity

biologic response modifiers (BRMs) A class of pharmacologic drugs used to enhance, direct, or restore the body's immune system

biotransformation The process by which the body chemically changes drugs into a form that can be excreted

bipolar disorder A disorder that involves swings between two moods, the manic and the depressive

Bishop score An objective measurement that assists in predicting whether labor induction may be successful; assess the readiness for labor induction

blackhead A type of noninflammatory acne lesion that is open

blepharitis Infection of the margins of the eyelid

blood-borne pathogens Microorganisms such as viruses or bacteria that can be spread through blood and body fluids

blood-brain barrier (BBB) A special endothelial lining in blood vessels in the brain where the cells are pressed tightly together (tight junctions)

blood dyscrasias Blood-cell disorders

bolus The first method used to deliver enteral feedings, by which 250 to 400 mL of solution is rapidly administered through a syringe into the tube four to six times a day

botanicals Additive substances that come from plants

bradycardia A pulse rate below 60 beats per minute

bradykinesia Slow movement

brand (trade) name Also known as the *proprietary name,* the name chosen by the drug company; usually a registered trademark

breakthrough bleeding An abnormal flow of blood from the uterus that occurs between menstrual periods

broad-spectrum antibiotics Drugs that can be effective against both gram-positive and gram-negative organisms

bronchial asthma Characterized by bronchospasm, wheezing, mucus secretions, and dyspnea; one of the lung diseases of chronic obstructive pulmonary disease (COPD)

bronchiectasis Abnormal dilation of the bronchi and bronchioles secondary to frequent infection and inflammation

bronchodilators Drugs that relax bronchial muscle and result in expansion of the bronchial air passages

bronchospasm Results when lung tissue is exposed to extrinsic or intrinsic factors that stimulate a bronchoconstrictive response

buccal Administered between the cheek and gum

C

cadaveric transplantation A healthy organ donated at the time of a person's death that is transplanted into the body of a patient with end-stage organ failure

calcium channel blockers (CCBs) Agents used for the treatment of stable and variant angina pectoris, certain dysrhythmias, and hypertension

cannabinoids The active ingredients in *Cannabis,* approved for clinical use in 1985 to alleviate nausea and vomiting resulting from cancer treatment

capillary leak syndrome A rare disorder from extravasation of plasma proteins and fluids in the extravascular space characterized by episodes of severe hypotension and multiorgan dysfunction

carbonic anhydrase inhibitors (CAIs)   Agents that decrease intraocular pressure by decreasing the production of aqueous humor

cardiac dysrhythmia (arrhythmia)   Any deviation from the normal rate or pattern of the heartbeat

cardiac glycosides   Drugs that inhibit the sodium-potassium pump, which results in an increase in intracellular sodium

catecholamines   Chemical structures of a substance, either endogenous or synthetic, that can produce a sympathomimetic response

cathartics   Agents used to elicit bowel movements

cation   A positive charge in ions

caudal block   An epidural block placed by administering a local anesthetic through the sacral hiatus

cell cycle–nonspecific (CCNS) drugs   Drugs that act during any phase of the cell cycle

cell cycle–specific (CCS) drugs   Drugs that exert their influence during a specific phase of the cell cycle

cellular checkpoints, cellular communication   Mechanism by which cell-to-cell communication occurs locally or remotely by signaling molecules to maintain homeostasis, regulate growth and division, develop and organize into tissues, and coordinate cellular functions

central nervous system (CNS)   A system that involves the brain and spinal cord and that regulates body functions

cerumen   Earwax

ceruminolytics   Topical otic agents that soften or break up cerumen

cervical ripening   Softening of the cervix just prior to labor induction

chalazion   Infection of the meibomian glands of the eyelids that may produce cysts, causing blockage of the ducts

chancre   A painless sore, typically at the site of infection, usually on the penis in men and outer genitals or inner vagina in women

chemical name   A name that describes the drug's chemical structure

chemoprotectant   An agent administered prior to certain chemotherapeutic drugs to prevent toxicity

chemoreceptor trigger zone (CTZ)   A major cerebral center that lies near the medulla

chemotherapy   The use of chemicals to kill cancer cells

chloasma   Hyperpigmentation of the skin

cholinergic agonists   Drugs that stimulate the parasympathetic nervous system

cholinergic antagonists (blocking agents)   Drugs that affect the parasympathetic nervous system

cholinergic crisis   Overdosing with acetylcholinesterase (AChE) inhibitors; may complicate myasthenia gravis

cholinergics   Medications that produce the same effects as the parasympathetic neurotransmitter acetylcholine

cholinesterase (ChE)   May destroy acetylcholine before it reaches the receptor or after it has attached to the site

cholinesterase inhibitors   Indirect-acting cholinergics that inactivate the enzyme cholinesterase, which typically breaks down acetylcholine

chronic bronchitis   A progressive lung disease caused by smoking or chronic lung infections

chronic obstructive pulmonary disease (COPD)   A major category of lower respiratory tract disorders, COPD is caused by airway obstruction with increased airway resistance of airflow to lung tissues

chronotropic   An action that decreases heart rate

chylomicrons   Large particles that transport fatty acids and cholesterol to the liver

clonic seizure   A convulsive seizure

cluster headache   Headache characterized by a severe, unilateral, nonthrobbing pain usually located around the eye

colloid   A solution that contains protein or other large molecular substances that increase osmolarity without dissolving in the solution

colony-stimulating factors   Proteins that stimulate or regulate the growth, maturation, and differentiation of bone marrow stem cells

combination chemotherapy   The use of two or more chemotherapy agents to treat cancer

comedones   Noninflammatory acne lesions that may be open or closed

common cold   The most prevalent type of upper respiratory infection

complementary health therapies   Combine traditional and conventional Western health practices

concept   A concept is related to the patient's problems, medications, or topics of care; it is derived after the analysis of the nurse's assessment data, will influence the delivery of the patient's care, and its focus is on the patient-centered model of care

congenital rubella syndrome   Transmission of the rubella virus to the fetus via the placenta

congestive heart failure (CHF)   Occurs when the heart muscle does not pump blood as well as it should

conjugate vaccines   Newer vaccines that require a protein or toxoid from an unrelated organism to link to the outer coating of the disease-causing microorganism

conjunctivitis   Inflammation of the membrane covering the eye and inner eyelids

constipation   The accumulation of hard fecal material in the large intestine

contact dermatitis   A common form of eczema that results when skin is exposed to irritants or allergens

continuous feedings   Feedings prescribed for the critically ill and for those who receive feedings into the small intestine

controlled substance   A drug or chemical that has the potential for abuse whose manufacture, possession, or use is regulated by government

corticosteroids   Natural and synthetic agents that suppress inflammation

cretinism   A congenital abnormality caused by severe hypothyroidism causing delayed physical and mental growth

Critical Path Initiative   A national strategy "to drive innovation in the scientific processes through which medical products are developed, evaluated, and manufactured"

cross-resistance   Tolerance, usually to a toxic substance, that is acquired not as a result of direct exposure but by exposure to a related substance

cross-sensitivity   Sensitivity to one substance that predisposes an individual to sensitivity to other substances related in chemical structure

cryotherapy   A procedure used to destroy tissue of both benign and malignant lesions through a freezing process

cryptorchidism   Undescended testis

cryptosporidiosis   Infection caused by the protozoan parasite *Cryptosporidium*

crystalloid   A solution containing fluids and electrolytes that can freely cross capillary walls

crystalluria   Crystals in the urine

cultural need   Refers to the nurse being alert to the patient's cultural expectations

culture   Learned beliefs and behaviors shared by a group of people

Cushing syndrome   An endocrine disorder of the adrenal glands causing adrenal hypersecretion of its hormones

cyclic method   A type of continuous feeding infused over 8 to 16 hours daily (day or night)

cyclins   A family of proteins that stimulate the cell to move through the cell cycle

cyclooxygenase (COX)   The enzyme responsible for converting arachidonic acid into prostaglandins and their products

cyclooxygenase 2 (COX-2) inhibitors   Newer nonsteroidal antiinflammatory drugs that block only COX-2 and not COX-1

cycloplegics   Drugs that paralyze the eye muscles of accommodation

cytokine release syndrome   A symptom complex associated with the use of anti-T–cell antibody infusions

cytomegalovirus (CMV)   Infection caused by a virus that infects the entire body

cytotoxic   The ability to directly damage or kill cells

cytotoxic therapy   A treatment that uses drugs to destroy cancer cells

Current Good Manufacturing Practices (CGMPs)   US Food and Drug Administration standards requiring that package labels give the quality and strength of all contents and that products be free of contaminants and impurities

D

decongestants   Drugs that stimulate the alpha-adrenergic receptors, producing vascular constriction (vasoconstriction) of the capillaries within the nasal mucosa

delayed puberty   Defined clinically by the absence or incomplete development of secondary sexual characteristics bounded by an age at which 95% of children of that sex and culture have begun sexual maturation

dependence   A condition in which larger and larger doses of a drug are needed to reproduce the initial response

dependent variable   A mathematical variable whose value is determined by that of one or more other variables in a function (outcome, such as clinical effect)

depolarization   Myocardial contraction

depression   A mood disorder that causes a persistent feeling of sadness and loss of interest

dermatome   A nerve region where the virus had lain dormant

diabetes insipidus (DI)   A rare condition in which the kidneys are not able to conserve water

diabetes mellitus   A chronic disease that results from deficient glucose metabolism caused by insufficient insulin secretion from the beta cells

diarrhea   Frequent liquid stool

Dietary Supplement Health and Education Act (DSHEA)   A US federal act that defined dietary supplements

diffusion   Movement across the cell membrane from an area of higher concentration to one of lower concentration

diluent   A liquid used to reconstitute a drug to form a solution

dimensional analysis   A calculation method using factors of units and conversions to multiple and divide to obtain the amount to administer

direct-acting cholinergic agonists   Drugs that act on receptors to activate a tissue response

disease-modifying antirheumatic drugs (DMARDs)   Drugs that help alleviate the symptoms of rheumatic arthritis; DMARDs are also used in the treatment of multiple sclerosis

distribution   Movement from the circulation into body tissues

diuresis   Increased urine flow

diuretics   Agents used to decrease hypertension and edema

dopamine   A neurotransmitter that helps control the brain's reward and pleasure centers

dopamine agonists   Drugs that stimulate dopamine receptors

dose-response relationship   The body's physiologic response to changes in drug concentration at the site of action

doubling time   A factor that plays a major role in how cancer cells respond to anticancer drugs

dromotropic   An action that decreases conduction of heart cells

drop factor   Number of drops per milliliter

drug diversion   The deliberate redirecting of a drug from a patient or facility to the employee for personal use

drug interaction   An altered or modified action or effect of a drug as a result of interaction with one or multiple drugs

drug label   A label containing printed information about a drug

drug reconciliation   The process of identifying the most accurate list of all medications a patient is taking at transitions in care

drug toxicity   A condition that occurs when drug levels exceed the therapeutic range

drusen   Deposits of extracellular material under the retina

DTaP   Diphtheria toxoid-, tetanus toxoid-, and acellular pertussis-containing vaccines help protect against diphtheria, tetanus, and pertussis, but they will not prevent all cases

duodenal ulcer   Caused by hypersecretion of acid from the stomach passing into the duodenum because of (1) insufficient buffers to neutralize gastric acid in the stomach, (2) a defective or incompetent pyloric sphincter, or (3) hypermotility of the stomach

duration of action   The length of time over which a drug exerts its therapeutic effect

dysfunctional uterine bleeding   Abnormal uterine bleeding in the absence of organic disease

dyskinesia   Impaired voluntary movement

dysmenorrhea   Painful periods

dyspareunia   Painful sexual intercourse

dysphoria   Deep depression

dysrhythmias   Irregular heartbeats

dystonia   Prolonged muscle contractions with twisting, repetitive movements

dystonic movement   Involuntary abnormal movement

E

e-cigarettes   Electronic cigarettes that aerosolize "e-juice," a mixture of flavorings, propylene glycol (a toxic component of antifreeze), glycerin, and nicotine

eclampsia   New-onset grand mal seizures in a patient with preeclampsia

ejaculatory dysfunction   Impaired ejection of seminal fluid from the male urethra

electroencephalogram (EEG)   An electrophysiologic monitoring method to record electrical activity of the brain

electrolytes   Substances that separate or dissociate into ions (charged particles) in solution

electronic intravenous device   An electronic device to deliver prescribed rate of intravenous drugs

emetics   Drugs used to induce vomiting

emollients   Lubricants and stool softeners used to prevent constipation

emphysema   A progressive lung disease caused by cigarette smoking, atmospheric contaminants, or lack of the alpha$_1$-antitrypsin protein that inhibits proteolytic enzymes that destroy alveoli

endometriosis   The abnormal location of endometrial tissue outside the uterus

endophthalmitis   Infection and inflammation of structures of the inner eye

endorphins   Neurohormones

enteral nutrition (EN)   Delivery of nutrition or fluid via a tube into the gastrointestinal (GI) tract, which requires a functional, accessible GI tract

epidural block   Placement of local anesthetic in the epidural space just posterior to the spinal cord or the dura mater

epigenetics   The study of environmental influences on genetics

episiotomy   An incision made to enlarge the vaginal opening to facilitate newborn delivery

erectile dysfunction   The inability to achieve or maintain an erection satisfactory for sexual performance

ergot alkaloids   One of a large group of alkaloids derived from fungi; acts by direct smooth muscle cell–receptor stimulation

ergotism   Signs of ergot toxicity

erythema multiforme   An erythematous macular, papular, or vesicular eruption that can cover the entire body

erythrocytic phase   Invasion of the red blood cells

erythropoietin (EPO)   A glycoprotein produced by the kidney stimulating red blood cell production in the bone marrow

erythropoietin-stimulating agents (ESAs)   Agents that stimulate red blood cell production in the bone marrow

esophageal ulcer   Results from reflux of acidic gastric secretions into the esophagus as a result of a defective or incompetent cardiac sphincter

essential hypertension   The most common type of hypertension, affecting 90% of persons with high blood pressure

estimated average requirement (EAR)   The daily intake of a specific nutrient estimated to meet the requirement in 50% of healthy people in an age- and sex-specific group

ethinyl estradiol   The most commonly used synthetic estrogen found in CHC products

ethnomedicine   Sometimes referred to as *folk medicine* or *traditional medicine,* a focus within medical anthropology that examines the ways in which people from different cultures conceptualize health and illness

ethnopharmacology   A subdivision of ethnomedicine that focuses on the use of herbs, powders, teas, and animal products as healing remedies

evaluation   The phase of the nursing process during which the nurse determines whether the goals and teaching objectives are being met

excipients   Fillers and inert substances such as simple syrup, vegetable gums, aromatic powder, honey, and various elixirs

excretion   Elimination of drugs from the body

exfoliative dermatitis   Characterized by desquamation, scaling, and itching of the skin

expectorants   Agents that loosen bronchial secretions so they can be eliminated by coughing

extrapyramidal syndrome   Any of a group of clinical disorders marked by abnormal involuntary movements, alterations in muscle tone, and postural disturbances

extravasation   Tissue injury due to drugs infiltering tissues

F

facilitated diffusion   Relies on a carrier protein to move drug from an area of higher concentration to an area of lower concentration

family-centered care   Essential to ensuring safety during and after health care interventions, especially drug administration

fasciculations   Involuntary muscle twitching

fat-soluble vitamins Vitamins stored in fatty tissue, liver, and muscle in significant amounts that are metabolized slowly and excreted in the urine at a slow rate; includes vitamins A, D, E, and K

fibrinolysis Fibrin breakdown

first-line drugs Those drugs chosen first for therapy

first-pass effect (or first-pass metabolism) When drugs are metabolized in the liver to an inactive form and are excreted, thus reducing the amount of active drug available to exert a pharmacologic effect

flatus Intestinal gas

folliculitis Inflammation of a hair follicle resulting from contact with an irritating substance or allergen

fraction of inspired oxygen (FiO$_2$) The fraction or percentage of oxygen in the space being measured

fractional equation The equation H/V = D/x to calculate the amount x to be administered, where H is the dosage on hand; V is the vehicle; D is the desired dose

free drugs Drugs able to exit blood vessels and reach their site of action to cause a pharmacologic response

free-flow The rate of administration of intravenous drugs infused rapidly without the use of an electronic infusion device

G

gastric mucosal barrier (GMB) A thick, viscous, mucous material that provides a barrier between the mucosal lining and acidic gastric secretions

gastric ulcer Frequently occurs because of a breakdown of the gastric mucosal barrier (GMB)

gastroesophageal reflux disease (GERD) Inflammation or erosion of the esophageal mucosa caused by a reflux of gastric acid content from the stomach into the esophagus

gastrostomy tube A gastrointestinal tube used for enteral tube feedings

generic name The official, nonproprietary name for a drug; the name not owned by any drug company and universally accepted as the official drug name

genomes A complete set of chromosomes that make up a cell's DNA

genotoxicity The ability of a compound to damage genetic information in a cell

gestational hypertension Elevated blood pressure after 20 gestational weeks in patients who were normotensive before pregnancy

gigantism Excessive growth during childhood

gingival hyperplasia Overgrowth of gums or reddened gums that bleed easily

glaucoma A group of eye conditions that damage the optic nerve

glucocorticoids Most potent endogenous cortisol produced by the adrenal cortex; exogenous drugs used to treat variety of medical conditions, including inflammation, allergy, and some autoimmune disorders

glycogenolysis Breakdown of glycogen increasing blood glucose

Good Clinical Practice (GCP) Consolidated Guideline An international ethical and scientific quality standard for designing, conducting, monitoring, auditing, recording, analyzing, and reporting clinical research

gout An inflammatory condition that attacks joints, tendons, and other tissues

gram The basic unit of measure used for weight (g, G)

granulocyte A type of white blood cell with small granules that contain proteins

granulocyte colony–stimulating factor (G-CSF) A glycoprotein produced by the macrophages, endothelium and other immune cells to stimulate the synthesis of neutrophils

granulocyte-macrophage colony–stimulating factor (GM-CSF) A glycoprotein secreted by immune cells that support survival, proliferation, and differentiation (maturation) of hematopoietic progenitor cells in the granulocyte-macrophage pathway

Graves disease The most common type of hyperthyroidism caused by hyperfunction of the thyroid gland

growth fraction A factor that plays a major role in how cancer cells respond to anticancer drugs

gynecomastia Mammary gland enlargement in men

H

half-life The time it takes for the amount of drug in the body to be reduced by half

hangover Residual drowsiness

healers Individuals who play a role in health practices worldwide; may include priests, shamans, bone setters, herbalists, curanderos, and midwives

health care–acquired infections Infections acquired while patients are hospitalized

heart block A delay in the normal flow of electrical impulses of the heart, often times causing bradycardia

heart failure A condition that occurs when the heart muscle (myocardium) weakens and enlarges and loses its ability to pump blood through the heart and into the systemic circulation

HELLP syndrome A sequela of preeclampsia defined by hemolysis, elevated liver enzymes, and low platelet count

helminthiasis Worm infection

helminths Large parasitic worms that live and lay eggs in warm, moist soil where sanitation and hygiene are poor

hepatotoxicity Liver toxicity

herb Any plant used for culinary or medicinal purposes

herd immunity Occurs when most of the community is immunized against contagious diseases, thus allowing protection of those not immunized

high-density lipoprotein (HDL) One of the five major groups of lipoproteins

high-sensitivity C-reactive protein (hsCRP) A test used to evaluate the risk of developing coronary artery disease

hirsutism Increased hair growth

histamine 2 (H$_2$) receptor antagonists Agents used to treat duodenal ulcers and prevent their return

homocysteine A naturally occurring amino acid found in blood plasma

hordeolum A local infection of eyelash follicles and glands on lid margins, also known as a *stye*

hormone therapy A therapy that significantly improves vasomotor symptoms and vaginal dryness, two frequently encountered symptoms of menopause; also decreases the risk for osteoporosis and osteoporotic fractures

household measurement A measuring system that uses inches and pounds

hybridoma technology A genetic process that makes monoclonal antibodies

hydantoins Inhibit sodium influx, stabilize cell membranes, reduce repetitive neuronal firing, and limit seizures

hydrochloric acid A strongly acidic solution of the gas hydrogen chloride in water

hyperalimentation A form of malnutrition in which the intake of nutrients is oversupplied

hypercalcemia A calcium excess (>10.2 mEq/L)

hypercapnia Increased carbon dioxide in the blood

hyperchloremia An elevated serum chloride level

hyperemesis gravidarum Severe nausea and vomiting during pregnancy

hyperglycemia Elevated blood glucose

hyperkalemia A serum potassium level above 5.0 mEq/L

hyperlipidemia A condition that occurs when there is an excess of one or more lipids in the blood

hypermagnesemia A magnesium excess

hypernatremia A serum sodium level above 145 mEq/L

hyperosmolar A fluid that contains more particles than water

hyperoxia Excessive oxygenation

hyperphosphatemia An excess of phosphorus

hypertension Blood pressure greater than 140/90 mm Hg

hypertensive crisis When systolic blood pressure exceeds 180 to 200 mm Hg

hyperthyroidism An increase in circulating T$_3$ and T$_4$ levels, which usually results from an overactive thyroid gland or excessive output of thyroid hormones from one or more thyroid nodules

hypertonic Describes solutions that exert greater osmotic pressure than extracellular fluid (ECF), resulting in a higher solute concentration than the serum

hypertrichosis Darkening of hair

hyperuricemia Elevated serum uric acid level

hypnotic effect Not hypnosis but a form of "natural" sleep

hypocalcemia A calcium deficit (<8.6 mEq/L)

hypocarbia Decreased carbon dioxide (CO$_2$)

hypochloremia A decreased serum chloride level

hypoglycemic reaction Occurs when more insulin is administered than is needed for glucose metabolism

hypogonadism The clearest indication for exogenous androgen therapy

hypokalemia Potassium deficit; occurs with serum levels below 3.5 mEq/L

hypomagnesemia Magnesium deficit

hyponatremia A serum sodium level below 135 mEq/L

hypoosmolar Describes fluid that contains fewer particles than water

hypophosphatemia Deficiency of phosphorus

hypophysis The pituitary gland

hypothyroidism A decrease in thyroid hormone secretion

hypotonic Describes solutions that exert less osmotic pressure than extracellular fluid (ECF), which allows water to move into the cell

hypovolemic shock A life-threatening condition caused by more than 20% (one fifth) of the body's blood or fluid supply

hypoxemia Inadequate oxygen in the blood

hypoxia Lack of oxygen to body tissues

I

idiopathic Of unknown cause

immune globulin The general term used for replacement therapy

immune reconstitution inflammatory syndrome (IRIS) A syndrome related to a disease- or pathogen-specific inflammatory response in patients with antiretroviral therapy being initiated or changed

immune response The reaction of the cells and fluids of the body to the presence of a substance not recognized as a constituent of the body itself

immunoglobulins Antibody proteins such as immunoglobulins G and M

immunomodulation The immune system's ability to kill abnormal cells

immunomodulators Agents used to treat moderate to severe rheumatoid arthritis by disrupting the inflammatory process and delaying disease progression; immunomodulators are also used in the treatment of multiple sclerosis

immunosuppression The use of multiple drugs to alter different aspects of the immune system

immunosuppressives Agents used to treat refractory rheumatoid arthritis that does not respond to antiinflammatory drugs; immunosuppressives are also used in the treatment of multiple sclerosis

implementation The part of the nursing process in which the nurse provides education, drug administration, patient care, and other interventions necessary to assist the patient in accomplishing the established goals

independent variable A variable independent of the other variables in an expression or function and whose value determines one or more of the values of the other variables (e.g., treatment, such as with a drug)

indirect-acting cholinergic agonists Agents that inhibit the action of the enzyme cholinesterase (ChE)

induction therapy Treatment that provides intense immunosuppression with drugs designed to diminish antigen presentation and T-cell response

infection Caused by microorganisms, which results in inflammation

infertility The inability to conceive a child after 12 months of unprotected sexual intercourse

infiltration Extravasation of intravenous fluids into the tissues

inflammation A response to tissue injury and infection

influenza A highly contagious viral infection, usually seasonal

informed consent Consent to medical treatment or participation in medical experiments after achieving an understanding of what is involved and being apprised of the risks

inhalation Administration of medication via the nasal route

inherent resistance Bacterial resistance can result naturally

inhibited sexual desire Decreased or lacking interest in sexual activity

inotropic Action that increases myocardial contraction stroke volume

insomnia The inability to fall asleep or remain asleep

instillations Liquid medications usually administered as drops, ointments, or sprays

insulin A protein secreted from the beta cells of the pancreas necessary for carbohydrate metabolism and that plays an important role in protein and fat metabolism

insulin shock Occurs when more insulin is administered than is needed for glucose metabolism

interferon alfa An interferon produced by white blood cells that inhibits viral replication, suppresses cell proliferation, and regulates immune response

interferon beta (IFN-β) A type I interferon produced by fibroblasts, macrophages, and epithelial cells

interferon gamma (IFN-γ) A type II interferon produced endogenously by activating T lymphocytes and natural killer cells (NKCs), and produced genetically from *Escherichia coli*

interferons (IFNs) A family of proteins that occur naturally in the body and can be produced in the laboratory to slow the growth of cancer cells

interleukins A group of signaling-molecule proteins produced by T lymphocytes

intermittent enteral feedings Feedings administered every 3 to 6 hours over 30 to 60 minutes by gravity drip or infusion pump

intermittent infusion Considered an inexpensive method for administering enteral nutrition (EN)

international normalized ratio (INR) The laboratory test most frequently used to report prothrombin time (PT) results

intradermal Administered for skin testing

intramuscular (IM) An administration route used for solutions that are more viscous and irritating for adults, children, and infants

intraocular pressure (IOP) The pressure within the eyeball that gives it a round, firm shape

intravenous More rapid injection method than intramuscular or subcutaneous routes

intravenous flow rate A rate of intravenous drug administration based on several factors

intravenous piggyback (IVPB) A method of administering diluted drugs in small volume of fluid as a secondary infusion

intravenous push (IVP) A method of administering intravenous drugs using a syringe

iron Vital for hemoglobin regeneration

ischemia Deficient blood flow

isoosmolar Fluid that has the same weight proportion of particles (e.g., sodium, glucose) and water

isotonic Describes solutions that have the same approximate osmolality as extracellular fluid (ECF) or plasma

J

jejunostomy tube A gastrointestinal route used for enteral tube feedings

Just & Safe Culture An approach that supports encouraging individuals to report drug errors so the system can be repaired and the problem can be fixed

justice Requires that the selection of research subjects be fair

K

Kaposi sarcoma A cancer that causes patches of abnormal tissue to grow under the skin; in the lining of the mouth, nose, and throat; in lymph nodes; and in other organs

keep vein open (KVO) An intravenous fluid infusion given at a slow rate to maintain patent intravenous site

keratin A protein that is part of the skin

keratitis Infection and inflammation of the cornea

keratolysis Horny cell cohesion due to bacterial growth

ketoacidosis Diabetic acidosis or diabetic coma

L

labor augmentation Stimulation of effective uterine contractions with oxytocin once labor has begun

labor induction The process of causing or initiating labor

lacrimal duct Tear ducts

lactation Production and release of milk by the mammary glands

latency The establishment and maintenance of latent infection in nerve cell ganglia proximal to the site of infection

latent stage A period of time after an infection during which symptoms are absent

latent tuberculosis infection A state of persistent immune response to stimulation by *Mycobacterium tuberculosis* antigens without evidence of clinically manifested active tuberculosis

laxatives Agents that promote a soft stool; cathartics result in a soft to watery stool with some cramping

lecithin/sphingomyelin (L/S) ratio Ratio of lecithin and sphingomyelin that measured in the amniotic fluid, predicting fetal lung maturity and risk for neonatal respiratory distress syndrome (RDS)

ligand-binding domain The site on the receptor to which drugs bind

lipodystrophy A disorder of adipose (fatty) tissue characterized by a selective loss of body fat

lipoprotein Special particles made up of droplets of fats surrounded by a single layer of phospholipid molecules

liposomes Synthetic fat globules containing drugs to increase the duration of therapeutic effects

liter The basic unit of measure for volume (L)

living-donor transplantation An operation in which a kidney or a portion of liver donated by a living person is transplanted into the body of a patient with end-stage kidney or liver disease

loading dose Administration of a large initial dose

low-density lipoprotein (LDL) A molecule that is a combination of lipid (fat) and protein; transports cholesterol from the liver to the tissues of the body

lymphokines Cytokines produced by T cells (lymphocytes) of the immune system; also called interleukins

M

macrodrip An intravenous set that delivers 10 to 20 drops per milliliter

macrophages Mature monocytes

macules Flat and nonpalpable skin lesions, usually less than 10 mm in diameter with varying colors

maximal efficacy The point at which increasing a drug's dosage no longer increases the desired therapeutic response

menarche The start of spontaneous menstruation

meningococcal vaccine Vaccines available that can help prevent meningococcal disease, which is any type of illness caused by Neisseria meningitidis bacteria

menopause The transitional process experienced by women as they move from the reproductive years into the nonreproductive stage of life

menorrhagia Heavy periods

mestranol An older form of estrogen found in higher-dose (≥50 mcg) oral combination products

metabolism The process by which the body chemically changes drugs into a form that can be excreted

metastasis The spread of the disease to other areas of the body

metastasizing Spreading to other parts of the body

meter Basic unit of measure for linear measurement (m, M)

metered-dose inhalers (MDIs) Handheld devices used to deliver a number of commonly prescribed asthma and bronchitis drugs to the lower respiratory tract

metric system A decimal system based on the power of 10

metrorrhagia Irregular bleeding between periods, usually heavy

microdrip An intravenous tubing set that delivers 60 drops per milliliter

microorganisms Microscopic organisms that include viruses, fungi, protozoa, and rickettsiae

micturition Urination

migraine headaches Characterized by a unilateral throbbing head pain accompanied by nausea, vomiting, and photophobia

mineralocorticoids A group of hormones, the most important being aldosterone, that regulate the balance of water and electrolytes (ions such as sodium and potassium) in the body

minerals Substances the body requires in small amounts, such as iron, copper, zinc, chromium, and selenium

minimum effective concentration The minimum amount of drug required for drug effect

miosis A constriction of the pupil and contraction of the ciliary muscle

mitosis The process by which the nucleus divides in eukaryotic organisms, producing two new nuclei genetically identical to the nucleus of the parent cell

mittelschmerz Midcycle menstrual pain usually associated with ovulation

Monitoring the Future project A project that tracks drug use in adolescents and young adults

monoamine oxidase inhibitors (MAO-Is) Agents that inactivate norepinephrine, dopamine, epinephrine, and serotonin

monoclonal antibodies Antibodies produced by a single clone of cells or a cell line and consisting of identical antibody molecules

mononucleosis A contagious viral infection affecting the lymph nodes

mTOR kinase inhibitors A class of drugs that inhibit the mechanistic target of rapamycin

mucolytics Agents that act as detergents to liquefy and loosen thick mucus secretions so they can be expectorated

multikinase inhibitors (MKIs) Chemicals that directly inhibit the activity of multiple kinase enzymes in cancer cells

multiple sclerosis (MS) A neuromuscular autoimmune disorder that attacks the myelin sheath of nerve fibers, causing lesions known as *plaques*

muscarinic receptors Receptors that stimulate smooth muscle and slow the heart rate

muscle relaxants Agents that reduce spasticity of muscles

muscle spasms Muscle contractions resulting from various causes, including injury or motor neuron disorders associated with conditions such as multiple sclerosis (MS), myasthenia gravis (MG), cerebral palsy, spinal cord injury, cerebrovascular accident, or hemiplegia

myasthenia gravis (MG) An acquired autoimmune disease that impairs the transmission of messages at the neuromuscular junction, resulting in fluctuating muscle weakness that increases with muscle use

myasthenic crisis Occurs when muscular weakness in the patient with myasthenia gravis becomes generalized

***Mycobacterium avium* complex (MAC)** A blood infection caused by bacteria related to *M. tuberculosis*

mydriasis A condition in which the pupils remain dilated for a prolong duration

mydriatics Agents that dilate the pupils

myelosuppression A condition that occurs when a significant decrease in bone marrow activity results in decreased white blood cells, platelets, and red blood cells

myocardial infarction (MI) Heart attack

myocardial ischemia Lack of blood supply to the heart muscle

myxedema Severe hypothyroidism in the adult

N

nadir The low point; in nursing, used to describe the point at which the blood count is at the lowest

narcolepsy A neurological disorder characterized by falling asleep during normal waking activities, such as while driving a car or talking with someone

narrow-spectrum antibiotics Tolerance (as of a virus) to a usually toxic substance (as an antibiotic) that is acquired, not as a result of direct exposure, but by exposure to a related substance

nasoduodenal/nasojejunal Gastrointestinal routes used for enteral tube feedings

nasointestinal tube A tube passed through the nose and down through the nasopharynx and esophagus into the intestine

natriuresis Sodium loss in the urine

natriuretic An agent with a sodium-losing effect

natural acquired active immunity Immunity that occurs from exposure to a pathogen or disease

necrosis Tissue death caused by disease or injury

neoadjuvant chemotherapy Treatment performed before surgical extraction of a tumor with the objective of reducing the tumor's size

nephrotoxicity Toxicity to the kidney

nerve block A pain management technique involving the injection of an anesthetic into the area surrounding an affected nerve

neurohypophysis The posterior pituitary gland

neuroleptic Refers to any drug that modifies psychotic behavior and exerts an antipsychotic effect

neuroleptic malignant syndrome (NMS) A rare but potentially fatal condition associated with antipsychotic drugs

neuropathic pain An unusual sensory disturbance that often involves neural supersensitivity

neurotransmitters Substances released as a result of stimulation, such as by amphetamines

neutrophils The most abundant white blood cells that take part in the inflammatory response system, whose main function it is to detect and destroy harmful bacteria

nicotinic receptors Receptors that affect the skeletal muscles

nitrates The first agents used to relieve angina

nociceptors Sensory receptors for pain

nonopioid analgesics Drugs that are less potent than opioid analgesics, used to treat mild to moderate pain

non–rapid eye movement (NREM) sleep A definite stage of sleep

nonselective A term used to describe drugs capable of affecting multiple receptors

nonspecific   A term used to describe drugs capable of affecting multiple receptor sites

nonsteroidal antiinflammatory drugs (NSAIDs)   Nonopioid analgesics taken for pain and inflammation

normoxemia   Oxygen saturation between 94% and 99% depending on the patient's diagnosis and physiologic state

nystagmus   Constant, involuntary, cyclical movement of the eyeball

O

occlusive   Obstructive

ocular drugs   Drugs designed to be applied to the eyes

off label   Use of a drug for some purpose for which it has not been approved

older adult   Person over the age of 65

oligomenorrhea   Very scant periods

oligospermia   Low sperm count

oliguria   A marked decrease in urine output

oncogene   A mutation in a proto-oncogene that affects cellular growth-control proteins and triggers unregulated cell division

onset   The time it takes for a drug to reach the minimum effective concentration (MEC) after administration

open-angle glaucoma   A condition in which the trabecular network is open but becomes clogged

ophthalmia neonatorum   An eye infection among newborns

ophthalmic drugs   Drugs designed to be applied to the eyes

opiates   Analgesic agents that decrease intestinal motility and thereby decrease peristalsis

opioid agonist-antagonists   Medications in which an opioid antagonist is added to an opioid agonist

opioid agonists   Drugs prescribed for moderate and severe pain

opioid antagonist   An agent that blocks the receptor and displaces any opioid that would normally be at the receptor

opportunistic infections   Infections that usually occur in the immunocompromised or debilitated population

oral antidiabetic drugs   Synthetic preparations that stimulate insulin release or otherwise alter the metabolic response to hyperglycemia

oral hypoglycemic drugs   Synthetic preparations that stimulate insulin release or otherwise alter the metabolic response to hyperglycemia

orthostatic hypotension   Low blood pressure that occurs when an individual assumes an upright position from a supine position

osmolality   Describes the concentration of fluids

osmolarity   Describes the concentration of a solution in terms of osmoles of solute per liter of solution

osmole   The number of solutes in a solution, expressed as a unit of measurement

osmotics   Hyperosmolar laxatives

osteopenia   Low bone mineral density

osteoporosis   Loss of bone mass that predisposes patients to fractures

otalgia   Ear pain

otitis externa (OE)   An infection of the external auditory canal

ototoxicity   Ear poisoning that results from exposure to drugs or chemicals that damage the inner ear or the vestibulocochlear nerve

ounces   A unit of measurement related to mass

over-the-counter (OTC)   Those drugs that have been found to be safe and appropriate for use without the direct supervision of a health care provider and are available for purchase without a prescription

P

pain threshold   The level of stimulus needed to create a painful sensation

pain tolerance   The amount of pain a person can endure without having it interfere with normal functioning

palliative chemotherapy   Treatment used to relieve symptoms associated with advanced disease

papules   Raised and palpable skin lesions less than 10 mm in diameter

parasympatholytics   Drugs that affect the parasympathetic nervous system

parasympathomimetics   Drugs that mimic the parasympathetic neurotransmitter acetylcholine

parathyroid hormone (PTH)   A hormone that regulates serum calcium levels

parenteral   Administered via injection

parenteral nutrition (PN)   Administration of nutrients by a route other than the gastrointestinal tract; also called *total parenteral nutrition* (TPN)

paresthesia   A burning or prickling sensation usually felt in the hands, arms, legs, or feet but can also occur in other parts of the body

Parkinson disease   A chronic, progressive neurologic disorder that affects the extrapyramidal motor tract, which controls posture, balance, and locomotion

Parkinsonism   A syndrome, or a combination of similar symptoms, whose major features include rigidity, bradykinesia, gait disturbances, and tremors

paroxysmal supraventricular tachycardia (PSVT)   A sudden, uncontrolled, rapid rhythm that exceeds 150 beats per minute in adults and originates above the ventricles

Partial agonist   Drugs that elicit only moderate activity when binding to receptors; they also prevent receptor activation by other drugs

partial thromboplastin time (PTT)   A blood test that evaluates how long it takes for blood to clot

passive immunity   Immunity that can be natural, in which case the body produces its own antibodies, or acquired—that is, the body receives antibodies from an outside source

passive transport   Transport that occurs through two processes, diffusion and facilitated diffusion

pathogen   A disease-producing microorganism

patient-controlled analgesia (PCA)   An alternative route for opioid administration for self-administered pain relief as needed

patient-problem   Defines the most important health problem the patient is experiencing and guides the development of the nursing plan of care

peak   The point at which a drug reaches its highest concentration in the blood

peak drug level   The highest plasma concentration of a drug at a specific time

pelvic inflammatory disease (PID)   An infection of the upper genital tract, usually the uterine endometrium, fallopian tubes, or ovaries

pepsin   A digestive enzyme activated at a pH of 2

peptic ulcer   A broad term for an ulcer that occurs in the esophagus, stomach, or duodenum within the upper gastrointestinal tract

peptides   Biologically occurring short chains of amino acid monomers linked by peptide (amide) bonds

percutaneous endoscopic gastrostomy (PEG) tube   A tube placed surgically, endoscopically, or radiologically for the purpose of delivering nutrition; requires an intact gastrointestinal system

perinatal transmission   Transmission at the time of delivery

peripheral vasodilators   Drugs that dilate the distal blood vessels and lower the blood pressure

pharmacodynamics   Mechanisms of action and effects of a drug on the body; includes the onset, peak, and duration of effect of a drug

pharmacogenetics   The study of genetic factors that influence an individual's response to a specific drug

pharmacogenomics   The study of how genetics play a role in a person's response to drugs

pharmacokinetics   The process of drug movement throughout the body necessary to achieve drug action

phenothiazines   Subdivided into three groups—aliphatic, piperazine, and piperidine—which differ mostly in their side effects

photochemotherapy   A combination of ultraviolet (UV) radiation and the psoralen derivative methoxsalen; used to decrease proliferation of epidermal cells

photophobia   Sensitivity to light

photosensitivity   A skin reaction caused by exposure to sunlight

phytomedicine   A type of medicine that focuses on the therapeutic value of plants

pinocytosis   A process by which cells carry a drug across their membrane by engulfing the drug particles in a vesicle

placebo   A pill or substance given to a patient like a drug but that can be expected to have no lasting physical effect on the patient

placebo effect   A drug response not attributed to the chemical properties of the drug

planning   The phase during which the nurse uses collected data to set goals or expected outcomes and interventions

plaques   Palpable skin lesions greater than 10 mm in diameter that are depressed or elevated when compared with the skin surface

Pneumocystis jiroveci **pneumonia (PJP)**   A fungal infection that shares biologic characteristics with protozoa that infect the lungs

polycystic ovarian syndrome (PCOS) A form of metabolic syndrome caused by the oversecretion of luteinizing hormone

polydipsia Increased thirst

polydrug use Use of more than one drug

polymorphisms DNA variants that occur within a specific population at a frequency greater than 1%

polyphagia Increased hunger

polypharmacy Use of multiple drugs and/or the administration of drugs above what is clinically warranted

polyuria Increased urine output

postexposure prophylaxis (PEP) The treatment regimen instituted after exposure to human immunodeficiency virus (HIV)

potassium-sparing diuretics Diuretics that promote potassium retention

potassium-wasting diuretics Diuretics that promote potassium excretion

potency Refers to the amount of drug needed to elicit a specific physiologic response

preeclampsia Gestational hypertension with or without proteinuria

preload Amount of blood in the ventricles of the heart at the end of diastole

premenstrual syndrome (PMS) A collection of cyclic physical symptoms and perimenopausal mood alterations

preterm labor (PTL) Cervical changes and uterine contractions that occur between 20 and 37 weeks of pregnancy

priapism Painful, continuous erection

primary infection An infection that occurs in immunocompetent persons

primary syphilis Presents with a sore, or chancre, at the site where the infection entered the body, typically the penis in men and outer genitals or inner vagina in women

Principle of Atraumatic Care Provision of therapy using interventions that minimize or eliminate psychological and physical distress experienced by patients, particularly children and their families

Prodrug A compound metabolized into an active pharmacologic substance

progenitor cells Early descendants of stem cells that can differentiate to form one or more kinds of cells but that cannot divide and reproduce indefinitely

progesterone The naturally occurring sex hormone produced in the ovaries

progestins Natural or synthetic hormones that have progesterone-like effects

progestogen Any synthetically produced progesterone compound

prolactin (PRL) A protein hormone of the anterior pituitary that induces lactation

prophylactic Drugs to prevent infection

prophylaxis Prevention

prostaglandin analogues First-line drugs used primarily in the treatment of open-angle glaucoma and ocular hypertension

prostaglandins Chemical mediators that have been isolated from the exudate at inflammatory sites

proteasome Multienzyme complexes that degrade proteins intracellularly

protein binding Describes how drugs are distributed in the plasma and bind with plasma proteins (albumin, lipoproteins, and alpha-1-acid-glycoprotein [AGP])

prothrombin time (PT) A laboratory test that measures the time it takes blood to clot in the presence of certain clotting factors

protocols Specific guidelines

proto-oncogenes Normal genes involved in cell differentiation and division; they regulate cell death

pseudoparkinsonism Frequently occurs as an adverse reaction to chlorpromazine, haloperidol, lithium, metoclopramide, methyldopa, and reserpine

psoralen and ultraviolet A (PUVA) Therapy that permits lower doses of methoxsalen and UVA to be given

psoriasis A multisystem disease with predominant skin and joint disorders, usually with chronic skin inflammation

psychomotor seizure Occurs in temporal lobe epilepsy; characterized by a temporary impairment of consciousness, loss of judgment, automatic behavior, and abnormal acts

psychosis Loss of contact with reality

puerperium The period from delivery until 6 weeks postpartum

pulse oximetry Provides a digital display of oxygen saturation

purgatives Harsh cathartics that cause a watery stool with abdominal cramping

R

rapid eye movement (REM) sleep The sleep stage during which people experience most of their recallable dreams, characterized by discernable eye movement

reactive depression Depression that usually has a sudden onset after a precipitating event

rebound nasal congestion Caused by frequent use of decongestants

receptors Found on cell surface membranes or within cells

recombinant DNA The genetic engineering process that combines two human DNA strands artificially

recombinant hepatitis B A three-dose series vaccine for hepatitis B virus (HBV) indicated for HBV prophylaxis in infants

Recombinant subunit vaccines the insertion of some of the genetic material of a pathogen into another cell or organism, where the antigen is then produced in massive quantities

recommended dietary allowance (RDA) The amount of vitamins, minerals, or other essential nutrients that should be ingested every day by a normal person engaged in average activities

repolarization Return of cell membrane potential to resting after depolarization

respect for persons Treating patients as independent persons who are capable of making decisions in their own best interests

respiratory distress syndrome (RDS) A syndrome that can occur because of immature lung development and breathing control and decreased airway muscle tone and surfactant level

restrictive lung disease A decrease in total lung capacity as a result of fluid accumulation or loss of elasticity of the lung

reward circuit A structure that regulates the ability to feel pleasure and other emotions, both positive and negative

Rh sensitization Development of protective antibodies against incompatible Rh-positive blood

$Rh_0(D)$ immune globulin A substance routinely administered to women with incompatible maternal/fetal blood mixing

rhinorrhea Watery nasal discharge

right assessment Requires the collection of appropriate baseline data before administration of a drug

right documentation Requires the nurse to record immediately the appropriate information about the drug administered

right dose Requires verification by the nurse that the dose administered is the amount ordered and that it is safe for the patient for whom it is prescribed

right drug Requires confirming that a drug is right for the patient prior to its administration

right evaluation Asks whether the medication did for the patient what it was supposed to do

right patient Requires confirmation of a patient's identity with two forms of identification before drug administration

right route Ordered by the health care provider, it indicates the mechanism by which the medication will enter the body

right time The time the prescribed dose is ordered to be administered

right to education Requires that patients receive accurate and thorough information about the drugs they are taking and how each drug relates to their particular condition

right to refuse Refers to the patient's right to decline medication

risk-benefit ratio Identifying physical, psychological, and social risks and weighing them against the benefits

root-cause analysis (RCA) A method of problem solving used to identify potential workplace errors

S

saddle block Anesthesia given at the lower end of the spinal column to block the perineal area

saluretic Sodium-chloride losing

SARS-CoV-2 Severe acute respiratory syndome coronavirus 2, the virus that causes coronavirus disease (COVID-19), a highly virulent and severe disease that most frequently affects the respiratory system, but also causes long-lasting cardiac, nervous, and renal system damage or death

schizophrenia A chronic psychotic disorder

secondary hypertension Hypertension related to renal and endocrine disorders

secondary intravenous line set An intravenous tubing to administer drugs by intravenous piggyback (IVPB)

secondary syphilis Disease characterized by a skin rash that appears 2 to 8 weeks after the chancre

sedation   A state of diminished physical and mental responsiveness

seizure   A disorder that results from abnormal electrical discharges from the cerebral neurons, characterized by a loss or disturbance of consciousness and usually involuntary, uncontrolled movements

seizure threshold   The point at which a seizure may be induced

selective chloride channel activators   A new category of laxatives used to treat idiopathic constipation in adults

selective serotonin reuptake inhibitors (SSRIs)   Agents that block the reuptake of serotonin into the nerve terminal of the central nervous system

sentinel event   An unanticipated event in a health care setting that results in death or serious harm to a patient unrelated to the natural course of the patient's illness

seroconversion   The acquisition of detectable levels of antibodies in the bloodstream

serotonin norepinephrine reuptake inhibitors (SNRIs)   Agents that inhibit the reuptake of serotonin and norepinephrine, increasing availability in the synapse

shingles   A painful vesicular rash along the region of skin innervated by the nerve root ganglia

side effects   Secondary effects of drug therapy

signal transduction   A mechanism by which cell-to-cell communication occurs locally or remotely by signal molecules sent to maintain homeostasis, regulate growth and division, develop and organize into tissues, and coordinate cellular functions

signal transduction inhibitors (STIs)   Agents that block signals to cancerous cells by blocking signals passed from one molecule to another

sinusitis   Inflammation of the mucous membranes of one or more of the maxillary, frontal, ethmoid, or sphenoid sinuses

sloughing   Formation of dead tissue that separates from living tissue

small-molecule compounds   Chemicals small enough to have an intracellular effect, targeting the internal structures of cells

spacer   A device used to enhance the delivery of medications from a metered-dose inhaler

spermatogenesis   Formation of spermatozoa

spinal anesthesia   A local anesthetic injected into the subarachnoid space below the first lumbar space (L1) in adults and the third lumbar space (L3) in children

spinal block   Results from the penetration of anesthetic into the subarachnoid space

status epilepticus   A rapid succession of epileptic seizures

steady state   The plateau drug level; occurs when the amount of drug being administered is the same as the amount of drug being eliminated

Stevens-Johnson syndrome   Skin eruptions, usually due to adverse reaction to drugs, resulting in large blisters in the mucosa, pharynx, eyes, and viscera

stocking-glove syndrome   A sign of neurotoxicity involving the fingers and toes

stress ulcer   An ulcer that usually follows a critical situation, such as extensive trauma or major surgery

subcutaneous   Injections given under the skin only in areas such as the upper outer aspect of the arms; the abdomen, at least 2 inches from the umbilicus; and the anterior thighs

sublingual   Given under the tongue

substance use disorder   A disorder evidenced by recurrent use of a substance such that it causes considerable impairment, including problems with health and an inability to keep up with family and work responsibilities

superinfection   A new infection in a patient with a preexisting infection

suppository   A solid medical preparation that is cone- or spindle-shaped for insertion into the rectum, globular or egg shaped for use in the vagina, or pencil shaped for insertion into the urethra

suppressor gene   A gene that suppresses the phenotypic expression of another gene

surfactant   A substance that decreases the surface tension of the alveoli to allow the lungs to fill with air and prevent the alveoli from deflating

suspension   A mixture containing solid particles suspended in a liquid

sympatholytics   Drugs that affect the sympathetic nervous system; also called *adrenergic blockers*

sympathomimetics   Drugs that affect the sympathetic nervous system; also called *adrenergic agonists*

syndrome of inappropriate antidiuretic hormone (SIADH)   A condition in which excessive water retention expands the intracellular and intravascular volume

synergistic effect   Describes what occurs when two or more drugs are given together

syringe   A drug dispensing system composed of a barrel, plunger, and tip

T

tachycardia   Heart rate greater than 100 beats per minute

tachyphylaxis   An acute, rapid decrease in response to a drug

tardive dyskinesia   A serious adverse reaction that occurs in approximately 20% to 30% of patients who have taken a typical antipsychotic drug for more than 1 year

targeted therapy   Therapy that directs the treatment according to the person's genomic interfering with specific molecules

Tdap   Tdap vaccine can protect adolescents and adults from tetanus, diphtheria, and pertussis

taxanes   A drug derived from a yew tree that blocks cell growth by stopping cell division

teratogenic   The disturbance of the development of an embryo or fetus

teratogens   Substances that cause developmental abnormalities

tertiary syphilis   Disease that occurs as early as 1 year after infection or at any time during an untreated person's lifetime

testosterone   The principal male sex hormone, an anabolic steroid

therapeutic drug monitoring (TDM)   Checking serum drug levels

therapeutic index (TI)   The relationship between the therapeutic dose of a drug (ED_{50}) and the toxic dose of a drug (TD_{50})

therapeutic range   A range of doses that produce a therapeutic response without causing significant adverse effect

therapeutic serum level   Refers to the dosage range, blood plasma, or serum concentration usually expected to achieve desired therapeutic effects

thromboembolectomy   A treatment to dissolve dangerous clots in blood vessels, improve blood flow, and prevent damage to tissues and organs

thromboembolism   A clot in a blood vessel

thrombolytics   Agents used to promote the fibrinolytic mechanism (converting plasminogen to plasmin, which destroys the fibrin in the blood clot)

thrombosis   The formation of a clot in an arterial or venous vessel

thyroid-stimulating hormone (TSH)   An endocrine hormone from the anterior pituitary gland that stimulates the thyroid gland to release thyroxine (T_4) and triiodothyronine (T_3)

thyrotoxicosis   The most common type of hyperthyroidism, caused by hyperfunction of the thyroid gland; also known as Graves disease

thyroxine (T_4)   A hormone produced by the thyroid gland that controls metabolism

tinea capitis   A fungal infection of the skin on the head

tinea pedis   A fungal infection of the feet, also called *athlete's foot*

tissue phase   Invasion of body tissue

titrated   Adjustment of drug administration according to protocol

tocolytic therapy   Drug therapy to decrease uterine muscle contractions

tolerable upper intake level (UL)   The maximum level of continuing daily nutrient intake likely to pose no risk to the health of most of those in the age group for which it has been established

tolerance   The need for a larger dose of a drug to obtain the original euphoria

tonic-clonic   Convulsive, as with a tonic-clonic seizure

tonic seizure   A seizure in which muscles initially stiffen before the sufferer loses consciousness

tonicity   Used primarily as a measurement of the concentration of intravenous solutions compared with the osmolality of body fluids

topical   Medication applied to the skin, often by painting or spreading it over an area and applying a moist dressing or leaving the area exposed to air

torsades de pointes   An unusual polymorphic ventricular tachycardia often associated with a prolonged QT interval

total parenteral nutrition (TPN)   The administration of nutrients by a route other than the gastrointestinal tract; also called *parenteral nutrition*

toxic epidermal necrolysis   A hypersensitive drug reaction causing a widespread detachment of the epidermis from underlying skin layers

toxoids Inactivated toxins that can no longer produce harmful diseases but do stimulate formation of antitoxins

toxoplasmosis A disease caused by the parasite *Toxoplasma gondii*

transcription factors Substances that enter the nucleus and signal the cell to begin mitosis

transdermal Across the skin; a term used to describe medication stored in a patch and placed on the skin to be absorbed to produce a systemic effect

transplant rejection Occurs when the immune system of the transplant recipient attacks the transplanted organ

trichinosis A disease caused by ingestion of raw or inadequately cooked pork that contains larvae of the *Trichinella spiralis* parasite

tricyclic antidepressants (TCAs) Drugs used to treat major depression

triiodothyronine (T₃) A hormone made by the thyroid gland for cellular metabolism

trough drug level The lowest plasma concentration of a drug, it measures the rate at which the drug is eliminated

tuberculin syringe A 1-milliliter syringe calibrated in hundredths of a milliliter

tuberculosis infection A bacterial infection caused by *Mycobacterium tuberculosis*

type 1 diabetes mellitus A chronic condition in which the pancreas produces little or no insulin

type 2 diabetes mellitus A chronic condition that affects the way the body metabolizes sugar

typical antipsychotics A drug class subdivided into *nonphenothiazines*—such as butyrophenones (which block only the neurotransmitter dopamine), dibenzoxazepines, dihydroindolones, and thioxanthenes—and *phenothiazines,* which, along with the thioxanthenes, block norepinephrine to cause sedative and hypotensive effects early in treatment

tyrosine kinase (TK) An enzyme that activates other substances by adding a phosphate group (PO₄) to them, a process known as *phosphorylation*

tyrosine kinase inhibitors (TKIs) Drugs that inhibit tyrosine kinases and primarily exert their effects on an enzyme known as *BCR-ABL tyrosine kinase*

U

unit International units to quantify the effect of a drug (u)

unit dose method Method of dispensing drugs in which drugs are individually wrapped and labeled for single-dose use for each patient

uricosurics Agents that increase the rate of uric acid excretion by inhibiting its reabsorption

urinary analgesics Drugs that relieve pain and burning in the urinary tract

urinary antiseptics/antiinfectives Drugs that prevent microbial infections of any part of the urinary tract

urinary stimulants Agents that increase the tone of urinary muscles

urinary tract infection (UTI) Microbial infection of any part of the urinary tract

urticaria Skin rash caused by an allergic reaction

US Food and Drug Administration (FDA) The US federal agency responsible for approving and regulating drugs

uterine contractility Tightening and shortening of uterine muscles during labor

uterine inertia Uterine inactivity or hypotonic contractions

uveitis Infection of the vascular layer of the eye (ciliary body, choroid, and iris)

V

vaccination Involves the administration of a small amount of antigen, which although capable of stimulating an immune response does not typically produce the disease

Valsalva maneuver A method to prevent air embolism during dressing and tubing changes in which patients are asked to turn their head in the opposite direction of the insertion site, take a deep breath, hold it, and bear down

Vaping Inhaling the aerosol (vapor) produced by an e-cigarette or similar device, (e.g., vape pen or an advanced personal vaporizer)

Varicella vaccine A vaccine administered that prevents chickenpox and is approved for use in susceptible children and adults

vertical transmission The passage of infecting organisms from mother to neonate

very-low-density lipoprotein (VLDL) Contains the highest amount of triglycerides

vesicant A substance that causes tissue injury

vesication The act of tissue blistering due to injury from a vesicant

vesicles Clear, fluid-filled blisters smaller than 10 mm in diameter

vial Small glass vacuum container with a self-sealing rubber top

vinca alkaloids Substances derived from the periwinkle plant

viral load A measurement of the amount of a virus circulating in the blood, usually stated in virus particles per milliliter

virilization The development of male secondary sex characteristics in women or hypogonadal males

virus An obligate intracellular organism that must reside within a living host cell to survive and reproduce

vitamin K A fat-soluble vitamin given to newborns to prevent vitamin K–deficiency bleeding

vomiting center A major cerebral center that causes vomiting when stimulated

W

water-soluble vitamins A group of vitamins that includes the B-complex vitamins and vitamin C

whitehead A type of noninflammatory acne lesion that is closed

window period The time delay from infection to a positive test result

withdrawal bleeding Monthly bleeding women experience while using a hormonal birth control method

withdrawal symptoms A wide range of physical or emotional disorders that include nervousness, headaches, and insomnia that occur when an individual who is addicted to a substance (such as drugs or alcohol) stops using the substance

World Health Organization (WHO) An agency of the United Nations with the purpose of monitoring communicable and noncommunicable disease outbreaks globally

X

xerophthalmia Dry eyes

Z

Zoster vaccine A vaccine administered to adults to prevent shingles

Z-track technique A technique recommended for administering intramuscular injections to help minimize local skin irritation by sealing the medication in the muscle tissue

INDEX

Note: H_2 blockers, 574–575

Note: interferon α, 454–455